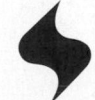

Stedman's

MEDICAL &
SURGICAL
EQUIPMENT
WORDS

FIFTH EDITION

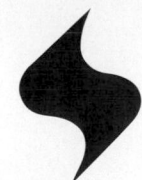

Stedman's

MEDICAL & SURGICAL EQUIPMENT WORDS

FIFTH EDITION

Wolters Kluwer | Lippincott Williams & Wilkins
Health

Philadelphia · Baltimore · New York · London
Buenos Aires · Hong Kong · Sydney · Tokyo

Wolters Kluwer | Lippincott Williams & Wilkins
Health
Philadelphia • Baltimore • New York • London
Buenos Aires • Hong Kong • Sydney • Tokyo

Publisher: Julie K. Stegman
Senior Product Manager: Eric Branger
Managing Editor: Cecilia González
Manufacturing Coordinator: Margie Orzech
Typesetter: Brighid Willson
Printer & Binder: Data Reproductions Corporation

Copyright © 2007 Wolters Kluwer Health I Lippincott Williams & Wilkins
351 West Camden Street
Baltimore, Maryland 21201-2436

Printed in the United States of America

Fifth Edition, 2007

Library of Congress Cataloging-in-Publication Data
Stedman's medical & surgical equipment words. — 5th ed.
    p. ; cm.
  Includes bibliographical references and index.
  ISBN-13: 978-0-7817-7522-9 (pbk.)
  ISBN-10: 0-7817-7522-1 (pbk.)
  1. Medical instruments and apparatus—Terminology. 2. Medical technology—
Terminology. I. Stedman, Thomas Lathrop, 1853-1938. II. Lippincott Williams &
Wilkins. III. Title: Stedman's medical and surgical equipment words. IV.
Title: Medical & surgical equipment words.
  [DNLM: 1. Equipment and Supplies—Terminology—English. W 15 S8126 2007]
  R123.S698 2007
  610.1'4—dc22

                                                                2007020544

Contents

Acknowledgments

An important part of our editorial process is the involvement of medical transcriptionists—as advisors, reviewers, and/or editors.

We extend special thanks to Jeanne Bock, CSR, MT, and to Kathy Hess, CMT, for editing the manuscript and for helping resolve many difficult questions. We are grateful to our Editorial Advisory Board members, including Darcy Johnson, Beverly Oberline, Kay Murphy, and Andrea Linderman, who were instrumental in the development of this reference. They recommended sources and shared their valuable judgment, insight, and perspective.

We extend thanks to Janet West for working on the appendices and to Jo-Ann Clarke for gathering sample reports.

Kathy Cadle played an integral role in the development process by reviewing the content files for format, updating the content, and providing a final quality check.

As with all our *Stedman's* word references, this resource incorporates the suggestions and expertise of our many contacts in the medical transcriptionist community. Thanks to all of our advisory board participants, reviewers, and editors; AAMT meeting attendees; and others who have written us with requests and comments—keep talking, and we'll keep listening.

Editors' Preface

We all know the worth of a good tool in your field of work is invaluable. A carpenter needs the very best carpentry tools to enable him to do his job; likewise, a medical language specialist needs the most accurate reference materials to do an excellent job. It is our hope and belief that *Stedman's Medical & Surgical Equipment Words, Fifth Edition*, will be that most excellent of references for your everyday needs.

When we began the task of updating this book, we made every effort to research the accuracy of the existing terms and to glean new equipment terms from all fields of medicine, with our goal being to have an up-to-date resource that would alleviate the necessity for users to reference other sources to confirm terms heard in the work setting. This process has been a challenging task, and the user will likely notice variations in hyphenation and capitalization of terms in this resource. These variations are reflective of the manufacturer's chosen spelling of terms, which are often within the trademarked name of the product.

In addition to an updated A–Z terminology section, this newest edition of *Stedman's Medical & Surgical Equipment Words, Fifth Edition*, has an improved illustration section, a nice selection of sample reports, and an updated listing of manufacturers and their Web sites.

Whether you are a medical transcriptionist, medical journal editor, court reporter, or other professional in the medical field who relies on accurate references, we believe this book will serve your needs.

Jeanne Bock, CSR, MT
Kathy Hess, CMT

Publisher's Preface

Stedman's Medical & Surgical Equipment Words, Fifth Edition, offers an authoritative assurance of quality and exactness to the wordsmiths of the healthcare professions—medical transcriptionists, medical editors and copyeditors, health information management personnel, court reporters, and the many other users and producers of medical documentation.

In *Stedman's Medical & Surgical Equipment Words, Fifth Edition*, users will find accurate and current terminology related to diagnosis, testing, treatment, procedures, and operations. This edition has been enhanced by carefully researching the accuracy of existing terms and by gleaning new medical and surgical equipment terms from all fields of medicine. The appendix sections, substantially enhanced over the previous edition, provide illustrations with useful captions and labels, sample reports, common terms by procedure, and common manufacturers and Web sites.

This new edition contains more than 8,000 new terms. The extensive A–Z list was developed from manufactures' literature, scientific reports, books, journals, CDs, and Web sites (please see list of References on page xvii).

We at Lippincott Williams & Wilkins strive to provide you with the most up-to-date and accurate word references available. Your use of this Word Book will prompt new editions, which we will publish as often as updates and revisions justify. We welcome your suggestions for improvements, changes, corrections, and additions—whatever will make this *Stedman's* product more useful to you. Please complete the postage-paid card in this book for future suggestions and recommendations, or visit us online at www.stedmans.com.

Explanatory Notes

Medical transcription is an art as well as a science. Both approaches are needed to correctly interpret the dictation of a physician, whose language is a product of education, training, and experience. This variety in medical language means that there are several acceptable ways to express certain terms, including jargon. *Stedman's Medical & Surgical Equipment Words, Fifth Edition*, provides variant spellings and phrasings for many terms. These elements, in addition to complete cross-indexing, make *Stedman's Medical & Surgical Equipment Words, Fifth Edition*, a valuable resource for determining the validity of terms as they are encountered.

Alphabetical Organization

Alphabetization of main entries is letter by letter as spelled, ignoring punctuation, spaces, prefixed numbers, or other characters. For example:

Jelm 2-way catheter
Jelonet dressing
JEM-100CX electron microscope

Terms beginning or ending with Greek letters show the Greek letters spelled out and listed alphabetically. For example:

alpha, α
a. bone substitute material
a. probe

In subentry alphabetization, the abbreviated singular form or the spelled-out plural form of the noun main entry word is ignored.

Format and Style

All main entries are in **boldface** to expedite locating a sought-after term, to enhance distinction between main entries and subentries, and to relieve the textual density of the pages.

Irregular plurals and variant spellings are shown on the same line as the singular or preferred form of the word. For example:

cannula, pl. cannulae, cannulas
guidewire, guide wire
lithotriptor, lithotripter

Capitalization
Trade/brand names (proprietary) and proper names (eponyms) begin with a capital letter.

Fahey pin
Javid shunt
Peri-Guard vascular graft

Product names that are represented in all upper case by the manufacturer are represented with an initial upper case in this book, as shown in bold below.

MAGNETOM Symphony MR scanner = **Magnetom Symphony MR scanner**
VISTA BRITE TIP guiding catheter = **Vista Brite Tip guiding catheter**
SUPRAMID EXTRA suture = **Supramid Extra suture**

Irregular capitalization used by the manufacturer is maintained as shown below.

FastStart HVPC pulsed stimulator
H-TRONplus insulin pump
MicroAir handheld nebulizer

Hyphenation
As a rule of style, multiple eponyms (e.g., Maloney-Hurst dilator) are hyphenated. Also, hyphens have been added between a manufacturer and

one or more eponyms (e.g., Leksell-Elekta stereotactic frame). Please note that in many cases, hyphenation is a question of style, not of accuracy, and thus is a matter of choice.

Possessives

Possessive forms have been dropped in this reference for the sake of consistency and conformance with the guidelines of the American Association for Medical Transcription (AAMT) and other groups. Please note, however, that in many cases, retaining the possessive, like hyphenating, is a question of style, not of accuracy, and thus is a matter of choice. To form the possessive of a word, simply add the apostrophe or apostrophe "s" to the end of the word.

Cross-indexing

The word list is in an index-like main entry–subentry format that contains two combined alphabetical listings:

(1) A *noun* main entry–subentry organization, which is typical of the A–Z section of medical dictionaries like *Stedman's*:

Sundt
S. carotid endartery shunt
S. slim-line graft clip
S. suction system

needle
caudal n.
Chiba n.
Sprotte spinal n.

(2) An *adjective* main entry–subentry organization, which lists words and phrases as you hear them. The main entries are the adjectives or modifiers in a multiword term. The subentries are the nouns around which the terms are constructed and to which the adjectives or modifiers pertain:

superconducting
s. magnet
s. open-magnet system
s. quantum interference device

straight
s. aneurysm clip
s. blade
s. guidewire

This format provides the user with more than one way to locate and identify a multiword term. For example:

Bowman	**stop**
B. needle stop	Bowman needle s.
external	**straightener**
e. straightener	external s.

It also allows the user to see together all terms that contain a particular descriptor, as well as all types, kinds, or variations of a noun entity. For example:

forceps	**perineal**
splinter f.	p. bandage
splitting f.	p. loop
spreading f.	p. pouch

Wherever possible, abbreviations are separately defined and cross-referenced. For example:

ALVAD
abdominal left ventricular assist device

abdominal
a. left ventricular assist device (ALVAD)

device
abdominal left ventricular assist d. (ALVAD)

References

In addition to the lists of our MT Editorial Advisory Board members (from their daily transcription work), we used the following sources for new terms in *Stedman's Medical & Surgical Equipment Words, Fifth Edition.*

Books

Stedman's Alternative Medicine Words, 2nd Edition. Baltimore: Lippincott Williams & Wilkins, 2005.

Stedman's Cardiology & Pulmonary Words, 4th Edition. Baltimore: Lippincott Williams & Wilkins, 2004.

Stedman's Dermatology & Immunology Words, 3rd Edition. Baltimore: Lippincott Williams & Wilkins, 2002.

Stedman's Emergency Medicine Words. Baltimore: Lippincott Williams & Wilkins, 2004.

Stedman's Endocrinology Words, 2nd Edition. Baltimore: Lippincott Williams & Wilkins, 2006.

Stedman's GI & GU Words, 4th Edition. Baltimore: Lippincott Williams & Wilkins, 2005.

Stedman's Neurology & Neurosurgery Words, 4th Edition. Baltimore: Lippincott Williams & Wilkins, 2006.

Stedman's OB-GYN & Pediatric Words, 4th Edition. Baltimore: Lippincott Williams & Wilkins, 2005.

Stedman's Oncology Words, 5th Edition. Baltimore: Lippincott Williams & Wilkins, 2006.

Stedman's Orthopaedic & Rehab Words, 5th Edition. Baltimore: Lippincott Williams & Wilkins, 2006.

Stedman's Pathology & Lab Medicine Words, 4th Edition. Baltimore: Lippincott Williams & Wilkins, 2005.

Stedman's Plastic Surgery/ENT/Dentistry Words, 4th Edition. Baltimore: Lippincott Williams & Wilkins, 2005.

Stedman's Radiology Words, 5th Edition. Baltimore: Lippincott Williams & Wilkins, 2006.

Stedman's Surgery Words, 3rd Edition. Baltimore: Lippincott Williams & Wilkins, 2006.

Web Sites

http://www.fda.gov/cdrh

http://www.hpisum.com

http://www.mdrweb.com

http://www.mtdaily.com

http://www.mtdesk.com

http://www.mtmonthly.com

Images

Agur, A. M. R., and M. J. Lee. *Grant's Atlas of Anatomy, 10th Edition.* Baltimore: Lippincott Williams & Wilkins, 1999.

Battista, K. From C. Oatis *Kinesiology: The Mechanics and Pathomechanics of Human Movement.* Baltimore: Lippincott Williams & Wilkins, 2003.

Beckmann, C. R. B., Ling, F. W., Laube, D. W., Smith, R. P., Barzansky, B. M., and Herbert, W. N. M. *Obstetrics and Gynecology, 4th Edition.* Baltimore: Lippincott Williams & Wilkins, 2002.

Caldwell, S. From *Stedman's Medical Dictionary, 27th Edition.* Baltimore: Lippincott Williams & Wilkins, 2000.

Crapo, J. D., Glassroth, J. Karlinsky, J. B., and King, T. E., Jr. *Baum's Textbook of Pulmonary Diseases, 7th Edition.* Baltimore: Lippincott Williams & Wilkins, 2004.

Hadry. N. O. From *Stedman's Medical Dictionary, 27th Edition.* Baltimore: Lippincott Williams & Wilkins, 2000.

Harwood-Nuss, A., Wolfson, A. B., et al. *The Clinical Practice of Emer-*

gency Medicine, 3rd Edition. Baltimore: Lippincott Williams & Wilkins, 2001.

LifeART Nursing Collection 3, CD-ROM. Baltimore: Lippincott Williams & Wilkins.

LifeART Pediatrics Collection 1, CD-ROM. Baltimore: Lippincott Williams & Wilkins.

LifeART Super Anatomy Collection 2, CD-ROM. Baltimore: Lippincott Williams & Wilkins.

LifeART Super Anatomy Collection 4, CD-ROM. Baltimore: Lippincott Williams & Wilkins.

LifeART Super Anatomy Collection 7, CD-ROM. Baltimore: Lippincott Williams & Wilkins.

LifeART Super Anatomy Collection 9, CD-ROM. Baltimore: Lippincott Williams & Wilkins.

Smeltzer, S. C., Bare, B. G. *Textbook of Medical-Surgical Nursing, 9th Edition.* Baltimore: Lippincott Williams & Wilkins, 2000.

Ward, L. From J. Fuller and J. Schaller-Ayers. *A Nursing Approach, 2nd Edition.* Philadelphia: J. B. Lippincott Company, 1994.

A2
A2 MicroArray system
A2 multipurpose catheter
A13 Sequel programmable behind-the-ear hearing instrument
A1, A2 Port multipurpose catheter
A1c At-Home testing kit
A1cNow glycemic monitoring device
A2008 ABGII hemodialysis machine
A675 Sequel Audio Vision hearing aid
Aagesen
A. disposable rasp
A. file
AAI
activating adjusting instrument
AAI pacemaker
AAI single-chamber pacemaker
AAI/AAIR pacemaker
Aalzet continuous infusion osmotic pump
Aaron cautery
Aastrom Replicell System
AAT
atrial triggered
AAT pacemaker
Abacus Concepts StatView 4.02 statistical analyzer
Abadie
A. enterostomy clamp
A. self-retaining retractor
ABaer infant hearing screening system
Abbe
A. flap
A. refractometer
Abbé condenser
Abbey needle holder
ABBI
advanced breast biopsy instrumentation
ABBI system
Abbokinase
A. catheter
A. Open-Cath
Abbott
A. brace
A. Cell-Dyn hematology analyzer
A. HCV EIA 2nd generation kit
A. HCV 2.0 test kit
A. infusion pump
A. LifeCare PCA Plus II infusion system
A. LifeCare pump
A. Lifeshield needleless system
A. tube
Abbott-Rawson gastrointestinal double-lumen tube

ABC
ABC anterior cervical plating system
ABC cervical plating system
ABC E-Plate
ABCFlex argon beam GI probe
abdominal
a. aortic counterpulsation device
a. bandage
a. belt
a. binder
a. brace
a. compression cylinder
a. left ventricular assist device (ALVAD)
a. packing
a. patch electrode
a. ring retractor
a. scissors
a. scoop
a. trocar
a. vascular retractor
a. zipper
abduction
a. cast
Cruiser hip a.
a. cushion
a. finger splint
a. knee separator
a. pillow
a. thumb splint
a. wedge
abductor
side-lying hip a.
Abee support
Abelson cricothyrotomy cannula
aberrant band
aberrometer
Hartmann-Shack wavefront a.
Shack-Hartmann a.
state-of-the-art a.
Tracey a.
Wasca a.
Z-View a.
Zywave II a.
ABG cement-free hip system
ABI
auditory brainstem implant
ABI model 373, 377 sequencing gel system
multichannel ABI
ABI Prism 3700 DNA analyzer
ABI Prism Dye Terminator Cycle Sequencing Ready Reaction Kit

ABI *(continued)*
    ABI Prism 3100 genetic analyzer
    ABI vest airway clearance system
AbioCor implantable replacement heart
Abiomed
    A. biventricular support system
    A. BVAD 5000 cardiac device
    A. implantable heart replacement
      device
ABL
    ABL 555 analyzer
    ABL 625 system
ABL520 blood gas measurement system
Ablaser laser delivery catheter
Ablatherm HIFU system
ablation
    a. catheter
    radiofrequency a. (RFA)
    transurethral needle a. (TUNA)
ablative device
ablator
    Concept a.
    endometrial a.
    radiofrequency a.
Ablatr temperature control device
Ablaza-Blanco aortic wall retractor
Ableware volumeter
AbMap electrophysiologic imaging
  system
Abocath catheter
abortion scoop
Aboulker stent
above-knee suction enhancement system
abrader
    cornea a.
    Dingman otoplasty cartilage a.
    Haverhill dermal a.
    Lieberman a.
Abraham
    A. contact lens
    A. peripheral button iridotomy lens
    A. YAG laser lens
Abrams
    A. biopsy needle
    A. needle
    A. pleural biopsy punch
Abrams-Lucas flap heart valve
Abramson catheter
abscess
    a. drainage catheter
    a. forceps
Abscession
    A. biliary drainage catheter
    A. fluid drainage catheter
abscission needle
absent pulmonary valve
Absolok endoscopic clip applicator
absolute
    A. absorbable interference screw

    A. absorbable screw
    A. biliary self-expanding stent
    A. biliary self-expanding stent
      system
absorbable
    a. clip
    a. collagen paste
    a. gelatin film
    a. gelatin film roll
    a. gelatin sponge
    a. implant
    a. mesh
    a. plate
    a. polyparadioxanone pin
    a. stent
    a. surgical suture
absorber
    Hollister wound exudate a.
    laser fume a.
Absorb-its material
absorptiometer
    Hologic 1000 QDR dual-energy a.
    Lunar DPX dual-energy a.
    QDR 1000 densitometer a.
    single-energy x-ray a.
absorptiometry
    dual-energy x-ray a. (DXA)
absorption
    a. powder
    a. spectrophotometer
A/B switch box
abuse
    InstaCheck Med+ immunoassay for
      drugs of a.
abutment
    Bio-Cera a.
    CeraOne a.
    custom healing a.
    Dalla Bona ball-and-socket a.
    dovetail stress broken a.
    Hex-Lock a.
    low-margin standard a.
    ProTect a.
    Spectra-System a.
    a. splint
    tooth-colored a.
    wide-diameter a.
    ZAAG a.
AC
  acromioclavicular
  anterior chamber
    AC IOL
    AC lens
    AC 3 plate reader
    AC tube inserter
Acaderm patch test
Acapella
    A. chest physical therapy device
Acat 1 intraaortic balloon pump

A

Acceava
A. hCG Basic
A. hCG Combo
A. Strep A
accelerator
alpha particle a.
Becker a.
Bevatron a.
A. cannula
dual-energy linear a.
electron linear a.
heavy-ion medical a.
high-energy bent-beam linear a.
A. II aspirator
linear a. (LINAC)
Mevatron 74 linear a.
Microtron a.
Mobetron mobile, self-shielded
electron a.
Philips linear a.
plasma prothrombin conversion a.
Siemens Mevatron 74 linear a.
a. tip
University of Florida linear a.
Varian a.
accelerometer
Caltrac a.
intracardiac a.
Koelner Vitaport a.
multiaxis a.
piezoelectric a.
triaxial a.
TriTrac-R3D a.
uniaxial a.
Accell
A. Connexus bone matrix
A. DBM 100 bone matrix
A. TBM bone matrix
A. total bone matrix
Accellon
A. Combi cervical biosampler
A. sampler
Accel stopcock
Accent balloon angioplasty catheter
Accent-DG balloon
Accents system
access
advanced venous a. (AVA)
A. AFP immunoassay analyzer
A-Port vascular a.
Check-Flo performer introducer set
for radial artery a.
E³xtreme A.
A. 2 immunoassay system
a. loop
A. MV system
Rapidpoint a.
a. set
AccessAED defibrillator

AccessALS defibrillator
Access-9 large-bore hemostasis valve
accessory, pl. **accessories**
Assura irrigation a.
Auto Glide walker a.
BabyFace 3D surface rendering a.
CUSALap ultrasonic a.
extravasation detection a.
a. eye implant
Isola spinal implant system a.
optical a.
AccessTrainer exerciser
Acclaim total elbow system
Accolade
A. C femoral component
A. hip prosthesis
A. TMZF femoral component
accommodating IOL
accommodative
a. brace
a. implant
a. orthosis
a. shoe
Accommodator arch support
Acco orthodontic appliance
Accor dental matrix
accordion
a. graft
a. implant
AccuAngle indicator
Accu-Back back support
Accu-Band
**Accu-Beam suction & irrigation
cannula**
AccuBrush dental brush
Accucap CO_2/O_2 monitor
Accu-Chek
A.-C. Active glucose meter
A.-C. Advantage glucose meter
A.-C. Advantage non-wipe blood
glucose monitoring system
A.-C. Comfort Curve test strip
A.-C. Compact glucose meter
A.-C. Complete blood glucose
monitoring system
A.-C. Complete glucose meter
system
A.-C. Easy glucose monitor
A.-C. II Freedom
A.-C. II Freedom blood glucose
monitor
A.-C. II glucometer
A.-C. III
A.-C. III blood glucose meter
A.-C. Instant glucose meter
A.-C. InstantPlus
A.-C. InstantPlus system
A.-C. SoftClix lancet device

Accu-Chek *(continued)*
    A.-C. Soft Touch lancing device
    A.-C. Voicemate glucose meter
Accucom cardiac output monitor
Accucore II biopsy needle
Accu-Cut
    A.-C. osteotomy guide
    A.-C. osteotomy guide system
Accuderm punch
accuDEXA
    a. bone densitometer
    a. bone mineral assessment device
    a. bone mineral density assessment
    system
Accudynamic adjustable damping
AccuFilm articulating film
Accufix
    A. II DEC pacing lead
    A. pacemaker
    A. pacemaker lead
Accuflate tourniquet
Accu-Flo
    A.-F. dural substitute
    A.-F. polyethylene bur hole cover
    A.-F. silicone rubber bur hole
    cover
AccuGage vessel calipers
Accugel lens
Accugraft
    A. ALIF allograft system
    A. allograft
    Puros A.
AccuGuide injection monitor
Accuguide syringe
Accuhair needle
Accuhaler
Accuject sterile disposable dental needle
AccuLase excimer laser
AccuLevel
Accu-Line
    A.-L. chamfer resection guide
    A.-L. distal femoral resection
    instrument
    A.-L. distal femoral resector
    A.-L. dual pivot
    A.-L. femoral resector
    A.-L. guide
    A.-L. knee instrument
    A.-L. knee instrumentation
    A.-L. patellar instrument
    A.-L. surgical marking pen
    A.-L. tibial resector
Accu-line
    A.-l. Products skin marker
    A.-l. surgical marker
Acculink
    A. modem
    A. self-expanding stent
AccuMap multifocal objective perimeter

AccuMark calibrated infant feeding tube
AccuMax
    A. bed
    A. self-adjusting pressure
    management mattress
Accu-Measure
    A.-M. personal body fat tester
    A.-M. skinfold calipers
AccuMeter
    Aware A.
    ChemTrak A.
    A. cholesterol test system
    A. HDL
Accunet
    A. distal protection device
    A. embolic protection system
Accu-o-Matic TENS unit
Accu-Patch
AccuPoint targeting sphere
AccuPressure heel cup
AccuProbe system
Accura hydrocephalus shunt
Accurate
    A. catheter
    A. Surgical and Scientific
    Instruments (ASSI)
Accuratome precurved papillotome
Accuray
    A. CyberKnife
    A. Neurotron 1000 machine
Accurbron
Accurette
    A. endometrial suction curette
    A. microcurettage
Accurox mask
Accurun 515 drug-resistant mutant control series
Accurus
    A. 2500 probe
    A. vitreoretinal surgical system
Accusat pulse oximeter
AccuScan CO$_2$ laser scanner
Accuscan Transducer 400
Accuscope II
Accu-Scope microscope
AccuSharp
    A. carpal tunnel release instrument
    A. endoscope
Accuson-128 color flow Doppler machine
Accu-Sorb gauze sponge
AccuSpan tissue expander
Accu-SPINA cervical decompression machine
Accustaple
AccuStat hCG pregnancy test
AccuSway balance measurement system
Accu-Temp cautery

Accutome
- A. black diamond blade
- A. low-speed diamond saw
- A. LRI diamond knife
- A. side-port diamond knife

Accutorr
- A. bedside monitor
- A. oscillometric device

Accutracker
- A. blood pressure device
- A. II ambulatory blood pressure monitor

AccuTrax peak flowmeter
AccuTread shoe
Accu-Tron microcurrent machine
Accuvac smoke evacuation attachment
AccuView model
Accu-Vu sizing catheter
Accuzyme
- A. enzymatic débrider
- A. enzymatic débriding agent

ACD
- arrhythmia control device

Ace
- A. adherent bandage
- A. aerosol cloud enhancer
- A. Autografter
- A. Autografter bone filter
- A. balloon
- A. bandage
- A. bone screw tack
- A. bone screw tacking kit
- A. brace
- A. cortical bone screw
- A. detachable mask
- A. fixed wire balloon catheter
- A. halo pelvic girdle
- A. longitudinal strips dressing
- A. Mark III halo
- A. OsteoGenic distractor
- A. pelvic stabilizer
- A. pin
- A. screw
- A. self-drilling bone screw system
- A. spica bandage
- A. TiMAX titanium captured hip screw
- A. titanium large fragment system
- A. TK2 hip screw system
- A. Trippi-Wells tong cervical traction
- A. Universal tong cervical traction
- A. wire tension assembly
- A. wrap

Ace-Colles
- A.-C. fixation
- A.-C. half ring

Ace-Fischer external fixator

acellular
- a. dermal allograft
- a. human dermal graft

Ace/Normed osteodistractor
acetabular
- a. angle guide
- a. component
- a. cup
- a. cup extractor
- a. endoprosthesis
- a. grater
- a. liner
- a. prosthesis
- a. prosthesis system
- a. prosthetic liner
- a. reconstruction plate
- a. reinforcement device
- a. reinforcement ring
- a. retractor
- a. round chisel
- a. shell guide

ACFS
- anterior cervical plate fixation system
- Dogbone ACFS

achalasia dilator
Achieve
- A. computer-assisted instrument
- A. off-pump system

Achiever
- A. balloon dilation catheter
- A. balloon dilator

Achilles
- A. boot
- A. densitometer
- A. heel pad

Achilles+
- A. ultrasonometer
- A. ultrasound bone densitometer

Achillon instrument guide
Achillotrain
- A. active Achilles tendon support
- Bauerfeind A.

achromatic lens
acid
- deoxyribonucleic a. (DNA)

acid-Schiff
- Alcian blue and periodic a.-S.

Acier stainless steel suture
AC-IOL
- anterior chamber intraocular lens

Acist contrast delivery injection system
ACIT system
Ackrad
- A. balloon-bearing catheter
- A. Bronchitrac L suction catheter
- A. H/S Elliptosphere catheter

ACL
- anterior cruciate ligament

ACL *(continued)*
>A. 100, 1000, 7000, 8000, 9000, 10000 advance coagulation analyzer
>A. drill
>A. drill guide
>A. graft knife
>A. guide set
>A. Lite functional knee brace

Acland
>A. clamp-applying forceps
>A. microvascular clamp

Acland-Banis arteriotomy set
Acland-Buncke counterpressor
ACL/PCL
>anterior cruciate ligament/posterior cruciate ligament

Acme
>A. articulator
>A. One Time enteral feeding bag

ACMI
>ACMI cautery
>ACMI cystoscopic tip
>ACMI cystourethroscope
>ACMI fiberoptic colonoscope
>ACMI fiberoptic esophagoscope
>ACMI fiberoptic proctosigmoidoscope
>ACMI gastroscope
>ACMI light source connector
>ACMI microlens Foroblique telescope
>ACMI monopolar electrode
>ACMI resectoscope
>ACMI Transvaginal Hydro laparoscope
>ACMI T-915, TX-915 fiberoptic sigmoidoscope

Acoma
>A. portable x-ray machine
>A. scanner

acorn
>a. cannula
>a. carver
>A. CorCap cardiac support device
>A. II nebulizer
>a. reamer

acorn-tipped
>a.-t. bougie
>a.-t. catheter

Acor Quikform I, II shoe
Acoustascope esophageal stethoscope
acoustic
>a. impedance probe
>a. microscope
>a. myograph
>a. otoscope
>a. respiratory motion sensor

acoustically transparent cradle

AcQsim CT simulator
Acra-clip system
Acra-Cut
>A.-C. spiral craniotome blade
>A.-C. wire pass drill

Acragun system
acridinium ester-labeled nucleic acid probe
Acro ComforT shoulder support
Acroflex artificial disc
AcroMed
>A. screw
>A. VSP fixation system
>A. VSP plate

acromioclavicular (AC)
acromionizer
>a. bur
>a. tip

Acrotorque hand engine
AcryDerm
>A. border island dressing
>A. hydrogel sheet
>A. Strands
>A. Strands absorbent wound dressing
>A. Strands filler

acrylic
>a. ball eye implant
>a. bite block
>a. bite wafer
>a. cap splint
>a. cement
>Durahue a.
>Duralay a.
>Dura-Liner a.
>a. ear splint
>fast-setting a.
>a. foldable intraocular lens
>a. graft
>a. hydroxyapatite implant
>a. implant material
>a. interocclusal splint
>a. jig
>a. mold
>a. palatal splint
>a. separator
>TMJ a.
>a. wafer temporomandibular joint splint
>a. wafer TMJ splint

Acryl-X orthopaedic cement removal system
AcrySof
>A. foldable intraocular lens
>A. haptic lens
>A. MA60 lens
>A. ReSTOR apodized diffractive optic posterior chamber intraocular lens

A. ReSTOR lens
A. single-piece IOL
ACS
Advanced Cardiovascular System
Alcon Closure System
automated corneal shaper
ACS Alpha balloon
ACS Amplatz guidewire
ACS anchor exchange device
ACS Angioject
ACS balloon catheter
ACS Concorde catheter
ACS Concorde OTW catheter
ACS Concorde over-the-wire
catheter system
ACS Endura coronary dilation
catheter
ACS Enhanced Torque 8/7.5-F
Taper Tip catheter
ACS extra-support guidewire
ACS Gemini prosthesis
ACS Gyroscan
ACS Hi-Torque Balance
middleweight guidewire
ACS Indeflator
ACS JL4 French catheter
ACS LIMA guidewire
ACS microglide wire
ACS Mini catheter
ACS Monorail catheter
ACS Multi-Link coronary stent
ACS Multi-Link coronary system
ACS Multi-Link Duet coronary
stent
ACS Multi-Link Duet stent
ACS Multi-Link RX Ultra
coronary stent system
ACS Multi-Link RX Ultra stent
ACS Multi-Link Tristar coronary
stent
ACS Multi-Link Tristar stent
ACS needle
ACS OTW Lifestream coronary
dilation catheter
ACS OTW Photon coronary
dilation catheter
ACS OTW Solaris coronary
dilation catheter
ACS percutaneous introducer set
ACS Photon coronary dilation
catheter
ACS Profile prosthesis
ACS RX Comet angioplasty
catheter
ACS RX Comet coronary dilation
catheter
ACS RX Comet VP coronary
dilation catheter
ACS RX Gemini catheter

ACS RX Lifestream catheter
ACS RX Multi-Link stent
ACS RX perfusion balloon catheter
ACS RX Rocket catheter
ACS RX Solaris coronary dilation
catheter
ACS 180 SE automated
chemiluminescent immunoassay
system
ACS Star prosthesis
ACS SULP II balloon
ACS Tourguide II guiding catheter
ACS Viking catheter
ACS:180 CK/MB analyzer
ACS-NT
Gyroscan ACS-NT
**ACST Tx2000 coronary dilation
catheter**
Ac·T
A. diff, Ac·T diff2 hematology
analyzer
A. 5 diff AL auto loader
hematology analyzer
A. 5 diff CP cap pierce
hematology analyzer
A. 5 diff OV open vial
hematology analyzer
A. series hematology analyzer
Act
A. joint support
A. knee support
A. Microcoil
A. MicroCoil delivery system
Actalyke activated clotting time test
Acticel wound dressing
Acticoat
A. burn dressing
A. composite dressing
A. foam dressing
A. silver-based burn dressing
A. 7 wound dressing
Acticon neosphincter
Actifoam
A. active hemostat
A. collagen sponge
A. hemostat
A. hemostat sponge
Actigraph
Mini-Motionlogger A.
Action
A. elbow wrap
A. Jr. wheelchair
A. ThumSling
A. traction system
A. wrist wrap
Actis
A. venous flow controller
A. VFC

Actisorb Silver 220 antimicrobial binding dressing
Activa
>A. Parkinson control system
>A. tremor control system

Activair battery
Activase
>Cathflo A.

activated
>a. balloon-expandable intravascular stent
>a. capsule endoscope

activating adjusting instrument (AAI)
activator
>Andresen a.
>Andresen-Haupl a.
>cutout a.
>palate-free a.
>Schwarz bow-type a.

active
>A. ankle brace
>A. Ankle support
>A. Can defibrillator lead system
>A. Cath catheter
>a. compression-decompression resuscitator
>a. fixation pacemaker lead
>A. Life convex 1-piece urostomy pouch with Durahesive skin barrier
>A. Life Flushaway 1-piece flushable closed-end pouch system
>A. Life 1-piece drainable pouch
>A. Life 1-piece opaque stoma cap
>A. Life 1-piece precut closed-end pouch
>a. MRI stent
>a. sock
>A. support and brace
>a. total PSA ELISA kit

Activent
>A. antimicrobial ventilation tube
>A. ear tube

Activin AB free beta-HCG ELISA test
Activitrax
>A. II pacemaker
>A. single-chamber responsive pacemaker
>A. variable-rate pacemaker

activity-guided pacemaker
Activity-Lite knee brace
activity-sensing pacemaker
Activskin support pantyhose
Activ slideboard
actocardiotocograph monitor
ACT-One coronary stent
Actros pacemaker
Actros+ pacemaker

actuator
>linear a.
>mechanical ventilator a.
>NYU-Hosmer prehension a.

AcuBase
>Omega A.

Acucair continuous airflow system
Acucare bed
Acucise
>A. access sheath
>A. balloon
>A. balloon catheter
>A. cutting balloon device
>A. endopyelotomy
>A. endopyelotomy catheter
>A. RP retrograde endopyelotomy catheter
>A. ureteral cutting cautery

AcuClip endoscopic multiple-clip applier
Acu-Derm TPN dressing
AcuDriver osteotome
ACU-dyne antiseptic
Acufex
>A. alignment guide
>A. ankle distractor
>A. arthroscope
>A. arthroscopic instrument
>A. bioabsorbable fixation device
>A. bioabsorbable Suretac suture
>A. bioabsorbable suture anchor
>A. curette
>A. curved basket forceps
>A. distractor pin
>A. drill
>A. drill guide
>A. Edge
>A. gouge
>A. grasper
>A. handle
>A. knee laxity arthrometer
>A. mallet
>A. meniscal basket
>A. microsurgical rear-entry to front-entry femoral guide system
>A. microsurgical tendon stripper
>A. MosaicPlasty instrument
>A. osteotome
>A. probe
>A. tensiometer
>A. T-Fix suture anchor

Acufex-Suretac implant
AcuFix anterior cervical plate system
Acuforce 7.0 therapy tool
Acu-Form flexible rod implant
acuity visual projector
Acu-Magnet
AcuMaster acupuncture needle

AcuMatch
- A. A, L, M series acetabular component
- A. integrated hip system
- A. M series modular femoral hip prosthesis

Acumed
- A. congruent clavicle plate
- A. great toe system
- A. suture anchor

AcuNav
- A. steerable phased vector-array ultrasound catheter probe
- A. ultrasound catheter

Acupoint stimulator
AcuPressor myotherapy tool
Acu-Pressure slipper
Acuprobe thermometer
acupuncture
- a. laser
- a. needle
- a. point skin patch

Acu-Ray x-ray unit
Acu-Razor blade
Acuscope microcurrent stimulator
AcuSnare
- A. polypectomy device
- A. snare

Acuson
- A. 128 apparatus
- A. cardiovascular system
- A. color Doppler
- A. Doppler ultrasound
- A. echocardiograph
- A. echocardiographic equipment
- A. 128EP imager
- A. 128EP scanner
- A. imaging system
- A. linear array
- A. linear array transducer
- A. model 128XP machine
- A. Sequoia 512 scanner
- A. transducer
- A. ultrasonoscope
- A. ultrasound
- A. ultrasound scanner
- A. V5M monitor
- A. V5M multiplane TEE transducer
- A. V5M multiplane transesophageal echocardiographic transducer
- A. V5M transesophageal echocardiographic monitor
- A. XP-128 echocardiographic system
- A. 128XP ultrasound system

AcuSpark piezoelectric device

Acustar
- A. I neurosurgical localization system
- A. surgical navigation system

acute
- a. ionization detector
- a. ventricular assist device (AVAD)

AcuTENS transcutaneous nerve stimulator
acute-tipped mammoscope
AcuTrainer
- A. bladder retraining device
- A. device
- A. handheld electronic device

Acutrak
- A. bone fixation system
- A. fusion system
- A. screw
- A. screw system
- A. small bone fixation system

Acutrol suture
Acutronic
- A. AMS automatic jet ventilator
- A. Mistral ventilator
- A. Monsoon ventilator

AcuVibe massager
Acuvue
- A. Advance contact lens
- A. bifocal lens
- A. brand toric contact lens
- A. 1-day disposable lens
- A. disposable contact lens
- A. etafilcon A lens
- A. toric contact lens
- A. 2-week UV-blocking disposable lens

ACX
- ACX balloon
- ACX II balloon catheter

AD 340 absorbance detector
ADAC
- ADAC Cirrus single-headed SPECT camera
- ADAC gamma camera
- ADAC MCD Vertex Plus MCD gamma camera
- ADAC Vertex dual-headed SPECT camera

Adair
- A. breast tenaculum
- A. uterine forceps

Adair-Allis tissue forceps
Adair-Veress needle
Adam and Eve rib belt splint
Adamount pocket mount
Adams
- A. clasp
- A. saw

Adams-DeWeese vena cava serrated clip

Adante
    A. Monorail catheter shaft
    A. PTCA balloon catheter
Adapta physical therapy table
adapter, adaptor
    Amsco Hall a.
    Biolase laser a.
    Bodai a.
    Briggs T a.
    catheter a.
    Ceralink slit lamp laser a.
    Christmas tree a.
    circuit a.
    C-mount a.
    coil machine a.
    Cook plastic Luer-Lok a.
    Cordis-Dow shunt a.
    ENTsol a.
    E-to-A a.
    Foregger-Racine a.
    Freestyle CAPD catheter a.
    friction-fit a.
    Grace plate 4-hole a.
    House a.
    Hudson a.
    Jacobs chuck a.
    Kaufman a.
    King connector a.
    KleenSpec otoscope a.
    large-bore Tuohy-Borst side-arm a.
    large spot slit lamp a.
    Lloyd a.
    Luer-Lok a.
    Luer suction cannula a.
    Mayfield a.
    Mayfield skull clamp a.
    Medi-Jector a.
    metal a.
    Passy-Muir O2 a.
    pediatric Racine a.
    Peep-Keep II a.
    peripheral interface a.
    portable radio a.
    power a.
    Protex swivel a.
    Ralks a.
    resectoscope a.
    rotating a.
    SACH foot a.
    sheath with side-arm a.
    Sheehy-Urban sliding lens a.
    Shiley pressure-relief a.
    side-arm a.
    side-port a.
    sleeve a.
    Storz catheter a.
    suction a.
    swivel a.
    T a.

    Telestill photo a.
    terminal electrode a.
    Trinkle chuck a.
    tubing a.
    Tuohy-Borst a.
    Universal T a.
    venous Y a.
    ventilation a.
    ventricle impedance a. (VIA)
    ventricle impedance a. (VIA)
    Venturi jet a.
    Venturi ventilation a.
    Volk retinal scale a.
    Volk Ultra Field aspherical lens a.
    Volk yellow filter a.
    Xanar laser a.
    Y a.
    Zeiss cine a.
Adapteur multifunctional drill guide
Adaptic
    A. dressing
    A. gauze
    A. gauze dressing
    A. II dental restorative material
    A. nonadhering dressing
    A. pack
    A. sponge
adaptive-rate pacemaker
adaptometer
    Collin 140 color a.
    color a.
    Feldman a.
    Goldmann-Weekers a.
adaptor (*var. of* adapter)
ADC
    analog-to-digital converter
    ADC Medicut shears
Adcon adhesive control gel
Adcon-L anti-adhesion barrier gel
Add-a-Cath
    A.-a-C. catheter
    Lawrence A.-a-C.
Add-A-Clamp
    Hex-Fix A.-A-C.
Add-On
    A.-O. Bucky digital x-ray image acquisition system
    A.-O. Bucky direct x-ray detector
    A.-O. Bucky image acquisition system
ADD side-directed probe
ADD'Stat laser
Addvent atrioventricular pacemaker
adenoid
    a. curette
    a. cutter
    a. forceps
    a. punch

adenoidectomy
    tonsillectomy and a. (T&A)
adenotome
    a. blade
    guillotine a.
    Kelly direct-vision a.
    LaForce a.
    Shambaugh reverse a.
Adeza TLi fetal fibronectin analysis
  system
adherent
    a. lens
    a. stent
    Tuf-Skin tape a.
adhesive
    a. absorbent dressing
    Aron Alpha a.
    autologous fibrin tissue a.
    BA bone cement a.
    a. band
    a. bandage
    Biobond tissue a.
    Biobrane a.
    biodendrimer a.
    BioGlue protein-based surgical a.
    biologic fibrogen a.
    bone cement a.
    Brown sterile a.
    Cel Touch a.
    Chewrite denture a.
    composite external fixator ring a.
    Coverlet a.
    Cover-Roll gauze a.
    cyanoacrylate tissue a.
    Dermabond topical skin a.
    a. drape
    fibrin glue a.
    fibrin sealant a.
    a. flange
    gelatin-resorcin-formalin tissue
     glue a.
    HA a.
    hydroxyapatite a.
    Hy-Tape a.
    Implast bone cement a.
    Indermil tissue a.
    Klutch denture a.
    LiquiBand tissue a.
    Mastisol liquid surgical a.
    methyl methacrylate cement a.
    Neuroacryl tissue a.
    Nexacryl tissue a.
    Nu-Hope a.
    Orthoset radiopaque bone
     cement a.
    Palacos cement a.
    a. plastic drape
    Scanpor acrylate a.
    silastic medical a.

    silicone a.
    stoma cap microporous a.
    Superglue a.
    surgical a.
    surgical appliance a.
    Surgical Simplex P a.
    a. system
    a. tape remover
    Tisseel biologic fibrogen a.
    tissue a.
    T-Stick a.
    Urihesive expandable a.
    Uro-Bond II brush-on silicone a.
    Zimmer low-viscosity a.
adhesive/sealant
    BioGlue a./s.
adhesive-type dressing
Adjustaback wheelchair backrest system
adjustable
    a. advanced reciprocating gait
     orthosis
    a. articulator
    a. breast implant
    a. cane
    a. cane board
    a. headrest
    a. leg and ankle repositioning
     mechanism
    a. ostomy appliance belt
    a. pedicle connector
    a. 2-point caliper sensory
     assessment device
    a. postoperative protective prosthetic
     socket
    a. pressure shunt
    a. skull traction tongs
    a. splint
    a. thigh antiembolism stocking
     (ATS)
    a. vaginal stent
adjustable-angle guide
adjustable-depth gauge needle
Adjusta-Rak hanger
Adjusta-Wrist
    A.-W. hinge
    A.-W. splint
adjuster
    Seibel paracentesis valve a.
    Serdarevic suture a.
Adkins strut
Adler tripronged lens error loupe
administration
    Veterans A. (VA)
adnexal forceps
adolescent
    a. condylar blade-plate
    a. vaginal speculum
Adolph Gasser camera system
adoptable baby cholangioscope

ADR Ultramark 4 ultrasound
Adson
- A. aneurysm needle
- A. bayonet dressing forceps
- A. bipolar forceps
- A. blunt dissecting hook
- A. bone rongeur
- A. brain-exploring cannula
- A. cerebellar retractor
- A. clamp
- A. clip-introducing forceps
- A. conductor
- A. cranial rongeur
- A. dissecting hook
- A. dressing forceps
- A. drill guide
- A. dural hook
- A. enlarging bur
- A. forceps
- A. ganglion scissors
- A. head rest
- A. hemilaminectomy retractor
- A. hemostatic forceps
- A. hook
- A. hypophysial forceps
- A. knot tier
- A. laminectomy chisel
- A. monopolar forceps
- A. needle holder
- A. perforating bur
- A. periosteal elevator
- A. pickup
- A. retractor
- A. scalp clip
- A. suction tube
- A. thumb forceps
- A. tissue forceps
- A. toothed forceps
- A. wire saw

Adson-Beckman self-retaining retractor
Adson-Brown
- A.-B. forceps
- A.-B. tissue forceps

adsorptive voltametry
ADS PLIF broach system
adult
- a. laryngoscope
- a. sigmoidoscope
- A. Star ultra-high-frequency ventilator

Advance
- A. Dynamicaire sleep surface
- A. EX self-adhesive urinary external catheter
- A. PS total knee prosthesis
- A. PS total knee system

advanced
- A. beta 200 otoscope

- a. breast biopsy instrumentation (ABBI)
- a. cardiac life support
- a. cardiovascular life support
- A. Cardiovascular System (ACS)
- A. Collection breast pump
- A. Instruments conductivity analyzer
- a. insulin infusion using a control loop
- a. life support
- A. NMR Systems scanner
- A. surgical suture applier
- a. trauma life support
- a. venous access (AVA)
- a. venous access device
- a. visual instrument system

advancement
- a. forceps
- a. needle

advancer
- Arrow A.
- rotator cuff a.

Advanta
- A. bed
- A. PTFE vascular graft

Advantage
- A. Fusion application
- GE RT 3200 A. II
- A. glucometer
- A. midurethral sling
- A. ultrasound

Advantage4D PET/CT applicator
AdvanTec Legacy
AdvanTeq II TENS unit
Advantim
- A. revision knee system
- A. total knee prosthesis
- A. total knee system
- A. unconstrained prosthesis

Advantx
- A. digital system
- A. LC+ cardiovascular imaging system
- A. LC/LP cardiac biplane system

Advantx-E Legacy system
Advent
- A. implant
- A. pachymeter

adventitial forceps
Advia
- A. 60, 120 automated cell counting instrument
- A. Centaur anti-HBs calibrator
- A. Centaur HBc IgM control material
- A. 1650 chemistry analyzer
- A. 120 hematology system

A

advisor
Schwinn Fitness A.
Advocate electric flexion distraction table
Aebli corneal scissors
AECD
automatic external cardioverter-defibrillator
Powerheart AECD
AED
automated external defibrillator
Star biphasic AED
AEDP
automated external defibrillator pacemaker
Aegis
A. ICD system
A. sonography management system
AEM
ambulatory electrogram monitor
analytical electron microscope
Aequalis
A. head
A. humeral head implant
A. humeral prosthesis
A. reamer
A. reversed shoulder prosthesis
A. stem
A. system
Aequitron
A. apnea monitor
A. pacemaker
A. ventilator
AER+ automatic endoscope reprocessor
AcrobiCycle
Universal A.
AeroChamber
A. face mask
A. nebulizer
A. pediatric spacer device
A. Plus valved holding chamber
A. spacer device
A. spacing device
A. VHC
Aerodose insulin inhaler
Aerodyne stationary bicycle
Aerodyn orthotic
AeroEclipse
A. aerosol delivery device
A. breath actuated nebulizer
AeroEtcher intraoral blaster device
AeroGear
A. asthma action kit
A. fanny pack
Aero-Kromayer lamp
AeroMat
A. balance beam
A. balance block
AeroNOx nitric oxide transport system

Aeroplast dressing
Aeroset clinical chemistry system
aerosol
a. barrier pipette tip
a. cloud enhancer
DEY albuterol inhalation a.
a. generator
a. inhalation monitor
a. mask
monodisperse a.
pirbuterol acetate inhalation a.
aerosolized bronchodilator
AeroSonic personal ultrasonic nebulizer
Aerospray
A. acid-fast bacteria slide stainer/cytocentrifuge
A. cytocentrifuge
A. hematology slide stainer/cytocentrifuge
AeroTech II nebulizer
AeroView optical intubation system
AERx
AERx diabetes management system
AERx drug delivery device
AERx electronic inhaler
AERx inhaler
AERx pain management system
AERx pulmonary drug delivery system
AES
antiembolic stocking
Auger electron spectroscope
Aescula
A. left ventricular lead
A. LV lead
Aesculap
A. ABC cervical plating system
A. argon ophthalmic laser
A. bipolar cautery
A. bipolar cautery forceps
A. drill
A. excimer laser
A. headholder
A. power shovel
A. saw
A. skull perforator
A. traction bow
Aesculap-Meditec
A.-M. excimer laser
A.-M. MEL60 system
Aesculap-Miethke valve
Aesculap-PM noncemented femoral prosthesis
Aesop
A. 2000, 3000 endoscopic stabilizer robot
A. Hermes-Ready system
aesthesiometer
Cochet-Bonnet a.

Aestiva/5 MRI anesthesia machine
AE surgical contraangle 20:1 press-button chuck
AF
    atrial fibrillation
AFB
    air-fluidized bed
Affinity
    A. anterior cervical cage system
    A. bed
    A. blood pump
    A. multimode plate reader
    A. oxygenator
    A. pacemaker
Affirm VP microbial identification system
Affymetrix GeneChip system
AFG
    ankle/foot gauntlet
AFO
    ankle-foot orthosis
    articulated AFO
    AFO brace
    AFO brace sock
    Littig strut AFO
    AFO posterior leaf-spring
    sliding AFO
    AFO standard shell
A-Focus steerable diagnostic catheter
A-Force dorsal night splint
AFP II pacemaker
aftercataract bur
After Five curette
afterload
    a. applicator
    a. colpostat
afterloader
    Fletcher a.
    Henschke a.
    Nucletron MicroSelectron/LDR
    remote a.
afterloading
    a. catheter
    a. probe
Ag-AgCl$_2$ electrode bipolar catheter
Agarloid hydrocolloid impression material
Agarwal
    A. irrigating phaco chopper
    A. nuclear manipulator globe
    stabilizer
agate burnisher
AGC
    anatomic graduated components
    AGC Biomet total knee system
    AGC femoral prosthesis
    AGC knee prosthesis
    AGC knee replacement system
    AGC Modular Tibial II component

    AGC porous anatomic femoral
    component
    AGC tibial prosthesis
Agee
    A. carpal tunnel release system
    A. device
    A. endoscope
    A. WristJack fracture reduction
    system
agent
    Accuzyme enzymatic débriding a.
    Albunex ultrasound imaging a.
    Amalgambond-Plus dentin
    bonding a.
    Coulter Clenz cleaning a.
    Durasphere injectable bulking a.
    enzymatic débriding a.
    Fibrimage diagnostic imaging a.
    Helitene absorbable collagen
    hemostatic a.
    Instat collagen absorbable
    hemostatic a.
    Panafil enzymatic débriding a.
    Panafil-White enzymatic
    débriding a.
    ProBond dentin bonding a.
    Santyl enzymatic débriding a.
Agfa
    A. ADC 70 storage phosphor
    system
    A. CR, PACS system
    A. Dentus M2 comfort intraoral
    radiograph film
    A. Dentus RP 6 blue-sensitive
    extraoral radiograph film
    A. Dentus ST8 G green-sensitive
    extraoral radiograph film
    A. LR 3300 laser imager
    A. Medical scanner
aggregate
    bone a.
aggregometer
    Chrono-log optical a.
    Chrono-log platelet a.
Aggressor meniscal blade
Agilis steerable introducer
Agility total ankle system
Agiltrac peripheral dilation catheter
AgiSite alginate wound cover
AGL-400
    Mira A.
Agnew
    A. canaliculus knife
    A. keratome
    A. tattooing needle
agraffe clamp
Agrikola
    A. eye speculum
    A. lacrimal sac retractor

A. refractor
A. tattooing needle
Agris-Dingman submammary dissector
AGV pars plana clip
AH-26 silver-free sealer
Ahmed
A. glaucoma artificial valve
A. glaucoma biplate valve
A. glaucoma drainage tube
A. glaucoma valve
A. glaucoma valve tube
A. shunt tube
Ahn thrombectomy catheter
AHP digital prosthesis
AHSC elbow prosthesis
AI
AI diagnostic ultrasound
AI 5200 diagnostic ultrasound system
AI 5200 S Open Color Doppler imaging system
AI 5200 S open color Doppler imaging system
AICD
automatic implantable cardiovascular defibrillator
Guardian AICD
AICD pacemaker
AICD plus Tachylog device
Ventak AICD
Ventak Mini II AICD
aid
air-conduction hearing a.
Argosy Cameo CIC hearing a.
A675 Sequel Audio Vision hearing a.
Audibel hearing a.
Audiotone hearing a.
BD Sensability breast self-examination a.
behind-the-ear hearing a.
BiCROS hearing a.
bone-anchored hearing a.
bone conduction hearing a.
Canal-Mate hearing a.
Carex ambulatory a.
CIC hearing a.
completely in-the-canal hearing a.
compression hearing a.
cryostat frozen sectioning a.
Crystal Tone I in-the-ear hearing a.
Dahlberg hearing a.
Digi-Sound hearing a.
Ear-Tronics hearing a.
extension a.
eyeglass hearing a.
Fonix hearing a.
hearing a.

in-the-canal hearing a.
in-the-ear hearing a.
ITE hearing a.
linear hearing a.
Lion hearing a.
low-vision a.
Magnatone hearing a.
Maico Gamma hearing a.
OrthoTurn standing transfer a.
Pacific Coast hearing a.
Panasonic hearing a.
postauricular hearing a.
Prisma digital hearing a.
prosthetic speech a.
Quantum hearing a.
ReSound CC4 hearing a.
ReSound Digital 2000 hearing a.
Rexton hearing a.
Sensability breast self-examination a.
Servox electronic speech a.
Servox Inton speech a.
sock a.
Songbird disposable hearing a.
speech a.
Starkey hearing a.
StraddleSitter seating a.
Tactaid hearing a.
Tactaid I vibrotactile a.
Trilogy I hearing a.
Tru-Canal hearing a.
Turn-Easy transfer a.
ultrasonic mobility a.
Ultra Voice speech a.
Unitron Esteem CIC hearing a.
walking a.
AID-Check monitor
Ailos nebulizer
AIM
AIM femoral nail system
AIM 7 thermocouple input module
aimer
Arthrotek femoral a.
aiming
a. bow
a. guide
air
a. aspirator needle
a. bag
a. band
a. bed
a. bicycle
a. chamber
a. clamp inflatable vessel occluder
a. cleaner
a. compression osteotome
a. compressor
a. cylinder
a. cystotome

air *(continued)*
>a. dermatome
>A. DonJoy patellofemoral brace
>a. drill
>a. entrainment face mask
>a. entrapment mask
>a. flow mat
>A. Force test grid target
>a. injection cannula
>a. medical transport
>a. pillow
>a. plethysmograph
>a. pressure dressing
>a. pressure splint
>A. Pulse sensory stimulator
>a. pump
>a. sampler
>a. saw
>a. splint
>A. Supply air purifier
>A. Supply wearable air purifier
>A. Temp Advantage back support belt
>A. Townsend brace
>a. trousers
>a. uterine displacer
>A. Viva
>a. walker

AIR1517 vacuum-formed static air wheelchair cushion
Air-Back spinal system
air-boot
>Jobst postoperative a.-b.

airbrush
Aircast
>A. Air-Stirrup leg brace
>A. ankle brace
>A. Cryo/Cuff
>A. Cryo/Cuff brace
>A. fracture brace
>A. knee system
>A. pneumatic air stirrup
>A. pneumatic air stirrup brace
>A. pneumatic walker
>A. Swivel-Strap
>A. Swivel-Strap brace
>A. walking brace

air-conduction hearing aid
air-core magnet
Airdance alternating overlay
air-displacement pipette
air-driven
>a.-d. artificial heart
>a.-d. bur
>a.-d. dermatome
>a.-d. oscillating saw

Air-Drop chiropractic table
Air-Dyne bicycle

Aire-Cuf
>A.-C. endotracheal tube
>A.-C. tracheostomy tube

Airex
>A. balance pad
>A. mat

air-filled balloon
AirFlex carpal tunnel splint
Air-Flex chiropractic table
AirFlo alternating pressure system
air-flow enclosure
air-fluidized bed (AFB)
airfuge
>Beckman a.

Airfuge ultracentrifuge
Airis II MRI system
Airkair seat cushion
Airlife
>A. cannula
>A. Dual Spray MiniSpacer
>A. MediSpacer

Airlift balloon retractor
Air-Limb amputation protector
Airlite
>A. alignable ankle block
>A. prosthesis
>A. support pad

Air-Lon tracheal tube brush
AirMax external nasal dilator
Air-O-Ease static air flotation mattress
Air-O-Pad pad
airplane
>a. cast
>a. shears
>a. splint
>a. splint shoulder brace

air-powered
>a.-p. drill
>a.-p. forceps
>a.-p. nebulizer

Airprene
>A. Action knee brace
>A. hinged knee prosthesis
>A. hinged knee support

air-puff tonometer
AirSep
>A. CPAP
>A. OxiScan oximetry recording, reporting, and archiving system
>A. Ultimate nasal seal gel insert

Airshields
>A. isolette
>A. jaundice meter

Airsoft dry replacement mattress
AirStance pylon
Air-Stirrup ankle training brace
Airstrip composite dressing
Airtrac ambulatory cervical/lumbar traction system

AirWatch asthma monitor
airway
>Berman a.
>Berman intubating pharyngeal a.
>binasal pharyngeal a.
>Combitube a.
>Concord/Portex a.
>Connell a.
>disposable a.
>double-lumen gastric laryngeal
> mask a.
>esophageal obturator a.
>Fastrach laryngeal mask a.
>Foerger a.
>Guedel a.
>intubating laryngeal mask a.
>laryngeal mask a.
>LMA disposable laryngeal mask a.
>LMA Fastrach laryngeal mask a.
>LMA ProSeal laryngeal mask a.
>nasopharyngeal a.
>oral pharyngeal a.
>oropharyngeal a.
>pharyngeal a.
>pharyngeal tracheal lumen a.
>Portex nasopharyngeal a.
>ProSeal laryngeal mask a.
>PtL a.
>Robertazzi nasopharyngeal a.
>rubber a.

AirZone peak flowmeter
AK-10 dialysis machine
Akahoshi
>A. acrylic intraocular lens forceps
>A. acrylic IOL loading forceps
>A. combo prechopper
>A. hybrid combo prechopper
>A. hydrodissection cannula
>A. implantation forceps
>A. nucleus completer
>A. nucleus manipulator
>A. nucleus ring sustainer
>A. nucleus separator
>A. nucleus splitter
>A. phaco prechopper
>A. prechopper forceps
>A. Universal prechopper

A-K diamond knife
Aker lens pusher
Akron tilt table
Akros
>A. DFD wheelchair wedge cushion
>A. extended care mattress
>A. mattress
>A. pressure mattress

AkroTech mattress
Akton pad
Akura partial depth astigmatic
** keratotomy marker**

Akutsu III total artificial heart
AL
>Amplatz left
> AL I, II guiding catheter

Alabama
>A. tying forceps
>A. University utility forceps

AlaBLOT kit
Aladdin
>A. infant flow system
>A. nasal CPAP system

Alamo alternating low air loss mattress
** overlay**
Alan-Thorpe lens
alar
>a. plate
>a. retractor
>a. screw

alar-columellar implant
alarm
>Bárány a.
>bed-wetting a.
>a. cushion
>enuresis a.
>glutaraldehyde a.
>Nite Train'r A.
>Silent Nite a.

AlaSTAT allergy immunoassay system
AlaTOP inhalant allergy screen
Albany eye guard
Albarran
>A. deflecting level
>A. laser cystoscope
>A. mechanism
>A. reflecting bridge

Albee
>A. bone graft
>A. hip arthrodesis
>A. lumbar spinal fusion
>A. olive-shaped bur

Albert
>A. Grass Heritage digital EEG
> system
>A. Grass Heritage digital PSG
> system
>A. Grass Heritage EEG system
>A. Grass neurodata system
>A. suture

Albert-Lembert suture
Albert-Smith pessary
albumin-coated vascular graft
albuminimeter
Albunex ultrasound imaging agent
Albustix reagent strip
Alcatel pacemaker
Alcian blue and periodic acid-Schiff
Alcock-Timberlake obturator
alcohol well

Alcon
- A. Accurus vitrectomy cutter
- A. AcrySof SA30AL single-piece lens
- A. A-OK crescent knife
- A. A-OK ShortCut knife
- A. A-OK slit knife
- A. aspirator
- A. Closure System (ACS)
- A. cryoextractor
- A. cryophake
- A. cryosurgical unit
- A. CU-15 needle
- A. cystotome
- A. Digital B ultrasound
- A. disposable drape
- A. EyeMap EH-290 corneal topography system
- A. hand cautery
- A. I-knife
- A. Infiniti system
- A. intraocular lens
- A. irrigating needle
- A. Legacy unit
- A. MA30BA optic AcrySof lens
- A. Master unit
- A. microsponge
- A. phacoemulsification unit
- A. portable autokeratometer
- A. reverse cutting needle
- A. spatula needle
- A. Surgical instrument
- A. suture
- A. taper cut needle
- A. taper point needle
- A. tonometer
- A. ultrasound pachymeter
- A. vitrectomy probe
- A. vitrector

AlcoSCRUB instant antiseptic hand cleanser
Alco-Sensor
aldehyde-tanned bovine carotid artery graft
Alden CDI orthotic
Aldrete needle
Aldridge rectus fascia sling
Aleo meter
AlereNet system
Alert catheter
Alexa
- A. 1000 breast diagnostic system
- A. 1000 breast lesion diagnostic device
- A. 1000 system

Alexander
- A. bone chisel
- A. chisel
- A. costal osteotome
- A. costal periosteotome
- A. elevator
- A. mastoid bone gouge
- A. rib stripper
- A. tonsil needle

Alexander-Ballen retractor
Alexander-Farabeuf
- A.-F. costal periosteotome
- A.-F. forceps
- A.-F. periosteotome
- A.-F. rasp

alexandrite laser (ALEXlazr)
Alexian Brothers overhead frame
ALEXlazr
- alexandrite laser
- Candela A.
- A. laser

Alfa-gliatest
- ELISA Kit A.-g.

Alfonso
- A. cutting platform
- A. diamond corneal transplant blade
- A. nucleus forceps
- A. nucleus ophthalmic trisector
- A. nucleus trisector
- A. pediatric eyelid speculum

Alfonso-McIntyre nucleus spoon
Alfred M. Large vena cava clamp
Alger brush
algesiometer, algesimeter
- Boas a.
- pressure a.
- vulvar a.

Al-Ghorab modification shunt
AlgiDerm
- A. alginate dressing
- A. alginate wound cover
- A. wound packing

alginate
- a. impression material
- a. wound cover
- a. wound dressing

AlgiSite alginate wound dressing
Algisorb wound dressing
Algo-1 automated auditory brainstem response device
Algo-2 hearing screening device
AlgoMed infusion system
algometer (*var. of* algesiometer)
Algo newborn hearing screener
Algosteril
- A. alginate dressing
- A. alginate wound cover

Alice4 sleep diagnostic system
AliCool splint spray
AliCork foot orthosis
Alien WildEyes lens

ALIF
    anterior lumbar interbody fusion
aligner
        Charnley femoral inlay a.
        femoral a.
        Geo-Matt 30-degree body a.
        incision a.
        orthodontic a.
        patellar a.
        tibial a.
alignment
        a. catheter
        a. guide rod
AliMed
        A. Conductive Patient Shifter
        A. diabetic night splint
        A. hemi-arm sling
        A. insert
        A. orthosis
        A. putty
        A. sensor floor mat
        A. turnbuckle elbow splint
        A. wrist/thumb support
AliMed-Freedom arthritis support
alimentary
        a. apparatus
        a. system
alimentation catheter
Alio
        A. capsulorrhexis forceps
        A. enclavation forceps
        A. iridectomy forceps
        A. MICS capsulorrhexis forceps
Alio-Kelman IOL hook
Alio-Prats irrigating chopper stinger
Alio-Rodriguez LASIK spatula
Aliplast
        A. blank
        A. custom-molded foot orthosis
        A. insole
        A. pad
Alisoft splinting material
AliStrap Velcro-type strapping
alkalimeter
All
        A. Access laser system
        A. Poly Deltafit keel
        A. Pupil II indirect ophthalmoscope
Alladin InfantFlow nasal continuous positive air pressure
all-alumina socket
Alldress
        A. composite dressing
        A. multilayered wound dressing
Allegiance nasal prongs
Allegra
        A. 64R high-speed refrigerated benchtop centrifuge

        A. 25R refrigerated benchtop centrifuge
        A. X-12, X-15R, X-22 benchtop centrifuge
Allegretto
        A. wave excimer laser
        A. Wave excimer laser system
        A. wave topolyzer
Allen
        A. anastomosis clamp
        A. applicator
        A. arthroscopic elbow positioner
        A. arthroscopic knee positioner
        A. arthroscopic wrist positioner
        A. diagnostic module
        A. eye implant
        A. fetal stethoscope
        A. figure
        A. hand/arm surgery table
        A. head screwdriver
        A. intestinal clamp
        A. laparoscopic stirrup
        A. orbital implant
        A. preschool card
        A. retractor
        A. shoulder/wrist arthroscopy traction system
        A. stereo separator
        A. stirrup
        A. strap
        A. traction system
        A. wrench
Allen-Brown shunt
Allender vertical laminar flow room
Allen-Schiötz plunger retractor tonometer
Allen-Thorpe
        A.-T. goniolens
        A.-T. gonioscopic prism
        A.-T. lens
Allen-type hex key
AllerCare allergy control product
Allergan
        A. AMO Array S155 lens
        A. Humphrey laser
        A. Humphrey lensometer
        A. Humphrey photokeratoscope
        A. Medical Optics photokeratoscope
Allergenco MK-3 spore trap
Allerprick needle
Allevyn
        A. adhesive foam dressing
        A. adhesive hydrocellular dressing
        A. cavity foam dressing
        A. foam
        A. hydrophilic polyurethane dressing
        A. island dressing
        A. island foam dressing

Allevyn *(continued)*
>A. Thin dressing
>A. tracheostomy foam dressing
>A. wound dressing

Allgöwer apparatus
Allgöwer-Donati suture
AllHear cochlear implant
Alliance
>A. integrated inflation system
>A. rehabilitation system

alligator
>a. bone-reduction forceps
>a. clip
>a. cup forceps
>a. ear forceps
>a. forceps
>a. grasping forceps
>a. jaws Olympus FG 6L grasping forceps
>a. pacing cable
>a. scissors

All-In-One laparoscopic electrode
all-in-the-bag intraocular lens
Allis
>A. catheter
>A. clamp
>A. delicate tissue forceps
>A. forceps
>A. hemostat
>A. intestinal forceps
>A. tissue forceps

Allis-Abramson breast biopsy forceps
Allis-Adair tissue forceps
Allis-Duval forceps
Allison
>A. clamp
>A. lung retractor
>A. lung spatula

AllKare protective barrier wipe
AlloAnchor
>A. RC allograft
>A. RC allograft device

Alloclassic hip system
AlloCraft
>A. bone spacer substitute
>A. PL allograft spacer

AlloDerm
>A. acellular dermal graft
>A. acellular dermal matrix
>Cymetra micronized A.
>A. onlay graft
>A. preserved human dermis
>A. processed tissue graft
>A. spacer graft
>A. strip
>A. tissue
>A. universal dermal tissue graft

Allofit acetabular cup system

Allofix
>A. freeze-dried bone
>A. freeze-dried cortical bone pin

AlloFuse DBM putty
allogeneic material
allograft
>Accugraft a.
>acellular dermal a.
>AlloAnchor RC a.
>AlloGro freeze-dried bone a.
>a. bone vise
>decalcified freeze-dried bone a.
>epithelium-derived orthotopic corneal a.
>fresh-frozen nonirradiated bone-patellar tendon-bone a.
>HTO wedge human donor tissue a.
>IBS a.
>intercalary a.
>living related conjunctival limbal a.
>MiCOR machine bone a.
>napkin ring calcar a.
>osteoarticular a.
>Puros Accugraft a.
>Red Cross freeze-dried a.
>Tutoplast processed a.

AlloGro
>A. bone graft material
>A. freeze-dried bone allograft

AlloMatrix
>A. bone graft putty
>A. injectable putty
>A. injectable putty bone graft substitute

AlloMune system
alloplastic
>a. graft material
>a. plate

Allo-Pro hip system
alloy
>amalgam a.
>Ceradelta a.
>Ceramalloy a.
>Cerapall a.
>cobalt-chromium-molybdenum a.
>Co-Span a.
>Degudent a.
>E-G a.
>Elgiloy metal a.
>Everest a.
>GM a.
>Hammond a.
>Leff a.
>vitallium a.

all-PMMA 1-piece C-loop intraocular lens
all-polyethylene socket
Allport
>A. clip applier

A. cutting bur
A. mastoid searcher
A. mastoid sound
A. retractor
Allport-Babcock searcher
all-purpose
    a.-p. boot (APB)
    A.-p. Boot Hi
All-Silicone Side-Eye EPT feeding tube
Allskin marker
All-Terrain balloon
all track wire (ATW)
All-Tronics scanner
Allurion foot prosthesis
Almacone II
Alm wound retractor
Alnico Magneprobe magnet alpha
**Aloe Vesta moisturizing skin care
    product**
Aloka
A. CL ultrasound
A. color Doppler
A. color Doppler system
A. linear ultrasound
A. MP-PN ultrasound probe
A. OB/GYN ultrasound
A. 650 scanner
A. SD ultrasound system
A. sector ultrasound
A. SSD-720 real-time scanner
A. SSD ultrasound system
A. SSD ultrasound system and
  probe
A. transducer
A. ultrasound
A. ultrasound linear scanner
A. 650 ultrasound scanner
A. ultrasound sector scanner
Alpern cortex aspirator/hydrodissector
alpha
A. Active pressure-relieving support
  surface
Alnico Magneprobe magnet a.
a. bone substitute material
a. cradle
A. cushion liner
A. Dx point-of-need test system
A. fiberoptic pocket otoscope
A. flat sheet
A. I penile implant
a. particle accelerator
a. probe
A. 1 pump
A. suction attachment block kit
Alphabed
alphabet board
alpha-BSM
    a.-BSM bone repair material
    a.-BSM bone substitute material

alpha-chymotrypsin cannula
AlphaCor
A. artificial cornea
A. hydrogel synthetic cornea
alpha-particle emitter
AlphaStar operating room table
Alphatec
A. mini lag-screw system
A. small fragment system
Alpine reusable leg bag
ALP Plus ankle brace
alprazolam
ALPS
    anterior locking plate system
      Amset ALPS
      ALPS container
      ALPS EasyLiner
Alps CustomPro custom liner
ALR cystoresectoscope
already-threaded suture
Alta
A. advance tibial/humeral rod
A. CFX reconstruction rod
A. condylar buttress plate
A. distal fracture plate
A. femoral bolt
A. femoral plate
A. humeral rod
A. intramedullary rod
A. modular trauma system
A. reconstruction rod
A. supracondylar screw
A. tibial/humeral rod
A. tibial nail
A. tibial rod
Altea
A. MicroPor
A. MicroPor laser
alternating pressure pad
alternative communication device
alternator
    film a.
Altertome
    Microvasive A.
ALTK system microkeratome
Alto
A. DR implantable cardioverter
  defibrillator
A. 2 implantable cardioverter
  defibrillator
A. VR implantable cardioverter-
  defibrillator
Alton
A. Deal pressure infuser
A. Dean blood/fluid warmer
Altra-Flux hemodialyzer
ALT ultrasound system
Alukart hemoperfusion cartridge
Alumafoam nasal splint

alumina
- a. cemented total hip prosthesis
- a. ceramic
- a. implant

alumina-on-alumina total hip prosthesis
aluminum
- a. eye shield
- a. finger cot splint
- a. Finn chamber
- a. oxide implant
- a. oxygen regulator

Aluwax impression wax
ALVAD
- abdominal left ventricular assist device
- ALVAD artificial heart

Alvarado
- A. collateral ligament protector
- A. knee holder
- A. legholder

Alvar condylar bolt
Alvarez prosthesis
alveolar arch acrylic splint
Alveolus stent technology system
AlveoSampler
- QuinTron A.

Alvis
- A. curette
- A. fixation forceps
- A. foreign body eye curette

Alvis-Lancaster sclerotome
Alzate catheter
Alzer Model 2001 osmotic minipump
Alzet continuous infusion osmotic pump
Alzheimer lamp
Alznner orthotic
AM
- ammeter

AM-50 portable air compressor
Amadeus
- A. epikeratome
- A. microkeratome
- A. ventilator

amalgam
- a. alloy
- a. burnisher
- a. carrier
- a. carver
- a. condenser
- Paragon a.
- a. plugger
- a. plugger elevator
- a. scraper

amalgamator
- Crown a.
- Dentomat a.
- Vari-Mix II a.

Amalgambond-Plus dentin bonding agent
Amazr catheter

Ambi
- A. compression hip screw system
- A. hip screw
- A. wrist brace

Ambicor
- A. inflatable prosthesis
- A. penile prosthesis

Ambler dilator
amblyoscope
- major a.
- Worth a.

Ambu
- A. bag
- A. CardioPump
- A. infant resuscitator
- A. respirator
- A. Spur disposable resuscitator

Ambu-E valve
ambulation training orthosis
ambulator
- Apex A.
- A. biomechanical footwear
- A. Bio-Rocker sole
- A. Chukka Boot
- A. conform footwear
- A. H1200 healing shoe

ambulatory
- a. electrogram monitor (AEM)
- household a.
- a. infusion management device
- a. measurement system
- a. nuclear detector
- A. shoe
- a. ventricular function probe

AMC
- AMC needle
- AMC total wrist prosthesis

Amcath catheter
Amdent ultrasonic scaler
AME
- AME bone growth stimulator
- AME microcurrent TENS unit
- AME PinSite shield
- AME pin site shield
- AME tongue retaining device

Ameflow device
Amelogen Plus radiopaque restorative material
Amenabar
- A. counterpressor
- A. lens

America
- United States of A. (USA)

American
- A. Catheter Corp. biopsy forceps
- A. Chiropractic College of Radiology adjusting table
- A. Endoscopy automatic reprocessor
- A. Endoscopy dilator

A. Heyer-Schulte-Radovan tissue expander prosthesis
A. Hydron instrument
A. Medical Optics (AMO)
A. Medical Optics Baron lens
A. Medical Source laparoscopic equipment
A. Medical Systems (AMS)
A. Medical Systems penile prosthesis
A. Medical Systems urethral sphincter
A. Optical coagulator
A. Optical ophthalmometer
A. Optical R-inhibited pacemaker
A. Pacemaker Corporation lead
A. Shared-CuraCare scanner
A. silk suture
A. Sterilizer operating table
A. tracheotomy tube

Amerigel topical ointment hydrogel dressing

Amersham

A. CDCS A-type needle
A. International ECL gene detection system
A. J tube
A. Life Science PCR product presequencing kit
A. Life Science Thermo Sequenase sequencing kit

Ames

A. Lab-Tek cryostat
A. ventriculoperitoneal shunt

Amfit

A. custom orthosis
A. digitizer
A. orthotic

Amico

A. extractor
A. nail nipper

Amicon D-20 filter
Amicus blood collection separator
Amigo mechanical wheelchair
Ami infant apnea monitor
amino acid analyzer
aminopropyltriethyoxysilane-coated glass slide
AMIS extension table
Amis 2000 respiratory mass spectrometer

AMK

AMK fixed bearing knee system
AMK total knee system
AMK unconstrained prosthesis

Amko vaginal speculum

AML

AML Plus prosthesis
AML total hip prosthesis

ammeter (AM)
AM-MI orthopaedic table
amnifocal lens
AmniHook amniotic membrane perforator
AmnioGraft wound dressing
amnioscope
amniotome

Baylor a.
Beacham a.

AMO

American Medical Optics
AMO Array foldable intraocular lens
AMO Array intraocular lens
AMO Array multifocal ultraviolet-absorbing silicone posterior chamber intraocular lens
AMO Array SA40N multifocal IOL
AMO Clariflex IOL
AMO HPF 500 pump
AMO intraocular lens
AMO Ioptex Model ACR 360 foldable acrylic lens
AMO Phacoflex II foldable intraocular lens
AMO PhacoFlex lens and inserter
AMO Prestige advanced cataract extraction system
AMO Prestige phaco system
AMO Sensar intraocular lens
AMO series 4 phaco handpiece
AMO Set-Up
AMO Sovereign compact WhiteStar system
AMO YAG 100 laser

A-mode echo-tracking device
Amoena breast form
Amoils epithelial scrubber
amorphous silicon filmless digital x-ray detection technology device
AmpErase electrocautery
amperometric meter
Amplatz

A. anchor system
A. angiography needle
A. aortography catheter
A. cardiac catheter
A. catheter
A. Clot Buster
A. coronary catheter
A. dilator
A. dilator set
A. exchange length wire
A. fascial dilator

Amplatz *(continued)*
A. femoral catheter
A. gooseneck microsnare
A. gooseneck snare
A. injector
A. left (AL)
A. left coronary catheter
A. left I, II catheter
A. retinal snare
A. right coronary catheter
A. right I, II catheter
A. Super Stiff catheter
A. Super Stiff guidewire
A. tapered extra-stiff wire guide
A. tapered movable core wire
A. Teflon sheath
A. thrombectomy device
A. torque wire
A. TractMaster system
A. tube guide
A. ultra-stiff wire guide
A. ventricular septal defect device
Amplatzer
A. device
A. duct occluder
A. septal occluder
Amplex guidewire
Amplicor
A. HIV-1 test kit
A. PCR kit
A. typing kit
amplification device
amplifier
Botox injection a.
endocardiographic a.
gradient a.
hearing aid a.
lock-in a.
NeuroProbe a.
Omniace RT3200N
electromyographic a.
power a.
pulse a.
Servo power a.
Servox a.
voltage a.
Ampliwax PCR gem
Ampoxen sling
amputation
a. knife
a. retractor
a. saw
a. screw
amputator
Smith intraocular capsular a.
amputee cushion
Amrex
A. muscle stimulator
A. therapeutic ultrasound

AMS
American Medical Systems
A. Ambicore penile prosthesis
A. 800 artificial urethral sphincter
A. autoclavable laparoscope
A. CX penile prosthesis cylinder
A. 700CX penile prosthesis
cylinder
A. 700CX-series penile prosthesis
A. disposable trocar
A. Hydroflex penile prosthesis
A. inflatable penile prosthesis
A. inflatable 700 penile prosthesis
A. malleable penile prosthesis
A. 3-piece inflatable penile
prosthesis
A. ProstaJect ethanol injection
system
A. Sphincter 800 urinary prosthesis
A. Ultrex penile prosthesis
A. urethral stent
Amsco
A. Hall adapter
A. headholder
A. hysteroscope
A. light
A. Orthairtome drill
Amset
A. ALPS
A. anterior locking plate system
A. R-F fixation system
A. R-F rod
A. R-F screw
Amsler
A. aqueous transplant needle
A. chart
A. grid
A. scleral marker
Amsoft lens
Amsterdam
A. biliary stent
A. ventilator
Amsterdam-type prosthesis
Amussat probe
AN69 membrane dialyzer
Anaconda
A. device
A. device and delivery system
anaerobic
a. Pulsator syringe
a. specimen collector
anal
a. dilator
a. EMG PerryMeter sensor
a. retractor
a. speculum
analgesia
WalkMed patient-controlled a.

**analgesic cell therapy implantable
 device**
analgizer
 Penthrane a.
analmoscope
analog
 a. rate meter
 a. video acquisition station
analog-to-digital converter (ADC)
analytical electron microscope (AEM)
Analytic Technology pulp tester
analyzer
 Abacus Concepts StatView 4.02
  statistical a.
 Abbott Cell-Dyn hematology a.
 ABI Prism 3700 DNA a.
 ABI Prism 3100 genetic a.
 ABL 555 a.
 Access AFP immunoassay a.
 ACL 100, 1000, 7000, 8000,
  9000, 10000 advance
  coagulation a.
 ACS:180 CK/MB a.
 Ac·T diff, Ac·T diff2
  hematology a.
 Ac·T 5 diff AL auto loader
  hematology a.
 Ac·T 5 diff CP cap pierce
  hematology a.
 Ac·T 5 diff OV open vial
  hematology a.
 Ac·T series hematology a.
 Advanced Instruments
  conductivity a.
 Advia 1650 chemistry a.
 amino acid a.
 Apec glucose a.
 Arthrodial Protractor range of
  motion a.
 Aution Max AX-4280 automated
  urine chemistry a.
 automated biochemical a.
 automated cerebral blood flow a.
 automatic a.
 automatic chemical a.
 automatic clinical a.
 automatic fluorescent image a.
 AVL Omni blood gas a.
 AVL Opti 1 portable blood gas a.
 AVL 9110 pH a.
 AxSYM a.
 Bayer DCA2000 a.
 Bayer Technicon H-2 a.
 Beckman Coulter CEQ8000
  fluorescent DNA a.
 Beckman ion-selective a.
 Beckman O$_2$ a.
 Beckman Synchron CX-7
  cholesterol a.

 BiliCheck bilirubin a.
 BiliChek bilirubin a.
 1620 blood gas a.
 840 blood gas a.
 BRACAnalyzer gene a.
 BVA-100 blood volume a.
 Capnomac infrared a.
 Capnomac multiple gas a.
 Careside a.
 CA-6000 spine motion a.
 Cat-a-Kit a.
 Cell Soft 2000 semen a.
 Cell Trak/DMS a.
 Cell Trak/S a.
 ChromaVision digital a.
 Clinitek 50 urine chemistry a.
 coagulation a.
 Cobas Fara centrifugal a.
 Cobas Fara H centrifugal a.
 Cobas fast centrifugal a.
 Cobas Helios differential a.
 Cobra Amplicor a.
 cooximeter a.
 Corning 170 blood gas a.
 CO Sleuth handheld carbon
  monoxide a.
 CO-stat end tidal breath a.
 Coulter Channelyser cell a.
 Coulter LH 500, 700, 750, 755,
  1500 Series hematology a.
 Coulter MAXM hematology a.
 Coulter STKS hematology a.
 C-Trak a.
 Delsa 440 SX Zeta potential a.
 Dicon ocular blood-flow a.
 digital dermoscopy a.
 DMI a.
 Dow hollow-fiber a.
 Elecsys 1010 a.
 Elecsys 2010 modular
  immunoassay a.
 Electra 1000C coagulation a.
 Elite Plus motion a.
 ERA 300 dual-chamber pacing
  system a.
 ESRA-10 erythrocyte sedimentation
  rate a.
 ESR-Auto Plus sedimentation
  rate a.
 Eye Scan corneal a.
 fast Fourier transformation
  spectrum a.
 FLx/TDx immunoassay a.
 Fourier transformation spectrum a.
 Friedmann visual field a.
 Futrex a.
 Galilei dual Scheimpflug a.
 GastrograpH Mark III pH a.
 GDx nerve fiber a.

analyzer *(continued)*
Gemini automated centrifugal a.
Gem Premier Plus blood
gas/electrolyte a.
GEM-Premier point-of-care blood a.
GenePhor DNA fragment a.
Gen-S hematology a.
Hamilton-Thorn motility a.
HemoCue B-Glucose a.
HemoCue blood glucose a.
HemoCue blood hemoglobin a.
Hitachi 704, 717, 736, 911 a.
Hitachi 747-100 cholesterol a.
Hitachi 747 CK/MB a.
HmX hematology a.
Humphrey field a. II
Humphrey Instruments vision a.
Humphrey lens a.
Humphrey visual field a.
IL Synthesis a.
immediate response mobile a.
(IRMA)
Immulite 2000 anti-HBc IgM a.
Immulite 2000 anti-HBs a.
Immulite 2000 chemiluminescent a.
Immulite Dynamic Duo a.
Immulite HBsAg immunoassay a.
immunoturbidimetry a.
IMx a.
Ionalyzer a.
i-STAT handheld a.
KC1 Delta coagulation a.
Keystone PF a.
Kodak Ektachem DT-60
cholesterol a.
Kodak Ektachem Vitros 250, 750,
950 cholesterol a.
Lactate Pro LT-1710 portable
lactate a.
laser microprobe mass a.
LeadCare handheld blood lead a.
LH 500, 750, 1500 series
hematology a.
LS 100Q/200/230 series laser
diffraction particle size a.
LS 13 320 series laser diffraction
particle size a.
Malvern a.
Marquette Series 8000 Holter a.
medical gas a.
Medigraphics 2000 a.
MicroLyzer Gas a.
miniature centrifugal fast a.
MiniOX IA oxygen a.
multichannel discrete a.
NE-8000 a.
nerve fiber a.
NordicTrack motion a.
Nova Celltrak 12 hematology a.

N5 submicron particle size a.
Octopus visual field a.
ocular blood flow a.
ocular response a.
Olympus AU5200 cholesterol a.
Olympus SP series image a.
Omni a.
Oncometrics Imaging Cyto-Savant
image a.
Opti 1 pH/blood gas a.
Opti 1 portable blood a.
Opti 1 portable pH/blood gas a.
Orion model EA 940 ion a.
Osteomeasure computer-assisted
image a.
oxygen a.
Pachymetric P55 a.
Packard Auto-Gamma 5650 a.
Paradigm ocular blood flow a.
Paramax a.
patient state a.
Pentra 60C+ a.
Piccolo blood chemistry a.
platelet function a. (PFA)
PocketChem UA a.
P55 pachymetric a.
PrinterNOx nitric oxide with
MKII a.
pulse-height a.
Radiometer ABL 500 blood gas a.
Rapidpoint 400 critical care a.
RapidVUE particle shape and
size a.
reflectance TS-200 spectrum a.
RJL model 10 bioelectrical
impedance a.
Sam Jr. posture a.
SA 3100 surface area and pore
size a.
sequential multiple a.
Serena Mx apnea recorder/a.
Serono SR1 FSH a.
Shimadzu DAR-2400 coronary
arteriographic a.
Siemens Somatom DRH CT a.
Sievers model 280 nitric oxide a.
simultaneous multiple a.
single-channel a.
Sonoclot coagulation a.
SPART a.
SRI automated immunoassay a.
STA a.
Stat Profile pHOx blood gas a.
Stratus II automatic a.
Stride A.
SureStep Pro glucose a.
Sweat-Chek conductivity a.
Synchron CX-5, CX-7
automated a.

Synchron LX20 pro chemical a.
Sysmex NE-8000 CBC a.
Sysmex XE-2100 hematology a.
Sysmex XT-2000i automated
  hematology a.
Tanita professional body
  composition a.
TDX a.
TDxFlx a.
thermal energy a.
tissue spectrum a. TS-200
Tomey retinal function a.
ultrasound bone a.
Urisys urine a.
Vi-Cell series cell viability a.
Vision a.
Vitalab ViVa clinical chemistry a.
Vitros a.
ViVa binocular infrared vision a.
Wescor Sweat-Chek conductivity a.
YSI STAT glucose and lactate a.

Analyze system
analyzing rod
**Anastomark flexible coronary graft
  marker**
anastomosis, pl. **anastomoses**
  a. apparatus
  a. clamp
  a. forceps
anastomotic button
anatomic
  a. expander
  a. graduated components (AGC)
  a. medullary locking hip system
  a. modular knee
  porous-coated a. (PCA)
  a. porous replacement hemispheric
    acetabular component
  A. Precoat hip prosthesis
**anatomical Tobin malar prosthetic
  implant**
Anatomotor traction/massage table
Ancap braided silk suture
anchor
  Acufex bioabsorbable suture a.
  Acufex T-Fix suture a.
  Acumed suture a.
  Anchorlok soft tissue a.
  Anspach suture a.
  Arthrex bone a.
  Arthrex TwistLoc suture a.
  AxyaWeld bone a.
  a. band
  Bio-Anchor suture a.
  Bio-FASTak a.
  Biologically Quiet Mini-Screw
    suture a.
  Biomet bone a.
  Bio-Phase suture a.

Bioraptor suture a.
BioROC EZ suture a.
BioSphere suture a.
Bio-Statak suture a.
BioZip suture a.
bone a.
Bone Bullet suture a.
Bone Button orthopaedic suture a.
buttress and button a.
Catera suture a.
A. catheter exchange device
Contack labral a.
Cope viscerotomy a.
Corkscrew suture a.
CurvTek drill bone a.
DePuy Mitek Contack labral a.
a. endosteal implant
esophageal Z stent with a.'s
E-Z ROC a.
FASTak suture a.
Fastin RC threaded a.
Fastin suture a.
Fastin threaded a.
GII Snap-Pak a.
GLS suture a.
Harpoon suture a.
a. hook
Howmedica bone a.
implantable bone a.
Innovasive bone a.
intraosseous suture a.
Isola spinal implant system a.
Kurer a.
Lemoine-Searcy a.
Linvatec bone a.
Mainstay urologic soft tissue a.
MicroLite suture a.
Micromax resorbable suture a.
Mini Bio-Phase suture a.
mini GLS a.
MiniMite suture a.
Mini-Revo Screws suture a.
Mini-Revo suture a.
Mini-ROC a.
Mitek absorbable bone a.
Mitek bone a.
Mitek Contack labral a.
Mitek Fastin threaded a.
Mitek GII easy a.
Mitek GII suture a.
Mitek GL a.
Mitek knotless a.
Mitek ligament a.
Mitek micro a.
Mitek Mini GII a.
Mitek Mini GLS a.
Mitek Panalok RC a.
Mitek rotator cuff a.
Mitek Tacit threaded a.

anchor *(continued)*
    Ogden bone a.
    Orthofix Ogden a.
    PaBA a.
    Panalok absorbable suture a.
    Panalok RC QuickAnchor Plus
      suture a.
    a. peg glenoid all-polyethylene
      prosthesis
    PLA a.
    A. plate
    PLLA a.
    press-in bone a.
    Quickanchor Plus small bone a.
    Radix a.
    Revo suture a.
    ROC a.
    RotorloC absorbable rotator cuff
      suture a.
    a. screw
    Sherlock threaded suture a.
    a. splint
    Statak suture a.
    Stealth a.
    Stryker BioZip suture a.
    Stryker Xcel suture a.
    Super Revo suture a.
    suture a.
    Tacit threaded a.
    Therap-Loop door a.
    ThRevo suture a.
    traction a.
    transvaginal bone a.
    UltraFix a.
    UltraFix MicroMite suture a.
    UltraFix MiniMite suture a.
    UltraFix RC suture a.
    UltraSorb suture a.
    a. washer
    Wright Medical bone a.
    Xcel suture a.
    ZAAG implant a.
    Zest implant a.
    Zimmer-Statak a.
anchored catheter
anchor/fixation
    Searcy a./f.
anchoring peg
Anchorlok
    A. soft tissue anchor
    A. soft tissue suture anchor system
Anchron biodegradable anchor system
ANCOR imaging system
Ancure
    A. endograft system
    A. system
    A. tube graft
Andersen Cascade impactor

Anderson
    A. acetabular prosthesis
    A. biopsy punch
    A. distractor
    A. fixation apparatus
    A. fixation device
    A. gastric tube
    A. leg-lengthening device
    A. 5-prong bear claw
    A. splint
Anderson-Adson self-retaining retractor
Anderson-Neivert osteotome
Andresen
    A. activator
    A. monoblock appliance
    A. removable orthodontic appliance
Andresen-Haupl activator
Andrews
    A. infant laryngoscope
    A. osteotome
    A. retractor
    A. spinal surgery frame
    A. spinal surgery table
    A. SST-3000 spinal surgery table
    A. suction tip
    A. tongue depressor
Andrews-Pynchon suction tube
Andries stethoscope
Androsov vascular stapler
Anel
    A. lacrimal probe
    A. syringe
AnemiaPro Self-Screening Kit
anemometer
    hot-wire a.
    mass-flow a.
aneroid
    a. chest bellows
    a. manometer
anesthesia
    a. bag
    barbiturate burst-suppression a.
    Hunstad system for tumescent a.
    a. needle
anesthesiometer
    Semmes-Weinstein pressure a.
anesthetic needle
Aneuroplastic resin
AneuRx
    A. bifurcated stent-graft system
    A. endograft
    A. IDS delivery system
    A. stent
    A. stent-graft
    A. stent graft system
aneurysm
    a. clamp
    a. clip
    a. clip applier

a. forceps
a. neck dissector
a. needle
aneurysmal
a. clip
a. coil
AneuVysion Assay prenatal genetic test
AngeCool
A. RF catheter
A. RF catheter ablation system
Angeflex defibrillation lead
Angeion 2000 ICD generator
AngeLase combined mapping-laser probe
Angelchik antireflux prosthesis
Angeles
University of California at Los A. (UCLA)
Angell
A. James dissector
A. James hypophysectomy forceps
Angell-Shiley
A.-S. bioprosthetic heart valve
A.-S. bioprosthetic valve
A.-S. xenograft prosthetic valve
angel wing guide
Ange-Med Sentinel ICD device
Anger
A. gamma camera system
A. scintillation camera
Angestat hemostasis introducer
Angetear tear-away introducer
Angiocath
A. Autoguard shielded IV catheter
A. catheter
A. flexible catheter
A. PRN catheter
angiocatheter
large-bore a.
a. with looped polypropylene suture
Angiocor prosthetic valve
Angioflow
A. high-flow catheter
A. meter system
angiographer
fluorescein a.
angiographic
a. balloon occlusion catheter
a. catheter
a. end-hole catheter
a. portacaval shunt
angiography
a. catheter
a. needle
Angioguard catheter device
Angioject
ACS A.

AngioJet
A. rapid thrombectomy system
A. rheolytic thrombectomy system
A. saline jet/vacuum device catheter
A. thrombectomy catheter
A. thrombectomy device
A. Xpeedior catheter
Angio-Kit catheter
Angiolink EVS closure device
Angiomat
A. 3000, 6000 contrast delivery system
A. Illumena contrast delivery system
A. Illumena injector
A. Illumena injector system
Angiomed
A. blue stent
A. Puroflex stent
Angiomedics catheter
angiopeptin-eluting stent
angioplasty
a. balloon
a. balloon catheter
Grüntzig balloon catheter a.
a. guiding catheter
percutaneous transluminal a. (PTA)
a. sheath
AngiOptic microcatheter
AngioRad
A. afterloader system
A. radiation system
angioscope
flexible a.
Olympus a.
angioscopic valvulotome
Angio-Seal
A.-S. carrier tube
A.-S. catheter
A.-S. closure device
A.-S. diagnostic device
A.-S. hemostasis system
A.-S. hemostatic puncture closure device
A.-S. system
A.-S. therapeutic device
A.-S. vascular closure device
Angiostar Plus vascular imaging equipment
AngioStent stent
AngioSURF system
angiotribe
Ferguson a.
a. forceps
angle
a. arch
ASSI Phaco Chopper 90-degree a.
A. basic E arch appliance

angle *(continued)*
- a. finder
- a. implant
- Konstram a.
- a. measurement device
- a. port pump
- RZ mandibular a.
- a. splint
- W&H Endodontic Contra A.

angled
- a. awl
- a. ball-end electrode
- a. balloon catheter
- a. biter
- a. cannula
- a. capsular forceps
- a. capsule forceps
- a. cartilage scissors
- a. clip
- a. Connor wand
- a. counterpressor
- a. DeBakey clamp
- a. decompression retractor
- a. delivery device
- a. discission hook
- a. dissector
- a. Glidewire
- a. guidewire
- a. iris hook and IOL dialer
- a. iris retractor
- a. iris spatula
- a. left cannula
- a. left/right cannula
- a. lens loupe
- a. Lowman-type bone clamp
- a. manipulator
- a. nucleus removal loupe
- a. peripheral vascular clamp
- a. pigtail catheter
- a. pleural tube
- 2-a. polypropylene loop
- a. probe
- a. right cannula
- a. ring curette
- a. sapphire knife
- a. stone forceps
- a. suction tube
- a. telescope
- a. vein retractor

angled-down forceps
angled-lens endoscope
angled-shaft endoscope
angled-up forceps
angle-fixated lens
Angle-Iron skull immobilizer
AngleLoop curette
angle-tip
- a.-t. electrode
- a.-t. Glidewire

- a.-t. guidewire
- a.-t. urethral catheter

Angstrom
- A. II ICD
- A. MD ICD
- A. MD implantable single-lead cardioverter-defibrillator

angular
- a. bolster
- a. elevator
- a. hinge clamp
- a. knife
- a. needle
- a. scissors
- a. screwing instrument

angulated
- ASSI breast dissector a.
- a. catheter
- a. iris spatula
- a. multipurpose catheter

angulator
animal beanbag exerciser
Animas
- A. R-1000 insulin pump
- A. R-1000 sensor

aniridia ring
Anis
- A. aspirating cannula
- A. capsule polisher
- A. corneal forceps
- A. corneal scissors
- A. irrigating vectis
- A. lens-holding forceps
- A. microforceps
- A. needle holder
- A. radial marker
- A. staple lens
- A. suture placement marker
- A. tying forceps

Ank-L-Aid brace
ankle
- a. air stirrup
- Buechel-Pappas total a.
- a. contracture orthosis
- C Stance a.
- a. disc device
- a. exercise machine
- a. guard
- a. hitch
- a. immobilizer
- A. Isolator
- A. Isolator ankle rehabilitator
- A. Isolator foot and ankle exerciser
- a. magnet
- a. orthosis (AO)
- a. rehabilitation pump
- R-Hab lighter weight a.
- a. splint

a. stabilizer
a. stirrup brace
a. stirrup splint
USMC multiaxis a.
a. weight
ankle-foot
a.-f. electrogoniometer
a.-f. orthosis (AFO)
a.-f. orthotic
a.-f. orthotic splint
a.-f. plastic orthosis
ankle/foot gauntlet (AFG)
ankleRAP postsurgical wound wrap
AnkleTough ankle rehabilitation system
ANMR Insta-scan MR scanner
Anna-Dote positioning support
AnnuloFlex flexible annuloplasty ring
AnnuloFlo
A. annuloplasty ring
A. annuloplasty ring system
anode tube
anomaloscope
Kamppeter a.
Nagel a.
Pickford-Nicholson a.
Spectrum color vision meter
712 a.
anophthalmic implant
anoscope
Bacon a.
Boehm a.
Brinkerhoff a.
Buie-Hirschman a.
Ferguson a.
fiberoptic a.
Hirschman a.
Ives a.
KleenSpec disposable a.
Otis a.
Pratt a.
Pruitt a.
rotating speculum a.
Sims a.
slotted a.
speculum a.
Welch Allyn a.
Anprolene sterilizer
Ansaldo ultrasound
Anspach
A. cranial perforator
A. craniotome
A. drill
A. 65K instrument system
A. 65K Universal instrument
system
A. suture anchor
Answer hip system
Ant-Cer dynamic cervical plate

antegrade
a. femoral nail
a. ureteral stent
antegrade/retrograde compression nail
Antense antitension device
antepartum monitor (APM)
anterior
a. anodal patch electrode
a. aspect esophageal sensor
a. bulbi camera
a. capsule forceps
a. capsule hydrodissector
a. cervical plate
a. cervical plate fixation system
(ACFS)
a. cervical plate system
a. chamber (AC)
a. chamber intraocular lens (AC-
IOL)
a. chamber irrigating cannula
a. chamber irrigating vectis
a. chamber irrigator
a. chamber maintainer
a. chamber synechia scissors
a. chamber tube shunt encircling
band
a. chamber washout cannula
a. cheek electrode
a. commissure laryngoscope
a. cruciate ligament (ACL)
a. cruciate ligament drill guide
a. cruciate ligament/posterior
cruciate ligament (ACL/PCL)
a. eye segment analysis system
a. forceps
a. internal fixation device
a. locking plate system (ALPS)
a. lumbar interbody fusion (ALIF)
a. quadrilateral triplane frame
a. vented gas forced fusion system
anterior-posterior cutting block
anteroposterior
a. control orthosis
a. cystoresectoscope
Anthony
A. cast boot
A. mastoid suction tube
A. orbital compressor
A. quadrisected minigraft dilator
Anthos ht II automatic photometer
Anthron
A. heparinized antithrombogenic
catheter
A. heparinized catheter
A. II catheter
anthropometer
anthropometric
a. calipers
a. total hip

Antia composite flap
antibacterial
    a. personal catheter
    a. pillow
antibiotic-coated stent
antibiotic-loaded
    a.-l. acrylic cement
    a.-l. acrylic cement total joint
      prosthesis
antibiotic removal device
antibody, pl. **antibodies**
antibody-coated suture
anticholinergic bronchodilator
antidecubitus
    a. mattress
    a. pad
Anti-DNaseB
    Immage A.-D.
antiembolic stocking (AES)
antiembolism stocking
antigen
antigravity suit
anti-G suit
antimicrobial
    a. catheter cuff
    a. MPM wound cleanser
    a. removal device
antimony
    a. monocrystalline electrode
    a. pH electrode
antiprotrusio cage
antireflux
    a. double-J stent
    a. prosthesis
antirestenotic stent
antirotation
    a. cable
    a. device
    a. guide
    proximal femoral nail a. (PFNA)
antisense RNA probe
antiseptic
    ACU-dyne a.
    Avagard instant hand a.
    a. dressing
antiseptic-impregnated central venous
  catheter
Antishear gel sheet
antishock
    a. pelvic clamp
    a. suit
Anti-Shox
    A.-S. foot cushion
    A.-S. gel insole
    A.-S. heel cup
    A.-S. orthosis
antisiphon
    a. device
    a. valve

antitachycardia pacemaker
antithrust seat
antitipper wheelchair
antitorque suture
antivibration glove
antra (*pl. of* antrum)
antral
    a. balloon
    a. curette
    a. drain
    a. trocar
antroscope
antrum, pl. **antra, antrums**
    a. exploring needle
    a. punch forceps
anular
    a. array transducer
    a. detector
    a. gouge
Anustim electronic neuromuscular
  stimulator
anvil
    Bunnell a.
Anywear shoe
AO
    ankle orthosis
      AO drill bit
      AO dynamic compression plate
      AO gouge
      AO guide pin
      AO mandibular system
      AO notched instrumentation
      AO reconstruction plate
      AO reduction forceps
      AO Reichert Instruments
        applanation tonometer
      AO Reichert Instruments binocular
        indirect ophthalmoscope
      AO Reichert Instruments Ful-Vue
        diagnostic unit
      AO Reichert Instruments lensometer
      AO Reichert Instruments Project-O-
        Chart
      AO rigid fixation
      AO rotary prism
      AO semitubular plate
      AO spongiosa screw
      AO spoon plate
      AO stopped drill guide
AOA
    atlanto-occipital articulation
      AOA cervical immobilization brace
      AOA halo cervical traction
AO/ASIF
    Association for Osteosynthesis/American
    Society of Internal Fixation
      AO/ASIF compression plate
      AO/ASIF screw

AO/ASIF titanium craniofacial system

AOO pacemaker

aortic

    a. aneurysm clamp
    a. aneurysm forceps
    a. arch cannula
    a. assist balloon introducer
    a. balloon pump
    a. bioprosthetic valve
    a. cannula clamp
    a. catheter
    a. connector system
    a. cross-clamp
    a. curette
    a. dilator
    a. occluder
    a. occlusion clamp
    a. perfusion cannula
    a. punch
    a. tube graft
    a. valve retractor
    a. valve rongeur

AO-Titanium microplate

AP

    Asia-Pacific
    AP nail
    AP portal

Apache CU Risk Predictor

APB

    all-purpose boot
    APB Hi all-purpose boot

APC

    APC hip retractor
    APC proximal femoral elevator

APC-3, APC-4 collimator

A-P cutting block

Apdyne phenol applicator kit

Apec glucose analyzer

aperture pad

apex

    A. Ambulator
    A. Ambulator shoe
    A. 409, 415 camera
    A. 409, 410, 415 ECT digital gamma camera
    A. insole
    a. locator
    A. Modular femoral stem system
    a. pin
    A. Plus excimer laser

Apexo elevator

Apfelbaum

    A. bipolar forceps
    A. micromirror

Apgar timer

apheresis catheter

API

    API osteotome
    API universal foam chin strap

apical axis guide

Apit electronic apex locator

aplanatic lens

Aplicap

    Espe Ketac-Bond A.
    Espe Photac-Bond A.

Apligraf

    A. graft
    A. Graftskin
    A. tissue-engineered skin

APL Plus ankle brace

APM

    antepartum monitor
    Nicolet VersaLab APM

APM-2000 vital signs monitor

apnea

    a. alarm mattress
    Bedbugg system for at-home diagnosis of sleep a.
    a. monitor

apochromatic lens

apodized diffractive IOL

Apofix

    A. cervical instrumentation
    A. interlaminar clamp

Apogee

    A. CX100, CX200 echocardiography system
    A. CX100 Interspec ultrasound machine
    A. RX400 diagnostic ultrasound system
    A. surgical mesh
    A. ultrasound device
    A. 800 ultrasound system
    A. vaginal vault prolapse repair system

Apollo

    A. DXA bone densitometer
    A. DXA bone densitometry system
    A. 95E tooth-whitening and curing system
    A. hip prosthesis
    A. hip system
    A. hot/cold pak
    A. knee prosthesis
    A. knee prosthesis system
    A. Light Systems
    A. TM electric flexion table
    A. total knee system

ApopTag Plus kit

A-Port

    A-P. implantable port
    A-P. vascular access

AP/PA portal

apparatus, pl. **apparatus, apparatuses**

apparatus *(continued)*
    Acuson 128 a.
    alimentary a.
    Allgöwer a.
    anastomosis a.
    Anderson fixation a.
    aspiration a.
    attachment a.
    automatic systematic
      desensitization a.
    Bárány alarm a.
    Bárány noise a.
    Barcroft a.
    Barcroft-Haldane a.
    Barcroft-Warburg a.
    Belzer a.
    Benedict-Roth a.
    biphase Morris fixation a.
    Bobrov a.
    Brown-Roberts-Wells a.
    Buck convoluted traction a.
    Buck extension a.
    Buck Redi-Traction a.
    C-arm fluoroscopic a.
    Charnley compression a.
    cryosurgical a.
    dental a.
    Desault a.
    Doppler a.
    electrooculogram a.
    experimental a.
    extension a.
    eye movement measuring a.
    Fell-O'Dwyer a.
    fixation a.
    fracture-banding a.
    Frigitronics nitrous oxide
      cryosurgery a.
    Georgiade visor halo fixation a.
    Gibson-Cooke sweat test a.
    Golgi a.
    Guthrie-Smith a.
    Haldane a.
    halo a.
    Hilal embolization a.
    hinged-distraction a.
    Hodgen a.
    Holman flushing a.
    Horsley-Clarke stereotactic a.
    Howard-Dolman a.
    isokinetic resistance a.
    Jackson-Rees a.
    Jaquet a.
    juxtaglomerular a.
    Kanavel a.
    Kandel stereotactic a.
    Kidde a.
    Killian suspension gallows a.
    Kinetron muscle strengthening a.

    Kirschner a.
    Kirschner traction a.
    Kroner a.
    Küntscher traction a.
    lacrimal a.
    Langendorff a.
    Leksell a.
    Lewy suspension a.
    LHE a.
    Light-Veley a.
    Lynch suspension a.
    Malgaigne a.
    Manifold II slot-blot a.
    masticatory a.
    Mayfield-Kees skull fixation a.
    McAtee a.
    McKesson pneumothorax a.
    mechanical joint a.
    MedX muscle testing a.
    mobile electroconvulsive therapy a.
    Nakayama anastomosis a.
    Neufeld a.
    optoelectric measuring a.
    Pearson flexed-knee a.
    Perroncito a.
    Philips Angiodiagnostics 96 a.
    Plummer-Vinson a.
    pneumothoracic a.
    portable insulin dosage-regulating a.
    Potain a.
    R&B portable pneumothorax a.
    Reichert-Mundinger a.
    Roger Anderson external fixation a.
    Roughton-Scholander a.
    Sandow a.
    Sayre suspension a.
    Scholander a.
    self-contained breathing a.
    self-contained underwater
      breathing a.
    Skatron a.
    spark-gap a.
    Spiegel-Wycis human a.
    spine a.
    stereotactic a.
    Stryker ConstaVac suction a.
    sucker a.
    suction a.
    surgical exhaust a.
    suspension a.
    temperature exchange a.
    Tobold laryngoscopic a.
    Todd-Wells a.
    traction a.
    triplanar protractor a.
    vacuum a.
    vacuum tube a.
    Van Slyke a.
    Venturi a.

Volkov-Oganesian-Povarov hinged
  distraction a.
V-Vac suction a.
Wagner a.
Wangensteen a.
Warburg a.
Watanabe a.
Wells stereotactic a.
Zander a.

AP-PA skull immobilizer
appendage clamp
appendectomy retractor
appendiceal retractor
applanation tonometer
applanator
  Johnston LASIK flap a.
applanometer
Applause Super-Hemi wheelchair
Applebaum incus replacement prosthesis
Apple Medical bipolar forceps
appliance
  Acco orthodontic a.
  Andresen monoblock a.
  Andresen removable orthodontic a.
  Angle basic E arch a.
  arch bar facial fracture a.
  Balters a.
  Begg light wire a.
  biphasic pin a.
  bite a.
  Case a.
  Crozat removable orthodontic a.
  dental speech a.
  double-band navel a.
  EMA a.
  E Merge Contour Grid eruption a.
  Erich facial fracture a.
  extraoral fracture a.
  facial fracture a.
  Fairdale orthodontic a.
  fixed a.
  FracSure a.
  Fränkel a.
  Gentle Touch colostomy a.
  Goldthwait fracture a.
  Hawley a.
  Herbst a.
  Hibbs fracture a.
  Hyrax a.
  ileostomy a.
  intraoral fracture a.
  Jelenko facial fracture a.
  Jewett fracture a.
  Jobst a.
  Joe-Hall-Morris biphasic a.
  Johnson twin-wire a.
  Joseph septal fracture a.
  Karaya adhesive ileostomy a.
  Kesling a.

Klearway oral a.
Latham a.
Level Anchorage a.
light wire a.
mandibular advancement a.
mandibular advancing oral a.
mandibular orthopaedic
  repositioning a.
mandibular repositioning oral a.
Marlen colostomy a.
microstomia prevention a.
monobloc-type a.
obturator a.
oral a.
Ormco a.
orthodontic a.
OSAP a.
ostomy a.
passive alveolar molding a.
prosthetic a.
Proxi-Floss cleaning a.
ribbon arch a.
Roger Anderson pin fixation a.
SACH orthopaedic a.
Skin Stretcher a.
Snoar a.
Snore-Ezzer oral a.
Snore Tec a.
soft ankle cushioned heel
  orthopaedic a.
surgical a.
therapeutic a.
TheraSnore oral a.
Unitck a.
Universal a.
vinyl palatal a.
Whitman fracture a.
Wilson fracture a.
Winter facial fracture a.
wire a.
W. W. Walker a.

application
  Advantage Fusion a.
  Hawkeye SPECT a.
  MCAS modular clip a.
  ultrathin needle brachytherapy-style
    delivery renal a.
applicator
  Absolok endoscopic clip a.
  Advantage4D PET/CT a.
  afterload a.
  Allen a.
  Bárány a.
  benzoin a.
  Betadine PrepStick Plus a.
  beta-ray a.
  beta therapy eye a.
  Bloedorn a.
  brachytherapy balloon a.

applicator *(continued)*
Brown a.
Brown-Dean cotton a.
Burnett a.
cesium a.
colpostat a.
Copalite a.
cotton a.
cotton-tipped a.
cymatic a.
Dean a.
Delrin a.
double-balloon a.
ear a.
Ernst radium a.
Falope ring a.
Filshie clip a.
Filshie clip minilaparotomy a.
Fletcher-Suit a.
a. forceps
Gass dye a.
global force a.
Grafco cotton-tip a.
Henschke seed a.
Holinger a.
infrared a.
intracavitary afterloading a.
intracavitary balloon a.
iontophoretic a.
Ivan laryngeal a.
Jackson laryngeal a.
Jobson-Horne cotton a.
Kevorkian-Younge uterine a.
Kyle a.
laryngeal a.
Lejeune cotton a.
LITT a.
Ludwig middle ear a.
Ludwig sinus a.
Mayfield clip a.
Mick seed a.
Mick TP-200 a.
microwave a.
minilaparotomy Falope ring a.
mini-ovoid a.
Miralva a.
Multifire clip a.
multiload occlusive clip a.
Nucletron a.
perfused needle a.
RapidMist metered-dose spray a.
resorbable thread clip a.
ring a.
Sawtell-Tobold laryngeal a.
small LITT a.
^{90}Sr-loaded eye a.
Stabiliplan orthovolt a.
standard LITT a.
Storz a.

strontium-90 ophthalmic beta-ray a.
Syed-Puthawala-Hedger
  esophageal a.
tandem a.
Uebe a.
Wang a.
**Applied Biosystems 340A nucleic acid
  extractor**
applier
AcuClip endoscopic multiple-clip a.
Advanced surgical suture a.
Allport clip a.
aneurysm clip a.
Autoclip a.
automatic Hemoclip a.
bayonet clip a.
clip a.
cotton-tipped a.
Crockard transoral clip a.
Endo Clip a.
endoscopic rotating clip a. (ERCA)
hemostatic clip a.
Hulka clip a.
Kaufman clip a.
Kerr clip a.
LDS clip a.
Ligaclip a.
Ligaclip MCA multiple-clip a.
Malis clip a.
Mayfield miniature clip a.
Mayfield temporary aneurysm
  clip a.
mini a.
Multifire Endo hernia clip a.
Olivecrona clip a.
PermaClip clip a.
pivot clip a.
Raney scalp clip a.
Sano clip a.
Spetzler clip a.
surgical clip a.
Vari-Angle clip a.
vascular clip a.
Weck clip a.
Yasargil aneurysm clip a.
Yasargil clip a.
Appolito suture
Appose skin stapler
apposition
a. forceps
stent a.
Appraise
A. clinical densitometer
A. monitor
approach
combined neurosurgical-external
  sinus a.
approximation forceps

approximator
Biemer a.
a. clamp
hook a.
Ikuta clamp a.
Kleinert-Kutz clamp a.
Lalonde tendon a.
Leksell sternal a.
Link a.
microanastomosis a.
Microspike a.
nerve a.
Neuromeet soft tissue a.
Pilling-Wolvek sternal a.
rib a.
sternal a.
Wolvek sternal a.

APR
APR acetabular prosthesis
APR femoral prosthesis
APR I femoral stem
APR II prosthesis

Aprema III device
ApriVera skin and hair cleanser
A-Probe
Soft-Touch A-P.

apron
Hottentot a.
lead a.
lead-rubber a.
perineal surgical a.

APS Hi-Lo electric lift table
Aptis distal radial ulna joint prosthesis
APU brace
aqua
a. PT dry physiotherapy
a. PT water massage
A. Spray wet nail débridement
system
A. Thermassage

AquaBodyCiser aquatic mat
Aquacel
A. AG wound dressing
A. Hydrofiber dressing
A. Hydrofiber wound dressing
A. wound packing and dressing

Aqua-Cel heating pad system
Aquaciser
A. hydrodynamic measurement
system
A. 100R underwater treadmill
system
A. underwater treadmill

Aquaflex
A. contact lens
A. gel pad
A. ultrasound gel pad

Aquaflo hydrogel wound dressing

AquaFlow collagen glaucoma drainage
device
AquaGaiter treadmill
Aquagel lubricating gel
AquaGuide ureteral access sheath
AquaJogger buoyancy belt
AquaLase
A. cataract removal system
A. liquefaction device

AQUALiner hydrophilic Ni-Ti alloy
guidewire
AquaMED
A. dry hydrotherapy equipment
A. hydrotherapy device

AquaMotion pool
Aquamount
Aquanex hydrodynamic measurement
system
AquaNot soft silicone custom-molded
earplug
Aquaphor
A. gauze
A. gauze dressing

Aquaplast
A. alloplastic material
A. cast
A. dressing
A. mask
A. mold
A. rapid-setting splint material
A. splint
A. splinting material

Aquarelle hydrogel nucleus viscoelastic
material
AquaRunners resistance footwear
Aqua-Seal chest drainage unit
AquaSense IOL
AquaSens FMS 1000 fluid monitoring
system
AquaShield
A. orthopaedic cast cover
A. reusable cast cover
A. reusable orthopaedic cast cover

Aquasight lens
Aquasil Smart Wetting impression
material
Aquasonic 100 ultrasound transmission
gel
Aquasorb
A. Border with Covaderm tape
A. hydrogel sheet
A. hydrogel wound dressing
A. transparent hydrogel dressing

AquaTack hydrocolloid barrier
Aquatech cast pad
Aquatherm bed pad
aquatic therapy pool
Aqua-Trainer
Aquatrek device

Aquatrend water workout station
Aqua/Whirl bath
aqueous
a. double-tubed valve shunt
a. transplant needle
a. tube shunt
Aquilion
A. combined CT-fluoroscopy scanner
A. plus V-detector CT scanner
AR-1, AR-2 diagnostic guiding catheter
arachnoid knife
arachnophlebectomy
a. needle
a. surgical device
Arbuckle sinus probe
arc
dynamic reference a.
a. guidance system
Leksell a.
shoulder ROM a.
xenon a.
Arc-22 catheter
arch
angle a.
a. bar
a. bar cutter
a. bar facial fracture appliance
a. binder
a. cushion
extramedullary alignment a.
FemoStop femoral artery compression a.
lingual a.
A. Rival foot orthotic
a. support
Wilson bimetric a.
Archer splinter forceps
Archimedean drill
archival system
archwire
Jarabak-type a.
Archxerciser foot exercise device
arcitome
Hanna a.
Arcitumomab diagnostic imaging system
ArCom
A. compression-molded polyethylene
A. processed polyethylene
arc-quadrant stereotactic system
ARC surgical wrist traction tower
Arctic
A. Blaze hot/cold pack
A. Sun temperature management system
arcuate skin stapler
area-specific curette
Arena hemodialysis device

Arenberg-Denver inner-ear valve implant
ArF
argon fluoride
ArF excimer laser
ArF excimer laser system
Arglaes
A. antimicrobial barrier film dressing
A. film dressing
A. powder
A. wound dressing
argon
a. beam coagulator
A. Beamer 2 device
a. blue laser
a. fluoride (ArF)
a. fluoride excimer laser
a. green laser
a. guidewire
a. ion laser
a. laser
a. laser photocoagulator
a. plasma coagulator
a. tuneable dye laser
argon/krypton laser
argon-pumped
a.-p. dye laser
a.-p. tunable dye laser
Argosy Cameo CIC hearing aid
Argus camera
Argyle
A. antireflux valve
A. arterial catheter
A. catheter
A. CPAP nasal cannula
A. Ingram trocar catheter
A. silicone Salem sump
A. trocar
A. trocar catheter
A. umbilical vessel catheter
Argyle-Salem sump antireflux valve
Argyle-Turkel safety thoracentesis system
Aria
A. coronary artery bypass graft
A. CPAP system
A. LX CPAP system
Ariat shoe
Ariel computerized exercise system
ARI Group I–IV filter
Aris transobturator tape
Arizona
A. ankle brace
A. Health Sciences Center-Volz hinge
A. universal leg support
Arjo loop sling
ARK-Juno refractor

Arloing-Courmont test
Arlt scoop
arm
  articulating a.
  a. board
  a. elevator sling
  a. ergometry treadmill
  flexible a.
  2-a. goniometer
  Heidelberg a.
  Huang Universal flexible a.
  Leonard a.
  Leyla flexible a.
  mechanical articulated a.
  MonitorMate monitor a.
  pediatric retractor adjustable a.
  PinPoint stereotactic a.
  a. positioner
  a. retractor
  scanning a.
  a. and shoulder immobilizer
  a. skate
  a. splint
  a. swathe
  Utah artificial a.
  Wiltmoser optical a.
  Yasargil Leyla retractor a.
Arm-a-Med endotracheal tube
armboard
  arterial catheter a.
armchair splint
armrest bolster
Armstrong
  A. CPR mask
  A. handheld pulse oximeter
  A. plate
  A. prosthesis
  A. tube
  A. tube line
  A. ventilation tube
Army
  A. chisel
  A. osteotome
Army-Navy retractor
Arndorfer
  A. capillary perfusion system
  A. pneumohydraulic capillary
    infusion system
Arnett LeFort implant
Arnett-TMP
  A.-TMP depth gauge
  A.-TMP system
Arnoff external fixation device
Arnold-Bruening syringe
Arnold lumbar brace
Arnott 1-piece all-PMMA intraocular
  lens
Aromamist steam tube
AromaScan aroma analysis device

Aroma-Stream diffuser
aromatherapy diffuser
Aromist Personal Steam Sauna
Aron Alpha adhesive
AROSupercut scissors
AR+ portable heart monitor
array
  Acuson linear a.
  A. 360, 360CE/CE-AL
    protein/drug/serology system
  Clarion HiFocus electrode a.
  convex a.
  epidural electrode a.
  A. foldable intraocular lens
  A. multifocal intraocular lens
  Nucleus Contour electrode a.
  a. processor
  subdural electrode a.
  A. ultrasound transducer
AR 1000 refractor
arrhythmia
  a. control device (ACD)
  a. mapping system
  a. mapping system catheter
  A. Net arrhythmia monitor
arrhythmogenic myocardial tissue
  ablation catheter
arrow
  A. absorbable meniscal repair
    device
  A. Advancer
  A. balloon wedge catheter
  A. Berman angiographic balloon
  Biofix meniscus a.
  Bionx a.
  a. blade
  A. Blue FlexTip
  A. Cannon catheter
  A. catheter
  A. Flex intraaortic balloon catheter
  A. FlexTip Plus catheter
  A. high-flow infusion set
  A. LionHeart left ventricular assist
    device
  A. 2-lumen hemodialysis catheter
  A. PICC
  A. PICC line
  a. pin clasp
  A. pneumothorax kit
  polylactic acid a.
  A. Pullback atherectomy catheter
  A. QuadPolar electrode catheter
  A. QuadPolar pulmonary artery
    catheter
  A. QuickFlash arterial catheter
  A. Raulerson introducer syringe
  A. Raulerson syringe
  A. sheath

arrow *(continued)*
    A. Twin Cath
    A. UserGard injection cap system
Arrow-Clarke thoracentesis device
Arrow-Fischell EVAN needle
ArrowFlex sheath
ARROWGard
    A. Blue antiseptic-coated catheter
    A. Blue hemodialysis catheter
    A. central venous catheter
ARROWgard
    A. Blue Line catheter
    A. Blue Plus multilumen central
    venous catheter kit
Arrow-Howes
    A.-H. multilumen catheter
    A.-H. quad-lumen catheter
arrow-shaft silicone punctal plug
Arrowsmith corneal marker
Arrow-Trerotola
    A.-T. percutaneous thrombectomy
    device
    A.-T. percutaneous thrombolytic
    device
    A.-T. PTD device
    A.-T. rotator drive unit
Arroyo
    A. encircling suture
    A. forceps
    A. implant
    A. protector
    A. trephine
Arruga
    A. capsule forceps
    A. elevator retractor
    A. encircling suture
    A. expressor
    A. forceps
    A. implant
    A. lacrimal trephine
    A. lens
    A. needle holder
    A. orbital retractor
Arruga-Moura-Brazil orbital implant
Arruga-Nicetic ophthalmology forceps
ArtAssist
    A. arterial assist device
    A. compression dressing/wrap
    A. leg compression dressing
Artecoll injectable microimplant
Artegraft natural collagen vascular graft
arterial
    a. cannula
    a. catheter
    a. catheter armboard
    a. clamp
    a. embolectomy catheter
    a. filter

    a. forceps
    a. graft prosthesis
    a. irrigation catheter
    a. line
    a. line pressure bag
    a. line transducer
    a. needle
    a. port catheter system
    a. puncture site closure device
    a. silk suture
arteriotomy scissors
arteriovenous (AV)
    a. catheter
Arthrex
    A. Banana SutureLasso
    A. Bio-Suturetak
    A. Bird-Beak device
    A. bone anchor
    A. coring reamer
    A. femoral guide
    A. instruments and systems
    A. meniscal dart
    A. meniscal dart gun
    A. penetrator
    A. sheathed interference screw
    A. tibial tunnel guide
    A. TransFix ACL reconstruction
    system
    A. TransFix biointerference screw
    A. TwistLoc suture anchor
    A. Viper suture passer
    A. zebra pin
arthritic shoe
arthritis sock
Arthro-BST arthroscopic probe
ArthroCare
    A. arthroscopic system
    A. Coblation-based cosmetic
    surgery system
    A. electrode
    A. multielectrode system
    A. thermal wand
    A. wand
arthrodesis
    Albee hip a.
    Elmslie triple a.
    Kapandji-Sauvé a.
    Lord total hip a.
    Spier elbow a.
arthrodial
    a. protractor
    A. Protractor range of motion
    analyzer
Arthro-Flo
    A.-F. arthroscopic irrigation system
    A.-F. irrigator
    A.-F. powered irrigation system
Arthroforce
    A. basket cutting forceps

A

A. hook scissors
A. III hand instrument
arthrogram
cine a.
Gordon-Broström single-contrast a.
triple-injection cine a.
Arthro-Knife sheathed arthroscopy knife
Arthro-Lok system of Beaver blades
arthrometer
Acufex knee laxity a.
Genucom a.
KT1000, 2000 knee ligament a.
Medmetric knee ligament a.
Medmetric KT1000 knee laxity a.
Robinson a.
Stryker a.
arthropathy
cuff tear a. (CTA)
arthroplasty
a. bur
cuff tear a. (CTA)
Global total shoulder a.
Gustilo-Kyle cementless total hip a.
A. Products Consultants foot and
   legholder
Putti-Platt a.
total articular replacement a.
Arthropor
A. acetabular cup
A. II acetabular prosthesis
ArthroProbe
A. arthroscopic laser
A. laser system
arthroscope
Acufex a.
Baxter angled a.
30-degree oblique a.
Downs a.
Eagle a.
fiberoptic a.
GoldenEye a.
Hopkins a.
Lumina rod lens a.
4M 30-degree a.
Medical Dynamics 5990 needle a.
Panoview a.
Richard Wolf a.
Sapphire View a.
spinal a.
Storz a.
Stryker a.
Trio a.
Watanabe a.
Wolf a.
Zimmer a.
arthroscopic
a. ankle holder
a. cannula
a. grabber

a. knife
a. legholder
a. monopolar thermal stabilization
   forefoot compression sleeve
a. pump
a. shaver
arthroscopy
Hawkeye suture needle for a.
a. knife
ArthroSew
A. arthroscopic suturing device
A. suturing system
Arthrosol dressing
Arthrotek
A. calibrated cylinder
A. Ellipticut hand instrument
A. femoral aimer
A. graft tensioner
A. meniscus staple
A. tibial fixation device
arthrotome
Hall a.
ArthroWand
Caps A.
A. device
A. disposable surgical wand
Eliminator A.
Microblator A.
RazorVac A.
Saber Bisector A.
A. tool
Arthur splinter forceps
articular insert
articulated
a. AFO
a. chin prosthesis
a. external fixator
a. minifixator
articulating
a. arm
a. paper forceps
articulation
atlanto-occipital a. (AOA)
DePuy Ultamet metal-on-metal a.
Ultamet metal-on-metal a.
articulator
Acme a.
adjustable a.
Balkwell a.
Bergström a.
Bonwill a.
Christensen a.
Denar a.
Dentatus a.
Evans a.
Galetti a.
Gariot a.
Granger a.
Gysi a.

articulator *(continued)*
    Hanau 130-21 a.
    Handy II a.
    hinge a.
    hinged a.
    Ney a.
    nonarcon a.
    plain-line a.
    semiadjustable a.
    Stuart a.
    Walker a.
    Whip-Mix a.
Articulator injection needle
articulostat
artificial
    a. cystine stone
    a. endplate
    a. eye
    a. heart
    a. hip joint
    a. intervertebral disc
    a. iris diaphragm implant
    a. iris implant
    a. joint implant
    a. larynx
    a. lung
    a. nose
    a. pacemaker
    a. pupil
    a. silicone retina
    a. skin
    a. sphincter
Artisan
    A. cement system
    A. IOL
    A. iris-fixated phakic IOL
    A. myopia lens
    A. surgical lead
Artoscan
    A. MRI scanner
    A. MRI system
Artscan
    A. 200 arthroscopic cartilage stiffness tester
    A. 200 arthroscopic cartilage stiffness testing device
ART transducer
arum fixation pin
Arvee model 2400 infant apnea monitor
Arx ceramic spinal spacer system
Arzbaecher pill electrode
Arzco
    A. model 7 cardiac stimulator
    A. pacemaker
    A. preamplifier
    A. Tapsul pill electrode
AS
    Auto Suture

AS-800
    AS-800 artificial sphincter
    AS-800 balloon
    AS-800 cuff
Asahi Prowater guidewire
Asap
    A. biopsy system
    A. channel-cut automated biopsy needle
    A. prostate biopsy needle
    A. Stacker automated multisample biopsy system
A-scan
    contact A-s.
    Ultra-Image A-s.
    Ultrascan Digital contact ultrasound A-s.
    A-s. ultrasonogram
Ascensia
    A. Autodisc test strip
    A. Breeze blood glucose monitoring system
    A. Breeze glucometer
    A. Breeze testing kit
    A. DEX2 diabetes care system
    A. Elite blood glucose monitoring system
    A. Elite test strip
    A. Elite XL diabetes blood glucose monitor
    A. Elite XL diabetes care system
    A. Microlet Adjustable lancing device
    A. Microlet Vaculance lancing device
Ascension
    A. MCP finger joint implant
    A. MCP total joint
    A. MCP total joint implant
    A. Neurolac nerve guide
    A. PIP total joint
    A. RADFx proximal radium fixation kit
Ascent
    A. guiding catheter
    A. total knee system
Asch septal forceps
Ascon instrument
ASDOS
    ASDOS umbrella
    ASDOS umbrella occluder
Asepticator unit
aseptic saw
Asepto bulb syringe
Aseptron II
Ash
    A. catheter
    A. septum-straightening forceps
Asher high-pull facebow

Asherman chest seal
Ashley breast prosthesis
Ashworth-Blatt implant
ASI
    ASI prostatic stent
    ASI Titan stent
Asia-Pacific (AP)
Asico
    A. capsulorrhexis forceps
    A. multiangled diamond knife
    A. multi incision system 10 facet
      blade
Asics Gel-MC shoe
ASID Bonz PP infusion pump
ASIF
    ASIF malleolar screw
    ASIF T plate
    ASIF twist drill
ASIS femoral head locator
Asissto-Seat
    Maddapult A.-S.
A·S·KMerit safety access kit
Ask-Upmark kidney
Aslan
    A. endoscopic scissors
    A. 2-mm minilaparoscope
asmaPLAN+ peak flowmeter
ASN
    automatic single needle
Asnis
    A. 3 cannulated screw system
    A. guided screw
    A. 2 guided screw
    A. 2 guided-screw system
    A. III cannulated screw
    A. pin
ASO ankle brace
Aspect computer
Aspen
    A. cervical collar
    A. cervical thoracic orthosis
    A. CTO
    A. digital ultrasound
    A. digital ultrasound system
    A. echocardiography system
    A. electrocautery
    A. Excalibur ESU
    A. laparoscopy electrode
    A. sonography unit
    A. ultrasound platform
    A. ultrasound system
AspenVac
    A. smoke evacuation system
    A. smoke evacuator
aspheric
    a. cataract lens
    a. implant
    a. lens
    a. viewing lens

aspherical ophthalmoscopic lens
aspirating
    a. cannula
    a. curette
    a. dissector
    a. lid speculum
    a. needle
    a. syringe
aspiration
    a. apparatus
    a. biopsy needle
    a. cannula
    a. catheter
    Integra Selector ultrasonic a.
    irrigation and a. (I&A, I/A)
    a. tube
    a. tulip device
aspirator
    Accelerator II a.
    Alcon a.
    Aspirette endocervical a.
    Care-e-Vac portable a.
    Castroviejo orbital a.
    Cavi-Pulse cavitation ultrasound
      surgical a.
    Cavitron a.
    Cavitron ultrasonic surgical a.
      (CUSA)
    Clerf a.
    Cogsell tip a.
    Cook a.
    Cooper a.
    CUSA Excel ultrasonic a.
    DeLee meconium trap a.
    DeVilbiss Vacu-Aide a.
    Dia pump a.
    Dieulafoy a.
    electric vacuum a.
    Endo-Assist sponge a.
    endocervical a.
    endometrial a.
    faucet a.
    Fibra Sonics phaco a.
    FirstCyte A.
    Flex-O-Jet a.
    Frazier suction-tip a.
    Frye a.
    Gesco a.
    Gomco uterine a.
    GynoSampler endometrial a.
    handgun a.
    Hu-Friedy suction-tip a.
    InDuct breast a.
    Ipas a.
    Kelman a.
    Legacy Series 2000
      Cavitron/Kelman
      phacoemulsifier a.
    Lukens a.

aspirator *(continued)*
    LySonix 250 a.
    manual vacuum a.
    meconium a.
    middle ear a.
    mucus a.
    nasal a.
    Nezhat-Dorsey a.
    Nugent soft cataract a.
    portable suction a.
    Potain a.
    red-tip a.
    Schueler Model 200 A.
    Selector ultrasonic a.
    Sharplan Ultra ultrasonic a.
    Sharplan USA ultrasonic surgical a.
    soft cataract a.
    Sonocut ultrasonic a.
    Sorensen a.
    Stat a.
    suction a.
    surgical a.
    Thorek gallbladder a.
    Topel endoscopic cyst a.
    Ultra-Lite portable a.
    ultrasonic surgical a.
    Ultra ultrasonic a.
    Universal a.
    uterine a.
    Vabra a.
    Vabra cervical a.
    Vac-Pak-II ultra-lite portable a.
    Vacu-Aide home-use a.
    vacuum a.
    Walker a.
    yellow-tip a.
aspirator/hydrodissector
    Alpern cortex a./h.
aSpire
    a. controlled release delivery
      system
    a. covered stent
Aspire continuous imaging system
Aspirette endocervical aspirator
ASPIRINcheck urine test
Aspisafe nasogastric tube
ASR
    ASR blade
    ASR scalpel
assembly, pl. **assemblies**
    Ace wire tension a.
    Brown-Roberts-Wells arc-ring a.
    Dentsleeve extruded silastic
      perfused manometric a.
    dilating catheter-gastrostomy tube a.
    infant nasal cannula a.
    Konigsberg 5-channel solid-state
      catheter a.
    linear array-hydrophone a.

    8-lumen catheter a.
    malleus-footplate a.
    malleus-stapes a.
    Massie nail a.
    purpose-built silicone rubber
      multilumen manometric a.
    standard silicone manometric a.
Asserachrom D-dimer kit
Assess
    A. esophageal testing kit
    A. peak flowmeter
ASSI
  Accurate Surgical and Scientific
    Instruments
    ASSI Accu-line surgical marking
      pen
    ASSI air injection cannula
    ASSI bipolar coagulating forceps
    ASSI breast dissector
    ASSI breast dissector angulated
    ASSI breast dissector spatulated
    ASSI capsulorrhexis forceps
    ASSI coagulator
    ASSI end-to-end
      vasoepididymostomy
    ASSI fixation hook
    ASSI IOL inserter forceps
    ASSI Microspike approximator
      clamp
    ASSI Phaco Chopper 90-degree
      angle
    ASSI Polar-Mate coagulator
    ASSI serrefine
    ASSI S&T microsurgical instrument
    ASSI triple marker
    ASSI tubing introducer forceps
    ASSI universal lens folding forceps
    ASSI wire pass drill
assist
    Columbus McKinnon lifting a.
    Elite posterior spring a.
    Thera-Band a.
    thumb interphalangeal extension a.
    Venturi exhalation a.
Assistant
    Carter Tubal A.
    A. Free calibrated femoral tibial
      spreader
    A. Free foot/ankle support
    A. Free hip surgery square frame
    A. Free hip surgery standard
      frame
    A. Free long prong collateral
      ligament retractor
    A. Free orthopaedic needle holder
    A. Free orthopaedic needle
      holder/scissors
    A. Free orthopaedic scissors

A. Free self-retaining hip surgery retractor system
A. Free Shubbs short prong collateral ligament retractor
A. Free Stulberg leg positioner
A. Free wide PCL retractor
assistive listening device
Association for Osteosynthesis/American Society of Internal Fixation (AO/ASIF)
Assura
    A. closed minipouch
    A. convex drainable pouch
    A. convex urostomy pouch
    A. deluxe irrigation set
    A. economy irrigation set
    A. irrigation accessory
    A. irrigation sleeve
    A. pediatric pouch
    A. pediatric skin barrier flange
    A. standard drainable pouch
    A. stoma cap
    A. stomy belt
Assurant balloon-expanded stent
Assure blood glucose monitoring system
Asta-Cath device
Astech peak flowmeter
Asthma Check peak flowmeter
AsthmaMentor peak flowmeter
AsthmaPACK personal asthma care kit
Asthmastik
astigmagraph
astigmatic
    a. dial
    a. lens
    a. marker
astigmatome
    Terry a.
    Terry-Schanzlin a.
Aston
    A. cartilage reduction
    A. cartilage reduction system
    A. nasal retractor
    A. submental retractor
Astra
    A. Tech dental implant
    A. Tech dental implant system
    A. T4, T6 pacemaker
AstraMax stereo topographer
AstraZeneca dental cartridge
Astro-Med Albert Grass Heritage digital EEG system
Astropulse cuff
Astro-Trace Universal adapter clip
ASVIP
    atrial synchronous ventricular inhibited pacemaker
    ASVIP pacemaker
asymmetrical gradient coil

asynchronous
    ventricular a. (VOO)
Atad
    A. cervical ripening device
    A. Ripener device
Atak knee brace
Atakr
    A. generator
    A. system
Atala-Shepard
    A.-S. coaxial balloon follower
    A.-S. coaxial balloon follower set
A-T antiembolism stocking
Atavi
    A. atraumatic spine fusion system
    A. atraumatic spine surgery system
    A. TiTLE rod fixation system
AtaxiTog
ATB PTA ablation catheter
Atec TriMark marker system
Aten olecranon screw
Athena high frequency mammography system
Athens suture spreader
atherectomy
    a. catheter
    a. device
    percutaneous a.
AtheroCath
    A. Bantam coronary atherectomy catheter
    DVI Simpson A.
    A. GTO coronary atherectomy catheter
    Simpson coronary A.
    Simpson peripheral A.
atherotome
AtheroTrack catheter
Athlete GT coronary guidewire
athletic brace
Athos laser
Atkins-Cannard tracheal tube
Atkinson
    A. corneal scissors
    A. introducer
    A. peribulbar needle
    A. prosthesis
    A. retrobulbar needle
    A. sclerotome
    A. short curved cystotome
    A. single-bevel blunt-tip needle
    A. tip peribulbar needle
    A. tube
Atkins-Tucker antiembolism stocking
ATL
    ATL HDI 5000 color Doppler
    ATL HDI 3000, 3500, 4000, 5000 ultrasound system

ATL *(continued)*
 ATL Mark 600 real-time sector
  scanner
 ATL Neurosector real-time scanner
 ATL real-time ultrasound
 ATL UltraMark 7
  echocardiographic device
 ATL UltraMark IV linear-array
  transducer
 ATL Ultramark ultrasound
 ATL UltraMark 9 ultrasound
  system
 ATL 3000 ultrasound device
 ATL ultrasound system
Atlanta-Scottish Rite
 A.-S. R. hip brace
 A.-S. R. Hospital orthosis
Atlantic
 A. overlap brace
 A. rim brace
Atlantis
 A. anterior cervical plate system
 A. cervical plate system
 A. SR intravascular ultrasound
  imaging catheter
 A. SR IVUS catheter
 A. Vision anterior cervical plate
  system
atlanto-occipital articulation (AOA)
atlas
 A. adjustable stand
 A. cable system
 A. corneal topographer
 A. DG balloon angioplasty catheter
 A. 2.0 diagnostic ultrasound system
 A. DR implantable cardioverter-
  defibrillator
 A. modular humeral prosthesis
 A. ophthalmic laser
 A. orthogonal percussion instrument
 Schaltenbrand-Wahren stereotactic a.
 stereotactic a.
 A. 995 topographer
 A. ULP balloon dilatation catheter
 A. Wire stone extractor
Atlas-Elite laser
Atlas-Storz eye magnet
AtLast blood glucose monitoring system
Atlee clamp
ATL-HDL color-flow Doppler scanner
atomic
 a. absorbance spectrophotometer
 a. absorption spectrometer
atomizer
 Jackson laryngeal a.
 laryngeal a.
Atomlab 200 dose calibrator
ATO walker
A-Trac atraumatic clamping system

Atrac-II double-balloon catheter
Atrac multipurpose balloon catheter
Atra-Grip clamp
Atraloc
 A. needle
 A. suture
Atraucan double-bevel spinal needle
Atrauclip hemostatic clip
atraumatic
 a. bowel clamp
 a. clamp
 a. forceps
 a. locking/grasping forceps
 a. needle
 a. Sprotte needle
 a. tip
 a. tissue forceps
ATR brace
atrial
 a. cannula
 a. demand inhibited pacemaker
 a. demand triggered pacemaker
 a. electrode
 a. fibrillation (AF)
 a. implantable cardioverter-
  defibrillator
 a. pacing wire
 a. septal defect occlusion system
 a. septal defect single disc closure
  device
 a. septal retractor
 a. septum defect occluder system
 a. synchronous noncompetitive
  pacemaker
 a. synchronous ventricular inhibited
  pacemaker (ASVIP)
 a. triggered (AAT)
 a. triggered noncompetitive
  pacemaker
 a. and ventricular implantable
  cardioverter-defibrillator
 A. View Ventak implantable
  cardioverter-defibrillator
atrial-based pacemaker
Atricor Cordis pacemaker
Atridox drug delivery system
Atrigel drug delivery system
atrioseptostomy catheter
atrioventricular
 a. junctional pacemaker
 a. sequential demand pacemaker
 a. tachycardia (AVT)
 a. valve ring
Atrioverter
 A. implantable atrial defibrillator
 A. implantable defibrillator device
 Metrix A.
 Metrix implantable A.
 A. system

Atrisorb
>A. bioabsorbable barrier
>A. FreeFlow GTR barrier

Atrium blood recovery system

atropine autoinjector

Atrostim phrenic nerve stimulator

ATS
>adjustable thigh antiembolism stocking
>ATS Open Pivot heart valve
>ATS 500/1500 tourniquet system

ATT-300 LAT traction table

Attache food scale

attachment
>Accuvac smoke evacuation a.
>a. apparatus
>bar-clip a.
>bar-sleeve a.
>Bivona tracheostomy tube with talk a.
>cerebellar a.
>closed-chain exercise a.
>Hader dental a.
>Hudson cerebellar a.
>Mayfield-Kees table a.
>MP videoendoscopic lens a.
>O-ring a.
>pathometer a.
>Planarm Haag Streit a.
>PRAFO PKA KAFO a.
>pyramid a.
>Roach ball precision a.
>specular a.
>Strauss dental a.
>Tach-EZ dental a.
>Tasserit shoulder a.
>Thomas splint with Pearson a.
>University Plate spinal a.

Attain
>A. bipolar over-the-wire lead
>A. Select guide catheter
>A. tube feeding formula

Attenborough total knee prosthesis

Attends
>A. beltless undergarment
>A. brief with Perma Dry Wings contoured incontinence brief
>A. pad and guard
>A. underpad

attic cannula

AttoFluor RatioVision

Attractor retrieval device

ATW
>all track wire
>ATW core wire
>ATW steerable guidewire

Atwood
>A. bridge remover
>A. crown remover

Audibel hearing aid

Audio Doppler D920

audiometer
>AudioScope 3 a.
>Békésy a.
>Crib-O-Gram neonatal screening a.
>GSI 16 a.
>MA 53 2-channel a.
>Madsen OB822 clinical a.
>Maico-MA 20 a.
>Pilot a.

AudioScope
>A. 3 audiometer
>Welch Allyn A.

Audiotone hearing aid

auditory
>a. brainstem implant (ABI)
>a. prosthesis
>a. response cradle
>a. tube

Auer rod

Aufranc
>A. cobra hip prosthesis
>A. cobra retractor
>A. osteotome

Aufranc-Turner hip prosthesis

Aufricht
>A. elevator
>A. fiberoptic light retractor
>A. glabellar rasp
>A. nasal rasp
>A. nasal retractor
>A. scissors

Auger-electron emitter

Auger electron spectroscope (AES)

augmentation
>PermaRidge alveolar ridge a.

augmentative communication device

Augustine
>A. boat nail
>A. guide and scope

Aura
>A. desktop laser
>A. Laser helical scanner
>A. Laser system
>A. Nd:YAG photodisruptor

AuRA cemented total hip system

aural
>a. forceps
>a. magnifier
>a. speculum
>a. thermometer

AuraMeter
>Cameron A.

Aureomycin suture

auricular prosthesis

Aurora
>A. dedicated breast MRI system
>A. diode-based dental laser system
>A. diode soft tissue laser

Aurora *(continued)*
- A. luminous acuity chart
- A. MR breast imaging system
- A. MR breast imaging system scanner

Aurous
- A. centimeter sizing catheter
- A. graduate sizing catheter

austenitic stainless steel

Austin
- A. knife
- A. Moore chisel
- A. Moore extractor
- A. Moore hip prosthesis
- A. Moore hook

Australian
- A. punch
- A. Special Plus wire

Auth Rotablator atherectomy catheter

Autima II dual-chamber cardiac pacemaker

Aution Max AX-4280 automated urine chemistry analyzer

auto
- A. Glide walker accessory
- a. injector
- A. Ref-keratometer instrument
- REMstar A.
- A. Sonix laparoscopic cutter/coagulator
- A. Suture (AS)
- A. Suture ABBI system
- A. Suture Multifire Endo GIA 30 stapler
- A. Suture Premium CEEA stapler
- A. Suture SFS stapler
- A. Suture stapler
- A. Suture surgical stapler
- A. Suture Surgiclip
- A. Syringe
- Tranquility A.

autoadhesive cellulose nitrate filter

AutoAdjust CPAP device

autoanalyzer
- Beckman 2 a.
- Hitachi 737, 747 a.
- Kodak Ektachem a.
- technetium H2 a.

Autoblock safety syringe

AutoCapture pacing system

Autocath bladder control device

AutoCAT intraaortic balloon pump

autoclave sterilizer

Autoclip applier

Autoclix fingerstick lancet device

Autocon electrosurgical unit

autocorrelator

AutoCorr portable pulse oximeter

Auto-Crane device

AutoCyte
- A. Image Analysis system
- A. Prep system

AutoDELFIA
- A. PRL molecule kit
- A. unconjugated E3 kit

autodistractor

AutoDriver screwdriver

Auto-Drive self-drilling screw

Autoflex II continuous passive motion unit

autofluorescent endsocopic system

autofluoroscope
- digital a.

autofunduscope

Autogenesis automator for Ilizarov screw

autogenic graft

autogenous
- a. corneal protector
- a. quadrupled hamstring tendon graft

autograft
- bone-patellar tendon-bone a.
- Epicel cultured epidermal a.

Autografter
- Ace A.

Autoguard shielded IV catheter

Autohaler

AutoIncisor

autoinfuser

Auto-Injector
- Lido-Pen A.-I.

autoinjector
- atropine a.
- PenInject 2.25 A.

autokeratometer
- Alcon portable a.

auto-kerato-refractometer
- Topcon KR-7000P a.-k.-r.

Autolance

AutoLensmeter

Autolet
- A. Clinisafe lancing device
- A. fingerstick device
- A. impression lancing device
- A. Lite lancing device
- A. Mini lancing device

AuTolo cure process

autoLog autotransfusion system

autologous
- a. blood management system
- a. fibrin tissue adhesive
- a. oral mucosal epithelium sheet

automated
- a. angle encoder system
- a. biochemical analyzer
- a. biopsy gun
- a. biopsy needle

a. cellular imaging system
a. cerebral blood flow analyzer
a. corneal shaper (ACS)
a. corneal shaper microkeratome
a. disposable keratome
a. endoscope reprocessor
a. endoscopic system for optimal
  positioning surgical robot
a. external defibrillator (AED)
a. external defibrillator pacemaker
  (AEDP)
a. gamma counter
a. hemisphere perimeter
a. laser-fluorescence sequencer
A. Quantification of After-Cataract
  automated analysis system
a. refractor
a. trephine
a. visual field
a. vitrector

automatic
a. analyzer
a. catheter
a. chemical analyzer
a. clinical analyzer
a. collimator
a. cranial drill
a. device
a. endoscopic reprocessor
a. external cardioverter-defibrillator
  (AECD)
a. external defibrillator
a. fluorescent image analyzer
a. gas sequencer
a. Hemoclip applier
a. implantable cardiovascular
  defibrillator (AICD)
a. implantable cardioverter-
  defibrillator
a. implantable defibrillator
a. intracardiac defibrillator
a. needle driver
a. oscillometric blood pressure
  monitor
a. positioning system
a. ratchet snare
a. screwdriver
a. single needle (ASN)
a. single-needle monitor
a. skin retractor
a. spring-loaded biopsy device
a. stapling device
a. suction device
a. systematic desensitization
  apparatus
a. tourniquet
a. transport ventilator
a. trephine

a. twin syringe injector
a. vehicle locator
Automator device
Autonomous Technologies laser
AutoPap
A. 300
A. automated screening device
A. 300 QC automatic Pap screener
A. 300 QC system
A. reader
autoperfusion
a. balloon
a. balloon catheter
Autophor femoral prosthesis
autophthalmoscope
autopsy, pl. **autopsies**
a. blade
a. handle
AutoPulse
A. CPR device
A. resuscitation system
autoradiographic film
Autoread centrifuge hematology system
Autoref keratometer
autorefractometer
Canon a.
autorefractor
6600 a.
Burton BAR-7 a.
Canon R-50+ a.
Hoya AR-570 a.
Nikon Retinomax K-Plus a.
Retinomax a.
Retinomax 2 a.
Retinomax cordless handheld a.
Shin-Nippon a.
Shin Nippon SRW-5000 a.
SureSight a.
Tomey a.
Topcon RM8000B table-mounted a.
Welch Allyn SureSight a.
autorefractor/keratometer
Retinomax K-Plus a./k.
auto-reinforced polyglycolide rod
AutoSet
A. CS device
A. Portable II
A. Portable II CPAP system
A. Portable II diagnosis and
  therapy device
AutoSPECT
autostainer
Biotek 1000 a.
Dako a.
autostapling device
Autostat ligating and hemostatic clip
Autosuture ProTack instrument
Autotechnicon
autotitration device

Autotome rotatable sphincterotome
autotopographer
Tomey a.
Autotransfuser
Biosurge Synchronous A.
autotransfusion
a. suction
a. system
Autotrans system
Autovac
A. autotransfusion canister
A. autotransfusion system
A. LF autotransfusion system
A. needle
A. TC orthopaedic autotransfusion system
Auvard weighted vaginal speculum
auxiliary
a. CT tabletop
a. lens
AV
arteriovenous
AV fistula needle
AV junctional pacemaker
AV synchronous pacemaker
A-V
A-V Impulse foot pump
A-V Impulse system
A-V Impulse System foot pump DVT prophylaxis device
A-V Impulse System foot wrap DVT prophylaxis device
AVA
advanced venous access
AVA 3Xi advanced venous access device
AVAD
acute ventricular assist device
Avagard instant hand antiseptic
Avanar
A. intravascular ultrasound catheter
A. IVUS catheter
Avance hearing enhancer
Avanta
A. implant
A. MCP joint implant finger prosthesis
A. metacarpophalangeal implant prosthesis
A. soft skeletal implant
A. uHead ulnar head implant
A. uHead ulnar head prosthesis
Avant Gauze nonwoven gauze
Avanti
A. introducer
A. J-20XP, J-25, J-30I, J-HC, J-E centrifuge
A. sheath
A. transradial sheath

Ava-Tex bone cement
Avaulta biosynthetic mesh
Avco
A. aortic balloon
A. balloon pump
AVE
AVE Bridge flexible balloon-expanded stent
AVE Bridge SE self-expanding stent
AVE Bridge stainless steel balloon-expandable stent
AVE GFX coronary stent
AVE Micro stent
AVE Microstent II stent
AVE S540, S670 stent
AVE stent
Avera breast imaging system
averager
multichannel signal a.
Averill press-fit prosthesis
Avian transport ventilator
Aviator RX balloon catheter
avidin-biotin complex immunodetection system
Avi lens system
Avina female urethral plug
Avitene
A. flour dressing
A. microfibrillar collagen
A. microfibrillar collagen hemostat
A. pack
Avit handpiece
Aviva mammography system
AVL
AVL Omni blood gas analyzer
AVL Opti 1 portable blood gas analyzer
AVL 9110 pH analyzer
AvocetPT rapid prothrombin time meter
Avogel hydrogel sheeting
Avosil scar gel
AvoSure
A. INR test device
A. PT monitor
Avotec MR-compatible liquid crystal display goggles
AVOXimeter
A. 4000 CO oximeter
A. 1000E whole blood oximeter
AV-Paceport thermodilution catheter
AVS spinal system
AVT
atrioventricular tachycardia
Aware
A. AccuMeter
A. AccuMeter rapid HIV test

awl
> angled a.
> bone a.
> Carroll a.
> Carter Rowe a.
> curved a.
> Ferran a.
> hemostat a.
> Kirklin sternal a.
> lacrimal a.
> Mark II Kodros radiolucent a.
> Mustarde a.
> pedicle a.
> pointed a.
> reaming a.
> rectangular a.
> Rush pin reamer a.
> starter a.
> Stedman a.
> sternum-perforating a.
> Swanson lunate a.
> Swanson scaphoid a.
> T-handle bone a.
> T-handled a.
> Uniflex distal targeting a.
> wire-passing a.
> Zelicof orthopaedic a.

Axcis
> A. percutaneous myocardial revascularization system
> A. PMR system

axe
> irrigating a.

Axel wire twister
Axer compression device
axes (*pl. of* axis)
Axhausen needle holder
axial
> a. anchor screw
> a. gradiometer
> a. plate
> a. resistance exerciser

axillary catheter
axiltraction
AxioCam camera
Axiom
> A. custom functional knee brace

> A. double sump pump
> A. drain
> A. modular knee system
> A. thoracic trocar
> A. total knee
> A. total knee system

Axios pacemaker
axis, pl. **axes**
> A. ankle brace
> A. 360-degree stabilization system
> A. fixation system
> 3-a. gradient coil
> a. traction forceps

axis-altering arthroereisis device
Axisonic II ultrasound
Axius vacuum 2 stabilizer
AxSYM
> A. analyzer
> A. free PSA test

Axtion foot prosthesis
Axxess
> A. spinal cord stimulation lead
> A. ureteral catheter

AxyaWeld
> A. bone anchor
> A. bone anchor system
> A. instrument
> A. J-tip suture welding system
> A. product line

Ayers
> A. cardiovascular needle holder
> A. spatula
> A. sphygmomanometer
> A. T-piece

Ayerst instrument
Aylesbury spatula
Ayre spatula
Azar
> A. cystotome
> A. lens
> A. lid speculum
> A. utility forceps

azathioprine
Aztec shoulder holder

Babbington-type nebulizer
Babcock
 B. clamp
 B. Endo-Grasper
 B. forceps
 B. intestinal forceps
 B. needle
 B. stainless steel wire
 B. thoracic tissue forceps
 B. wire-cutting scissors
Babcock-Vital
 B.-V. atraumatic forceps
 B.-V. tissue forceps
BABE OB ultrasound reporting system
babies (*pl. of* baby)
Babinski percussion hammer
BA bone cement adhesive
baby, pl. babies
 b. Adson forceps
 B. Air mesh netting
 b. Balfour retractor
 b. Crile forceps
 B. Dopplex 3000 antepartum fetal
  monitor
 b. Lane forceps
 b. Metzenbaum scissors
 b. Mixter forceps
 b. mosquito forceps
 b. Overholt forceps
 b. pylorus clamp
 b. scope
 B. Sense monitor
 b. Tischler biopsy punch
 b. Weitlaner self-retaining retractor
BabyBeat ultrasound instrument
BABYbird
 B. II respirator
 B. II ventilator
 B. respirator
BabyFace
 B. 3D surface rendering accessory
 B. 3D surface rendering accessory
  device
Babyhaler spacer device
Babylog
 B. 8000 oscillator
 B. 8000 respirator
babyPAC ventilator
Babystart
 B. fertility test kit
 B. ovulation test
Babytherm
 B. IC
 B. IC gel mattress

BacFix system
back
 b. board
 b. brace
 B. Bubble gravity traction unit
 B. Bull lumbar support cushion
 B. Bull lumbar support system
 b. clamp
 B. Hammer muscle stimulator
 b. range of motion device
 b. range of motion instrument
 B. Revolution Stick
 B. Revolution Stick exercise
 B. Revolution System
 B. Revolution traction/exercise unit
 B. Seat torso-wrap brace
 B. Specialist chiropractic table
 B. Specialist electric table
 B. Specialist manual table
 b. table
 B. Trainer spinal exercise system
back-and-forth vibrating cannula
Backbar device
backbiter
 b. instrument
 MicroFrance pediatric b.
backbiting
 b. bone punch
 b. forceps
backboard
 half b.
 long b.
 short b.
 short wooden b.
 vest-type b.
BackCycler continuous passive motion
  device
Back-Ease aromatherapy hot/cold pack
Backhaus
 B. clamp
 B. dilator
 B. forceps
 B. towel clamp
 B. towel clip
Backhaus-Kocher towel clamp
Backhaus-Roeder forceps
Back-Huggar
 Bodyline B.-H.
 B.-H. lumbar support
 B.-H. lumbar support cushion
backing
 Hahnenkratt b.
Backjoy seat
back-leg-chest dynamometer

Backlund
    B. biopsy needle
    B. stereotactic instrument
BackMaster device
Backnobber II massage tool
backRAP postsurgical wound wrap
back-stop laser probe
Backstroke
    The B.
BackStrong lumbar extension machine
BackThing lumbar support
BackTracker
backward-biting ostrum punch
backward-cutting knife
Bacon
    B. anoscope
    B. bone rongeur
    B. cranial bone rongeur
BacStop dental antiretraction check
    valve
BacT/Alert
    B. automated blood culture system
    B. automated microbial detection
        system
    B. microbial detection system
Bactec
    B. automated blood culture system
    B. blood culture system
    B. blood culturing system
    B. 9000 MB system
    B. MGIT 960
bacterial filter
Bactigras
    B. dressing
    B. gauze
Bactiseal antimicrobial-impregnated
    catheter system
Bactrol Plus quality control culture
Bactron 1.5 anaerobic chamber
Badal stimulus system
badge
    film b.
Badger drill bit
Badgley laminectomy retractor
Bad Wildungen Metz spine system
Baer
    B. bone-cutting forceps
    B. bone rongeur
    B. rib shears
Baerveldt
    B. glaucoma drainage implant
    B. glaucoma implant
    B. glaucoma implant tube
    B. seton implant
    B. shunt
    B. shunt tube
baffle
    fabric b.
    Gore-Tex b.

baffled jet nebulizer
bag
    Acme One Time enteral feeding b.
    air b.
    Alpine reusable leg b.
    Ambu b.
    anesthesia b.
    arterial line pressure b.
    Bard Dispoz-A-Bag leg b.
    Bardex b.
    Barnes b.
    Belly B.
    Belly Bag urine storage b.
    bile b.
    biohazard b.
    Boardshield disposable backboard b.
    Bogota b.
    breath b.
    breathing b.
    Bunyan b.
    Capno-Flo single-patient
        resuscitation b.
    Cardiff resuscitation b.
    Champetier de Ribes b.
    CLO Cool B.
    Coloplast b.
    Coloplast colostomy b.
    Coloplast urine leg b.
    colostomy b.
    containment b.
    Conveen bedside drainage b.
    Conveen deluxe contoured leg b.
    coudé b.
    Curity leg b.
    Davol b.
    Davol feeding b.
    DeRoyal Surgical grab b.
    dialysate b.
    Dobbhoff enteral feeding b.
    Douglas b.
    drainage b.
    Endobag specimen b.
    Endo Catch b.
    EndoMate grab b.
    Endopouch Pro specimen-
        retrieval b.
    Endosac specimen b.
    Endo-Sock specimen retrieval b.
    Entri-Pak enteral feeding b.
    eXtract specimen b.
    exudate disposal b.
    Foley hemostatic b.
    Freedom T-tap leg b.
    Frenta enteral feeding b.
    Gambro freezing b.
    Gamow b.
    gauze tissue b.
    GEM nonlatex medical b.
    Grafco colostomy b.

B

Hagner hemostatic b.
Hagner urethral b.
hemostatic b.
Heyer-Schulte disposal b.
Hollister colostomy b.
Hollister drainage b.
Hollister urostomy b.
Hope resuscitation b.
hydrostatic b.
ice b.
ileostomy b.
Infusible pressure infusion b.
Infu-Surg pressure infuser b.
intestinal b.
intracervical b.
isolation b.
Karaya seal ileostomy stomal b.
Keofeed enteral feeding b.
Lahey b.
Lapides collecting b.
Lapides ileostomy b.
latex b.
Le B.
Lifesaver disposable resuscitator b.
manual resuscitation b.
Marlen ileostomy b.
Marlen leg b.
b. and mask
micturition b.
Mikulicz b.
millinery b.
3M limb isolation b.
Mosher b.
night drainage b.
nylon tissue biopsy b.
ostomy b.
Pearman transurethral hemostatic b.
pneumatic b.
3-point spreader b.
4-point spreader b.
Polar enteral feeding b.
Politzer air b.
prostatectomy b.
rebreathing b.
replacement collection b.
Rusch b.
Rusch leg b.
Rutzen ileostomy b.
severance transurethral b.
Shea-Anthony b.
short-tip hemostatic b.
sleeve b.
Speci-Gard specimen transport b.
sterile isolation b.
stomal b.
SureGrip breathing b.
Sur-Fit colostomy b.
Sur-Fit urinary drainage b.
Tedlar b.

The Deluxe Button B.
Top-Fill enteral feeding b.
Uri-Drain leg b.
urinary leg b.
Urocare latex reusable leg b.
Uro-Safe vinyl disposable leg b.
Versi-Splint carry b.
Vi-Drape bowel b.
Void-Ease urine collection b.
Voorhees b.
VPI urinary leg b.
zinc-free plastic b.
BagEasy disposable manual resuscitator
bag-fixated intraocular lens
Baggish
  B. hysteroscope
  B. injection tube
Bagley helical basket
bag-mask device
Bagolini lens
bag-valve
  b.-v. device
  b.-v. device to tracheostomy tube
  b.-v. mask
  b.-v. resuscitator
  b.-v. unit
bag-valve-mask (B-V-M)
  b.-v.-m. device
Baha
  B. osseointegrated bone conduction
    implant
  B. system
Bahnson aortic clamp
Bahnson-Brown forceps
Baikoff lens
Bailey
  B. aortic clamp
  B. aortic valve rongeur
  B. baby rib contractor
  B. catheter
  B. chalazion forceps
  B. conductor
  B. Gigli saw guide
  B. lacrimal cannula
  B. rib contractor
  B. rib spreader
  B. saw guide
  B. wire saw
Bailey-Gibbon rib contractor
Bailey-Glover-O'Neill commissurotomy knife
Bailey-Lovie test chart
Bailey-Williamson obstetrical forceps
Bailliart
  B. goniometer
  B. ophthalmodynamometer
  B. tonometer
bail-lock brace
Baim pacing catheter

Bainbridge
- B. intestinal clamp
- B. intestinal forceps
- B. thyroid forceps

Bain circle

Bair
- B. Hugger
- B. Hugger blanket
- B. Hugger convective warming unit
- B. Hugger fluid warming device
- B. Hugger forced-air warmer
- B. Hugger infant warming device
- B. Hugger patient heating unit
- B. Hugger patient warming blanket
- B. Hugger patient warming system
- B. Hugger warming blanket
- B. Hugger warming body cover

Baird
- B. chalazion forceps
- B. Electric System Power Plus electrosurgical unit

BAK
- BAK cage
- BAK fusion cage
- BAK interbody fusion system

BakVista radiolucent interbody fusion system

BAK-1 interbody fusion system

BAK/C
- BAK/C cervical interbody fusion implant
- BAK/C interbody fusion system

Bakelite cystoscopy sheath

Baker
- B. jejunostomy tube
- B. punch
- B. self-sumping tube

Baker-Cummings punch

Baker-David clamp

Bakes
- B. dilator
- B. probe

BAK/Proximity interbody fusion implant

BAK/T thoracic interbody fusion system

balafilcon A contact lens

balance
- b. beam scale
- b. board
- b. bridge
- B. hip prosthesis
- Humphriss binocular b.
- B. Master
- B. Master-training and assessment system
- B. Master training and assessment system
- b. pad
- b. padding orthosis
- Secure B.

balanced
- b. forearm orthosis
- B. Knee system
- b. suspension traction
- b. traction device

balancer
- MMS-900 microscope b.

Baldwin
- B. butterfly ventilation tube
- B. perineum needle

Balectrode
- B. pacing catheter
- B. pacing probe

Balfour
- B. bladder blade
- B. center blade
- B. pediatric abdominal retractor
- B. self-retaining retractor

Balkan fracture frame

Balkin Up and Over contralateral introducer with radiopaque band

Balkwell articulator

ball
- birthing b.
- Body B.
- Bouncewell medicine b.
- b. burnisher
- burst resistance fitness b.
- carotid b.
- cauterizing b.
- B. coagulator
- cold-weld femoral b.
- cotton b.
- b. dissector
- b. electrode
- Electrodes b.
- Esmarch b.
- Ex-Balls medicine b.
- ExerFlex b.
- Finger Fitness Spring B.
- Fitness B.
- b. forceps
- Gertie b.
- Gripp squeeze b.
- gym b.
- Gymnastik b.
- Gymnic Plus exercise b.
- hand exercise b.
- b. heart valve
- HeavyMed b.
- Jurgan pin b.
- B. knee lock
- Ledraplastic exercise b.
- massage b.
- medicine b.
- New Versaback gym b.
- parietal b.
- PhysioGymnic exercise b.
- Physio-Roll VisuaLiser exercise b.

Pinky b.
B. reusable electrode
R-Value exercise b.
silastic b.
sinoatrial b.
Slo-Mo b.
squeeze b.
Super Pinky b.
Swiss b.
Thera-Band exercise b.
TheraGym exercise b.
therapy b.
b. tipped scissors
tissue link floating b.
B. valve
b. valve prosthesis
Vari-Firm Medicine B.
vestibular b.
b. wedge
Wooden Wobble balance b.
ball-and-cage prosthesis
ball-and-socket ankle prosthesis
Ballen-Alexander orbital retractor
ball-end elevator
Ballenger
B. ethmoid curette
B. gouge
B. nasal knife
B. sponge forceps
B. swivel knife
Ballenger-Lillie mastoid bur
ballistic energy generator
ballistocardiograph
Ballobes gastric balloon
balloon
Accent-DG b.
Ace b.
ACS Alpha b.
ACS SULP II b.
Acucise b.
ACX b.
air-filled b.
All-Terrain b.
angioplasty b.
b. angioplasty catheter
antral b.
Arrow Berman angiographic b.
AS-800 b.
autoperfusion b.
Avco aortic b.
Ballobes gastric b.
Bandit b.
Bardex b.
Bard temporary pacing electrode
  catheter with b.
barium enema retention b.
barostat b.
barostatic b.
b. biliary catheter

BioEnterics intragastric b. (BIB)
Blue Max high-pressure b.
Brandt cytology b.
Brighton epistaxis b.
b. catheter
catheter b.
b. catheter sealing device
centering b.
compliant b.
Cook b.
Cordis Powerflex angioplasty b.
counterpulsation b.
cryoplasty b.
cutting b.
cylindrical b.
DASH extraction b.
Datascope b.
detachable silicone b.
b. dilatation catheter
b. dilating catheter
b. dilator
Dispatch b.
b. dissector
doughnut-shaped b.
Duralyn b.
Dynasty b.
elastomeric b.
electrode b.
electrodetachable b.
Eliminator dilatation b.
b. embolectomy catheter
endocapsular b.
Epistat b.
epistaxis b.
esophageal b.
Express b.
extraction b.
Extractor 3-lumen retrieval b.
Extractor XL triple-lumen
  retrieval b.
Falcon Omniflex b.
fixed-wire b.
b. flotation catheter
b. flotation pacing catheter
fluid-filled b.
Fogarty b.
Foley b.
Force b.
Fox postnasal b.
French Swan-Ganz b.
Garren-Edwards gastric b.
gastric b.
Gau gastric b.
Grüntzig b.
GuardWire distal b.
Guidant b.
Hartzler Micro II b.
Hartzler Micro II angioplasty b.
Helix b.

balloon *(continued)*
Helmstein b.
high-compliance latex b.
high-pressure Blue Max b.
Honan b.
Hunter-Sessions b.
hydrostatic b.
b. imaging catheter
inflated b.
Inoue self-guiding b.
Integra II b.
intraaortic b.
intraaortic counterpulsation b.
intragastric b.
intraocular b.
Kay b.
Kaye nephrostomy tamponade b.
kissing b.
Kontron intraaortic b.
laser b.
latex b.
Lo-Fold b.
Lo-Profile b.
low-compliance b.
low-compliance, fixed diameter b.
low-profile angioplasty b.
LPS b.
Magic B1 b.
Mansfield b.
Medtronic Evergreen b.
metrizamide-filled b.
Micross SL b.
Microvasive retrieval b.
Microvasive Rigiflex through-the-scope b.
Microvasive Rigiflex TTS b.
Monorail Speedy b.
Multi-Link Tristar b.
nasomaxillary b.
NC b.
noncompliant b.
nondetachable b.
nondetachable endovascular b.
nondetachable occlusive b.
occlusion b.
b. occlusion-aspiration embolus entrapment device
Olbert b.
Omega-NV b.
Omniflex b.
Opta 5 angioplasty b.
Optiplast Centurion b.
Origin b.
Origin PDB 1000 b.
Orion b.
Owens b.
Panther b.
PE b.
pediatric b.

Penta b.
percutaneous transluminal angioplasty b.
PET b.
Piccolino b.
pillow-shaped b.
Pivot b.
POC b.
polyethylene terephthalate b.
polyolefin copolymer b.
polyvinyl chloride b.
positron emission tomography b.
postnasal b.
preperitoneal distension b.
preperitoneal dilator b.
pressure-detachable silicone b.
ProCross Rely b.
Provocative sensitivity b.
b. PTA catheter
pulmonary b.
b. pump
Quantum TTC biliary b.
QuickFurl SL b.
radiofrequency b.
radiofrequency hot b.
Ranger b.
Raptor PTCA b.
Rashkind b.
rectal b.
retrieval b.
right ventricular copulsation b.
Rigiflex b.
Rigiflex achalasia b.
Rigiflex TTS b.
Schwarten Microglide LP b.
Sci-Med Express Monorail b.
scintigraphic b.
self-sealing latex b.
Sengstaken b.
Sengstaken-Blakemore esophageal b.
b. septostomy catheter
Shadow b.
Shea-Anthony b.
b. shunt
Simpson PET b.
Simpson positron emission tomography b.
sinus b.
sizing b.
Slalom b.
Soft-Wand atraumatic tissue manipulator b.
Solo b.
Solstice b.
Spacemaker II b.
Spears laser b.
Stack autoperfusion b.
Stealth catheter b.
stone-retrieval b.

surgical b.
Surpasse b.
Symmetry angioplasty b.
b. tamponade
Target Therapeutics Stealth
  angioplasty b.
Taylor gastric b.
TEGwire b.
Ten b.
Thermachoice uterine b.
through-the-scope b.
transluminal b.
trefoil Schneider b.
Tri-Ex triple-lumen extraction b.
Tyshak b.
UltraFuse b.
ultrasmall-shafted b.
Ultrathin Diamond b.
Ultraxx nephrostomy b.
USCI PET b.
b. valvuloplasty catheter
water displacing b.
b. wedge pressure catheter
Wilson-Cook dilating b.
Wilson-Cook gastric b.
windowed esophageal b.
wire-guided hydrostatic b.
Xomed dual-chamber b.

balloon-expandable
  b.-e. flexible coil stent
  b.-e. intravascular stent
  b.-e. metallic stent
  b.-e. stent
  b.-e. tracheal stent
balloon-flotation pacing catheter
balloon-imaging catheter
ballooning esophagoscope
Balloon-on-a-Wire
  B.-o.-a-W. cardiac device
  B.-o.-a-W. dilatation system
balloon-tipped
  b.-t. angiographic catheter
  b.-t. flow-directed catheter
  b.-t. thermodilution catheter
ball-tip
  b.-t. coagulating electrode
  b.-t. microcatheter
  b.-t. nerve hook
ball-tipped seeker
ball-type
  b.-t. disc prosthesis
  b.-t. retractor
Balmoral shoe
Baloser hysteroscope
Balser hook plate
Balshi packer
Balters appliance

Baltherm
  B. catheter
  B. thermodilution catheter
Baltimore Therapeutic Equipment Work Simulator
Banaji
  B. irrigation cannula
  B. LASIK cannula
  B. LASIK irrigating cannula
  B. spatula
banana
  b. Beaver blade
  b. finger extension splint
  b. plug dipolar generator
  B. SutureLasso
band
  aberrant b.
  adhesive b.
  air b.
  anchor b.
  anterior chamber tube shunt
    encircling b.
  Balkin Up and Over contralateral
    introducer with radiopaque b.
  belly b.
  big b.
  Broca diagonal b.
  Can-Do exercise b.
  copper b.
  Cosgrove-Edwards annuloplasty b.
  Dentaform b.
  distal thigh b.
  DOC B.
  dynamic orthotic cranioplasty b.
  EasyBand telemetrically adjustable
    gastric b.
  elastic rubber b.
  encircling b.
  Exerband therapy b.
  exercise b.
  Falope ring tubal occlusion b.
  Fit-Lastic therapy b.
  fracture b.
  Fränkel head b.
  GelBand arm b.
  Gennari b.
  Hahnenkratt matrix b.
  Harris b.
  isotropic b.
  Jobst air b.
  Johnson dental b.
  Ladd b.
  Lap-Band adjustable gastric b.
    (LAGB)
  latex O b.
  b. ligator device
  Lukens orthodontic b.
  Magill orthodontic b.
  Marlex b.

band *(continued)*
matrix b.
Mersilene b.
metal b.
orthodontic b.
parietal b.
Parma b.
patellar b.
PDS b.
pelvic b.
Pepper Medical tube neck b.
proximal thigh b.
Q b.
reelin immunoreactive b.
Remak b.
Rep Band exercise b.
Resist-A-Band exercise b.
Resist-A-Tube exercise b.
b. saw
scleral expansion b.
Securline blood b.
silastic b.
silicone elastomer b.
Simonart b.
snap gauge b.
Storz b.
Swedish Adjustable Gastric B.
T b.
tennis elbow arm b.
Thera-Band Max b.
Thera-Band therapy b.
Tofflemire matrix b.
tooth b.
tourniquet b.
tracheal b.
transcallosal b.
True Blue exercise b.
T-type matrix b.
vessel b.
Vesseloops rubber b.
Watzke b.
Xercise b.
Zipper Medical tracheostomy tube
neck b.

bandage
abdominal b.
Ace b.
Ace adherent b.
Ace spica b.
adhesive b.
Band-Aid b.
BandNet ready-to-use precut b.
barrel b.
Barton b.
binocular b.
Borsch b.
Bulkee II gauze b.
Buller b.
butterfly b.

capeline b.
Cellamin resin plaster of Paris b.
Cellona resin plaster of Paris b.
Champ elastic b.
circular b.
ClearSite b.
Coban b.
Coban cohesive medium stretch b.
cohesive b.
collodion-treated self-adhesive b.
Comperm tubular elastic b.
compression b.
Comprilan b.
Conco elastic b.
Conform stretch b.
b. contact lens
Coplus cohesive medium stretch b.
cotton elastic b.
cotton-wool b.
Cover-Roll stretch b.
cravat b.
crepe short stretch b.
crucial b.
Curad b.
demigauntlet b.
Dressinet netting b.
D-Stat clamp accessory b.
D-Stat dry b.
D-Stat 2Dry b.
D-Stat flowable b.
D-Stat radial b.
DuoDERM SCB sustained
compression b.
Duracast plaster b.
Dyna-Flex elastic b.
Dyna-Flex Layer Three b.
Dyna-Flex Layer Two b.
elastic b.
elastic foam b.
Elastikon b.
Elastomull elastic gauze b.
Elastoplast b.
Elset long stretch b.
Esmarch b.
eye b.
Fabco gauze b.
fiberglass b.
figure-of-8 b.
First Aid triple-antibiotic b.
fixation b.
flat eye b.
flexible b.
Flexicon gauze b.
Flexilite conforming elastic b.
FoamTrac traction b.
B. Gard cast protector
gauntlet b.
gauze b.
Gauztape b.

Gauztex b.
Gelocast b.
Gibney fixation b.
Gibson b.
Hamilton b.
hammock b.
HemCon b.
Hollister medial adhesive b.
Hueter b.
Hydron burn b.
Isoplast adhesive short stretch b.
Kerlix b.
Kerlix gauze b.
Kling b.
Kling gauze b.
Kold Wrap cold compression b.
Larrey b.
4-layer b.
Leukotape P stretch b.
Liquiderm liquid adhesive b.
Lister b.
long stretch b.
Maisonneuve b.
many-tailed b.
Marlex b.
Martin b.
3M Clean Seals waterproof b.
Medi-Band b.
Medicopaste b.
moleskin b.
monocular b.
MPM b.
Nylexogrip cohesive long stretch b.
oblique b.
occlusive b.
2-octylcyanoacrylate topical b.
Orthoflex elastic plaster b.
Ortho-Trac adhesive skin
  traction b.
perineal b.
plano T b.
plaster b.
plaster of Paris b.
b. plaster shears
Plast-O-Fit thermoplastic b.
polyurethane b.
POP b.
pressure b.
Priessnitz b.
Profore 4-layer b.
protective b.
QwikStrip adhesive b.
recurrent b.
Redigrip pressure b.
Robert Jones b.
roller b.
rubber-reinforced b.
scarf b.
b. scissors

scultetus b.
self-adherent b.
Setopress high-compression b.
Seutin b.
short stretch b.
Shur-Band self-closure elastic b.
Silesian b.
sling-and-swathe b.
Sof-Band bulky b.
Sof-Kling conforming b.
b. soft contact lens
Spandage tubular stretch b.
spica b.
spiral b.
spiral reverse b.
spray b.
starch b.
Stegman-Tromovitch b.
Steri-Strips b.
stockinette amputation b.
SurePress high-compression b.
Sureseal pressure b.
suspensory b.
T b.
4-tailed b.
Telfa 4 x 4 b.
Thera-Boot b.
Thermophore b.
ThrombiGel b.
Thrombix b.
thumb spica b.
triangular b.
Tricodur compression support b.
Tricodur Epi compression b.
Tricodur Omos compression b.
Tricodur Talus compression b.
Tricoplast adhesive elastic b.
Tru-Support EW b.
Tru-Support SA b.
TubeGauz b.
TubeGauz seamless tubular knitted
  cotton b.
TubiFast b.
Tubigrip b.
Tubigrip circumferential elastic b.
Tubigrip elastic support b.
Tubipad b.
tubular elastic b.
tumescent absorbent b.
Ulcosan Unna boot with inelastic
  zinc plaster b.
Unna boot b.
Velpeau b.
Viscopaste PB7 zinc paste b.
Webril b.
wet b.
woven elastic b.
Y b.
zinc oxide b.

Band-Aid
    B.-A. bandage
    B.-A. brand surgical dressing
    B.-A. composite dressing
bander
Band-It
    B.-I. magnetic elbow support
    B.-I. tennis elbow strap
Bandit
    B. balloon
    B. catheter
    B. PTCA catheter
Bandito
    B. endoscopic ligator
    B. single-band ligator
BandNet ready-to-use precut bandage
bandpass filter
Bane
    B. bone rongeur
    B. mastoid rongeur
    B. rongeur forceps
Bane-Hartmann bone rongeur
Bangerter
    B. angled iris spatula
    B. iris spatula
    B. muscle forceps
banjo curette
bank
    bone b.
Bankart
    B. rasp
    B. rectal retractor
    B. retractor
    B. shoulder prosthesis
    B. shoulder repair set
    B. tack
    B. tack implant
Banner
    B. enucleation snare
    B. forceps
    B. snare enucleator
Bannon-Klein implant
Bansal
    B. LASIK cannula
    B. LASIK forceps
Bantam
    B. CDH prosthesis
    B. wire-cutting scissors
Banyan emergency kit
BAPS ankle system
BAR
    biofragmentable anastomotic ring
    Valtrac BAR
bar
    arch b.
    Berens prism b.
    Bill traction b.
    Brookdale b.
    calcaneonavicular b.

clasp b.
cross b.
Denis Browne b.
dental arch b.
distraction b.
b. drill
Dynamic Mesh craniomaxillofacial
    preangled connecting b.
Erich dental arch b.
Erich malleable arch b.
Erich-Winter arch b.
Essig arch b.
exercise grab b.
1-b. external fixator
facial fracture appliance dental
    arch b.
Fillauer b.
fixed arch b.
fracture b.
Gerster traction b.
grab b.
Greenberg b.
Hader implant b.
Hahnenkratt lingual b.
hex b.
intramedullary b.
Jelenko arch b.
Jewett b.
Joseph septal b.
Kazanjian T b.
Kennedy b.
leading b.
Leyla b.
Leyla self-retaining tractor b.
lingual b.
Livingston intramedullary b.
locking b.
LockJaw arch b.
longitudinal spinal b.
lumbrical b.
mandibular arch b.
maxillary arch b.
occlusal rest b.
orbital b.
palatal b.
Passavant b.
physial b.
plastic premilled b.
posterior thigh b.
b. prism
retention b.
Roger Anderson fixation b.
screw alignment b.
side-cutting Swanson b.
Simonart b.
spondylitic b.
spondylotic b.
Sports-Grip b.
spreader b.

stabilizing b.
stall b.
strut b.
T b.
tarsal b.
Thera-P exercise b.
Tommy trapeze b.
traction b.
trapeze b.
unilateral b.
unsegmented b.
valgus b.
Winter arch b.

4-bar
4-b. external fixation device
4-b. linkage prosthetic knee
mechanism
4-b. polycentric knee prosthesis

Bara-Med
bar-and-shoe orthosis
Bárány
B. alarm
B. alarm apparatus
B. applicator
B. chair
B. noise apparatus
B. noise apparatus whistle
B. noise box
B. speculum

Barbara needle
barbed
b. broach
b. plastic washer
b. snare
b. stapler

Barbie retractor
barbiturate burst-suppression anesthesia
barb-tip lead
bar-clip attachment
Barcroft apparatus
Barcroft-Haldane apparatus
Barcroft-Warburg apparatus
Bard
B. absorption dressing
B. adhesive and barrier film
remover
B. AlgiDERM dressing
B. AlgiDERM rope
B. alligator cup
B. ambulatory PCA device
B. automatic reprocessor
B. biopsy needle
B. Biopty cut needle
B. Biopty gun
B. BladderScan
B. BladderScan bladder volume
instrument
B. button
B. catheter strap

B. cervical cannula
B. Clamshell septal occluder
B. Clamshell septal umbrella
B. closed-end adhesive pouch
B. coil stent
B. Commander PTCA guidewire
B. Companion papillotome
B. CPS system
B. Crurasoft patch
B. Cunningham incontinence clamp
B. Director guidewire
B. disposable male external
catheter
B. Dispoz-A-Bag leg bag
B. drainage adhesive pouch
B. Edwards outflow tract fabric
B. EndoCinch endoscopic suturing
system
B. evacuator
B. extension tubing
B. flexible endoscopic injection
system
B. gastrostomy catheter
B. gastrostomy feeding tube
B. implant
B. irrigation sleeve
B. leg bag holder
B. male external catheter
B. Memotherm colorectal stent
B. Monopty reusable core biopsy
instrument
B. needle
B. oval cup
B. PCA pump
B. PDA Umbrella
B. PEG
B. PEG tube
B. percutaneous cardiopulmonary
support system
B. Precisor direct bite forceps
B. protective barrier film
B. rotary atherectomy system
(BRAS)
B. Safety Excalibur catheter
B. Saxx stent
B. security pouch
B. self-adhesive fecal containment
device
B. soft double-pigtail stent
B. Sperma-Tex preshaped mesh
B. Stinger S ablation catheter
B. temporary pacing electrode
catheter with balloon
B. tip
B. Touchless intermittent catheter
B. universal Foley catheter sterile
insertion tray
B. urethral catheter sterile tray
B. Urolase

Bard (*continued*)
- B. Urolase fiber laser system
- B. Ventralex hernia patch
- B. Visilex mesh
- B. XT coronary stent

Bardco catheter
Bardeleben bone-holding forceps
Bardex
- B. all silicone sterile Foley catheter
- B. bag
- B. balloon
- B. catheter
- B. I.C. sterile Foley catheter
- B. Lubricath Foley catheter
- B. silicone Foley catheter

Bardex-Foley catheter
Bard-Marlex mesh
Bard-Parker
- B.-P. autopsy blade
- B.-P. blade
- B.-P. forceps
- B.-P. handle
- B.-P. keratome
- B.-P. knife
- B.-P. razor
- B.-P. scalpel
- B.-P. surgical blade
- B.-P. trephine

BardPort
- B. implanted port
- B. low-profile port
- B. MRI full-size port

Bard-Stiegmann-Goff variceal ligation kit
Bard-U-Cath self-adhering male external catheter
bare-metal stent
Bareskin knee positioner
bariatric mat table
BariKare bed
barium enema retention balloon
Barkan
- B. goniolens
- B. gonioscopic lens
- B. goniotomy knife
- B. infant implant
- B. light

Barker needle
Barnard mitral valve prosthesis
Barnes
- B. bag
- B. common duct dilator

Barnes-Crile hemostatic forceps
Barnes-Hind ophthalmic dressing
Barnhart 1/2 universal curette
Barnhill adenoid curette
baromacrometer

Baron
- B. lens
- B. suction tube

Baron-Frazier suction tube
baroreceptor
- cardiac b.

barospirator
barostat
- b. balloon
- electronic b.
- rectal b.
- Synectics visceral stimulator electronic b.

barostatic balloon
Barouk
- B. button space
- B. cannulated bone screw
- B. microstaple
- B. spacer

Barr
- B. crypt hook
- B. fistular probe
- B. rectal speculum

Barracuda flexible cystoscopic hot biopsy forceps
Barraquer
- B. applanation tonometer
- B. baby needle holder
- B. blade
- B. cannula
- B. cilia forceps
- B. conjunctival forceps
- B. corneal dissector
- B. corneal knife
- B. corneoscleral scissors
- B. cyclodialysis spatula
- B. eye needle holder
- B. eye shield
- B. eye speculum
- B. forceps
- B. hemostatic mosquito forceps
- B. implant
- B. iris scissors
- B. iris spatula
- B. irrigator spatula
- B. keratoplasty knife
- B. lens
- B. microkeratome
- B. needle
- B. needle carrier
- B. needle holder
- B. needle holder clamp
- B. operating room tonometer
- B. sable brush
- B. silk suture
- B. solid speculum
- B. sweep
- B. trephine

B. vitreous strand scissors
B. wire speculum
Barraquer-Carriazo microkeratome
Barraquer-Colibri
   B.-C. eye speculum
   B.-C. forceps
   B.-C. speculum
Barraquer-Katzin forceps
Barraquer-Troutman needle holder
Barraquer-von Mandach capsule forceps
Barraya tissue forceps
barrel
   b. bandage
   b. bur
   b. crawl
   b. guide
   guide b.
   Opti-Vue plastic b.
Barrett
   B. hydrodelineation cannula
   B. irrigating lens manipulator
   B. uterine tenaculum
barrier
   Active Life convex 1-piece
    urostomy pouch with Durahesive
    skin b.
   AquaTack hydrocolloid b.
   Atrisorb bioabsorbable b.
   Atrisorb FreeFlow GTR b.
   bioabsorbable adhesion b.
   calcium sulfate bone graft b.
   Capset bone graft b.
   Capset calcium sulfate bone
    graft b.
   contrast absorption b.
   DermaMend b.
   b. drape
   Durahesive skin b.
   external urethral b.
   ferric hyaluronate adhesion b.
   b. gown
   Guidor matrix b.
   Interceed absorbable adhesion b.
   Interceed TC7 absorbable
    adhesion b.
   b. laparoscopy drape
   B. laparoscopy LAVH pack
   b. lower extremity sheet
   Marlen SkinShield adhesive skin b.
   b. membrane
   Nu-Hope adhesive waterproof
    skin b.
   b. pack
   B. phaco extracapsular pack
   b. sheet
   Sil-K OB b.
   space-maintaining b.
   sterile field b.

TC7 adhesion b.
VitaCuff tissue interface b.
Barron
   B. alligator forceps
   B. artificial anterior chamber
   B. disposable artificial anterior
    chamber
   B. disposable trephine
   B. donor corneal punch
   B. donor punch
   B. epikeratophakia trephine
   B. marking corneal punch
   B. pump
   B. radial vacuum trephine
   B. stainless steel base
Barron-Hessburg corneal trephine
Barr-Shuford speculum
bar-sleeve attachment
bar-supported overdenture
Bart abdominoperineal unit
Barth mastoid curette
Bartholin gland catheter
bar-to-bar clamp
Barton
   B. bandage
   B. dressing
   B. forceps
   B. obstetrical forceps
Barton-Mayo tracheostoma button
BAS-300 transurethral thermotherapy
  device
basal
   b. block cervical saddle
   b. body thermometer
base
   Barron stainless steel b.
   fixation b.
   b. plate
   Plexiglas b.
   Profix nonporous tibial b.
   b. station
baseball
   b. finger splint
   b. suture
base-down prism
Baseline
   B. Bubble inclinometer
   B. dynamometer
basic
   Acceava hCG B.
   b. frame (type IV)
   b. hand splint
   OneTouch B.
basilar block skull positioner
basin
   catch b.
   emesis b.
Basis breast pump

B

basket
        Acufex meniscal b.
        Bagley helical b.
        biliary stone b.
        Cook N-Circle tipless bone b.
        Councill stone b.
        b. cutting forceps
        DASH tipless extraction b.
        Dormia biliary stone b.
        Dormia gallstone b.
        Dormia stone b.
        Eliminator stone extraction b.
        Ellik kidney stone b.
        Escape nitinol stone retrieval b.
        Expand212 helical stone b.
        b. forceps
        gallstone b.
        Gemini paired wire helical b.
        Glassman b.
        helical b.
        Highflex large stone retrieval b.
        Hobbs stone b.
        Howard stone b.
        instrument b.
        Johns Hopkins stone b.
        Johnson ureteral stone b.
        laser lithotriptor b.
        Meditech multipurpose b.
        Meditech stone b.
        Memory b.
        minihelical b.
        Moss-Harms b.
        nitinol b.
        NTrap stone retrieval b.
        Olympus stone retrieval b.
        parrot-beak b.
        Positrap miniretrieval b.
        b. punch forceps
        Pursuer CBD helical stone b.
        Pursuer minihelical stone b.
        retrieval b.
        Segura CBD b.
        Segura-Dretler laser b.
        sphincterotomy b.
        spiral b.
        sterilizing b.
        Stokes b.
        stone b.
        stone-retrieval b.
        b. stretcher
        Sur-Catch NT stone retrieval b.
        ultrasonic cleaner b.
        ureteral stone b.
        VPI stone b.
        walker b.
        Wilson-Cook stone b.
        6-wire spiral-tip Segura b.
basket-style scleral supporter speculum
basket-type crushing forceps

basolateral membrane transport system
Bassett electrical stimulation device
Bassini needle
Basswood splint
basting suture
Batchelor plaster hip spica cast
Bateman
        B. UPF II bipolar knee system
        B. UPF II shoulder prosthesis
Bates-Jensen pressure ulcer status tool
bath
        Aqua/Whirl b.
        b. blanket
        Charcot b.
        Dickson paraffin b.
        electric cabinet b.
        Finsen b.
        immersion b.
        Para-Care paraffin therapy b.
        B. respirator
        sitz b.
        Thermasplint heating b.
Bathlifter
        Leo B.
Batson vertebral brain system
batten
        b. graft
        lateral b.
battery, pl. batteries
        Activair b.
        button b.
        Duracell Activair hearing aid b.
        external pacemaker b.
        hearing aid b.
        lithium iodine b.
        Panasonic hearing aid b.
        Renata b.
battery-operated breast pump
battery-powered
        b.-p. endoscope
        b.-p. instrument
batting
        cotton b.
Batt tip
batwing
        b. catheter
        b. dissector
Batzdorf
        B. cervical wire passer
        B. cervical wire twister
Baudelocque pelvimeter
Bauer
        B. retractor
        B. sponge forceps
Bauerfeind
        B. Achillotrain
        B. ankle brace
        B. Comprifix knee brace
        B. malleolic ankle orthosis

B. OmoTrain active shoulder
support
B. silicone heel pad
B. SofSpot heel cup
B. support
**Baumanometer standard mercury
sphygmomanometer**
Baumgartner needle holder
Baum-Hecht tarsorrhaphy forceps
Baumrucker-DeBakey clamp
Baumrucker urinary incontinence clamp
Baum tonsillar needle holder
Bausch
B. & Lomb manual keratometer
B. & Lomb Optima lens
B. & Lomb Surgical L161U lens
B. & Lomb-Thorpe slit-lamp
Baxa oral dispenser
Baxter
B. angled arthroscope
B. CA-210 filter
B. disposable blade
B. Health Care Continu-Flo
infusion device
B. hemodialyzer
1550 B. hemodialyzer
B. infuser
B. Interline IV system
B. PCA pump
B. personal Von-Loc ice pack
B. PMT device
B. surgical clipper
B. VAMP
B. V. Mueller catheter
B. V. Mueller laparoscopic
instrumentation
B. volumetric infusion pump
bay
Trach-Mist aerosol drainage b.
Bayer
B. AG II chemistry analyzer
system
B. DCA2000 analyzer
B. glucometer
B. Technicon H-2 analyzer
B. Technicon H1 automated flow
cytometer
B. Versant HCV RNA 2.0 assay
test kit
Baylor
B. amniotic perforator
B. amniotome
B. autologous transfusion system
B. cardiovascular sump tube
Baylor-Video Acuity Testing
Bayne Pap brush
bayonet
b. bipolar forceps
b. clip applier

b. curette
b. forceps
b. handle
b. knife
Lucae b.
b. monopolar forceps
b. needle holder
b. osteotome
b. root tip forceps
b. scissors
bayonet-point wire
bayonet-tip electrode
Bazooka support surface bed
BB
blow bottle
body belt
**B&B Trachguard antidisconnection
device**
BCA-1 protein assay kit
BCD Plus cardioplegic unit
BCI
BCI Capnocheck DualStream
capnograph
BCI 3301 handheld pulse oximeter
BClear system
BCNU-impregnated polymer wafer
BCP
biphasic calcium phosphate
BCP bone graft
OsSatura BCP
BD
Becton-Dickinson
BD BBL CultureSwab Plus
collection and transport system
BD Beaver safety knife system
BD bone marrow biopsy needle
BD Insyte Autoguard shielded
intravenous catheter
BD K-3000 microkeratome
BD Lancet device
BD needle
BD Phoenix automated
microbiology system
BD Potain thoracic trocar
BD prism
BD ProbeTec ET system
BD Safety-Gard needle
BD SafetyGlide shielding
hypodermic needle
BD safety knife
BD Sensability breast self-
examination aid
BD Xstar blade
BD-CHEK intestinal inflammation kit
BDH prosthesis
BDP pad
Beacham amniotome
beach chair positioner
Beachcomber waterproof prosthesis

B

Beacon surgical line
bead
    Chelex b.
    glass b.
    hydroxyapatite b.
    immunomagnetic b.
    IOBeads magnetic b.
    magnetic b.
    methyl methacrylate b.
    packed b.
    Percoll b.
    polyacrylamide b.
    Sephadex b.
    Septobal b.
bead-blasted prosthesis
beaded guidewire
beaded-tip scissors
bead-loaded wire
beaked forceps
Beall
    B. circumflex artery scissors
    B. disc heart valve
    B. mitral valve prosthesis
    B. prosthetic valve
    B. valve
Beall-Surgitool
    B.-S. ball-cage prosthetic valve
    B.-S. disc prosthetic valve
beam
    AeroMat balance b.
    CO_2 b.
    continuous-wave laser b.
    coplanar b.
    helium-neon b.
    He-Ne b.
    4-b. laser Doppler probe
    load b.
    pencil electron b.
    probe b.
    split b.
    b. splitter
    The Summit HeNe aiming b.
    Visx Star Reticule aiming b.
Beamer
    B. injection stent
    B. injection stent system
beam-splitter
bean forceps
Bear
    B. 1, 2 adult volume ventilator
    B. Cub infant ventilator
    B. Hugger warming blanket
    B. NUM-1 tidal volume monitor
    B. respirator
    B. ventilator
Beard cystotome
Beardsley
    B. cecostomy trocar

    B. intestinal clamp
    B. intestinal forceps
bearing
    ceramic b.
    Steinmann pin with ball b.
    unipolar b.
Beasley-Babcock tissue forceps
BeasyTrans transfer device
Beath pin
Beaufort seating orthosis
Beaupre cilia forceps
Beaver
    B. Arthro-Lok blade
    B. blade
    B. cataract knife
    B. clear cornea incision system
    B. discission blade
    B. dissector
    B. ES miniblade
    B. handle
    B. keratome
    B. keratome blade
    B. knife
    B. miniblade
    B. Ocu-1 curved cystotome
    B. retractor
    B. ring cutter
    B. Xstar knife
Beaver-DeBakey blade
beavertail
    b. burnisher
    b. retractor
    b. tip
Bebax
    B. Bootie
    B. orthosis
Bechert
    B. lens-holding forceps
    B. nucleus rotator
    B. 1-piece all-PMMA intraocular
    lens
Bechert-Kratz cannulated nucleus
  retractor
Bechert-McPherson tying forceps
Bechert-Sinskey needle holder
Bechtol shoulder prosthesis
Beck
    B. abdominal scoop
    B. aorta forceps
    B. vascular clamp
Becker
    B. accelerator
    B. brace
    B. breast prosthesis
    B. corneal section spatulated
    scissors
    B. dissector cannula
    B. flat dissector tip
    B. goniogram

B

    B. gonioscopic prism
    B. Greater Grater dissecting cannula
    B. hand prosthesis
    B. 655 motion control limiter
    B. orthopaedic spinal system (BOSS)
    B. orthopaedic spinal system orthotic device
    B. orthopaedic thermoformable ankle system
    B. round dissector tip
    B. septal scissors
    B. tissue expander
    B. tissue expander/breast prosthesis
    B. tissue expander prosthesis
    B. twist dissector tip
    B. vibrating cannula system
Becker-Parkin pliers
Becker-Rojas Sub-Sonic surgical system
Beckman
    B. adenoid curette
    B. airfuge
    B. 2 autoanalyzer
    B. Coulter CEQ8000 fluorescent DNA analyzer
    B. Coulter QuickStart
    B. ICS Nephelometer system
    B. ion-selective analyzer
    B. JE-10X elutriation rotor
    B. J-6M centrifuge
    B. nasal scissors
    B. nasal speculum
    B. O_2 analyzer
    B. Synchron CX-7 cholesterol analyzer
    B. UV spectrophotometer
Beckman-Adson laminectomy retractor
Beckman-Eaton laminectomy retractor
Beckman-Weitlaner laminectomy retractor
Beck-Potts aortic and pulmonic clamp
Beck-Schenck tonsillar snare
Beck-Steffee total ankle prosthesis
Becton Colles fracture plate
Becton-Dickinson (BD)
    B.-D. guidewire
    B.-D. needle
    B.-D. Teflon-sheathed needle
bed
    AccuMax b.
    Acucare b.
    Advanta b.
    Affinity b.
    air b.
    air-fluidized b. (AFB)
    BariKare b.
    Bazooka support surface b.
    Betabed b.

BioDyne b.
Biologics Airlift b.
Biomet b.
Burke bariatric treatment system powered bariatric b.
Chick-Foster orthopaedic b.
circle b.
CircOlectric b.
Clini-Care b.
Clini.Dyne b.
Clini.Float b.
Clinitron b.
Clinitron air b.
Clinitron air-fluidized b.
dynamic b.
electric b.
Fisher b.
Flexicair b.
Flexicair II low-air-loss therapy unit b.
Flexicair MC3 low-air-loss therapy unit b.
Fluid-Air Plus b.
Foster b.
fracture b.
fusion b.
Gatch b.
Gelastic b.
head of b.
high air-loss b.
high muscular resistance b.
hospital b.
hydrostatic b.
hyperbaric b.
Isoflex b.
Keane mobility b.
KinAir b.
KinAir III, TC low-air-loss b.
Lapidus b.
low air-loss b.
Lumex shower b.
Magnum 800 b.
Magnum bariatric patient system b.
Medicus b.
Medline Alpha subacute care b.
Mega-Air b.
Mega Tilt and Turn b.
obese b.
Ohio b.
Orthoderm consummate air therapy b.
Plastazote foot b.
pulsating low-air-loss b.
Restcue b.
Roho b.
Roto Kinetic b.
Roto-Rest b.
Sanders b.
sawdust b.

bed (*continued*)
    skeletal b.
    Skytron b.
    Skytron air-fluidized b.
    SMI 3000, 5000 b.
    Spa B.
    Stress Echo b.
    Stryker b.
    Stryker CircOlectric b.
    Swinger car b.
    TheraPulse pulsating air
      suspension b.
    Tilt and Turn Paragon b.
    TriaDyne b.
    Ultra Dream Ride car b.
    water b.
Bed-Bar support rail
Bedbugg
    B. sleep apnea system
    B. system for at-home diagnosis
      of sleep apnea
Bedfont
    B. carbon monoxide monitor
    B. EC60 Gastrolyzer hydrogen
      monitor
Bedge
    B. antireflux mattress
    B. pillow
bedpan
bedside
    b. air chair
    b. monitor
    b. scale
    b. spirometer
    b. sterile drainage collection system
bed-wetting alarm
Beebe
    B. hemostatic forceps
    B. lens
    B. loupe
    B. wire-cutting scissors
Beehler irrigating pupil expander
Beer
    B. blade
    B. canaliculus knife
    B. cataract knife
    B. knife
Beeson
    B. cast spreader
    B. plaster spreader
Begg
    B. light wire appliance
    B. straight-wire combination bracket
behind-the-ear (BTE)
    b.-t.-e. hearing aid
    b.-t.-e. listening device
Behler
    B. LASIK enhancement hook
    B. LASIK retreatment hook

Békésy audiometer
Belin needle holder
bell
    Gomco b.
    Gomco circumcision b.
    Hydro-Tone B.
    b. rasp
    b. stethoscope
    B. suture
Bellavar medical support stocking
bellied bougie
bellows
    aneroid chest b.
    B. cryoextractor
Bellucci
    B. alligator scissors
    B. ear forceps
    B. scissors
belly
    B. Bag
    B. Bag urine storage bag
    b. band
Belmont collar
below-knee
    b.-k. cast
    b.-k. prosthesis
    b.-k. walking cast
    b.-k. walking plaster
Belscope
    B. blade
    B. laryngoscope
belt
    abdominal b.
    adjustable ostomy appliance b.
    Air Temp Advantage back
      support b.
    AquaJogger buoyancy b.
    Assura stomy b.
    Black hernia b.
    body b. (BB)
    Carabelt therapeutic b.
    cast b.
    Coloplast ostomy b.
    compression b.
    ComPressor pelvic compression b.
    Cool-Flex A/K suspension b.
    gait b.
    Hackett sacral b.
    Hackett sacroiliac cinch b.
    Little Ones Sur-Fit pediatric
      appliance b.
    magnetic support b.
    Marsupial b.
    maternity Si-Loc sacroiliac b.
    Max-Support abdominal
      retraction b.
    Meek pelvic traction b.
    pelvic traction b.
    Posey b.

Pouchkins pediatric ostomy b.
Reed cast b.
sacroiliac cinch b.
safety b.
Sam Sling pelvic b.
Saunders sacroiliac b.
Schiek B.
Serola sacroiliac b.
Si-Loc sacroiliac b.
Soma sacroiliac stabilization b.
Spine Power pelvic stabilizer b.
S'port Max sacroiliac b.
Sports Plus II back b.
TES b.
Thera-Band Aqua B.
traction b.
Tri-Flex auxiliary suspension b.
Universal pelvic traction b.
waist b.

belt-position booster seat
Belzer apparatus
Belz lacrimal sac rongeur
Bemis
B. air purifier
B. suction canister
Bence Jones cylinder
bench
Ensolite padded transfer b.
Invacare vinyl transfer b.
meditation b.
Paramount 3-way press b.
pelvic b.
b. scale calorimeter
Winco adjusting b.
Benchekroun hydraulic ileal valve
Bend-A-Boot foot splint
bender
Bunnell knuckle b.
cast b.
French rod b.
plate b.
rod b.
Tessier bone b.
Watt stave b.
bending pliers
Benedict operating gastroscope
Benedict-Roth
B.-R. apparatus
B.-R. calorimeter
B.-R. spirometer
Benefoot & Birkenstock orthotic sandal
Benephit
B. CV infusion system
B. HF infusion system
B. PV infusion system
Bengolea arterial forceps
Béniqué
B. catheter

B. dilator
B. sound
Benjamin
B. binocular laryngoscope
B. binocular slimline laryngoscope
B. pediatric laryngoscope
B. pediatric operating laryngoscope
B. tube
Benjamin-Havas fiberoptic light clip
Benjamin-Lindholm microsuspension laryngoscope
Ben-Jet tube
Bennett
B. basic hand splint
B. bone elevator
B. bone retractor
B. Cascade II Servo controlled heated humidifier
B. cilia forceps
B. contour mammography system
Nellcor Puritan B.
B. orthosis
B. respirator
B. tibial retractor
B. twin
B. ventilator
Benoist penetrometer
Benson baby pylorus separator
bent
b. blunt blade
b. blunt needle
b. Hohman retractor
b. infusion cannula
b. malleable retractor
b. reform implant
Bentle button
Bentley
B. autotransfusion system
B. Duraflo II
B. transducer
Bentson
B. exchange length wire
B. exchange straight guidewire
B. floppy-tip guidewire
B. floppy-tipped guidewire
B. Plus cerebral wire guide
Bentson-Hanafee-Wilson catheter
Bentson-style guidewire
Bentson-type Glidewire guidewire
Benzaquen-Chajchir extraction/reinjection system
benzene scintillator
benzoin applicator
Béraud valve
Berchtold cautery
Berens
B. blade
B. cataract knife
B. conical implant

B

71

Berens *(continued)*
- B. corneal dissector
- B. corneal transplant forceps
- B. corneal transplant scissors
- B. corneoscleral punch
- B. dilator
- B. electrode
- B. expressor
- B. glaucoma knife
- B. iridocapsulotomy scissors
- B. keratoplasty knife
- B. lens expressor
- B. lens loupe
- B. lid everter
- B. lid retractor
- B. marking calipers
- B. mastectomy skin flap retractor
- B. muscle clamp
- B. muscle forceps
- B. orbital compressor
- B. partial keratome
- B. prism
- B. prism bar
- B. ptosis forceps
- B. ptosis knife
- B. pyramidal implant
- B. refractor
- B. scleral hook
- B. spatula
- B. speculum
- B. suturing forceps
- B. tonometer

Berens-Rosa scleral implant
Berenstein guiding catheter
Berens-Tolman ocular hypertension indicator
Bergen retractor
Bergh ciliary forceps
Bergland-Warshawski phaco/cortex kit
Bergman
- B. mallet
- B. plaster saw

Bergmann Optical laser scanner
Bergström
- B. articulator
- B. needle

Bergstrom cannula
Bergström-Stille muscle cannula
Beriplast fibrin sealant
Berke
- B. cilia forceps
- B. clamp
- B. double-end lid everter
- B. ptosis clamp
- B. ptosis forceps

Berkefeld filter
Berkeley
- B. Bioengineering ptosis forceps
- B. scarifier

- B. suction curette
- B. suction machine
- B. Vacurette

Berkeley-Bonney retractor
Berkovits-Castellanos hexapolar electrode
Berlind-Auvard vaginal speculum
Berliner
- B. neurological hammer
- B. percussion hammer

Berman
- B. airway
- B. angiographic catheter
- B. foreign body locator
- B. intubating pharyngeal airway

Bernays sponge
Bernay uterine packer
Bernstein
- B. catheter
- B. gastroscope
- B. nasal retractor

Bertillon cephalometer
Bertin hip retractor
Best bite block
BeStent
- B. balloon-expandable stent
- B. 2 coronary stent
- B. Rival coronary stent system
- B. Rival stent
- B. 2 with Discrete Technology coronary stent system

Bestfoam insole
Bestneb nebulizer
beta
- B. Pile II, III splint strap
- b. ray microscope
- b. scintillation counter
- b. therapy eye applicator

beta-actin cDNA probe
Betabed bed
Beta-Cap
- B.-C. catheter closure
- B.-C. II closure

Beta-Cath
- B.-C. system
- B.-C. system catheter

Betacel-Biotronik pacemaker
Betadine
- B. PrepStick Plus
- B. PrepStick Plus applicator

Beta-Rail catheter
beta-ray applicator
Betaseron needle-free delivery system
BetaSorb device
Bethea sheet holder
Bethune-Coryllos rib shears
Bethune rib shears
BetterBinder back support
Bettman-Fovash thoracotome
Bevalac system

Bevatron accelerator
bevel
    Menghini-type coring b.
beveled
    b. chisel
    b. needle
    b. thin-walled needle
    b. trocar
bevel-point Rush pin
Beverly referential valve
Beyer
    B. bone rongeur
    B. laminectomy rongeur
BF+ bone void filler
BF large core bronchoscope
BFO
    BFO Kit
    BFO orthosis
bG
    blood glucose
    Chemstrip bG
BGC
    BGC matrix collagen
    BGC matrix hydrocolloid
    BGC matrix hydrocolloid dressing
BGS
    bone graft substitute
B-H forceps
BHTU microscope
BIAcore system
Biad
    B. camera
    B. SPECT imaging system
Biafine wound dressing emulsion
Bianchi valve
biangled hook
Bi-Angular shoulder prosthesis
biarticular
    b. bone-cutting forceps
    b. bone shears
bias
    B. stockinette
    b. wrap
bias-cut stockinette dressing
Biaxial Weave composite prosthesis
Biax total wrist system
BIB
    BioEnterics intragastric balloon
    BIB system
bibeveled cutting instrument
bibulous dressing
bicanalicular silicone tube
BICAP
    bipolar circumactive probe
    BICAP bipolar hemostasis probe
    BICAP cautery
    BICAP II cautery
    BICAP monopolar

    BICAP probe
    BICAP unit
Bicarbon Sorin valve
biceps
    B. bipolar coagulator
    b. elevator
Bicer-Val prosthetic valve
Bichat
    B. deep cheek pad
    B. tunic
Bickel
    B. intramedullary nail
    B. intramedullary rod
BiCoag forceps
Bicol collagen sponge
Bicon
    B. dental implant
    B. integrated abutment crown
biconcave
    b. contact lens
    b. lens
    b. washer
bicondylar ankle prosthesis
Bicon-Plus cup
biconvex intraocular lens
Bicor
    B. catheter
    B. Top
bicortical superior border screw
bicoudé catheter
BiCROS hearing aid
bicurved needle
bicycle
    Aerodyne stationary b.
    air b.
    Air-Dyne b.
    Collins b.
    b. dynamometer
    b. ergometer
    MedGraphics CPE 2000
      electronically braked b.
    Monark b.
    New Schwinn 900 b.
    New Schwinn elliptical b.
    recumbent b.
    Schwinn Airdyne b.
    Schwinn Spinner b.
    Schwinn 900 stationary b.
    Tredex powered b.
bicylindrical lens
Bident electrosurgical system
Bidet toilet insert
bidirectional
    b. Glenn shunt
    b. 4-pole Butterworth high-pass
      digital filter
    b. shunt
    b. telescopic distractor

B

Biemer
  B. approximator
  B. vessel clip
Bier
  B. amputation saw
  B. lumbar puncture needle
Bierer ovum forceps
Bierman needle
Bietti lens
bifid hook
bifilar needle electrode
bifocal
  b. demand DVI pacemaker
  executive b.
  b. eye implant
  b. glasses
  b. intracorneal lens
  b. lens
  b. multiplane rectal transducer
  b. spectacles
bifoil balloon catheter
bifurcated
  b. aortofemoral prosthesis
  b. blade-plate
  b. drain extension
  b. J-shaped tined atrial pacing and
  defibrillation lead
  b. retractor
  b. seamless prosthesis
  b. stent
  b. vascular graft
bifurcation prosthesis
big band
Bigliani/Flatow
  B. complete shoulder
  B. shoulder system
Bihrle
  B. dorsal clamp
  B. dorsal clamp T-C needle holder
Bike ankle brace
bikini
  disposable b.
BiLAP
  B. bipolar cautery
  B. bipolar cautery unit
  B. bipolar cutting probe
  B. bipolar laparoscopic probe
  B. bipolar needle electrode
bilateral
  b. breast coil
  b. breast pump
  b. pleural tube
  b. variable screw placement system
  b. ventricular assist device
    (BIVAD)
bilayered
  b. cellular matrix
  b. skin substitute
Bilbao-Dotter tube

bileaflet
  b. prosthesis
  b. tilting-disc prosthetic valve
bile bag
bilevel
  b. chisel
  b. positive airway pressure
    (BiPAP)
  b. positive pressure device
bili
  b. light
  B. mask
  b. mask eye shield
biliary
  b. balloon catheter
  b. balloon probe
  b. drainage catheter
  b. duct balloon dilator
  b. endoprosthesis
  b. retractor
  b. stent
  b. stone basket
BiliBed
  B. phototherapy system
  B. phototherapy unit
Bilibed
BiliBlanket Plus phototherapy system
BiliBottoms
BiliCheck
  B. battery-powered system
  B. bilirubin analyzer
  B. breath analyzer device
  B. test
BiliChek bilirubin analyzer
Bili-Labstix
Bililite
**biliopancreatic diversion with duodenal
  stent**
bilirubin blanket
bilirubinometer
  BiliTest transcutaneous b.
  direct-reading b.
  transcutaneous b.
  Unistat b.
**Bilitec 2000 intraluminal fiberoptic
  probe**
BiliTest transcutaneous bilirubinometer
Bili-Timer
Billeau
  B. ear loupe
  B. ear wax curette
  B. wax curette
**Billingham-Bookwalter rectal fenestrated
  blade**
Billroth uterine tumor forceps
Bill traction bar
Bilok interference screw
**Bilson fixable-removable cross arch bar
  splint**

bilumen mammary implant
Bi-Metric hip prosthesis
Bimler elastic plate
binasal
  b. cannula
  b. pharyngeal airway
  b. prongs
binaural stethoscope
Binax
  B. Now *Legionella* urine antigen test
  B. Now *Streptococcus pneumoniae* antigen test
  B. Now urinary antigen test
Bindazyme ANA screening ELISA kit
binder
  abdominal b.
  arch b.
  breast b.
  cloth b.
  compression b.
  Dale abdominal b.
  Dale surgical b.
  Orthomatrix b.
  Osteograf b.
  Scultetus b.
  B. submalar implant
binding
  table b.
Bing stylet
Binkhorst
  B. collar stud lens implant
  B. hooked cannula
  B. irrigating cannula
  B. 2-loop intraocular lens implant
  B. 4-loop iris-fixated implant
  B. 2-loop lens
  B. modified J-loop intraocular lens
  B. tip
Binkhorst-Fyodorov lens
binocular
  b. bandage
  b. fixation forceps
  b. indirect ophthalmocmicroscope
  b. indirect ophthalmomicroscope
  b. indirect ophthalmoscope
  b. loupe
  b. microscope
  b. ophthalmoscope
binophthalmoscope
binoscope
Bio
  B. Core therapeutic mattress
  B. Flote air flotation system
  B. Gard Plus
Bio-1000 knee brace system
bioabsorbable
  b. adhesion barrier
  b. Dexon suture

  b. interference screw
  b. mesh scaffold
  b. sheath-delivered vascular device
  b. staple
bioaccumulator
BioAction great toe implant
bioactive
  b. bone cement
  b. glass ceramics
  b. implant
  b. material
Bio-Anchor suture anchor
bioartificial
  b. liver device
  b. liver support device
  b. liver support system
BioBands bracelet
BioBarrier
  B. membrane
  B. membrane-guided tissue regeneration system
Biobond tissue adhesive
Bio-Boot
Biobrane
  B. adhesive
  B. dressing
  B. experimental skin substitute
  B. glove
  B. glove dressing
  B. glove graft
  B. graft material
  B. sheet
  B. skin substitute
  B. wound dressing
Biobrane/HF
  B./HF dressing
  B./HF skin substitute
BioBypass gene-based drug delivery product
Biocare dental implant
BioCast wrist/hand orthosis
biocavity laser
Biocell
  B. anatomical reconstructive mammary implant
  B. RTV breast implant
  B. RTV implant
  B. smooth surface implant
  B. textured shell surface implant
  B. textured silicone
Bio-Cera abutment
Bioceram
  B. 2-stage series II
  B. 2-stage series II endosteal dental implant
bioceramic
  b. implant
  b. implant material
Bioceram type S

Bio-Chromatic hand prosthesis
Biocide
Bioclad with pegs reinforced acetabular
   prosthesis
BioCleanse tissue sterilization process
Bioclusive
   B. dressing
   B. MVP Select transparent dressing
   B. MVP transparent film
   B. transparent dressing
Biocol dressing
biocompatible
   b. membrane
   b. nonresorbable glass ceramics
   b. spacing material
   b. stent
BioCompression Pneumatic Sleeve
biocompression pneumatic sleeve
Biocontrol Technology/Coratomic lead
Biocor
   B. 200 high-performance
     oxygenator
   B. porcine stented aortic valve
   B. porcine valve
   B. softshell venous reservoir
Biocoral
   B. graft
   B. implant
BioCore collagen dressing
Bio-Corkscrew
   headed B.-C.
Biocryl TCP/PLA screw
BioCuff
   B. bioresorbable screw and spiked
     washer implant
   B. C bioresorbable cannulated
     screw
   B. C bioresorbable cannulated
     screw and spike washer implant
   B. C bioresorbable spike washer
     implant
BioCurve saline-filled breast implant
biodegradable
   b. calcium phosphate cement
   b. collagen plug
   b. fixation device
   b. fixation instrumentation
   b. implant
   b. plate
   b. polylactide screw
   b. polymer scaffold
   b. scaffold
   b. stent
   b. surgical tack
   b. synthetic polymer
Biodel implant
biodendrimer adhesive
Bio-Dermal Hydrogel kit

Biodex
   B. Balance System
   B. cycle ergometer
   B. gait trainer
   B. isokinetic dynamometer
   B. isokinetic testing machine
   B. Multi-Joint System 3 MVP
   B. System
   B. target balance trainer
   B. Unweighing Support System
BioDiamond
   B. F stent
   B. Micro stent
   B. S rapid exchange PTCA
     catheter
BioDIMENSIONAL
   B. saline-filled implant
   B. system
BioDisc spinal disc repair system
BiodivYsio
   B. added support stent
   B. AS PC-coated stent
   B. OC over-the-wire stent
   B. open cell stent
   B. PC stent
   B. small vessel stent
   B. stent
   B. SV PC-coated stent
BioDyne bed
bioelectric field enhancement
BioElectric Shield
BioEnterics intragastric balloon (BIB)
bioerodible mucoadhesive
Bio-Esthetic abutment system
Bio-Eye hydroxyapatite ocular implant
Bio-FASTak
   B.-F. anchor
   B.-F. suture
biofeedback
   B. 5DX device
   b. electroencephalograph
   b. instrumentation
biofilm
Biofilter cardiovascular
   hemoconcentrator
Bio-Fit total hip system
Biofix
   B. absorbable rod
   B. absorbable screw
   B. arrow gun
   B. biodegradable implant
   B. fixation rod
   B. meniscus arrow
   B. stent
   B. system pin
BIOflex
   B. magnet back support
   B. magnetic counterforce brace
   B. medical magnet

B. orthotic
B. penile orthotic
Biofoot orthotic
Bio-Form glove
biofragmentable anastomotic ring (BAR)
Biogel
B. Diagnostic surgical gloves
B. M surgical gloves
B. Neotech surgical gloves
B. orthopaedic surgical glove
B. Reveal glove
B. Reveal/Indicator surgical gloves
B. Reveal puncture indication
system
B. Sensor surgical glove
B. Super-Sensitive surgical gloves
B. surgeons' glove
Bio-Gel HTP
Bio-Gen urine test strip
Bio-Gide
B.-G. resorbable barrier membrane
B.-G. resorbable bilayer membrane
Bioglass
B. bone graft substitute material
low-surface reactive B.
B. synthetic bone graft particulate
Bio-Glide
Import vascular access port
with B.-G.
BioGlide catheter
BioGlue
B. adhesive/sealant
B. glue
B. protein-based surgical adhesive
B. surgical patch
Biograft
Dardik B.
B. graft
Meadox Dardik B.
Biogran resorbable synthetic bone graft
Biographer
GlucoWatch B.
biograph molecular imaging system
Bio-Groove
B.-G. acetabular prosthesis
B.-G. HA hip stem
B.-G. HA hip system
B.-G. hip
B.-G. Macrobond HA femoral
prosthesis
Bio-Guard spectrum antimicrobial
bonded catheter
biohazard bag
bioimpedance electrocardiograph
bioimplant
DynaGraft b.
OrthoBlast osteoinductive b.
bioincompatible membrane

Bio-Interference
B.-I. screwdriver
B.-I. tibial screw
Bioject jet injector
Biojector
B. 2000 jet injector
B. 2000 needle-free injection
management system
Biokinetics pedobarograph
Bio-kinetics reader
BioKnit garment electrode
Biolab
Malakit *Helicobacter pylori* B.
Biolase
B. laser adapter
B. TwiLite laser system
Biolectron bone growth stimulator
Biolex
B. hydrogel dressing
B. impregnated dressing
B. impregnated gauze
B. wound cleanser
B. wound glue
Biolite ventilation tube
biological
b. aortic valve
b. tissue valve
Biologically
B. Quiet interference screw
B. Quiet Mini-Screw suture anchor
B. Quiet stapler
BioLogic-DTPF system
BioLogic-DT system
biologic fibrogen adhesive
BioLogic-HT system
Biologics Airlift bed
Biolox-forte ball head
BIOM
BIOM lens
BIOM noncontact panoramic
viewing system
BIOM noncontact wide-angle
viewing system
biomagnet
biomagnetic
b. insole
b. support
biomagnetometer
Magnes b.
BiomarC tissue marker
BioMask
biomaterial
carbon-based b.
ceramic b.
collagen-based b.
DualMesh Plus b.
Emerge b.
Gore-Tex DualMesh b.
Gore-Tex DualMesh Plus b.

B

biomaterial *(continued)*
>Gore-Tex Mycromesh b.
>Gore-Tex Mycromesh Plus b.
>inert allograft b.
>Mycromesh b.
>Mycromesh Plus b.
>polymeric b.
>polymethylmethacrylate b.
>technical b.

Biomatrix ocular implant
biomechanical ankle platform system
Biomedics contact lens
Bio-Medicus
>B.-M. arterial catheter
>B.-M. centrifugal pump
>B.-M. percutaneous cannula set
>B.-M. pump

biomedium
>Dynafill graft b.

Bio-Med pediatric ventilator
BioMed TENS unit
biomembrane
BioMend
>B. collagen membrane
>B. periodontal material

BioMerieux Vitek system
biomesh
>PelviSoft acellular collagen b.

Biomet
>B. AGC knee component
>B. AGC knee prosthesis
>B. AGC primary and posterior stabilized component
>B. ankle arthrodesis nail
>B. Ascent total knee
>B. Ascent total knee system
>B. bed
>B. Bi-Polar component
>B. bone anchor
>B. button
>B. cement removal hand chisel
>B. custom implant
>B. Finn salvage/oncology knee reconstruction system
>B. fracture brace
>B. Genus uni knee system
>B. hip
>B. hip prosthesis
>B. M2A metal-on-metal articulation for hip replacement system
>B. MARS acetabular component
>B. Maxim knee system
>B. Maxim total knee system
>B. plug
>B. Repicci II unicompartment knee component
>B. revision acetabular component
>B. revision hip stem
>B. revision knee system

B. Second Assistant knee positioner
>B. shoulder component
>B. staple
>B. total toe prosthesis
>B. trigger finger release knife
>B. Ultra-Drive cement remover
>B. Ultra-Drive ultrasonic revision system

biometer
>Ophthasonic Ultrasonic B.
>UV b.

Biometric prosthesis
biometry probe
biomicroscope
>Haag-Streit slit-lamp b.
>high-frequency ultrasound b.
>Nikon FS-3 photo slit-lamp b.
>slit-lamp b.
>ultrasonic b.

biomicroscopic indirect lens
biomicroscopy
>ultrasound b. (UBM)

Bio-Modular
>B.-M. shoulder prosthesis
>B.-M. total shoulder system

Bio-Moore endoprosthesis
Bionaire Air Cleaner
Bionic
>B. Ear
>B. ear prosthesis
>B. eye microdetector subretinal implant

Bionicare
>B. stimulator
>B. 1000 stimulator system

Bionix nasal speculum
Bionx
>B. absorbable cannulated screw
>B. arrow
>B. self-reinforced PLLA smart screw
>B. servohydraulic testing machine

bioocclusive dressing
Bio-Optics
>B.-O. Bambi cell analysis system
>B.-O. Bambi image analysis system
>B.-O. camera
>B.-O. specular microscope

Bio-Oss
>B.-O. collagen
>B.-O. corticalis bone graft material
>B.-O. freeze-dried demineralized bone
>B.-O. maxillofacial bone filler
>B.-O. spongiosa block
>B.-O. spongiosa bone graft material
>B.-O. synthetic bone

Biopatch antimicrobial foam wound dressing
Bio-Pen biometric ruler
Bio-Phase suture anchor
biophotometer
Biophysic
- B. Medical YAG laser
- B. Ophthascan S instrument

Bioplant
- B. hard tissue replacement synthetic bone
- B. HTR synthetic bone

Bioplastique
- B. augmentation material
- B. injectable microimplant
- B. polymer

Bioplate screw fixation system
biopolymeric vascular graft
Biopore
- B. membrane
- B. membrane device
- B. TM lead

biopotential skin electrode
BioPress plate
BioPro ceramic TARA head
bioprosthesis
- Carpentier-Edwards Duraflex low-pressure porcine mitral b.
- Carpentier-Edwards Perimount RSR pericardial b.
- Carpentier-Edwards porcine b.
- Freestyle aortic root b.
- Freestyle stentless b.
- Hancock II porcine b.
- Hancock M.O. II porcine b.
- Medtronic Intact porcine b.
- Mosaic cardiac b.
- pericarbon b.
- Perimount RSR pericardial b.
- porcine b.
- SJM X-Cell cardiac b.
- Toronto SPV b.
- X-Cell cardiac b.

bioprosthetic heart valve
biopsy, pl. **biopsies**
- b. cannula
- CT-guided stereotactic b.
- b. forceps
- b. gun
- b. loop electrode
- minimally invasive breast b.
- b. needle
- Pipelle b.
- b. probe
- b. punch
- b. punch forceps
- b. specimen forceps
- b. suction curette

- b. telescope
- Tru-Cut needle b.

Biopsys mammotome
bioptic
- b. amorphic lens system
- b. telescope

bioptome
- cardiac b.
- Caves-Schultz b.
- Cordis b.
- King b.
- King cardiac b.
- Konno b.
- Mansfield b.
- Scholten endomyocardial b.
- Stanford b.

Biopty
- B. biopsy gun
- B. cut needle
- B. gun

Biopty-Cut biopsy needle
Bio-Pump pump
Bio-Rad Model 5000 titanium system
Bioraptor suture anchor
Biorate pacemaker
BioRCI bioabsorbable screw
bioreactor
- magnetic resonance imaging-compatible hollow-fiber b.
- MRI-compatible hollow-fiber b.

bioresorbable
- b. drug delivery system
- b. implant
- b. stent

BioROC EZ suture anchor
Bio-R-Sorb resorbable poly-L-lactic acid ministaple
Biosafe
- B. PSA4 screen
- B. TSH test

biosampler
- Accellon Combi cervical b.

BioScrew absorbable interference screw
Biosearch
- B. anal biofeedback device
- B. 7000 enteral feeding pump
- B. female intermittent urinary catheter
- B. male intermittent urinary catheter
- B. needle

Biosense
- B. NOGA catheter-based endocardial mapping system
- B. Webster Navistar Thermocool catheter

Biosense-guided laser myocardial revascularization
Bioshaf automated 1-step fertility kit

BioSkin
>B. DP wrist support
>B. Q knee brace

BioSling bioabsorbable urethral sling
BioSole-GEL orthotic
BioSorb
>B. collagen resorbable membrane
>B. endoscopic browlift screw
>B. FX dental implant
>B. resorbable urology stent
>B. suture

BioSorbFX SR self-reinforced plate and screw
Biosound
>B. AU3, AU4, AU5 system
>B. Genesis II scanning system
>B. high-resolution ultrasound
>B. II ultrasound unit
>B. ultrasound unit

BioSource Cytoscreen SAA kit
Biospan
>B. anatomical tissue expander
>B. breast tissue expander

BioSpec
>B. MR imaging system
>B. MR imaging system scanner

BioSphere
>B. suture anchor
>B. suture anchor implant

Bio-Statak suture anchor
Biostator
Biostent biliary stent
Biosteon wedge interference screw
BioStim Digital NMS muscle stimulator
BioStinger
>B. absorbable meniscal implant
>B. fixation system
>B. low-profile fixation device

BioStinger-V bioabsorbable meniscal repair device
Biostop G cement restrictor
Biosurge Synchronous Autotransfuser
Bio-Suturetak
>Arthrex B.-S.

Biosyn synthetic monofilament suture
Biosystems feeding tube
Biotek 1000 autostainer
Bio-Tek EIx800 plate reader
biotelemetry system
Biotene
>B. Dry Mouth Kit
>B. Ultra Soft Toothbrush

Biotens neurostimulator
biothesiometer
>penile b.

Biothotic
>B. foot orthosis
>B. orthotic
>B. orthotic mold

Biotrack coagulation monitor
BioTrainer exercise meter
Biotronik
>B. lead
>B. pacemaker

Bio-Vascular prosthetic valve
Bio-Vent implant
Biovert
Biovue catheter
Bio-Wick sock
BioWrap lumbosacral/sacral support
BI-OX III ear oximeter
BioZ
>B. heart monitor
>B. hemodynamic monitoring system
>B. noninvasive cardiac function monitoring system
>B. system

BioZ.com cardiac output monitor
BioZip suture anchor
BioZ.pc system
BioZtect sensor
BIP
>BIP biopsy instrument
>BIP high-speed multibiopsy needle

BiPAP
>bilevel positive airway pressure
>BiPAP Duet LX
>BiPAP Duet LX CPAP system
>BiPAP machine
>BiPAP mask
>BiPAP Pro II with heated humidification
>BiPAP S/T-D 30 system
>BiPAP S/T-D ventilatory support system
>BiPAP unit
>BiPAP Vision system

biparietal suture
biphase
>Hall-Morris b.
>b. Morris fixation apparatus

biphasic
>b. calcium phosphate (BCP)
>b. pin
>b. pin appliance
>b. system

bipivotal hinge knee brace
biplanar
>b. fixator
>b. transducer

biplane
>b. DSA unit
>b. image intensifier system
>b. intracavitary probe
>b. sector probe
>b. system
>b. TEE transducer

bipolar
- b. bayonet forceps
- b. cable
- b. catheter
- b. cautery
- b. cautery probe BP-7350A
- b. cautery scissors
- b. circumactive probe (BICAP)
- b. coagulating forceps
- b. coagulator
- b. coaptation forceps
- b. connection cord
- b. cutting forceps
- b. cutting loop
- b. depth electrode
- b. diathermy adapter clip
- b. diathermy forceps tip
- b. electrocautery
- b. electrocautery forceps
- b. electrode
- b. electrosurgical scissors
- b. electrosurgical unit
- B. EndoStasis probe
- b. forceps
- b. generator
- b. glass electrode
- b. hemostasis probe
- b. hip arthroplasty component
- b. irrigating forceps
- b. irrigating stylet
- b. laparoscopic forceps
- b. long-shaft forceps
- b. magnet
- b. myocardial electrode
- b. needle
- b. needle electrode
- b. pacemaker
- b. pacing electrode catheter
- b. radiofrequency surgical ablation instrument
- b. sphincterotome
- b. stimulating electrode
- b. suction forceps
- b. traction splint
- b. urological loop

BiPort hemostasis introducer sheath kit
BIPP
  bismuth-iodoform-paraffin paste
  BIPP ribbon gauze
Bircher-Ganske meniscal cartilage forceps
Bircher meniscus knife
Birch-Hirschfeld lamp
bird
- B. Ascension ventilator
- B. & Cronin wrist brace
- B. machine
- B. Mark 8 respirator
- B. OP cup

- b.'s eye catheter
- b.'s nest filter
- b.'s nest IVC filter
- B. vacuum extractor

birdcage
- b. head coil
- b. resonator
- b. splint

Birkenstock
- B. Blue Footbed arch support
- B. high-flange arch support
- B. shoe

Birkett hemostatic forceps
Birkhauser eye testing chart
Birmingham Hip resurfacing system
Birtcher hyfrecator
birth cushion
birthing
- b. ball
- b. chair

BIS
  Bispectral Index Sensor
  BIS Sensor
  BIS Sensor Plus
bisected minigraft dilator
Bi-Set catheter
Bishop
- B. chisel
- B. mastoid gouge
- B. putty
- B. retractor
- B. sphygmoscope
- B. tendon tucker
- B. tissue forceps

Bishop-Harmon
- B.-H. anterior chamber irrigating cannula
- B.-H. crisscross forceps
- B.-H. iris forceps
- B.-H. knife
- B.-H. ophthalmic forceps

bismuth-germanate detector
bismuth-iodoform-paraffin paste (BIPP)
BiSNARE bipolar polypectomy snare
Bi-Soft lens
Bispectral
- B. Index Sensor (BIS)
- B. Index System

bispherical lens
Bisping electrode
bisque-baked prosthesis
Bissinger detachable bipolar coagulation forceps
bistoury
- b. blade
- Jackson b.
- Jackson tracheal b.
- b. knife
- straight b.

Biswas Silastic vaginal pessary
bit
> AO drill b.
> Badger drill b.
> cannulated drill b.
> diamond b.
> drill b.
> drill guide with drill b.
> hip fracture compaction drill b.
> Howmedica Microfixation System
>   drill b.
> Leibinger Micro System drill b.
> Luhr Microfixation System drill b.
> Storz Microsystems drill b.
> Synthes Microsystems drill b.

bite
> b. appliance
> b. biopsy forceps
> b. block
> b. force transducer
> b. protector
> b. stick
> B. Wafer denture bite wax

biteplate
biter
> angled b.
> Stille bone b.
> suction b.

biterminal electrode
biting forceps
Bitome
> B. bipolar sphincterotome
> B. bipolar system
> B. catheter

Bitpad digitizer
Bitumi monobjective microscope
BIVAD
> bilateral ventricular assist device
>   BIVAD bilateral left and right
>   ventricular assist device

bivalved
> b. anal speculum
> b. overlap brace
> b. pancake plaster hand cast
> b. retractor

bivalve nasal splint implant
biventricular
> b. assist device
> b. pacing wire

Bivona
> B. epistaxis catheter
> B. foam cuff
> B. Fome-Cuf tube
> B. Medical Technologies
>   customized tracheostomy tube
> B. OptiVox Electrolarynx
> B. tracheostomy tube

> B. tracheostomy tube with talk
>   attachment
> B. TTS tracheostomy tube

Bivona-Colorado voice prosthesis
Bizzarri-Giuffrida laryngoscope
Bjerrum
> B. scotometer
> B. screen

Björk
> B. diathermy forceps
> B. prosthesis
> B. rib drill

Björk-Shiley
> B.-S. aortic valve prosthesis
> B.-S. convexoconcave 60-degree
>   valve prosthesis
> B.-S. convexoconcave disc
>   prosthetic valve
> B.-S. floating disc prosthesis
> B.-S. graft
> B.-S. heart valve holder
> B.-S. heart valve sizer
> B.-S. mitral prosthesis
> B.-S. mitral valve
> B.-S. monostrut valve

Björk-Stille diathermy forceps
BK prosthesis
BKS refractive system
black
> B. Beauty ureteral stent
> b. braided nylon suture
> b. braided silk suture
> b. hatchet
> b. hernia belt
> b. light fluorescent lamp
> B. Max high-speed drill
> B. Max mid-size knee component
> B. rasp
> b. ray lamp
> b. silk bridle suture
> b. silk sling suture

blackened speculum
Blackstone anterior cervical plate
black/white occluder
bladder
> b. blade
> b. catheter
> b. evacuator
> gel-filled b.
> b. neck support pessary
> b. neck support prosthesis
> b. pacemaker
> b. replacement urinary pouch
> b. retractor
> b. sound

BladderManager
> B. portable ultrasonic device
> B. portable ultrasound scanner
> B. ultrasound device

BladderScan
>Bard B.
>B. BVI2500
>B. BVI2500 ultrasound scanner
>B. monitor
>B. ultrasound

blade
>Accutome black diamond b.
>Acra-Cut spiral craniotome b.
>Acu-Razor b.
>adenotome b.
>Aggressor meniscal b.
>Alfonso diamond corneal
> transplant b.
>arrow b.
>Arthro-Lok system of Beaver b.'s
>Asico multi incision system 10
> facet b.
>ASR b.
>autopsy b.
>Balfour bladder b.
>Balfour center b.
>banana Beaver b.
>Bard-Parker b.
>Bard-Parker autopsy b.
>Bard-Parker surgical b.
>Barraquer b.
>Baxter disposable b.
>BD Xstar b.
>Beaver b.
>Beaver Arthro-Lok b.
>Beaver-DeBakey b.
>Beaver discission b.
>Beaver keratome b.
>Beer b.
>Belscope b.
>bent blunt b.
>Berens b.
>Billingham-Bookwalter rectal
> fenestrated b.
>bistoury b.
>bladder b.
>bone saw b.
>Bookwalter-Cook anorectal b.
>Bookwalter malleable retractor b.
>Bookwalter-Mayo b.
>Bookwalter-Parks anal sphincter b.
>Bovie b.
>breakable b.
>broken razor b.
>Brown dermatome b.
>capsulotomy b.
>carbon steel b.
>cartilage shaver b.
>Caspar b.
>cast b.
>Castroviejo razor b.
>cataract b.
>cervical biopsy b.

>chisel b.
>chondroplastic b.
>chondroplasty Beaver b.
>circular b.
>clear cornea b.
>ClearCut dual-bevel b.
>CLM articulating laryngoscope b.
>Cloward single-tooth retractor b.
>Converse retractor b.
>Cottle nasal knife b.
>crescent b.
>crescentic b.
>Curdy b.
>Curdy-Hebra b.
>curved b.
>curved meniscotome b.
>Davis b.
>Deaver b.
>Deaver-type b.
>DeBakey b.
>DeBakey-Beaver b.
>Denis Browne pediatric abdominal
> retractor b.
>Derma b.
>dermatome b.
>diamond crescent b.
>diamond wafering b.
>Dingman mouthgag tongue
> depressor b.
>double-angled b.
>double-vector b.
>dull-sided diamond b.
>Duotrak b.
>Dyonics arthroscopic b.
>Edge coated b.
>b. electrode
>electrosurgical b.
>E-Mac laryngoscope b.
>Endo-Assist retractable b.
>EpiVision b.
>expandable b.
>eye b.
>Feather carbon breakable b.
>fiberoptic laryngoscope b.
>Field b.
>fine b.
>Flagg b.
>Flagg stainless steel
> laryngoscope b.
>folding b.
>Fugo b.
>Genesis diamond b.
>Gigli saw b.
>Gill b.
>Gillette Blue B.
>Gott-Balfour b.
>Gott-Harrington b.
>Goulian b.
>Grieshaber b.

blade *(continued)*
  GS-9 b.
  GSA-9 b.
  Guedel laryngoscope b.
  b. handle
  Hebra b.
  hemilaminectomy b.
  Hemostatix scalpel b.
  Henley retractor b.
  Hibbs b.
  Hibbs spinal retractor b.
  b. holder
  Horgan center b.
  House detachable b.
  House knife b.
  House ophthalmic b.
  Incisor arthroscopic b.
  infant urethrotome b.
  jigsaw b.
  K b.
  Katena double-edged sapphire b.
  Keeler retractable b.
  Kellan sutureless incision b.
  keratome Beaver b.
  Kjelland b.
  Knapp b.
  b. knife
  knife b.
  Komet K-2000 surgical saw b.
  K-2000 surgical saw b.
  LaForce adenotome b.
  lamellar b.
  laminectomy b.
  lancet b.
  Lange b.
  laryngoscope b.
  Lieberman-type speculum reversible
    thin solid b.
  Lieberman-type speculum thin
    solid b.
  Lieberman-type speculum with
    Kratz open wire b.
  Lieberman wire aspirating speculum
    with V-shape b.
  Linvatec débrider b.
  Lite b.
  Lundsgaard b.
  MacIntosh b.
  MacIntosh fiberoptic
    laryngoscope b.
  Magnum Tiger b.
  malleable b.
  Martin b.
  Martinez corneal trephine b.
  Mastel trifaceted diamond b.
  McPherson-Wheeler b.
  meniscectomy b.
  Merlin arthroscopy b.
  Merlin bendable b.

  Meyerding retractor b.
  M4-400 freedom b.
  microplaner b.
  Micro-Sharp b.
  microvitreoretinal b.
  Miller b.
  Miller b. #0, #1
  miniature b.
  mini-meniscus b.
  3M Maxi Driver b.
  mouthgag tongue depressor b.
  multiincision 10-facet diamond b.
  MVR b.
  Myocure b.
  myringotomy b.
  myringotomy knife b.
  narrow Assistant Free retractor b.
  nasal knife b.
  nasal saw b.
  notchplasty b.
  ophthalmic b.
  Optimum b.
  orbit b.
  oscillating b.
  Otocap myringotomy b.
  Oxiport laryngeal b.
  Padgett dermatome b.
  Parker-Bard b.
  Paufique b.
  pediatric Hendren retractor b.
  pediatric mastoid retractor b.
  Personna prep b.
  Personna steel b.
  Personna surgical b.
  plasma b.
  PowerCut drill b.
  Prizm keratome b.
  3-pronged rake b.
  5-prong rake b.
  Rad airway laryngeal b.
  RADenoid adenoidectomy b.
  ramus b.
  razor b.
  rectangular b.
  replaceable b.
  retractable b.
  retractor b.
  retrograde Beaver b.
  Rhein 3D trapezoid diamond b.
  ribbon b.
  ring tongue b.
  rosette b.
  rosette Beaver b.
  Rubin b.
  Satterlee bone saw b.
  b. scalpel
  Schanz Scheie b.
  Scheie b.
  scimitar b.

scleral b.
sclerotome b.
self-retaining retractor b.
semilunar-tip b.
b. septostomy catheter
serrated b.
Sharpoint spoon b.
Sharpoint V-lance b.
Sharptome crescent b.
shoulder b.
sickle b.
sickle-shaped Beaver b.
side b.
side-cutting b.
Skimmer laryngeal b.
slimcut b.
slit b.
snub-nose diamond b.
spear b.
spinal retractor b.
spoon b.
Sputnik Russian razor b.
stab incision angled b.
stainless steel b.
Stealth DBO diamond b.
sterile electrodermatome b.
sternal retractor b.
Storz disposable b.
straight b.
Stryker b.
Superblade b.
Superblade No. 75 b.
SuperCut b.
surgical saw b.
Surgistar ophthalmic b.
Swann-Morton surgical b.
Swiss b.
Synovator arthroscopic b.
synovectomy b.
tapered b.
Taylor spinal retractor b.
Temperlite saw b.
The Edge coated b.
Thornton arcuate b.
Thornton tri-square b.
Tiger b.
tongue retractor b.
Tooke b.
trapezoid b.
trephine b.
Tricut b.
trifacet b.
triradial resector b.
Troutman b.
Turner-Warwick b.
Typhoon cutter b.
Typhoon microdebrider b.
UltraEdge keratome b.

ultrathin surgical b.
Universal nasal saw b.
urethrotome b.
vectis b.
V-lance b.
Weck b.
Weck-Prep b.
Weinberg b.
Welch Allyn laryngoscope b.
wire side b.
Wisconsin b.
Wisconsin laryngoscope b.
X-Acto b.
Yu-Holtgrewe malleable b.
Ziegler b.
Zimmer Gigli saw b.

bladebreaker
Castroviejo b.
razor b.
Troutman b.

bladed
2-b. dilator
3-b. clamp

blade-form
b.-f. device
b.-f. implant

blade-plate, bladeplate
adolescent condylar b.-p.
bifurcated b.-p.
Blair talar body fusion b.-p.
Blair tibiotalar arthrodesis b.-p.
Blanchard traction device b.-p.
fixed-angle AO b.-p.
Giebel b.-p.
pediatric b.-p.
semitubular b.-p.

Blade-Vent implant system
Blair
B. cleft palate clamp
B. cleft palate elevator
B. knife
B. nasal chisel
B. 4-prong retractor
B. retractor
B. talar body fusion blade-plate
B. tibiotalar arthrodesis blade-plate

Blair-Brown
B.-B. graft
B.-B. implant

Blair-Ivy loop
Blake
B. dressing forceps
B. ear forceps
B. gallstone forceps
B. inverted orthotic
B. silicone drain
B. uterine curette

Blakemore-Sengstaken tube

Blakesley
  B. ethmoid forceps
  B. grasper
Blakesley-Weil upturned ethmoid forceps
Blalock
  B. pulmonary artery clamp
  B. pulmonary artery forceps
  B. shunt
Blalock-Taussig shunt
Blanchard
  B. hemorrhoid forceps
  B. traction device
  B. traction device blade-plate
blank
  Aliplast b.
  implant b.
  Nickelplast b.
  Plastazote b.
Blanke inverted tibialis posterior tendon orthotic
blanket
  Bair Hugger b.
  Bair Hugger patient warming b.
  Bair Hugger warming b.
  bath b.
  Bear Hugger warming b.
  bilirubin b.
  CareDrape b.
  circulating water b.
  cooling b.
  forced air b.
  Gaymar water-circulating b.
  Hollister Hot/Ice knee b.
  Hot/Ice System III knee b.
  hypothermia b.
  magnetic b.
  Rowe b.
  b. suture
  thermal space b.
Blauth knee prosthesis
Blaydes
  B. corneal forceps
  B. lens-holding forceps
Blazer RPM navigation and ablation catheter
BLB mask
bleb cup
Bledsoe
  B. Achilles boot
  B. adjustable post-op brace
  B. cast brace
  B. conformer diabetic boot
  B. fracture brace
  B. knee brace
bleed-back valve
bleeding needle
Bleier clip

blender
  Virtis b.
Blenderm
  B. tape
  B. tape dressing
blend tool
blepharochalasis forceps
blepharoplasty scissors
blepharostat
  Goldman scleral fixation ring and b.
  McNeill-Goldman b.
blind
  b. endosonography probe
  b. loop
  b. medullary nail
blinded acupuncture needle
Blinkeze eyelid external lid weight
Bliskunov implantable femoral distractor
BlisterFilm
  B. transparent film
  B. transparent wound dressing
Blitz suture retriever
block
  acrylic bite b.
  AeroMat balance b.
  Airlite alignable ankle b.
  anterior-posterior cutting b.
  A-P cutting b.
  Best bite b.
  Bio-Oss spongiosa b.
  bite b., biteblock
  bone b.
  Brightbill corneal cutting b.
  Cerrobend b.
  Cerrobend trim b.
  corneal b.
  cutting b.
  4-in-1 cutting b.
  cutting Delrin b.
  cutting Teflon b.
  Dembone demineralized cortical dental b.
  disposable Styrofoam b.
  dual lateral skull b.
  Ethox bite b.
  Fine folding b.
  B. fixator
  functional grip pushup b.
  Greco cutting b.
  hand b.
  hydroxyapatite b.
  HyProCure sinus tarsi implant b.
  lead b.
  methyl methacrylate b.
  OB-10 Comfort bite b.
  Omni Bloc bite b.
  Oxyguard endoscopy bite b.
  paraffin b.

PED b.
pelvic b.
Perspex b.
Plexiglas tissue equivalency b.
punch b.
push-up b.
shielding b.
shock b.
silicone b.
Southern Eye Bank corneal
 cutting b.
Teflon b.
tibial augmentation b.
tibial cutting b.
TruBlock BGS b.
unidirectional b.
unifascicular b.
yoke b.

blocker
hook b.

Bloedorn applicator
Blom-Singer
B.-S. esophagoscope
B.-S. tracheoesophageal prosthesis
B.-S. valve
B.-S. voice prosthesis

blood
b. agar plate
b. cell separator
b. flow enhancement device
b. flowmeter
b. flow probe
1620 b. gas analyzer
840 b. gas analyzer
b. glucose (bG)
b. glucose reagent strip
b. perfusion monitor
b. pressure cuff
b. pressure recorder
b. pressure transducer
b. pump

blood-contactin catheter
blood-containment needle
bloodless circumcision clamp
Bloodshot WildEyes lens
BloodSTOP EX hemostatic gauze
Bloodwell-Brown forceps
Bloodwell forceps
Bloomberg
B. SuperNumb anesthetic ring
B. trabeculotome set

bloomer
Kins pull-on waterproof b.

Bloom programmable stimulator
Blount
B. brace
B. epiphysial staple
B. knee retractor
B. laminar spreader

Blount-Schmidt-Milwaukee brace
blow bottle (BB)
blow-by ventilator
blower
Cardiovations CO2 b.
CO_2 b.
DeVilbiss powder b.
powder b.

B&L pinch gauge
Blucher low-quarter shoe
blue
B. Brand Therapy Putty
b. Cook sheath
b. filtering lens
b. filtration hydrophobic IOL
B. FlexTip catheter
b. light-absorbing intraocular lens
B. Line cuffed endotracheal tube
B. Line orthotic
B. Line ThumbStay splint
B. Line Uno splint
B. Line wrist control splint
b. litmus paper
B. Max balloon catheter
B. Max high-pressure balloon
B. Max high-pressure reinforced
 polyethylene balloon catheter
b. opaque Herrick lacrimal plug
b. ring pessary
b. twisted cotton suture
B. Vista

blue-black monofilament suture
blue-filtering IOL
Bluemle pump
**Bluetooth remote wireless technology
 microphone**
Blumenthal
B. anterior chamber maintainer
B. bone rongeur
B. conjunctiva dissector
B. dissector
B. push-pull irrigating cystotome

**Blu-Mousse polyvinyl registration
 material**
blunt
b. bullet-tip cannula
b. dissecting hook
b. elevator
b. forceps
b. hook
b. hook dissector
b. iris hook
b. K-wire
b. lacrimal probe
b. Metzenbaum scissors
b. needle
b. nerve hook
b. nose hemostat
b. obturator

blunt *(continued)*
    b. palpator
    b. probe
    b. rake retractor
    b. ring curette
    b. suction tube
    b. trocar
blunt-end sialogram needle
Bluntport disposable trocar
blunt-tipped
    b.-t. epidural needle
    b.-t. extraction cannula
    b.-t. obturator
    b.-t. Vannas scissors
blunt-tip probe
BLU-U blue light photodynamic therapy illuminator
Blythemobile
B-mode
    B-m. handpiece
    B-m. ultrasound
BMP cabling and plating system
BMSI 5000 electroencephalograph
Boa Duel TLSO
board
    adjustable cane b.
    alphabet b.
    arm b., armboard
    back b.
    balance b.
    broad-based cane b.
    Competitive Ankle B.
    cutting b.
    English cane b.
    Euroglide MKII slide b.
    Flexisplint flexed arm b.
    full spine b.
    Gibson-Ross b.
    glider cane b.
    graft b.
    grid maze b.
    Hadfield hand b.
    J b.
    manipulation b.
    memory b.
    papoose b.
    pivoting surgical arm b.
    powder b.
    prone b.
    quad b.
    recumbent infant b.
    right-angled isosceles triangle b.
    Rock ankle exercise b.
    rocker b.
    Rock & Roller exercise b.
    scooter b.
    spine b.
    b. splint

    Spri Xercise b.
    string drawing b.
    SummaSketch III digitizing b.
    tape b.
    Targa+ image capture b.
    tilt b.
    transfer b.
    vestibular b.
    wobble b.
BoarderAnkle brace
Boardshield disposable backboard bag
Boas algesiometer
boat hook
bobbin myringotomy tube
Bobechko
    B. sliding barrel hook
    B. spreader
Boberg-Ans
    B.-A. lens
    B.-A. lens implant
Bobrov apparatus
Bock knee prosthesis
Bodai adapter
Bodenstab tourniquet
Bodi
    B. Dynamic orthosis
    B. knee extension orthosis
Bodian lacrimal pigtail probe
bodies (*pl. of* body)
BOD incubator
Bodkin thread holder
Bodnar retractor
body, pl. **bodies**
    B. Armor short leg walker
    B. Armor walker cast
    B. Ball
    b. belt (BB)
    b. coil
    b. cooling unit
    b. exhaust suit
    B. Gard neoprene support
    B. Glove orthopaedic product
    Howell-Jolly b.
    b. jacket
    b. jacket cast
    b. logic rehabilitation system
    B. Masters MD 510 hi-lo pulley system
    b. mechanics examination chart
    Ortho-Mold lumbar b.
    b. piercing instrument
    b. positioner
    B. Response system
    B. Sport ankle brace
    B. Sticks massager
    b. table
BodyBilt chair
Bodyblade

BodyCushion
  B. positioner
  SwimEx aquatic therapy B.
BodyForm thoracolumbar plate
BodyGem metabolism monitor
BodyIce
  B. cold pack
  B. cold pack wrap
  B. wrap
Bodyline
  B. Back-Huggar
  Satalite cushion by B.
  B. sleeper mattress overlay
  B. sports brace
Bodynapper comfort pillow
Body-Solid exercise equipment
BodyTable
  HiLo B.
  TouchAmerica B.
BodyWrap premium overlay
Boehm
  B. anoscope
  B. proctoscope
  B. rectal diagnostic and treatment
  set
  B. sigmoidoscope
Boehringer
  B. Autovac autotransfusion system
  B. kit
  B. Mannheim DIG-nucleic detection
  kit
  B. Mannheim DIG-oligonucleotide
  tailing kit
  B. suction regulator
Boer craniotomy forceps
Boerma obstetrical forceps
Boettcher
  B. forceps
  B. tonsil scissors
Bogota bag
Böhler
  B. clamp
  B. exerciser
  B. extension bow
  B. hip nail
  B. iron
  B. nail
  B. os calcis clamp
  B. pin
  B. plaster cast breaker
  B. reducing fracture frame
  B. rongeur
  B. tongs
  B. traction bow
  B. tractor
  B. wire splint
Böhler-Braun
  B.-B. fracture frame

  B.-B. leg sling
  B.-B. splint
Böhler-Knowles hip pin
Böhler-Steinmann pin
Boies
  B. cutting forceps
  B. nasal fracture elevator
Boies-Lombard mastoid rongeur
Bojrab Hapex universal prosthesis
Bold compression screw
Bolero lift bath trolley
Boley gauge
Bolin wedge filter system
bollard device
Bollinger knee brace
Boloxie OT Prehension Game
bolster
  angular b.
  armrest b.
  breast b.
  b. buddy
  knee b.
  knee arthrography b.
  retention suture b.
  roll control b.
  b. suture
  Teflon felt b.
  Telfa b.
  tie-over b.
bolt
  Alta femoral b.
  Alvar condylar b.
  bone lock b.
  cannulated b.
  Hardinge expansion b.
  hexhead b.
  Hubbard b.
  I b.
  ICP Camino b.
  Nylok b.
  Philly b.
  Richmond b.
  slotted b.
  solid hex b.
  tibial b.
  transfixion b.
  trochanteric b.
  Wilson b.
  wire fixation b.
  Zimmer tibial b.
Bolton forceps
bolus
  b. dressing
  standardized constant b.
Bonaccolto
  B. cup jaws forceps
  B. fragment forceps
  B. jeweler's forceps

B

Bonaccolto *(continued)*
  B. magnet tip forceps
  B. utility and splinter forceps
Bondek absorbable suture
Bondeze resin
bonding
  In-Ceram Alumina b.
  In-Ceram Cerestore b.
  In-Ceram Empress b.
  In-Ceram Fortress b.
  In-Ceram Optec b.
  In-Ceram Spinell b.
  Poly-Lock b.
bone
  b. abduction instrument
  b. aggregate
  Allofix freeze-dried b.
  b. anchor
  b. awl
  b. bank
  Bio-Oss freeze-dried
    demineralized b.
  Bio-Oss synthetic b.
  Bioplant hard tissue replacement
    synthetic b.
  Bioplant HTR synthetic b.
  b. block
  B. Bullet suture anchor
  b. bur
  B. Button orthopaedic suture
    anchor
  b. calipers
  b. cement
  b. cement adhesive
  b. chisel
  b. collector
  b. conduction hearing aid
  b. crusher
  b. curette
  b. cutter
  Dembone demineralized human b.
  Dembone freeze-dried b.
  demineralized b.
  b. densitometer
  b. dowel
  b. elevator
  endochondral b.
  b. estimator
  b. extension clamp
  b. extractor
  b. femoral plug
  b. file
  b. fixation device
  b. fixation kit
  b. fixation wire
  b. flap fixation plate
  b. forceps
  b. formation marker
  b. gouge

  b. graft holder
  b. grafting material
  b. graft plug
  b. graft punch
  b. graft shoe horn
  b. graft substitute (BGS)
  b. growth stimulator
  b. hand drill
  b. holder
  b. hole punch
  hollow b.
  b. hook
  b. hook with cable/wire hole
  b. implant material
  b. injection gun
  Lambone cortical b.
  Lambone demineralized laminar b.
  Lambone freeze-dried b.
  b. lavage
  b. lever
  b. lock bolt
  b. mallet
  b. marrow biopsy needle
  b. marrow transplant unit
  b. morphogenic protein
  b. mulch screw
  Osteomin freeze-dried b.
  b. paste
  b. peg
  B. Plast bone replacement material
  b. plate
  b. plug extractor
  b. prosthesis
  b. punch forceps
  b. punch rongeur
  b. rasp
  b. reamer
  b. resorption marker
  b. retractor
  b. saw
  b. saw blade
  b. scalpel
  b. screw
  b. screw depth gauge
  b. screw targeter
  b. skid
  b. staple system
  b. substitute material (BSM)
  b. tack system
  b. tamp
  Tutoplast b.
  Vitoss synthetic b.
  b. wax
  b. wax suture
  b. weapon
  b. wedge
  b. window
  b. wire guide
bone-anchored hearing aid

B

bone-biting
    b.-b. forceps
    b.-b. rongeur
BoneCollector bone fillings harvest collector
bone-cutting
    b.-c. forceps
    b.-c. rongeur
Bone-Dri femoral surgical wick
bone-holding
    b.-h. clamp
    b.-h. forceps
Boneloc cement
Bone-Lok device
bone-measuring calipers
Bone-Mill
    R. Quétin B.-M.
bone-patellar tendon-bone autograft
BonePlast bone void filler
bone-reduction forceps
BoneSource hydroxyapatite cement
bone-splitting forceps
bone-tendon graft material
Bonfiglio
    B. bone graft
    B. bone replacement material
Bongort
    B. 1-piece drainable pouch
    B. 1-piece ostomy pouch
Bonn
    B. iris forceps
    B. iris hook
    B. iris scissors
    B. microiris hook
    B. suturing forceps
Bonnano catheter
Bonnet
    Hydro B.
Bonnie balloon catheter
Bonopty needle system
Bonwill articulator
Boo-Boo Pacs
book
    B. Butler book-grip device
    Ishihara test chart b.
Bookler
    B. swivel-ball laparoscope holder
    B. swivel-ball laparoscopic instrument holder
Bookwalter
    B. malleable retractor blade
    B. retractor
    B. retractor system
    B. ring retractor
    B. Rotilt ratchet mechanism
    B. Wishbook adjustable frame
Bookwalter-Cook anorectal blade
Bookwalter-Goulet retractor
Bookwalter-Hill-Ferguson rectal retractor

Bookwalter-Mayo blade
Bookwalter-Parks anal sphincter blade
Bookwalter-St. Mark deep pelvic retractor
Boolean operator
boomerang
    b. bladder needle
    b. needle holder
Boost demineralized bone matrix
Booster clip
boot
    Achilles b.
    all-purpose b. (APB)
    Ambulator Chukka B.
    Anthony cast b.
    APB Hi all-purpose b.
    Bledsoe Achilles b.
    Bledsoe conformer diabetic b.
    b. brace
    Bunny B.
    cast b.
    Chukka b.
    Circulator b.
    clamshell AFO b.
    compression b.
    Conformer diabetic b.
    ConvaTec Unna-Flex elastic Unna b.
    cradle b.
    Cryo/Cuff b.
    Cryo/Cuff pressure b.
    De Lorme b.
    derotation b.
    Dome-Paste b.
    DonJoy MaxTrax diabetic walker b.
    Duke b.
    external sequential pneumatic compression b.
    fluid barrier b.
    fracture b.
    gelatin compression b.
    Gelocast Unna b.
    Gibney b.
    Hang Ups gravity b.
    Heelift suspension b.
    Heelift traction b.
    HighTide diabetic b.
    hyperbaric b.
    In-Bed AFO b.
    IPC b.
    Jobst b.
    Junod b.
    L'Nard b.
    Lunax B.
    Markell brace b.
    Markell open-toe b.
    MaxTrax diabetic walker b.
    Moon B.

boot *(continued)*
    Multi Podus b.
    O_2 B.
    Ongoing Ambulating AFO b.
    open-heeled Unna b.
    pneumatic compression b.
    PNS Unna b.
    primer flexible Unna b.
    primer modified Unna b.
    quadriceps De Lorme b.
    Rik FootHugger fluid heel b.
    Rooke perioperative b.
    sheepskin b.
    SlimLine cast b.
    Sorrel-type snowboard b.
    Spenco b.
    Tenderwrap Unna b.
    Unna b.
    Unna-Flex elastic Unna b.
    Venodyne b.
    weight b.
    Wilke b.
Boothby mask
Bootie
    Bebax B.
Boplant
    B. graft
    B. Surgibone bovine bone
      substitute
borazone blade cutting machine
Borchardt olive-shaped bur
Bordeaux prosthesis
Bores
    B. corneal fixation forceps
    B. optic zone marker
    B. radial marker
    B. twist fixation ring
    B. U-shaped forceps
boron counter
Boros esophagoscope
Borsch
    B. bandage
    B. dressing
Borst side-arm introducer set
Bosch ERG 500 ergometer
Bosker
    B. TMI reconstruction system
    B. transmandibular implant
BOSS
    Becker orthopaedic spinal system
Boston
    B. brace system
    B. 7 contact lens
    B. elbow system
    B. Envision contact lens
    B. EO, ES contact lens
    B. II, IV contact lens
    B. overlap brace
    B. postoperative hip orthosis

    B. RXD contact lens
    B. scoliosis brace
    B. soft body jacket
    B. soft corset
    B. thoracic splint
    B. trephine
    B. XO contact lens
Bosworth
    B. coracoclavicular screw
    B. screwdriver
    B. temporary crown
    B. tongue depressor
Botox
    B. injection amplifier
    B. injection amplifier brace
bottle
    blow b. (BB)
    Castaneda b.
    disposable b.
    ENTsol refillable b.
    hot water b.
    McGaw plastic b.
    Mead Johnson b.
    Nalgene PETG media b.
    night drain b.
    Nu-Hope urine collection b.
    Nursette prefilled disposable b.
    Plasma-Plex b.
    transgrow b.
    urinary night drainage b.
    water b.
2-bottle thoracic drainage system
Bottoms-Up posture system
Botvin iris forceps
Boucheron ear speculum
Bouchut laryngeal tube
bougie
    acorn-tipped b.
    bellied b.
    b. à boule
    bulbous b.
    conic b.
    cylindrical b.
    dilating b.
    b. dilator
    ear b.
    elastic b.
    elbowed b.
    EndoLumina b.
    EndoLumina illuminated b.
    esophageal mercury-filled b.
    filiform b.
    Fort urethral b.
    Friedman-Otis b. à boule
    fusiform b.
    Gruber b.
    Hegar intrarectal b.
    Holinger infant b.
    Hurst b.

Hurst mercury-filled esophageal b.
Hurst-type b.
Jackson steel-stem woven
  filiform b.
Klebanoff common duct b.
LeFort filiform b.
Maloney b.
Maloney tapered mercury-filled
  esophageal b.
mercury b.
mercury-filled esophageal b.
mercury-weighted rubber b.
olive-tipped b.
Otis b. à boule
Plummer b.
polyvinyl b.
rosary b.
Rusch b.
Savary-Gilliard Silastic flexible b.
Savary-Gilliard wire-guided b.
spiral-tipped b.
through-the-scope b.
Tucker b.
Tucker retrograde b.
Wales rectal b.
wax b.
whip b.
wire-guided polyvinyl b.
yellow-eyed dilating b.

bougienage
transgastric esophageal b.
Bouncewell medicine ball
Bourassa catheter
Bourdon
B. gauge
B. tube
B. tube pressure gauge
Bourns
B. electronic adult respirator
B. infant respirator
B. infant ventilator
Bourns-Bear I ventilator
Boutin thoracoscope
boutonniere splint
Bovie
B. blade
B. cauterization
B. cautery
B. coagulating forceps
B. conization electrode
B. electrocautery
B. electrocautery device
B. electrocautery unit
B. 1250 electrosurgical device
B. electrosurgical unit
B. holder
B. liquid conductor
B. needle
B. retinal detachment unit

Ritter B.
underwater B.
B. unit
B. wet-field cautery
bovine
b. collagen implant
b. collagen material prosthesis
b. collagen plug device
b. heart valve
b. heterograft
b. pericardial valve
b. pericardium dural graft
b. pericardium strip
bow
Aesculap traction b.
aiming b.
B. & Arrow cannulated drill guide
Böhler extension b.
Böhler traction b.
extension b.
Framer finger extension b.
Hanau face b.
harelip traction b.
Kirschner extension b.
Kirschner wire traction b.
lip traction b.
Logan lip traction b.
Schwarz finger extension b.
traction b.
bowel
b. forceps
b. grasper
b. retractor
Bowen
B. double-bladed scalpel
B. resin
Bower PEG tube
Bowins suction
bowl
b. curette
Ganzfeld b.
Latham b.
Prism mixing b.
rubber spa b.
Bowlby arm splint
bowleg brace
Bowling lens
Bowman
B. cataract needle
B. lacrimal probe
B. needle stop
B. probe
B. stop needle
B. tube
box, pl. **boxes**
A/B switch b.
Bárány noise b.
bronchoscopic battery b.
BTE bolt b.

B

box *(continued)*
    carpal b.
    b. curette
    head b.
    Hogness b.
    mammographic view b.
    B. osteotome
    steam b.
    sterilizer b.
    Storz light b.
    SunBox light b.
    switch b.
boxing strip
box-joint forceps
boxwood mallet
Boyce needle holder
Boyd
    B. orbital implant
    B. perforator
    B. side plate
    B. surgical light
Boyden
    B. chamber
    B. chamber assay device
Boyes-Goodfellow hook
Boyle-Davis mouthgag
Boyle uterine elevator
Boynton needle holder
Boys-Allis tissue forceps
Boys-Smith laser lens
Bozeman
    B. forceps
    B. LR dressing forceps
    B. speculum
    B. uterine dressing forceps
    B. uterine forceps
    B. uterine packing forceps
Bozeman-Douglas dressing forceps
Bozeman-Fritsch catheter
Bozeman-Wertheim needle holder
BP-7350A
    bipolar cautery probe B.
BP Cuff pressure infuser
B-plus Fix
BPXG body plethysmograph
bra
    lead b.
Braasch
    B. bulb ureteral catheter
    B. direct catheterization cystoscope
Braasch-Kaplan direct-vision cystoscope
BRACAnalyzer gene analyzer
Bracco system
brace
    Abbott b.
    abdominal b.
    accommodative b.
    Ace b.
    ACL Lite functional knee b.

Active ankle b.
Active support and b.
Activity-Lite knee b.
AFO b.
Aircast Air-Stirrup leg b.
Aircast ankle b.
Aircast Cryo/Cuff b.
Aircast fracture b.
Aircast pneumatic air stirrup b.
Aircast Swivel-Strap b.
Aircast walking b.
Air DonJoy patellofemoral b.
airplane splint shoulder b.
Airprene Action knee b.
Air-Stirrup ankle training b.
Air Townsend b.
ALP Plus ankle b.
Ambi wrist b.
Ank-L-Aid b.
ankle stirrup b.
AOA cervical immobilization b.
APL Plus ankle b.
APU b.
Arizona ankle b.
Arnold lumbar b.
ASO ankle b.
Atak knee b.
athletic b.
Atlanta-Scottish Rite hip b.
Atlantic overlap b.
Atlantic rim b.
ATR b.
Axiom custom functional knee b.
Axis ankle b.
back b.
Back Seat torso-wrap b.
bail-lock b.
Bauerfeind ankle b.
Bauerfeind Comprifix knee b.
Becker b.
Bike ankle b.
BIOflex magnetic counterforce b.
Biomet fracture b.
BioSkin Q knee b.
bipivotal hinge knee b.
Bird & Cronin wrist b.
bivalved overlap b.
Bledsoe adjustable post-op b.
Bledsoe cast b.
Bledsoe fracture b.
Bledsoe knee b.
Blount b.
Blount-Schmidt-Milwaukee b.
BoarderAnkle b.
Bodyline sports b.
Body Sport ankle b.
Bollinger knee b.
boot b.
Boston overlap b.

Boston scoliosis b.
Botox injection amplifier b.
bowleg b.
Brite-Life wrist b.
cage-back b.
Caligamed b.
Camp b.
Cam Walker ankle b.
Cam Walker leg b.
Can Am b.
canvas b.
Carpal Lock CTS b.
Carpal Lock wrist b.
CASH b.
cast b.
Castaway leg b.
cast boot b.
cast boot polypropylene hip
  abduction b.
CDO b.
Centec Formfit ankle b.
Centec Propoint knee b.
cervical collar b.
chairback b.
Charleston b.
Charleston nighttime bending b.
Charleston scoliosis b.
Cheetah ankle b.
CI functional knee b.
Cinch Lock CTS b.
clamshell b.
Clinch Lock CTS wrist b.
CM-Band 505N b.
CM-Band silicone rubber b.
collar b.
Collum CMC thumb b.
Combined Instabilities functional
  knee b.
contraflexion b.
controlled position b.
Cook walking b.
cool CPB b.
Cooper ankle b.
Cotrel-Dubousset orthopaedic b.
Counter Rotation System b.
Count'R-Force arch b.
CRM rehab b.
CRS b.
Cruiser hip abduction b.
Cruiser OA b.
CTEV b.
CTi b.
C.Ti.2 knee b.
CTi2 knee b.
custom-fitted b.
cutout patellar b.
Dalco Astro ankle b.
Darco back b.
DarcoGel ankle b.

Defiance functional knee b.
Dennison cervical b.
DePuy fracture b.
derotation b.
3D fracture walker b.
DonJoy b.
DonJoy ALP b.
DonJoy Drytex Wraparound
  Playmaker knee b.
DonJoy Female Fource custom
  knee b.
DonJoy Female Fource OTS
  knee b.
DonJoy GoldPoint knee b.
DonJoy Legend ACL knee b.
DonJoy Opal knee b.
DonJoy 4-point Super Sport
  knee b.
DonJoy Quadrant shoulder b.
DonJoy Universal ankle b.
double Becker ankle b.
doughnut support b.
b. drill
dropfoot b.
Drytex RocketSoc ankle b.
Drytex Wraparound Playmaker
  knee b.
dual-lock ankle b.
Dura-Flex back b.
dynamic hinge elbow fracture b.
Easy Lok ankle b.
Easy-On elbow b.
Eclipse Gel ankle b.
economy ROM b.
EconoSoc ankle b.
Edge knee b.
elastic-hinge knee b.
elastic knee sleeve b.
Elite knee b.
English b.
Exotec b.
Extreme Select ligament b.
EZ ROM postoperative knee b.
felt b.
Female Fource custom knee b.
Female Fource OTS knee b.
figure-of-8 b.
Fisher b.
Flagg fiberglass knee b.
Flex Foam b.
flexor hinge hand splint b.
FlexTech knee b.
Floam ankle stirrup b.
Florida back b.
Florida cervical b.
Florida contraflexion b.
Florida extension b.
Florida hyperextension b.
Florida J-24, J-35, J-45, J-55 b.

brace *(continued)*
  Florida postfusion b.
  Florida spinal b.
  foot-ankle b.
  footdrop b.
  Frazer wrist b.
  Friedman splint b.
  functional electronic peroneal b.
  functional fracture b.
  furniture b.
  Futuro wrist b.
  gaiter b.
  gait lock splint b.
  Galveston metacarpal b.
  Generation II 3DX b.
  Generation II knee b.
  Generation II Unloader ADJ
    knee b.
  Generation II Unloader Select
    knee b.
  Genutrain knee b.
  GII Unloader ADJ knee b.
  GII Unloader OA b.
  Gillette b.
  GLS b.
  GoldPoint ACL functional knee b.
  GoldPoint hinged knee b.
  GoldPoint PCL functional knee b.
  Goldthwait b.
  Guilford cervical b.
  halo b.
  hand b.
  H buttress support
    patellofemoral b.
  head b.
  high-tide walking b.
  hinged knee b.
  Hi-Top foot/ankle b.
  horseshoe patellofemoral b.
  Hudson b.
  Hudson TLSO b.
  hyperextension b.
  Ilfeld b.
  InCare b.
  Industrial Work b.
  Inner Lok ankle b.
  internal tibial torsion b.
  Intrepid functional knee b.
  I-Plus System humeral fracture b.
  I-Plus System ulnar fracture b.
  ischial weightbearing b.
  IsoDyn knee b.
  Jace knee b.
  Jewett-Benjamin cervical b.
  Jewett contraflexion b.
  Jewett hyperextension b.
  Jewett postfusion b.
  J-59 Florida b.
  Jones b.

  Joseph nasal b.
  J-55 postfusion b.
  Juzo b.
  Juzo Patellaligner b.
  Kallassy b.
  Key wrist b.
  Kicker Pavlik harness hip
    abduction b.
  King cervical b.
  Klenzak b.
  knee cage b.
  knee MD b.
  KneeRanger hinged knee b.
  Knight b.
  Knight-Taylor b.
  KS 5 ACL b.
  KSO b.
  Kuhlman cervical b.
  Küntscher-Hudson b.
  Kydex b.
  kyphosis b.
  lace-on b.
  lace-up RocketSoc ankle b.
  leaf-spring b.
  left long leg b.
  leg b.
  Legend ACL functional knee b.
  Legend PCL functional knee b.
  Lerman hinge b.
  Liberty CMC thumb b.
  ligamentous control b.
  limb b.
  long double upright b.
  long leg b.
  Lorenz b.
  Lovitt-Uhler modification of Jewett
    postfusion b.
  low-tide walking b.
  LSU reciprocation-gait orthosis b.
  lumbosacral b.
  Lyman-Smith toe drop b.
  Magnetic Support b.
  M-Brace knee b.
  McClintoch b.
  McCollough internal tibial
    torsion b.
  McDavid knee b.
  McKee b.
  MCL b.
  MC walker b.
  Medical Design b.
  Medipedic Multicentric knee b.
  Miami fracture b.
  Miami TLSO scoliosis b.
  Milwaukee b.
  Milwaukee scoliosis b.
  Minerva cervical b.
  MKS II knee b.
  Monarch knee b.

Moon Boot b.
MTA b.
Mueller ATF ankle b.
Mueller hinged knee b.
Mueller Lite ankle b.
Mueller orthopaedic shoulder b.
Mueller Ultralite b.
Mueller wrap-around knee b.
Multi-Lig knee b.
Multi-Lock knee b.
Nakamura b.
neck b.
neoprene hinged knee b.
neoprene Osgood-Schlatter knee b.
neoprene wrist b.
Nevin ankle b.
New England scoliosis b.
Newport MC hip orthosis b.
Nextep knee b.
nonweightbearing b.
no-stretch RocketSoc b.
OAdjuster knee b.
OA knee b.
OAsys knee b.
offloading knee b.
Omni knee b.
Orthotech Controller knee b.
Ortho Tech performer knee b.
OS-5/Plus 2 knee b.
osteoarthritic knee b.
osteoarthritis padded night
  sleeve b.
out-of-cast ankle b.
outside-the-boot b.
oyster-shell b.
Pacesetter knee b.
Palumbo knee b.
Palumbo stabilizing b.
Palumbo stabilizing knee b.
pantaloon b.
parachutist ankle b.
Patellaligner knee b.
patellar stabilizing b.
patellofemoral b.
pediatric PRAFO b.
pelvic b.
Performer Ultralight knee b.
PFT traction b.
Phelps b.
piano-wire dorsiflexion b.
Playmaker functional knee b.
Playmaker knee b.
PlayTuf knee b.
PMT halo system b.
PneuGel ankle b.
Pneu Knee b.
Pneu-trac neck b.
4-point cervical b.
4-point IROM b.

6-point knee b.
4-point SuperSport functional
  knee b.
Polaris knee rehab b.
2-poster b.
postoperative flexor tendon
  traction b.
Pro-8 ankle b.
Procase Ankle-Lock b.
Proline Stomatex shoulder b.
PTB b.
Push medical b.
Quadrant advanced shoulder b.
QualCare knee b.
Raney flexion jacket b.
range-of-motion b.
ratchet-type b.
Rehab TROM b.
Rhino Triangle b.
Rhino Triangle polypropylene hip
  abduction b.
Richie b.
rigid postoperative b.
Risser b.
Ritchie b.
RocketSoc ankle b.
Rolyan D-ring wrist b.
Rolyan TakeOff Sprint b.
ROM knee b.
ROM walker b.
Sarmiento b.
SAS II b.
Sawa shoulder b.
SCOI shoulder b.
scoliosis overlap b.
Scottish Rite b.
Selectively Lockable knee b.
short leg caliper b.
shoulder subluxation inhibitor b.
SmartBrace b.
SmartWrap elbow b.
snap-lock b.
SofTec rigid b.
SOMI b.
SOMI Jr. b.
Speed b.
Spinal Technology bivalve
  TLSO b.
SpineCor nonrigid b.
Sports-Caster I, II knee b.
SSI b.
Stardox wrist b.
Stealth knee b.
sternooccipital-mandibular
  immobilization b.
Stimprene electrotherapy b.
stirrup b.
stop action b.
straight walker b.

brace *(continued)*
    Strap Lok ankle b.
    Stromgren ankle b.
    Stubbs 4-way clavicle b.
    Sully shoulder stabilizer b.
    Sure Step ankle b.
    Swede-O Ankle Lok b.
    Swede-O Universal b.
    Swivel-Strap ankle b.
    System-Loc back b.
    Taylor-Knight b.
    Taylor spine b.
    telescoping b.
    Teurlings wrist b.
    The Richie b.
    Thermoskin b.
    Thomas cervical collar b.
    Thomas walking b.
    thoracolumbar standing orthosis b.
    toedrop b.
    total anatomical hinge knee b.
    Townsend knee b.
    Townsend Rebel convertible b.
    Tracker knee b.
    Tri-Angle shoulder abduction b.
    TROM knee b.
    Tru-Fit b.
    turnbuckle ankle b.
    turnbuckle knee b.
    UCLA functional long leg b.
    Ultrabrace b.
    unilateral calcaneal b.
    Unloader ADJ unloader b.
    Unloader Bi-ComPF knee b.
    Unloader Express unloader b.
    Unloader Select unloader b.
    Unloader Spirit knee b.
    Value Walker b.
    Verlow b.
    walking b.
    Warm Springs b.
    weightbearing b.
    Wheaton Pavlik harness b.
    Wilke boot b.
    Williams back b.
    Wilmington scoliosis b.
    Wrist Restore b.
    Yale b.
    Zinco Air Cam b.
    Zinco Airprene b.
    Zinco Cam Walker b.
    Zinco Castaway D b.
    Zinco Hi-Top b.
    Zinco Minerva cervical b.
    Zinco Multi-Lig knee b.
    Zinco Pin Cam Walker b.
brace/corset
    Hoke lumbar b./c.

bracelet
    BioBands b.
    MedicAlert b.
    Nussbaum b.
    Q-Ray b.
    ^{89}Sr b.
brachial coronary catheter
BrachySeed
    B. brachytherapy seed
    B. palladium-103 seed
    B. Pd-103 implant
brachytherapy balloon applicator
BrachyVision brachytherapy planning system
Bracken
    B. fixation forceps
    B. iris forceps
    B. irrigating cannula
bracket
    Begg straight-wire combination b.
    Broussard b.
    curved-base Lewis b.
    Cusp-Lok b.
    Hanson speed b.
    Lee b.
    Lewis b.
    Lewis vertical slot b.
    ligatureless b.
    metal frame reinforced plastic b.
    molar b.
    orthodontic b.
    plastic b.
    Siamese twin b.
    single width b.
    steel-slotted plastic b.
    Steiner b.
    b. table
    torqued slot b.
    twin edgewise b.
bracketed splint
Brackett dental probe
Brackmann
    B. II EMG system
    B. suction irrigator
Braden flushing reservoir
Bradley femoral canal preparation scraper
Bradshaw-O'Neill aorta clamp
Brady balanced suspension splint
Bragg-Paul respirator
braid
    carbon fiber lamination b.
braided
    b. diagnostic catheter
    b. Ethibond suture
    b. Mersilene suture
    b. Nurolon suture
    b. nylon suture
    b. occlusion device

b. polyamide suture
b. polyester fiber
b. polyester suture
b. polyglactin suture
b. silk suture
b. titanium cable
b. Vicryl suture
b. wire
b. wire suture

brain
b. biopsy cannula
b. biopsy needle
b. clip
b. clip carrier
b. clip forceps
b. depressor
b. dressing forceps
b. exploring cannula
b. probe
b. retractor
b. scissors
b. spatula
b. spatula forceps
b. tissue forceps
b. trocar
b. tumor forceps

BrainLAB VectorVision neuronavigation system
BrainSCAN computer planning system
Braithwaite skin graft knife
brake lever extension
Bralon braided nylon suture
branch
septal perforator b.
Brand
B. tendon-holding forceps
B. tendon-passing forceps
Brandel cell harvester
Brandt cytology balloon
Brandy
B. scalp stretcher
B. scalp stretcher II, front closure
B. scalp stretcher I, rear closure
Brånemark
B. endosteal implant
B. implant system
B. osseointegration implant
Brannock
B. Device shoe sizer
B. foot measuring device
Brantigan interbody fusion cage
Bra Pocket pump holder
BRAS
Bard rotary atherectomy system
brass
b. scleral plug
b. wire
Brasseler Optipost

Braun
B. cranioclast
B. episiotomy scissors
B. frame
B. obstetrical hook
B. stent
B. tympanic thermometer
B. uterine depressor
Braun-Schroeder single-tooth tenaculum
Braun-Stadler episiotomy scissors
Braunstein fixed calipers
Braunwald-Cutter
B.-C. ball valve prosthesis
B.-C. valve
Braunwald heart valve
Braun-Wangensteen graft
Bravo Catheter-Free pH testing system
Brawner orbital implant
breakable blade
breakaway
b. lap cushion
b. pin
BreakAway absorptive wound dressing
breaker
Böhler plaster cast b.
cast b.
Castroviejo blade b.
Troutman-Barraquer miniblade b.
Wölfe-Böhler cast b.
Breakstone lithotriptor
Breas
B. PV10 CPAP device
B. ventilator
breast
b. binder
B. Biopsy Guard
b. bolster
B. Cancer System 2100
b. cone
b. implant
b. implant protector
b. localization needle
b. plate
b. prosthesis
b. sizer
b. tenaculum
B. Vest
B. Vest Exi-Dry 1-piece wound dressing
BreastAlert
B. differential temperature sensor
B. DTS screening device
BreastCheck
BreastExam
breast-mound form
BreastScan IR system
breath
b. bag
B. Tracker

B

Breathe
 B. Easy foam pad
 B. Right nasal strip
 B. Right nasal strips
 B. with EEZ nasal dilator
Breathe-Easy nasal splint
Breather
 The Sports B.
breathing
 b. bag
 b. pacemaker
breath-operated inhaler
BreathTek UBT *H. pylori* test
Brecht feeder
Bredall amalgam plugger
breeder reactor
Breeze
 B. E150 ventilation system
 B. respirator
Breg pain care infusion pump
Breisky-Navratil straight retractor
Breisky vaginal retractor
Bremer
 B. AirFlo halo vest
 B. AirFlo vest
 B. halo
 B. halo cervical traction
 B. halo crown
 B. halo crown cervical collar
 B. halo crown system
 B. halo crown traction
 B. halo crown traction set
 B. halo system
Brems astigmatism marker
Brener carotid shunt
Brennen biosynthetic surgical mesh
Brent pressure earring
brephoplastic graft
Brescia-Cimino shunt
Brevi-Kath epidural catheter
Brevio nerve conduction monitor
Brewer vaginal speculum
Brewster phrenic retractor
bridge
 Albarran reflecting b.
 B. Assurant biliary stent delivery
  system
 balance b.
 ceramometal implant b.
 B. deep surgery forceps
 double b.
 B. extra-support over-the-wire renal
  stent system
 B. hemostatic forceps
 B. Hip system
 1-horn b.
 Maryland b.
 muscle b.

 pediatric b.
 retention suture b.
 Rochette b.
 Short b.
 b. splint
 Trestle prostatic b.
 3-unit anterior b.
 3-way b.
 B. X3 renal stent system
bridged loop-gap resonator
bridging plate
bridle
 control b.
 b. suture
brief
 Attends brief with Perma Dry
  Wings contoured incontinence b.
 ConQuest male continence system
  supporter b.
 First Quality full-fit b.
 Harmonie Classic Plus b.
 Kim Care contour b.
 Kins all-in-1 cotton b.
 MaxiCare adult disposable
  contoured b.
 PrimeTime Plus adult disposable b.
 Promise b.
 Protection Plus b.
 SlimLine disposable b.
 Soft & Silent vinyl pull-on b.
 Soft & Silent vinyl snap-on b.
 Ultra-Fit b.
Brierley
 B. capsulorrhexis cannula
 B. chamber maintainer
 B. nucleus splitter
Briggs T adapter
Brigham thumb tissue forceps
Brightbill corneal cutting block
Brighton epistaxis balloon
Brilliance 109 MP PC monitor
Brimms Quik-Fix denture repair kit
Brinkerhoff
 B. anoscope
 B. rectal speculum
Brinker tissue retractor
Brink PeriPyriform implant
**Brisman-Nova carotid endarterectomy
 shunt**
Bristol disc prosthesis
Bristol-Myers system
Bristow rasp
Brite
 B. Lite III light
 B. Tip catheter
 B. Tip guide catheter
 B. Tip guiding catheter
Brite-Life wrist brace

BriteSmile
    B. laser tooth-whitening system
    B. teeth-whitening laser device
Britt
    B. argon/krypton laser
    B. argon pulsed laser
    B. BL-12 laser
    B. krypton laser
BRK series transseptal needle
broach
    barbed b.
    Charnley femoral b.
    chipped-tooth b.
    endodontic b.
    b. extractor
    femoral b.
    glenoid fin b.
    intramedullary b.
    Koenig metatarsal b.
    metacarpal b.
    metatarsal stem b.
    orthopaedic b.
    phalangeal b.
    root canal b.
    square-hole b.
    starter b.
    Swanson metatarsal b.
    tibial b.
broad AO dynamic compression plate
broad-based
    b.-b. cane
    b.-b. cane board
broad-toed shoe
Broca diagonal band
Brockenbrough curved needle
Brodie knee
broken razor blade
Brombach perimeter
Brompton Hospital retractor
bronchial
    b. catheter
    b. dilator
    b. tube
bronchial-grasping forceps
Bronchitrac L flexible suction catheter
bronchoalveolar lavage
Broncho-Cath double-lumen endotracheal tube
bronchocele sound
bronchodilator
    aerosolized b.
    anticholinergic b.
    Inhal-Aid b.
    Marax b.
    Maxi-Myst b.
bronchofiberscope
    Pentax b.
Broncho pulmonary disposable biopsy forceps

bronchopulmonary lavage
bronchoscope
    BF large core b.
    double-channel irrigating b.
    Dumon b.
    Dumon-Harrell b.
    Dumon laser b.
    fiberoptic b.
    flexible fiberoptic b.
    Foregger b.
    foroblique b.
    Fujinon EB-410S b.
    Fujinon flexible b.
    Haslinger b.
    Holinger b.
    Holinger infant b.
    Holinger ventilating fiberoptic b.
    hook-on b.
    infant b.
    Jackson standard b.
    Jackson staple b.
    Kernan-Jackson b.
    Michelson b.
    Moersch b.
    Negus b.
    Olympus fiberoptic b.
    open-tube rigid b.
    Pentax b.
    Pilling b.
    respiration b.
    Safar b.
    Savary b.
    single-channel fiberoptic b.
    Storz b.
    Storz infant b.
    ventilation b.
    white-light b.
    Yankauer b.
bronchoscopic
    b. battery box
    b. brush
    b. face shield
    b. spectacles
    b. sponge
    b. sponge carrier
    b. telescope
bronchoscopy disposable suction tube
bronchospirometer
bronchospirometric catheter
bronchus-grasping forceps
Bronkhorst High Tec controller
Bronkometer
Brookdale bar
Brooke Army Hospital splint
Brooker
    B. double-locking unreamed tibial nail
    B. wire
Brooker-Wills nail

Brookfield viscometer
Brooks shoe
broomstick cast
Brophy
    B. dressing forceps
    B. scissors
    B. tenaculum retractor
    B. tissue forceps
Broselow
    B. chart
    B. emergency tape
    B. pediatric resuscitative tape
    B. tape
Broselow-Hinkle pediatric emergency
  system
Broselow-Luten pediatric system
Broussard bracket
Broviac
    B. atrial catheter
    B. catheter
    B. hyperalimentation catheter
    B. long-term catheter
brow
    b. lift suspension screw
    b. tape
Browlift bone bridge system
Brown
    B. air dermatome
    B. applicator
    B. dermatome blade
    B. electric dermatome
    B. insertion forceps
    B. interchangeable lid speculum
    B. limbal relaxing incision guide
    B. periosteotome
    B. pocket starter
    B. rasp
    B. side-grasping forceps
    B. sphenoid cannula
    B. sterile adhesive
    B. tissue forceps
    B. uvula retractor
Brown-Adson
    B.-A. forceps
    B.-A. side-grasping forceps
    B.-A. tissue forceps
Brown-Bovari machine
Brown-Buerger
    B.-B. cystoscope
    B.-B. forceps
Brown-Cushing forceps
Brown-Davis mouthgag
Brown-Dean cotton applicator
Browne splint
Brown-Grabow capsulorrhexis cystotome
  forceps
Brown-McHardy pneumatic dilator
Brown-Mueller
    B.-M. T-bar fastener

    B.-M. T-fastener
    B.-M. T-fastener set
Brown-Roberts-Wells (BRW)
    B.-R.-W. apparatus
    B.-R.-W. arc-ring assembly
    B.-R.-W. base ring
    B.-R.-W. CT stereotactic guide
    B.-R.-W. floor stand
    B.-R.-W. frame
    B.-R.-W. head frame
    B.-R.-W. stereotactic frame
    B.-R.-W. stereotactic system
Brown-Sharp gauge suture
Broyle
    B. esophagoscope
    B. retrograde cystoscope
Brüel
    B. & Kjaer axial transducer
    B. & Kjaer transvaginal ultrasound
      probe
    B. & Kjaer ultrasound
    B. & Kjaer 1860 ultrasound
      machine
    B. & Kjaer ultrasound scanner
Bruening
    B. chisel
    B. ear snare
    B. esophagoscope
    B. esophagoscopy forceps handle
    B. forceps
    B. nasal snare
    B. otoscope set
    B. pneumatic otoscope
    B. septal forceps
    B. tongue depressor
    B. tonsillar snare
Bruker
    B. AMX 300 NMR spectrometer
    B. Biospec system
    B. console
    B. CSI Omega MR system
    B. minispec measuring device
    B. PC-10 relaxometer
    B. relaxometer
    B. scanner
    B. S 200 MR system
    B. TC-10 relaxometer
Brun
    B. bone curette
    B. mastoid curette
Brunetti chisel
Brunner
    B. intestinal forceps
    B. ligature set
    B. rib shears
    B. tissue forceps
Brunton otoscope
brush
    AccuBrush dental b.

Air-Lon tracheal tube b.
Alger b.
Barraquer sable b.
Bayne Pap b.
b. biopsy kit
bronchoscopic b.
bur b.
Castaneda thrombolytic b.
Cohort bone b.
Combo Cath wire-guided
  cytology b.
contour instrument cleaning b.
Cragg-Castaneda thrombolytic b.
Cragg thrombolytic b.
Cytobrush S b.
cytological b.
cytology b.
Cytolong b.
denture b.
Edwards-Carpentier aortic valve b.
endometrial b.
Endovations disposable cytology b.
flexible retinal b.
FoamCare double scrub b.
Gill biopsy b.
Glassman b.
Haidinger b.
Hobbs sheath b.
intramedullary b.
manual dermatome b.
mechanical epithelial b.
Mill-Rose cytology b.
nylon scrub b.
ophthalmic sable b.
Oral-B soft foam interdental b.
OTW thrombolytic b.
Plak-Vac oral suction b.
polishing b.
polypropylene hand b.
protected specimen b.
rectal snare stem b.
rotating b.
rotating wire b.
sable b.
scraping b.
scrub b.
soft scrub b.
stomach b.
Stormby b.
Suction oral b.
Thomas b.
tracheal tube b.
Wilson-Cook cytology b.

BRVO knife
BRW
  Brown-Roberts-Wells
  BRW CT stereotaxic guide
  BRW head ring halo
  BRW stereotactic system

Bryan
  B. cervical disc prosthesis
  B. cervical disc system
Bryant traction
Brymill
  B. CryAc cryosurgical unit
  B. cryosurgical probe
  B. 30 cryosurgical unit
B-scan
  contact B-s.
  Humphrey B-s.
  B-s. ultrasonogram
BSD-300 device
B&S gauge suture
BSM
  bone substitute material
BST-CarGel
BTA S-2000 biofeedback system
BTE
  behind-the-ear
  BTE assembly tree
  BTE bolt box
  BTE dynamic lift
  BTE listening device
  BTE work simulator
BTF-37 arterial blood filter
bubble
  gastric b.
  Guibor Expo eye b.
  b. humidifier
  b. oxygenator
Bubble-Jet
  Puritan B.-J.
buccal
  b. cortical plate
  b. fat extractor
  b. fat extractor tip
  b. retractor
Buchbinder Thruflex Over-the-Wire
  catheter
Buchwald tongue depressor
Buchwalter retractor
Buck
  B. bone curette
  B. convoluted traction apparatus
  B. convoluted traction device
  B. ear curette
  B. ear probe
  B. earring curette
  B. extension
  B. extension apparatus
  B. femoral cement restrictor
    inserter
  B. myringotomy knife
  B. neurological hammer
  B. percussion hammer
  B. periosteal elevator
  B. plug
  B. Redi-Traction apparatus

Buck *(continued)*
    B. traction
    B. traction stockinette
    B. wax curette
bucket
    kick b.
    Lenox b.
Buck-Gramcko
    B.-G. bone lever
    B.-G. gouge
buckle
    Miragel episcleral b.
    scleral b.
    segmental b.
    wire-fixation b.
Buckley chisel
Bucky
    B. diaphragm
    B. digital x-ray device
    B. film
    B. grid
    oscillating B.
    upright B.
Bucy-Frazier suction cannula
Bud
    B. bur
    B. drainage catheter
Budde
    B. halo neurosurgical retractor
    B. halo retractor system
    B. halo ring
    B. halo ring retractor
buddy
    bolster b.
    ostomy Shadow B.
    b. splint
    b. strap
    Wheelchair B.
BuddyWrap
    FoamWrap B.
Budin
    B. hammertoe splint
    B. toe splint
Buechel-Pappas
    B.-P. integrated hip replacement
      system
    B.-P. total ankle
    B.-P. total ankle prosthesis
    B.-P. total ankle replacement
      system
Buedding squeegee cortex extractor and
    polisher
Buehler Isomet low-speed saw
buffing sponge
Bugbee
    B. electrocautery
    B. electrode
    B. fulgurating electrode

buggy
    cruiser b.
    Maclaren mobile b.
Buhl spirometer
Buie
    B. biopsy forceps
    B. fistula probe
    B. fulguration electrode
    B. pile clamp
    B. rectal injection cannula
    B. rectal suction tube
    B. sigmoidoscope
Buie-Hirschman anoscope
Builder Grip hand exerciser
build-up implant
Bülau trocar
bulb
    b. dynamometer
    phototherapy b.
    self-inflating b.
    b. syringe
    b. and thumb screw valve
    b. ureteral catheter
bulbous bougie
bulbous-tip
    b.-t. ear syringe
    b.-t. stiff malleable cannula
Bulkee II gauze bandage
bulky
    b. compressive dressing
    b. dressing
    b. hand dressing
    b. pressure dressing
Bullard intubating laryngoscope
bulldog
    b. clamp
    b. clamp-applying forceps
    b. scissors
    vascular b.
Buller
    B. bandage
    B. eye shield
bullet
    b. forceps
    b. probe
bullet-shaped cannula
bullet-tip
    b.-t. catheter
    b.-t. dilator
Bullseye femoral guide
Bumm uterine curette
Bumpa Bed crib bumper pad
bumper
    Cloverleaf internal b.
    dome-shaped internal b.
    PEG b.
    b. wedge
Bunge evisceration spoon

bunion
>	b. dissector
>	b. shield

Bunker implant

Bunnell
>	B. active hand and finger splint
>	B. anvil
>	B. digital exertion measurer
>	B. dissecting probe
>	B. dressing
>	B. finger extension splint
>	B. finger loop
>	B. forwarding probe
>	B. knuckle bender
>	B. reverse knuckle-bender splint
>	B. safety-pin splint
>	B. suture
>	B. tendon needle
>	B. tendon passer
>	B. tendon stripper
>	B. wire pull-out suture

Bunny
>	B. Boot
>	B. Boot foot splint

Bunsen burner

Bunt forceps holder

Bunyan bag

bur, burr
>	acromionizer b.
>	Adson enlarging b.
>	Adson perforating b.
>	aftercataract b.
>	air-driven b.
>	Albee olive-shaped b.
>	Allport cutting b.
>	arthroplasty b.
>	Ballenger-Lillie mastoid b.
>	barrel b.
>	bone b.
>	Borchardt olive-shaped b.
>	b. brush
>	Bud b.
>	carbide finishing b.
>	coarse carbide cone b.
>	coarse-olive b.
>	cone b.
>	conical b.
>	corneal foreign body b.
>	countersink b.
>	cranial b.
>	cross-cut straight fissure b.
>	curetting b.
>	cutting b.
>	cylinder b.
>	cylindrical b.
>	decortication b.
>	dental b.
>	dentate b.
>	denture vulcanite b.

dermabrasion b.
D'Errico enlarging drill b.
D'Errico perforating drill b.
diamond b.
3-in-1 diamond b.
diamond barrel b.
diamond-coated b.
diamond-dusted b.
diamond finishing b.
Doyen cylindrical b.
Doyen spherical b.
b. drill
Dyonics arthroplasty b.
EF Cutter Ergo Toothing b.
end-cutting fissure b.
endodontic b.
enlarging b.
excavating b.
Fantastic Burr nail b.
Feldman b.
fenestration b.
Ferris-Smith-Halle sinus b.
FG diamond b.
fine olive b.
finish b.
finishing b.
Fisch cutting b.
fissure b.
flame b.
flame-tip b.
fluted finishing b.
foreign body b.
Frey-Freer b.
Gates-Glidden b.
gold b.
guarded b.
Hall bone b.
handpiece round b.
Happy podiatric b.
high-speed diamond 3-tiered depth
	cutting b.
high-speed diamond wheel b.
high-speed 2-grit b.
high-speed tungsten carbide b.
high-torque b.
Hudson b.
Hudson bone b.
Hudson brace b.
Hudson conical b.
Hudson cranial b.
Hu-Friedy dental b.
inverted cone b.
Jordan-Day cutting b.
Jordan-Day fenestration b.
Jordan-Day polishing b.
Jordan perforating b.
lacrimal sac b.
large nail spicule b.
Le Blond R diamond dental b.

bur *(continued)*
    Lee diamond b.
    Lempert diamond-dust polishing b.
    Lempert fenestration b.
    Lindemann b.
    long coarse b.
    low-speed Christmas tree diamond b.
    low-speed tapered carbide b.
    Martin b.
    Masseran trepan b.
    mastoid b.
    McKenzie enlarging b.
    medium carbide cone b.
    medium fine b.
    Micro-Aire b.
    motorized b.
    Mueller b.
    neurosurgical b.
    olive-shaped b.
    orthopaedic b.
    Osteon b.
    Oto-Flex carbide b.
    Oto-Flex diamond b.
    oval b.
    oval cutting b.
    Parapost b.
    paronychia b.
    pear b.
    pear-shaped b.
    perforating b.
    pilot b.
    pineapple contouring b.
    plug-finishing b.
    podiatric b.
    Podi-Burr nail b.
    pointed cone b.
    polishing b.
    rhinoplasty diamond b.
    right ankle b.
    rosehead b.
    Rosen b.
    Rotablator rotating b.
    round b.
    round cutting b.
    round diamond b.
    Shannon b.
    short coarse b.
    short fine b.
    side-cutting b.
    side-cutting Swanson b.
    sinus b.
    skull b.
    slotting b.
    small nail spicule b.
    sphenoidal b.
    spherical b.
    spiral fluted tungsten carbide b.
    S.S. White J-Notch surgical handpiece b.
    S.S. White 100 K surgical handpiece b.
    Starlite Omni-AT b.
    Stille b.
    Storz corneal b.
    straight fissure b.
    straight shank b.
    Stryker b.
    SuperCut diamond b.
    surgical b.
    tapered fissure b.
    tungsten carbide b.
    ultrasonic oscillating b.
    vulcanite b.
    water-cooled power b.
    wheel b.
    wire-passing b.
    Wittmann patch artificial b.
    Zimmer b.

Buratto
    B. contact lens spoon and spatula
    B. flap forceps
    B. flap protector
    B. forceps
    B. III acrylic implantation forceps
    B. irrigating cannula
    B. LASIK forceps
    B. LASIK irrigating cannula
    B. ophthalmic forceps

Burbank carotid shunt

Burch
    B. calipers
    B. fixation pick
    B. pick

Burch-Greenwood tendon tucker
Burch-Schneider antiprotrusio cage
Burdick ECG machine
Burette multiple patient delivery system
Burford-Finochietto
    B.-F. rib retractor
    B.-F. rib spreader
Burford rib spreader
Burhenne steerable catheter
burhole button
Burian-Allen
    B.-A. bipolar contact lens electrode
    B.-A. contact lens
    B.-A. contact lens electrode
Burkard
    B. sampling device
    B. spore trap
Burke bariatric treatment system powered bariatric bed
Burker Avance spectrometer
Bürker chamber

B

burner
  Bunsen b.
  Fischer b.
Burnett
  B. applicator
  B. BiDirectional TMJ device
  B. cylinder
  B. power tip
burnisher
  agate b.
  amalgam b.
  ball b.
  beavertail b.
  fishtail b.
  fissure b.
  flat b.
  gold b.
  straight b.
Burns Unifile
burr (*var. of* bur)
Burron Discofix stopcock
burst
  b. pacemaker
  b. resistance fitness ball
Burton
  B. BAR-7 autorefractor
  B. osteotome
Busch umbilical cord scissors
Buselmeier shunt
Busenkell posterior hip retractor
Bush
  B. DL ureteral illuminating catheter
  B. DL ureteral illuminating catheter set
  B. SL ureteral illuminating catheter
  B. SL ureteral illuminating catheter set
bushing
  patellar planer b.
  Uniflex drill b.
buster
  Amplatz Clot B.
  Moss Suction B.
Butterfield cystoscope
butterfly
  b. bandage
  b. catheter
  B. cushion
  B. cushion with strap
  b. drain
  b. dressing
  b. heart valve
  b. intravenous tube drain
  b. needle
  b. needle infusion port
Butterworth bidirectional 4-pole high-pass digital filter
button
  anastomotic b.

Bard b.
Barton-Mayo tracheostoma b.
b. battery
Bentle b.
Biomet b.
burhole b.
Charnley suture b.
coronary artery b.
Davy surgical b.
b. electrode
Endo b.
feeding b.
fixation b.
gastrostomy b.
Graether collar b.
Groningen b.
Helsper laryngectomy b.
b. hook
b. infuser
Jaboulay b.
Kazanjian tooth b.
Kistner tracheal b.
Lee lingual b.
ligament b.
b. lip lens manipulator
Microvasive One-Step b.
Moore tracheostomy b.
Murphy b.
nasal septal perforation b.
One-Step gastric b.
B. One-Step gastrostomy device
Panje voice b.
patellar b.
periosteal b.
peritoneal b.
polyethylene b.
polyethylene collar b.
polypropylene b.
pull-out b.
Sheehy collar b.
silastic b.
silastic septal b.
silicone b.
B. Spacer
Spitzy b.
stoma b.
subdural b.
Surgitek b.
suture b.
Teflon collar b.
Todd bur hole b.
tracheal b.
tracheostomy b.
voice b.
Wisconsin b.
buttoned device
button-end knife
buttonhook
button-tip manipulator

button-type G tube
buttress
>b. and button anchor
>b. graft
>mechanical b.
>b. pad
>b. pin
>b. plate
>pretibial b.
>rotator cuff b.
>Teflon pledget suture b.
>B. thread screw

buttressed hook
buttress-type plate
butyl cyanoacrylate glue
Buxton uterine clamp
Buyes air-vent suction tube
Buzard-Thornton fixation ring
BV2 needle
BVA-100 blood volume analyzer
BVI2500
>BladderScan B.

BVM
>BVM device
>BVM resuscitator

B-V-M
>bag-valve-mask
BVS-5000 biventricular support system
BVS pump
BWM spine system
Bx
>Bx Isostent
>Bx Sonic over-the-wire stent
>Bx Velocity coronary artery stent
>Bx Velocity stent
>Bx Velocity stent with Raptor OTW delivery system
>Bx Velocity with Hepacoat on Raptor stent system

bypass
>b. machine
>b. Speedy balloon catheter
Byrd EndoPlastic retractor
Byrel SX pacemaker
Byron infiltrator

C

C clamp
C knife
C oxygen cylinder
C Stance ankle

C-2

C-2 hip system
C-2 OsteoCap hip prosthesis

C-150 LXP EBT scanner

CA

C. cellulose acetate membrane hollow-fiber dialyzer
C. monitor

CA110 dialyzer
CA-5000 drill-guide isometer
CA-6000 spine motion analyzer
CAAS QCA system

cabin

magnetic shielded c.

cabinet

grid c.
Waldmann UV5000 c.

cable

alligator pacing c.
antirotation c.
bipolar c.
braided titanium c.
chrome-cobalt c.
coaxial c.
Dall-Miles c.
ESI Lite-Pipe fiberoptic c.
European/German bipolar c.
fiberoptic light c.
FlexStrand c.
Gallie fusion-using c.
c. graft
Howmedica cerclage c.
internal fiberoptic c.
interspinous c.
OxyLead interconnect c.
SecureStrand c.
Sof'Wire c.
Songer c.
c. tie
titanium c.

Cable-Ready cable grip system
cable-twister orthosis

Cabot

C. cannula
C. Medical Corporation diagnostic laparoscope
C. Medical Corporation operating laparoscope
C. Medical Corporation videoscope
C. trocar

CAD

computer-aided detection
RapidScreen digital CAD
RapidScreen RS-2000 CAD

cadaveric knee
caddie (*var. of* caddy)
CADD-Plus

CADD-P. external volumetric programmable pump
CADD-P. intravenous infusion pump

CADD-Prizm pain control system
CADD-TPN

CADD-TPN ambulatory infusion system
CADD-TPN pump

caddy, caddie

SwingAlong walker c.
tip cleaner c.

Cadence tiered therapy defibrillator system
Cadet

C. high-voltage can implantable cardioverter-defibrillator
C. V-115 implantable cardioverter-defibrillator

cadmium iodide detector
Cadwell 5200A somatosensory evoked potential unit device
CADx SecondLook system
Caffinière prosthesis

cage

antiprotrusio c.
BAK c.
BAK fusion c.
Brantigan interbody fusion c.
Burch-Schneider antiprotrusio c.
carbon fiber-composite c.
carbon fiber-reinforced c.
c. catheter device
DePuy AcroMed Harms c.
elastic knee c.
Faraday c.
fusion c.
Harms c.
InterFix RP threaded spinal fusion c.
InterFix titanium threaded spinal fusion c.
Link acetabular c.
lumbar I/F C.
lumbar intersomatic fusion expandable c.
metallic c.
Moss c.

cage *(continued)*
 Novus LC threaded interbody fusion c.
 Novus LT titanium threaded interbody fusion c.
 Ocelot stackable c.
 osseocartilaginous thoracic c.
 protrusio c.
 Pyramesh c.
 Ray TFC threaded fusion c.
 Ray threaded fusion c.
 Recovery protrusio c.
 Rotafix lumbar c.
 SL c.
 stereolithography c.
 Swedish knee c.
 thoracic c.
 threaded fusion c.
 threaded interbody fusion c.
 titanium c.
 titanium mesh c.
 trapezoidal metal c.
cage-back brace
caged
 c. ball heart valve
 c. ball valve prosthesis
Caire
 C. Sprint portable liquid oxygen device
 C. Stroller portable liquid oxygen device
Cairns
 C. hemostatic forceps
 C. scalp retractor
CairPad incontinence pad
cake mix kit
Cal-20 central dialysate preparation unit
Calandruccio
 C. clamp
 C. external fixation system
 C. II compression device
 C. nail
 C. triangular compression fixation device
Calasept
 C. medicament delivery system
 C. sealer
Calcanea calcaneal fracture plate
calcaneal
 c. spreader
 c. spur cookie orthosis
calcaneonavicular bar
calcar
 c. planer
 c. replacement femoral prosthesis
 c. replacement stem
Cal-Chex for Cell-Dyn whole blood calibrator

calcified tissue scissors
calciobiotic root canal sealer
Calcitek
 C. drill
 C. implant
 C. implant system
 C. retaining screw
Calcitite bone graft
calcium
 c. alginate dressing
 c. alginate swab
 c. hydroxyapatite pellet
 c. phosphatase bone paste
 c. phosphate ceramic implant
 c. sodium alginate wound dressing
 c. sulfate bone graft barrier
 c. sulfate bone void filler
Calculair spirometer
calculator
 pediatric IOL c.
Calcusplit pneumatic lithotriptor
Calcutript
 C. electrohydraulic lithotriptor
 Karl Storz C.
Caldwell
 C. hanging cast
 C. needle/cannula Quick-Tap paracentesis system
 C. protection
 C. suction trephine
calf
 c. bone dowel
 c. compression unit
Calgiswab dressing
Calgitrol calcium alginate wound dressing with maltodextrin
Calhoun-Hagler lens needle
Calhoun needle
calibrated
 c. depth gauge
 c. monofilament
 c. probe
 c. tris-acryl gelatin microsphere
 c. V-Lok cuff
calibration ruler
calibrator
 Advia Centaur anti-HBs c.
 Atomlab 200 dose c.
 Cal-Chex for Cell-Dyn whole blood c.
 digital isotope c.
 dose c.
 isotope c.
 keratometer c.
 radioisotope c.
 Vitros Immunodiagnostic Products anti-HBc c.
 Vitros Immunodiagnostic Products HBsAg Reagent Pack and C.

calices (*pl. of* calix)
California
    C. hatchet
    University of Southern C. (USC)
Caligamed
    C. ankle orthosis
    C. brace
caliper orthosis
calipers
    AccuGage vessel c.
    Accu-Measure skinfold c.
    anthropometric c.
    Berens marking c.
    bone c.
    bone-measuring c.
    Braunstein fixed c.
    Burch c.
    Castroviejo c.
    dial c.
    Digimatic c.
    digital c.
    EKG c.
    electronic c.
    eye c.
    Fat-O-Meter skinfold c.
    FatTrack Digital body fat c.
    FatTrack skinfold c.
    Harpenden c.
    Harpenden skinfold c.
    House strut c.
    Jameson c.
    John Green c.
    Kapp Surgical Instrument total
     hip c.
    Ladd c.
    Lafayette skinfold c.
    Lange skinfold c.
    Machemer c.
    McGaw skinfold c.
    Mendez degree c.
    middle ear c.
    Mitutoyo Digimatic c.
    Mitutoyo digital c.
    ophthalmic c.
    Prader c.
    restraint c.
    ruler c.
    skinfold c.
    Stahl c.
    Storz c.
    strut c.
    Tenzel c.
    Thorpe c.
    tonsillar c.
    Townley c.
    Vernier c.
    x-ray c.
calix, calyx, pl. **calices, calyces**

    C. 2 fluoroscopic tracking module
    c. tube
Callahan fixation forceps
Call-Press graft press
Calnan-Nicolle
    C.-N. metatarsophalangeal prosthesis
    C.-N. synthetic joint prosthesis
calomel electrode
calorimeter
    bench scale c.
    Benedict-Roth c.
    Deltatrac II indirect c.
calorimetry
    indirect c.
Calot jacket
Caltrac accelerometer
Caluso PEG gastrostomy tube
calvarial
    c. clamp
    c. hook
Calvitron hair replacement system
calyces (*pl. of* calix)
Calypso
    C. lift
    C. Rely catheter
    C. Rely PTCA balloon angioplasty
     catheter
calyx (*var. of* calix)
Cam
    C. Lock knee joint
    C. vision stimulator
    C. Walker ankle brace
    C. Walker ankle walker
    C. Walker leg brace
Camber axis hinge
Cambridge
    C. acuity card
    C. Biotech HIV-1 urine Western
     blot test
    C. electrocardiograph
Cameco
    C. syringe holder
    C. syringe pistol
    C. syringe pistol aspiration device
camera, pl. **camerae, cameras**
    ADAC Cirrus single-headed
     SPECT c.
    ADAC gamma c.
    ADAC MCD Vertex Plus MCD
     gamma c.
    ADAC Vertex dual-headed
     SPECT c.
    Anger scintillation c.
    anterior bulbi c.
    Apex 409, 415 c.
    Apex 409, 410, 415 ECT digital
     gamma c.
    Argus c.
    AxioCam c.

camera *(continued)*
  Biad c.
  Bio-Optics c.
  Canon CF-60U, CF60Z fundus c.
  Carl Zeiss Jena Retinophot
    fundus c.
  CCD c.
  Ceraspect c.
  CFA digital c.
  CF-60DSi fundus c.
  charge-coupled device
    monochrome c.
  charge-coupled device TV c.
  charge-coupled device video c.
  CID c.
  Cidtech c.
  cine c.
  Circon-ACMI MicroDigital-I c.
  Circon video c.
  Coburn c.
  coincidence gamma c.
  coincident gamma c.
  color fundus c.
  CompuCam digital intraoral c.
  CooperVision c.
  CR6-45NMf retinal c.
  crystal gamma c.
  CTI-Siemens 933/8-12 PET c.
  data c.
  Dental Pro II c.
  Digirad gamma c.
  DigiScope c.
  Dine Digital Macro c.
  Docustar fundus c.
  Donaldson fundus c.
  DSI c.
  DSX Sopha c.
  dual-head coincidence c.
  dual-head gamma c.
  dual single-crystal gamma c.
  3Dx digital stereo disc c.
  DyoCam arthroscopic view c.
  electron diffraction c.
  Elscint Apex 409-AG ECT c.
  Elscint Apex 009 Precursor c.
  Elscint dual-detector cardiac c.
  Elscint dual-head helix c.
  endo-c.
  Endocam digital c.
  EndoView c.
  Eyecor c.
  fiberoptic digital fundus c.
  field-of-view c.
  fundus c.
  gamma c.
  gamma scintillation c.
  Gammatone II gamma c.
  gantry-free gamma c.
  Garcia-Ibanez M picture c.

  GE 400AC/T; STAR II c.
  GE gamma c.
  GE Maxicamera gamma c.
  Genesys Vertex variable-angle
    gamma c.
  GE Neurocam c.
  GE single-detector SPECT-
    capable c.
  GE Starcam single-crystal
    tomographic scintillation c.
  Haifa c.
  handheld fundus c.
  Handy nonmydriatic video
    fundus c.
  Handy video fundus c.
  3-head c.
  4-head c.
  Helix c.
  Hitachi SPECT 2000H-40 c.
  Holofax Oxford retroillumination
    cataract c.
  hybrid PET/SPECT c.
  infrared c.
  Insight digital c.
  integral uniformity scintillation c.
  isocon c.
  Israel c.
  Keeler c.
  Kowa angiographic c.
  Kowa hand c.
  Kowa PRO II retinal c.
  Kowa RC-XV fundus c.
  large field-of-view gamma c.
  Leicaflex c.
  Macro-5 c.
  MedX c.
  MLR+ c.
  multicrystal gamma c.
  multiple-headed gamma c.
  Multispect 3 c.
  multiwire gamma c.
  Neitz CT-R cataract c.
  Nidek 3Dx stereo c.
  Nidek 3Dx stereodisk c.
  Nikon D100 digital c.
  Nikon digital c.
  Nikon microprocessor-controlled c.
  Nikon Retinopan fundus c.
  NM-1000 digital nonmydriatic
    fundus c.
  nuclear medicine c.
  Olympus OM-1 reflex c.
  Olympus operating c.
  Olympus OTV-S series
    miniature c.
  Orthicon c.
  PhotoScreener pediatric c.
  Picker c.
  pinhole c.

Pixsys FlashPoint c.
positron c.
positron scintillation c.
Prism 2000XP gamma c.
PULSEcdc compact gamma c.
radioisotope c.
radionuclide c.
RC-2 fundus c.
Reflec UV instant c.
Reichert c.
RetCam 120 fiberoptic fundus c.
retinal c.
retinal fundus c.
Retinopan 45 c.
Reveal MLR+ c.
Reveal single lens reflex c.
R&F c.
rotating gamma c.
Scanditronix 1024-7B c.
Scheimpflug c.
Scinticore multicrystal
  scintillation c.
scintillation c.
Shimadzu HeadTome Set-031 c.
Siemens gamma c.
Siemens Orbiter gamma c.
Siemens Orbiter large field-of-
  view c.
single-crystal gamma c.
single-head rotating gamma c.
SKYLight gantry-free nuclear
  medicine gamma c.
slip-ring c.
Sopha DSX1 c.
Sopha Medical gamma c.
Sophy c.
SP6 c.
spectacle-mounted c.
Spot RT Monochrome Kodak KAI-
  2000 CCD digital c.
Starcam large field of view
  gamma c.
stereoscopic fundus c.
SteriCam endoscopic c.
Storz Laparocam c.
Strichman SME-810 c.
Stryker chip c.
Technicare c.
telecentric fundus c.
TeliCam intraoral c.
time-of-flight positron emission
  tomographic c.
Topcon 50IA c.
Topcon SL-45 c.
Topcon TRC-501A fundus c.
Topcon TRC-50IX ICG-capable
  fundus c.
Topcon TRC-SS2 stereoscopic
  fundus c.

Topcon TRC-50VT retinal c.
Topcon TRC-50X retinal c.
Topcon TRV-50VT fundus c.
Toshiba GGA 9300 c.
Trionix c.
Trionix-Triad c.
triple-head gamma c.
Urban microsurgery closed-circuit
  color TV c.
variable-angle gamma c.
Vertex c.
6-c. Vicon motion capture system
video display c.
video pill c.
Vision c.
Visucam C fundus c.
Visucam nonmydriatic fundus c.
Yashica Dental Eye II c.
Zeiss fundus c.
Zeiss-Nordenson fundus c.
Zeiss operating c.
camera/microscope
  Coolscope digital c./m.
camera-processor
cameras (*pl. of* camera)
Cameron
  C. AuraMeter
  C. electrosurgical unit
  C. elevator
  C. fracture device
  C. omniangle gastroscope
Cameron-Haight elevator
Cameron-Miller
  C.-M. electrocoagulation unit
  C.-M. type monopolar forceps
Cameron-Myers vaginoscope
Camey
  C. reservoir
  C. urinary pouch
cam-guided trephine
Camino
  C. intracranial catheter
  C. intracranial pressure monitoring
    device
  C. intracranial pressure monitoring
    system
  C. intraparenchymal fiberoptic
    device
  C. micromanometer catheter
  C. microventricular bolt catheter
  C. monitor
  C. OLM intracranial pressure
    monitoring kit
  C. postcraniotomy subdural pressure
    monitoring kit
  C. subdural screw
  C. transducer catheter
Cammann stethoscope
Camo disposable dental splint

C

113

camouflage prosthesis
Campbell
    C. nerve root retractor
    C. periosteal elevator
    C. slit-lamp
Campbell-Boyd tourniquet
Camp brace
campimeter
    stereo c.
Camp-Sigvaris stocking
CamStar
    C. exercise machine
    C. power leg press
Camwrap plastic covering
can
    C. Am brace
    Contour high-voltage c.
    pacemaker c.
Canadian
    C. hip disarticulation prosthesis
    C. knee orthosis
canal
    completely in c. (CIC)
    C. Finder system
    c. knife
    C. Master drill
    c. reamer
canalicular scissors
canaliculus knife
Canal-Mate hearing aid
cancellous
    c. bone screw
    c. pin
    c. screw
candela
    C. AlexLAZR
    C. laser
    C. MDA-200 Lasertripter
    C. miniscope
    C. Model MDL 2000 laser
    C. 405-nm pulsed dye laser
    C. ScleroLaser
    C. ScleroLaser laser
    C. SPTL laser
    c. videoimaging system
candle
    cesium c.
    urethral c.
    vaginal c.
Can-Do exercise band
candy
    c. cane cannula
    c. cane stirrup
cane
    adjustable c.
    broad-based c.
    Double Duty c.
    English c.
    glider c.

    large-base quad c.
    Liberty walking stick c.
    MAFO c.
    narrow-base quad c.
    offset c.
    single-base c.
    small-base quad c.
    Thera c.
    wide-base quad c.
Canfield
    C. facial plastics garment
    C. shoe
canister
    Autovac autotransfusion c.
    Bemis suction c.
    coil c.
    Lipovacutainer c.
    reusable Sorensen c.
    Sep-T-Vac suction c.
    Vac-U-Port suction c.
Cannon
    C. catheter
    C. curette
Cannon-type stripper
Cannu-Flex guidewire
cannula, pl. **cannulae, cannulas**
    Abelson cricothyrotomy c.
    Accelerator c.
    Accu-Beam suction & irrigation c.
    acorn c.
    Adson brain-exploring c.
    air injection c.
    Airlife c.
    Akahoshi hydrodissection c.
    alpha-chymotrypsin c.
    angled c.
    angled left c.
    angled left/right c.
    angled right c.
    Anis aspirating c.
    anterior chamber irrigating c.
    anterior chamber washout c.
    aortic arch c.
    aortic perfusion c.
    Argyle CPAP nasal c.
    arterial c.
    arthroscopic c.
    aspirating c.
    aspiration c.
    ASSI air injection c.
    atrial c.
    attic c.
    back-and-forth vibrating c.
    Bailey lacrimal c.
    Banaji irrigation c.
    Banaji LASIK c.
    Banaji LASIK irrigating c.
    Bansal LASIK c.
    Bard cervical c.

Barraquer c.
Barrett hydrodelineation c.
Becker dissector c.
Becker Greater Grater dissecting c.
bent infusion c.
Bergstrom c.
Bergström-Stille muscle c.
binasal c.
Binkhorst hooked c.
Binkhorst irrigating c.
biopsy c.
Bishop-Harmon anterior chamber
 irrigating c.
blunt bullet-tip c.
blunt-tipped extraction c.
Bracken irrigating c.
brain biopsy c.
brain exploring c.
Brierley capsulorrhexis c.
Brown sphenoid c.
Bucy-Frazier suction c.
Buie rectal injection c.
bulbous-tip stiff malleable c.
bullet-shaped c.
Buratto irrigating c.
Buratto LASIK irrigating c.
Cabot c.
candy cane c.
Caps-Lock shoulder c.
cardiovascular c.
Castroviejo cyclodialysis c.
CellFriendly c.
cervical c.
Chang hydrodissection c.
Cimochowski cardiac c.
Circon-ACMI c.
c. clamp
clysis c.
coaxial irrigation/aspiration c.
Cobra c.
Cobra+ c.
Cobra K c.
Cobra K+ c.
Cobra LASIK irrigating c.
Cohen-Eder uterine c.
Cohen uterine c.
Coleman aspiration c.
Coleman infiltration c.
Concorde disposable suction c.
Concorde suction c.
contour ERCP c.
Cook c.
Core Dynamics disposable c.
coronary artery c.
coronary perfusion c.
cortex-aspirating c.
cortical cleaving hydrodissector c.
Corydon expression c.
Corydon hydroexpression c.

Cosmetech c.
cricothyrotomy c.
curved cricothyrotomy c.
c. cushion
cyclodialysis c.
dacryocystorhinostomy c.
Day attic c.
DeCamp viscoelastic c.
De La Vega vitreous aspirating c.
Dexide disposable c.
Dishler irrigation c.
Dishler-type LASIK irrigating c.
disposable cystotome c.
DLP aortic root c.
double irrigating/aspirating c.
double-lumen irrigation c.
Dougherty anterior chamber c.
Dow Corning c.
ear c.
egress c.
Eichen irrigating c.
Elsberg brain-exploring c.
EndoForehead c.
endometrial c.
Endo-Pool suction c.
Endotrac c.
Entree thoracoscopy c.
ERCP c.
Eriksson muscle biopsy c.
Ethicon disposable c.
exploring c.
extractor/injector c.
fallopian c.
Fasanella lacrimal c.
Fazio-Montgomery c.
Feaster K7-5460 hydrodissecting c.
Fem-Flex II femoral cannulae
femoral artery c.
femoral perfusion c.
Fisher ventricular c.
flap dissector c.
flattened irrigating c.
Fletcher-Pierce c.
Flexicath silicone subclavian c.
Fluoro Tip ERCP c.
flute c.
Franklin-Silverman biopsy c.
Frazier suction c.
Freeman positioning c.
frontal sinus c.
Fukasaku anesthesia c.
gallbladder c.
Gans cyclodialysis c.
Gass cataract aspirating c.
Gass retinal detachment c.
Gass vitreous aspirating c.
G-bevel c.
Genitor mini-intrauterine
 insemination c.

115

cannula *(continued)*

Gesco c.
Gess I/A c.
Gill double I&A c.
Gills double Luer-Lok c.
Gills-Welsh aspirating c.
Gills-Welsh irrigating c.
Gimbel fountain c.
Girard irrigating c.
Goddio disposable c.
Goldstein c.
Goldstein irrigating c.
Goldstein lacrimal c.
golf tee hollow titanium c.
golf tee UAL c.
goniotomy knife c.
Gonzalez specialized dissecting c.
Gott c.
Grafco c.
Gram c.
gravity infusion c.
Gregg c.
Grizzard subretinal fluid c.
Grüntzig femoral stiffening c.
c. guard
Guell irrigation c.
Guell LASIK c.
Guell LASIK irrigating c.
guiding c.
Gulani triple function LASIK c.
Harvard c.
Hasson c.
Hasson balloon uterine elevator c.
Hasson open laparoscopy c.
Hasson stable access c.
Healon aspirating c.
Heartport endovenous drainage c.
Heyner double c.
high-flow coaxial c.
Hilton self-retaining infusion c.
Hilton sutureless infusion c.
Hoffer forward-cutting knife c.
3-hole aspiration c.
Holinger c.
hollow c.
Hulka uterine c.
HUMI c.
Hunt-Reich c.
hydrodissection c.
I/A c.
I&A coaxial c.
iliofemoral c.
Illouz c.
Illouz suction c.
indwelling c.
infiltration c.
inflow c.
infusion c.
infusion/infiltration c.

inhalation c.
injection c.
Interlink c.
Interlink threaded lock c.
intraarterial c.
intracardiac c.
Intraducer peritoneal c.
intragastric c.
intraocular lens c.
intrauterine balloon c.
intrauterine balloon-type c.
intrauterine insemination c.
introducer c.
Ipas flexible c.
iris hook c.
irrigating/aspirating c.
irrigating J-hook c.
irrigation/aspiration c.
I-tech c.
IUI disposable c.
Jacobs c.
Jarit air injection c.
Jarit disposable c.
Jensen capsule polisher c.
Jensen-Thomas I&A c.
Jetco spray c.
J-hook c.
Johnson double c.
Johnson hydrodelineation c.
Johnson hydrodissection c.
J-shaped I&A c.
J-shaped irrigating/aspirating c.
Judd c.
Kahn c.
Kahn trigger c.
Kahn uterine c.
Kanavel brain exploring c.
Kara cataract aspirating c.
Karickhoff double c.
Karman c.
Katena c.
KDF-2.3 intrauterine
 insemination c.
Kellan hydrodissection c.
Kelman cyclodialysis c.
Khouri hydrodissection c.
Kidde uterine c.
Killian antral c.
Killian nasal c.
Klein c.
Klein curved c.
Knolle anterior chamber
 irrigating c.
Knolle-Pearce c.
Kraff cortex c.
Krause nasal snare c.
lacrimal irrigating c.
Lamprey c.
Landers subretinal aspiration c.

Landolt c.
LaparoSAC single-use obturator and c.
laparoscopic c.
large antral c.
large-bore c.
large egress c.
laryngeal c.
laser-assisted intrastromal keratomileusis c.
lens c.
Leon cobra c.
Lewicky threaded infusion c.
Lichtwitz antral c.
Lifemed c.
ligature c.
Lillie attic c.
Lindeman self-retaining uterine vacuum c.
Linvatec c.
liquid vitreous aspirating c.
Litwak c.
Look I&A coaxial c.
Lübke uterine vacuum c.
Luer tracheal c.
Lukens c.
lumen c.
LV apex c.
Makler c.
Malström-Westman c.
Manche irrigation c.
Manche-type LASIK irrigating c.
Marlow disposable c.
Maumenee knife goniotomy c.
maxillary sinus c.
Mayo coronary perfusion c.
Mayo-Ochsner c.
McCain TMJ c.
McGoon c.
McIntyre anterior chamber c.
McIntyre-Binkhorst irrigating c.
McIntyre coaxial c.
McIntyre lacrimal c.
mediastinal c.
Medicut c.
Meditech flexible stiffening c.
Menghini c.
Mercedes c.
Mercedes tip c.
metal c.
metallic tip c.
microaire c.
middle ear suction c.
Mladick concave c.
Mladick convex c.
Montgomery tracheal c.
Morris flexible c.
Narins c.
nasal c.

nasal snare c.
Nichamin hydrodissection c.
Nichamin LASIK irrigating c.
nucleus delivery c.
O'Gawa cataract aspirating c.
olive-tip c.
Olympus disposable c.
outflow c.
outlet c.
Packo pars plana c.
Pautler infusion c.
PeaceKeeper c.
Pearce coaxial I&A c.
Pearce coaxial irrigating/aspirating c.
Peczon I&A c.
Pereyra ligature c.
perfluorocarbon coaxial I/A c.
perfusion c.
Pettigrove irrigation c.
Pettigrove LASIK irrigating c.
pickle fork c.
Pierce coaxial I&A c.
Pinto c.
Pinto superficial dissection c.
plastic c.
polyethylene c.
Polystan perfusion c.
portal c.
Post washing c.
power c.
pyramid c.
quad-ported LASIK irrigating c.
Quickdraw venous c.
Rabinov c.
Rainin air injection c.
Ramirez Silastic c.
Ramirez telescoping c.
Randolph cyclodialysis c.
Ranfac c.
RAP c.
reciprocating c.
rectal injection c.
reel aspiration c.
remote access perfusion c.
Rhein aspiration c.
Rhein irrigation c.
Robles cutting point c.
Roper alpha-chymotrypsin c.
Rosenberg dissecting c.
Rubenstein LASIK c.
Rubenstein-type LASIK irrigating c.
Rycroft c.
saber-toothed c.
saphenous vein c.
Sarns aortic arch c.
Sarns soft-flow aortic c.
Sarns 2-stage c.
Sarns venous drainage c.

C

cannula *(continued)*
Scheie anterior chamber c.
Scott c.
Sedan c.
Seibel LASIK flap irrigator and squeegee c.
Seibel LASIK flap squeegee c.
self-retaining infusion c.
self-retaining irrigating c.
self-sealing c.
Semm uterine vacuum c.
Shahinian lacrimal c.
shark-mouth c.
shark-tip c.
Sheets irrigating vectis c.
Shepard incision irrigating c.
Shepard radial keratotomy irrigating c.
side-cutting c.
side-port c.
sidewall infusion c.
silicone c.
Silver c.
Simcoe cortex extractor aspiration c.
Simcoe double-barreled c.
Simcoe II PC double c.
Simcoe nucleus delivery c.
Simcoe reverse aperture c.
Simcoe reverse I&A c.
Sims c.
single-holed suction c.
single-lumen c.
sinus antral c.
sinus irrigating c.
Skillern sphenoid c.
Slade formed irrigation c.
Sluijter-Mehta SMK-C10 c.
small-bore c.
small egress c.
smooth c.
Softclamp arterial return c.
Softip oxygen nasal c.
soft-tipped c.
soft tissue shaving c.
Solos disposable c.
SpaceSEAL balloon tip c.
spatula c.
spatula-tip c.
Spencer c.
sphenoidal c.
stable access c.
2-stage Sarns c.
step-down c.
Steriseal disposable c.
Storz disposable c.
Storz needle c.
straightening c.
straight lacrimal c.

StraightShot arterial c.
subclavian c.
subretinal aspiration c.
subretinal fluid c.
sub-Tenon anesthesia c.
suction c.
suprapatellar c.
suprapubic c.
surgical c.
Swets goniotomy knife c.
Tandem XL triple-lumen ERCP c.
Tenner lacrimal c.
thin disposable c.
Thomas I&A c.
Thurmond nucleus-irrigating c.
Tibbs arterial c.
tiger-tip c.
c. tip
Toledo V-dissector c.
Toomey angled c.
Toomey G-bevel c.
Toomey standard c.
Tornambe infusion c.
tracheal c.
tracheostomy c.
tracheotomy c.
transseptal c.
transzonular vitreal injection c.
Trendelenburg c.
Trevisani c.
TriEye c.
trigeminus c.
trigger c.
triport c.
triport sub-Tenon anesthesia c.
Troutman c.
Troutman alpha-chymotrypsin c.
trumpet c.
TruPro lacrimal c.
tubal insufflation c.
Tulevech lacrimal c.
Tulip c.
tumescent infiltrator c.
Uldall subclavian hemodialysis c.
ultrasonic c.
Unitech Toomey c.
Unitri c.
Universal c.
urethral instillation c.
urethrographic c.
USCI c.
U-shaped c.
uterine self-retaining c.
uterine vacuum c.
Vabra c.
vacuum c.
vacuum uterine c.
Van Alyea frontal sinus c.
Vancaillie uterine c.

Vance prostatic aspiration c.
VC2 atrial caval c.
vein graft c.
Veirs c.
vena cava c.
Venflon c.
venoclysis c.
venous c.
ventricular c.
Veress laparoscopic c.
Vidaurri double irrigation c.
Vidaurri LASIK c.
viscocanalostomy c.
Viscoflow c.
Visitec anterior chamber c.
Visitec I&A c.
Visitec irrigating/aspirating c.
Vitalcor cardioplegia infusion c.
vitreous aspirating c.
vitreous-aspirating c.
Von Eichen antral c.
Wallace Flexihub central venous
   pressure c.
washout c.
2-way cataract aspirating c.
Webb c.
Weck disposable c.
Weil lacrimal c.
Wells Johnson c.
Welsh cortex stripper c.
Welsh flat olive-tip double c.
West c.
West lacrimal c.
Wisap disposable c.
c. with locking dilator
c. with preloaded guidewire
Wolf disposable c.
Wolf drainage c.
Ximed disposable c.
Yamagishi viscocanalostomy c.
cannular scissors
cannulated
   c. bolt
   c. bronchoscopic forceps
   c. cancellous lag screw
   c. cortical step drill
   c. drill
   c. drill bit
   c. 4-flute reamer
   c. hemi-implant (CHI)
   c. nail
   c. obturator
   C. Plus screw system
   c. screw
   c. screwdriver
   c. wire threader
cannulation catheter
cannulatome
   Cotton c.

Canon
   C. automatic keratometer
   C. autorefraction keratometer
   C. autorefractometer
   C. CF-60U, CF60Z fundus camera
   C. perimeter
   C. R-5+ Auto Ref-Keratometer
   C. R-50+ autorefractor
   C. refractor
   C. RO-4000, -5000 slit-lamp
   C. scanner
   C. SLO scanning laser
      ophthalmoscope
Can-Opt
   C.-O. dual-lumen ERCP system
   C.-O. stand-alone dual-lumen ERCP
      catheter
canopy ventilation monitor
canted finger hook
cantilever external fixator
Cantor intestinal tube
canvas brace
Canyons irrigation syringe
CAP
   conservative anatomic prosthesis
cap
   Active Life 1-piece opaque
      stoma c.
   C.'s ArthroWand
   C.'s ArthroWand device
   Assura stoma c.
   Carnation corn c.'s
   cervical c.
   Cloward drill guard c.
   Coloplast stoma c.
   compliance c.
   digit c.
   endoscopic suction c.
   Gelfilm c.
   Interlink injection c.
   Navigus cranial base and c.
   nerve c.
   Oves cervical c.
   plastic end c.
   ProtectaCap c.
   Silipos mesh c.
   c. splint
   stockinette c.
   Sur-Fit flange c.
   Sur-Fit Natura flange c.
   syringe c.
   Universal reducer c.
   Zang metatarsal c.
capability, pl. **capabilities**
   snap-off c. (SOC)
capacitive sensor
capacitor
   MOS c.
Capasee diagnostic ultrasound system

C

capeline bandage
Capello
    C. press-fit prosthesis
    C. slim-line abduction pillow
Capener
    C. coil splint
    C. finger splint
    C. gouge
cap-fitted
    c.-f. endoscope
    c.-f. panendoscope
capillary, pl. **capillaries**
    c. bed shunt
    c. flow dialyzer
    c. microscope
    C. System slide holder
    c. tube
    c. tube plasma viscosimeter
Capintec
    C. instant gamma counter
    C. nuclear Vest monitor
Capiox-E bypass system oxygenator
Capiox hollow flow oxygenator
capitonnage suture
Caplan nasal bone scissors
Capless polyaxial pedicle screw system
Capner boutonniere splint
Capnocheck
    C. handheld capnometer
    C. II CO_2/pulse oximeter
    C. Plus NIPB monitor
    C. quantitative capnometer
Capno-Flo single-patient resuscitation bag
Capnogard capnograph monitor
capnogram
capnograph
    BCI Capnocheck DualStream c.
    Clarity c.
    Microcap handheld c.
    Microstream c.
    Nellcor N-2500 c.
    Novametrix Tidal Wave handheld c.
    SC-300 portable c.
    SC-210 sidestream c.
    Tidal Wave handheld c.
Capnomac
    C. infrared analyzer
    C. multiple gas analyzer
    C. Ultima monitor
capnometer
    Capnocheck handheld c.
    Capnocheck quantitative c.
    Datex Normocap infrared c.
    MicroSpan c.
    sidestream c.
CapnoProbe sublingual CO_2 system

Capnostat CO_2 sensor
capped lead
caprolactam suture
Caprosyn monofilament suture
Capset
    C. bone graft barrier
    C. calcium sulfate bone graft barrier
Caps-Lock
    C.-L. shoulder cannula
    C.-L. shoulder cannula system
capsular
    c. forceps
    c. plug
    c. retraction device
    c. tension ring
    c. tension segment
capsular-style lens
capsule
    c. applier system
    Crosby c.
    Crosby-Kugler biopsy c.
    Crosby-Kugler pediatric c.
    dental c.
    c. forceps
    c. fragment forceps
    c. fragment spatula
    Heyman-Simon c.
    M2A swallowable imaging c.
    pH-sensitive radiotelemetry c.
    Pillcam ESO video c.
    c. polisher
    radioisotope c.
    c. retractor
    Sitzmarks radiopaque marker in gelatin c.
    SmartPill pH.p c.
    Watson c.
capsule-grasping forceps
capsulorrhexis forceps
capsulotome
capsulotomy
    c. blade
    c. forceps
    c. scissors
CapSure
    C. cardiac pacing lead
    C. continence shield
    C. electrode
    C. SP lead
    C. VDD lead
CapSureFix lead
Captiflex polypectomy snare
Captivator polypectomy snare
Captura
    C. helical stone extractor
    C. 3-prong grasper
Carabelli tube

Carabelt
C. lower back support
C. therapeutic belt
Carapace disposable face shield
carbide finishing bur
carbide-jaw forceps
Carb-N-Sert needle holder
CarboFlex odor-control dressing
CarboMedics
C. bileaflet prosthetic heart valve
C. cardiac valve prosthesis
C. Top-Hat supraannular valve
C. valve device
carbon
c. arc lamp
C. Copy high-performance foot prosthesis
C. Copy II foot prosthesis
C. Copy II Light foot
C. Copy II Light prosthesis
C. Copy II light prosthesis
C. Copy II lightweight prosthesis
c. dioxide (CO_2)
c. dioxide generator
c. dioxide laser
c. dioxide laser scalpel
c. dioxide laser scanner system
c. fiber-composite cage
c. fiber lamination braid
c. fiber-reinforced cage
c. fiber-reinforced polyethylene
c. implant
c. monoxide (CO)
c. monoxide oximeter
c. steel blade
carbon-based biomaterial
CarbonX active heel
Carboplast
C. II composite
C. II sheeting
C. II sheet orthotic material
Carborundum grinding wheel
Carbo-Seal
C.-S. ascending aortic prosthesis
C.-S. graft material
Carbo-Zinc skin barrier material
Carcon stent
card
Allen preschool c.
Cambridge acuity c.
CloneSaver c.
digital acuity c.
ecarin clotting time test c.
ECT test c.
ECT time test c.
Guthrie c.
Hemoccult II c.
Howell phoria c.
Jaeger acuity c.

memory exercise c.
microendoscopic test c.
MIM c.
pace c.
reduced Snellen c.
Snellen near-vision c.
Teller acuity c.
TruZone asthma action plan wallet c.
Cardak introducer
Carden bronchoscopy tube
cardiac
c. apnea monitor
C. Assessment System for Exercise (CASE)
C. Assist intraaortic balloon catheter
c. automatic resuscitative device
c. balloon pump
c. baroreceptor
c. bioptome
c. catheter
c. conduction system
C. Control Systems lead
c. defibrillator
c. event monitor
FluoroPlus C.
c. infant catheter
c. monitor
c. monitor strip
c. output recorder
c. pacemaker
C. Pacemaker, Inc. (CPI)
c. probe
c. pulse duplicator
C. Reader IQC test strip
c. resynchronization therapy defibrillator (CRT-D)
c. resynchronization therapy pacemaker (CRT-P)
c. retraction clip
c. sling
C. STATus CK-MB test
c. stretch device
c. tamponade
c. trauma
c. valve dilator
C. View probe
CardiArc
C. cardiac SPECT system
C. SPECT imaging device
C. SPECT scanner
Cardica PAS-Port system
Cardiff resuscitation bag
Cardima Pathfinder mapping microcatheter
cardinal suture
CardioBeeper CB-12L cardiac monitor

Cardioblate
    C. BP, RF surgical ablation
       system
    C. RF generator
    C. surgical ablation pen
    C. surgical ablation system
CardioCamera imaging system
Cardiocap
    C. II pressure monitor
    C. 5-patient monitor
Cardiocap/5 monitor
Cardiocare stethoscope
CardioCoil self-expanding coronary stent
Cardio-Control pacemaker
Cardio-Cool myocardial protection pouch
Cardio-Cuff
Cardio Data MK3 Holter scanner
CardioDiary
cardiodilator
cardioesophageal junction dilator
CardioFix pericardium patch
Cardioflon suture
CardioGenesis
    C. PMR system
    C. TMR system
cardiogenic sheath
CardioGram
cardiokymograph (CKG)
CardioLab 2000 single monitor EP system
Cardiology II stethoscope
Cardiomarker catheter
Cardiomatic electrocardiograph
CardioMed
    C. Bodysoft epidural catheter
    C. endotracheal ventilation catheter
    C. thermodilution catheter
Cardiomemo device
Cardiometrics
    C. FloWire Doppler echo crystal
    C. FloWire guidewire
cardiomyostimulator
Cardionyl suture
CardioPass
    C. coronary artery bypass graft
    C. layered microporous small-bore vascular graft
cardioplegic needle
Cardiopoint cardiac surgery needle
cardiopulmonary
    c. bypass pump
    c. exercise
    c. support
    c. support system
CardioPump
    Ambu C.
CardioRhythm generator
Cardioscint nuclear detector

cardioscope U system
CardioSEAL
    C. device
    C. occluder
    C. septal occluder
    C. septal occlusion system
    C. septal occlusion system with QWIKLoad
CardioSearch sensor
Cardioserv defibrillator
cardiospasm dilator
CardioSync cardiac synchronizer
cardiotachometer
CardioTek electrophysiologic tracer system
Cardiotest portable electrograph
cardiotomy reservoir
cardiovascular
    C. Angiography Analysis System
    c. bulldog clamp
    c. cannula
    c. clamp
    c. computed tomographic scanner
    c. monitor
    c. needle holder
    c. retractor
    c. scissors
Cardiovations CO2 blower
cardioverter
    Lown c.
    Lyra 2020 implantable c.
cardioverter-defibrillator
    Alto VR implantable c.-d.
    Angstrom MD implantable single-lead c.-d.
    Atlas DR implantable c.-d.
    atrial implantable c.-d.
    atrial and ventricular implantable c.-d.
    Atrial View Ventak implantable c.-d.
    automatic external c.-d. (AECD)
    automatic implantable c.-d.
    Cadet high-voltage can implantable c.-d.
    Cadet V-115 implantable c.-d.
    Contour LTV-135D implantable c.-d.
    Contour MD implantable single-lead c.-d.
    Contour V-145D implantable c.-d.
    CPI PRx implantable c.-d.
    Endotak nonthoracotomy implantable c.-d.
    external c.-d. (ECD)
    Gem III AT implantable c.-d.
    Gem II VR implantable c.-d.
    implantable c.-d. (ICD)
    implantable automatic c.-d.

InSync implantable c.-d.
Intermedics Res-Q implantable c.-d.
internal c.-d.
Jewel AF implantable c.-d.
Lumos implantable c.-d.
Lyra 2020 implantable c.-d.
Medtronic external c.-d.
Medtronic PCD implantable c.-d.
Micron Res-Q implantable c.-d.
Mini II, II+ automatic
  implantable c.-d.
MycroPhylax implantable c.-d.
nonthoracotomy lead implantable c.-d.
Phylax AV dual-chamber
  implantable c.-d.
Phylax 06 implantable c.-d.
Powerheart automatic external c.-d.
Profile MD implantable c.-d.
programmable c.-d. (PCD)
PRx implantable c.-d.
Res-Q ACD implantable c.-d.
Res-Q Micron implantable c.-d.
Sentinel 2010 implantable c.-d.
Siemens Siecure implantable c.-d.
Telectronics ATP implantable c.-d.
tiered-therapy implantable c.-d.
Transvene nonthoracotomy
  implantable c.-d.
Ventak A-V III DR automatic
  implantable c.-d.
Ventak Mini II and III automatic
  implantable c.-d.
Ventak Prizm 2 automatic
  implantable c.-d.
Ventak PRx c.-d.
ventricular implantable c.-d.
Ventritex Angstrom MD
  implantable c.-d.
Ventritex Cadence implantable c.-d.
wearable c.-d.
cardiovirus
Cardiovit
C. AT-10 ECG/spirometry
  combination system
C. AT-10 monitor
C. AT-series ECG
Cardona threading forceps
CareDrape blanket
Care-e-Vac portable aspirator
Careside analyzer
CAREvent
C. ALS handheld resuscitator
C. BLS handheld resuscitator
Carex ambulatory aid
Carey-Coons
C.-C. biliary endoprosthesis kit
C.-C. biliary stent
C.-C. soft stent

C.-C. soft stent biliary
  endoprosthesis
Ca-Rezz moisture barrier cream
Carl
C. Zeiss instrument
C. Zeiss Jena Retinophot fundus
  camera
C. Zeiss lens
C. Zeiss lensometer
C. Zeiss tonometer
C. Zeiss YAG laser
Carle analytic gas chromatograph
Carlens
C. double-lumen endotracheal tube
C. mediastinoscope
C-arm
DEC 9800 plus cardiac mobile C-a.
C-a. DSA system
C-a. fluoroscope
C-a. fluoroscopic apparatus
C-a. fluoroscopy unit
C-a. image intensifier
C-a. portable x-ray unit
Siremobil Iso-C3d isocentric C-a.
Carmalt
C. forceps
C. hemostat
C. splinter forceps
Carmault clamp
Carmeda
C. BioActive Surface
C. BioActive surface extracorporeal
  circuit
Carmel clamp
Carmody-Batson elevator
Carmody-Brophy forceps
carmustine wafer
Carnation corn caps
Carolon
C. AFO sock
C. life support antiembolism
  stocking
C. multi-layer stocking system
Carones
C. LASEK pump
C. LASEK spatula
carotid
c. artery clamp
c. ball
c. sheath
c. stent
Carotid-Wallstent Monorail
carpal
c. box
C. Care carpal tunnel exerciser
C. Lock cock-up splint
C. Lock cock-up wrist splint
C. Lock CTS brace

carpal *(continued)*
   C. Lock wrist brace
   C. Lock wrist splint
   c. lunate implant
   C. Trac traction device
   c. tunnel glove
   c. tunnel release system device
   C. Tunnel Stretch exerciser
   c. tunnel surgery relief kit
Carpal-Lock wrist support
Carpel
   C. speculum
   C. trabeculectomy punch
Carpentier
   C. pericardial valve
   C. ring
Carpentier-Edwards
   C.-E. aortic valve prosthesis
   C.-E. bioprosthetic valve
   C.-E. Duraflex low-pressure porcine
      mitral bioprosthesis
   C.-E. glutaraldehyde-preserved
      porcine xenograft prosthesis
   C.-E. mitral annuloplasty valve
   C.-E. pericardial valve
   C.-E. Perimount mitral valve
   C.-E. Perimount RSR pericardial
      bioprosthesis
   C.-E. Physio annuloplasty ring
   C.-E. porcine bioprosthesis
   C.-E. porcine prosthetic valve
   C.-E. porcine supraannular valve
   C.-E. SAV aortic porcine
      bioprosthesis valve
**Carpentier-McCarthy-Adams IMR
   ETlogix annuloplasty ring**
carpometacarpal (CMC)
carposcope
Carpuject
   C. syringe
   C. syringe system
Carpule needle
CarraFilm
   C. transparent film
   C. transparent film dressing
   C. wound dressing
CarraGauze
   C. hydrogel wound dressing pad
   C. impregnated gauze
   C. packing strip
CarraSmart
   C. foam
   C. foam dressing
   C. gel
CarraSorb
   C. H
   C. H alginate wound cover
   C. H calcium alginate wound
      dressing

   C. hydrogel dressing
   C. M
   C. M freeze-dried gel wound
      dressing
Carrasyn
   C. hydrogel
   C. hydrogel wound dressing
   C. V viscous hydrogel wound
      dressing
Carrel-Lindbergh pump
Carrel mosquito forceps
Carriazo-Barraquer
   C.-B. instrument set
   C.-B. microkeratome
Carriazo-Pendular microkeratome
Carrie car seat
carrier
   amalgam c.
   Barraquer needle c.
   brain clip c.
   bronchoscopic sponge c.
   clamp c.
   Converta-Litter c.
   DeBakey ligature c.
   DeBakey-Semb ligature c.
   Deschamps ligature c.
   double-headed stereotactic c.
   ear snare wire c.
   Endo-Assist disposable ligature c.
   Endo-Assist endoscopic ligature c.
   Endo Close suture c.
   Favaloro-Semb ligature c.
   fiberoptic light c.
   Finochietto clamp c.
   foil c.
   gauze pad c.
   Goldwasser suture c.
   Jackson sponge c.
   Kilner suture c.
   Lahey ligature c.
   laryngeal sponge c.
   ligature c.
   light c.
   linear in-line ligature c.
   London College foil c.
   Madden ligature c.
   Mayo goiter ligature c.
   Miya hook ligament c.
   Miya hook ligature c.
   nasal snare wire c.
   Pereyra-Raz ligature c.
   Raz double-prong ligature c.
   sigmoidoscope light c.
   sponge c.
   suture c.
   tendon c.
   Thermafil plastic c.
   c. tube
   Yasargil ligature c.

Carrington Dermal wound gel
Carrion-Small penile implant
Carr-Locke injection needle
Carroll
>C. awl
>C. bone-holding forceps
>C. dressing forceps
>C. hand retractor
>C. skin hook
>C. tendon-pulling forceps
>C. tendon retriever
>C. tissue forceps

Carroll-Bennett finger retractor
carrot finger orthosis
Carson
>C. internal/external endopyelotomy stent
>C. Zero Tip balloon dilatation catheter
>C. Zero Tip balloon dilation catheter

cart
>crash c.
>Harloff c.
>MedGraphics CPX/D metabolic c.
>metabolic c.
>Reach & Roll c.
>resuscitation c.
>SensorMedics 2900 metabolic c.

Cartella eye shield
Carter
>C. foam pillow
>C. immobilization cushion
>C. intranasal splint
>C. pillow
>C. Rowe awl
>C. sphere
>C. sphere introducer
>C. submucous curette
>C. Tubal Assistant

Carter-Thomason
>C.-T. CloseSure System
>C.-T. CloseSure System XL
>C.-T. port closure device
>C.-T. suture passer

cartesian reference coordinate system
cartilage
>c. clamp
>c. crusher
>c. elastic pullover kneecap splint
>c. forceps
>c. implant
>c. knife
>c. scissors
>c. shaver blade
>c. stripper

cartilage-holding forceps
cartilaginous dorsal implant
Cartman lens insertion forceps

Carto EP navigation system
cartridge
>Alukart hemoperfusion c.
>AstraZeneca dental c.
>Clark hemoperfusion c.
>Dimension RxL PSA Flex reagent c.
>ELAD c.
>Genotropin 2-chamber c.
>HDL direct test prefilled c.
>LDL direct test prefilled c.
>Monarch C c.
>serum pregnancy assay c.
>sorbent dialysis c.

Cartwright heart prosthesis
carver
>acorn c.
>amalgam c.
>dental wax c.
>G-C wax c.
>Hollenback c.
>modeling c.

Cary
>C. 118C spectrophotometer
>C. 100 UV-Vis spectrophotometer

CAS
>CAS DNA staining kit
>CAS 200 image cytometer

CAS-8000V general angiography positioner
Cascade
>C. impactor
>C. Up and About system

CASE
>Cardiac Assessment System for Exercise
>>CASE computerized exercise ECG system

case
>C. appliance
>Cloward PLIF c.
>Codman dilator c.
>Contique contact lens c.
>C. enamel cleaver
>C. 16 exercise system
>eyeglass c.
>M6/C cylinder carrying c.

Casebeer capsulorrhexis forceps
CA-series dialyzer
Casey pelvic clamp
CASH
>cruciform anterior spinal hyperextension
>>CASH brace

casing
>silastic electrode c.

Caspar
>C. alligator forceps
>C. anterior instrumentation
>C. blade
>C. cervical plate

125

Caspar *(continued)*
    C. cervical retractor
    C. cervical screw
    C. disc space spreader
    C. distractor
    C. drill
    C. headholder
    C. plating
    C. retraction post
    C. retractor
    C. rongeur
    C. vertebral body spreader
Caspari
    C. shuttle
    C. suture punch
CASS
    computer-assisted stereotactic surgery
    CASS whole-brain mapping system
Casselberry suture punch
cassette
    c. cup collecting device
    Curix film screen c.
    film screen c.
    Kodak X-Omatic C-1 c.
Cassi rotational core biopsy device
cast
    abduction c.
    airplane c.
    Aquaplast c.
    Batchelor plaster hip spica c.
    below-knee c.
    below-knee walking c.
    c. belt
    c. bender
    bivalved pancake plaster hand c.
    c. blade
    Body Armor walker c.
    body jacket c.
    c. boot
    c. boot brace
    c. boot polypropylene hip
      abduction brace
    c. brace
    c. breaker
    broomstick c.
    Caldwell hanging c.
    Comfort C.
    cotton c.
    C. Cozy
    dermoplasty c.
    Equalizer short leg walking c.
    Frejka c.
    C. Gard cast protector
    gel c.
    gravity equinus c.
    Gypsona c.
    Hexcelite c.
    hinged c.

hip spica c.
c. immobilizer
Jones compression c.
c. knife
c. liner
long above-elbow c.
long arm navicular c.
long below-elbow c.
long leg cylinder c.
long leg plaster c.
long leg walking c.
medium below-elbow c.
Minerva c.
Muenster c.
Munster c.
negative impression c.
Orfizip knee c.
Orfizip wrist c.
Orthoplast slipper c.
c. padding
Petri c.
plaster of Paris c.
polysiloxane c.
pontoon spica c.
POP c.
Risser-Cotrel body c.
Risser localizer c.
Risser localizer scoliosis c.
Sarmiento c.
c. saw
semirigid fiberglass c.
c. shoe
short above-elbow c.
short arm cylinder c.
short arm navicular c.
short below-elbow c.
short leg cylinder c.
short leg nonwalking c.
short leg nonweightbearing c.
short leg plaster c.
short leg walking c.
slipper c.
spica c.
c. spreader
SP Walker c.
standard above-elbow c.
sugar-tong c.
thumb spica c.
total contact c.
Velpeau c.
walking heel c.
zipper c.
CastAlert device
Castanares facelift scissors
Castaneda
    C. bottle
    C. thrombolytic brush
    C. vascular clamp

Castaway
  C. leg brace
  C. leg walker
castbelt
Castech extremity support
CastGuard guard
Castillo catheter
casting
  Cerrobend c.
  focused rigidity c. (FRC)
  c. wax sheet
Castle
  C. examination light
  C. surgical light
Castmate plaster bandage dressing
cast-molded PMMA intraocular lens
Castorit investment material
Castroviejo
  C. acrylic implant
  C. anterior synechia scissors
  C. blade breaker
  C. bladebreaker
  C. blade holder
  C. calipers
  C. capsule forceps
  C. clip-applying forceps
  C. compressor
  C. corneal dissector
  C. corneal-holding forceps
  C. corneal scissors with inside
   stop
  C. corneal section scissors
  C. corneal transplant marker
  C. corneal transplant scissors
  C. corneal transplant trephine
  C. corneoscleral punch
  C. cyclodialysis cannula
  C. cyclodialysis spatula
  C. discission knife
  C. double-end lacrimal dilator
  C. electro keratome
  C. electrokeratotome
  C. enucleation snare
  C. eye speculum
  C. eye suture forceps
  C. fixation forceps
  C. forceps
  C. iridocapsulotomy scissors
  C. keratoplasty scissors
  C. lacrimal dilator
  C. lacrimal sac probe
  C. lens loupe
  C. lens spoon
  C. lid clamp
  C. lid forceps
  C. lid retractor
  C. needle driver
  C. needle holder
  C. needle holder clamp

  C. orbital aspirator
  C. razor
  C. razor blade
  C. refractor
  C. scleral fold forceps
  C. scleral shortening clip
  C. snare enucleator
  C. speculum
  C. suture forceps
  C. suturing forceps
  C. synechia scissors
  C. synechia spatula
  C. transplant-grafting forceps
  C. twin knife
  C. tying forceps
  C. vitreous aspirating needle
  C. wide-grip handle forceps
Castroviejo-Arruga capsular forceps
Castroviejo-Barraquer needle holder
Castroviejo-Colibri corneal forceps
Castroviejo-Kalt eye needle holder
Castroviejo-Mayo needle holder
Castroviejo-Troutman scissors
Castroviejo-Vannas capsulotomy scissors
catadioptric lens
Cat-a-Kit analyzer
Catalano intubation set
Catalyst
  C. anterior instrument set
  C. machine
Catamaran swim plug
cataract
  c. aspirating needle
  c. blade
  c. knife
  c. knife guard
  c. mask ring
  c. needle
  c. pencil
  c. probe
  c. scissors
  c. spoon
Catarex cataract removal system
catch basin
Catera suture anchor
Cateye
  C. Ergociser
  C. treadmill
catgut
  c. needle
  Rica surgical c.
  SMIC surgical c.
  c. suture
Cath
  Arrow Twin C.
  Freedom C.
Cathcart orthocentric hip prosthesis
Cathcor LX hemodynamic recording system

Cathelin segregator
catheter
A1, A2 Port multipurpose c.
Abbokinase c.
Ablaser laser delivery c.
ablation c.
Abocath c.
Abramson c.
abscess drainage c.
Abscession biliary drainage c.
Abscession fluid drainage c.
Accent balloon angioplasty c.
Accurate c.
Accu-Vu sizing c.
Ace fixed wire balloon c.
Achiever balloon dilation c.
Ackrad balloon-bearing c.
Ackrad Bronchitrac L suction c.
Ackrad H/S Elliptosphere c.
acorn-tipped c.
ACS balloon c.
ACS Concorde c.
ACS Concorde OTW c.
ACS Endura coronary dilation c.
ACS Enhanced Torque 8/7.5-F
  Taper Tip c.
ACS JL4 French c.
ACS Mini c.
ACS Monorail c.
ACS OTW Lifestream coronary
  dilation c.
ACS OTW Photon coronary
  dilation c.
ACS OTW Solaris coronary
  dilation c.
ACS Photon coronary dilation c.
ACS RX Comet angioplasty c.
ACS RX Comet coronary
  dilation c.
ACS RX Comet VP coronary
  dilation c.
ACS RX Gemini c.
ACS RX Lifestream c.
ACS RX perfusion balloon c.
ACS RX Rocket c.
ACS RX Solaris coronary
  dilation c.
ACS Tourguide II guiding c.
ACST Tx2000 coronary dilation c.
ACS Viking c.
Active Cath c.
Acucise balloon c.
Acucise endopyelotomy c.
Acucise RP retrograde
  endopyelotomy c.
AcuNav ultrasound c.
ACX II balloon c.
Adante PTCA balloon c.
c. adapter

Add-a-Cath c.
Advance EX self-adhesive urinary
  external c.
A-Focus steerable diagnostic c.
afterloading c.
Ag-AgCl$_2$ electrode bipolar c.
Agiltrac peripheral dilation c.
Ahn thrombectomy c.
Alert c.
alignment c.
AL I, II guiding c.
alimentation c.
Allis c.
Alzate c.
Amazr c.
Amcath c.
Amplatz c.
Amplatz aortography c.
Amplatz cardiac c.
Amplatz coronary c.
Amplatz femoral c.
Amplatz left coronary c.
Amplatz left I, II c.
Amplatz right coronary c.
Amplatz right I, II c.
Amplatz Super Stiff c.
A2 multipurpose c.
anchored c.
AngeCool RF c.
Angiocath c.
Angiocath Autoguard shielded
  IV c.
Angiocath flexible c.
Angiocath PRN c.
Angioflow high-flow c.
angiographic c.
angiographic balloon occlusion c.
angiographic end-hole c.
angiography c.
AngioJet saline jet/vacuum
  device c.
AngioJet thrombectomy c.
AngioJet Xpeedior c.
Angio-Kit c.
Angiomedics c.
angioplasty balloon c.
angioplasty guiding c.
Angio-Seal c.
angled balloon c.
angled pigtail c.
angle-tip urethral c.
angulated c.
angulated multipurpose c.
Anthron heparinized c.
Anthron heparinized
  antithrombogenic c.
Anthron II c.
antibacterial personal c.

antiseptic-impregnated central venous c.
aortic c.
apheresis c.
AR-1, AR-2 diagnostic guiding c.
Arc-22 c.
Argyle c.
Argyle arterial c.
Argyle Ingram trocar c.
Argyle trocar c.
Argyle umbilical vessel c.
arrhythmia mapping system c.
arrhythmogenic myocardial tissue ablation c.
Arrow c.
Arrow balloon wedge c.
Arrow Cannon c.
Arrow Flex intraaortic balloon c.
Arrow FlexTip Plus c.
ARROWGard Blue antiseptic-coated c.
ARROWGard Blue central venous c.
ARROWGard Blue hemodialysis c.
ARROWGard Blue Line c.
ARROWGard central venous c.
Arrow-Howes multilumen c.
Arrow-Howes quad-lumen c.
Arrow 2-lumen hemodialysis c.
Arrow Pullback atherectomy c.
Arrow QuadPolar electrode c.
Arrow QuadPolar pulmonary artery c.
Arrow QuickFlash arterial c.
arterial c.
arterial embolectomy c.
arterial irrigation c.
arteriovenous c.
Ascent guiding c.
Ash c.
aspiration c.
ATB PTA ablation c.
atherectomy c.
AtheroCath Bantam coronary atherectomy c.
AtheroCath GTO coronary atherectomy c.
AtheroTrack c.
Atlantis SR intravascular ultrasound imaging c.
Atlantis SR IVUS c.
Atlas DG balloon angioplasty c.
Atlas ULP balloon dilatation c.
Atrac-II double-balloon c.
Atrac multipurpose balloon c.
atrioseptostomy c.
Attain Select guide c.
Aurous centimeter sizing c.
Aurous graduate sizing c.

Auth Rotablator atherectomy c.
Autoguard shielded IV c.
automatic c.
autoperfusion balloon c.
Avanar intravascular ultrasound c.
Avanar IVUS c.
Aviator RX balloon c.
AV-Paceport thermodilution c.
axillary c.
Axxess ureteral c.
Bailey c.
Baim pacing c.
Balectrode pacing c.
balloon c.
c. balloon
balloon angioplasty c.
balloon biliary c.
balloon dilatation c.
balloon dilating c.
balloon embolectomy c.
balloon flotation c.
balloon flotation pacing c.
balloon-flotation pacing c.
balloon imaging c.
balloon-imaging c.
balloon PTA c.
balloon septostomy c.
balloon-tipped angiographic c.
balloon-tipped flow-directed c.
balloon-tipped thermodilution c.
balloon valvuloplasty c.
balloon wedge pressure c.
Baltherm c.
Baltherm thermodilution c.
Bandit c.
Bandit PTCA c.
Bardco c.
Bard disposable male external c.
Bardex c.
Bardex all silicone sterile Foley c.
Bardex-Foley c.
Bardex I.C. sterile Foley c.
Bardex Lubricath Foley c.
Bardex silicone Foley c.
Bard gastrostomy c.
Bard male external c.
Bard Safety Excalibur c.
Bard Stinger S ablation c.
Bard Touchless intermittent c.
Bard-U-Cath self-adhering male external c.
Bartholin gland c.
batwing c.
Baxter V. Mueller c.
BD Insyte Autoguard shielded intravenous c.
Béniqué c.
Bentson-Hanafee-Wilson c.
Berenstein guiding c.

C

catheter *(continued)*

Berman angiographic c.
Bernstein c.
Beta-Cath system c.
Beta-Rail c.
Bicor c.
bicoudé c.
bifoil balloon c.
biliary balloon c.
biliary drainage c.
BioDiamond S rapid exchange
  PTCA c.
BioGlide c.
Bio-Guard spectrum antimicrobial
  bonded c.
Bio-Medicus arterial c.
Biosearch female intermittent
  urinary c.
Biosearch male intermittent
  urinary c.
Biosense Webster Navistar
  Thermocool c.
Biovue c.
bipolar c.
bipolar pacing electrode c.
bird's eye c.
Bi-Set c.
Bitome c.
Bivona epistaxis c.
bladder c.
blade septostomy c.
Blazer RPM navigation and
  ablation c.
blood-contactin c.
Blue FlexTip c.
Blue Max balloon c.
Blue Max high-pressure reinforced
  polyethylene balloon c.
Bonnano c.
Bonnie balloon c.
Bourassa c.
Bozeman-Fritsch c.
Braasch bulb ureteral c.
brachial coronary c.
braided diagnostic c.
Brevi-Kath epidural c.
Brite Tip c.
Brite Tip guide c.
Brite Tip guiding c.
bronchial c.
Bronchitrac L flexible suction c.
bronchospirometric c.
Broviac c.
Broviac atrial c.
Broviac hyperalimentation c.
Broviac long-term c.
Buchbinder Thruflex Over-the-
  Wire c.
Bud drainage c.

bulb ureteral c.
bullet-tip c.
Burhenne steerable c.
Bush DL ureteral illuminating c.
Bush SL ureteral illuminating c.
butterfly c.
bypass Speedy balloon c.
Calypso Rely c.
Calypso Rely PTCA balloon
  angioplasty c.
Camino intracranial c.
Camino micromanometer c.
Camino microventricular bolt c.
Camino transducer c.
Cannon c.
cannulation c.
Can-Opt stand-alone dual-lumen
  ERCP c.
cardiac c.
Cardiac Assist intraaortic balloon c.
cardiac infant c.
Cardiomarker c.
CardioMed Bodysoft epidural c.
CardioMed endotracheal
  ventilation c.
CardioMed thermodilution c.
Carson Zero Tip balloon
  dilatation c.
Carson Zero Tip balloon
  dilation c.
Castillo c.
catheter introducing forceps c.
Cath-Finder c.
Cath-Guide closed suction c.
Cathlon IV c.
Cathmark suction c.
Caud-A-Kath epidural c.
Cayote OTW balloon c.
CCOmbo c.
cecostomy c.
Celsius c.
central venous c.
central venous pressure c.
Centurion PTA balloon dilatation c.
Centurion PTA dilatation c.
cephalad c.
Cereblate c.
cerebral ablation c.
C-Flex c.
C-flex c.
Cheetah angioplasty c.
Chemo-Port c.
Chilli cooled-tip ablation c.
Cholangiocath c.
cholangiography c.
ChronoFlex c.
Chubby balloon c.
cisterna magna c.
Clark expanding mesh c.

Clark helix c.
Clark rotating cutter c.
Clay Adams PE-series c.
Clear Advantage latex-free c.
Clear Advantage silicone male c.
ClearWay irrigating PTFE
 balloon c.
CliniCath peripherally inserted c.
Clisco covered needle c.
closed end-hole c.
Cloverleaf c.
Cloverleaf EP c.
coaxial c.
coaxillary directed c.
Cobe-Tenckhoff peritoneal
 dialysis c.
Cobra 1, 2 c.
Cobra diagnostic c.
Cobra over-the-wire balloon c.
cobra-shaped c.
Codman-Holter c.
c. coil
coil c.
Coil-Cath c.
coil-tipped c.
colon motility c.
combination biliary brush c.
Comet c.
Comfort Cath I, II c.
Conceptus Soft Seal cervical c.
Conceptus Soft Torque uterine c.
Conceptus VS c.
condom c.
conductance c.
cone tip c.
conical c.
Conquest balloon dilatation c.
Conquest PTA balloon dilatation c.
continuous irrigation c.
contrast-filled c.
Conveen curved/tapered
 intermittent c.
Conveen female intermittent c.
Conveen Security+ self-sealing male
 external c.
Cook c.
Cook Cardiovascular infusion c.
Cook-Cope type loop c.
Cook cystotomy c.
Cook mini-compression balloon c.
Cook Spectrum c.
Cook TPN c.
Cooled ThermoCath treatment c.
Cool Tip c.
Cope locking loop c.
Cope loop c.
Cope loop nephrostomy c.
Corcath c.
Cordis Brite Tip guiding c.

Cordis Ducor I, II, III c.
Cordis Ducor I, II, III coronary c.
Cordis Ducor pigtail c.
Cordis guiding c.
Cordis Predator PTCA balloon c.
Cordis Titan balloon dilatation c.
Cordis-Webster ablation c.
Cordis-Webster diagnostic/ablation
 deflectable tip c.
Cordis-Webster mapping c.
Corflo percutaneous access c.
coronary angiographic c.
coronary dilatation c.
coronary guiding c.
coronary perfusion c.
coronary sinus thermodilution c.
Cotton graduated dilation c.
coudé c.
coudé suction c.
coudé-tip demeure c.
coudé urethral c.
Councill c.
Councill retention c.
Cournand Tip Arrow QuadPolar
 electrode c.
Coxeter prostatic c.
Cragg-McNamara multiple side-hole
 infusion c.
Cragg-McNamara valved infusion c.
CRE balloon c.
Crista Cath 20-pole deflectable c.
CritiCath PA c.
CritiCath thermodilution c.
Critikon balloon temporary
 pacing c.
Critikon balloon-tipped end-hole c.
Critikon balloon wedge pressure c.
CrossPoint TransAccess c.
CrossSail coronary dilatation c.
cryoablation c.
cup c.
Curl Cath c.
curved c.
cutdown c.
cutting balloon c.
CVP c.
CVS c.
Cynosar c.
Cystocath c.
Dacron c.
Dacron sleeve c.
Damato curved c.
c. damping
DASH ERCP c.
Datascope c.
Datascope CL-II percutaneous
 translucent balloon c.
Datascope DL-II percutaneous
 translucent balloon c.

catheter *(continued)*

Datascope intraaortic balloon pump c.
Datascope true sheathless c.
Davis c.
Davol sterile red rubber c.
Dawson-Mueller drainage c.
decapolar electrode c.
decompression c.
deflectable quadripolar c.
DeKock 2-way bronchial c.
DeLee infant c.
DeLee suction c.
DeLee tracheal c.
Dentsleeve single multilumen extrusion c.
DeOrio intrauterine insemination c.
de Pezzer c.
Derek Harwood-Nash c.
Desai VectorCath mapping c.
Dewan suprapubic urodynamics c.
diagnostic ultrasound imaging c.
Dialy-Nate c.
dialysis c.
dilating pressure balloon c.
dilation balloon c.
dilator c.
DirectFlow arterial c.
directional atherectomy c.
Dispatch infusion c.
Dispatch over-the-wire c.
disposable c.
distal c.
DLP cardioplegic c.
DLP infant ventricular c.
DLP left atrial pressure monitoring c.
dog-leg c.
Dome Port c.
Doppler coronary c.
Dormia stone basket c.
Dorros infusion and probing c.
Dotter c.
Dotter caged-balloon c.
Dotter coaxial c.
double-balloon triple-lumen c.
double-chip micromanometer c.
double-current c.
double-J c.
double-J indwelling c.
double-J stent c.
double-J ureteral c.
double-lumen c.
double-lumen balloon c.
double-lumen Broviac c.
double-lumen central venous c.
double-lumen Hickman c.
double-lumen Hickman-Broviac c.
double-lumen injection c.

double-lumen silastic c.
double-lumen subclavian c.
double-lumen Swan-Ganz c.
double-thermistor coronary sinus c.
Dover 100% silicone Foley c.
Dover Teflon-coated latex Foley c.
Dover Texas Catheter Disposable Male C.
Dowd II prostatic balloon dilatation c.
drainage c.
Drew-Smythe c.
drill-tip c.
D114S balloon c.
dual balloon perfusion c.
dual-lumen c.
dual-lumen silicone hemodialysis/apheresis c.
dual-sensor micromanometric high-fidelity c.
Dualtherm dual-thermistor thermodilution c.
Ducor angiographic c.
Ducor-Cordis pigtail c.
Duett c.
duodecapolar c.
Duo-Flow c.
DuPen long-term epidural c.
DURAglide 3 stone balloon c.
DVI Simpson AtheroCath c.
EAC c.
EASI c.
Easy Rider neurovascular c.
E-cath c.
EchoMark c.
EchoMark angiographic c.
EchoMark salpingography c.
Echotip Soft-Pass embryo transfer c.
EDM infusion c.
Edwards c.
Ehrlich c.
EID percutaneous central venous large-bore c.
Ekos ultrasound c.
elastomer c.
elbowed c.
Elecath electrophysiologic stimulation c.
electrode c.
electrohemostasis c.
electrothermal c.
El Gamal coronary bypass c.
El Gamal guiding c.
Eliminator balloon c.
embolectomy c.
Embryon GIFT c.
Embryon HSG c.
Encapsulon epidural c.

en chemise c.
Endeavor nondetachable silicone
  balloon c.
end-hole c.
end-hole balloon-tipped c.
end-hole fluid-filled c.
end-hole pigtail c.
end-hole ureteral c.
EndoClamp-ST II aortic c.
EndoCPB c.
Endopledge sinus c.
endoscopic retrograde
  cholangiopancreatography c.
EndoSonics balloon dilatation c.
EndoSonics IVUS/balloon
  dilation c.
Endosound endoscopic ultrasound c.
Endotak C lead c.
endotracheal c.
Endovent pulmonary c.
Enforcer balloon dilation c.
Enhanced Torque guiding c.
EnSite multielectrode array
  transvenous c.
Envoy guide c.
Envy c.
Epistat double balloon c.
Epistat II nasal c.
Epistat nasal c.
Eppendorf c.
EPT-Dx steerable diagnostic c.
EPTFE ventricular shunt c.
EP-XT steerable c.
Equinox occlusion balloon c.
ERCP c.
Erythroflex hydromer-coated central
  venous c.
esophageal balloon c.
esophageal manometry c.
esophageal perfusion c.
e-TRAIN 110 AngioJet c.
eustachian c.
Evert-O-Cath drug delivery c.
exdwelling ureteral occlusion
  balloon c.
expandable access c.
Explorer 360-degree rotational
  diagnostic c.
Explorer 360-degree rotational
  diagnostic EP c.
Explorer pre-curved diagnostic
  EP c.
Explorer ST fixed curve
  diagnostic c.
Expo angiographic c.
Expo diagnostic c.
Export c.
Express PTCA c.
extended-curve thermistor c.

extended wear self-adhering urinary
  external c.
external biliary drainage c.
external ureteral c.
Extra Back-up guiding c.
Extractor 3-lumen retrieval
  balloon c.
Extreme II peripheral excimer
  laser c.
4-eye c.
6-eye c.
E-Z Cath c.
Falcon coronary c.
Falcon single-operator exchange
  balloon c.
fallopian c.
Fasguide c.
Fast-Cath hemostasis introducer c.
Fast-Cath introducer c.
FasTracker c.
FasTracker-18 infusion c.
faucial eustachian c.
Feldman aortic stenosis c.
female c.
femoral cerebral c.
femoral guiding c.
femoral hemodialysis c.
fenestrated c.
Feth-R-Kath epidural c.
fiberoptic c.
fiberoptic oximeter c.
fiberoptic pressure c.
filiform c.
filiform-tipped c.
fine-bore c.
Finesse guiding c.
Finesse large-lumen guiding c.
Fino DVT c.
fixed-wire coronary balloon c.
flat-blade-tipped c.
Flex-Cath double-lumen intraaortic
  balloon c.
flexible balloon-tipped c.
flexible metal c.
flexible plastic c.
flexible plastic suction c.
flexible Teflon c.
Flexima biliary drainage c.
Flexima ureteral c.
Flexi-Tip ureteral c.
Flexxicon Blue dialysis c.
Flexxicon II PC internal jugular c.
floating c.
flotation c.
flow-assisted short-term balloon c.
flow-directed balloon
  cardiovascular c.
flow-directed balloon-tipped c.
flow-directed end-hole c.

C

catheter *(continued)*
    flow-directed thermodilution c.
    FloWire Doppler c.
    flow-oximetry c.
    Flow Rider flow-directed c.
    Flow Rider neurovascular c.
    fluid-filled c.
    fluid-filled balloon cardiovascular c.
    fluid-filled balloon-tipped flow-directed c.
    fluid-filled pigtail c.
    Focus PV c.
    Fogarty adherent clot c.
    Fogarty arterial embolectomy c.
    Fogarty arterial irrigation c.
    Fogarty atrioseptostomy c.
    Fogarty balloon c.
    Fogarty balloon biliary c.
    Fogarty balloon embolectomy c.
    Fogarty dilation c.
    Fogarty embolectomy c.
    Fogarty embolus c.
    Fogarty graft thrombectomy c.
    Fogarty occlusion c.
    Fogarty Thru-Lumen c.
    Fogarty vascular c.
    Fogarty venous irrigation c.
    Fogarty venous thrombectomy c.
    Folatex c.
    Foley c.
    Foley balloon c.
    Foley cone-tip c.
    Foley 3-way c.
    Foltz c.
    Foltz-Overton cardiac c.
    Force balloon dilatation c.
    ForeRunner coronary sinus guiding c.
    Fountain infusion system and c.
    Fox PTA c.
    Franz monophasic action potential c.
    Freedom external c.
    French c.
    French angiographic c.
    French Cope loop nephrostomy c.
    French curve out-of-plane c.
    French double-lumen c.
    French Foley c.
    French Gesco c.
    French SAL c.
    French shaft c.
    French sizing of c.
    French Teflon pyeloureteral c.
    French tip c.
    Friend c.
    Friend-Hebert c.
    Fritsch c.
    fused-tip c.
    FX miniRAIL RX PTCA c.
    Gambro c.
    Ganz-Edwards coronary infusion c.
    Garceau ureteral c.
    gastroenterostomy c.
    gastrojejunostomy c.
    gastrostomy c.
    Gauder Silicon PEG c.
    Gazelle balloon dilatation c.
    Gensini coronary arteriography c.
    Gensini Teflon c.
    Gentle-Flo suction c.
    Gesco c.
    Gibbon urethral c.
    Gilbert-type Bardex Foley c.
    Gizmo c.
    Glidecath hydrophilic coated c.
    GlideCath hydrophilic coated c.
    Glidecath XP c.
    Glide Cobra c.
    Glidewire c.
    Glidex coated Percuflex c.
    Glo-tip biliary c.
    G91-9215 monocrystant antimony pH c.
    Goeltec c.
    Gold Probe bipolar hemostasis c.
    Gold Probe Direct bipolar hemostasis c.
    Gold Probe electrohemostasis c.
    Goldstein sonohysterography c.
    Goodale-Lubin c.
    Goodale-Lubin cardiac c.
    Gore-Tex c.
    Gore-Tex peritoneal c.
    Gorlin pacing c.
    Gould PentaCath 5-lumen thermodilution c.
    graduated c.
    Graft ACE fixed-wire balloon c.
    graft-seeking c.
    Graham c.
    Greenfield c.
    Greenfield caval c.
    Grollman pigtail c.
    Grollman pulmonary artery-seeking c.
    Groshong c.
    Groshong distal-valve c.
    Groshong double-lumen c.
    Grüntzig arterial balloon c.
    Grüntzig balloon c.
    Grüntzig balloon angiography c.
    Grüntzig balloon dilatation c.
    Grüntzig-Dilaca c.
    Grüntzig Dilaca c.
    Grüntzig G, S dilating c.
    Grüntzig steerable c.
    Guardian c.

Guidant guiding c.
c. guide
c. guidewire
guiding c.
Guyon ureteral c.
H1 c.
H-1 c.
Haas intrauterine insemination c.
Hagner bag c.
Hakim c.
Halo XP electrophysiology c.
Hancock coronary perfusion c.
Hancock embolectomy c.
Hancock fiberoptic c.
Hancock hydrogen detection c.
Hancock luminal electrophysiologic
  recording c.
Hancock thermodilution c.
Hancock wedge pressure c.
Hands-Off thermal dilution c.
Hartmann eustachian c.
Hartzler ACS coronary dilation c.
Hartzler ACX II c.
Hartzler balloon c.
Hartzler LPS dilatation c.
Hartzler Micro-600 c.
Hartzler Micro II c.
Hartzler Micro XT c.
Hartzler RX-014 balloon c.
Hartzler Ultra-Lo-Profile c.
Hatch c.
headhunter visceral angiography c.
Hearport EndoClamp-ST II
  aortic c.
Heartport DirectFlow arterial c.
Heartport EndoClamp-ST aortic c.
Heartport endocoronary sinus c.
Heartport Endopledge sinus c.
Heartport endovascular c.
Heartport Endovent pulmonary c.
Heimlich c.
helical PTCA dilatation c.
helium-filled balloon c.
Helix PTCA dilation c.
hemodialysis c.
HemoGlide long-term
  hemodialysis c.
Hemoject injection c.
HemoSplit c.
HemoSplit hemodialysis c.
HemoSplit long-term dialysis c.
hemostatic c.
Heyer-Schulte c.
Hickman c.
Hickman-Broviac c.
Hickman indwelling right atrial c.
Hickman long-term c.
Hickman tunneled indwelling c.
high-density sector basket c.

high-fidelity micromanometric c.
high-flow c.
high-speed rotation dynamic
  angioplasty c.
Hilal modified headhunter c.
His bundle c.
Hi-Torque Floppy guide c.
Hobbs dilatation balloon c.
hockey-stick c.
Hohn central venous c.
1-hole angiographic c.
1-hole angioplastic c.
Hollister external c.
Hollister self-adhesive c.
Holter distal peritoneal c.
Holter-Hausner c.
Holter lumboperitoneal c.
Holter ventricular c.
hooked c.
Hopkins hook-guiding c.
Howmedica slit c.
HP Sonos imaging c.
H/S Elliptosphere c.
c. hub
HUI c.
Huibregtse-Katon ERCP c.
HUMI c.
Hurwitz c.
Hurwitz dialysis c.
HydraGlide XL small-caliber
  silicone chest tube c.
HydroCath c.
Hydrolyser hydrodynamic
  thrombectomy c.
Hydrolyser percutaneous
  thrombectomy c.
hydromer-coated central venous c.
hydrophilic-coated guiding c.
hydrostatic balloon c.
hysterosalpingography c.
IAB c.
ICE c.
ICP c.
ILUS c.
Imager II angiographic c.
Imager Torque selective c.
impeller basket c.
implantable access c.
implantable cardioverter-
  defibrillator c.
Impra peritoneal c.
Impulse angiographic c.
Impulse diagnostic c.
indwelling c.
indwelling Foley c.
indwelling subclavian c.
indwelling venous c.
infant female c.
infant male c.

C

catheter *(continued)*
inferior vena cava c.
Infiniti c.
inflatable Foley bag c.
infratympanic c.
Infusaid c.
InfusaSleeve II c.
Infuse-A-Cath c.
Infuse-a-Port c.
infusion c.
Ingram c.
injection c.
injection electrode c.
Inoue balloon c.
Inquiry fixed curve diagnostic c.
Inquiry His diagnostic c.
Inquiry H steerable diagnostic c.
inside-the-needle c. (INC)
inside-the-needle infusion c.
Insyte Autoguard IV shielded c.
Intact c.
Integra c.
Intellicath pulmonary artery c.
intercostal c.
internal/external c.
internal mammary artery c.
interventional c.
intraaortic balloon c.
intraarterial chemotherapy c.
intracardiac c.
IntraCardiac Echocardiography
  IVUS c.
Intracath c.
intracoronary guiding c.
intracoronary perfusion c.
intracranial pressure c.
Intraducer peritoneal c.
intraductal imaging c.
IntraEAR Microdose Cath c.
intraluminal ultrasound c.
intramedullary c.
intrapleural c.
intrathecal c.
intraurethral prostatic bridge c.
intrauterine c. (IUC)
intrauterine insemination c.
intrauterine pressure c.
intravascular ultrasound c.
intravenous pacing c.
intravenous ultrasound c.
intraventricular pressure
  monitoring c.
Intrepid balloon c.
Intrepid percutaneous transluminal
  coronary angioplasty c.
Intrepid PTCA c.
Introcan Safety IV c.
introducer c.
c. introducer

irrigated coiled c.
irrigating c.
irrigation c.
Itard eustachian c.
ITC radiopaque balloon c.
IUI c.
IV c.
IVUS c.
Jackman coronary sinus
  electrode c.
Jackman orthogonal c.
Jackson-Pratt c.
Jacques c.
Javid c.
JB1 c.
jejunostomy c.
Jelco c.
Jelco intravenous c.
Jelm 2-way c.
Jinotti dual-purpose c.
JL c.
JL4, JL5 c.
Jography angiographic c.
Johnson transtracheal oxygen c.
Josephson quadripolar c.
Josephson Tip Arrow QuadPolar
  electrode c.
Joseph urodynamics c.
Jostra c.
JR c.
JR4, JR5 c.
Judkins c.
Judkins coronary c.
Judkins curve LAD c.
Judkins curve LCX c.
Judkins curve STD c.
Judkins 4 diagnostic c.
Judkins guiding c.
Judkins left c.
Judkins left coronary c.
Judkins pigtail left
  ventriculography c.
Judkins right coronary c.
Judkins torque-control c.
Judkins USCI c.
jugular venous c.
J-Vac c.
Karmen c.
Katzen long balloon dilatation c.
Kaufman c.
Kaye tamponade balloon c.
KDF-2.3 intrauterine c.
Kearns bag c.
Kendall double-lumen c.
Kendall Foley c.
kidney internal splint/stent c.
kidney internal stent c.
Kimball c.
King guiding c.

King multipurpose c.
King multipurpose coronary
  graft c.
kink-resistant peritoneal c.
Kish urethral illuminated c.
Koala intrauterine pressure c.
Konigsberg c.
Kontron balloon c.
Kumpe c.
Labcath c.
Labotect c.
LacriCATH balloon c.
LacriCATH lacrimal duct c.
lacrimal balloon c.
Lahey c.
Landmark midline c.
Lane gastroenterostomy c.
Lane rectal c.
Langston dual-lumen c.
laparoscopic cholangiography c.
Lapides c.
Lapras c.
large-bore c.
large-bore suction c.
large-lumen c.
laser delivery c.
Laserprobe c.
Lasso c.
latex c.
lavaging c.
L-Cath peripherally inserted
  neonatal c.
LeFort male c.
LeFort urethral c.
left coronary c.
left heart c.
left Judkins c.
left ventricular sump c.
c. leg strap
Lehman aortographic c.
Lehman pancreatic manometry c.
Lehman ventriculography c.
Leonard c.
LeRoy ventricular c.
LeVeen c.
Levin c.
Levin tube c.
Lifecath c.
LifeJet c.
Lifemed c.
Lifestream coronary dilation c.
Lincoff balloon c.
Livewire TC ablation c.
Livewire TC steerable
  electrophysiology c.
Lloyd bronchial c.
Lloyd double c.
Lloyd esophagoscopic c.
long ACE fixed-wire balloon c.

long Brite Tip guiding c.
Longdwel Teflon c.
long skinny over-the-wire
  balloon c.
long-term internal jugular c.
Lo-Profile II c.
Lo-Profile II balloon c.
Lo-Profile steerable dilatation c.
low-profile balloon-positioning c.
low-speed rotation angioplasty c.
Lucae eustachian c.
Luma-Cath fixed-curve diagnostic c.
Luma-Cath steerable curve
  diagnostic c.
Lumaguide c.
Lumax fiberoptic c.
Lumax Flex guiding c.
lumbar drainage c.
lumbar peritoneal c.
lumbar subarachnoid c.
8-lumen manometric c.
4-lumen polyvinyl manometric c.
Lunderquist c.
Mach 1 guide c.
Madduri urethrogram c.
Magill endotracheal c.
Maglinte enteroclysis c.
magnet-tipped flexible c.
Mahurkar c.
Mahurkar curved extension c.
Mahurkar dual-lumen femoral
  dialysis c.
male c.
Malecot c.
Malecot 2-wing c.
Malecot 4-wing c.
Malecot nephrostomy c.
Malecot reentry c.
Malecot self-retaining urethral c.
Malecot silastic c.
Malecot suprapubic c.
Malecot suprapubic cystostomy c.
Mallinckrodt angiographic c.
Mallinckrodt vertebral c.
Maloney c.
MammoSite radiation therapy
  system c.
manometer-tipped c.
manometric c.
Mansfield balloon dilatation c.
Mansfield orthogonal electrode c.
Mansfield Scientific dilatation
  balloon c.
Mansfield-Webster deflectable
  curved c.
mapping c.
mapping/ablation c.
Marathon guiding c.
marker c.

C

catheter *(continued)*
Mark IV Moss decompression-feeding c.
Marlin thoracic c.
mastoid c.
Maverick balloon c.
Maverick 2 Monorail c.
Maverick OTW c.
MaxForce balloon dilatation c.
MaxForce TTS biliary balloon dilatation c.
MaxForce TTS high-performance balloon dilatation c.
Maxi LD PTA dilation c.
McCarthy c.
McGoon coronary perfusion c.
McIntosh double-lumen hemodialysis c.
Meadox Surgimed c.
measuring-mounting c.
Medena continent ileostomy c.
mediastinal c.
Medicut c.
Medina ileostomy c.
MediPort c.
Meditech balloon c.
Meditech steerable c.
Medrad angiographic c.
Medtronic c.
Medtronic balloon c.
Medtronic Transvene 6937 electrode c.
Medtronic Zuma guiding c.
MegaSonics PTCA c.
Melker cuffed emergency cricothyrotomy c.
Memokath c.
memory c.
Mentor c.
Mentor coudé c.
Mentor Foley c.
Mentor nonhydrophilic PVC c.
Mentor Self-Cath soft c.
Mentor straight c.
Mentor UroSan external c.
Mercator atrial high-density array c.
Mercier c.
metal ball-tip c.
metallic-tip c.
Metras c.
Metricath 1000 console c.
Metricath measurement c.
Mewi-5 side-hole infusion c.
Mewissen infusion c.
Microdose Cath c.
microendoscopic optical c.
MicroFerret-18 infusion c.
Micro-Guide c.

micromanometer c.
micromanometer-tipped c.
MicroMewi multiple side-hole infusion c.
Micro-Soft Stream side-hole infusion c.
Micross dilatation c.
microtip c.
microtip sensor c.
microtip transducer c.
Micro-Transducer c.
MicroVac c.
Microvasive balloon c.
midline c.
midstream aortogram c.
Mikaelsson c.
Mikro-Tip micromanometer tipped c.
Millar Doppler c.
Millar micromonometer c.
Millar MPC-500 c.
Millar pigtail angiographic c.
Millar urodynamic c.
Millenia balloon c.
Millenia PTCA c.
Miller-Abbott c.
Miller septostomy c.
MiniBard c.
Mini-Profile c.
Minispace IUI c.
Mirage over-the-wire balloon c.
Missouri c.
Mistifier spray c.
modified aspirating c.
Molina needle c.
Monorail angioplasty c.
Monorail aspiration c.
Monorail imaging c.
Monorail Piccolino c.
More-Flow long-term high-flow c.
Moss decompression feeding c.
Moss Suction Buster c.
Motarjeme c.
MPA1 c.
MPA2 c.
MR-trackable intramyocardial injection c.
MS Classique balloon dilatation c.
MTC c.
Mullins transseptal c.
multiaccess c.
multielectrode c.
multielectrode basket c.
multielectrode impedance c.
Multiflex c.
multilayer design c.
multilumen manometric c.
multiple side-hole infusion c.
multiplex c.

multipolar electrode c.
multipolar impedance c.
multipurpose c.
multisensor c.
multi-sideport infusion c.
multislit c.
mushroom c.
mushroom-tip c.
MVP c.
Namic c.
NarrowFlex intraaortic balloon c.
nasal c.
nasobiliary c.
nasocystic c.
nasopancreatic c.
nasotracheal c.
nasovesicular c.
National Institutes of Health left
  ventriculography c.
National Institutes of Health
  marking c.
NavAblator c.
Navarre universal drainage c.
Naviport deflectable-tip guiding c.
Navistar c.
Navistar Thermocool c.
NBIH c.
NC Bandit c.
NC Raptor over-the-wire coaxial
  PTCA dilatation balloon c.
NC Raptor PTCA dilatation c.
NC Stormer Zipper MX
  noncompliant balloon dilatation c.
Nd:YAG laser c.
Neal c.
c. needle
needle-tip c.
Nélaton c.
Nélaton urethral c.
Neo-Sert umbilical vessel c.
NephroMax balloon c.
nephrostomy c.
Neptune high-pressure PTCA
  balloon c.
NeuroVasx submicroinfusion c.
Newton c.
Nexus 2 linear ablation c.
Niagara temporary dialysis c.
NIH cardiomarker c.
Ninja FX series over-the-wire
  coaxial PTCA dilatation
  balloon c.
nondetachable balloon c.
nondetachable silicone balloon c.
nonflow-directed c.
nontunneled c.
Norton flow-directed Swan-Ganz
  thermodilution c.
Nova thermodilution c.

Novoste c.
NuMed intracoronary Doppler c.
Nutricath c.
Nycore pigtail c.
Nylex diagnostic c.
Nylex flush angiographic c.
nylon c.
Oasis thrombectomy c.
Oasis triple-lumen c.
occlusion c.
octapolar c.
Odman-Ledin c.
Olbert balloon c.
olive-tipped c.
Olympix II PTCA dilatation c.
Olympus PW-1L wash c.
Olympus PW-5V spray c.
Olympus spray c.
Omega NV angioplasty c.
Omega NV polyethylene balloon c.
OmniCath atherectomy c.
Omni Flush c.
Omni Selective 0-3 c.
On-Command c.
one-hole angiographic c.
one-hole angioplastic c.
Onik-Cohen percutaneous access c.
On-Q Soaker c.
open-ended ureteral c.
OpenSail balloon c.
OpenSail coronary dilatation c.
Opta 5 c.
Opta Pro PTA balloon dilatation c.
Opta Pro PTA dilatation c.
Optical c.
Opticath oximeter c.
Opti-Flow dialysis c.
Opti-Plast balloon dilatation c.
Opti-Plast XT balloon c.
Optiva c.
Oracle Focus imaging c.
Oracle Focus PTCA c.
Oracle intravascular ultrasound c.
Oracle MegaSonics c.
Oracle Micro Plus c.
Oracle Micro Plus PTCA c.
Oracle PTCA c.
Orbiter woven atrial mapping
  diagnostic c.
Oreopoulos-Zellerman c.
OTW HighSail coronary
  dilatation c.
OTW perfusion c.
Outback LTD reentry c.
over-the-needle infusion c.
over-the-wire PTCA balloon c.
Owens balloon c.
Owens Lo-Profile dilatation c.
oximetric c.

C

catheter *(continued)*
oximetry c.
PA c.
Pace bipolar pacing c.
pacemaker c.
Paceport c.
pacing c.
ParCA c.
Parodi c.
partially implantable c.
PAS Port c.
Passage biliary dilatation c.
Passport Balloon-on-a-Wire
dilatation c.
PE c.
pectoral c.
pediatric balloon c.
pediatric Foley c.
pediatric pigtail c.
peel-away banana c.
peel-off c.
PE-MT balloon dilatation c.
PE-MV balloon dilatation c.
pennate suction c.
PENSIL c.
Pentalumen c.
PE Plus II peripheral balloon c.
Percor Stat-DL intraarotic
balloon c.
Percuflex c.
Percuflex nephrostomy c.
percutaneous central venous c.
percutaneous cholecystotomy c.
percutaneous drainage c.
percutaneous femoral venous c.
percutaneous intraaortic balloon
counterpulsation c.
percutaneous nephrostomy
Malecot c.
percutaneous radiofrequency c.
percutaneous rotational
thrombectomy c.
percutaneous transhepatic biliary
drainage c.
percutaneous transhepatic pigtail c.
percutaneous transluminal coronary
angioplasty c.
Performa diagnostic c.
perfusion c.
perfusion balloon c.
Periflow peripheral balloon
angioplasty infusion c.
peripheral atherectomy c.
peripheral long-line c.
peripherally inserted c.
peripherally inserted central c.
(PICC)
peripherally inserted central
venous c. (PICVC)

peripheral vein c.
peritoneal dialysis c.
peritoneal reflux control c.
permanent silicone c.
PermCath c.
PermCath dual-lumen c.
Per-Q-Cath percutaneously inserted
central venous c.
Personal Catheter 100% silicone
intermittent c.
pervenous c.
Pezzer c.
Pezzer mushroom-tipped c.
Pezzer self-retaining urethral c.
Pezzer suprapubic cystostomy c.
Pharmaseal c.
pheresis c.
Philips follower dilator and c.
Phoenix Anti-Blok ventricular c.
Piccolino Monorail c.
pigtail c.
pigtail nephrostomy c.
pigtail rotation c.
Pinkerton balloon c.
Pipelle endometrial suction c.
plastic Tiemann c.
Pleur-evac chest c.
Pleurx c.
Pleurx indwelling pleural c.
Pleurx pleural c.
c. plug
plugged telescoping c.
pneumatic balloon c.
POC Bandit c.
PolarCath balloon c.
Polaris-Dx steerable diagnostic c.
Polaris LE c.
Polaris X steerable diagnostic c.
Poly-Cath c.
polyethylene c.
polyethylene intravenous c.
polypropylene c.
Polystan venous return c.
PolyTech nonlatex urinary
external c.
polyurethane c.
polyurethane nasoenteric c.
polyvinyl chloride c.
Pop-On self-adhering male
external c.
Port-A-Cath c.
Port-A-Cath implantable c.
portal c.
Portex chorionic villus sampling c.
position-sensing c.
Positrol II c.
Positrol USCI c.
Possis AngioJet Xpeedior c.
postprostatectomy hemostatic c.

Pourchez XpressO hemodialysis c.
Powerflex Extreme PTA balloon c.
Powerflex P3 high-pressure
 balloon c.
PowerPICC power injector
 peripherally inserted central c.
Predator PTCA c.
preshaped c.
Prevail steerable c.
Prima Laser c.
Pro-Bal protected balloon-tipped c.
c. probe
probe balloon c.
c. probe ultrasound
probing sheath exchange c.
Procath electrophysiology c.
ProCross Rely over-the-wire
 balloon c.
Profile Plus balloon dilatation c.
Proflex 5 c.
PRO infusion c.
Pronto-Short extraction c.
Pronto V3 extraction c.
Prostaprobe c.
prostatic bridge c.
Prowler Plus c.
Pruitt irrigation c.
Pruitt occlusion c.
PTBD c.
PTCA c.
PTHC c.
PU c.
Pudenz-Heyer vascular c.
Pudenz peritoneal c.
Pudenz ventricular c.
pulmonary arterial c.
pulmonary artery c.
pulmonary flotation c.
pulmonary thermodilution c.
pulmonary triple-lumen c.
pulse spray c.
Pulse-Spray/PRO infusion c.
Pursuit balloon angioplasty c.
pusher c.
push-pull c.
PVC c.
pyeloureteral c.
quadripolar diagnostic c.
quadripolar diagnostic
 electrophysiology c.
quadripolar electrode c.
quadripolar pacing c.
quadripolar steerable electrode c.
quadripolar steerable
 mapping/ablation c.
quadripolar thermocouple-equipped
 ablation c.
Quantum Maverick balloon c.
quick c.

Quick-Cross c.
QuickFlash arterial c.
Quinton c.
Quinton central venous c.
Quinton dual-lumen c.
Quinton-Mahurkar dual-lumen
 peritoneal c.
Quinton peritoneal c.
Quinton PermCath c.
Raaf dual-lumen c.
Racz Tun-L-Kath c.
radial arterial c.
radial artery c.
Radii-T c.
radiofrequency-generated thermal
 balloon c.
radiopaque ERCP c.
radiopaque silastic c.
RadPICC c.
railway c.
Raimondi c.
Raimondi peritoneal c.
Raimondi ventricular c.
Ranfac cholangiographic c.
Ranfac disposable
 cholangiography c.
Ranger over-the-wire balloon c.
rapid exchange balloon c.
rapid exchange Flowtrack c.
Rapid Transit c.
Raptor PTCA dilatation c.
Raptorrail PTCA dilatation c.
Rashkind septostomy balloon c.
rat-tail c.
RC1, RC2 c.
Rebar-18 micro c.
recessed balloon septostomy c.
rectal c.
Reddick cystic duct
 cholangiogram c.
Redha-cut c.
Rediguard IAB c.
red Robinson c.
red rubber c.
red rubber Robinson c.
reference c.
Reflexion steerable c.
Ref-Star EP c.
Release c.
Reliance urinary control insert c.
Rentrop c.
reperfusion c.
Replogle suction c.
Resolution ultrasonic c.
Response electrophysiology c.
retention c.
retrograde occlusion balloon c.
retroperfusion c.
RF-generated thermal balloon c.

C

catheter *(continued)*
RF Marinr c.
rheolytic c.
rheolytic thrombectomy c.
Rhythm c.
right-angle chest c.
right coronary c.
right heart c.
right Judkins c.
right ventricular ejection fraction c.
rigid suction c.
Rigiflex ABD balloon dilatation c.
Rigiflex biliary balloon dilatation c.
Rigiflex esophageal TTS balloon c.
Rigiflex OTW balloon dilatation c.
Rigiflex TTS balloon c.
Rigiflex TTS balloon dilatation c.
Ring biliary drainage c.
Ring-McLean c.
Ritchie c.
RMI antegrade cardioplegia c.
Robinson c.
Robinson urethral c.
Rob-Nel c.
Rochester Medical self-adhering
    male external c.
Rochester Medical 100% silicone
    Foley c.
Rosch hepatic c.
Rotablator burr c.
rotatable pigtail c.
rotational dynamic angioplasty c.
Rothbarth Uni-Flo infusion c.
Roubin infusion c.
round-tip c.
Royal Flush angiographic flush c.
Royal Flush pigtail c.
Royal Flush Plus high-flow
    angiographic flush c.
R1 rapid exchange balloon
    dilatation c.
rubber c.
rubber-shod c.
ruler c.
Rusch c.
Rusch coudé c.
Rusch external c.
Rusch-Foley c.
Rutner wedge c.
RX CrossSail coronary dilatation c.
RX perfusion c.
RX Streak balloon c.
Sable PTCA balloon c.
Sacks QuickStick c.
Sacks Single-Step c.
Safe-Steer support c.
SAL c.
Saratoga sump c.
Sarns wire-reinforced c.

Savvy PTA dilatation c.
Schmitz-Rode c.
Schneider Guider c.
SchonCath chronic dialysis c.
Schoonmaker multipurpose c.
Schrötter c.
Scimed angioplasty c.
Scimed guiding c.
scleral buckling c.
Scoop 1, 2 c.
Scoop model polyurethane
    intratracheal c.
Scoop transtracheal c.
Security+ self-sealing Urisheath
    external c.
Self-Cath closed system c.
Self-Cath coudé tipped c.
Self-Cath HydroGel c.
Self-Cath soft c.
Self-Cath straight-tipped female c.
Self-Cath straight-tipped pediatric c.
Self-Cath straight-tipped soft c.
self-drainage c.
self-guiding c.
self-retaining c.
self-retaining Cope loop pigtail c.
Sellheim uterine c.
semipermeable hollow-fiber c.
semirigid c.
Sensation intraaortic balloon c.
sensing c.
Sentron pigtail microtip-
    manometer c.
Sentry balloon c.
septostomy balloon c.
Seroma-Cath c.
Seroma-Cath wound drainage c.
serrated c.
S.E.T. thrombectomy system c.
S-G c.
Shadow over-the-wire balloon c.
shaft c.
c. sheath
Sheldon c.
shellac-covered c.
shepherd's hook c.
shepherd's hook-shaped
    angiographic c.
Sherpa guiding c.
Shiley c.
Shiley guiding c.
Shiley irrigation c.
short monorail imaging c.
sidewinder diagnostic c.
sidewinder percutaneous intra-aortic
    balloon c.
Siegel-Cohen dilating c.
silastic c.
silastic Foley c.

silastic mushroom c.
silicone c.
silicone elastomer infusion c.
silicone epistaxis c.
silicone Robinson c.
silicone rubber Dacron-cuffed c.
silver c.
silver-coated c.
SilverHawk c.
SIM 2 c.
Simmons c.
Simmons II, III c.
Simmons sidewinder c.
Simmons-type sidewinder c.
Simplastic c.
Simpson atherectomy c.
Simpson AtheroCath c.
Simpson coronary AtheroCath c.
Simpson directional atherectomy c.
Simpson-Robert c.
Simpson-Robert ACS dilatation c.
single-curved Cobra c.
single-lumen balloon stone
  extractor c.
single-lumen Broviac silicone c.
single-lumen infusion c.
single-stage c.
single-use c.
Skene c.
Skinny balloon c.
Skinny dilatation c.
Slalom PTA balloon dilatation c.
Slalom PTA dilatation c.
SmartCath esophageal balloon c.
Smart position-sensing c.
Smec balloon c.
snare c.
Soaker c.
Soehendra graduated dilating c.
Soehendra Universal c.
soft c.
Soft-Cell c.
Soft-Cell permanent dual-lumen c.
Softip c.
Softip diagnostic c.
Softouch diagnostic c.
Softouch spinal angiography c.
Soft-Pass embryo transfer c.
Soft-Tip c.
Soft Torque uterine c.
Soft-Vu angiographic c.
Soft-Vu Omni flush c.
Solera thrombectomy c.
solid-state esophageal manometry c.
solid-state manometry c.
solid-tip c.
Solo c.
SoloPass c.
Sones c.

Sones coronary c.
Sones Hi-Flow c.
Sones woven Dacron c.
Sonicath endoluminal ultrasound c.
Sonicath imaging c.
Sonicath intravascular ultrasound c.
Soules intrauterine insemination c.
Spectranetics c.
Spectranetics C rapid-exchange
  laser c.
Spectraprobe-PLS laser
  angioplasty c.
Spectrum silicone Foley c.
spinal c.
SpineCATH intradiscal c.
spiral-tipped c.
split-sheath c.
Spring c.
Spyglass angiography c.
Stack perfusion c.
Stack perfusion coronary
  dilatation c.
Stamey c.
Stamey-Malecot c.
Stamey open-tip ureteral c.
Stamey percutaneous suprapubic c.
standard ERCP c.
standard Lehman c.
Stargate falloposcopy c.
Stealth angioplasty balloon c.
steerable decapolar electrode c.
steerable guidewire c.
steering c.
Steerocath c.
Steerocath-Λ ablation c.
Steerocath-Dx octapolar and valve
  mapping c.
Steerocath-Dx special procedure
  octa c.
Steerocath-T temperature ablation c.
stenting c.
Steri-Cath c.
Stertzer brachial c.
stimulating c.
Stinger M ablation c.
Stinger S ablation c.
Stinger SM ablation c.
Stormer OTW balloon dilatation c.
Storz-DeKock 2-way bronchial c.
straight end-hole c.
straight flush percutaneous c.
straight side-hole c.
straight tipped c.
Stretta c.
subclavian apheresis c.
subclavian dialysis c.
subclavian hemodialysis c.
subclavian vein access c.
submicroinfusion c.

catheter *(continued)*

Sub-4 small vessel balloon dilatation c.
suction c.
Suction Buster c.
Sugita c.
sump drainage c.
sump pump c.
Super Torque braided angiographic c.
Super Torque Plus c.
support c.
SupraFoley c.
suprapubic c.
Supreme electrophysiology c.
SureCath port access c.
Sure Seal Golden Drain c.
Surflo Teflon IV c.
surgically implanted hemodialysis c.
Surpass PTCA perfusion c.
Swan-Ganz c.
Swan-Ganz balloon c.
Swan-Ganz balloon flotation c.
Swan-Ganz bipolar pacing c.
Swan-Ganz flow-directed c.
Swan-Ganz guidewire TD c.
Swan-Ganz pacing TD c.
Swan-Ganz pulmonary artery c.
Swan-Ganz thermodilution c.
swan-neck Missouri c.
swan-neck pediatric Coil-Cath c.
SynchroMed infusion system intraspinal c.
Syntel latex-free embolectomy c.
synthetic 5-channel water-perfused motility c.
systemic arterial c.
TADcath temporary transvenous defibrillation c.
Talon balloon dilatation c.
Tandem thin-shaft transureteroscopic balloon dilatation c.
tapered c.
tapered-tip hydrophilic-coated push c.
Taut cholangiographic c.
Taut cystic duct c.
Taut M55, M56, M57 c.
TEC extraction c.
TEC guide c.
TEC-guide c.
Tefcat intrauterine insemination c.
Teflon c.
Teflon guiding c.
Teflon injection c.
Teflon needle c.
Teflon pyeloureteral c.
Teflon-tipped c.
telescoping plugged c.

Tempo diagnostic c.
temporary pacing c.
Tempo selective and flush c.
Temp Tip drainage c.
Tenckhoff c.
Tenckhoff 2-cuff c.
Tenckhoff peritoneal dialysis c.
Tenckhoff renal dialysis c.
Ten-Ten duodecapolar diagnostic c.
Terumo SP coaxial c.
Tesio c.
tethered c.
tetrapolar esophageal c.
Texas condom c.
Texas-style 2-piece c.
Thermachoice c.
thermistor c.
thermodilution c.
thermodilution balloon c.
thermodilution Swan-Ganz c.
thin-walled c.
thin-wall introducer c.
ThoraCath c.
thoracic c.
thrombectomy c.
Thrombolizer c.
thrombosuction c.
through-the-needle c.
Tiemann coudé c.
Tiemann-Foley c.
TigerTail ureteral c.
c. tip
tip-deflecting c.
c. tip occluder
Tis-U-Trap endometrial suction c.
Titan Mega XL PTCA dilatation c.
TLC Baxter balloon c.
Tomac c.
Tomac-Nélaton c.
tonsil-tip c.
toposcopic c.
Torcon blue c.
Torcon NB Advantage coronary angiographic c.
Torcon NB selective angiographic c.
Toronto-Western c.
torque c.
torque control balloon c.
torque-control balloon c.
torque tube c.
Total Abscession drainage c.
Total Cross balloon c.
totally implantable c.
Tourguide guiding c.
Trabucco double balloon c.
tracer c.
tracheal c.

Trach-Eze closed suction c.
Tracker 10 c.
Tracker Excel c.
Tracker infusion c.
Tracker Soft Stream sidehole
  microinfusion c.
Tracker-18 Soft Stream sidehole
  microinfusion c.
Tracker-18 Unibody c.
Trakstar balloon c.
transanal c.
transcervical Foley c.
transcervical tubal access c.
transcutaneous extraction c.
transducer c.
transducer-tipped c.
transfemoral endoaortic occlusion c.
transhepatic c.
translumbar inferior vena cava c.
transluminal angioplasty c.
transluminal endarterectomy c.
transnasal intraduodenal feeding c.
transoral c.
Transport dilation balloon c.
Transport drug delivery c.
transseptal c.
transthoracic c.
transtracheal oxygen c.
transurethral c.
transvenous pacemaker c.
TRAX c.
trefoil balloon c.
Trilogy low-profile balloon
  dilatation c.
triple-lumen c.
triple-lumen Arrow c.
triple-lumen balloon flotation
  thermistor c.
triple-lumen biliary manometry c.
triple-lumen central c.
triple-lumen manometry c.
triple-thermistor coronary sinus c.
tripolar Damato curved c.
tripolar electrode c.
tripolar with Damato curve c.
Trip tonometry c.
Trocath peritoneal dialysis c.
True Sheathless intraaortic
  balloon c.
TTS c.
T-tube c.
Tun-L-Kath epidural c.
tunneled c.
Tuohy c.
Turbo Tracker c.
Tygon c.
Tyshak c.
Tyshak balloon valvuloplasty c.
Uldall subclavian hemodialysis c.

ULP c.
Ultra 8 balloon c.
UltraCross profile imaging c.
Ultraflex self-adhering male
  external c.
UltraFuse infusion c.
Ultra ICE c.
ultra low-profile fixed-wire balloon
  dilation c.
Ultramer c.
ultrasound ablation c.
c. ultrasound probe
ultrasound-tipped c.
Ultrathin balloon c.
umbilical artery c.
umbilical vein c.
umbilical venous c.
UMI c.
Uni-Fuse infusion c.
Universal drainage c.
Uresil biliary c.
Uresil embolectomy-
  thrombectomy c.
Uresil irrigation c.
Uresil occlusion balloon c.
ureteral dilation c.
ureteral occlusion c.
ureteral occlusion balloon c.
urethral c.
urethrographic c.
urinary c.
Urocare Foley c.
Urocath external c.
Urocath molded latex male
  external c.
urodynamic c.
urological c.
UroMax II high-pressure balloon c.
Uro-San Plus external c.
USCI c.
USCI Bard c.
USCI guiding c.
USCI Mini-Profile balloon
  dilatation c.
USCI Positrol coronary c.
uterine cornual access c.
uterine ostial access c.
Vabra c.
vacuum aspiration c.
valve-ended c.
Valve Mapper Steerocath-Dx
  mapping c.
valvuloplasty balloon c.
Van c.
Van Aman pulmonary pigtail c.
van Andel dilating c.
Van Buren c.
Van Sonnenberg gallbladder c.
Van Sonnenberg sump c.

catheter *(continued)*

Van Tassel c.
Vantex central venous c.
Variflex c.
Vas-Cath c.
vascular access c.
Vaxcel c.
Vaxcel dialysis c.
Vaxcel peripherally inserted c.
Vaxcel peripherally inserted
central c.
Vaxcel Plus chronic dialysis c.
V-Cath c.
vector phased-array ultrasound
tipped c.
Vector-X coronary guiding c.
Venaport coronary sinus guiding c.
venous c.
venous irrigation c.
venous thrombectomy c.
venting c.
Ventra c.
ventricular c.
ventriculoatrial shunt c.
ventriculography c.
Veripath peripheral guiding c.
vertebrated c.
vessel-sizing c.
Viatrac 14 Plus peripheral
dilation c.
Vietnam c.
Viggo Spectramed c.
Viking Bard c.
Viking coronary guiding c.
Visa II ST PTCA balloon c.
Vision PTCA c.
Vista Brite Tip guiding c.
Vista Brite Tip large-lumen
guiding c.
Vitesse Cos laser c.
Vitesse E2 rapid-exchange c.
Viva Primo balloon c.
Vivonex jejunostomy c.
VNUS Closure c.
VNUS Restore c.
vortex effect c.
VPI nonadhesive condom c.
VTC biliary c.
Vueport balloon-occlusion
guiding c.
waist of c.
Walther female c.
washing c.
Watanabe c.
water-infusion esophageal
manometry c.
water-perfused manometry c.
wave guide c.
2-way c.

3-way Foley c.
3-way irrigating c.
Weber rectal c.
Weber winged c.
Webster coronary sinus c.
Webster halo c.
Webster orthogonal electrode c.
wedge pressure balloon c.
whalebone filiform c.
whistle-tip c.
whistle-tip Foley c.
whistle-tip ureteral c.
White LuMax guiding c.
White vessel sizing c.
Wholey balloon occlusion c.
wick c.
wicking c.
Willscher c.
Wilson-Cook fine-needle
aspiration c.
Wilson-Cook Quantum TTC
esophageal balloon dilatation c.
Wilton Webster coronary sinus
thermodilution c.
Wilton Webster thermodilution flow
and pacing c.
winged c.
4-wing Malecot retention c.
wire stylet c.
Wiseguide guide c.
Wolf nephrostomy c.
Word Bartholin gland c.
WorkHorse percutaneous
transluminal angioplasty balloon c.
woven Dacron c.
WovenFlexie diagnostic c.
Xpeedior c.
Yankauer c.
Yankauer eustachian c.
Yankauer tonsil-tip suction c.
Z cardiac c.
Zimmon c.
Zucker cardiac c.
Zuma guiding c.
Zynergy Zolution
electrophysiology c.

catheter-based

c.-b. sensor
c.-b. ultrasound probe

catheter-borne sector transducer
catheter-delivered platinum coil
catheter-introducing forceps
catheterization

subclavian approach for cardiac c.
Y wave pressure on right atrial c.

catheterizing Foroblique telescope
catheter/stent

Schoborg nephrostomy c./s.

catheter-tip
  c.-t. micromanometer system
  c.-t. occluder
Cath-Finder
  C.-F. catheter
  C.-F. catheter tracking system
Cathflo Activase
Cath-Gard
  C.-G. catheter contamination shield
  TwistLock C.-G.
Cath-Guide closed suction catheter
CathLink 20 implanted port
Cath-Lok catheter locking device
Cathlon IV catheter
Cathmark suction catheter
cathode
  c. ray oscilloscope
  c. ray tube (CRT)
CathScanner ultrasound imaging system
Cath-Secure
  C.-S. catheter holder
  C.-S. Dual Tab holder
  C.-S. tape
Cath-Strip catheter fastener
CathTrack catheter locator system
Catlin
  C. amputating knife
  C. amputation knife
Catrix wound dressing
cat's
  C.'s Paw exerciser
  C.'s Paw retractor
CatsEye digital camera system
Cattell T tube
Caud-A-Kath epidural catheter
caudal
  c. hook
  c. needle
Cauer chalazion forceps
caulking gun
Causse
  C. partial ossicular replacement
    prosthesis
  C. piston
cauterization
  Bovie c.
cauterizer
cauterizing ball
cautery
  Aaron c.
  Accu-Temp c.
  ACMI c.
  Acucise ureteral cutting c.
  Aesculap bipolar c.
  Alcon hand c.
  Berchtold c.
  BICAP c.
  BICAP II c.
  BiLAP bipolar c.

bipolar c.
Bovie c.
Bovie wet-field c.
cold c.
Colorado c.
Colorado tip c.
Concept disposable c.
Concept handheld c.
Corrigan c.
cutting c.
Davis-Bovie c.
disposable c.
electrocautery c.
c. electrode
eraser c.
eraser-tip c.
fine micropoint c.
Geiger c.
Gonin c.
Hildreth c.
Hotsy high-temperature c.
L-shaped c.
MegaDyne c.
Mentor wet-field c.
Mira c.
monopolar c.
Mueller c.
National c.
needlepoint c.
ocular c.
Op-Temp c.
Paquelin c.
pencil c.
pencil-tip c.
Prince c.
right-angle bipolar c.
SLT laser c.
c. snare
Souttar c.
suction c.
Todd c.
unipolar c.
Valleylab c.
von Graefe c.
Wadsworth-Todd eye c.
Walker c.
wet-field c.
Wills Hospital eye c.
Ziegler c.
caval snare
Cavanaugh-Wells tonsillar forceps
Caverject
CaverMap surgical device
cavernospongiosum shunt
Caves-Schultz bioptome
Cavi-Endo ultrasonic system
Cavi-Jet dental prophylaxis device
Cavilon diabetes foot care kit

C

Cavi-Pulse cavitation ultrasound surgical aspirator
Cavitec cavity liner
cavities (*pl. of* cavity)
Cavitron
    C. aspirator
    C. I&A handpiece
    C. irrigation/aspiration system
    C. laser
    C. phacoemulsification unit
    C. Phaco-Emulsifier
    C. SPS ultrasonic scaler
    C. ultrasonic surgical aspirator (CUSA)
    C. ultrasonic system
Cavitron-Kelman irrigation/aspiration system
cavity, pl. **cavities**
    pulp c.
    C. SpineWand
cavus foot support
Cayote OTW balloon catheter
CB
    CB Diode/532 laser
    CB Erbium/2.94 laser
    CB MercuRay maxillofacial imaging system
C&B-Metabond adhesive resin cement
C.B.T.
    C.B.T. conductive stretcher pad
    C.B.T. nonconductive stretcher pad
    C.B.T. Siderail bumper pad
CCD
    CCD camera
    CCD detector
    CCD Spirette
CCK femoral stem provisional guide
C-clamp
    Fukushima C-c.
CCOmbo catheter
CCS endocardial pacing lead
CD
    CD Horizon Eclipse spinal system
    CD Horizon Legacy spinal system
    CD Horizon M8 multiaxial screw
    CD Horizon Sextant percutaneous screw-rod system
    CD Horizon Sextant rod insertion set
    CD Horizon Sextant system
C-D
    C-D fixation device
    C-D hook
    C-D instrumentation
    C-D instrumentation device
CD-5 needle
CD8 AIS CELLector
C-Dak dialyzer

CDBR respiratory muscle training
CDI
    Cotrel-Dubousset instrumentation
    CDI 2000 blood gas monitor
    CDI 2000 blood gas monitoring system
cDNA probe
CDO
    crossed delivery for osteoplasty
    CDO brace
    CDO system
CDRPan digital x-ray system
CE-24 needle
CE-2 cryostat
CEA-Scan
Cebotome
    C. bone cement drill
    C. osteotome
Cecar electrode
cecostomy catheter
CEEA stapler
Ceegraph 128 EEG system
CeeOn
    C. Edge
    C. Edge foldable IOL
    C. foldable lens
    C. heparin surface-modified lens
    C. intraocular lens
    C. model 920 foldable intraocular lens
Cel Touch adhesive
Celay
    C. InCeram crown
    C. milling unit
    C. system
    C. Tech light-curing resin
Celect vena cava filter
Celestin
    C. endoprosthesis
    C. esophageal tube
    C. prosthesis
    C. tube
celiac clamp
celioscope
celioscopy
Celita
    C. elite knife
    C. sapphire knife
cell
    c. analysis system
    c. cushion
    Immuno-trol c.
    C. Lab IC 100 image cytometer
    C. Proliferation kit
    C. Recovery System
    C. Saver
    C. Saver autologous blood recovery system

C. Saver 4 cardiopulmonary bypass blood centrifuge and washing equipment
C. Saver Haemolite
C. Saver Haemonetics autotransfusion system
C. Saver Haemonetics Autotransfusion system
C. Soft 2000 semen analyzer
C. Soft system
Stem-Trol control c.
C. Trak/DMS analyzer
C. Trak/S analyzer

Cellamin resin plaster of Paris bandage
cell-coated stent
Cell-Dyn
C.-D. 1200, 3200, 4000 automated cell-counting instrument
C.-D. Sapphire hematology instrument
C.-D. SlideMaker/Stainer
C.-D. SMS

Cellect
C. graft preparation device
C. Selective Retention device

CELLector
CD8 AIS C.

CellFIT acquisition system
CellFriendly cannula
Cellona resin plaster of Paris bandage
cellophane dressing
CellPlant stent
CellPrep sample preparation system
cell-seeded stent
CellSpray spray-on skin
Cell-Tak autologous fibrin
Cell-Track
celltrifuge
CritSpin c.
c. device

cellular
c. debris centrifuge polarizing microscope
c. wrinkle filler

celluloid implant material
cellulose surgical sponge
Celluron dental roll
Cellvizio-GI endoscopic imaging system
Cell-VU disposable semen analysis chamber
celoscope
Celsite implanted port
Celsius
C. catheter
C. Control intravascular cooling catheter system
C. thermometer

Cemax/Icon
C./I. PACS system
C./I. scanner

cement
acrylic c.
antibiotic-loaded acrylic c.
Ava-Tex bone c.
bioactive bone c.
biodegradable calcium phosphate c.
bone c.
Boneloc c.
BoneSource hydroxyapatite c.
C&B-Metabond adhesive resin c.
Cemex Genta bone c.
c. centralizer
Ceramlin dental c.
Ceramsave dental c.
Cobalt G-HV high-contrast bone c.
Cobalt HV high-contrast bone c.
composite dental c.
Concert spine VR bone c.
copper phosphate c.
c. curette
dental c.
DePuy CMW 1 bone c.
dermatome c.
Diaket root canal c.
Duall 88 c.
Durelon dental c.
Eastman dental c.
Endurance bone c.
Freegenol c.
glass ionomer c.
Howmedica Simplex P c.
hydroxyapatite c.
hydroxyapatite-coated porous alumni c.
Implast bone c.
inorganic dental c.
Ketac Fil c.
Ketac Silver c.
Kirkland c.
KyphX HV-R bone c.
low-viscosity bone c.
master c.
modified zinc oxide-eugenol c.
Nogenol dental c.
Norian SRS c.
organic dental c.
Orthocomp c.
orthodontic c.
orthopaedic c.
Orthoset radiopaque bone c.
Osteobond copolymer bone c.
Palacos radiopaque bone c.
Palacos R bone c.
polycarboxylate c.
polymethylmethacrylate bone c.
pressurized c.

cement *(continued)*
>Pronto c.
>prosthetic antibiotic-loaded
>>acrylic c.
>radiopaque bone c.
>c. removal hand chisel
>resin c.
>c. restrictor
>c. restrictor inserter
>Shofu dental c.
>silicate c.
>Simplex P bone c.
>SmartSet HV bone c.
>c. spacer inserter
>c. spatula
>SRS/CRS c.
>SRS injectable c.
>Sulfix-6 c.
>SuperEBA c.
>Surgical Simplex P bone c.
>Surgical Simplex P radiopaque
>>bone c.
>temporary dental c.
>tooth c.
>Torbot c.
>TotalBond 4-Meta c.
>unmodified zinc oxide-eugenol c.
>VersaBond medium-viscosity
>>bone c.
>Vitrebond c.
>Wacker Sil-Gel 604 silicone c.
>Zimmer bone c.
>zinc phosphate c.

cemental spike
cementless
>c. prosthesis
>c. Sportorno hip arthroplasty stem
>>device

Cemex
>C. Genta bone cement
>C. system

CEM handswitching nosecone
Cencit
>C. facial scanner
>C. imaging system
>C. surface scanner

Cenflex central monitoring system
CenSlide 2000 urinalysis system
Centauri Er:YAG dental laser system
Centec
>C. Formfit ankle brace
>C. Propoint knee brace

center
>Veterans Administration
>>Prosthetics C. (VAPC)

center-action forceps
CenterFlex graft
centering
>c. balloon

>c. drill
>c. ring

Centermark vascular access device
CenterPointLock 2-piece ostomy system
centigrade thermometer
centimeter subtraction ruler
Centimist nebulizer
Centocor CA 125 radioimmunoassay kit
central
>c. blunt-tipped mammoscope
>c. caged ball occluder valve
>c. caged disc occluder valve
>c. core wire
>c. DXA bone densitometry system
>c. hyperalimentation
>c. line
>c. retinal lens
>c. retinal vein occlusion knife
>c. terminal electrode
>c. venous access device
>c. venous catheter
>c. venous line
>c. venous pressure
>c. venous pressure catheter

Centralign precoat hip prosthesis
centralizer
>cement c.
>Integral distal c.
>PMMA c.

Centrax bipolar system
Centrica rotational core biopsy system
Centricon-10 filter
Centriflow membrane cone
centrifugal pump
centrifuge
>Allegra 64R high-speed refrigerated
>>benchtop c.
>Allegra 25R refrigerated
>>benchtop c.
>Allegra X-12, X-15R, X-22
>>benchtop c.
>Avanti J-20XP, J-25, J-30I, J-HC,
>>J-E c.
>Beckman J-6M c.
>CritSpin microhematocrit c.
>CytoFuge 2 c.
>Eppendorf 5702 c.
>Ficoll-Hypaque density gradient c.
>HemataSTAT Easy Read c.
>J6-HC, J6-MC, J6-MI high
>>capacity c.
>MicroMax c.
>MicroPrep 2 c.
>c. microscope
>PK110 c.
>Spinchron DLX, 15 series c.
>Stat-60 c.
>StatSpin Express 2 c.

StatSpin MP c.
StatSpin MP multipurpose c.
Centrix-type syringe
Centronic 200 MGA respiratory mass spectrometer
Centry dialysis unit
Centurion
    C. needleless catheter extension
    C. PTA balloon dilatation catheter
    C. PTA dilatation catheter
    C. SES microkeratome
    C. SiteGuard MVP transparent film
    C. SorbaView composite dressing
    C. SorbaView window dressing
Century
    C. bicarbonate dialysis control unit
    C. birthing chair
    C. heart-lung machine
    C. urodynamics chair
CEP
    CEP 12 SpectrumOrange DNA probe kit
    CEP X, Y SpectrumOrange DNA probe kit
cephalad catheter
cephalometer
    Bertillon c.
cephalometric
    c. protractor
    c. viewer
cephalostat
    Porta-Stat c.
cephalotribe
    Tarnier c.
Ceprate
    C. SC Instrument II
    C. SC stem cell concentration system
CEQ 8000, 8800 genetic analysis system
CerAdapt
Ceradelta alloy
Cera-Fine
Ceralas
    C. I laser
    C. PDT 633 diode laser system
Ceralink slit lamp laser adapter
Ceramalloy alloy
ceramic
    alumina c.
    c. bearing
    c. biomaterial
    chairside economical restoration of esthetic c.
    c. endosteal implant
    c. femoral head prosthesis
    c. implant
    machinable apatite-free glass c.
    c. magnet

    c. ossicular prosthesis
    c. vertebral spacer
ceramics
    bioactive glass c.
    biocompatible nonresorbable glass c.
Ceramion prosthesis
Ceramlin dental cement
ceramometal implant bridge
Ceramsave dental cement
CeraOne
    C. abutment
    C. abutment implant
    C. implant system
Cerapall alloy
Cerasorb resorbable synthetic bone void filler
Ceraspect camera
Ceravital incus replacement prosthesis
cerclage
    Howmedica c.
    McDonald c.
    c. wire
    c. wire twister
cerebellar
    c. attachment
    c. electrode
    c. retractor
Cereblate catheter
cerebral
    c. ablation catheter
    c. angiography needle
    c. function monitor
    c. retractor
Cercbrograph
cerebrospinal fluid shunt
Cerrobend
    C. block
    C. casting
    C. trim block
cerumen curette
Cervex-Brush
    C.-B. cervical cell collector
    C.-B. cervical cell sampler
cervical
    c. AOA halo traction
    c. biopsy blade
    c. biopsy curette
    c. biopsy forceps
    c. block kit
    c. cannula
    c. cap
    c. clamp
    c. collar
    c. collar brace
    c. cone knife
    c. cushion
    c. dilator
    c. disc retractor

C

cervical *(continued)*
  c. drill
  c. immobilization device (CID)
  c. mallet
  c. orthosis (CO)
  c. pedicle screw
  c. pillow
  c. plate
  c. punch
  c. punch forceps
  c. range-of-motion device
  c. range-of-motion instrument
  c. rest
  c. roll
  c. rongeur
  c. saddle
  c. skull pillow
  c. sleep pillow
  c. suture
  c. suture needle
  c. tenaculum
  c. thoracic orthosis
cervical/lumbar hammer
Cervical-Stim cervical bone growth stimulator
cervical-thoracic-lumbar orthosis
cervical-thoracic-lumbar-sacral orthosis
cervicothoracic
  c. jacket
  c. orthosis (CTO)
cervicothoracolumbosacral orthosis
Cer-View lateral vaginal retractor
CerviFix system
CerviSoft cytology collection device
Cervitrak device
Cervive anterior cervical plating system
cesarean forceps
cesium
  c. applicator
  c. candle
  c. cylinder
  c. needle
  c. source
cesium-137 wire
CF-200Z Olympus colonoscope
CF-60DSi fundus camera
CFA digital camera
CFC BioScanner system
CFC-free product
CF indicator system chloride patch
C-Flex
  C-F. Amsterdam stent
  C-F. catheter
  REMstar Plus with C-F.
  REMstar Pro with C-F.
  C-F. supine cervical traction
  C-F. ureteral stent

C-flex
  C-f. catheter
  C-f. stent
CFS
  contoured femoral stem
  CFS hip prosthesis
CF100TL
  Olympus C.
CF-UM3 echocolonoscope
CFV wrist component
^{14}C-glycocholate breath test
CGR biplane angiographic system
C-guide
  screw placement C-g.
Chadwick scissors
Chaffin-Pratt drain
chain
  c. saw
  wheelchair c.
chair
  Bárány c.
  bedside air c.
  birthing c.
  BodyBilt c.
  Century birthing c.
  Century urodynamics c.
  combination stretcher c.
  Combisit surgeon's c.
  computerized rotary c.
  dynamic integrated stabilization c.
  EasyChair massage c.
  ergonomically correct c.
  EZ Rider support c.
  fluoroscopic imaging c.
  Gardner c.
  geriatric c.
  Invacare padded shower c.
  invalid c.
  Kaleidoscope c.
  Midmark 413 power female procedure c.
  mobile air c.
  OB/GYN c.
  Orthokinetics travel c.
  Pogon c.
  Portal Pro 2 treatment c.
  recliner air c.
  reclining c.
  shower c.
  Sirocco evacuation c.
  sit/stand c.
  stair c.
  STC 900-series travel c.
  Vess c.
  videofluoroscopic imaging c.
chairback
  c. brace
  c. lumbosacral orthosis
ChairCiser adjustable exerciser

chairside economical restoration of esthetic ceramic
Chajchir dissector
chalazion
  c. clamp
  c. curette
  c. forceps
  c. knife
  c. trephine
Challenger digital applanation tonometer
chamber
  AeroChamber Plus valved
    holding c.
  air c.
  aluminum Finn c.
  anterior c. (AC)
  Bactron 1.5 anaerobic c.
  Barron artificial anterior c.
  Barron disposable artificial
    anterior c.
  Boyden c.
  Bürker c.
  Cell-VU disposable semen
    analysis c.
  drill c.
  drip c.
  dual c.
  EasiVent valved holding c.
  Finn c.
  Fisher-Paykel MR290 water-feed c.
  flush c.
  Fuchs-Rosenthal c.
  hydraulic c.
  hyperbaric c.
  hyperbaric oxygen c.
  Hyper-Oxy portable hyperbaric c.
  Makler counting c.
  Makler reusable semen analysis c.
  Microcell c.
  MoistAir humidifying c.
  moisture c.
  Monoplace hyperbaric c.
  MR 290 humidification c.
  multicorneal perfusion c.
  multiplace c.
  multiwire proportional c.
  OptiChamber valved holding c.
  parallel-plate flow c.
  Petroff-Hauser counting c.
  plasma clot diffusion c.
  portable topical hyperbaric oxygen
    extremity c.
  Pudenz flushing c.
  reentrant well c.
  respiratory c.
  Sechrist monoplace hyperbaric c.
  Shandon Cytospin c.
  Sigma II Dualplace hyperbaric c.
  Sigma 34 monoplace hyperbaric c.

  Symphony I/C graft c.
  Ussing c.
  valved holding c. (VHC)
  Van der Bend c.
  well-type ionization c.
Chamberlen obstetrical forceps
ChamberLift 2000 patient lift system
Chameleon Cooler
chamfer
  c. guide
  c. reamer
Chamois
  C. swab
  C. underpad
Champ
  C. CTS cold therapy wrap
  C. elastic bandage
  C. Insulated Propac II
Champetier de Ribes bag
Champion
  C. Power Sox
  C. stent system
Championnière
  C. bone drill
  C. forceps
Champy miniplate rigid fixation system
Chana EZ clean reamer handle
chandelier illumination system
Chandler
  C. bone elevator
  C. iris forceps
  C. knee retractor
  C. spinal perforating forceps
  C. unreamed interlocking tibial nail
  C. V-pacing probe
Chang
  C. combination phaco chopper
  C. combo chopper
  C. hydrodissection cannula
  C. pin clamp
  C. Quick Chop combo
  C. Quick Chop combo ophthalmic
    instrument
changer
  film c.
  Littmann Galilean magnification c.
  Puck film c.
  Sanchez-Perez cassette c.
  Schonander film c.
  tracheal tube c.
  tube c.
channel
  c. dissector
  c. retractor
2-channel
  2-c. Badal optical system
  2-c. phased-array RF receiver coil
    system

4-channel
4-c. Aesculap ventriculoscope
4-c. transcranial Doppler monitor
8-channel
8-c. muscle stimulator
8-c. whole-head magnetometer
Chan wrist rest
Chaoul voltage x-ray tube
Chaput tissue forceps
charcoal filter
Charcot
C. bath
C. restraint orthotic walker
Charcot-Bottcher filament
Chardack-Greatbatch
C.-G. implantable cardiac pulse
generator
C.-G. pacemaker
Chardack Medtronic pacemaker
char-free carbon dioxide laser
charge-coupled
c.-c. device
c.-c. device endoscope
c.-c. device monochrome camera
c.-c. device scanner
c.-c. device TV camera
c.-c. device video camera
c.-c. device videocamera
Charité
C. artificial disc
C. artificial disc system
Charles
C. anterior segment sleeve
C. flute needle
C. handheld infusion lens
C. infusion sleeve
C. intraocular lens
C. vacuuming needle
Charleston
C. brace
C. nighttime bending brace
C. scoliosis brace
Charnley
C. acetabular cup
C. acetabular scraper
C. bone curette
C. cemented hip prosthesis
C. centering ring
C. compression apparatus
C. deepening reamer
C. expanding reamer
C. external fixation clamp
C. external fixation device
C. femoral broach
C. femoral condyle radius gauge
C. femoral inlay aligner
C. femoral inlay guillotine
C. femoral prosthesis neck punch
C. flat-back femoral component

C. foam suture pad
C. hip prosthesis
C. horizontal retractor
C. implant
C. initial incision retractor
C. introducer
C. knee retractor
C. offset-bore cup
C. self-retaining retractor
C. socket gauge
C. starting drill
C. suction drain
C. suture button
C. suture forceps
C. taper reamer
C. template
C. tibial onlay jig
C. total hip prosthesis
C. trochanter holder
C. trochanter reamer
C. wire-holding forceps
C. wire passer
C. wire tightener
Charnley-Hastings prosthesis
Charnley-Howorth Exflow system
Charnley-Mueller hip prosthesis
Charriere
C. amputation saw
C. aseptic metacarpal saw
C. bone saw
chart
Amsler c.
Aurora luminous acuity c.
Bailey-Lovie test c.
Birkhauser eye testing c.
body mechanics examination c.
Broselow c.
contemporary nearpoint c.
cross-Polaroid projection c.
ETDRS acuity c.
Ferris c.
Hawley c.
illiterate E c.
Jaeger eye c.
Jaeger reading c.
Landolt-C acuity c.
Lea Symbol c.
Lebensohn c.
Lighthouse ET-DRS acuity c.
logMAR c.
Mentor B-VAT visual acuity c.
Pelli-Robson letter c.
Regan low-contrast acuity c.
sclerotome pain c.
Snellen c.
Snellen acuity c.
tumbling E c.
Vistech wall c.
Welch Allyn SureSight eye c.

Chaston eye pad
Chatillon
    C. digital force gauge
    C. dolorimeter
Chattanooga
    C. Balance system
    C. traction
    C. traction device
Chaussier tube
Chavasse strabismus hook
Chayes handpiece
Chayet corneal marker
Chayet-type corneal LASIK marker
CHD prosthesis
Cheatle sterilizing forceps
Checkerboard wheelchair cushion
Check-Flo
    C.-F. introducer
    C.-F. performer introducer set for
      radial artery access
    C.-F. sheath obturator
Checklist
Checkmate
    C. gamma brachytherapy system
    C. gamma radiation system
    C. system
check socket
check-valve sheath
cheek retractor
Cheetah
    C. angioplasty catheter
    C. ankle brace
cheiroscope
Chelex
    C. bead
    C. resin
Chelsea-Eaton anal speculum
chemical
    c. agent monitor
    c. detection equipment
chemiluminescent
    c. probe
    c. substrate kit
ChemMate capillary gap slide
ChemoBloc vial venting system
chemonucleolysis table
Chemo-Port
    C.-P. catheter
    C.-P. perivena catheter system
      device
    C.-P. vascular access system
chemosterilized graft
Chemstrip
    C. bG
    C. dipstick
    C. LN dipstick
    C. MatchMaker blood glucose
      meter

ChemTrak
    C. AccuMeter
    C. AccuMeter theophylline test
CHEMXpress system
Cherf
    C. cast stand
    C. legholder
Chermel
    C. bone gouge
    C. osteotome
Cheron uterine dressing forceps
Cherry
    C. osteotome
    C. traction tongs
chest
    c. dressing
    c. shell
    c. strap
    c. tube
chest-band transmitter
Chevalier
    C. Jackson esophagoscope
    C. Jackson gastroscope
    C. Jackson laryngeal speculum
Chewrite denture adhesive
Cheyne
    C. dissector
    C. periosteal elevator
CHI
    cannulated hemi-implant
    CHI system
Chiba
    C. biopsy needle
    C. eye needle
    C. needle
Chicco breast pump
Chick
    C. CLT operating frame
    C. CLT operating table
    C. sterile dressing
    C. surgical table
chicken-bill rongeur forceps
Chick-Foster orthopaedic bed
Chick-Langren table
Chiesi powder inhaler
child
    c. esophagoscope
    C. intestinal forceps
children
    C.'s EarPlanes earplug
    C.'s Hospital brain spatula
    C.'s Hospital intestinal forceps
    c.'s mat
    Total Knee for C.
child-resistant container
child-restraint device
Childs-Phillips intestinal plication needle

C

Chilli
C. cooled ablation system
C. cooled-tip ablation catheter
Chill Tip cooling handpiece
chin
extended anatomical c.
c. implant
c. support
China ink
Chinese
C. fingertrap suture
C. fingertrap traction device
C. fingertrap tube
ChinUpps cervicofacial support
Chin-Up strip
Chiou SP tube introducer
chip
chlorhexidine c.
Dembone demineralized
  cancellous c.
Dembone demineralized cortical c.
Dembone demineralized
  corticocancellous c.
DNA microarray c.
chipped-tooth broach
Chiroflex C11UB lens
Chiroflow
C. adjustable back support
C. back rest
Chiro-Manis chiropractic table
Chiron
C. ACS microkeratome
C. automated corneal shaper
C. Hansatome
C. Hansatome microkeratome
C. RIBA HCV test system second
  generation
chiropractic
c. mattress
c. table
chiroscope
Chiroslide
C. Jamar hand dynamometer
C. measuring device
Chirotech x-ray system
chirped-pulse amplification system
chisel
acetabular round c.
Adson laminectomy c.
Alexander c.
Alexander bone c.
Army c.
Austin Moore c.
beveled c.
bilevel c.
Biomet cement removal hand c.
Bishop c.
c. blade
Blair nasal c.

bone c.
Bruening c.
Brunetti c.
Buckley c.
cement removal hand c.
Clev-Dent-Wakefield c.
Cloward spinal fusion c.
Converse c.
Converse guarded c.
Converse guarded nasal c.
Converse nasal c.
cornea c.
Cottle c.
Cottle antral c.
Cottle curved c.
Cottle nasal c.
Councilman c.
curved c.
Dautrey c.
Derlacki-Shambaugh c.
D'Errico lamina c.
disarticulation c.
dissecting c.
double-guarded c.
double safe-sided c.
c. elevator
ethmoidal c.
Farrior-Derlacki c.
Faulkner-Browne c.
fishtail c.
Fomon c.
Fomon nasal c.
fracture c.
Freer c.
Freer bone c.
Freer lacrimal c.
Freer nasal c.
Freer submucous c.
French c.
frontal sinus c.
Gardner bone c.
Goldman guarded c.
gold-paneled c.
gooseneck c.
guarded c.
Hajek c.
Hajek septal c.
Halle c.
Harmon c.
Hatch c.
Henderson bone c.
Hibbs bone c.
hollow c.
Holmes c.
Joseph c.
Keyes bone-splitting c.
Killian frontal sinus c.
Kilner c.
lacrimal sac c.

Lambert-Lowman c.
Lambotte bone c.
laminectomy c.
Lebsche sternal c.
Lexer c.
Lorenz c.
Lowman c.
Lowman-Hoglund c.
Lucas c.
MacAusland c.
Magnum c.
Mannerfelt c.
Martin cartilage c.
mastoid c.
McIndoe nasal c.
meniscotomy c.
Metzenbaum c.
middle ear c.
Miles bone c.
monoangle c.
mortising c.
nasal c.
orthopaedic c.
Partsch c.
Partsch bone c.
Passow c.
Pearson c.
Pick c.
pterygoid c.
Puka c.
Rollet c.
Rubin nasal c.
Schwartze c.
septal c.
Sheehan c.
single safe-sided c.
sinus c.
Skoog nasal c.
Smillie cartilage c.
Smillie meniscectomy c.
Smith-Petersen c.
spinal fusion c.
splitting c.
stapes c.
Stille bone c.
straight c.
submucous c.
c. tip
Trautmann c.
twin-pattern c.
unibevel c.
U.S. Army bone c.
Virchow c.
vulcanite c.
West bone c.
West lacrimal c.
West nasal c.
White bone c.
ChiselTip suction cautery device

chisel-tip wire
Chito-Seal topical hemostasis pad
chlorhexidine chip
chloridometer
    coulometric c.
Cho/Dyonics 2-portal endoscope
Choice
    Medi-Jector C.
    C. PT exchange wire
    C. PT guidewire
    C. PT plus wire
choice
    Medi-Jector C.
Cholangiocath catheter
cholangiocatheter
cholangioclamp
cholangiography
    c. catheter
    c. clamp
cholangiograsper
    Storz c.
cholangiopancreatogram
    endoscopic retrograde c. (ERCP)
cholangioscope
    adoptable baby c.
    Olympus CHF-Q10 c.
    prototype c.
cholecystostomy tube
choledochocystonephrofiberscope
choledochofiberscope
    Olympus CHF-BP30
      transduodenal c.
    Olympus URF-P2
      translaparoscopic c.
choledochoscope
    fiberoptic c.
    Olympus CHF-P20 c.
    Olympus XCHF-37 c.
choledochoscope-nephroscope
    Storz c.-n.
cholesterol
    C. Manager
    c. 1, 2, 3 noninvasive testing
    device
CholesTrak
Chondrogel
chondroplastic blade
chondroplasty Beaver blade
chondrotome
    Stryker c.
Cho-Pat
    C.-P. Achilles tendon strap
    C.-P. dual action knee strap
    C.-P. elbow strap
    C.-P. ITB strap
    C.-P. knitted compression support
CHOP frame
Cho 2-portal Dyonics endoscope

C

chopper
    Agarwal irrigating phaco c.
    Chang combination phaco c.
    Chang combo c.
    combination phaco c.
    Davidoff ambidextrous nucleus c.
    Dodick-Kammann bimanual c.
    Dodick nucleus irrigating c.
    dull-tipped horizontal c.
    Fine irrigating reverse actuating
      splitting c.
    Fine-Nagahara phaco c.
    Fine sideport actuating quick c.
    Fukasaku snap & split-tip
      irrigating c.
    Inamura race c.
    irrigating c.
    Katena MicroFinger tip irrigating c.
    Koch c.
    Koch-Minami c.
    Lane quick c.
    Langerman bidirectional phaco c.
    Langerman bi-directional phaco c.
    McIlwain tissue c.
    Minardi phaco c.
    Miyoshi c.
    Nagahara karate c.
    Nagahara phaco c.
    Nagahara quick c.
    Nichamin I and II nucleus
      quick c.
    Nichamin I, II nucleus quick c.
    Nichamin quick c.
    Nichamin triple c.
    Nichamin vertical c.
    Olson phaco c.
    Olson quick c.
    Seibel nucleus c.
    Seibel vertical safety quick c.
    Shepherd Tomahawk c.
    Steinert double-ended claw c.
    Steinert II claw c.
    Sung reverse nucleus c.
    Tsuneoka irrigating c.
chopper/manipulator
    Universal phaco c./m.
Chorus
    C. DDD pacemaker
    C. RM rate-responsive dual-
      chamber pacemaker
Choyce
    C. lens-inserting forceps
    C. Mark VIII implant
    C. Mark VIII lens
Choyce-Tennant lens
Christensen
    C. articulator
    C. TMJ prosthesis system
Christmas tree adapter

Christoudias fascial closure device
ChromaMeter CR-200 handheld
    colorimeter
Chromaser dermatology laser
chromated catgut suture
chromatograph
    Carle analytic gas c.
    column c.
    gas c.
    high-performance liquid c.
    high-pressure liquid c.
    ion c.
    QuinTron Microlyzer 12 c.
    solid-phase extraction c.
    thin-layer c.
    Varian gas c.
chromatoptometer
chromatoskiameter
ChromaVision digital analyzer
chrome-cobalt
    c.-c. cable
    c.-c. screw
Chromel-Alumel thermocouple
chromic
    c. blue dyed suture
    c. catgut suture
    c. collagen suture
    c. gut suture
    c. suture
chromicized catgut suture
chromium-cobalt alloy implant
chromoendoscope
chromophore-enhanced laser welding
Chromos imager system
ChromoVision video system
chronaximeter
Chronicle implantable hemodynamic
    monitor
Chronicure
    C. protein hydrolysate powder
    C. wound dressing
ChronoFlex catheter
Chrono-log
    C.-l. optical aggregometer
    C.-l. platelet aggregometer
chronolog
    nebulizer c.
Chronos 04 pacemaker
CHRYS CO$_2$ laser
CHS
    compression hip screw
Chubby balloon catheter
chuck
    AE surgical contraangle 20:1 press-
      button c.
    EA surgical contraangle 10:1 press-
      button c.
    E/200 contraangle 1:5 press-
      button c.

F/KM surgical contraangle 40:1
  press-button c.
gold-handled c.
Jacobs T-handled c.
pin c.
press-button c.
T-handle Jacob c.
Trinkle c.

Chu foldable lens cutter
Chukka boot
Chulalongkorn University vacuum device
Church deep surgery scissors
Chuter endovascular device
Chux incontinent dressing
Ciaglia
  C. Blue Rhino percutaneous
    tracheostomy introducer set
  C. percutaneous tracheostomy
    introducer
  C. percutaneous tracheostomy
    introducer set

Ciba-Corning 2500 co-oximeter
CibaSoft Visitint contact lens
Ciba TearSaver punctal gauging system
Cibathin lens
CIC
  completely in canal
  CIC hearing aid
  CIC listening device
Cica-Care
  C.-C. adhesive silicone gel
  C.-C. silicone gel sheet dressing
  C.-C. topical gel sheeting
  C.-C. wound dressing
Cicherelli bone rongeur
CID
  cervical immobilization device
  CID camera
CIDA foam
CIDS
  continuous insulin delivery system
Cidtech camera
CIF4 needle
CIF needle
CI functional knee brace
cigarette drain
Cilco
  C. argon laser
  C. Frigitronics laser
  C. Hoffer Lascridge
  C. krypton laser
  C. YAG laser
ciliary neurotrophic factor capsule protein eye implant
cilium, pl. **cilia**
  c. pacemaker
  cilia suture forceps
CIMA*flex* 411 foldable silicone lens

Cimino
  C. arteriovenous shunt
  C. AV shunt
  C. dialysis shunt
  C. fistula
Cimino-Brescia arteriovenous fistula
Cimochowski cardiac cannula
cinch
  C. bladder neck suspension anchor
    system
  C. instant suction B.K. prosthesis
  C. instant suction prosthesis
  joint c.
  C. Lock CTS brace
Cincinnati Sub-Zero (CSZ)
cine
  c. arthrogram
  c. camera
  c. CT scanner
  c. scan
cinearthrography
  triple-injection c.
Cinelli osteotome
Cineloop
  C. image review ultrasound system
  C. memory function
  C. ultrasound
cine-MRI
CineView Plus Freeland system
Cintor
  C. bone rongeur
  C. knee prosthesis
Cionni capsular tension ring
CipherGen Express software biomarker analysis system
Circadia dual-chamber rate-adaptive pacemaker
circadian
  c. event recorder
  c. pacemaker
CircAid elastic stocking
Circe device
circle
  Bain c.
  c. bed
  c. knife
  pediatric c.
  Randot c.
Circline magnifier
circline magnifier
CircOlectric bed
Circon
  C. ACMI diagnostic laparoscope
  C. video camera
  C. videocamera
Circon-ACMI
  C.-ACMI cannula
  C.-ACMI electrohydraulic
    lithotriptor probe

C

Circon-ACMI *(continued)*
  C.-ACMI endoscope
  C.-ACMI hysteroscope
  C.-ACMI lithotriptor
  C.-ACMI MicroDigital-I camera
  C.-ACMI miniscope
  C.-ACMI trocar
  C.-ACMI ureteroscope
  C.-ACMI USL-2000 rigid device
CircPlus
  C. bandage/wrap system
  C. leg compression dressing
  C. wrap
circuit
  c. adapter
  Carmeda BioActive surface
    extracorporeal c.
  FilterLine c.
  Intertech anesthesia breathing c.
  Intertech nonrebreathing modified
    Jackson-Rees c.
  Jackson-Rees c.
  low-flow c.
  Magill c.
  multipurpose breathing c.
  phototube output c.
  Pulmanex PAC pulmonary assist c.
  quad resonance NMR probe c.
  sensing c.
  shunting c.
  timing c.
Circulaire
  C. aerosol drug delivery device
  C. aerosol drug delivery system
  C. inhaled medication delivery
    device
Circul'Air shoe process system
circular
  c. anal dilator
  c. bandage
  c. blade
  c. cup bronchoscopic biopsy
    forceps
  c. external fixator
  c. fine-wire external fixator
  c. fixation device
  c. intraluminal stapler
  c. mechanical stapler
  c. polarized volume head coil
  c. stapler
  c. stapling device
  c. suture
circularly polarized coil
circulating water blanket
circulator
  C. boot
  C. boot system
  sequential c.

Circulon
  C. dressing
  C. leg compression dressing
  C. System Step 1, 2 venous ulcer
    kit
  C. wrap
circumaortic
  c. venous collar
  c. venous ring
circumcision
  c. clamp
  Mogen c.
circumcisional
  c. shield
  c. suture
circumdental wire
circumductor table
circumferential
  c. dedicated knee coil
  c. dressing
  c. extremity coil
circumflex artery scissors
Circumstraint restraint
CirKuit-Guard
  C.-G. device
  C.-G. pressure relief valve
Cirrus
  C. composite prosthetic foot
  C. foot prosthesis
  C. foot prosthetic
cisternal-peritoneal shunt
cisternal-pleural shunt
cisterna magna catheter
Citelli
  C. punch forceps
  C. rongeur
  C. sphenoid rongeur
Citroclear
Civiale forceps
CKG
  cardiokymograph
CKS knee system
CLA echoendoscope
Claes scleral depressor
clamp
  Abadie enterostomy c.
  Acland microvascular c.
  Adson c.
  agraffe c.
  Alfred M. Large vena cava c.
  Allen anastomosis c.
  Allen intestinal c.
  Allis c.
  Allison c.
  anastomosis c.
  aneurysm c.
  angled DeBakey c.
  angled Lowman-type bone c.
  angled peripheral vascular c.

angular hinge c.
antishock pelvic c.
aortic aneurysm c.
aortic cannula c.
aortic occlusion c.
Apofix interlaminar c.
appendage c.
approximator c.
arterial c.
ASSI Microspike approximator c.
Atlee c.
Atra-Grip c.
atraumatic c.
atraumatic bowel c.
Babcock c.
baby pylorus c.
back c.
Backhaus c.
Backhaus-Kocher towel c.
Backhaus towel c.
Bahnson aortic c.
Bailey aortic c.
Bainbridge intestinal c.
Baker-David c.
Bard Cunningham incontinence c.
Barraquer needle holder c.
bar-to-bar c.
Baumrucker-DeBakey c.
Baumrucker urinary incontinence c.
Beardsley intestinal c.
Beck-Potts aortic and pulmonic c.
Beck vascular c.
Berens muscle c.
Berke c.
Berke ptosis c.
Bihrle dorsal c.
3-bladed c.
Blair cleft palate c.
Blalock pulmonary artery c.
bloodless circumcision c.
Böhler c.
Böhler os calcis c.
bone extension c.
bone-holding c.
Bradshaw-O'Neill aorta c.
Buie pile c.
bulldog c.
Buxton uterine c.
C c.
Calandruccio c.
calvarial c.
cannula c.
cardiovascular c.
cardiovascular bulldog c.
Carmault c.
Carmel c.
carotid artery c.
c. carrier
cartilage c.

Casey pelvic c.
Castaneda vascular c.
Castroviejo lid c.
Castroviejo needle holder c.
celiac c.
cervical c.
chalazion c.
Chang pin c.
Charnley external fixation c.
cholangiography c.
circumcision c.
Clark c.
Clevis c.
coarctation c.
Collins umbilical c.
colon c.
columella c.
contour block c.
Cooley anastomosis c.
Cooley aortic c.
Cooley aortic aneurysm c.
Cooley-Beck vessel c.
Cooley bronchus c.
Cooley bulldog c.
Cooley cross-action bulldog c.
Cooley-Derra anastomosis c.
Cooley iliac c.
Cooley patent ductus c.
Cooley pediatric vascular c.
Cooley peripheral vascular c.
Cooley renal artery c.
Cooley-Satinsky c.
Cooley vena cava c.
Cope crushing c.
Cope modification of Martel
  intestinal c.
Cosgrove c.
Cottle columella c.
cotton-roll rubber dam c.
Craafoord aortic c.
Craafoord coarctation c.
Crawford c.
Crile c.
Crile appendiceal c.
Crile hemostatic c.
cross-action towel c.
crushing c.
Crutchfield c.
Crutchfield carotid artery c.
Cunningham urinary incontinence c.
curved-8 c.
curved cardiovascular c.
curved Mayo c.
curved mosquito c.
Cygnet flexible c.
cystic duct catheter c.
Dandy c.
Dardik c.
D'Assumpcão marking c.

clamp *(continued)*
David-Baker lip c.
Davidson c.
Davidson pulmonary vessel c.
DeBakey aortic c.
DeBakey aortic aneurysm c.
DeBakey aortic exclusion c.
DeBakey arterial c.
DeBakey-Bahnson vascular c.
DeBakey-Bainbridge vascular c.
DeBakey bulldog c.
DeBakey-Crafoord vascular c.
DeBakey cross-action bulldog c.
DeBakey-Derra anastomosis c.
DeBakey-Harken auricular c.
DeBakey-Howard aortic
  aneurysm c.
DeBakey-Kay aortic c.
DeBakey-McQuigg-Mixter
  bronchial c.
DeBakey pediatric c.
DeBakey peripheral vascular c.
DeBakey ring-handled bulldog c.
DeBakey-Satinsky vena cava c.
DeBakey tangential occlusion c.
DeMartel-Wolfson anastomosis c.
Demos tibial artery c.
Dennis intestinal c.
Derra anastomosis c.
Derra aortic c.
Derra vena cava c.
Desmarres c.
Desmarres lid c.
DeWeese vena cava c.
Diethrich aortic c.
Diethrich bulldog c.
Dingman bone and cartilage c.
Dingman cartilage c.
disposable muscle biopsy c.
dissecting c.
distraction c.
Dixon-Thomas-Smith intestinal c.
double c.
double-angled c.
double approximating c.
double towel c.
Downes lid c.
Doyen intestinal c.
drape c.
dreamer c.
duckbill c.
ductus c.
Duval lung c.
Edna towel c.
Edwards c.
endoaortic c.
enterostomy c.
Erhardt lid c.
Ewing lid c.

exclusion c.
extension bone c.
extracutaneous vas fixation c.
Farabeuf-Lambotte bone-holding c.
Favaloro proximal anastomosis c.
Favorite c.
Fehland intestinal c.
Fehland right-angled colon c.
femoral c.
Ferrier 212 gingival c.
ferrule c.
fine-tooth c.
fine-toothed c.
Finochietto arterial c.
Finochietto bronchial c.
Fitzgerald aortic aneurysm c.
flexible aortic c.
flexible retractor pressure c.
flexible retractor sliding c.
flexible vascular c.
flow-regulator c.
Fogarty c.
Fogarty Hydragrip c.
c. forceps
Forrester c.
Foss anterior resection c.
Foss intestinal c.
Frazier-Adson osteoplastic flap c.
Frazier-Sachs c.
full-curved c.
Furniss-Clute duodenal c.
Gandy c.
Gant c.
Garcia aortic c.
Gaskell c.
gastric c.
gastroenterostomy c.
gastrointestinal c.
Gemini c.
Gerster bone c.
GI c.
gingival c.
Gladstone-Putterman transmarginal
  rotation entropion c.
Glassman c.
Glassman bowel atraumatic c.
Glassman intestinal c.
Glassman noncrushing
  gastroenterostomy c.
Glassman noncrushing
  gastrointestinal c.
Glover auricular c.
Glover bulldog c.
Glover curved c.
Glover-DeBakey c.
Glover patent ductus c.
Glover spoon-shaped anastomosis c.
Glover-Stille c.
Glover vascular c.

goiter c.
Goldblatt c.
Goldstein Microspike
  approximator c.
Gomco c.
Gomco bell c.
Gomco bloodless circumcision c.
Gomco circumcision c.
Gomco umbilical c.
Goodwin bone c.
Grafco incontinence c.
Grafco umbilical cord c.
graft c.
Grant abdominal aortic
  aneurysmal c.
grasping c.
Gray c.
Greenberg c.
Green bulldog c.
Green lid c.
Gregory carotid bulldog c.
Gregory external c.
Gregory stay suture c.
Gregory vascular miniature c.
Grover c.
gut c.
Guyon kidney c.
Guyon-Péan vessel c.
Guyon vessel c.
Haberer intestinal c.
Halifax interlaminar c.
Halsted c.
Halsted curved mosquito c.
Halsted straight mosquito c.
Harken auricular c.
Harrington hook c.
Harrington-Mixter thoracic c.
Harrington rod c.
Hartmann c.
Hatch c.
Hausmann vascular c.
Haverhill c.
Hayes anterior resection c.
Hayes colon c.
Hayes intestinal c.
Heaney c.
Heartport endoaortic c.
hemorrhoidal c.
hemostatic c.
Hendren c.
Hendren megaureter c.
Hendren ureteral c.
Henley subclavian artery c.
Henley vascular c.
Herrick kidney c.
Herrick pedicle c.
Hex-Fix Universal swivel c.
Hibbs c.
hilar c.

Hirsch mucosal c.
Hoffmann c.
Hoffmann ligament c.
Hoff towel c.
Hohmann c.
c. holder
Hollister c.
Holter pump c.
hook c.
Hopkins aortic occlusion c.
Hopkins hysterectomy c.
Hudson c.
Hufnagel aortic c.
Hunt c.
Hunt colostomy c.
Hurwitz intestinal c.
hysterectomy c.
ICSI Massachusetts c.
iliac c.
incontinence c.
c. insert
interlaminar c.
intestinal anastomosis c.
intestinal occlusion c.
intestinal resection c.
intestinal ring c.
Intrack XT c.
isoelastic rip c.
ivory rubber dam c.
Jackson bone c.
Jacobs c.
Jacobson bulldog c.
Jacobson microbulldog c.
Jacobson vessel c.
Jako c.
Jansen c.
Jarit anterior resection c.
Jarit cartilage c.
Jarit intestinal c.
Jarvis pile c.
Javid bypass c.
Javid carotid c.
Johns Hopkins bulldog c.
Johns Hopkins coarctation c.
Johns Hopkins modified Potts c.
Johnston c.
Jones thoracic c.
Jones towel c.
Joseph septal c.
Judd c.
Judd-Allis c.
Julian-Damian c.
Kalt needle holder c.
Kane umbilical cord c.
Kantor circumcision c.
Kantrowitz hemostatic c.
Kantrowitz thoracic c.
Kapp-Beck bronchial c.
Kapp-Beck coarctation c.

C

clamp *(continued)*
Kapp-Beck colon c.
Kaufman kidney c.
Kay aortic anastomosis c.
Kelly c.
Kelsey pile c.
Kern bone-holding c.
Khan-Jaeger c.
Khodadad c.
kidney pedicle c.
Kindt arterial c.
Kindt carotid artery c.
King c.
Kleinert-Kutz c.
Knutsson penile c.
Koala vascular c.
Kocher c.
Kocher intestinal c.
Kolodny c.
Ladd lid c.
Lahey c.
Lahey bronchial c.
Lahey thoracic c.
Lalonde bone c.
Lalonde oblique fracture large
  bone c.
Lalonde oblique fracture medium
  bone c.
Lalonde oblique metacarpal fracture
  bone c.
Lalonde small bone c.
Lambert aortic c.
Lambert-Kay aortic c.
Lambert-Kay vascular c.
Lambert-Lowman bone c.
Lambotte bone-holding c.
Lamis patellar c.
c. lamp
Lane bone-holding c.
Lane gastroenterostomy c.
Lane intestinal c.
Lane towel c.
laparoscopic Allis c.
Large vena cava c.
Lee bronchus c.
Lee microvascular c.
Lees vascular c.
Lees wedge resection c.
Leland-Jones vascular c.
Lem-Blay circumcision c.
Lewin bone-holding c.
lid c.
Liddle aorta c.
ligament c.
Lillie rectus tendon c.
Lindner anastomosis c.
Linnartz intestinal c.
Linnartz stomach c.
Linton tourniquet c.

lion-jaw c.
lip c.
liver-holding c.
Lloyd-Davies c.
lobster-type c.
locking c.
Lockwood c.
Lorna nonperforating towel c.
Lowman bone-holding c.
Lowman-Hoglund c.
lung exclusion c.
Macdonald gastric c.
Madden intestinal c.
Maingot c.
Malgaigne c.
Malis hinge c.
marginal c.
marking c.
Martel c.
Martel intestinal c.
Martin cartilage c.
Martin muscle c.
Mason vascular c.
Masters intestinal c.
Masterson pelvic c.
Masters-Schwartz intestinal c.
Masters-Schwartz liver c.
Mastin muscle c.
Matthew cross-leg c.
Mattox aorta c.
Mayfield aneurysm c.
Mayfield head c.
Mayfield 3-pin skull c.
May kidney c.
Mayo-Guyon kidney c.
Mayo-Guyon vessel c.
Mayo kidney c.
Mayo-Lovelace spur crushing c.
Mayo-Robson intestinal c.
Mayo vessel c.
McCleery-Miller intestinal
  anastomosis c.
McCullough hysterectomy c.
McDonald gastric c.
McDougal prostatectomy c.
McGuire c.
McKenzie c.
McLean c.
McNealey-Glassman-Mixter c.
McQuigg c.
meatal c.
medial malleolar/small bone
  fragment c.
Meeker gallstone c.
Meeker right-angle c.
megaureter c.
meniscal c.
metal wing c.
microarterial c.

microbulldog c.
Microspike approximator c.
microvascular c.
Mikulicz peritoneal c.
Millard c.
Millin T c.
miniature bulldog c.
Mixter ligature-carrier c.
Mogen c.
Mogen circumcision c.
Mohr pinchcock c.
Moreno gastroenterostomy c.
mosquito c.
mosquito hemostatic c.
mosquito lid c.
mouse-tooth c.
Moynihan c.
Moynihan towel c.
Mueller vena cava c.
multipurpose c.
muscle c.
muscle biopsy c.
Myles hemorrhoidal c.
Naraghi-DeCoster reduction c.
needle holder c.
neonatal vascular c.
nephrostomy c.
nerve-approximating c.
noncrushing bowel c.
noncrushing intestinal c.
noncrushing vascular c.
nonperforating towel c.
Noon AV fistula c.
Nussbaum intestinal c.
OBrien bone c.
occluding c.
occlusive c.
Ochsner c.
O'Connor lid c.
Olivecrona aneurysm c.
Olsen cholangiogram c.
ossicle-holding c.
osteoplastic flap c.
padded c.
parametrium c.
Parker-Kerr intestinal c.
partial occlusion c.
patellar cement c.
patent ductus c.
Payr gastrointestinal c.
Payr pylorus c.
Payr resection c.
Payr stomach c.
Péan hemostatic c.
Péan hysterectomy c.
Péan intestinal c.
Péan vessel c.
pediatric bulldog c.
pediatric vascular c.

pedicle c.
Peers towel c.
pelvic c.
Pemberton spur-crushing c.
penile c.
Pennington c.
Percy c.
peripheral vascular c.
peritoneal c.
phalangeal c.
Phaneuf c.
Phillips rectal c.
pile c.
pin c.
pinchcock c.
pin-to-bar c.
Pitanguy marking c.
placental c.
Plastibell circumcision c.
point-of-reduction c.
Potts aortic c.
Presbyterian Hospital occluding c.
Presbyterian Hospital tubing c.
Prince muscle c.
Providence c.
Providence Hospital c.
ptosis c.
Pudenz-Heyer c.
pulmonary arterial c.
pulmonary embolism c.
pulmonary nodulectomy c.
pulmonary vessel c.
pulmonic stenosis c.
Putterman levator resection c.
Putterman ptosis c.
pylorus c.
Rankin anastomosis c.
ratchet c.
Rayport muscle c.
recession c.
rectal c.
Reich-Nechtow c.
renal artery c.
renal pedicle c.
resection c.
Rica vessel c.
right-angle c.
right-angle colon c.
ring-handled bulldog c.
ring-jawed holding c.
Robin chalazion c.
Rochester Kocher c.
Rochester Péan c.
Roeder towel c.
root rubber dam c.
rubber dam c.
rubber-sheathed c.
rubber shod c.
Ruel aorta c.

clamp *(continued)*

Rumel rubber c.
saddle c.
Sarot arterial c.
Sarot bronchus c.
Satinsky c.
Satinsky anastomosis c.
Satinsky aortic c.
Satinsky pediatric c.
Satinsky vascular c.
Satinsky vena cava c.
Schaedel cross-action towel c.
Schlein c.
Schlesinger c.
Schnidt c.
Schoemaker intestinal c.
Schwartz c.
Scoville-Lewis c.
Sehrt c.
self-retaining c.
Selverstone carotid artery c.
Semb bronchus c.
septal c.
serrefine c.
sesamoid c.
Sevrain cranial c.
SGIA knifeless c.
Sheldon c.
Sheth adnexa hysterectomy c.
shutoff c.
side biting c.
Sideris c.
sidewinder aortic c.
sigmoid anastomosis c.
single c.
Singley intestinal ring c.
sizing c.
skull c.
Slim Fit flex c.
Slocum meniscal c.
slotted nerve c.
sponge c.
spoon anastomosis c.
spur-crushing c.
S-shaped peripheral vascular c.
S.S. White c.
stainless steel c.
Steinhauser bone c.
stenosis c.
Steri-Clamp c.
Stille c.
Stimson pedicle c.
stomach c.
Stone intestinal c.
Storey c.
straight mosquito c.
Strelinger colon c.
St. Vincent tube c.

Subramanian classic miniature aortic c.
Sugita head c.
suprahepatic caval c.
suture c.
Swan aortic c.
swan-neck c.
swivel c.
T c.
tangential occlusion c.
temporalis transfer c.
tenacular c.
tension c.
thoracic c.
Thumb-Saver introducer c.
tissue occlusion c.
tonsil c.
tonsillar c.
towel c.
trochanter-holding c.
truncus c.
tube-occluding c.
tubing c.
turkey-claw c.
Ulrich bone-holding c.
umbilical c.
umbilical cord c.
Universal wire c.
upper occlusive c.
ureteral c.
urethrographic cannula c.
urinary incontinence c.
uterine c.
vaginal cuff c.
Varco dissecting c.
vas c.
VascuClamp minibulldog vessel c.
VascuClamp vascular c.
vascular c.
vasovasostomy c.
vena cava c.
Verbrugge bone c.
Verbrugge bone-holding c.
Vermont spinal fixator c.
vessel c.
vessel-occluding c.
vestibular c.
von Petz c.
von Petz intestinal c.
Vorse-Webster c.
VSF c.
vulsellum c.
Wadsworth lid c.
Walton cartilage c.
Wangensteen anastomosis c.
Wangensteen patent ductus c.
Weber aortic c.
Weck c.
wedge resection c.

Wells pedicle c.
Wertheim-Cullen kidney pedicle c.
Wertheim kidney pedicle c.
White c.
whole-cell patch c.
Wikström gallbladder c.
Wikström-Stilgust c.
Willett c.
Williams c.
Wilson c.
Winston cervical c.
wire-tightening c.
Wolfson intestinal c.
Wylie carotid artery c.
Wylie J c.
X c.
Yasargil carotid c.
Yellen c.
Young renal pedicle c.
Z c.
Zachary-Cope c.
Zeppelin c.
Zeppelin S vaginal hysterectomy c.
Zinnanti c.
Zipser meatal c.
Zipser penile c.

clamshell
c. AFO boot
c. brace
C. device
C. double umbrella occluder
C. II device
c. prosthesis
C. septal occluder
c. septal umbrella

Clar head light

ClariFlex
C. foldable IOL
C. foldable silicone intraocular lens
C. lens
C. OptiEdge foldable intraocular lens

Clarion
C. CII behind-the-ear sound processor
C. CII Bionic Ear system
C. CII BTE sound processor
C. cochlear implant system
C. hearing implant
C. HiFocus electrode
C. HiFocus electrode array
C. multistrategy cochlear implant
C. Platinum BTE sound processor

Clarity
C. capnograph
C. multiparameter monitoring system

clariVit
c. central mag lens

c. central magnification vitrectomy lens
c. wide-angle lens
c. wide-angle vitrectomy lens

Clark
C. capsule fragment forceps
C. clamp
C. common duct dilator
C. expanding mesh catheter
C. eye speculum
C. helix catheter
C. hemoperfusion cartridge
C. hemoperfusion system
C. oxygen electrode
C. probe
C. rotating cutter catheter
C. speculum
C. vein stripper

Clarke
C. ligator scissor forceps
C. stereotactic instrument

Clarke-Reich knot pusher

Clark-type polarographic electrode

Clarus
C. model 5169 peristaltic pump
C. peristaltic pump
C. SpineScope

clasp
Adams c.
arrow pin c.
c. bar
Crozat c.
Epi-Sport epicondylitis c.
eyelet c.
c. knife
preformed c.

Classic II stethoscope

Classon pediatric scissors

CLAVE needleless system

Clave needleless system

clavicle orthosis

claw
Anderson 5-prong bear c.
c. forceps
c. retractor

clawed pedicle hook

Clay Adams PE-series catheter

Clayman
C. intraocular lens
C. iris hook
C. lens-holding forceps
C. lens implant forceps
C. lens-inserting forceps
C. lid retractor

Clayman-Knolle irrigating lens loop

Clayton
C. osteotome
C. prosthesis

CLBF-100 blood flowmeter

C

cleaner
> air c.
> Bionaire Air C.
> Proxi-Floss interproximal c.
> unclassified air c.
> VT Mercury Vac organic mercury vacuum c.

Cleanlet lancet
cleanser
> AlcoSCRUB instant antiseptic hand c.
> antimicrobial MPM wound c.
> ApriVera skin and hair c.
> Biolex wound c.
> Clinical Care wound c.
> Curaklense wound c.
> Curasol wound c.
> Debrisan wound c.
> Dermagran wound c.
> DermaMend wound c.
> Dey-Wash skin wound c.
> DiaB Klenz wound c.
> Elta Dermal wound c.
> Gentell wound c.
> Hibiclens antiseptic/antimicrobial skin c.
> Hyperion wound c.
> Lobana wound c.
> MicroKlenz wound c.
> MPM antimicrobial wound c.
> Optipore Sponge wound c.
> Puri-Clens wound c.
> Restore wound c.
> Saf-Clens wound c.
> Sea-Clens wound c.
> SeptiCare wound c.
> Septi-Soft skin care c.
> Shur-Clens wound c.
> SilqueClenz skin c.
> SkinTegrity wound c.
> Techni-Care wound c.
> UltraKlenz wound c.
> wound c.

cleanup
> Wizard MagneSil PCR c.
> Wizard MagneSil sequencing c.

Cleanwheel
> C. disposable neurological pinwheel
> C. presterilized disposable device

clear
> C. Advantage latex-free catheter
> C. Advantage silicone male catheter
> C. Advantage spirometry filter
> c. cornea angled CVD diamond knife
> c. cornea blade
> c. PVC tube and connector kit

> c. sterile premium tubing
> C. View hydrophilic shield

ClearChart digital acuity system
ClearCRIT microhematocrit tube
ClearCut
> C. dual-bevel blade
> C. dual-bevel line knife
> C. 2 electrosurgical handpiece
> C. 2 instrument
> C. ophthalmic dual-bevel knife
> C. SatinSlit knife

Clearfix
> C. meniscal dart
> C. meniscal screw
> C. screw

Clearglide precision bipolar device
Clearpath corneal diamond knife
ClearPlan Easy fertility monitor
Clearpro suction socket
CLeaRS cardiac lead removal system
ClearSite
> C. bandage
> C. borderless dressing
> C. hydrogauze dressing
> C. hydrogel absorptive borderline wound dressing
> C. hydrogel sheet
> C. impregnated gauze
> C. wound dressing

ClearView
> C. C. Diff A test
> C. contact lens
> C. intracoronary shunt
> C. intravascular arteriotomy shunt
> C. model
> C. uterine manipulator

ClearWay irrigating PTFE balloon catheter
Cleasby
> C. spatula
> C. spatulated needle

cleaver
> Case enamel c.
> fiber c.
> Haefliger c.
> Orton enamel c.

cleft
> c. palate elevator
> c. palate forceps
> c. palate knife
> c. palate needle
> c. palate prosthesis
> c. palate rasp

C-Leg
> C-L. lower limb prosthesis
> C-L. System artificial leg

Clemetson uterine forceps
Clerf
> C. aspirator

C. cancer cell collector
C. dilator
C. forceps
C. laryngeal saw
C. laryngectomy tube
C. laryngoscope
C. needle holder
Clerf-Arrowsmith safety pin closer
clerical spectacles
Clev-Dent excavator
Clev-Dent-Wakefield chisel
Clevedon positive pressure respirator
Cleveland
C. bone-cutting forceps
C. bone rongeur
Clevis clamp
Clevisphere ankle joint
clicker
compression c.
Clickhaler
Click'X
climber
Fitstep II stair c.
Sprint C.
Clinac 600SR stereotactic radiation treatment system
Clinch Lock CTS wrist brace
clinical
c. bone sonometer
C. Care wound cleanser
c. electromagnetic flowmeter
c. electromagnetic flowmeter clip
C. HandMaster system
Clini-Care
C.-C. bed
C.-C. low-air-loss system
CliniCath peripherally inserted catheter
Clinicel silicon gel-filled cushion
clinic exolever elevator
Clini.Dyne bed
Clini.Float
C. bed
C. flotation therapy bed system
Cliniguard pad
Clinisert mattress
Cliniset infusion set
Clinitek 50 urine chemistry analyzer
Clinitemp fever detector
Clinitron
C. air bed
C. air-fluidized bed
C. bed
C. Elexis air-fluidized therapy unit
C. II air-fluidized therapy unit
C. uplift air-fluidized therapy unit
clinometer
clinoscope
clip
absorbable c.

Adams-DeWeese vena cava serrated c.
Adson scalp c.
AGV pars plana c.
alligator c.
aneurysm c.
aneurysmal c.
angled c.
c. applier
Astro-Trace Universal adapter c.
Atrauclip hemostatic c.
Autostat ligating and hemostatic c.
Backhaus towel c.
Benjamin-Havas fiberoptic light c.
Biemer vessel c.
bipolar diathermy adapter c.
Bleier c.
Booster c.
brain c.
cardiac retraction c.
Castroviejo scleral shortening c.
clinical electromagnetic flowmeter c.
cranial aneurysm c.
crankshaft c.
cross-legged c.
curved c.
Cushing c.
DeWeese-Hunter c.
double tantalum c.
Drake aneurysm c.
Drake fenestrated c.
Drake-Kees c.
Duraclose scleral c.
ear c.
Elgiloy c.
Elgiloy-Heifitz aneurysm c.
encircling c.
Endo GIA surgical c.
Ethicon c.
Federov 4-loop iris c.
Feldstein blepharoplasty c.
fenestrated aneurysm c.
ferromagnetic intracerebral aneurysm c.
Filshie c.
Filshie female sterilization c.
Flexi-Seal fecal collector & tail c.
Fogarty spring c.
c. force meter
c. forceps
Friedman tantalum c.
gate c.
c. gauge
c. graft
Greyhound adjustable spring c.
Hader bar c.
Halberg c.
Heath c.

clip *(continued)*

Hegenbarth c.
Heifitz c.
Heifitz-Weck c.
hemostasis scalp c.
hemostasis silver c.
hemostatic c.
holding c.
Horizon surgical ligating and marking c.
Hulka c.
Hulka-Clemens c.
Indiana Tome c.
inferior vena cava c.
jaw spring c.
Kapp c.
Khodadad c.
laparoscopic tie c.
Lapra-Ty c.
lens c.
LeRoy infant scalp c.
Ligaclip surgical c.
L-shaped aneurysm c.
magazine c.
magnetic resonance-compatible c.
Mayfield-Kees c.
McDermott c.
McFadden-Kees c.
McKenzie hemostasis c.
McKenzie silver brain c.
McKenzie V c.
metal c.
metallic c.
Michel c.
Michel scalp c.
Michel skin c.
Michel suture c.
microanastomosis c.
microbulldog c.
microvascular c.
Miles vena cava c.
mini-Sugita c.
Moretz c.
nonferromagnetic c.
nose c.
Novaclip atraumatic spring c.
Olivecrona silver c.
C. On torquer
Opticaid spring c.
palmar c.
partial occlusion inferior vena cava c.
Perneczky aneurysm c.
pivot aneurysm c.
plastic scalp c.
primary c.
Raney c.
Raney scalp c.
c. remover

retractor c.
right-angle booster c.
scalp hemostasis c.
Scanlan aneurysm c.
Schaedel c.
scleral shortening c.
Scoville c.
Security carpal tunnel release system c.
silver c.
skin c.
Smith c.
Spetzler titanium aneurysm c.
spring c.
sternal c.
straight aneurysm c.
suction tube c.
Sugita c.
Sugita aneurysm c.
Sugita cross-legged c.
Sugita temporary straight c.
Sundt booster c.
Sundt cross-legged c.
Sundt-Kees aneurysm c.
Sundt-Kees booster c.
Sundt-Kees encircling patch c.
Sundt-Kees graft c.
Sundt-Kees Slimline c.
Sundt slim-line graft c.
Sundt straddling c.
surgical c.
Surgiclip c.
tantalum c.
tantalum hemostasis c.
Teflon c.
temporary vascular c.
temporary vessel c.
titanium c.
titanium aneurysm c.
Tomac c.
towel c.
triangular encompassing c.
U c.
umbilical c.
Uni-Shunt right-angle c.
V c.
Vari-Angle c.
vascular c.
vena cava c.
vessel c.
vitallium c.
von Petz suture c.
Wachenfeldt suture c.
2-way towel c.
Weck c.
Weck Hemoclip c.
window c.
wing c.
wound c.

Yasargil-Aesculap spring c.
Yasargil cross-legged c.
Yasargil titanium aneurysm c.
Zimmer c.

clip-applier
Sundt aneurysm c.-a.

clip-applying aneurysm forceps
clip-bending forceps
clip-cutting forceps
clip-introducing forceps
cliplamp
mini c.

Clip-Lite clip-on headlight
clip-on/tie-on occluder
clipper
Baxter surgical c.

clip-reinforced cotton sling
clip-removing forceps
ClipTip reusable sensor
Clirans T-series dialyzer
Clisco covered needle catheter
clitoral therapy device
CLM articulating laryngoscope blade
CLO
CLO Cool Bag
CLO Cool Wand
CLO Recirculating Slim Pack

clog
Hollander c.
Markell Mobility Health C.
wooden postoperative c.

CloneSaver card
C-loop posterior chamber lens
closed
c. Cotrel-Dubousset hook
c. cnd-hole catheter
c. Küntscher nail
c. minipouch
c. suction drain
c. suction tube
c. unlocked nail

closed-chain exercise attachment
closed-circuit
c.-c. spirometer
c.-c. television vision enhancement
system

closed-loop
c.-l. device
c.-l. EndoButton
c.-l. infrared video tracking system
c.-l. system
c.-l. system passing electrode

closer
Clerf-Arrowsmith safety pin c.
c. forceps
Perclose C.
C. percutaneous suture-mediated
closure device

safety pin c.
C. stapler

CloseSure
C. procedure kit
C. System
C. System XL

closing forceps
Clo-Sur
C.-S. PAD closure device
C.-S. PAD nonwoven hydrophilic
wound dressing

closure
Beta-Cap catheter c.
Beta-Cap II c.
Brandy scalp stretcher II, front c.
Brandy scalp stretcher I, rear c.
C. catheter/radiofrequency generator
compression skullcap c.
c. device
Duo-Lock curved tail c.
facial compression finger c.
facial compression skullcap c.
Lowsley retractor with hand-
sutured c.
Steri-Strips skin c.
Sur-Fit irrigation sleeve tail c.
Sur-Fit Natura irrigation sleeve
tail c.
Suture Strip Plus wound c.
The VAC Vacuum Assisted C.
vacuum-assisted c. (VAC)
VasoSeal Elite vascular c.

clot
C. Buster Amplatz thrombectomy
device
c. forceps
C. Stop drain

cloth
c. binder
Dacron c.

Cloutier unconstrained knee prosthesis
cloverleaf
C. catheter
C. EP catheter
C. internal bumper
c. met foot pad
c. nail
c. pin
c. pin extractor
c. rod

Cloward
C. anterior fusion kit
C. blade retractor
C. bone graft impactor
C. bone punch
C. brain retractor
C. cervical dislocation reducer
C. cervical drill guard
C. cervical drill tip

C

Cloward (*continued*)
  C. cervical retractor
  C. cervical retractor set
  C. crossbar handle
  C. curette
  C. depth gauge
  C. double-hinged cervical retractor
    handle
  C. dowel cutter
  C. dowel ejector
  C. drill guard cap
  C. drill guide
  C. drill shaft
  C. dural hook
  C. dural retractor
  C. hammer
  C. instrument
  C. intervertebral disc rongeur
  C. nerve root retractor
  C. osteophyte elevator
  C. periosteal elevator
  C. pituitary rongeur
  C. PLIF case
  C. PLIF II kit
  C. posterior lumbar interbody
    fusion kit
  C. self-retaining retractor
  C. single-tooth retractor blade
  C. spanner wrench
  C. spinal fusion chisel
  C. spinal fusion osteotome
  C. spreader
  C. surgical saddle
  C. tissue retractor
ClozeX needleless wound closure device
CLR 2940 erbium laser
CLS
  CLS hip stem
  CLS hip system
clubfoot splint
Clyburn Colles fracture fixator
clysis cannula
CMA 600 neuromonitoring system
C-Max
  C-M. cutting loop
  C-M. cutting loop electrode
CM-Band
  CM-B. 505N brace
  CM-B. silicone rubber brace
CMC
  carpometacarpal
  CMC splint
CMC-III
  Malis irrigating bipolar CMC-III
CMI
  CMI vacuum delivery system
  CMI vacuum extractor
CMI-Mityvac cup
CMI-O'Neil cup

C-mount adapter
CMS AccuProbe 450 system
CMSI warming system
CMV
  cool mist vaporizer
CMW cement gun
CO
  carbon monoxide
  cervical orthosis
    CO Sleuth
    CO Sleuth carbon monoxide
      monitor
    CO Sleuth handheld carbon
      monoxide analyzer
CO_2
  carbon dioxide
    CO_2 beam
    CO_2 blower
    CO_2 cylinder
    CO_2 FeatherTouch SilkLaser
    CO_2 generator
    CO_2 laser
    CO_2 laser probe
    CO_2 powered gun system
    CO_2 Sharplan laser
    CO_2 waveform
Coach incentive spirometer
Coag-a-Mate
    C.-a.-M. coagulometer
    C.-a.-M. prothrombin device
CoaguChek
  C. aPTT testing system
  C. portable prothrombin time
    device
  C. Pro/DM coagulometer
  C. Pro/DM monitor
  C. Pro/DM system
  C. self-testing device
coagulating
  c. electrode
  c. forceps
  c. suction cannula connection cord
coagulation
  c. analyzer
  c. aspirator tube
  c. electrode
  c. forceps
  c. probe
  c. suction tube
coagulator
  American Optical c.
  argon beam c.
  argon plasma c.
  ASSI c.
  ASSI Polar-Mate c.
  Ball c.
  Biceps bipolar c.
  bipolar c.
  Codman-Mentor wet-field c.

cold c.
Concept bipolar c.
Cosman c.
Elmed BC 50 M/M digital
  bipolar c.
Erbe Unit argon plasma c.
Erbe Unit argon plasma c.
Fabry c.
Fukushima monopolar malleable c.
Grieshaber microbipolar c.
Hildreth c.
Hyfrecator c.
infrared c.
Jarit bipolar c.
Karl Storz c.
Malis CMC-II bipolar c.
Malis CMC-II PC bipolar c.
Malis solid-state c.
Mentor wet-field cordless c.
Meyer-Schwickerath c.
microwave tissue c.
Polar-Mate c.
Polar-Mate bipolar c.
Ramirez EndoForehead suction c.
Redfield IRC 2100 infrared c.
solid-state c.
Storz microsurgical bipolar c.
suction c.
Walker c.
wet-field c.
xenon arc c.
Zeiss c.

coagulometer
Coag-a-Mate c.
CoaguChek Pro/DM c.
Coaguloop resection electrode
Coakley
C. antral trocar
C. nasal speculum
C. sinus curette
C. tenaculum
coaptation
c. bipolar forceps
c. splint
coarctation
c. clamp
c. forceps
coarse carbide cone bur
coarse-olive bur
Coat-A-Count neonatal 17
  hydroxyprogesterone kit
coated
c. biopsy forceps
c. polyester suture
c. prosthesis
c. Vicryl Rapide suture
c. Vicryl suture

coater
Hummer V Sputter c.
Polaron sputter c.
coating
coaxial
c. cable
c. catheter
C. Endostat
c. I&A nylon connector
c. irrigation/aspiration cannula
c. micropuncture introducer set
c. micropuncture needle set
C. Multicolor LIO
c. needle electrode
c. sheath cut biopsy needle
c. snare
coaxillary directed catheter
Coballoy twist drill
cobalt
c. alloy stent
c. blue light
C. G-HV high-contrast bone
  cement
C. HV high-contrast bone cement
C. knife
c. megavoltage machine
C. scalpel
cobalt-60 eye plaque
cobalt-chrome
c.-c. alloy and polyethylene
  implant
c.-c. head
cobalt-chromium
c.-c. alloy prosthesis
c.-c. head
c.-c. implant
cobalt-chromium-molybdenum
c.-c.-m. alloy
c.-c.-m. alloy metal implant
cobalt-chromium-tungsten-nickel alloy
  metal implant
Coban
C. bandage
C. cohesive medium stretch
  bandage
C. dressing
C. elastic dressing
C. tape
C. wrap
Cobas
C. Fara centrifugal analyzer
C. Fara H centrifugal analyzer
C. fast centrifugal analyzer
C. Helios differential analyzer
Cobb
C. bone curette
C. curette
C. periosteal elevator
C. spinal curette

C

Cobb *(continued)*
    C. spinal elevator
    C. spinal gouge
Cobbett skin graft knife
Cobb-Ragde needle
Cobe
    C. AV fistular needle
    C. AV shunt
    C. blood cell separator
    C. 2991 cell processor
    C. Centrysystem dialyzer 400 HG
    C. CML oxygenator
    C. 2991 computerized centrifuge
      system
    C. double blood pump
    C. Optima hollow-fiber membrane
      oxygenator
    C. Spectra apheresis system
    C. staple gun
Cobed tube
Cobe-Stöckert
    C.-S. heart-lung console
    C.-S. heart-lung machine
**Cobe-Tenckhoff peritoneal dialysis
  catheter**
coblation
    C. spinal surgery system
    tonsillar c.
Coblation-based spinal surgery system
Coblator II surgery system
Cobra
    C. Amplicor analyzer
    C. auto-gamma counter
    C. cannula
    C. 1, 2 catheter
    C. diagnostic catheter
    C. K+ cannula
    C. K cannula
    C. K+ cannula tip
    C. LASIK irrigating cannula
    C. Master
    C. over-the-wire balloon catheter
Cobra+
    Cobra+ cannula
    Cobra+ cannula tip
cobra-head
    c.-h. drill
    c.-h. plate
    c.-h. retractor
cobra-shaped catheter
Coburn
    C. anterior chamber intraocular
      lens implant
    C. camera
    C. intraocular lens
    C. irrigation/aspiration system
    C. lensometer
    C. refractor
    C. tonometer

coccyx cushion
Cochet-Bonnet aesthesiometer
cochlea
    Contigen Bard c.
cochlear
    c. implant
    c. stimulator
cock
    stop c.
cock-up
    c.-u. arm splint
    c.-u. wrist support
cocoon dressing
Co-Cr-Mo
    C.-C.-M. pin
    C.-C.-M. prosthesis
Codemaster defibrillator
Code-On Immunoslide stainer
Codivilla
    C. extension
    C. graft
Codman
    C. Accu-Flow shunt
    C. ACP system
    C. anterior cervical plating system
    C. Bactiseal antimicrobial
      impregnated catheter system
    C. Cranioplastic Type 1 Slow Set
    C. dilator case
    C. disposable ICP lock
    C. external drainage ventricular set
    C. Hakim programmable valve
    C. ICP monitoring line
    C. IMA kit
    C. intracranial pressure monitor
    C. Medos programmable valve
    C. neurological headrest system
    C. ovary forceps
    C. scissors
    C. Ti-frame posterior fixation
      system
    C. ventricular silicone
Codman-Holter catheter
Codman-Kerrison laminectomy rongeur
Codman-Leksell laminectomy rongeur
Codman-Mentor wet-field coagulator
CoEase viscoelastic
Coecal
Coe-Comfort tissue conditioner
Coe investment material
Coe-Pak periodontal dressing
COER-24 delivery system
Coe-Rect denture reliner
Coe-Soft denture reliner
coffin-type transpalatal wire
Cofield 2 total shoulder system
Coflex
    C. adherent wrap

C. dressing
C. flexible wrap
Cogan-Boberg-Ans lens implant
Cogent
C. light
C. LightWear headlight
C. XL illuminator
Cogsell tip aspirator
CO$_2$Guard
Cohan needle holder
Cohan-Vannas iris scissors
Cohan-Westcott scissors
Cohen
C. corneal forceps
C. periosteal elevator
C. retractor
C. rongeur
C. uterine cannula
Cohen-Eder uterine cannula
Coherent
C. 920 argon/dye laser
C. argon laser photocoagulator
C. CO$_2$ surgical laser
C. 5000C UltraPulse laser
C. EPIC laser
C. 7910 laser
C. LaserLink slit-lamp
C. Medical YAG laser
C. model 90-K laser
C. Novus Omni multiwavelength laser
C. photocoagulator
C. radiation argon/krypton laser
C. radiation argon model 800 laser
C. radiation Fluorotron
C. Schwind Keraton 2 laser
C. Selecta 7000 laser
C. UltraPulse 5000C laser
C. UltraPulse CO$_2$ laser
C. VersaPulse device
cohesive
c. anatomic silicone gel breast implant
c. bandage
c. dressing
Cohn cardiac stabilizer
Cohney scissors
Cohort
C. anterior plate system
C. bone brush
C. bone screw
C. spinal impactor
coil
aneurysmal c.
asymmetrical gradient c.
3-axis gradient c.
bilateral breast c.
birdcage head c.
body c.

c. canister
catheter c.
c. catheter
catheter-delivered platinum c.
circularly polarized c.
circular polarized volume head c.
circumferential dedicated knee c.
circumferential extremity c.
collagen-filled interlocking detachable c.
conventional head c.
Cook detachable PDA c.
coupled array c.
crossed c.
custom-curved c.
Dacron fiber-coated c.
Dacron-fibered platinum c.
DCS-10, DCS-18 mechanically detachable platinum c.
dedicated phased-array c.
detachable c.
detachable embolization c.
detachable platinum c.
distal shocking c.
double breast c.
DuctOcclud c.
electrically detachable c.
c. electrode
electro-detachable platinum c.
2-element phased-array c.
4-element phased array c.
elliptical end-capped quadrature radiofrequency c.
embolization c.
endoanal c.
endoesophageal MRI c.
endorectal c.
endorectal-pelvic phased-array c.
endoscopic quadrature radiofrequency c.
endovaginal c.
endovascular c.
extremity c.
fat-suppressed body c.
figure-of-8 c.
flexible radiofrequency c.
flexible surface c.
free fibered c.
GDC 360-degree detachable c.
GDC-10 soft c.
Gianturco c.
Gianturco occlusion c.
Gianturco steel c.
Gianturco-Wallace-Anderson c.
Gianturco wool-tufted wire c.
Golay gradient c.
gonion gradient c.
Gore torso array MRI surface c.
gradient c.

coil *(continued)*
    gradient sheet c.
    Guglielmi detachable c. (GDC)
    head c.
    helical c.
    Helmholtz double-surface c.
    Helmholtz head c.
    high-speed gradient c.
    Hilal c.
    Hipper twist release c.
    immediately detachable c.
    Intercept vascular internal MR c.
    interlocking detachable c.
    intraurethral c.
    Ivalon wire c.
    Jackson c.
    liver c.
    local gradient c.
    c. machine adapter
    Macroduct c.
    Margulies c.
    Matrix2 detachable c.
    Maxwell c.
    MDS c.
    mechanically detachable platinum c.
    Medrad MRInnervu endorectal colon probe c.
    micronester platinum embolization c.
    modified birdcage c.
    multiply tuned c.
    nester c.
    occlusion c.
    opposed loop-pair quadrature magnetic resonance c.
    opposed loop-pair quadrature NMR c.
    orthogonal radiofrequency c.
    orthogonal square Helmholtz c.
    pelvic phased-array c.
    phased-array receiver c.
    phased-array torso c.
    planar circular c.
    platinum c.
    platinum embolization c.
    posterior neck surface c.
    prolapse c.
    pushable c.
    quadrature birdcage c.
    quadrature body c.
    quadrature cervical spine c.
    quadrature head c.
    quadrature radiofrequency receiver c.
    quadrature surface c.
    quadrature terminal latency surface c.
    quadrature transmit/receive head c.
    radiofrequency c.
    radiofrequency head c.
    receive-only circular surface c.
    RF c.
    right ventricular c.
    saddle c.
    send-receive phased-array extremity c.
    sensing c.
    shielded gradient c.
    shim c.
    shoulder surface c.
    solenoid surface c.
    spring c.
    steel embolization c.
    c. stent
    Stylet internal esophageal MRI c.
    surface c.
    Surgi-Vision MRI c.
    switchable c.
    Tornado embolization c.
    torso phased-array c.
    transmit-receive c.
    transverse gradient c.
    TriSpan detachable c.
    twist-release c.
    c. vascular stent
    VortX vascular occlusion c.
    VortXX c.
    wrist quadrature phased-array surface c.
    Yasargil-Leyla brain retractor z-gradient c.
    z-gradient c.
Coil-Cath catheter
coiled spring
coilette
    FLX flexible treatment c.
coil-tipped catheter
coincidence gamma camera
coincident gamma camera
Co$_2$ject system
Colapinto
    C. compression device
    C. needle
    C. sheath
    C. transjugular biopsy set
Colclough laminectomy rongeur
cold
    c. beam laser
    c. biopsy forceps
    c. cautery
    c. coagulator
    C. Compress mask
    c. cup biopsy forceps
    c. knife
    c. knife hook
    c. pack
    c. pad
    c. quartz lamp

c. quartz lamp germicidal lamp
c. scissors

Coldhot pack
cold-mist humidifier
cold-weld femoral ball
Cole
C. duodenal retractor
C. endotracheal tube
C. orotracheal tube
C. uncuffed endotracheal tube

Coleman
C. aspiration cannula
C. infiltration cannula
C. microinfiltration system
C. retractor

Colibri forceps
Colin STBP-780 stress test blood pressure monitor
CollaCote collagen wound dressing
collagen
c. absorbable suture
Avitene microfibrillar c.
BGC matrix c.
Bio-Oss c.
CosmoDerm 1, 2 human-based c.
CosmoPlast human-based c.
Cymetra c.
Dermalogen human c.
c. dressing
Fibracol c.
c. hemostatic material
c. implant
InterGard knitted c.
Isolagen human c.
matrix c.
c. mediated closure device
Medifil c.
c. membrane
microfibrillar c.
Phonagel c.
c. plug
c. plug device
c. scaffold
c. shield
Skin Temp c.
c. sponge
Vocalogen c.
Woun'Dres c.
ZCI c.

collagenase
Cordase injectable c.

collagen-based biomaterial
collagen-filled interlocking detachable coil
collagen-impregnated Dacron
CollagENT wand
Collagraft
C. bone graft matrix
C. bone graft substitute

Collamer
C. intraocular lens
C. 1-piece intraocular lens
C. 3-piece intraocular lens

CollaPlug
C. absorbable collagen dressing
C. collagen material
C. wound dressing

collapsible tissue retractor
collar
Aspen cervical c.
Belmont c.
c. brace
Bremer halo crown cervical c.
cervical c.
circumaortic venous c.
cone c.
Cowboy c.
c. and crown scissors
c. dressing
Exo-Static cervical c.
foam c.
Georgiade visor cervical c.
hard c.
hard cervical c.
Headmaster c.
heated tracheostomy c.
high-humidity tracheostomy c.
Houston halo traction cervical c.
implant c.
intramedullary c. (IMC)
MAC cervical c.
Marlin cervical c.
Mayo rigid cervical c.
Miami acute care cervical c.
Miami J cervical c.
Minerva c.
molded Thomas c.
Nec-Loc cervical c.
Newport c.
Philadelphia c.
Philadelphia cervical c.
Philadelphia rigid c.
Philly Bloc-Head cervical c.
Philly 1-piece cervical c.
pillow c.
Plastazote cervical c.
plastic c.
plastizote cervical c.
Pneu-trac cervical c.
c. prosthesis
rigid c.
c. scissors
soft cervical c.
StediSpine c.
tension c.
Thomas rigid c.
tracheostomy c.

collar *(continued)*
    Tuxedo c.
    wire frame c.
collar-button iris retractor
**collared press-fit femoral stem
implantation**
collarless
    c. polished taper
    c. stem
**Collastat OBP microfibrillar collagen
hemostat**
CollaTape
    C. tape
    C. wound dressing
CollectFirst system
collecting tube
collection
    Macroduct system for sweat
      stimulation and c.
    c. trap
collector
    anaerobic specimen c.
    bone c.
    BoneCollector bone fillings
      harvest c.
    Cervex-Brush cervical cell c.
    Clerf cancer cell c.
    Conveen drip c.
    Cytobrush cell c.
    Cytobrush Plus cell c.
    Cytopick endocervical and
      uterovaginal cell c.
    drainable fecal c.
    Endocell endometrial cell c.
    fetal incontinence c.
    Flexi-Seal fecal c.
    Grass force displacement fluid c.
    Leukotrap red cell c.
    Little Ones pediatric urine c.
    Lukens c.
    Misstique female external
      urinary c.
    Papette cervical c.
    Papette cervical cell c.
    Sheehy Pate C.
    stool c.
    Uterobrush endometrial sample c.
    Wallach-Papette disposable cervical
      cell c.
    wound drainage c.
    Xomed sinus secretion c.
College
    C. forceps
    C. Park TruStep foot
    C. Park TruStep foot prosthesis
    C. pliers
Colles
    C. external fixation frame
    C. splint

Collier-Crile hemostatic forceps
Collier needle holder
collimation scintillation detector
collimator
    APC-3, APC-4 c.
    automatic c.
    c. cone
    converging c.
    converging-hole c.
    diverging c.
    Eureka c.
    external c.
    fan-beam c.
    focusing c.
    c. helmet
    high-resolution c.
    high-resolution fan-beam c.
    high-resolution multileaf c.
    high-resolution parallel hole c.
    high-sensitivity c.
    LEAP c.
    LEUHR fan-beam c.
    LEUHR parallel-hole c.
    Leur-par c.
    long-bore c.
    low-energy c.
    Machlett c.
    medium-energy c.
    Micro-Cast c.
    micromultileaf c.
    multihole c.
    multileaf c.
    multirod c.
    parallel-hole medium-sensitivity c.
    Picker Dyna Mo c.
    pinhole c.
    single-hole c.
    slant hole c.
    slit c.
    Sophy high-resolution c.
    thick-septa c.
    thin-septa c.
    ultra high-resolution parallel-hole c.
Collin
    C. abdominal retractor
    C. amputating knife
    C. 140 color adaptometer
    C. intestinal forceps
    C. knife
    C. lung-grasping forceps
    C. mesher
    C. osteoclast
    C. pelvimeter
    C. rib shears
    C. tissue forceps
    C. tongue forceps
    C. tongue-seizing forceps
    C. uterine-elevating forceps
    C. vaginal speculum

Collin-Duval intestinal thumb forceps
Collings
 C. electrode
 C. electrosurgery knife
Collin-Hartmann retractor
Collin-Pozzi uterine forceps
Collins
 C. bicycle
 C. dynamometer
 C. respiratometer
 C. Survey spirometer
 C. umbilical clamp
Collis-Taylor retractor
Collis TDR instrument
collodion dressing
collodion-treated self-adhesive bandage
Collostat hemostatic sponge
Collum CMC thumb brace
Collyer pelvimeter
colmascope
colometrometer
colon
 c. clamp
 c. motility catheter
colonic
 c. insufflator
 c. stent
 c. Z-stent
colonofiberscope
colonoscope, coloscope
 ACMI fiberoptic c.
 CF-200Z Olympus c.
 double-channel c.
 Evis 200I c.
 Fujinon EC-130LT c.
 Fujinon EC-200LT c.
 Fujinon EC-410MP c.
 Fujinon EC-300MS c.
 Fujinon EC series video c.
 Fujinon FE-100LR c.
 Innoflex variable-stiffness c.
 Machida FCS-ML II magnifying c.
 magnifying c.
 Olympus CF-HM series
  magnifying c.
 Olympus CF-MB/LB c.
 Olympus CF-MB-M c.
 Olympus CF-MB series c.
 Olympus CF24OZI c.
 Olympus CF-PL series c.
 Olympus CF-P20S fiberoptic c.
 Olympus CF-1T100L c.
 Olympus CF-T series c.
 Olympus CF-UM3 c.
 Olympus CF-VL series c.
 Olympus CF-200Z c.
 Olympus EVIS video c.
 Olympus PCF-100, -130
  pediatric c.

 Olympus PCF series pediatric c.
 Olympus SIF-M magnifying c.
 PCF-140L pediatric c.
 Pentax FC series c.
 Pentax VSB-P2900 pediatric c.
 single-channel c.
 standard c.
 Toshiba TCE-M series c.
 Welch Allyn video c.
colonoscopy
 Virtual Vision audiovisual system
  for EGD and c.
ColonoSight system
Coloplast
 C. bag
 C. closed pouch
 C. colostomy bag
 C. deluxe irrigation kit
 C. drainable pouch
 C. economy irrigation set
 C. hospital irrigation set
 C. irrigation faceplate
 C. irrigation kit
 C. ostomy belt
 C. 1-piece closed pouch with filter
 C. 1-piece Conseal plug
 C. 2-piece Conseal plug
 C. 1-piece small drainable pouch
 C. 2-piece small drainable pouch
 C. 2-piece small urostomy pouch
 C. 1-piece standard drainable
  pouch
 C. 2-piece sterile post-op set
 C. 2-piece stoma cap with filter
 C. skin barrier paste
 C. skin barrier ring
 C. stoma cap
 C. stoma cone
 C. transparent irrigation sleeve
 C. urine leg bag
 C. wafer
color
 c. adaptometer
 c. bar Schirmer strip
 c. bar Schirmer tear test
 c. Doppler
 c. Doppler scan
 c. Doppler ultrasound
 c. fundus camera
Colorado
 C. cautery
 C. electrocautery tip
 C. microdissection needle
 C. MicroNeedle
 C. MicroNeedle needle electrode
 C. needle
 C. 2 spinal system
 C. tip cautery

C

ColorCards
    Everyday Objects C.
ColorChecker
    Macbeth C.
color-coded
    c.-c. guidewire
    c.-c. therapy putty
color-contrast microscope
colored contact lens
color-flow Doppler
Colorfrost disposable microscope slide
colorimeter
    ChromaMeter CR-200 handheld c.
    differential scanning c.
colorimetric detector
Colormark slide
ColorMax color vision enhancement lens
ColorPAC toxin A test
ColorpHast Indicator Strips
colorvascular Doppler ultrasound
ColorZone
    C. Management system
    C. tape
coloscope (*var. of* colonoscope)
Coloscreen VPI
colostomy
    c. bag
    c. rod
    Ultra Duet C.
Colour-Quad-System imaging system
Colpacs pack
colpomicrohysteroscope
colposcope
    CooperSurgical overhead c.
    Cryomedics c.
    CS1500 articulating arm video-ready c.
    CS500 articulating arm zoom c.
    CS200 upright post zoom c.
    Frigitronics c.
    Leisegang c.
    MM-6000 c.
    Opmi c.
    OZM c.
    Wallach ZoomStar c.
    Zeiss c.
    ZoomScope c.
colpostat
    afterload c.
    c. applicator
    dome c.
    FSD c.
    Henschke c.
Coltene
    C. direct inlay system
    C. impression material
    C. inlay system
    C. oven

Coltex impression material
Columbia
    C. scaler
    C. 13/14 universal curette
Columbus
    C. McKinnon Hugger device
    C. McKinnon lifting assist
columella clamp
columellar implant
column
    c. chromatograph
    contrast c.
    DEAE-Sephacel ion exchange c.
    disposable PD-10 c.
    immunoadsorption c.
    NHS-activated HiTrap affinity c.
    PD-10 disposable Sephadex G-25 c.
    Prosorba c.
    Sephadex G-25 c.
Colvard handheld infrared pupillometer
Colver tonsil-seizing forceps
comb
    toe c.
Combi
    C. 40 cochlear implant
    C. 40+ cochlear implant system
Combicath
CombiDERM
    C. ACD hydrocolloid
    C. ACD hydrocolloid dressing
    C. nonadhesive absorbent dressing
Combiguard II irrigation splash guard
Combilight PDD 5133 laparoscope
Combiline System
combination
    c. biliary brush catheter
    c. cone/tube irrigator kit
    c. cone/tube stoma irrigator drain film-screen c.
    c. gel and inflatable mammary prosthesis
    Grafton bone matrix/marrow c.
    c. needle electrode
    c. phaco chopper
    c. stretcher chair
combined
    c. CT-fluoroscopy scanner
    C. Instabilities functional knee brace
    c. magnetic field system
    c. neurosurgical-external sinus approach
    c. wire guide bone elevator
Combisit surgeon's chair
Combison 530 3D sonographer
Combitip Plus pipette tip
Combitrans transducer

Combitube
C. airway
C. airway device
C. endotracheal tube
esophageal tracheal C.

combo
Acceava hCG C.
C. Cath wire-guided cytology brush
Chang Quick Chop c.

Comed
C. footgear
C. postoperative shoe
C. postsurgical footgear

comedo extractor

Comet catheter

Comfeel
C. contour dressing
C. hydrocolloid
C. hydrocolloid dressing
C. Plus pressure relief dressing
C. Plus triangle dressing
C. powder
C. Purilon dressing
C. Ulcus dressing
C. Ulcus occlusive dressing

Comfit
C. endotracheal tube
C. endotracheal tube holder

comfort
C. Ag prosthetic sock
C. Care bed system
C. Cast
C. Cast casting system
C. Cast stirrup
C. Cath I, II catheter
C. Club tub pillow
C. Cool neoprene support
C. Cool thumb abduction strap
C. Cool thumb CMC restriction splint
C. Cool wrist and thumb CMC restriction splint
c. leg bag strap
C. n' Care Seamfree sock
C. Plus cushion
C. Rite footwear
C. Take-Along wheelchair cushion
C. wrist immobilizer

ComfortClassic nasal mask

ComfortCuff blood pressure cuff

comforter
C. splint
Thermo hand c.
Thermo knee c.

ComfortFull nasal mask

ComfortGel nasal mask

Comf-Orthotic
C.-O. 3/4-length insole
C.-O. sports replacement insole
C.-O. wool felt insole

ComfortScan system

ComfortSeal mask

Comfortseat
Flo-Fit C.

Comfort-U total body pillow

ComfortWalk
C. foot system
C. prosthetic foot

ComfortWalk$_2$ prosthetic foot

ComfortWear pouch cover

Comfy
C. elbow orthosis
C. elbow splint
C. knee orthosis
C. toilet lift seat
C. walker

Command
C. hip instrumentation system
C. Instrument System surgical instrument
C. joint replacement instrument system

Commander angioplasty guidewire

commissure laryngoscope

committed mode pacemaker

common
c. duct-holding forceps
c. duct probe
c. pH electrode

CO$_2$mmO$_2$n sensor transcutaneous gas electrode

Compac microcentrifuge

compact
C. II desktop spirometer
c. plating system (CPS)

Compaction pliers

compactor
McSpadden c.
Micro-Flow c.

Compafill MH dental restorative material

CompAire Elite compressor nebulizer system

Compak-200 mini-excimer

Compalay dental restorative material

Compamolar dental restorative material

Companion
C. feeding pump
C. 314, 318 nasal CPAP system
C. 2 self-monitoring blood glucose device

company
Direct Optical Research C. (DORC)
United States Catheter & Instruments C. (USCI)

comparison eyepiece

C

compass
C. arc-quadrant stereotactic system
C. frame-based stereotactic system
C. hinge
C. Hinge external fixator
Mastel diamond c.
C. stereotactic frame
C. stereotactic system
Compat 199205 enteral feeding pump
Compeed
C. protective dressing
C. skin protector dressing
compensated sheath
compensating eyepiece
compensator
GDx-variable corneal c.
multivane intensity modulation c.
scattering foil c.
time gain c.
Compere fixation wire
Comperm tubular elastic bandage
Competitive Ankle Board
**complementary metal oxide
semiconductor**
**Complement C31 desArg Biotrack RIA
system**
complete
c. denture prosthesis
C. implant
C. Ophthalmic Analysis System
c. pacemaker patient testing system
C. stent delivery platform
Tenax-XR C.
c. upper and lower dentures
completely
c. in canal (CIC)
c. in-the-canal hearing aid
c. in-the-canal listening device
completer
Akahoshi nucleus c.
complex
C. Cu3 dressing
oligometric c.
c. platinum microcoil
retractor-endoscope c.
compliance
c. cap
c. matching stent
compliant
c. balloon
c. prestress system
component
Accolade C femoral c.
Accolade TMZF femoral c.
acetabular c.
AcuMatch A, L, M series
acetabular c.
AGC Modular Tibial II c.
AGC porous anatomic femoral c.

anatomic graduated c.'s (AGC)
anatomic porous replacement
hemispheric acetabular c.
Biomet AGC knee c.
Biomet AGC primary and posterior
stabilized c.
Biomet Bi-Polar c.
Biomet MARS acetabular c.
Biomet Repicci II unicompartment
knee c.
Biomet revision acetabular c.
Biomet shoulder c.
bipolar hip arthroplasty c.
Black Max mid-size knee c.
CFV wrist c.
Charnley flat-back femoral c.
custom-designed swan-neck
femoral c.
Definition PM femoral implant c.
dorsi stop c.
Duramer polyethylene c.
Durasul prosthetic c.
femoral head implant c.
Freeman femoral c.
Harris-Galante hip replacement
acetabular c.
Harris-Galante I porous-coated
acetabular c.
Harris-Galante porous acetabular c.
Harris-Galante porous-coated
femoral c.
Healey revision acetabular c.
HGP II acetabular c.
Hoffmann II compact external
fixation c.
hybrid fixation of hip
replacement c.
Immunotech immunoassay c.
Interlok primary femoral c.
Isola spinal implant system c.
Judet impactor for acetabular c.
Kirschner Universal self-centering
captive-head bipolar c.
Kudo elbow c.
Lubinus acetabular c.
Mallory-Head Interlok primary
femoral c.
MARS revision acetabular c.
Meridian PA femoral c.
Meridian ST femoral implant c.
Meridian TMZF femoral c.
Metasul hip joint c.
monoblock femoral c.
Morse taper lock of modular hip
implant c.
neck c.
NexGen c.
NexGen knee c.
Ogee acetabular c.

Omnifit HA femoral c.
Opti-Fix femoral c.
Osteolock acetabular c.
Osteolock HA femoral c.
Osteonics Omnifit-HA c.
PCA hip c.
PFC c.
polyethylene liner implant c.
Precision Osteolock femoral c.
press-fit condylar c.
press-fit femoral c.
Profix porous femoral c.
QSAC acetabular c.
quadrant-sparing acetabular c. (QSAC)
Reliance CM femoral implant c.
roof-reinforcement ring hip arthroplasty c.
Rothman Institute porous femoral c.
2-c. sealant
Smith & Nephew reflection acetabular cup implant c.
Sofamor-Danek c.
Springlite G foot c.
Springlite II foot c.
S-ROM modular femoral c.
stem c.
sternal attachment c.
straight stem femoral c.
supracondylar barrel/plate c.
Taperloc femoral c.
Tharies femoral resurfacing c.
Tharies hip c.
thoracic extension c.
Ti-Bac acetabular c.
trial c.
Tri-Con c.
Tri-Spike acetabular c.
Ultima C femoral c.
Vision acetabular c.
vitallium mesh c.
Vitalock cluster acetabular c.
Vitalock solid-back acetabular c.
wheelchair seating c.
Zimmer NexGen LPS knee femoral c.

composite
Carboplast II c.
c. cultured skin
c. dental cement
dentin-bonded resin c.
c. dressing
c. external fixator ring adhesive
c. polymer stent
c. prosthesis
Sepramesh biosurgical c.
c. spring elastic splint

compound
c. curved rasp
Dermatex c.
c. dressing
Finite dental glazing c.
c. lens
Microfil silicone-rubber injection c.
OCT c.
Pediplast moldable footcare c.
c. spectacles
c. suture
compress
Cool Tops c.
Kold Wrap freezable c.
compressed
c. air-powered dermatome
c. Ivalon patch graft
compressible acrylic intraocular lens
compression
c. bandage
c. belt
c. binder
c. boot
c. clicker
c. device
c. dressing
c. earring
c. forceps
c. garment
c. girdle
c. glove
c. hearing aid
c. hip screw (CHS)
c. hook
c. instrumentation posterior construct
c. paddle
c. plate
c. pump
c. rod
c. skullcap closure
c. sleeve shin splint
c. spring
c. stocking
c. U rod
c. U-rod instrumentation
compression-molded PMMA intraocular lens
compressive
c. internal fixating device
c. plastic splint
compressor
air c.
AM-50 portable air c.
Anthony orbital c.
Berens orbital c.
Castroviejo c.
Conn aortic c.
continuous air c.

C

compressor *(continued)*
    Deschamps c.
    DeVilbiss Pulmo-Aide I.T c.
    Easy Air 15 c.
    Easy Neb c.
    enucleation c.
    external inflatable c.
    Freeway Lite portable aerosol c.
    orbital c.
    Pari Proneb Turbo c.
    Pulmo-Mist c.
    Puritan all-purpose c.
    screw c.
    Sehrt c.
    shot c.
    tonsillar c.
compressor/nebulizer
    Pulmo-Aide aerosol c./n.
    PulmoMate aerosol c./n.
ComPressor pelvic compression belt
Comprifix
    C. active ankle support
    C. ankle splint
Compriform support stocking
Comprilan
    C. bandage
    C. wrap
Compro Plus Knee support
Compton
    C. suppression spectrometer
    C. suppression system
CompuCam digital intraoral camera
Compudriver digital torque-meter
Compumedics P-series sleep monitoring system
Compu-Neb ultrasonic nebulizer
Compuscan Hittman computerized electrocardioscanner
Compuscan-P pachymeter
computed
    C. Anatomy Corneal Modeling System
    c. tomography (CT)
computer
    Aspect c.
    image reconstruction c.
    c. navigation system
    on-demand analgesia c.
    Sequential Multiple Analyzer C. (SMAC)
    sequential multiple analyzer plus c.
    thermodilution cardiac output c.
computer-aided
    c.-a. detection (CAD)
    c.-a. fluency establishment trainer
    c.-a. sensory evaluator
computer-assisted
    c.-a. neurosurgical navigational system
    c.-a. stereotactic surgery (CASS)
    c.-a. videokeratoscope
computer-controlled
    c.-c. infusion pump
    c.-c. neurological stimulation system
    c.-c. neurological stimulation system cone
computerized
    c. bedside transfusion identification system
    c. corneal topographer
    c. image analysis system
    c. isokinetic dynamometer
    c. morphometric system
    c. pattern generator
    c. rotary chair
    c. sleep analysis system
    c. speech laboratory
Comtesse medical support stocking
concave
    c. dental mirror
    c. gouge
    c. lens
    c. loading socket
    c. mirror
    c. obturator
    c. sheath
    c. skull disc
concavoconcave lens
concavoconvex lens
concentrator
    Keystone Plus oxygenator c.
    Millennium oxygen c.
    NewLife Elite c.
    NewLife oxygen c.
    Puritan Bennett Aeris 590 oxygen c.
    SolAiris III oxygen c.
    SolAiris III, V oxygen c.
    speed vacuum c.
    stem cell c.
concentric
    c. needle
    c. needle electrode
Concentrix
    C. dual aspiration pump system
    C. Fluidics
Concept
    C. ablator
    C. bipolar coagulator
    C. CTS Relief Kit
    C. disposable cautery
    C. handheld cautery
    C. II rowing ergometer
    C. shaver
Conceptus
    C. fallopian tube catheterization system
    C. Robust guidewire

C. Soft Seal cervical catheter
C. Soft Torque uterine catheter
C. VS catheter
Concert spine VR bone cement
concha-mastoid suture
conchotome
    Hartmann nasal c.
    Henke-Stille c.
    Olivecrona c.
    Stille c.
    Watson-Williams c.
    Weil-Blakesley c.
Concise
    C. cementing sculp
    C. compression hip screw
    C. compression hip screw system
    C. Plus hCG urine test
    C. resin
    C. side plate
Conco elastic bandage
Concorde
    C. disposable skin stapler
    C. disposable suction cannula
    C. implant and implement system
    C. lumbar implant
    C. suction cannula
Concord/Portex airway
condenser
    Abbé c.
    amalgam c.
    dark-field c.
condensing lens
conditioner
    Coe-Comfort tissue c.
    Shuttle cardiomuscular c.
condom
    c. catheter
    c. catheter collecting system
    female c.
    male c.
    c. urinal
conductance catheter
conductive hydrogel wound dressing
conductor
    Adson c.
    Bailey c.
    Bovie liquid c.
    Gigli saw c.
    Kanavel c.
    Martel c.
    Xomed Audiant bone c.
conduit
    Neurotube bioabsorbable nerve c.
    polyglycolic acid c.
    Rastelli c.
    C. TCP graft material
    C. TCP granule
condylar
    c. cuff

c. implant
c. lag screw plate
c. neck retractor
condyle rod
cone
    c. biopsy needle
    breast c.
    c. bur
    Centriflow membrane c.
    C. checkers game
    c. collar
    collimator c.
    Coloplast stoma c.
    computer-controlled neurological
      stimulation system c.
    hand c.
    hard sonolucent plastic c.
    McIntyre truncated c.
    nose c.
    Placido 25-ring c.
    Posey palm c.
    prosthetic c.
    C. ring curette
    28-ring Placido c.
    Samsung Medical Center-type
      collimator c.
    shielded open-end c.
    C. skull punch
    SMC-type collimator c.
    C. splint
    stacking c.
    stoma c.
    Stone C.
    C. suction biopsy curette
    c. tip catheter
    C. ventricular needle
    Visi-Flow stoma c.
coned heparin tip
Confide HIV test kit
confidence ring
confocal
    c. laser scanning microscope
    c. laser scanning ophthalmoscope
    c. microscope
    c. optics
    c. scanning laser ophthalmoscope
    c. scanning laser polarimeter
Conform
    C. dressing
    C. II with Heel-Ease Nature Sleep
      pressure pad
    C. stretch bandage
Conformant
    C. contact layer sheet
    C. 2 nonadherent transparent
      wound veil
    C. wound dressing
**Conforma 3000 proton beam treatment
system**

C

conformer
>C. diabetic boot
>McGuire c.
>Moore-Wilson hyperopic c.
>silicone c.
>Universal c.

Conformexx biliary stent
ConfoScan
>C. 3 microscope
>C. slit corneal confocal microscope
>C. 2.0 slit corneal confocal microscope

congenital
>c. portacaval shunt
>c. subluxated crystalline lens

congruous cup-shaped reamer
conical
>c. bur
>c. catheter
>c. centrifuge tube
>c. implant
>c. inserter tip
>c. nut wrench
>c. probe

conical-tip electrode
conic bougie
conization
>c. electrode
>c. instrument

conjunctival
>c. fixation forceps
>c. scissors

conjunctiva spreader
Conmed
>C. Aspen Excalibur-Plus electrosurgical unit
>C. electrosurgical pencil

Conn aortic compressor
connecting
>c. plate
>c. tubing

connection
>c. cord
>internal hex-thread c.
>Luer c.

connector
>ACMI light source c.
>adjustable pedicle c.
>coaxial I&A nylon c.
>domino spinal instrumentation c.
>drain-to-wall suction c.
>dual bypass c.
>extension tubing with c.
>c. forceps
>Holter c.
>intrinsic transverse c.
>Karl Storz light source c.
>Luer c.
>Luer-Lok c.

>Luer-Lok jet ventilator c.
>Machida light source c.
>McIntyre nylon cannula c.
>Olympus light source c.
>pedicle c.
>Pentax light source c.
>plastic c.
>Prolene hernia system c.
>Pudenz c.
>quick c.
>SidePort AutoControl airway c.
>straight c.
>Symmetry bypass system aortic c.
>T c.
>tandem c.
>transverse c.
>tube c.
>Tuohy-Borst c.
>Uni-Gard piggyback c.
>Universal c.
>venous Y c.
>wire loop c.
>c. with lock washer
>Y c.
>Y-port c.

Connell
>C. airway
>C. suture

Con-Nex reamer
Connor
>C. angled wand
>C. capsulorrhexis peeler forceps
>C. curved wand
>C. straight irrigating wand
>C. straight nonirrigating wand
>C. wand

conoidal ankle prosthesis
ConQuest
>C. female continence system pressure pad with preattached flange
>C. incontinence system
>C. male continence system condom catheter with preattached flange
>C. male continence system leg bag kit
>C. male continence system supporter brief

Conquest
>C. balloon dilatation catheter
>C. meniscal crescent punch
>C. PTA balloon dilatation catheter
>C. suture retriever

Conrad-Crosby bone marrow biopsy needle
conservative anatomic prosthesis (CAP)
Conserve hip system
conserver
>EX-2000 DeVilbiss c.

Hideaway oxygen c.
Oxymatic electronic oxygen c.
PulseDose EX2000D oxygen c.
Walkabout oxygen c.

console
Bruker c.
Cobe-Stöckert heart-lung c.
c. compression garment
Dissectron ultrasonic neurosurgical
  aspirator c.
Hitachi EUB-515C ultrasound c.
Marconi Medical Systems c.
Siemens Satellite CT evaluation c.

constant
c. current stimulator
c. passive-motion machine (CPMM)
c. tension splint

Consta Vac autoreinfusion system

constrained
c. hinged knee prosthesis
c. nonhinged knee prosthesis
c. Wallgraft endoprosthesis

constriction ring

construct
compression instrumentation
  posterior c.
double-rod c.
Edwards modular system
  compression c.
Edwards modular system
  kyphoreduction c.
Edwards modular system
  neutralization c.
Edwards modular system rod-
  sleeve c.
Edwards modular system
  scoliosis c.
Edwards modular system standard
  sleeve c.
hook-to-screw L4-S1 compression c.
iliosacral and iliac fixation c.
pedicle screw c.
reconstructive cell/polymer c.
rigid cantilever beam c.
rod-hook c.
screw-to-screw compression c.
segmental compression c.
single-rod c.
Texas Scottish Rite Hospital
  double-rod c.
tissue-engineered c.
titanium c.
triplane c.
TSRH double-rod c.
TSRH pedicle screw-laminar
  claw c.
upper cervical spine anterior c.
upper cervical spine posterior c.
Wiltse system double-rod c.

Wiltse system H c.
Wiltse system single-rod c.

Constructa-Foam

Contack labral anchor

contact
c. A-scan
c. bandage lens
c. B-scan
c. B-scan ultrasonography
c. compressive forceps
c. glasses
c. hysteroscope
C. Laser convex probe
C. Laser round probe
C. Laser scalpel
c. laser vaporization
c. lens
c. lens training mirror
c. low-vacuum lens
c. probe
c. shield
c. side field lens
C. SPH cups system

contact-layer wound dressing

contact-tip laser system

container
ALPS c.
child-resistant c.
Cryocyte freezing c.
cryogenic storage c.
instrument retrieval c.
Mini-Bag Plus c.
non-child-resistant c.
quartz-glass c.
Quickbox c.
Safe-T-Flex enteral feeding c.
screw-cup c.

containment bag

Contak
C. CD CRTD Easytrak system
C. CD ventricular resynchronization
  pacemaker
C. Renewal 3 cardiac
  resynchronization therapy
  defibrillator
C. Renewal 3 CRTD system

contemporary nearpoint chart

ContiCath catheter system

Contigen
C. Bard cochlea
C. Bard collagen implant

contiguous spinal fluid reservoir

Contimed
C. II measuring unit
C. II pelvic floor muscle monitor

continuous
c. air compressor
c. bar retainer
c. clip forceps

C

187

continuous *(continued)*
    c. insulin delivery system (CIDS)
    c. irrigation catheter
    c. microinfusion device
    c. passive motion (CPM)
    c. passive motion device
    c. positive airway pressure (CPAP)
    c. subcutaneous insulin infusion pump
    c. suction tube
continuous-flow Wolfe resectoscope
continuously perfused probe
continuous-wave
    c.-w. argon laser
    c.-w. arthroscopy pump
    c.-w. CO_2 laser
    c.-w. diode laser
    c.-w. Doppler
    c.-w. high-frequency Doppler ultrasound system
    c.-w. laser beam
    c.-w. laser system
    c.-w. photocoagulator
Continuum
    C. bipolar acetabular head
    C. elliptical acetabular cup
    C. hip stem
    C. knee system
    C. knee system implant
    C. polyethylene acetabular cup
    C. P/S total knee
    C. total knee base plate
    C. unconstrained prosthesis
Contiplex catheter set
Contique contact lens case
ContiRing
contour
    C. back cushion
    c. block clamp
    c. defect molding kit
    C. Emboli artificial embolization device
    c. ERCP cannula
    C. Genesis UAL system
    C. Genesis ultrasonic-assisted lipoplasty system
    C. high-voltage can
    C. high-voltage can ICD
    C. II ICD
    c. instrument cleaning brush
    C. laser
    C. LT V-135D ICD
    C. LTV-135D implantable cardioverter-defibrillator
    C. MD implantable single-lead cardioverter defibrillator
    C. MD implantable single-lead cardioverter-defibrillator

    C. Meniscus Arrow bioresorbable repair system
    C. Profile Natural saline breast implant
    C. Profile silicone breast implant prosthetic buttock c.
    c. scalp retractor
    C. SE microsphere
    C. spine system
    C. tilting compression mammography system
    C. V-145D ICD
    C. V-145D implantable cardioverter-defibrillator
contoured
    c. anterior spinal plate
    c. anterior spinal plate drill guide
    c. femoral stem (CFS)
    c. washer
contourer
    prosthesis c.
contraceptive
    c. film
    c. implant
    Lea's shield female barrier c.
contractor
    Bailey baby rib c.
    Bailey-Gibbon rib c.
    Bailey rib c.
    Finochietto-Burford rib c.
    Finochietto infant rib c.
    Lemmon rib c.
    Medicon c.
    rib c.
    Scanlan-Crafoord c.
    Sellors rib c.
    surgical c.
contraflexion brace
Contrajet ERCP contrast delivery system
contrast
    c. absorption barrier
    c. column
contrast-filled catheter
Contraves stand
Contreet hydrocolloid nonadhesive foam dressing
control
    c. adjustment strap
    c. bridle
    C. cable and wire system
    intravascular accurate c. (IVAC)
    pronation/spring c. (PSC)
    c. wire
    C. Wire guidewire
controlled
    c. drain
    c. position brace
    c. radial expansion

controller
    Actis venous flow c.
    Bronkhorst High Tec c.
    flow c.
    Imed Gemini PC-2 volumetric c.
    mass flow c.
    pressure c.
    shoulder c.
    C. shoulder orthosis
    Siepser endocapsular c.
    vacuum c.
    viscous fluid c.
    volume c.
ControlWire guidewire
Contura medicated dressing
ConvaTec
    C. ostomy pouch
    C. Unna-Flex elastic Unna boot
    C. urostomy pouch
Conve back support
Conveen
    C. bag hanger
    C. bedside drainage bag
    C. curved/tapered intermittent
      catheter
    C. deluxe contoured leg bag
    C. drip collector
    C. female intermittent catheter
    C. leg bag strap
    C. net pant
    C. Security+male external catheter
      & liner
    C. Security+ self-sealing male
      external catheter
    C. self-sealing Urisheath
conventional
    c. cutting needle
    c. head coil
    c. processor
    c. shell implant
    c. single-axis knee prosthesis
    c. static scanner
    c. stent
    c. transmission electron microscope
convergent
    C. color Doppler
    c. lens
Converge porous acetabular system
converging collimator
converging-hole collimator
convergiometer
Converse
    C. blade retractor
    C. chisel
    C. double-ended alar retractor
    C. double-ended retractor
    C. guarded chisel
    C. guarded nasal chisel
    C. hinged skin hook

    C. nasal chisel
    C. nasal knife
    C. nasal retractor
    C. nasal root rongeur
    C. nasal saw
    C. nasal speculum
    C. nasal tip scissors
    C. needle holder
    C. osteotome
    C. periosteal elevator
    C. plastic surgery scissors
    C. rasp
    C. retractor blade
    C. sweeper curette
Converse-Gillies needle holder
Converse-Lange rongeur
Converse-MacKenty elevator
Converse-Wilmer conjunctival scissors
Converta-Litter carrier
converter
    analog-to-digital c. (ADC)
    D/A c.
    digital-to-analog c.
    motion-compensating format c.
    real-time format c.
    time-to-pulse height c.
convertible
    c. fin
    c. telescope
    C. trocar system
Convertors surgical drape
convex
    c. array
    c. lens
    c. mirror
    c. probe
    c. rasp
convexoconcave
    c. heart valve
    c. lens
convexoconvex lens
Convo-Gel cushion
convoluted
    c. foam mattress
    c. mattress pad
    c. wheelchair cushion
convolution mask
Conway lid retractor
Conzett goniometer
Cook
    C. aspirator
    C. balloon
    C. biopsy gun
    C. cannula
    C. Cardiovascular infusion catheter
    C. catheter
    C. Celect vena cava filter
    C. continence cuff
    C. continence ring

C

Cook (*continued*)
    C. cystotomy catheter
    C. detachable PDA coil
    C. drainage pouch set
    C. endoscopic curved needle driver
    C. enforcer
    C. eye speculum
    C. flexible biopsy forceps
    C. FlexStent
    C. FlexStent stent
    C. intracoronary stent
    C. locking stylet
    C. Logic coronary stent
    C. micropuncture introducer
    C. mini-compression balloon
      catheter
    C. N-Circle tipless bone basket
    C. osteotome
    C. pacemaker
    C. Peel-Away introducer
    C. peel-away sheath
    C. percutaneous entry needle
    C. plastic Luer-Lok adapter
    C. rectal retractor
    C. rectal speculum
    C. Spectrum catheter
    C. speculum
    C. stent
    C. stent positioner
    C. stereotactic guide
    C. straight guidewire
    C. Stratasis urethral sling
    C. tissue morcellator
    C. TPN catheter
    C. ureteral stent
    C. urological trocar
    C. walking brace
Cook-Amplatz dilator
Cook-Cope type loop catheter
cookie
    c. cutter
    c. cutter-type areolar marker
    Gelfoam c.
    C. Insert
    metatarsal c.
cool
    C. Comfort cold pack
    c. CPB brace
    c. Irom splint
    c. mist vaporizer (CMV)
    c. pack
    C. Tip catheter
    C. Tops compress
    C. Touch laser
Cooled ThermoCath treatment catheter
cooler
    Chameleon C.
    Hot/Ice cold therapy c.

Cooley
    C. anastomosis clamp
    C. aortic aneurysm clamp
    C. aortic clamp
    C. aortic forceps
    C. arteriotomy scissors
    C. atrial retractor
    C. atrial valve retractor
    C. bronchus clamp
    C. bulldog clamp
    C. cardiovascular scissors
    C. coarctation forceps
    C. cross-action bulldog clamp
    C. dilator
    C. forceps
    C. graft suction tube
    C. iliac clamp
    C. neonatal instrument
    C. patent ductus clamp
    C. pediatric vascular clamp
    C. peripheral vascular clamp
    C. renal artery clamp
    C. rib retractor
    C. rib shears
    C. sump tube
    C. U suture
    C. vascular tissue forceps
    C. vena cava clamp
Cooley-Baumgarten wire twister
Cooley-Beck vessel clamp
Cooley-Bloodwell-Cutter valve
Cooley-Bloodwell mitral valve prosthesis
Cooley-Cutter disc prosthetic valve
Cooley-Derra anastomosis clamp
Cooley-Merz sternum retractor
Cooley-Satinsky clamp
Cool-Flex A/K suspension belt
CoolGlide aesthetic laser system
Coolidge
    C. transformer
    C. x-ray tube
cooling
    c. blanket
    c. helmet
    c. machine
Coolscope digital camera/microscope
CoolSorb absorbent cold transfer
    dressing
CoolSpot skin-cooling device
cool-tip laser
Cool-tip RF system
CoolTouch
    C. Nd:YAG laser
    C. 1320nm laser system
    C. Varia laser
Coombs bone biopsy system
Coonrad-II prosthesis

Coonrad-Morrey
    C.-M. implant
    C.-M. total elbow prosthesis
Coonrad/Morrey total elbow system
Coons/Carey endoprosthesis
Coons Super Stiff long tip guidewire
Cooper
    C. ankle brace
    C. aspirator
    C. Clear DW contact lens
    C. disc cryostat
    C. implant
    C. irrigating/aspirating unit
    C. 2000, 2500 laser
    C. Laser Sonics laser
    C. nasal ganglia guide
    C. Toric contact lens
Cooper-Rand intraoral artificial larynx
CooperSurgical (CS)
    C. overhead colposcope
CooperVision
    C. argon laser
    C. camera
    C. diagnostic imaging refractor
    C. fragmatome
    C. I&A machine
    C. imaging perimeter
    C. irrigating needle
    C. irrigation/aspiration handpiece
    C. irrigation/aspiration unit
    C. microscope
    C. ocutome
    C. PMMA-ACL Flex lens
    C. refractive surgery photokeratoscope
    C. spatulated needle
    C. ultrasound
    C. vitrector
    C. YAG laser
CooperVision-Cilco-Kelman multiflex all-PMMA intraocular lens
Coordinate complete revision knee system
co-oximeter
    Ciba-Corning 2500 c.-o.
    IL-282 c.-o.
cooximeter analyzer
Copalite applicator
Cope
    C. biopsy needle
    C. crushing clamp
    C. gastrointestinal suture anchor set
    C. locking loop catheter
    C. loop catheter
    C. loop nephrostomy catheter
    C. loop nephrostomy tube
    C. mandrel guidewire
    C. modification of Martel intestinal clamp

    C. nitinol mandril wire guide
    C. pleural biopsy needle
    C. viscerotomy anchor
    C. wire
Copeland
    C. fetal scalp electrode
    C. humeral resurfacing head
    C. implant
    C. intraocular lens implant
    C. radial panchamber UV lens
    C. streak retinoscope
Copilot bleed-back control valve
coplanar beam
Coplus cohesive medium stretch bandage
copolymer
    c. ankle-foot orthosis
    c. foam
copper
    c. band
    c. band-acrylic splint
    c. bromide laser
    c. grid
    c. mallet
    c. phosphate cement
    c. T 380A IUD
    c. vapor laser
    c. vapor pulsed laser
Copper-7 intrauterine device
copper-clad steel needle
copper-constantan thermocouple
copy tool
coquille plano lens
Corail
    C. HA-coated stem
    C. HA-coated stem hip implant
    C. hip system
    C. press-fit prosthesis
Coratomic R wave inhibited pacemaker
Corazonix Predictor
Corbett bone rongeur
Corboy
    C. hemostat
    C. needle holder
Corcath catheter
cord
    bipolar connection c.
    coagulating suction cannula connection c.
    connection c.
    diathermy c.
    Racestyptine c.
Cordase injectable collagenase
Cordguard
    C. II
    C. umbilical cord sampler
Cordigital
    C. MicroER recorder
    C. MicroLR recorder

Cordis
- C. Ancar pacing lead
- C. Atricor pacemaker
- C. bioptome
- C. Bioptome sheath
- C. Brite Tip guiding catheter
- C. coaxial microcatheter
- C. CrossFlex coronary stent
- C. Ducor I, II, III catheter
- C. Ducor I, II, III coronary catheter
- C. Ducor pigtail catheter
- C. endovascular system
- C. guiding catheter
- C. implantable drug reservoir device
- C. injector
- C. LC multipurpose stent system
- C. Mini stent system
- C. multipurpose access port
- C. Palmaz Corinthian stent
- C. Palmaz Schatz long medium stent
- C. Powerflex angioplasty balloon
- C. Predator PTCA balloon catheter
- C. Secor implantable pump
- C. sheath
- C. Smart nitinol stent
- C. tantalum coil stent
- C. Titan balloon dilatation catheter

Cordis-Dow shunt adapter
Cordis-Hakim shunt
Cordis-Webster
- C.-W. ablation catheter
- C.-W. diagnostic/ablation deflectable tip catheter
- C.-W. mapping catheter

cordless
- c. dermatome
- c. monocular indirect ophthalmoscope

Cordostat
Foley C.

cordotomy

core
- C. bone biopsy needle
- C. Dynamics disposable cannula
- C. Dynamics disposable trocar
- C. Hibak Rest
- C. Lobak Rest
- C. Max-Relax cushion
- nitinol wire c.
- c. reamer
- C. Reflex wrist support
- C. Sitback Rest
- C. Slimrest
- C. Universal elastic knee support
- C. Universal elbow support
- C. Universal rib support

Core-Check tympanic thermometer
Coremetrics fetal apnea monitor
Coretemp deep tissue thermometer
CoreTherm high-energy device
Core-Vent
- C.-V. implant
- C.-V. implant system

Corex instrument
Corey ovum forceps
Corfit System 7000-series lumbosacral support
Cor-Flex wire guide
Corflo
- C. enteral feeding tube
- C. PEG tube
- C. percutaneous access catheter

Corflo-Cubby low-profile gastrostomy device
Corin
- C. hip arthroplasty system
- C. total hip

coring biopsy gun
Corinthian stainless steel balloon-expandable stent
Corival 400 ergometer
cork
- c., leather, and elastic orthotic sheet c.

Corkscrew
- C. Parachute
- C. rotator cuff repair system
- C. suture anchor

Cormed ambulatory infusion pump
cornea
- c. abrader
- AlphaCor artificial c.
- AlphaCor hydrogel synthetic c.
- c. chisel

cornea-holding forceps
corneal
- c. block
- c. contact lens electrode
- c. débrider
- c. erysiphake
- c. fascia lata spatula
- c. fixation forceps
- c. foreign body bur
- c. hook
- c. implant
- c. knife
- c. knife dissector
- c. lens
- c. light shield
- c. microscope
- c. needle
- c. pachymeter
- c. prosthesis forceps
- c. prosthesis trephine
- c. punch

c. section spatulated scissors
c. shaper microkeratome
c. splinter forceps
c. spud
c. topography system (CTS)
c. transplant centering ring
c. transplant marker
c. transplant scissors
c. tube
c. utility forceps

CorneaScope 9-ring photokeratoscope
CorneaSparing LTK system
Corneometer
corneoscleral
c. forceps
c. punch
c. scissors

corner
C. plug
c. retractor
C. tampon

Cornet forceps
Corning
C. 170 blood gas analyzer
C. implant

Corometrics
C. Doppler scanner
C. fetal monitor
C. Gold Quik Connect spiral electrode tip
C. maternal/fetal monitor
C. 118 maternal/fetal monitor
C. Medical Systems Inc. fetal monitoring system
C. monitor

Corometrics-Aloka echocardiograph machine
Coronado vacuum fixation device
coronary
c. anastomotic shunt
c. angiographic catheter
c. angiography analysis system
c. artery button
c. artery cannula
c. artery forceps
c. artery probe
c. artery scissors
c. dilatation catheter
c. dilator
c. guiding catheter
c. perfusion cannula
c. perfusion catheter
c. perfusion tip
c. sinus thermodilution catheter
c. wire

Coroskop Plus cardiac angiography system

Corpak
C. enteral Y extension set
C. weighted-tip self-lubricating tube

Corps
United States Marine C. (USMC)

Correct-a-Prizm
Correct-a-Prizmbar
corrected cosmetic contact shell eye implant
corrective
c. shoe
c. soft dressing

CorRestore
C. implantable patch
C. system

Corrigan cautery
corrugated forehead retractor
Corrxit foot and ankle orthosis
corset, corsette
Boston soft c.
dorsal lumbar c.
c. front
lumbar c.
lumbodorsal support c.
lumbosacral c.
surgical c.
Warm 'n' Form lumbosacral c.

Corson
C. myoma grasping forceps
C. needle
C. needle electrosurgical probe

Cortac monitoring electrode
cortex, pl. **cortices**
c. extractor
c. screw

cortex-aspirating cannula
Cortexplorer cerebral blood flow monitor
cortical
c. ASIF screw
c. bone screw
c. cleaving hydrodissector
c. cleaving hydrodissector cannula
c. electrode
c. incision coronary dilator
c. oral plate
c. pin
c. screw

cortices (*pl. of* cortex)
COR/T implant
Cortomic pacemaker
Cortoss bone void filler
corundum ceramic implant material
Corvac integrated serum separator tube
Corvita
C. endoluminal graft
C. endoprosthesis stent graft
C. endovascular graft
C. stent

Corwin
C. knife handle
C. wire twister
Corydon
C. expression cannula
C. hydroexpression cannula
Coryllos-Bethune rib shears
Coryllos retractor
Coryllos-Shoemaker rib shears
Corzyme kit
CoSeal
C. fibrin glue
C. resorbable synthetic sealant
Cosgrove
C. clamp
C. mitral valve retractor
C. retractor
Cosgrove-Edwards
C.-E. annuloplasty band
C.-E. annuloplasty system
Cosman
C. coagulator
C. ICP Tele-Sensor system
Cosman-Roberts-Wells (CRW)
C.-R.-W. stereotactic head frame
C.-R.-W. stereotactic ring
C.-R.-W. stereotactic system
Cosmederm-7
Cosmetech cannula
cosmetic contact shell implant
CO₂SMO
CO₂SMO capnograph/pulse oximeter
CO₂SMO Plus continuous
noninvasive respiratory profile
monitor
CosmoDerm
C. 1, 2 human-based collagen
C. 1, 2 human-based collagen
implant
Cosmolon closure for splint
CosmoPlast
C. human-based collagen
C. human-based collagen implant
Cosmos
C. 283 DDD pacemaker
C. II DDD pacemaker
C. II multiprogrammable dual-
chamber cardiac pulse generator
C. II pulse generator
Co-Span alloy
costal periosteotome
COSTART system
CO-stat end tidal breath analyzer
costotome
cot
EZ-Pro R4 ambulance c.
finger c.
Kenwood finger c.
MX-Pro R3 ambulance c.

rectal finger c.
rubber finger c.
Cotrel
C. pedicle screw
C. traction
Cotrel-Dubousset
C.-D. closed hook
C.-D. distraction system
C.-D. dynamic transverse traction
device
C.-D. hook-rod
C.-D. instrumentation (CDI)
C.-D. orthopaedic brace
C.-D. pediatric rod
C.-D. pedicle screw instrumentation
C.-D. pedicular instrumentation
C.-D. screw-rod system
C.-D. spinal instrumentation
C.-D. system
Cottingham punch
Cottle
C. alar protector
C. alar retractor
C. angular scissors
C. antral chisel
C. biting forceps
C. bone crusher
C. bulldog scissors
C. chisel
C. columella clamp
C. crossbar chisel osteotome
C. curved chisel
C. dissector
C. dorsal scissors
C. double-edged nasal knife
C. double hook
C. dressing scissors
C. heavy septal scissors
C. knife guide
C. knife guide and retractor
C. lower lateral forceps
C. mallet
C. modified knife handle
C. nasal-biting rongeur
C. nasal chisel
C. nasal hook
C. nasal knife
C. nasal knife blade
C. nasal rasp
C. nasal retractor
C. nasal scissors
C. nasal speculum
C. osteotome
C. periosteal elevator
C. 4-prong retractor
C. protected knife handle
C. rasp
C. saw
C. septal elevator

C. septal speculum
C. sharp-prong retractor
C. single-prong tenaculum
C. skin elevator
C. skin hook
C. soft palate retractor
C. tenaculum hook
C. thumb hook retractor
C. Universal nasal saw
C. upper lateral retractor
Cottle-Arruga cartilage forceps
Cottle-Jansen
C.-J. rongeur
C.-J. rongeur forceps
Cottle-Joseph
C.-J. hook
C.-J. retractor
C.-J. saw
Cottle-Kazanjian
C.-K. bone-cutting forceps
C.-K. nasal-cutting forceps
C.-K. nasal forceps
C.-K. rongeur
Cottle-MacKenty
C.-M. elevator
C.-M. elevator rasp
Cottle-Medicon osteotome
Cottle-Neivert retractor
cotton
c. applicator
c. ball
c. batting
c. bolster dressing
C. cannulatome
c. cast
c. elastic bandage
c. elastic dressing
c. glove
C. graduated dilation catheter
c. nonabsorbable suture
c. pledget
C. sphincterotome
c. suture
cotton-ball
c.-b. dressing
c.-b. sponge
cotton-covered tourniquet
Cotton-Huibregtse
C.-H. biliary stent set
C.-H. double pigtail stent
Cotton-Leung
C.-L. biliary stent
C.-L. biliary stent set
cottonoid
c. dissector
neurosurgical c.
c. patty
c. pledget
cotton-roll rubber dam clamp

cotton-tipped
c.-t. applicator
c.-t. applier
Cottontome
cotton-wadding dressing
cotton-wool bandage
cottony
c. Dacron
c. Dacron hollow suture
couch
Siemens c.
couching needle
couch-mounted head frame
coudé
c. bag
c. catheter
c. fulgurating electrode
c. suction catheter
c. urethral catheter
coudé-tip demeure catheter
coulometric
c. chloridometer
c. meter
Coulter
C. Channelyser cell analyzer
C. Clenz cleaning agent
C. counter
C. Epics Elite flow cytometer
C. Epics flow cytometer
C. Epics 700-series flow cytometer
C. Epics V flow cytometer
C. LH 500, 700, 750, 755, 1500 Series hematology analyzer
C. MAXM hematology analyzer
C. MD 16 hemocytometer
C. reticONE system
C. STKS hematology analyzer
CoumaCare Coumadin management system
coumarin flashlamp pumped pulsed dye laser
Coumatrak prothrombin time device
Councill
C. catheter
C. retention catheter
C. stone basket
C. stone dislodger
C. stone scoop
C. ureteral dilator
C. ureteral stone extractor
Councilman chisel
Council-tip tube
Counsellor vaginal mold
Counter rotation system brace
counter
automated gamma c.
beta scintillation c.
boron c.
Capintec instant gamma c.

counter *(continued)*
    Cobra auto-gamma c.
    Coulter c.
    event/episode c.
    gamma ray c.
    gamma well c.
    Geiger c.
    Geiger-Müller c.
    ionization c.
    joule c.
    Linson electronic cell c.
    LKB/Wallac automatic gamma c.
    LKB/Wallac scintillation c.
    Multisizer 3 Coulter c.
    pacing c.
    pill c.
    RackBeta liquid scintillation c.
    scintillation c.
    Sysmex NE8000 cell c.
    Sysmex R-1000 reticulocyte c.
    time-based c.
    Top-Count microplate
      scintillation c.
    whole-body c.
    Wizard gamma c.
    Z1, Z2 series Coulter c.
countercurrent heat exchanger
counterforce strap
counteroccluder
Counterpoint electromyograph
counterpressor
    Acland-Buncke c.
    Amenabar c.
    angled c.
counterpulsation
    c. balloon
    percutaneous intraaortic balloon c.
counterrotational splint
Counter Rotation System brace
countersink bur
counting
    liquid scintillation c.
Count'R-Force arch brace
Coupland
    C. elevator
    C. nasal suction tube
coupled array coil
coupler
    Ferrier c.
    Natus Ear C.
    Precise anastomotic c.
coupling head
Cournand
    C. arterial needle
    C. needle
    C. Tip Arrow QuadPolar electrode
      catheter
Cournand-Grino angiography needle
Cournand-Potts needle

Covaderm
    C. composite wound dressing
    C. Plus adhesive barrier dressing
    C. Plus V.A.D. dressing
Coventry screw
cover
    Accu-Flo polyethylene bur hole c.
    Accu-Flo silicone rubber bur
      hole c.
    AgiSite alginate wound c.
    AlgiDerm alginate wound c.
    alginate wound c.
    Algosteril alginate wound c.
    AquaShield orthopaedic cast c.
    AquaShield reusable cast c.
    AquaShield reusable orthopaedic
      cast c.
    Bair Hugger warming body c.
    CarraSorb H alginate wound c.
    ComfortWear pouch c.
    Curasorb zinc alginate wound c.
    Dermacea alginate wound c.
    E-Z Flap bur hole c.
    FyBron alginate wound c.
    Gentell alginate wound c.
    Hollister replacement filters
      pouch c.
    Kalginate alginate wound c.
    Kold Wrap general use sterile
      burn dressing & emergency
      wound c.
    Maxorb alginate wound c.
    Medipore dressing c.
    MIP reusable c.
    Nu-Hope pouch c.
    Overcast cast c.
    OxiLink oximeter probe c.
    PolyMem alginate wound c.
    protective mattress c.
    Restore alginate wound c.
    c. screw
    SeaSorb alginate wound c.
    Sheathes ultrasound probe c.
    ShowerSafe waterproof cast and
      bandage c.
    Show'rbag cast and dressing c.
    silastic bur hole c.
    soft cosmetic c.
    Sorbsan alginate wound c.
    Spenco top c.
    Springlite polyolefin BK c.
    Springlite polyurethane AK, BK
      conical c.
    Tegagen HG, HI alginate
      wound c.
    titanium mini bur hole c.
covered
    c. biliary metal stent
    c. Gianturco stent

c. self-expanding prosthesis
c. stent
c. Z-stent
covering
    Camwrap plastic c.
    Permalume c.
Coverlet
    C. adhesive
    C. adhesive dressing
    C. composite dressing
    C. O.R. adhesive surgical dressing
    C. Strips wound dressing
Cover-Roll
    C.-R. adhesive gauze
    C.-R. dressing
    C.-R. gauze
    C.-R. gauze adhesive
    C.-R. stretch bandage
Coverslipper
    Jung CV 5000 Robotic C.
Cover-Strip wound closure strip
Covertell composite secondary dressing
CovRSite dressing
Cowboy collar
cowhorn explorer
Co-Wrap dressing
Cox
    C. II ocular laser shield
    C. metatarsal spreader
    C. rapid dry heat transfer sterilizer
    C. sterilizer and incinerator unit
Coxeter prostatic catheter
Cox-Uphoff implant
CozMore insulin technology system
Cozy
    Cast C.
CP2 inflatable cold pack
CPAP
    continuous positive airway pressure
    AirSep CPAP
    CPAP kit
    lightweight and portable Sullivan nasal CPAP
    CPAP machine
    NightBird nasal CPAP
    Phantom nasal mask CPAP
    Revitalizer Soft-Start nasal CPAP
    Sullivan III CPAP
    Tranquility Quest CPAP
    CPAP ventilator
CPD Commander combined air/fluid exchange and silicone oil delivery system
C-PET scanner
CPHV OptiForm mitral valve
CPI
    Cardiac Pacemaker, Inc.
    CPI endocardial defibrillation rate-sensing pacing lead

CPI Endotak transvenous electrode
CPI Microthin DI, DII lithium-powered programmable pacemaker
CPI Mini device
CPI PRx implantable cardioverter-defibrillator
CPI Ventak AICD device
CPI/Guidant
    CPI/G. lead
    CPI/G. pacemaker
CPI-PRx pulse generator
CPM
    continuous passive motion
    CPM device
    CPM exerciser machine
    CPM machine
CPMM
    constant passive-motion machine
CPR Micromask
CPS
    compact plating system
    Inion CPS
    CPS modular air cranioclast
    CPS system
    CPS unitized air cranioclast
CPT
    CPT hip system
    CPT prosthesis
    CPT revision tamp
C-QUR bioabsorbable surgical mesh
CR49
    RIGScan CR49
CR-39 nuclear tract detector
CR6-45NMf retinal camera
cracker
    Dodick nucleus c.
    Ernest nucleus c.
    LeVeen plaque c.
    Newsom side-port nucleus c.
    nucleus c.
cradle
    acoustically transparent c.
    alpha c.
    c. arm sling
    auditory response c.
    c. boot
    Criss Cross c.
    CT scan c.
    foot c.
    Posey bed c.
    Spectrum DG-P pediatric c.
Crafoord
    C. aortic clamp
    C. arterial forceps
    C. coarctation clamp
    C. lobectomy scissors
    C. thoracic scissors
Crafoord-Sellors hemostatic forceps

Cragg
   C. endoluminal graft
   C. EndoPro stent-graft
   C. Endopro system
   C. Endopro System I covered stent
   C. Endopro System I stent
   C. FX-wire
   C. stent
   C. thrombolytic brush
Cragg-Castaneda thrombolytic brush
Cragg-McNamara
   C.-M. multiple side-hole infusion catheter
   C.-M. valved infusion catheter
Craig
   C. abduction splint
   C. biopsy needle
   C. headrest holder
   C. septal forceps
   C. septum bone-cutting forceps
Craigie tube
Craig-Scott orthosis
Cramer wire splint
Crampton-Tsang percutaneous endoscopic biliary stent set
Crane
   C. dental pick
   C. elevator
   C. mallet
cranial
   c. aneurysm clip
   c. bur
   c. drill
   c. forceps
   c. helmet
   c. Jacobs hook
   c. molding device
   c. molding helmet
   c. orthosis
   c. osteosynthesis system
   c. perforator
   c. pin
   c. plating system
   c. retractor
cranioblade
   Spiral Flute c.
CranioCap custom-made cranial orthosis
craniocervical plate
cranioclast
   Braun c.
   CPS modular air c.
   CPS unitized air c.
   Tarnier c.
craniofacial instrumentation
CranioFIX device
craniomandibular orthopaedic repositioning device

craniomaxillofacial
   c. mesh
   c. plating system
Cranioplastic
   C. acrylic cranioplasty material
   C. material dressing
   C. powder
cranioplasty
   dynamic orthotic c. (DOC)
craniosacral table
craniotome
   Anspach c.
   Midas Rex c.
craniotomy scissors
craniotribe
cranium clip-applying forceps
crank
   c. frame retractor
   c. table
crankshaft clip
crash cart
cravat bandage
Crawford
   C. aortic retractor
   C. clamp
   C. forceps
   C. hook
   C. lacrimal intubation set
   C. needle
   C. tube
crawl
   barrel c.
CR Bard Urolase
cream
   Ca-Rezz moisture barrier c.
   Prudoxin c.
   SoftGUARD hand c.
   Thera-Gesic c.
C-reamer
Creative diabetic sock
CRE balloon catheter
Credo razor
Creed dissector
Crego
   C. elevator
   C. periosteal elevator
   C. retractor
Cremer-Ikeda
   C.-I. papillotome
   C.-I. sphincterotome
crenulated tantalum wire
crepe
   c. bandage dressing
   c. short stretch bandage
crescent
   c. blade
   C. Complete Sleeper pillow
   c. CVD diamond knife
   C. memory pillow

C. pillow
c. scleral tunneler
c. snare
crescentic blade
Crescent-Pillo pillow
crest buttress pad
crib
c. splint
TiMesh mandibular c.
Cribier-Edwards aortic percutaneous heart valve
Crib-O-Gram neonatal screening audiometer
Cricket recording pulse oximeter
cricothyrotomy cannula
Crile
C. angle retractor
C. appendiceal clamp
C. arterial forceps
C. clamp
C. forceps
C. gall duct forceps
C. gall hemostat
C. gasserian ganglion knife
C. gasserian ganglion knife and dissector
C. hemostat
C. hemostatic clamp
C. hemostatic forceps
C. malleable retractor
C. needle holder
C. nerve hook
C. right-angle retractor
Crile-Murray needle holder
Crile-Rankin forceps
Crile-Wood needle holder
Crile-Wood-Vital needle holder
crimped
c. Dacron prosthesis
c. wire prosthesis
crimper
c. forceps
Francis-Gray wire c.
Juers wire c.
McGee wire c.
pin c.
wire c.
crimping forceps
crimp stop
Criss
C. Cross cradle
C. Cross Cradle
C. Cross Cradle device
Crista Cath 20-pole deflectable catheter
Cristobalite investment material
Critic-Aid skin paste
critical
c. care mattress

c. care unit
c. care ventilator
criticality locket dosimeter
Criticare
C. comprehensive vital sign monitor
C. $ETCO_2/SpO_2$ monitor
C. 507N noninvasive blood pressure monitor
C. 507O pulse oximeter/NIBP monitor
C. pulse oximeter
C. 503 pulse oximeter
C. 507-series noninvasive blood pressure monitor
C. 507S vital sign monitor
CritiCath
C. PA catheter
C. thermodilution catheter
CritiCore monitoring system
Critikon
C. automated blood pressure cuff
C. balloon temporary pacing catheter
C. balloon-tipped end-hole catheter
C. balloon wedge pressure catheter
C. guidewire
CritiView bedside patient monitoring device
Crit-Line
C.-L. fluid monitor
C.-L. III TQA fluid management and access device
C.-L. instrument
Crit-Scan noninvasive hematocrit measurement device
CritSpin
C. celltrifuge
C. microhematocrit centrifuge
CRM
CRM cup
CRM rehab brace
CRM stem
CRM system
Crockard
C. hard palate retractor
C. transoral clip applier
Crock-Yamagishi system
crocodile biopsy forceps
croissant tissue expander
Cronin
C. palate elevator
C. palate knife
C. silastic mammary prosthesis
Crookes
C. glasses
C. lens
Crookes-Hittorf tube
Crosby capsule

C

Crosby-Kugler
  C.-K. biopsy capsule
  C.-K. pediatric capsule
cross
  c. bar
  C. scleral trephine
  C. Top replacement oxygen sensor
cross-action
  c.-a. capsule forceps
  c.-a. towel clamp
crossbar
cross-bracing
  spinal rod c.-b.
  Wiltse system c.-b.
cross-clamp
  aortic c.-c.
cross-connector
  Crossover c.-c.
cross-cut straight fissure bur
Crosseal fibrin sealant
crossed
  c. coil
  c. delivery for osteoplasty (CDO)
  c. Kirschner wire
  c. loop resonator
Crossfire polyethylene material
CrossFlex
  C. coil stent
  C. LC coronary artery stent
  C. LC stainless steel laser-cut
    coronary stent
Cross-Jones
  C.-J. disc prosthetic valve
  C.-J. disc valve prosthesis
  C.-J. mitral valve
cross-legged clip
crosslink
  Edwards modular system rod c.
  Galveston fixation with TSRH c.
  c. gamma
  C. plate
  C. plate spinal system
  Texas Scottish Rite Hospital c.
  TSRH c.
crosslinked
  c. EVA copolymer foam
  c. poly glaucoma filtration device
Crossover
  C. cross-connector
  C. cross-connector system
CrossPoint TransAccess catheter
cross-Polaroid projection chart
CrossSail coronary dilatation catheter
cross-slot screwdriver
cross-table leg immobilizer
crosstalk pacemaker
Crosswire
  C. nitinol hydrophilic guidewire
  C. PTCA guidewire

crotchless compression garment
Crouch corneal protector
Croupette child tent
croup tent
Crowe
  C. pilot point
  C. pilot point on Steinmann pin
Crowe-Davis
  C.-D. mouthgag
  C.-D. mouth retractor
crown
  C. amalgamator
  Bicon integrated abutment c.
  Bosworth temporary c.
  Bremer halo c.
  Celay InCeram c.
  freestanding single c.
  C. high-profile cushion
  C. mattress system
  C. needle
  NuSmile primary c.
  C. Quadro cushion
  c. saw
  c. scissors
  stainless steel c.
  C. stent
**Crown-A-Matic crown and bridge
  remover**
crown-crimping pliers
Crozat
  C. clasp
  C. removable orthodontic appliance
CRS
  CRS brace
  CRS tibial torsion system
**CRS-series alternating overlay with
  pump**
C-R syringe
CRT
  cathode ray tube
CRT-D
  cardiac resynchronization therapy
    defibrillator
CrTmEr:YAG laser
CRT-P
  cardiac resynchronization therapy
    pacemaker
crucial bandage
cruciate
  c. condylar unconstrained prosthesis
  c. ligament guide
  c. punch
cruciate-retaining prosthesis
cruciate-sacrificing prosthesis
cruciform
  c. anterior spinal hyperextension
    (CASH)

c. anterior spinal hyperextension orthosis

c. screwdriver

cruiser

c. buggy

C. hip abduction

C. hip abduction brace

C. OA brace

Crurasoft patch

crusher

bone c.

cartilage c.

Cottle bone c.

Lieberman phaco c.

Lowsley stone c.

Mayo-Lovelace spur c.

ultrasonic stone c.

crushing clamp

crutch, pl. **crutches**

c. and belt femoral closed nail

EuroCuff forearm c.

c. glasses

Hardy aluminum c.

iWALKfree hands-free c.

Kenny c.

Lofstrand c.

Warm Springs c.

crutched

c. stick-type biliary duct stent

c. stick-type polyurethane endoprosthesis

Crutchfield

C. carotid artery clamp

C. clamp

C. skeletal traction

C. skeletal traction tongs

Crutchfield-Raney drill

CRVO knife

CRW

Cosman-Roberts-Wells

CRW stereotactic system

CRx Diamond valve

Cryer

C. dental elevator

C. root elevator

C. Universal forceps

cryoablation

c. catheter

c. probe

Cry-O-Cadet

Cryocare

C. cardiac surgical system

C. cryoablation system

cryocatheter

Freezor c.

CryoCor cryoablation system

Cryo/Cuff

Aircast C./C.

C./C. ankle dressing

C./C. boot

C./C. compression dressing

C./C. compression support

C./C. knee compression dressing system

C./C. pressure boot

Cryocup ice massager

Cryo-Cut microtome

Cryocyte freezing container

cryoenucleator

cryoextractor

Alcon c.

Bellows c.

Keeler c.

Kelman c.

Thomas c.

cryogenic

c. probe

c. storage container

CryoGuide ultrasound guidance system

cryogun

Wallach LL100 cryosurgical c.

CryoHit

C. cryotherapy device

C. tumor ablation system

CryoLife

C. homograft

C. valvular graft

CryoLife-O'Brien valve

cryomagnet

CryoMed 1010A freezer

Cryomedical Sciences AccuProbe 450 system

Cryomedics

C. colposcope

C. disposable LLETZ electrode

C. electrosurgery system

CryoNeedle

SeedNet gold ultrathin C.

cryopencil

Mira endovitreal c.

cryopexy probe

cryophake

Alcon c.

Kelman c.

cryoplasty balloon

cryopreserved homograft valve

cryoprobe

Erbe c.

Frigitronics c.

intravitreal c.

Lee c.

Linde c.

Rubinstein c.

Thomas c.

cryoptor

Thomas c.

cryoretractor

Cryo rubber mold

CryoSeal
    C. fibrin sealant system
    C. FS system
cryostat
    Ames Lab-Tek c.
    CE-2 c.
    Cooper disc c.
    c. frozen sectioning aid
    Tissue Tek-II c.
Cryo-Surg
    C.-S. cryosurgical system
    C.-S. liquid nitrogen spray unit
cryosurgical
    c. apparatus
    c. instrument
    c. unit
cryosystem
    Keeler-Amoils ophthalmic c.
cryotherapy
    freeze-thaw c.
    c. probe
    c. system
    c. wrap
cryotome
cryotube
    Nunc c.
Cryo-Vac-A cryostat vacuum system
CryoValve-SG
CryoVein
cryovial tube
crypt hook
cryptoscope
    Satvioni c.
crystal
    C. adjusting table
    Cardiometrics FloWire Doppler
      echo c.
    c. gamma camera
    piezoelectric c.
    C. polymer gel
    C. Tone I in-the-ear hearing aid
Crystalens IOL
CrystaLens model AT-45 implant
CrystalEyes endoscopic video system
crystalline
    c. lens
    c. phosphor detector
CS
    CooperSurgical
CS1500 articulating arm video-ready colposcope
CS200 upright post zoom colposcope
CS500 articulating arm zoom colposcope
CS-5 cryosurgical system
CS-9000 densitometer
C-Scan
    C-S. color-ellipsoid topometer
    Technomed C-S.

CSCT-2000 electromagnetic device
CSF
    C. reservoir
    C. T-tube shunt
C-shaped plate
CSI toric contact lens
CSM Stretta system
C-sponge
C-Stem triple taper stabilized hip implant
CSV Bovie electrosurgical unit
CSZ
    Cincinnati Sub-Zero
CT
    computed tomography
      CT body scanner
      CT 200 corneal topographer
      CT densitometer
      CT Max 640 scanner
      CT scan cradle
      CT scan gantry
      CT Twin scanner
CT-10 computerized tonometer
CT1 suture
CT9000, 9800 scanner
CTA
    cuff tear arthropathy
    cuff tear arthroplasty
CT-based CAD/CAM revision femoral implant
CTDx electrostimulation system
C-Tek anterior cervical plate system
CTEV brace
CTE:YAG laser
CT-guided stereotactic biopsy
CTI
    CTI cyclotron
    CTI 933/04 ECAT scanner
    CTI 931 PET scanner
    CTI positron emission tomography
      scanner
C.Ti.2 knee brace
CTi2 knee brace
CTi brace
CTI-Siemens 933/8-12 PET camera
CT/MRI-compatible stereotactic head frame
CTNF capsule protein eye implant
CTO
    cervicothoracic orthosis
      Aspen CTO
C-Trak
    C-T. analyzer
    C-T. handheld gamma detector
    C-T. handheld gamma probe
    C-T. probe
    C-T. surgical guidance system
CTRS device

CTS
    corneal topography system
        CTS gauge
        CTS Gripfit splint
        CTS Relief kit
C-TUB instrument receptacle
C-type acupuncture needle
Cu-7 intrauterine device
CU-8 needle
cube
    foam c.
    Gelfoam c.
    c. pessary
    porous calcium phosphate c.
    Rancho c.
    Temper Foam c.
    tumbling E c.
CUBEx multifunctional step
Cub R-200 enteral feeding pump
Cuda shaver
Cue fertility monitor
Cueva
    C. cranial nerve electrode
    C. cranial nerve electrode
        monitoring device
cuff
    antimicrobial catheter c.
    AS-800 c.
    Astropulse c.
    Bivona foam c.
    blood pressure c.
    calibrated V-Lok c.
    ComfortCuff blood pressure c.
    condylar c.
    Cook continence c.
    Critikon automated blood
      pressure c.
    Dacron c.
    Dinamap blood pressure c.
    Ducker-Hayes nerve c.
    c. electrode
    elephant c.
    endotracheal tube c.
    Ethox c.
    Finapres finger c.
    finger c.
    hand c.
    Honan c.
    inflatable tourniquet c.
    inflatable tracheal tube c.
    joint distraction c.
    Kendall endotracheal tube c.
    Kidde tourniquet c.
    C. Link orthopaedic device
    neonatal c.
    nerve c.
    oscillometric blood pressure c.
    pneumatic c.
    Portex XL endotracheal tube c.

    pressure c.
    push c.
    Push-Ease Quad C.
    Rusch endotracheal tube c.
    Safe-Cuff blood pressure c.
    Salubria nerve c.
    shoulder c.
    c. sphygmomanometer
    sphygmomanometer c.
    Steri-Cuff disposable tourniquet c.
    supracondylar c.
    suprapatellar c.
    c. tear arthropathy (CTA)
    c. tear arthroplasty (CTA)
    tourniquet c.
    tracheal tube c.
    vaginal c.
    VitaCuff c.
    V-Lok disposable blood pressure c.
cuffed
    c. endotracheal tube
    c. esophageal endoprosthesis
    c. ET tube
    c. tracheostomy tube
cuff-type inactive electrode
CUI
    C. artificial breast prosthesis
    C. gel mammary prosthesis
cuirass
    c. respirator
    c. ventilator
cul-de-sac irrigation T tube
culdoscope
Culler
    C. fixation forceps
    C. hook
    C. iris spatula
    C. lens spoon
    C. muscle hook
    C. rectus muscle hook
Culp biopsy needle
culture
    Bactrol Plus quality control c.
culturette
    mini-tip c.
Cummings folding forceps
Cummins disc prosthesis
Cun-Meter
Cunningham-Cotton
    C.-C. sleeve
    C.-C. sleeve coaxial dilator
Cunningham urinary incontinence clamp
cup
    AccuPressure heel c.
    acetabular c.
    Anti-Shox heel c.
    Arthropor acetabular c.
    Bard alligator c.
    Bard oval c.

cup *(continued)*
Bauerfeind SofSpot heel c.
Bicon-Plus c.
c. biopsy forceps
Bird OP c.
bleb c.
c. catheter
Charnley acetabular c.
Charnley offset-bore c.
CMI-Mityvac c.
CMI-O'Neil c.
Continuum elliptical acetabular c.
Continuum polyethylene
   acetabular c.
CRM c.
c. curette
DePuy Solution System
   acetabular c.
DePuy Tri-Lock interlocking
   acetabular c.
dry c.
Duraloc acetabular c.
ear c.
Essential Energy c.
eye c.
Flo-Trol drinking c.
c. forceps
Galin bleb c.
Ganz c.
Gap c.
Gemini c.
Harris-Galante c.
Hedrocel c.
heel c.
Hemisphere modular c.
HGP II acetabular c.
ileostomy c.
Instead feminine protection c.
Integrity acetabular c.
Interseal acetabular c.
iodine c.
jumbo acetabular c.
Kennedy spillproof c.
Lineage acetabular c.
Lord c.
magnetic c.
Malmstrom c.
Malström c.
McBride c.
McKee-Farrar acetabular c.
Mityvac obstetric vacuum
   extractor c.
Mityvac Super M c.
monolithic A1203 c.
multipolar bipolar c.
nasal suction c.
New England Baptist acetabular c.
ocular c.
Omnifit acetabular c.

ophthalmic c.
optics c.
Opti-Fix acetabular c.
Opti-Fix II acetabular c.
patella c.
PCA acetabular c.
c. pessary
Polysorb heel c.
porous-coated acetabular c.
c. positioner
PQ premium heel c.
prophy c.
prosthesis c.
prosthetic c.
Reflection I, V, FSO acetabular c.
Restoration GAP acetabular c.
Riecken PQ premium heel c.
screw-in ceramic acetabular c.
silastic obstetrical vacuum c.
Silipos silicone wonder c.
slit-lamp c.
Smith-Petersen c.
Solution System acetabular c.
Sorbothane II heel c.
S-ROM acetabular c.
stainless steel c.
suction c.
Tender Touch vacuum birthing c.
Titan hip c.
trial acetabular c.
Tri-Lock acetabular c.
Trilogy acetabular c.
Tuli heel c.
Tuli Pro heel c.
Tuli rubber heel c.
University of California
   Biomechanics Laboratory heel c.
vacuum c.
vitallium c.
wet c.
Wonder-Cup heel c.
Wonder-Spur heel c.
zinc-free plastic specimen c.
ZTT acetabular c.
ZTT I, II c.
cupboard
RF-shielded c.
cupped
c. curette
c. forceps
cuprophane membrane
cup-shaped
c.-s. curette forceps
c.-s. electrode
Curad
C. bandage
C. surgical adhesive dressing
Curaderm
C. hydrocolloid

C. hydrocolloid dressing
C. hydrocolloid dressing material
Curafil
    C. gel wound dressing
    C. hydrogel dressing
    C. hydrogel-impregnated gauze
    C. impregnated gauze
Curafoam
    C. foam dressing
    C. foam wound dressing
    C. island dressing
    C. wound dressing
Curagel
    C. hydrogel dressing
    C. hydrogel island wound dressing
    C. hydrogel sheet
    C. wafer
Curaklense wound cleanser
curare
Curasol
    C. hydrogel dressing
    C. impregnated gauze
    C. sterile wound dressing
    C. wound cleanser
Curasorb
    C. calcium alginate dressing
    C. zinc alginate dressing
    C. zinc alginate wound cover
Curdy
    C. blade
    C. sclerotome
Curdy-Hebra blade
C-urea breath test
CureLight
    C. Broadband red light
    C. lamp
curette, curet
    Accurette endometrial suction c.
    Acufex c.
    adenoid c.
    After Five c.
    Alvis c.
    Alvis foreign body eye c.
    angled ring c.
    AngleLoop c.
    antral c.
    aortic c.
    area-specific c.
    aspirating c.
    Ballenger ethmoid c.
    banjo c.
    Barnhart 1/2 universal c.
    Barnhill adenoid c.
    Barth mastoid c.
    bayonet c.
    Beckman adenoid c.
    Berkeley suction c.
    Billeau ear wax c.
    Billeau wax c.

biopsy suction c.
Blake uterine c.
blunt ring c.
bone c.
bowl c.
box c.
Brun bone c.
Brun mastoid c.
Buck bone c.
Buck ear c.
Buck earring c.
Buck wax c.
Bumm uterine c.
Cannon c.
Carter submucous c.
cement c.
cerumen c.
cervical biopsy c.
chalazion c.
Charnley bone c.
Cloward c.
Coakley sinus c.
Cobb c.
Cobb bone c.
Cobb spinal c.
Columbia 13/14 universal c.
Cone ring c.
Cone suction biopsy c.
Converse sweeper c.
cup c.
cupped c.
Daubenspeck bone c.
Dawson-Yuhl-Cone c.
de Cornier endometrial suction c.
dental c.
dermal c.
diagnostic c.
disc c.
disposable c.
disposable vacuum c.
double-ended c.
double-ended bone c.
double-ended dental c.
double-ended stapes c.
down-biting Epstein c.
ear c.
endaural c.
endocervical biopsy c.
endodontic c.
endometrial c.
Endosampler disposable endometrial
  biopsy c.
Epstein c.
ethmoidal c.
extended shank Gracey c.
eye c.
Farrior ear c.
Faulkner c.
Faulkner ethmoidal c.

C

curette *(continued)*
    fenestration c.
    fine c.
    fine angled c.
    fine bone c.
    flat back c.
    c. forceps
    foreign body c.
    fossa c.
    Fox c.
    Fox dermal c.
    frontal sinus c.
    Fukushima ring c.
    Garcia-Rock endometrial biopsy c.
    Gills-Welsh c.
    Goldman c.
    Gracey Deep Pocket c.
    Greene endocervical c.
    Greene uterine c.
    Gross ear c.
    Gusberg cervical biopsy c.
    Gusberg cervical cone c.
    Halle bone c.
    Halle ethmoidal c.
    Halle sinus c.
    Hardy bayonet c.
    Hardy hypophysial c.
    Hardy ring c.
    Harrison-Shea c.
    Hartmann adenoidal c.
    Hatfield bone c.
    Heaney endometrial biopsy c.
    Heaney uterine c.
    Heath c.
    Heath chalazion c.
    Hebra c.
    Hebra chalazion c.
    Hebra corneal c.
    Helix endocervical c.
    Helix uterine biopsy c.
    Hibbs c.
    Hibbs bone c.
    Hibbs spinal c.
    hook-type dermal c.
    horizontal ring c.
    Hough c.
    House ear c.
    House stapes c.
    hypophysial c.
    Ingersoll adenoid c.
    Innomed bone c.
    intervertebral c.
    irrigating uterine c.
    Jacobson c.
    Jansen bone c.
    Jones adenoid c.
    Jordan-Rosen c.
    Juers ear c.
    Kelly c.

    Kelly-Gray uterine c.
    Kerpel bone c.
    Kevorkian c.
    Kevorkian endocervical c.
    Kevorkian endometrial c.
    Kevorkian-Younge endocervical biopsy c.
    Kevorkian-Younge uterine c.
    Kirkland c.
    Kraff capsule polisher c.
    Kuhn-Bolger angled c.
    Kuhn-Bolger frontal recess c.
    Langer c.
    large bowel c.
    large uterine c.
    Latitude c.
    Laufe aspirating c.
    Laufe-Novak diagnostic c.
    Lempert bone c.
    Lempert endaural c.
    Lempert fine c.
    long-handle c.
    loop c.
    Lucas alveolar c.
    Luer bone c.
    Lynch c.
    Magnum c.
    Malis c.
    Marino rotatable transsphenoidal horizontal ring c.
    Marino rotatable transsphenoidal vertical ring c.
    Marino transsphenoidal c.
    Maroon lip c.
    Martin dermal c.
    Martini bone c.
    mastoid c.
    Mayfield spinal c.
    McCain TMJ c.
    Meigs endometrial c.
    Meigs uterine c.
    meniscal c.
    Meyhoefer bone c.
    Meyhoefer chalazion c.
    MicroLoop c.
    Microsect c.
    middle ear ring c.
    Milan uterine c.
    Mi-Mark disposable endocervical c.
    miniature Gracey c.
    modified Gracey c.
    Moe bone c.
    Molt c.
    Mosher ethmoid c.
    Mueller c.
    nasal c.
    Novak c.
    Novak biopsy c.
    Novak uterine c.

optical aspirating c. (OAC)
orthopaedic c.
oval c.
oval window c.
ovum c.
periapical c.
Piffard dermal c.
Pipelle de Cornier endometrial suction c.
Pipelle endometrial c.
pituitary c.
placental c.
plastic c.
polyvinyl c.
Pratt ethmoid c.
Ray pituitary c.
Read facial c.
Récamier uterine c.
rectal c.
Reu c.
reverse-angle skid c.
reverse-curve adenoid c.
Rhoton blunt-ring c.
Rica ear c.
right-angle c.
rigid c.
ring c.
ring bayonet Rand c.
Rosenmüller c.
rotatable transsphenoidal horizontal ring c.
rotatable transsphenoidal vertical ring c.
ruptured disc c.
Safe Ear c.
saw-toothed c.
scarifying c.
Schede bone c.
Schroeder uterine c.
Scoville ruptured disc c.
serrated c.
Shambaugh adenoidal c.
Shapleigh c.
Shapleigh wax c.
sharp dermal c.
sharp loop c.
Shea c.
Sheehy-House c.
Simon bone c.
Simon cup uterine c.
sinus c.
Skeele c.
Skeele chalazion c.
Skeele corneal c.
Skeele eye c.
Skillern sinus c.
soft rubber c.
sonic c.
spinal fusion c.

sponge ear c.
spoon c.
Spratt bone c.
Spratt ear c.
Spratt mastoid c.
stapes c.
Statak c.
St. Clair-Thompson c.
stirrup-loop c.
stout-neck c.
straight c.
straight ring c.
submucous c.
suction c.
suction tip c.
surgical c.
Synthes facial c.
T-handle c.
T-handled cup c.
Thomas uterine c.
tonsillar c.
Townsend endocervical biopsy c.
toxemia c.
transsphenoidal c.
Ultra-Cut Cobb c.
Unimar Pipelle c.
up-angled c.
uterine c.
uterine biopsy c.
uterine irrigating c.
uterine suction c.
Vabra suction c.
Vacurette suction c.
vacuum c.
vertical ring c.
Vision Curvette c.
Visitec capsule polisher c.
Volkmann bone c.
Volkmann oval c.
Walker ruptured disc c.
Walsh dermal c.
wax c.
Whitney single-use plastic c.
Williger bone c.
Wolff dermal c.
Yankauer c.
Yankauer ear c.
Yasargil c.
Z-Sampler endometrial suction c.

curetting bur
curing light
Curity

C. ABD absorptive dressing
C. ABD pad
C. cover sponge
C. disposable laparotomy sponge
C. gauze sponge
C. irrigation tray
C. leg bag

Curix
- C. Capacity Plus film processing system
- C. film screen cassette
- C. Ultra UV-L film

Curl Cath catheter

Curran knife needle

Curry
- C. intravascular retriever set
- C. needle

Curschmann trocar

Curtinova hydrocolloid dressing

curve
- ventricular function c. (VFC)

curved
- c. awl
- c. blade
- c. cardiovascular clamp
- c. catheter
- c. chisel
- c. clip
- c. Connor wand
- c. conventional microscissors
- c. cricothyrotomy cannula
- c. dissecting forceps
- c. electrode
- c. explorer
- c. gouge
- c. hemostat
- c. intraluminal stapler
- c. iris forceps
- c. iris scissors
- c. J exchange wire
- c. Kelly hemostat
- c. knot-tying forceps
- c. laryngeal mirror
- c. laser probe
- c. magnifying mirror
- c. Maryland forceps
- c. Mayo clamp
- c. meniscotome blade
- c. microbipolar forceps
- c. microneedle holder
- c. mosquito clamp
- c. mosquito hemostat
- c. needle spud
- c. operating scissors
- c. osteotome
- c. retinal probe
- c. slim-diameter tip
- c. suture needle
- c. tapered Tefcor movable core wire guide
- c. tenotomy scissors
- c. tip jeweler's bipolar forceps
- c. tipped spatula
- c. transjugular needle
- c. turbinate scissors
- c. turbinectomy scissors
- c. tying forceps

curved-8 clamp

curved-array
- c.-a. echoendoscope
- c.-a. transducer

curved-base Lewis bracket

curved-on-flat scissors

curved-tipped spatula

curvilinear
- c. chin implant
- c. scanning echoendoscope

CurvTek
- C. drill bone anchor
- C. system
- C. TSR bone drill

CUSA
- Cavitron ultrasonic surgical aspirator
- CUSA CEM system
- CUSA electrosurgical module
- CUSA Excel ultrasonic aspirator
- CUSA laparoscopic tip
- CUSA system 200 straight autoclavable handpiece

CUSALap
- C. accessory needle
- C. ultrasonic accessory

Cusco vaginal speculum

Cushing
- C. angled decompression retractor
- C. bayonet forceps
- C. bipolar neurosurgical forceps
- C. bivalve retractor
- C. bone rongeur
- C. brain forceps
- C. clip
- C. disc rongeur
- C. dressing forceps
- C. dural hook
- C. forceps
- C. intervertebral disc rongeur
- C. Little Joker elevator
- C. nerve retractor
- C. perforator drill
- C. periosteal elevator
- C. pituitary rongeur
- C. saw guide
- C. spatula spoon
- C. straight retractor
- C. subtemporal retractor
- C. suture
- C. thumb forceps
- C. tissue forceps
- C. vein retractor

Cushing-Brown tissue forceps

Cushing-Kocher retractor

Cushing-Landolt transsphenoidal speculum

Cushing-Taylor carbide-jaw forceps

cushion

abduction c.
Airkair seat c.
AIR1517 vacuum-formed static air wheelchair c.
Akros DFD wheelchair wedge c.
alarm c.
amputee c.
Anti-Shox foot c.
arch c.
Back Bull lumbar support c.
Back-Huggar lumbar support c.
birth c.
breakaway lap c.
Butterfly c.
cannula c.
Carter immobilization c.
cell c.
cervical c.
Checkerboard wheelchair c.
Clinicel silicon gel-filled c.
coccyx c.
Comfort Plus c.
Comfort Take-Along wheelchair c.
Contour back c.
Convo-Gel c.
convoluted wheelchair c.
Core Max-Relax c.
Crown high-profile c.
Crown Quadtro c.
Disc-O-Sit Jr. c.
Dry Flotation wheelchair c.
Easebak lumbar support c.
Easy Up c.
EcstaSeat seat c.
enhancer c.
EZ-Dish pressure relief c.
Ezo denture c.
Ficoll c.
Flexseat c.
Flo-Fit c.
foam c.
foam wedge wheelchair c.
foot c.
GasBGon filter seat c.
gel c.
Geo-Matt contour c.
Geo-Matt gel c.
Geo-Matt PRT c.
Geo-Matt wheelchair c.
Healthier seating c.
heel c.
HeelCare c.
Hudson Hydrofloat c.
hydrofloat c.
Invacare Comfort-Mate extra c.
invalid c.
Isch-Dish Plus c.
J2 c.
Jay basic c.
Jay Combi c.
Jay Rave c.
Jay Triad c.
Jay Xtreme c.
laptop c.
latex c.
latex wheelchair c.
lumbar support c.
MaxiFloat wheelchair c.
Medline gel/foam wheelchair c.
Medline Lap-pal safety c.
Memory II c.
Passavant c.
Pediplast c.
pommel c.
Position Plus c.
Postura wheelchair c.
Posture Curve lumbar c.
Posture Wedge seat c.
pressure-relief c.
Prop'R Toes hammertoe c.
Quadtro c.
ring c.
Roho high-profile c.
Roho Pack-It c.
Sacral DISH pressure relief back c.
Samadhi c.
Sat-A-Lite contoured wedge seat c.
scintimammography prone breast c.
Shockmaster heel c.
Side Rester c.
Sit-Straight wheelchair c.
SkareKare silicon gel-filled c.
Skil-Care c.
Skil-Care Alarm c.
Snug denture c.
Sof-Care chair c.
Sof-Care Plus c.
Sorbothane heel c.
Sullivan bubble c.
Temper Foam c.
Tempur-Med wheelchair c.
T-Foam c.
T-Gel c.
The Corner c.
trilaminate c.
Vac-Lok c.
Vac-Lok immobilization c.
Viscoheel K heel c.
Viscoheel N c.
Viscoheel SofSpot viscoelastic heel c.
ViscoSpot heel c.
Waffle seating c.
wheelchair c.
Xact positioning c.

Cusp-Lok
- C.-L. bracket
- C.-L. cuspid traction system

Custodis
- C. implant
- C. sponge
- C. suture

custom
- c. drill guide
- c. healing abutment
- c. healing orthotic
- c. tip
- c. total alloplastic TMJ reconstruction prosthesis
- C. Ultrasonic automatic reprocessor

custom-contoured implant

CustomCornea
- C. wavefront measurement system
- C. wavefront system

custom-curved coil

custom-designed swan-neck femoral component

custom-fitted brace

customized jig

custom-made
- c.-m. insert
- c.-m. shoe

custom-molded
- c.-m. orthotic
- c.-m. shoe

custom-threaded prosthesis

cut
- c. biopsy needle
- horizontal gantry c.
- c. taper needle

Cutalon nylon polyamide surgical suture

cutaneous
- c. punch
- c. thoracic patch electrode

cutdown catheter

cuticle
- c. nipper
- c. scissors

Cutifilm
- C. Plus
- C. Plus composite dressing
- C. Plus waterproof wound dressing

Cutinova
- C. alginate dressing
- C. cavity dressing
- C. cavity wound filler
- C. cavity wound filling material
- C. foam dressing
- C. Hydro
- C. hydroactive dressing
- C. Hydro dressing
- C. thin dressing
- C. thin hydrocolloid
- C. thin hydrocolloid dressing

Cutiplast sterile wound dressing

Cutler
- C. implant
- C. lens spoon

cutout
- c. activator
- c. knee support
- c. patellar brace
- c. table

cutter
- adenoid c.
- Alcon Accurus vitrectomy c.
- C. aortic valve prosthesis
- arch bar c.
- Beaver ring c.
- bone c.
- Chu foldable lens c.
- Cloward dowel c.
- cookie c.
- Dedo-Webb c.
- diamond pin c.
- distal end c.
- double-action c.
- dowel c.
- electronic vitreous c.
- Endopath ETS-Flex endoscopic articulating linear c.
- Endopath EZ35 endoscopic linear c.
- endoscopic linear c.
- Expand-O-Graft c.
- EZ45 thoracic linear c.
- fascial c.
- finger ring c.
- flat-end c.
- full-radius c.
- Gator meniscal c.
- Guilford-Wright wire c.
- guillotine-type c.
- high-speed c.
- hollow c.
- Horsley bone c.
- Horsley spine c.
- Hough Teflon c.
- Howmedica Microfixation System plate c.
- HSV Lightning vitrectomy c.
- C. implant
- infusion suction vitreous c.
- Jarit pin c.
- Kalish Duredge wire c.
- Katena soft IOL c.
- Kirschner wire c.
- Kleinert-Kutz bone c.
- Koo foldable intraocular lens c.
- Koo foldable IOL c.
- Leibinger Micro System plate c.

Lempert malleus c.
lens glide c.
Lindemann bone c.
linear-array staple c.
linear staple c.
Luhr microfixation system plate c.
Machemer vitreous c.
Maguire-Harvey vitreous c.
malleus c.
Martin diamond wire c.
meniscal c.
Microvit c.
Millennium vitreous c.
milling c.
M-Pact cast c.
Nu-Hope hole c.
plate c.
plug c.
Polaris reusable c.
Proximate linear c.
Redi-Vac cast c.
rib c.
ring c.
Rochester harvest bone c.
Rochester recipient bone c.
rod c.
rotating-type c.
round end c.
side-cut pin c.
Sklar pin c.
soft IOL c.
Spartan jaw wire c.
stent c.
Storz Microsystems plate c.
Stryker cast c.
surgical c.
suture c.
Synthes Microsystems plate c.
T-C pin c.
Tolentino vitreous c.
Utrata foldable lens c.
vitreoretinal infusion c.
vitreous infusion suction c.
wire c.
Wister wire/pin c.

cutter/coagulator
Auto Sonix laparoscopic c./c.

Cutter-Smeloff
C.-S. aortic valve prosthesis
C.-S. cardiac valve prosthesis
C.-S. disc valve
C.-S. mitral valve

cutting
c. balloon
c. balloon catheter
c. balloon device
c. block
c. board
c. bur

c. cautery
c. Delrin block
c. forceps
c. jig
c. loop
c. loop electrode
c. LR needle
c. needle
c. Teflon block

cuvette
dye c.

CV-1 videoscope
CV232 square-round-edge IOL
CVA Sling
CVD
CVD black diamond keratome line
CVD diamond knife
C-Vest radiation detector system
CVIS
CVIS imaging device
CVIS information system
CVP catheter
CVS catheter
C-Walk foot 1C40 prosthetic foot
CXM prosthesis
CX Plus prosthesis
cyanoacrylate
c. glue
c. tissue adhesive
c. tissue glue

CyberKnife
Accuray C.
C. Express device
C. planning system
C. robotic radiosurgery system
C. SRS image-guided stereotactic
radiosurgery precision radiotherapy
system
C. stereotactic
radiosurgery/radiotherapy system
C. stereotactic radiosurgery system

Cyberonics vagus nerve stimulator electrode
Cybertach
C. automatic-burst atrial pacemaker
C. 60 bipolar pacemaker
Cybertech 1000 back support
Cyberware
C. 3030 digitizer
C. 3D scanning system
C. 3030RGB digitizer
Cybex
C. back rehabilitation equipment
C. cycle ergometer
C. ergometer
C. I, II+ exercise system
C. II, II+ isokinetic exerciser
C. II isokinetic dynamometer
C. isokinetic dynamometer

C

Cybex *(continued)*
    C. 340 isokinetic rehabilitation and testing system
    C. machine
    C. torso rotation testing and rehabilitation unit
    C. training system
    C. trunk extension flexion unit
Cybon surgical navigation tool
cycle
    Ergociser exercise c.
    Exer-Pedic c.
    Power Trainer c.
    recumbent c.
    Saratoga c.
    Schwinn bi-directional Windjammer upper body c.
    Stratagene SCS-96 thermocycler c.
    upper body c.
CycleBeads fertility device
cycler
    thermal c.
cyclodialysis
    c. cannula
    c. spatula
cyclodiathermy electrode
cycloergometer
cyclohexane scintillator
cyclophorometer
cyclotron
    CTI c.
    medical c.
    multiparticle c.
Cyfra 21-1 IRMA kit
Cygnet
    C. flexible clamp
    C. Laboratories fetal monitoring system
Cygnus
    C. PFS image-guided system
    C. transdermal fentanyl device
cylinder
    abdominal compression c.
    air c.
    AMS CX penile prosthesis c.
    AMS 700CX penile prosthesis c.
    Arthrotek calibrated c.
    Bence Jones c.
    c. bur
    Burnett c.
    cesium c.
    CO_2 c.
    C oxygen c.
    Delclos c.
    dome c.
    drill stop c.
    Feldenkrais c.
    Fletcher-Delclos dome c.
    gas c.

    high-pressure inflatable prosthesis c.
    inflated rubber c.
    Mentor Bioflex c.
    Mitroflow PeriPatch c.'s
    3-month postoperative refractive c.
    M6 oxygen c.
    oxygen (size D, E, M, G, and H) c.
    pneumatic c.
    suction c.
    TPS-coated c.
    Ultrex c.
    vaginal c.
cylinder-type implant
cylindrical
    c. balloon
    c. bougie
    c. bur
    c. diffuser
    c. dowel
    c. lens
    c. sponge
cylindric lens
Cylos pacemaker
cymatic
    c. applicator
    c. device
Cymetra
    C. collagen
    C. micronized AlloDerm
    C. nonsurgical soft tissue replacement material
Cynosar catheter
Cynosure long-pulse infrared laser
Cypher sirolimus-eluting coronary stent
cystenterostome
    diathermic c.
cystic
    c. duct catheter clamp
    c. duct forceps
    c. duct scoop
cystitome *(var. of* cystotome)
Cystocath catheter
cystofiberscope, cystofibroscope
    Olympus CYF-3 OES c.
Cysto Flex stent
cystogastrotome
cystometer
    Lewis c.
    Lewis recording c.
cystonephroscope
cystoresectoscope
    ALR c.
    anteroposterior c.
    Damon-Julian c.
    Julian c.
cystoscope
    Albarran laser c.
    Braasch direct catheterization c.

Braasch-Kaplan direct-vision c.
Brown-Buerger c.
Broyle retrograde c.
Butterfield c.
French c.
InjecTx c.
Judd c.
Kelly c.
Kidd c.
Laidley double-catheterizing c.
Lowsley-Peterson c.
McCarthy-Campbell miniature c.
McCarthy foroblique
  panendoscope c.
McCrea c.
Miller c.
Morganstern continuous-flow
  operating c.
National general purpose c.
Nesbit c.
Olympus fiberoptic c.
Storz c.
Wappler c.
Young c.
cystoscopic
c. forceps
c. fulgurating electrode
cystoscopy table
cystotome, cystitome
air c.
Alcon c.
Atkinson short curved c.
Azar c.
Beard c.
Beaver Ocu-1 curved c.
Blumenthal push-pull irrigating c.
double-cutting sharp c.
Drews c.
formed nonirrigating c.
Graefe c.
Graefe flexible c.
guarded irrigating c.
Holth c.
irrigating c.
Kelman air c.
Kelman double-bladed c.
Kelman knife c.
Kelman knife-cannula c.
kibisitome c.
Knapp c.
knife c.
Knolle-Kelman cannulated c.
Knolle-Kelman sharp c.
Kratz c.
Lewicky formed c.
Lieppman sharp c.
Look c.
McIntyre guarded c.
McIntyre reverse c.

Mendez c.
Mendez ultrasonic c.
Neuhann c.
Nevyas double sharp c.
reverse c.
Sharp point-tip c.
side-cutting irrigating c.
Visitec double-cutting c.
von Graefe c.
Wheeler c.
Wilder c.
Worth c.
cystourethrogram
voiding c. (VCUG)
cystourethroscope
ACMI c.
microlens c.
O'Donoghue c.
Wappler microlens c.
cyst puncture device
cytobrush
C. cell collector
C. Plus
C. Plus cell collector
C. Plus endocervical cell sampler
C. Plus GT
C. S brush
C. spatula
Zelsmyr c.
Cytocare Prolase II
cytocentrifuge
Aerospray c.
CytoFuge 2 c.
Cytopro c.
Cyto-Tek c.
cytochemical probe
CytoFluor II fluorometer
cytofluorometer
CytoFuge
C. 2 centrifuge
C. 2 cytocentrifuge
cytokeratin filament
cytological brush
cytology brush
Cytolong brush
cytometer
Bayer Technicon H1 automated
  flow c.
CAS 200 image c.
Cell Lab IC 100 image c.
Coulter Epics Elite flow c.
Coulter Epics flow c.
Coulter Epics 700-series flow c.
Coulter Epics V flow c.
Dickinson FACS 400-series flow c.
Epics C flow c.
Epics Elite flow c.
Epics Profile flow c.
Epics 700-series flow c.

cytometer *(continued)*
 Epics V flow c.
 Epics XL flow c.
 FACSCalibur flow c.
 FACScan flow c.
 FACSort flow c.
 FACStar Plus flow c.
 FACSVantage flow c.
 flow c.
 HmX Hematology flow c.
 Maxm hematology flow c.
 Ortho System 20 flow c.
Cytomics FC 500 series flow cytometry system
Cytopick endocervical and uterovaginal cell collector

Cytoplast
Cytopro cytocentrifuge
CytoRich
 C. cervical cytology monolayer system
 C. cervical cytology slide
Cyto-Tek cytocentrifuge
Czaja-McCaffrey rigid stent introducer/endoscope
Czapski microscope
Czermak keratome
Czerny
 C. rectal speculum
 C. suture
Czerny-Lembert suture

D
dual
    D syringe
1D35
    Dynamic Motion Foot 1D35
2D
    2-dimensional
       2D B-mode ultrasound machine
       2D Doppler
       2D flat plate
       2D linear plating system
       2D railed plate
3D
    3-dimensional
       3D Accuscan facial implant
       3D flat Lactosorb plate
       3D fracture walker brace
       3D hexahedral element
       3D i-Scan ophthalmic ultrasound
       3D laparoscope
       3D MRA slab
       3D plate
       3D plating system
       3D railed plate
       3D stainless steel knife
       3D surface digitizer scanner
       3D worker's back support
D920
    Audio Doppler D920
D114S balloon catheter
D2L OTW balloon dilatation catheter with extended pressure range
da
    da Vinci femtosecond surgical laser
    da Vinci robotic surgical system
    da Vinci surgical system
Dacomed
    D. Catalyst VCD
    D. snap gauge
D/A converter
Dacron
    D. arterial prosthesis
    D. bifurcation prosthesis
    D. bolstered suture
    D. catheter
    D. cloth
    collagen-impregnated D.
    cottony D.
    D. cuff
    D. fiber
    D. fiber-coated coil
    D. implant
    D. intracardiac patch
    knitted D.
    D. knitted graft

    D. mesh
    D. netting
    D. onlay patch-graft
    D. patch
    D. preclotted graft
    D. prosthesis
    D. retraction tape
    D. sleeve catheter
    D. stent
    D. synthetic ligament
    D. synthetic ligament material
    D. traction suture
    D. tray
    D. tube graft
    D. tubular graft
    D. velour graft
    D. vessel prosthesis
Dacron-backed implant
Dacron-coated microcoil
Dacron-covered
    D.-c. stent
    D.-c. stent graft
Dacron-fibered platinum coil
Dacron-impregnated silastic sheet
dacryocystorhinostomy cannula
Dafilon suture
Dagrofil suture
Dahlberg hearing aid
Daig
    D. ESI-II, DSI-III screw-in lead pacemaker
    D. sheath
Dailies contact lens
daily
    D. cataract needle
    d. wear contact lens
Daisy I&A instrument
Dako
    D. autostainer
    D. fast red substrate system
    D. hepatocyte immunostain
    D. HercepTest
    D. large volume LSAB2 alkaline phosphatase kit
DakoCytomation EGFR pharmDx colorectal cancer diagnostic kit
Dalco Astro ankle brace
Dale
    D. abdominal binder
    D. drainage bulb and G-tube holder
    D. femoropopliteal anastomosis forceps
    D. first rib rongeur
    D. Foley catheter holder

D

215

Dale *(continued)*
　D. gastrostomy tube holder
　D. nasal dressing holder
　D. oxygen cannula support
　D. secondary wound dressing and holder
　D. surgical binder
　D. tapeless wound dressing holder
　D. tracheostomy tube holder
　D. ventilator tubing support
Dale-Schwartz tube
Dalkon
　D. shield
　D. shield intrauterine device
Dalla Bona ball-and-socket abutment
Dallas lens-inserting forceps
Dall-Miles
　D.-M. cable
　D.-M. cable/crimp cerclage system
　D.-M. cable grip system
　D.-M. cerclage wire
dam
　nonlatex dental d.
Damato curved catheter
Damon-Julian cystoresectoscope
damping
　Accudynamic adjustable d.
　catheter d.
Dana Diabecare insulin pump
DANA shoulder prosthesis
dancer's pad
Dan chalazion forceps
Dandy
　D. clamp
　D. hemostatic forceps
　D. nerve hook
　D. neurosurgical scissors
　D. scalp hemostat
　D. scalp hemostatic forceps
　D. suction tube
　D. trigeminal scissors
Danek
　D. cervical fusion plate
　Medtronic Sofamor D.
　D. self-retaining retractor
Daniel
　D. EndoForehead instrument
　D. grasper
Dannheim eye implant
Danniflex
　D. CPM exerciser
　D. CPM machine
Dansac
　D. colostomy irrigation set
　D. Contour 1 mini 1-piece pouch
　D. Contour 1 oval 1-piece pouch
　D. irrigation system
　D. standard F 1-piece pouch
Dansko shoe

Dantec
　D. 12-channel Urocolor video system
　D. Etude uroflow transducer
　D. Menuet system
　D. rotating disc flowmeter
　D. Urodyn 1000 flowmeter
　D. Urodyn uroflowmeter
DAR breathing system
Darby surgical shoe
d'Arcet metal
Darco
　D. back brace
　D. Body Armor Hi
　D. Body Armor Lo
　D. Body Armor short leg walker
　D. foot splint
　D. Medical-Surgical shoe
　D. Medical-Surgical shoe and toe alignment splint
　D. moldable insole
　D. OrthoWedge healing shoe
　D. Softie shoe
　D. surgical shoe
　D. wedge shoe
DarcoGel ankle brace
Dardenne nucleus forceps
Dardik
　D. Biograft
　D. clamp
　D. umbilical graft
dark-field condenser
Darox cutaneous thoracic patch electrode
Darrach retractor
d'Arsonval galvanometer
dart
　Arthrex meniscal d.
　Clearfix meniscal d.
Dasco Pro angle finder
Dascor disc arthroplasty system
DASH
　DASH ERCP catheter
　DASH extraction balloon
　DASH sphincterotome
　DASH system
　DASH tipless extraction basket
Dasher guidewire
Dash single-chamber rate-adaptic pacemaker
DAS single-pass dialyzer
D'Assumpcão marking clamp
D'Assumpeau rhytidoplasty marker
data
　d. camera
　d. collection system
data-acquisition system
DataHand system

Datascope
D. Accutor bedside monitor
D. balloon
D. catheter
D. CL-II percutaneous translucent balloon catheter
D. DL-II percutaneous translucent balloon catheter
D. intraaortic balloon pump catheter
D. pulse oximeter
D. 300 pulse oximeter
D. System 90 intraaortic balloon pump
D. true sheathless catheter

Datex
D. infrared CO_2 monitor
D. model CH-S-23 pulse oximeter
D. Normocap infrared capnometer
D. Ultima spirometer

Datex-Ohmeda ventilator
DaTSCAN imager
Daubenspeck bone curette
daughter endoscopic retrograde cholangiopancreatoscopy system

Dautrey
D. chisel
D. osteotome

David-Baker
D.-B. eyelid retractor
D.-B. lip clamp

Davidoff ambidextrous nucleus chopper
David rectal speculum

Davidson
D. clamp
D. pulmonary vessel clamp
D. scapular retractor
D. syringe
D. thoracic trocar

Davidson-Mathieu-Alexander periosteal elevator
Davidson-Mathieu rib rasp
Davidson-Sauerbruch-Doyen periosteal elevator
Davidson-Sauerbruch rib rasp

Daviel
D. cataract spoon
D. lens scoop
D. lens spoon
D. scoop
D. spoon

Davis
D. blade
D. brain spatula
D. catheter
D. diathermy forceps
D. double-ended retractor
D. dura dissector
D. forceps

D. foreign body spud
D. graft
D. interlocking sound
D. knife needle
D. loop stone dislodger
D. percussion hammer
D. periosteal elevator
D. pillar retractor
D. rhytidectomy scissors
D. ring mouthgag
D. saw guide
D. self-retaining scalp retractor
D. spud
D. sterilizing forceps
D. thoracic tissue forceps
D. trephine

Davis-Bovie cautery
Davis-Crowe mouthgag
Davis-Geck suture

Davol
D. bag
D. colon tube
D. dermatome
D. feeding bag
D. feeding tube
D. irrigation system
D. sterile female catheterization kit
D. sterile irrigation tray
D. sterile red rubber catheter
D. tunneler

Davol-Simon dermatome
Davy surgical button
DAWSkin
Dawson-Mueller drainage catheter

Dawson-Yuhl
D.-Y. impactor
D.-Y. periosteal elevator
D.-Y. rongeur forceps
D.-Y. suction tube

Dawson-Yuhl-Cone curette
Dawson-Yuhl-Kerrison rongeur forceps
Dawson-Yuhl-Key elevator
Dawson-Yuhl-Leksell rongeur forceps

Day
D. attic cannula
D. ear hook

daylight processor
DayTimer carpal tunnel support
Daytona cervical orthosis
dBA scale
DBM
demineralized bone matrix
DBX
demineralized bone matrix
DBX bone paste
DBX bone putty
DBX bone void filler
DC-101 chiropractic table

DCI-S automated coronary analysis system
D-Core support pillow
DCS-10, DCS-18 mechanically detachable platinum coil
DCS pin
DC SQUID sensor
DDD
    dual-sensing, dual-pacing, dual-mode DDD pacemaker
DDI mode pacemaker
DDMS
    diamond-dusted membrane scraper
        Synergetics DDMS
DDP table
DDSA
    Integris V3000 DDSA
DDT lock screw inserter
DDV ligator
de
    De Alvarez forceps
    de Cornier endometrial suction curette
    de la Caffinière trapeziometacarpal prosthesis
    De La Cruz piston
    de la Plaza transconjunctival retractor
    De La Vega lens pusher
    De La Vega vitreous aspirating cannula
    De Lorme boot
    De Mayo hip positioner
    De Mayo 2-point discrimination device
    De Mayo suture passer
    de Pezzer catheter
    de Pezzer drain
    De Vega prosthesis
    de Wecker iris scissors
    de Wecker scissors
DEAE-Sephacel ion exchange column
Dean
    D. applicator
    D. bone rongeur
    D. capsulotomy knife
    D. dissecting scissors
    D. iris knife
    D. knife holder
    D. knife needle
    D. periosteal elevator
    D. rongeur
    D. scissors
    D. tonsil hemostat
    D. tonsillar forceps
    D. tonsillar knife
    D. tonsillar scissors
Deane unconstrained knee prosthesis
Dean-Shallcross tonsil-seizing forceps

Deaver
    D. blade
    D. operating scissors
    D. pediatric retractor
    D. retractor
Deaver-type blade
DeBakey
    D. aortic aneurysm clamp
    D. aortic clamp
    D. aortic exclusion clamp
    D. arterial clamp
    D. arterial forceps
    D. Atraugrip forceps
    D. ball valve prosthesis
    D. blade
    D. bulldog clamp
    D. chest retractor
    D. cross-action bulldog clamp
    D. dissecting forceps
    D. endarterectomy scissors
    D. femoral bypass tunneler
    D. forceps
    D. graft
    D. implant
    D. infant and child rib spreader
    D. ligature carrier
    D. needle
    D. pediatric clamp
    D. peripheral vascular clamp
    D. pickup
    D. prosthetic valve
    D. rib spreader
    D. ring-handled bulldog clamp
    D. tangential occlusion clamp
    D. thoracic forceps
    D. tissue forceps
    D. VAD
    D. VAD continuous-axial-flow pump
    D. vascular dilator
    D. vascular forceps
    D. Vasculour-II vascular prosthesis
DeBakey-Adson suction tube
DeBakey-Bahnson vascular clamp
DeBakey-Bainbridge vascular clamp
DeBakey-Balfour retractor
DeBakey-Beaver blade
DeBakey-Colovira-Rumel thoracic forceps
DeBakey-Cooley retractor
DeBakey-Craford vascular clamp
DeBakey-Derra
    D.-D. anastomosis clamp
    D.-D. anastomosis forceps
DeBakey-Diethrich
    D.-D. coronary artery forceps
    D.-D. vascular forceps
DeBakey-Harken auricular clamp

DeBakey-Howard aortic aneurysm
  clamp
DeBakey-Kay aortic clamp
DeBakey-Kelly hemostatic forceps
DeBakey-McQuigg-Mixter bronchial
  clamp
DeBakey-Metzenbaum scissors
DeBakey-Mixter thoracic forceps
DeBakey-NASA axial-flow ventricular
  assist device
DeBakey-Péan cardiovascular forceps
DeBakey-Potts scissors
DeBakey-Rankin hemostatic forceps
DeBakey-Reynolds anastomosis forceps
DeBakey-Rumel thoracic forceps
DeBakey-Satinsky vena cava clamp
DeBakey-Semb ligature carrier
DeBakey-Surgitool prosthetic valve
DeBastiani
  D. distractor
  D. external fixator
  D. fixation
Debioclip single-dose delivery system
debonded femoral stem prosthesis
debonding pliers
Debove tube
débridement needle
débrider
  Accuzyme enzymatic d.
  corneal d.
  Panafil enzymatic d.
  Panafil-White enzymatic d.
  Santyl enzymatic d.
  Sauer corneal d.
Debrisan
  D. dressing
  D. wound cleanser
debris-retaining acetabular reamer
Debut ear piercing kit
decalcified freeze-dried bone allograft
decalcifier
  Surgipath D. I, II
Decal Plus
DeCamp viscoelastic cannula
decapolar electrode catheter
decelerator
  graduated electronic d.
decentered spectacles
deck plate
decoder
decompression
  d. catheter
  interspinous process d. (IPD)
  laser disc d.
  vertebra axial d.
  vertebral axial d. (VAX-D)
decompressive
  d. chest tube
  d. retractor

decompressor
  Savage intestinal d.
decontaminating room
decortication bur
DEC 9800 plus cardiac mobile C-arm
DeCube
  D. mattress
  D. therapeutic mattress
  D. therapeutic surface
decubitus
  d. boot shoe
  d. pad
dedicated
  d. Doppler probe
  d. head scanner
  d. mammography system
  d. PET scanner
  d. phased-array coil
  d. push enteroscope
Dedo laser laryngoscope
Dedo-Pilling laryngoscope
Dedo-Webb cutter
Dee elbow hinge
deep
  d. abdominal ring
  d. blunt rake retractor
  d. brain lead
  d. retractor
  d. surgery forceps
  d. vessel forceps
deepening reamer
DeepLight glaucoma treatment system
Defiance functional knee brace
defibrillation
  d. paddle
  d. patch
defibrillator
  AccessAED d.
  AccessALS d.
  Alto DR implantable
    cardioverter d.
  Alto 2 implantable cardioverter d.
  Atrioverter implantable atrial d.
  automated external d. (AED)
  automatic external d.
  automatic implantable d.
  automatic implantable
    cardiovascular d. (AICD)
  automatic intracardiac d.
  cardiac d.
  cardiac resynchronization therapy d.
    (CRT-D)
  Cardioserv d.
  Codemaster d.
  Contak Renewal 3 cardiac
    resynchronization therapy d.
  Contour MD implantable single-lead
    cardioverter d.
  Endotak lead d.

defibrillator *(continued)*
  FirstSave automated external d.
  ForeRunner d.
  fully automated d.
  Gem DR implantable d.
  Gem II DR dual-chamber d.
  Guidant d.
  Heart Aid 80 d.
  HeartStart MRx d.
  Heartstream FR2+ d.
  Hewlett-Packard d.
  Hewlett-Packard Codemaster XL d.
  d. implant
  implantable d.
  implantable atrial d. (IAD)
  Intec implantable d.
  Jewel AF implantable d.
  Lifepak d.
  LifeVest wearable d.
  manual d.
  Marquette Responder 1500
    multifunctional d.
  Medtronic Gem automatic
    implantable d.
  Medtronic Jewel Plus Active
    Can d.
  Medtronic Micro Jewel d.
  Metrix implantable atrial d.
  Micro Jewel d.
  Odam d.
  pacer-cardioverter d.
  d. paddle
  PD 2000 d.
  Photon Micro DR/VR implantable
    cardioverter d.
  Porta Pulse 3 portable d.
  Powerheart external d.
  public access d.
  semiautomated external d.
  shock-advisory d.
  transvenous implantable d.
  Ventak Mini III implantable d.
  Ventak Prizm dual-chamber
    implantable d.
  Ventak Prizm implantable d.
  Zoll M-series critical care
    transport d.
defibrillator/monitor
  Lifepak 12 d./m.
**Definition PM femoral implant
  component**
Definity contact lens
deflectable quadripolar catheter
deflector
Deflux
  D. injectable implant
  D. system implant
Defourmentel bone rongeur
Defyne urethral assist device

degradable polyglycolide rod
degree
  4M 30-d. arthroscope
  4-d.-of-freedom manipulator
  70-d. telescope
30-degree
  30-d. oblique arthroscope
  30-d. telescope
45-degree
  45-d. bent reform implant
  45-d. spinal wedge
6 degrees of freedom electrogoniometer
Degudent alloy
dehumidifier
  Gobi d.
  Grand Sahara d.
  Mojave-Mini d.
Deitz
  D. incision depth gauge
  D. ophthalmic gauge
Dejerine-Davis percussion hammer
Dejerine percussion hammer
DeJuan ophthalmic pick forceps
Deklene
  D. II cardiovascular suture
  D. polypropylene suture
Deknatel
  D. K-needle
  D. orthopaedic autotransfusion
    system
  D. silk suture
  D. wound closure tape
  D. wound tape
DeKock 2-way bronchial catheter
Del
  D. Mar Avionics 3-channel
    recorder
  D. Mar Avionics scanner
Delaborde tracheal dilator
Delaborde-Trousseau tracheal dilator
Delaire mask
Delaney phrenic retractor
Delarnette scanner
DeLaura knee prosthesis
DeLaura-Verner knee prosthesis
Delbet-Reverdin needle
Delbet splint
Delclos
  D. cylinder
  D. ovoid
DeLee
  D. cervical forceps
  D. corner retractor
  D. fetal stethoscope
  D. infant catheter
  D. meconium trap aspirator
  D. obstetrical forceps
  D. pelvimeter
  D. suction catheter

D. suction device
D. tracheal catheter
D. Universal retractor
DeLee-Breisky pelvimeter
DeLee-Hillis fetal stethoscope
DeLee-Simpson forceps
delicate
d. grasping forceps
d. intervertebral disc rongeur
d. needle holder
d. operating scissors
Delitala T pin
delivery
d. assistance sleeve
d. guidewire
d. wire
Dell
D. astigmatism marker
D. fixation ring
Della Badia laparoscopic suturing device
Delm imaging system
DeLorme table
Delrin
D. applicator
D. disc heart valve
D. frame of valve prosthesis
D. heart valve
Delrin-handle bone saw
Delsa 440 SX Zeta potential analyzer
delta
D. CTA reverse shoulder system
D. 32 digital stereotactic system
D. Recon proximal drill guide
d. rod
D. shunt
D. 32 TACT 3-dimensional breast imaging system
D. valve
D. walker
D. wire grasper
Deltafit keel
Delta-Lite
D.-L. casting tape
D.-L. FlashCast
DELTAmanager MedImage system
Delta-Rol cast padding
Deltatrac
D. II indirect calorimeter
D. II metabolic monitor
Deltec-Pharmacia CADD pump
Deltec portable external infusion device
Deltoid-Aid
D.-A. arm counterbalance system
D.-A. arm support
Deltran disposable transducer
deluxe
d. head halter
d. leg bag strap

demand
d. cardiac pacemaker
d. flow machine
demand-valve ventilation device
demarcator
flap d.
Pitanguy flap d.
Demariniff protractor
DeMartel wire saw
DeMartel-Wolfson
D.-W. anastomosis clamp
D.-W. clamp holder
Dembone
D. cortical bone powder
D. demineralized cancellous chip
D. demineralized cortical chip
D. demineralized cortical dental block
D. demineralized cortical granule
D. demineralized cortical powder
D. demineralized cortical powder Pastegraft
D. demineralized cortical powder Pulvograft
D. demineralized corticocancellous chip
D. demineralized human bone
D. freeze-dried bone
D. graft
Demel
D. wire-tightening forceps
D. wire-twisting forceps
demigauntlet
d. bandage
d. dressing
demineralized
d. bone
d. bone matrix (DBM, DBX)
d. cortical bone powder
d. flexible laminar bone strip
demodulator
demonstration
d. eyepiece
d. ophthalmoscope
Demos tibial artery clamp
Denar articulator
denatured homograft
Denck esophagoscope
Denham
D. external fixation device
D. pin
Denhardt-Dingman mouthgag
Denhardt mouthgag
Denis
D. Browne bar
D. Browne clubfoot splint
D. Browne hip splint
D. Browne pediatric abdominal retractor blade

D

Denis *(continued)*
D. Browne pediatric retractor
D. Browne pouch
D. Browne splint
D. Browne tonsil forceps
D. forceps
Denlan magnifying loupe
DenLite illuminated handheld mirror
Dennen forceps
Dennis
D. colorectal tube
D. dissecting scissors
D. intestinal clamp
Dennison cervical brace
Densitometer
densitometer
accuDEXA bone d.
Achilles d.
Achilles+ ultrasound bone d.
Apollo DXA bone d.
Appraise clinical d.
bone d.
CS-9000 d.
CT d.
DEXAscan bone d.
Discovery bone d.
DPX Bravo bone d.
DPX-IQ d.
dual-energy x-ray absorptiometry d.
dual-photon d.
DXA d.
dynamic spiral CT lung d.
Expert bone d.
Expert-XL d.
hair d.
Hoefer GS 300 laser d.
Hologic 2000 d.
Hologic 1000 QDR d.
Hologic QDR 4500 DXA bone d.
imaging d.
Lunar DPX d.
Lunar Expert d.
Norland bone d.
Norland XR26 bone d.
OsteoAnalyzer d.
OsteoGram 2000 d.
OsteoView digital bone d.
pDEXA x-ray peripheral bone d.
PIXI bone d.
PIXI peripheral d.
Prodigy bone d.
QDR-1500, -2000 bone d.
Sahara portable bone d.
single-photon d.
Victoreen digital d.
video d.
Dentacam
Dentaflex wire
Dentaform band

dental
d. amalgam packer
d. antisnoring device
d. apparatus
d. arch bar
d. bur
d. capsule
d. cement
d. curette
d. diode laser
d. dressing forceps
d. drill
d. excavator
d. explorer
d. implant
d. implant cover screw
d. pick
d. pliers
D. Pro II camera
d. retractor
d. rongeur
d. scaler
d. sealant
d. shield
d. speech appliance
d. wax
d. wax carver
Dentalaser
Multi-Operatory D.
dentate bur
Dentatus
D. articulator
D. screw
DentCAM
Dentemp filling material
DentiCAD system
Dentifix home denture repair kit
dentin-bonded resin composite
DentiPatch lidocaine transoral delivery system
Dento-Infuser
Dentomat amalgamator
Dentsleeve
D. device
D. extruded silastic perfused manometric assembly
D. pneumohydraulic perfusion system
D. single multilumen extrusion catheter
D. sleeve sensor
Dentsply
D. FlexoFiles
D. implant system
denture
d. brush
complete upper and lower d.'s
full lower d.
full upper d.

implant-retained d.
maxillary removable implant-
retained d.
partial lower d.
partial upper d.
removable partial d.
soft-lined d.
unilateral removable partial d.
d. vulcanite bur

Dentus x-ray film
Dent-X intraoral x-ray unit
Denucath
Denver
D. ascites shunt
D. hydrocephalus shunt
D. hydrocephalus shunt system
D. nasal splint
D. percutaneous access kit
D. peritoneovenous shunt
D. pleuroperitoneal shunt
D. Pleurx pleural catheter/home
drainage kit
D. shunt
D. valve

DeOrio intrauterine insemination
catheter
deoxyribonucleic
d. acid (DNA)
d. acid synthesizer

DePaul tube
depilatory dermal forceps
deployment
stent d.

depolarizing electrode
depressor
Andrews tongue d.
Bosworth tongue d.
brain d.
Braun uterine d.
Bruening tongue d.
Buchwald tongue d.
Claes scleral d.
Flynn scleral d.
Israel tongue d.
Kocher d.
Lewis tongue d.
metal tongue d.
O'Connor d.
O'Connor scleral d.
oral screw tongue d.
orbital d.
Schepens scleral d.
Schocket scleral d.
scleral d.
Simcoe scleral d.
Sims uterine d.
Spaide scleral d.
Tobold tongue d.
tongue d.

torque d.
Weider tongue d.
Wilder scleral d.
wood tongue d.

depth
d. electrode
d. gauge
d. inlay shoe
D. orthopaedic shoe
d. plate

Depthalon monitoring electrode
DePuy
D. Acclaim total elbow system
D. Ace Pe.R.I. tongs
D. acetabular liner
D. acetabular lining
D. Ace TiMAX Pe.R.I. small
fragment lower extremity plate
system
D. AcroMed Harms cage
D. AML hip
D. Biax total wrist system
D. Casting FRC system
D. CMW 1 bone cement
D. coaptation splint
D. Control cable and wire system
D. C-Stem triple taper stabilized
hip implant
D. Endurance all-polyethylene
acetabular cup system
D. fracture brace
D. FRS screw
D. FRS SOC pin
D. FRS standard staple
D. FRS twist-off screw
D. fusion and reconstruction
system
D. Global Advantage CTA humeral
head
D. Global Advantage shoulder
eccentric humeral head
D. Global FX shoulder fracture
system
D. Global shoulder glenoid
component with fin
D. graft preparation table
D. hip prosthesis with Scuderi
head
D. interference screw
D. LCS mobile-bearing knee
D. Marathon crosslinked
polyethylene liner
D. Mitek Biocryl TCP/PLA screw
D. Mitek Contack labral anchor
D. Mitek Rigidfix anterior cruciate
ligament cross-pin system
D. Orthogenesis LPS
D. Pinnacle acetabular cup system
D. Poly-Dial constrained liner

D

DePuy (*continued*)
   D. Preservation unicompartmental knee system
   D. Prodigy total hip system
   D. Replica total hip system
   D. Rockwood AC screw
   D. Rockwood clavicle pin
   D. Solution System acetabular cup
   D. Summit tapered hip system
   D. support
   D. total hip system
   D. Tri-Lock interlocking acetabular cup
   D. Ultamet metal-on-metal articulation
DePuy-Pott splint
DePuy-Weiss tonsillar needle
Derby nail
Derek Harwood-Nash catheter
Derf eye needle holder
Derlacki-Hough mobilizer
Derlacki-Juers headholder
Derlacki-Shambaugh chisel
Derma
   D. blade
   FotoFinder D.
   D. K combination Er:YAG & CO_2 laser
   D. K combination laser
   D. K laser
   D. K laser system
   D. 20 laser
   D. 20 laser system
Dermabond
   D. topical skin adhesive
   D. wound closure device
dermabrader
   diamond d.
   high-speed d.
   HydroBrader irrigating/aspirating d.
   Iverson d.
   sandpaper d.
dermabrasion bur
dermacarrier
Dermacea
   D. alginate dressing
   D. alginate wound cover
DermaCol hydrocolloid wound dressing
DermaFilm dressing
Dermafit massage mat
Derma-Gel hydrogel sheet
DermaGlide needle
Dermagraft
   D. dermal substitute
   D. graft
   D. skin device
   D. skin substitute
   D. wound healing device

Dermagraft-TC temporary skin substitute
Dermagran
   D. hydrogel dressing
   D. hydrogel wound dressing
   D. hydrophilic gauze dressing
   D. impregnated gauze
   D. ointment wound dressing
   D. wound cleanser
   D. zinc-saline hydrogel wound dressing
Dermagran-B hydrophilic wound dressing
dermal
   d. curette
   d. elevator
   d. interposition splint
   d. regeneration template
   d. suture
Dermalase laser system
Dermalene polyethylene suture
Dermalogen
   D. human collagen
   D. material
Dermalon cuticular suture
DermaMend
   D. barrier
   D. cavity foam dressing
   D. foam
   D. foam wound dressing
   D. hydrogel dressing
   D. island foam dressing
   D. wound cleanser
Dermanet
   D. contact layer sheet
   D. contact layer wound dressing
Dermaphot system
Dermapor glove
DermaPulse
DermaScan
DermaSeptic device
Dermasil impression material
DermaSite transparent film dressing
DermaSof gel sheeting
Dermasoft mattress
Dermasorb hydrocolloid/alginate wound dressing
DermAssist
   D. filler
   D. gel/gauze dressing
   D. glycerin hydrogel dressing
   D. hydrocolloid
   D. hydrocolloid dressing
   D. hydrocolloid dressing material
   D. hydrogel packing strip
   D. impregnated gauze
   D. transparent film
   D. transparent site dressing
   D. wound filling material

Derma-Tattoo surgical tattoo
Dermatell
    D. hydrocolloid
    D. hydrocolloid dressing
    D. hydrocolloid dressing material
DermaTemp
    D. DT-1000 infrared temperature
      scanner
    D. infrared thermographic sensor
Dermatex compound
dermatologic ultraviolet light
dermatome
    air d.
    air-driven d.
    d. blade
    Brown air d.
    Brown electric d.
    d. cement
    compressed air-powered d.
    cordless d.
    Davol d.
    Davol-Simon d.
    drum d.
    drum-type d.
    Duval disposable d.
    electric d.
    electricity-driven d.
    Goulian d.
    Hall d.
    Hood manual d.
    Jordan-Day d.
    manual d.
    Meek-Wall d.
    Padgett d.
    Padgett-Hood d.
    Padgett manual d.
    Reese d.
    Schink d.
    sick d.
    Simon d.
    single-use d.
    Tanner-Vandeput mesh d.
    Weck d.
    Zimmer d.
dermatoscope
    handheld d.
Dermatron
Derma-Wand
    D.-W. device
    D.-W. germicidal lamp
Dermicare hypoallergenic paper tape
Dermicel
    D. dressing
    D. hypoallergenic cloth tape
    D. hypoallergenic knitted tape
    D. Montgomery strap
    D. tape
Dermiclear tape
Dermiform hypoallergenic knitted tape

dermis
    AlloDerm preserved human d.
    human fibroblast-derived d.
dermis-fat passer
Dermiview hypoallergenic transparent
    tape
DermMaster first macroabrasion system
dermohygrometer
Dermo-Jet high-pressure injector
dermometer
Dermophase dressing
Dermoplast-Plastazote orthosis
dermoplasty cast
Dermostat implant
Dero
    D. hole-in-1 prosthetic sock
    D. hole-in-toe prosthetic sock
derotation
    d. boot
    d. brace
derotational pin
derotator splint
DeRoyal
    D. laparotomy sponge
    D. LMB finger splint
    D. mattress overlays
    D. Surgical grab bag
Derra
    D. anastomosis clamp
    D. aortic clamp
    D. valve dilator
    D. vena cava clamp
Derra-Cooley forceps
D'Errico
    D. dressing forceps
    D. enlarging drill bur
    D. hypophysial forceps
    D. lamina chisel
    D. perforating drill bur
    D. retractor
    D. tissue forceps
D'Errico-Adson retractor
Desai
    D. VectorCath mapping catheter
    D. VectorCath mapping system
Desault apparatus
Descemet membrane punch
Deschamps
    D. compressor
    D. ligature carrier
    D. ligature needle
    D. needle
desiccation-fulguration needle
desiccation needle
DesignLine orthotic
Design Veronique compression wear
Desilets-Hoffman
    D.-H. catheter introducer
    D.-H. introducer

D

Desilets-Hoffman *(continued)*
    D.-H. introducer set
    D.-H. sheath
Desilets introducer system
Desjardins
    D. forceps
    D. gall duct probe
    D. gallstone forceps
    D. gallstone scoop
desk
    Posture-Rite lap d.
Desk-Rest arm support
Desmarres
    D. chalazion forceps
    D. clamp
    D. corneal dissector
    D. eyelid retractor
    D. fixation pick
    D. knife
    D. lamellar dissector
    D. lid clamp
    D. lid elevator
    D. lid retractor
    D. lid speculum
    D. paracentesis needle
    D. refractor
    D. retractor
desmin filament
destructive obstetrical hook
detachable
    d. balloon-modified reducing stent
    d. coil
    d. embolization coil
    d. platinum coil
    d. silicone balloon
    d. stretcher frame
Detachol adhesive remover
detection
    computer-aided d. (CAD)
detector
    acute ionization d.
    AD 340 absorbance d.
    Add-On Bucky direct x-ray d.
    ambulatory nuclear d.
    anular d.
    bismuth-germanate d.
    cadmium iodide d.
    Cardioscint nuclear d.
    CCD d.
    Clinitemp fever d.
    collimation scintillation d.
    colorimetric d.
    CR-39 nuclear tract d.
    crystalline phosphor d.
    C-Trak handheld gamma d.
    dielectric track d.
    digital amorphous silicon flat-panel d.
    digital x-ray d.

diode d.
Doppler blood flow d.
Doppler ultrasonic blood flow d.
Doptone fetal pulse d.
DTX series multimode d.
EarCheck Pro otitis media d.
Easy Cap II CO_2 d.
electrical resistance d.
electrochemical d.
electron capture d.
element-specific d.
emission spectrometric d.
flame ionization d.
flame photometric d.
flat-plate d.
fluorescence d.
forward fluorescence d.
gamma probe radiation d.
Geiger-Müller d.
glass tract d.
high-purity germanium d.
HPGe d.
Innova 4100 flat-panel d.
Isometer bone graft placement site d.
kinestatic charge d.
LD 400 luminescence d.
mass spectrophotometric d.
multihead d.
NaI d.
Navigator gamma ray d.
Neoprobe 1000, 1500 portable radioisotope d.
Neoprobe radioactivity d.
nitrogen-phosphorus d.
passive track d.
Pediatric Ingesta Scan metal d.
Pedi-cap d.
phase-sensitive d.
photoionization d.
pulsed ultrasonic velocity d.
quadrature phase d.
radiation d.
rature d.
Revolution XR/d digital d.
semiconductor d.
Si d.
slot-scanning d.
sodium d.
sodium iodide d.
solid-state nuclear track d.
d. system
thermal conductivity d.
thermoluminescence d.
Thoravision selenium x-ray d.
tissue-equivalent d.
TubeChek esophageal intubation d.
ultraviolet d.
VEST ambulatory nuclear d.

Wang-Binford edge d.
Waters M-440 fixed
  wavelength d.
DET fluorescein strip
Detroit Receiving Hospital razor
**detunable elliptic transmission line
  resonator**
deuterium-tritium generator
Deutschman cataract knife
developer
  Hemoccult Sensa d.
Devex spinal system
device
  abdominal aortic counterpulsation d.
  abdominal left ventricular assist d.
    (ALVAD)
  Abiomed BVAD 5000 cardiac d.
  Abiomed implantable heart
    replacement d.
  ablative d.
  Ablatr temperature control d.
  Acapella chest physical therapy d.
  Accu-Chek SoftClix lancet d.
  Accu-Chek Soft Touch lancing d.
  accuDEXA bone mineral
    assessment d.
  Accunet distal protection d.
  Accutorr oscillometric d.
  Accutracker blood pressure d.
  acetabular reinforcement d.
  A1cNow glycemic monitoring d.
  Acorn CorCap cardiac support d.
  ACS anchor exchange d.
  Acucise cutting balloon d.
  Acufex bioabsorbable fixation d.
  AcuSnare polypectomy d.
  AcuSpark piezoelectric d.
  acute ventricular assist d. (AVAD)
  AcuTrainer d.
  AcuTrainer bladder retraining d.
  AcuTrainer handheld electronic d.
  adjustable 2-point caliper sensory
    assessment d.
  advanced venous access d.
  AeroChamber pediatric spacer d.
  AeroChamber spacer d.
  AeroChamber spacing d.
  AeroEclipse aerosol delivery d.
  AcroEtcher intraoral blaster d.
  AERx drug delivery d.
  Agee d.
  AICD plus Tachylog d.
  Alexa 1000 breast lesion
    diagnostic d.
  Algo-1 automated auditory
    brainstem response d.
  Algo-2 hearing screening d.
  AlloAnchor RC allograft d.
  alternative communication d.

ambulatory infusion management d.
Ameflow d.
AME tongue retaining d.
A-mode echo-tracking d.
amorphous silicon filmless digital
  x-ray detection technology d.
Amplatzer d.
Amplatz thrombectomy d.
Amplatz ventricular septal defect d.
amplification d.
Anaconda d.
analgesic cell therapy
  implantable d.
Anchor catheter exchange d.
Anderson fixation d.
Anderson leg-lengthening d.
Ange-Med Sentinel ICD d.
Angioguard catheter d.
AngioJet thrombectomy d.
Angiolink EVS closure d.
Angio-Seal closure d.
Angio-Seal diagnostic d.
Angio-Seal hemostatic puncture
  closure d.
Angio-Seal therapeutic d.
Angio-Seal vascular closure d.
angled delivery d.
angle measurement d.
ankle disc d.
Antense antitension d.
anterior internal fixation d.
antibiotic removal d.
antimicrobial removal d.
antirotation d.
antisiphon d.
Apogee ultrasound d.
Aprema III d.
AquaFlow collagen glaucoma
  drainage d.
AquaLase liquefaction d.
AquaMED hydrotherapy d.
Aquatrek d.
arachnophlebectomy surgical d.
Archxerciser foot exercise d.
Arena hemodialysis d.
Argon Beamer 2 d.
Arnoff external fixation d.
AromaScan aroma analysis d.
arrhythmia control d. (ACD)
Arrow absorbable meniscal
  repair d.
Arrow-Clarke thoracentesis d.
Arrow LionHeart left ventricular
  assist d.
Arrow-Trerotola percutaneous
  thrombectomy d.
Arrow-Trerotola percutaneous
  thrombolytic d.
Arrow-Trerotola PTD d.

D

device *(continued)*

ArtAssist arterial assist d.
arterial puncture site closure d.
Arthrex Bird-Beak d.
ArthroSew arthroscopic suturing d.
Arthrotek tibial fixation d.
ArthroWand d.
Artscan 200 arthroscopic cartilage stiffness testing d.
Ascensia Microlet Adjustable lancing d.
Ascensia Microlet Vaculance lancing d.
aspiration tulip d.
assistive listening d.
Asta-Cath d.
Atad cervical ripening d.
Atad Ripener d.
atherectomy d.
ATL UltraMark 7 echocardiographic d.
ATL 3000 ultrasound d.
atrial septal defect single disc closure d.
Atrioverter implantable defibrillator d.
Attractor retrieval d.
augmentative communication d.
AutoAdjust CPAP d.
Autocath bladder control d.
Autoclix fingerstick lancet d.
Auto-Crane d.
Autolet Clinisafe lancing d.
Autolet fingerstick d.
Autolet impression lancing d.
Autolet Lite lancing d.
Autolet Mini lancing d.
automatic d.
automatic spring-loaded biopsy d.
automatic stapling d.
automatic suction d.
Automator d.
AutoPap automated screening d.
AutoPulse CPR d.
AutoSet CS d.
AutoSet Portable II diagnosis and therapy d.
autostapling d.
autotitration d.
AVA 3Xi advanced venous access d.
A-V Impulse System foot pump DVT prophylaxis d.
A-V Impulse System foot wrap DVT prophylaxis d.
AvoSure INR test d.
Axer compression d.
axis-altering arthroereisis d.

BabyFace 3D surface rendering accessory d.
Babyhaler spacer d.
Backbar d.
BackCycler continuous passive motion d.
BackMaster d.
back range of motion d.
bag-mask d.
bag-valve d.
bag-valve-mask d.
Bair Hugger fluid warming d.
Bair Hugger infant warming d.
balanced traction d.
balloon catheter sealing d.
balloon occlusion-aspiration embolus entrapment d.
Balloon-on-a-Wire cardiac d.
band ligator d.
Bard ambulatory PCA d.
Bard self-adhesive fecal containment d.
4-bar external fixation d.
Bassett electrical stimulation d.
BAS-300 transurethral thermotherapy d.
Baxter Health Care Continu-Flo infusion d.
Baxter PMT d.
B&B Trachguard antidisconnection d.
BD Lancet d.
BeasyTrans transfer d.
Becker orthopaedic spinal system orthotic d.
behind-the-ear listening d.
BetaSorb d.
bilateral ventricular assist d. (BIVAD)
bilevel positive pressure d.
BiliCheck breath analyzer d.
bioabsorbable sheath-delivered vascular d.
bioartificial liver d.
bioartificial liver support d.
biodegradable fixation d.
Biofeedback 5DX d.
Biopore membrane d.
Biosearch anal biofeedback d.
BioStinger low-profile fixation d.
BioStinger-V bioabsorbable meniscal repair d.
BIVAD bilateral left and right ventricular assist d.
biventricular assist d.
BladderManager portable ultrasonic d.
BladderManager ultrasound d.
blade-form d.

Blanchard traction d.
blood flow enhancement d.
bollard d.
bone fixation d.
Bone-Lok d.
Book Butler book-grip d.
Bovie electrocautery d.
Bovie 1250 electrosurgical d.
bovine collagen plug d.
Boyden chamber assay d.
braided occlusion d.
Brannock foot measuring d.
Breas PV10 CPAP d.
BreastAlert DTS screening d.
BriteSmile teeth-whitening laser d.
Bruker minispec measuring d.
BSD-300 d.
BTE listening d.
Buck convoluted traction d.
Bucky digital x-ray d.
Burkard sampling d.
Burnett BiDirectional TMJ d.
buttoned d.
Button One-Step gastrostomy d.
BVM d.
Cadwell 5200A somatosensory
  evoked potential unit d.
cage catheter d.
Caire Sprint portable liquid
  oxygen d.
Caire Stroller portable liquid
  oxygen d.
Calandruccio II compression d.
Calandruccio triangular compression
  fixation d.
Cameco syringe pistol aspiration d.
Cameron fracture d.
Camino intracranial pressure
  monitoring d.
Camino intraparenchymal
  fiberoptic d.
Caps ArthroWand d.
capsular retraction d.
CarboMedics valve d.
cardiac automatic resuscitative d.
cardiac stretch d.
CardiArc SPECT imaging d.
Cardiomemo d.
CardioSEAL d.
Carpal Trac traction d.
carpal tunnel release system d.
Carter-Thomason port closure d.
cassette cup collecting d.
Cassi rotational core biopsy d.
CastAlert d.
Cath-Lok catheter locking d.
CaverMap surgical d.
Cavi-Jet dental prophylaxis d.
C-D fixation d.

C-D instrumentation d.
Cellect graft preparation d.
Cellect Selective Retention d.
celltrifuge d.
cementless Sportorno hip
  arthroplasty stem d.
Centermark vascular access d.
central venous access d.
cervical immobilization d. (CID)
cervical range-of-motion d.
CerviSoft cytology collection d.
Cervitrak d.
charge-coupled d.
Charnley external fixation d.
Chattanooga traction d.
Chemo-Port perivena catheter
  system d.
child-restraint d.
Chinese fingertrap traction d.
Chiroslide measuring d.
ChiselTip suction cautery d.
cholesterol 1, 2, 3 noninvasive
  testing d.
Christoudias fascial closure d.
Chulalongkorn University
  vacuum d.
Chuter endovascular d.
CIC listening d.
Circe d.
Circon-ACMI USL-2000 rigid d.
Circulaire aerosol drug delivery d.
Circulaire inhaled medication
  delivery d.
circular fixation d.
circular stapling d.
CirKuit-Guard d.
Clamshell d.
Clamshell II d.
Cleanwheel presterilized
  disposable d.
Clearglide precision bipolar d.
clitoral therapy d.
closed-loop d.
Closer percutaneous suture-mediated
  closure d.
closure d.
Clo-Sur PAD closure d.
Clot Buster Amplatz
  thrombectomy d.
ClozeX needleless wound
  closure d.
Coag-a-Mate prothrombin d.
CoaguChek portable prothrombin
  time d.
CoaguChek self-testing d.
Coherent VersaPulse d.
Colapinto compression d.
collagen mediated closure d.
collagen plug d.

D

device *(continued)*

Columbus McKinnon Hugger d.
Combitube airway d.
Companion 2 self-monitoring blood glucose d.
completely in-the-canal listening d.
compression d.
compressive internal fixating d.
continuous microinfusion d.
continuous passive motion d.
Contour Emboli artificial embolization d.
CoolSpot skin-cooling d.
Copper-7 intrauterine d.
Cordis implantable drug reservoir d.
CoreTherm high-energy d.
Corflo-Cubby low-profile gastrostomy d.
Coronado vacuum fixation d.
Cotrel-Dubousset dynamic transverse traction d.
Coumatrak prothrombin time d.
CPI Mini d.
CPI Ventak AICD d.
CPM d.
cranial molding d.
CranioFIX d.
craniomandibular orthopaedic repositioning d.
Criss Cross Cradle d.
CritiView bedside patient monitoring d.
Crit-Line III TQA fluid management and access d.
Crit-Scan noninvasive hematocrit measurement d.
crosslinked poly glaucoma filtration d.
CryoHit cryotherapy d.
CSCT-2000 electromagnetic d.
CTRS d.
Cueva cranial nerve electrode monitoring d.
Cuff Link orthopaedic d.
Cu-7 intrauterine d.
cutting balloon d.
CVIS imaging d.
CyberKnife Express d.
CycleBeads fertility d.
Cygnus transdermal fentanyl d.
cymatic d.
cyst puncture d.
Dalkon shield intrauterine d.
DeBakey-NASA axial-flow ventricular assist d.
Defyne urethral assist d.
DeLee suction d.

Della Badia laparoscopic suturing d.
Deltec portable external infusion d.
demand-valve ventilation d.
De Mayo 2-point discrimination d.
Denham external fixation d.
dental antisnoring d.
Dentsleeve d.
Dermabond wound closure d.
Dermagraft skin d.
Dermagraft wound healing d.
DermaSeptic d.
Derma-Wand d.
Deyerle fixation d.
Deyo d.
Diagnodent laser d.
Digiflator digital inflation d.
digital Add-On Bucky x-ray d.
Digit-Grip d.
Digitrapper Mk III reflux testing d.
Dilamezinsert d.
Dinamap automated blood pressure d.
directional atherectomy d.
DirectRay direct-to-digital image capture d.
DirectRay direct-to-digital x-ray capture d.
DisCoVisc ophthalmic viscosurgical d.
Disk-Criminator nerve stimulation measuring d.
displacement sensing d.
Dispo-sand d.
distal targeting d.
distraction d.
Diva laparoscopic morcellator d.
Donnez endometrial ablation d.
Doppler d.
double-balloon d.
double-disc ASD closure d.
double-umbrella d.
Douek-Med ear d.
DPAP Stealth d.
DPAP Stealth positive airway pressure d.
Dressflex orthotic d.
Dr. Grip writing d.
Duett arterial closure d.
Duett arterial puncture site closure d.
Duett closure d.
Duett diagnostic d.
Duett therapeutic d.
Duett vascular sealing d.
Dunn fracture d.
Durathane cardiac d.
Dwyer d.

dynamic cooling d.
dynamic orthotic cranioplasty d.
dynamic transverse traction d.
DynaVox 2 communication d.
DynaWell medical compression d.
Eagle inflation d.
Easy-Pull sock aide d.
Echocheck hearing screening d.
Econo-Cerv traction d.
Econolith d.
Eder cord blood collection d.
Edwards AVA high-flow d.
Edwards modular system sacral
  fixation d.
EEA stapling d.
EGTA d.
Elbow-Up Protector elbow
  suspension d.
electrical stimulation d.
electric suction d.
electroacupuncture d.
Electro-Acuscope d.
electrocoagulation biterminal d.
electronic infusion d.
electronic portal imaging d.
Electronics electrical stimulation d.
El Gamal cardiac d.
emergency infusion d.
Enclose anastomosis assist d.
Enclose II anastomosis assist d.
Enclose proximal anastomotic
  assist d.
Encore Orthopedics d.
Endermologie noninvasive body
  contouring d.
Endo Babcock surgical grasping d.
Endo-Bender bending d.
Endo Catch II d.
Endo GIA stapling d.
Endo Grasp d.
EndoLift d.
EndoPearl bioabsorbable d.
EndoPearl fixation d.
endoscopically deliverable tissue-
  transfixing d.
endoscopic hemoclip d.
Endoscrub d.
Endoskeleton TA structural d.
Endostaple d.
Endo Stitch laparoscopic
  suturing d.
end-to-end anastomosis stapling d.
Envision TD ophthalmic drug
  delivery d.
EOA d.
EpiPen injection d.
EpiPen-Jr injection d.
Epi-Stay d.

Epos Ultra extracorporeal shock
  wave therapy d.
Equinox EEG acquisition d.
ErecAid vacuum erection d.
Ergolift d.
Eros-CTD eroscillator d.
Eros-CTD female sexual therapy d.
esophageal detection d.
esophageal detector d.
evacuation d.
Everest disposable inflation d.
Evershears surgical instrument d.
EVS mechanical closure d.
ExacTech glucose measuring d.
Exeter intramedullary bone plug d.
EX-FI-RE external fixation d.
eXit disposable puncture closure d.
Exogen 2000 noninvasive low-
  intensity pulsed ultrasound d.
expanded foam immobilization d.
extended collection d.
exterior pelvic d.
external counterpressure d.
external tachyarrhythmia control d.
external vascular compression d.
extracorporeal assist d.
extracorporeal liver assist d.
  (ELAD)
extracorporeal organ bioartificial
  liver d.
extraction atherectomy d.
ExtreSafe phlebotomy d.
extrication d.
E-Z Flex jaw exercising d.
EZ Hold manual compression d.
E-Z Lets II lancing d.
EZLoc femoral fixation d.
EZ-Trac orthopaedic suspension d.
fail-safe d.
FastOut d.
fecal containment d. (FCD)
feeding tube attachment d.
FemCap barrier contraceptive d.
Femcept d.
FemoStop inflatable pneumatic
  compression d.
ferromagnetic monitoring d.
fiberoptic delivery d.
FilterWire distal embolic
  protection d.
FilterWire distal protection d.
Finesse cardiac d.
finger photoplethysmographic d.
Finn chamber patch test d.
Fischer-Leibinger bur hole-mounted
  fixation d.
fixation d.
flexible delivery d.
flexible endoscopic suturing d.

D

device *(continued)*

flexible Olympus GF-eUM3 d.
Flexible Sew-Right d.
Flexible Ti-Knot d.
Flexi-Trak skin anchoring d.
floating alveolar d.
FlossBrite dental floss d.
Flotem IIe fluid-warming d.
flow-controlled d.
FloWire ultrasound d.
flow restricted oxygen-powered
  ventilation d.
flow-restricted oxygen-powered
  ventilation d.
Flowtron DVT compression d.
Flowtron thigh-high d.
flushing d.
Flutter mucus clearance d.
Flutter therapeutic d.
FM wireless assistive listening d.
FNA-21 fine-needle aspiration d.
fog reduction/elimination d.
FootFlex performance stretching d.
foot orthotic d.
forced air active cooling d.
forearm lift assist adjustable
  spring-loaded d.
ForeRunner automatic external
  defibrillator d.
Fox internal fixation d.
fracture fixation d.
frameless stereotactic d.
FrameLock reference-arc fixation d.
Fromm triangle orthopaedic d.
Galtac d.
galvanic skin response d.
gastroesophageal antireflux d.
Gastro-Port II feeding d.
GDC SynerG detachment d.
Gelbfish-Endovasc d.
Genotropin Pen 5 growth hormone
  delivery d.
Gensini cardiac d.
Gentle-Lance lancet d.
geometric d.
Georgiade fixation d.
Gerster traction d.
Gianturco-Grifka vascular
  occlusion d.
GIA stapling d.
Giliberty d.
glaucoma drainage d.
GlideCath torque d.
Glucoband electronic scanning d.
Glucolet Automatic lancing d.
Glucolet lancet d.
GlucoWatch glucose monitoring d.
Goetz cardiac d.
Golgi d.

Goodale-Lubin cardiac d.
Gore thyroplasty d.
Gould polygraph gastric motility
  measuring d.
Goulter d.
Graftmaster d.
Grass pressure-recording d.
gravimetric d.
gravitational d.
Green Sleeve compression d.
Grip-Ease d.
grip torque d.
GSI 60 distortion product
  otoacoustic emission d.
G-suit d.
Guidant-CPI d.
Guyuron endoscopic access d.
GynoSampler endometrial
  sampling d.
Haemolance Plus lancet d.
halo craniomaxillofacial fixation d.
halo femoral traction d.
halo gravity traction d.
halo hoop d.
handheld flutter d.
Hand Helper d.
Handisol phototherapy d.
hand-operated suction d.
HandPort hand assist d.
hand-powered suction d.
Hare splint d.
Hare traction d.
Harmony surgical suction d.
Harrington fixation d.
Harrington-Kostuik distraction d.
Harrington rod instrumentation
  distraction outrigger d.
head fixation d.
head-mounted d.
hearing protection d.
heart assist d.
Heartflo anastomotic d.
HeartMate implantable ventricular
  assist d.
Hemoband hemostasis d.
hemoclipping application d.
HemoCue AB hemoglobin
  measurement d.
hemostatic occlusive leverage d.
hemostatic puncture closure d.
Hemovac suction d.
Hepatix d.
Hershey left ventricular assist d.
Hexascan Mark I, II model robotic
  scanning d.
Heyer-Schulte antisiphon d.
Hi-Per cardiac d.
hipGRIP body positioning d.
HiSonic-TRD d.

HiSonic ultrasonic bone conduction hearing d.
Hoffmann external fixation d.
Hoffmann mini-lengthening fixation d.
Hoffmann traction d.
Hoffmann-Vidal external fixation d.
Hollister circumcision d.
Hollister collecting d.
Horizon CPAP d.
horizontal drain attachment d.
horizontal tube attachment d.
hot/ice cold therapy cooler therapy d.
Hotline fluid warming d.
Howmedica external bone-lengthening d.
H2 Score office-based diagnostic d.
HSRA d.
HX-5/6-1 endoscopic clipping d.
Hybrid Capture 2 d.
HydroKeratome d.
HylaSine d.
ICD-ATP d.
iFind handheld d.
Ikuta fixation d.
ILA-series stapling d.
Ilizarov d.
Imed infusion d.
implantable bone anchor d.
implantable middle ear hearing d.
implantable vascular access d. (IVAD)
implantable venous access d.
ImPulse electronic oxygen-conserving d.
inductive coupling d.
indwelling transcutaneous vascular access d. (ITVAD)
In-Exsufflator respiratory d.
InfaMyst aerosol spray d.
infection-prevention d.
Infiltrator local drug delivery d.
InFuse bone graft/LT-Cage lumbar tapered fusion d.
infusion d.
Innovasive d.
InPath cervical cancer screening d.
input d.
InspirEase d.
Inspiron small inspiratory training d.
Insta-Mold ear protection d.
Insta-Nerve d.
insufflation d.
Insuflon insulin delivery d.
InSync cardiac resynchronization d.
Intelect laser system d.
Interceptor wire distal protection d.

Inter Fix RP threaded spinal fusion d.
Inter Fix RP threaded spinal fusion cage d.
Inter Fix threaded spinal fusion cage d.
internal cervical d.
internal fixation d.
interrogation d.
interspinous spacer d.
InterStim d.
in-the-ear listening d.
In-Time retrieval d.
intraaortic balloon assist d.
intraaortic balloon counterpulsation d.
Intracell mechanical muscle d.
Intracell myofascial trigger-point d.
intracervical d. (ICD)
intracranial pressure monitoring d.
intramedullary fixation d.
intraoperative d.
intraoral titanium mandibular distraction d.
IntraSonix TULIP laser d.
intrauterine d. (IUD)
intrauterine contraception d.
intravenous accurate control d.
InvertaChair traction d.
inverted buttoned d.
Irrijet DS wound irrigation d.
Isobar barostat distension d.
IsoCode Stix d.
Isolator endoscopic ablation d.
i-STAT bedside blood testing d.
ITE listening d.
IVAC d.
Jace W550 CPM d.
Jacobson resonator d.
JAS elbow motion d.
Jewel AF implantable arrhythmia management d.
Jewel atrial fibrillation dual-chamber d.
Kaneda anterior spine stabilizing d.
Kaneda distraction d.
KangarooWeb abdominal retraction d.
Kaufman incontinence d.
Kendall sequential compression d.
Kendrick extrication d.
Kennedy ligament augmentation d.
Kerboull acetabular reinforcement d.
Kerraboot d.
Kessler fixation d.
keyed filling d.
Kin-Con d.
kinetic continuous passive motion d.

D

device *(continued)*
kinetic rehabilitation d.
King cardiac d.
King interlocking d.
Kirschner d.
Kirsch stapling d.
knee height measuring d.
Kostuik-Harrington d.
KRD L2000 rehab d.
Kronner external fixation d.
Kuhlman cervical traction d.
Küntscher traction d.
LactoSorb resorbable fixation d.
language acquisition d.
Laparofan pneumoperitoneum d.
Laparomed cholangiogram d.
Laparomed suture applier d.
Lap Disc hand access d.
Laser Lancet laser d.
Lasette laser lancing d.
Lasette Plus assisted blood
  sampling d.
Lawrence d.
LazerSmile tooth-whitening d.
lead locking d.
left ventricular assist d. (LVAD)
Legasus support CPM d.
legGRIP body positioning d.
leg-holding d.
Lehman cardiac d.
Leinbach d.
Leksell stereotactic d.
Leonard arm d.
Lewy suspension d.
Libbe lower bowel evacuation d.
LifeSpex d.
ligament augmentation d. (LAD)
ligation d.
Light Talker d.
linear stapling d.
Link Orthopaedics d.
Linx guidewire extension cardiac d.
Lippes loop intrauterine d.
liquefaction d.
LiteGait partial weightbearing gait
  therapy d.
Lite Touch lancing d.
Lock Clamshell d.
locking d.
Look micropuncture d.
lumbar tapered cage lumbar
  tapered fusion d.
Luque fixation d.
Lymphapress d.
LySonix 2000 ultrasound d.
Macroplastique implantable d.
Magna-Finder locating d.
magnetic induction d.
magnetic jaw tracking d.

Makler insemination d.
malleable microsurgical suction d.
MammoReader mammogram d.
MammoSite RTS balloon
  interstitial d.
Mammotome core biopsy d.
mandibular advancement d.
mandibular positioning d.
Margulies intrauterine d.
M.A.T. postoperative comfort d.
Max30 inflation d.
Mayo elbow distraction d.
M-Brace posterior dynamic
  stabilization d.
McAtee olecranon compression
  screw d.
McCleery-Miller locking d.
McKeever patellar resurfacing d.
McLaughlin osteosynthesis d.
3M CTRS d.
M-cup vacuum extraction d.
MDILog therapy monitoring d.
measuring d.
mechanical d.
mechanical support d.
Medelec 5-channel
  neurophysiological d.
Medicamat ultrasound d.
Medicon ultrasonic liposuction d.
Medilog 9000 polysomnography d.
MediPort infusion vascular
  access d.
MediRule II measuring d.
Medtronic Activa tremor control
  therapy d.
Medtronic defibrillator implant
  support d.
Medtronic external tachyarrhythmia
  control d.
Medtronic-Hall d.
Medtronic-Hancock d.
Medtronic Hemopump cardiac
  assist d.
Medtronic Inspire implantable d.
Medtronic Jewel AF implantable
  arrhythmia management d.
Medtronic Jewel 7219C, D d.
Medtronic Octopus tissue
  stabilizing d.
Medtronic tremor control
  therapy d.
MedX physical therapy d.
MelaFind handheld imaging d.
Mentor ultrasound d.
Menuet Compact urodynamic
  testing d.
Merry Walker ambulation d.
Metrecom d.

MicroDigitrapper-S apnea
screening d.
MicroFET2 muscle testing d.
Microgyn II urinary incontinence d.
Microjet-based cutting and
débriding d.
MicroMed DeBakey ventricular
assist d.
Microsampler d.
MicroStim 100 TENS d.
MicroTymp tympanometric d.
Microvasive biliary d.
Microvasive Gold probe bipolar
electrocautery d.
Microvena retrieval d.
Miltner constraint compliance d.
miniature ultrasound suction d.
Minnesota thermal disc temperature
testing d.
Mirena intrauterine d.
Mission vacuum constriction d.
Mission vacuum erection d.
Mitek QuickAnchor d.
3M microvascular anastomotic
coupling d.
Mobilimb CPM d.
Mobin-Uddin umbrella
endoluminal d.
Molteno double-plate drainage d.
Molteno implant drainage d.
Molteno single-plate drainage d.
Monarch 25 inflation d.
Monojector fingerstick d.
Morwel ultrasound d.
motorized transducer pullback d.
MTI PhotoScreener vision
screening d.
Mucat cervical sampling d.
mucus clearance d.
Mueller fixation d.
Mullins cardiac d.
multiband ligating d.
Multifire Endo GIA stapling d.
multileaf collimator d.
multiple parameter telemetry d.
Multispatula cervical sampling d.
muscle and neurological stimulation
electrotherapy d.
Myocor Coapsys pacing assist d.
myReader low-vision auto-
reading d.
Nachlas-Linton esophagogastric
balloon tamponade d.
nail-bending d.
nail-mounted compression d.
Nasal-Aire I, II continuous positive
airway pressure d.
Nauth traction d.
NB200 vascular access d.

Needle-Ease d.
Needle-Pro needle protection d.
needlescope d.
negative pressure d.
NeoDisc cervical replacement d.
NeoNaze d.
Nervoscope d.
Neufeld d.
Neuro-Aide testing d.
neurocalometer thermography d.
Neurometer CPT
electrodiagnostic d.
Niplette d.
Nite Train'r enuresis
conditioning d.
Nit-Occlud d.
Nitrospray Plus cryosurgical d.
Nogier auriculotherapy d.
noise reduction d.
nonferromagnetic positioning d.
nonthoracotomy system
antitachycardia d.
notcher d.
Novacor Diasys cardiac d.
Novacor Diasys left ventricular
assist d.
Novacor left ventricular assist d.
Novo-10a CBF measuring d.
NovolinPen d.
Novus 3000 photocoagulation d.
NTrap endoscopic entrapment and
extraction d.
NuPulse d.
Nu-Trake cricothyrotomy d.
Nycore cardiac d.
OAT d.
oblique prism d.
O₂ disposable boot d.
Ogden Anchor soft tissue d.
Olcott torque d.
Olympia Vacpac support d.
Olympus clip-fixing d.
Olympus LUS-1 rigid d.
Olympus LUS-2 ultrasonic energy
rigid d.
Olympus UES series snare
cautery d.
Ommaya reservoir d.
Omni-Flexor d.
Omniscience valve d.
Omnisense multisite QUS d.
One Step Button gastrostomy d.
OnTrak TestTcard drug testing d.
Opal RF needle ablation d.
Oppociser exercise d.
OptiChamber drug-holding d.
OralScreen rapid oral fluid
screening and test d.
oral temperature d.

235

device *(continued)*
OraSure d.
OraSure collection d.
OraSure HIV-1 oral specimen
collection d.
OraSure salivary collection d.
Original Jacknobber II muscle-
massage d.
Orion d.
Orthofix external fixation d.
Orthofix ISKD d.
Orthofix lengthening d.
orthopaedic fixation d.
orthotic d.
OssaTron d.
OssaTron noninvasive extracorporeal
shock wave therapy d.
OsteoAnalyzer d.
OsteoAnalyzer bone densitometry d.
Osteomark NTx point-of-care d.
OsteoView d.
OsteoView x-ray d.
output d.
Oxford uncompartmental d.
OxiMax pulse oximetry d.
oxygen disposable boot d.
Oxylator EM-100 emergency
resuscitation d.
Oxymizer d.
palatal lifting d.
Palpagraph breast mapping d.
Panoramic200 ultra-widefield
ophthalmic imaging d.
Panosol II home phototherapy d.
Papette d.
ParaGard intrauterine d.
Parascan scanning d.
Parham-Martin fracture d.
Passager d.
passive motion d.
Pathfinder irrigation d.
patient self-administration d.
Pavcnik Monodisk d.
PCA Plus infusion d.
PC Polygraf HR d.
PDN d.
pegboard lateral positioning d.
Penlet II Automatic blood
sampling d.
Pennig minifixator d.
Perclose arterial closure d.
Perclose closure d.
Perclose diagnostic d.
Perclose/Prostar d.
Perclose PVS d.
Perclose suture d.
Perclose therapeutic d.
Perclose vascular closure d.
Percuss-O-Matic jackhammer d.

Percusurg distal protection d.
PercuSurge recovery system d.
percutaneous arterial closure d.
percutaneous atherectomy d.
percutaneous suture-mediated
arteriotomy closure d.
percutaneous suture-mediated
closure d.
percutaneous thrombolytic d.
percutaneous ventricular assist d.
(pVAD)
PerDUCER percutaneous pericardial
access d.
PerfectCapsule irrigation d.
Perfect Pupil expansion d.
peripheral indwelling intermediate
infusion d.
personal heart d.
PET balloon atherectomy d.
PGK stereotactic d.
phased-array ultrasonographic d.
Philips Integris 3000 biplane digital
subtraction angiography d.
phonologic acquisition d.
PhotoDerm PL pulsed light d.
PhotoDerm PL, VL pulsed light d.
PhotoDerm VL d.
Piccolino Monorail balloon d.
Pierce-Donachy Thoratec ventricular
assist d.
Piezosurgery d.
Pigg-O-Stat immobilization d.
Pillo-Boot lower leg positioning d.
Pisces spinal cord stimulation d.
Pivot Pole walking d.
Plastibell circumcision d.
plastizote orthotic d.
plate-guided distraction d.
Pleur-evac d.
PlexiPulse intermittent pneumatic
compression d.
PLM d.
pneumatic peripheral circulation
improvement d.
POCT d.
PodoFlex reflexology d.
Polar Bair forced-air active
cooling d.
Polar Care 500 cryotherapy d.
Poly CS d.
portable aerosol delivery d.
portable monitoring d.
portable suction d.
Port-A-Cath d.
Portex Thermovent heat and
moisture d.
Portnoy DPV d.
PortSaver PercLoop d.
Positrol cardiac d.

posterior reduction d.
Pos-T-Vac vacuum erection d.
PPCID sequential foot
  compression d.
precalibrated pointing d.
Premium CEEA circular stapling d.
Pressurefuse automatic constant
  pressure d.
pressure-specified sensory d.
Prestige Lite Touch lancing d.
Prima total occlusion d.
ProCon incontinence d.
Profile-II ER drug screening d.
Progestasert intrauterine d.
ProLumen thrombectomy d.
pronation spring-control d.
prone cranial support d.
Pronex patient-controlled pneumatic
  traction d.
Pron-Pillo head positioning d.
Pro/Pel coating cardiac d.
Prostar Plus percutaneous
  closure d.
Prostar Plus percutaneous vascular
  surgical d.
Prostar-Techstar suture-mediated
  closure d.
Prostar XL hemostatic puncture
  closure d.
Prostar XL percutaneous closure d.
Prostar XL 8, 10 suture-mediated
  closure d.
Prostathermer d.
Prostatron transurethral
  thermotherapy d.
prosthetic d.
ProTack tacking d.
ProTime INR test d.
Protocult stool sampling d.
ProTrac cruciate reconstruction
  measurement d.
ProTrac measurement d.
pullback atherectomy d.
pulsatile assist d.
pulse oximetry d.
PulStarFRAS d.
pyrolytic carbon d.
pyxigraphic d.
Q-Maxx side-firing laser d.
Quantum biliary inflation d.
Quantum inflation d.
Quartzo d.
Quengel d.
QuicKlamp hemostasis d.
QuickLance lancing d.
radiant heat d.
radiative hyperthermia d.
radiofrequency diathermy d.
RadStat hemostasis d.

Rancho ankle-foot control d.
Rapid Rhino d.
Rashkind cardiac d.
Rashkind double umbrella d.
Rashkind hooked d.
rate-adaptive d.
Redi-Trac traction d.
Reichert-Mundinger stereotactic d.
Relia-Flow d.
ReliefBand electrostimulating d.
ReSound Digital 5000 hearing d.
RESPeRATE interactive
  breathing d.
Respiradyne pulmonary function d.
Res-Q arrhythmia control d.
retaining d.
retrieval d.
Rezaian external fixation d.
Rezaian interbody d.
Rheolog d.
rheolytic mechanical
  thrombectomy d.
Richards lag screw d.
Richards lag screw compression d.
Richard Wolf model 2271.004
  ultrasonic energy rigid d.
Riechert-Mundinger stereotactic d.
right ventricular assist d. (RVAD)
right ventricular wall d.
rigid internal fixation d.
Rigiflator handheld
  inflation/deflation d.
RigiScan d.
ring-type rigidity measuring d.
Rinn XCP radiographic
  paralleling d.
RMC knee replacement d.
robotic-automated assist d.
Rochester bone trephine d.
Roeder manipulative aptitude
  test d.
roentgen knife stereotactic
  radiosurgical d.
Roger Anderson external
  fixation d.
Roger Anderson stabilization d.
Roll-A-Bout mobility d.
RollerBack self-massage d.
Rolz d.
root-form d.
rope stretching d.
Rotablator atherectomy d.
RotaLink Plus rotational
  atherectomy d.
rotational atherectomy d.
roticulator stapling d.
RVAD centrifugal right ventricular
  assist d.
Safeguard post-hemostasis d.

D

device *(continued)*

Safe-T Mate anti-rollback d.
SAFHS ultrasound d.
Saf-T-Coil intrauterine d.
Sarns ventricular assist d.
scaling d.
scavenging d.
ScopeGuide magnetic resonance imaging d.
ScopeGuide MRI d.
Scopette d.
Scully Hip S'port d.
Scully Hip S'port hip d.
sealed capsule irrigation d.
Sebbin ultrasound d.
Second Look breast imaging d.
Select-Lite lancing d.
Senso listening d.
Sentinel ICD d.
Sepacell RZ-2000 d.
sequential compression d. (SCD)
Serena Mx handheld apnea detection d.
Servo Screen 390 ventilator monitoring d.
Servox d.
seton drainage d.
Sew-Right suturing d.
Sgarlato d.
shear-off d.
Shiley saphenous vein irrigation and pressurization d.
Shug male contraceptive d.
Sideris adjustable buttoned d.
Siemens Magnetom Vision whole-body MR d.
Silent Night diagnostic and screening d.
SilverHawk d.
single-needle d.
single-use d.
Skinscan d.
SkinTech medical tattooing d.
Sleeper Gripper prosthetic d.
Slot distraction d.
SmartFlow multiple-lesion d.
SmartSuction Harmony surgical suction d.
SMEI ultrasound d.
Smoke Controller d.
snare d.
Snore Guard mandibular repositioning d.
Snorenomor d.
Sock-Assist d.
Soehendra stent retrieval d.
Sofamor spinal d.
Sofamor spinal instrumentation d.
SofPulse d.

SofTouch vacuum erection d.
Soft Touch lancet d.
SOLEutions custom orthotic d.
SOLEutions Prefab orthotic d.
SomaSensor d.
SomnoStar apnea testing d.
Sonic Air 1500 d.
Sonoblate ablation d.
Sonoline Sierra ultrasound imaging d.
SonoSite 180 hand-carried ultrasound d.
Sonotron electronic therapeutic d.
Sony Promavica still capture d.
Spa Touch hair removal d.
Spencer incontinence d.
Spenco orthotic d.
Spider embolic protection d.
spinal fusion d.
Spitz-Holter flushing d.
Sport-Rite Olympian d.
Sport-Rite Runner d.
SporTX stimulation d.
spot film d.
StairClimber assist d.
stapling d.
StarBurst Flex RFA d.
StarBurst SDE RFA d.
StarBurst Semi-Flex RFA d.
StarBurst XLi-enhanced RFA d.
StarBurst XLi RFA d.
StarBurst XL RFA d.
STARFlex d.
Statak soft tissue attachment d.
Statak suturing d.
static topical occlusive hemostatic pressure d.
StatLock catheter securement d.
Status Cup Plus drug testing d.
Stellbrink fixation d.
stent-anchoring d.
Step d.
stereotactic d.
stereotactic vacuum-assisted biopsy d.
stereotaxic d.
stereotaxic positioning d.
Steri-Oss dental implant d.
Steri-Oss implant d.
St. Jude cardiac d.
stoma measuring d.
Stone clamp-locking d.
Stone Cone nitinol stone retrieval d.
STOP nonsurgical permanent contraception d.
Stratagene CastAway sequencing d.
Stress-Ray varus-valgus d.
Stryker d.

Stryker knee joint laxity d.
STx lumbar traction d.
STx Saunders lumbar disc d.
subcutaneous peritoneal
administration d.
subcutaneous tunneling d.
Sub-Q-Set subcutaneous continuous
infusion d.
suction d.
Sukhtian-Hughes fixation d.
Sullivan III nasal continuous
positive air pressure d.
superconducting quantum
interference d.
Super-9 guiding cardiac d.
Super Pinky d.
SuperQuad assistive d.
SuperStitch d.
SuperStitch closure d.
Sure-Closure d.
SureSight vision screening d.
Suretac bioabsorbable shoulder
fixation d.
Surgicutt incision d.
Surgiflex Wave suction-irrigation d.
Surgitron 3000 ultrasound d.
Surveyor recording d.
Sutter d.
Sutter-CPM knee d.
Suture Assistant endoscopic
suturing d.
SuturTek 360-degree fascia
closure d.
SVAB d.
Swedish Helparm d.
Swiss Lithoclast Master d.
Symbion cardiac d.
Symbion pneumatic assist d.
Symphonix Vibrant Soundbridge
hearing d.
Synergist vacuum erection d.
Syvek Patch closure d.
Tacticon peripheral neuropathy
screening d.
Tandem cardiac d.
Tanner mesher d.
Tano d.
Taperseal hemostatic d.
targeted cryoablation d.
TA stapling d.
T-bar immobilization d.
Teaser d.
TEC atherectomy d.
TechMate 500 automatic
immunostaining d.
Techstar d.
Techstar percutaneous closure d.
Techstar suturing closure d.
Tekscan in-shoe monitoring d.

Telangitron d.
Telectronics Guardian ATP 4210 d.
telescoping tubular d.
Telos radiographic stress d.
temperature and galvanic skin
response biofeedback d.
temporary endoprosthetic d.
Tenderlett d.
Tenderlett Jr. lancing d.
Tenderlett Plus fingerstick blood
collection d.
Tenderlett Toddler lancing d.
terminal d.
Texas Scottish Rite Hospital
corkscrew d.
Texas Scottish Rite Hospital mini-
corkscrew d.
T-fastener d.
T-Fix absorbable meniscal repair d.
The Closer arterial puncture site
closure d.
Thera-Band therapy d.
Thera-Putty therapy d.
TheraSnore d.
ThermaCool TC radiofrequency d.
ThermaStim muscle warming d.
TherMatric hyperthermia d.
TherMatrx TMx-2000 d.
Thermedics cardiac d.
Thermedics left ventricular assist d.
Thermex-II transurethral prostate
heating d.
Thermocardiosystems left ventricular
assist d.
Thermo Cardiosystems left
ventricular assist d.
thermocouple d.
The Rope stretch-and-traction d.
The Rope stretching d.
Thoratec biventricular assist d.
Thoratec cardiac d.
Thoratec implantable vascular
access d.
Thoratec right ventricular assist d.
Thoratec ventricular assist d.
thread-locking d.
Threshold inspiratory muscle
trainer d.
Threshold PEP d.
Threshold positive expiratory
pressure d.
Thumper d.
Tibbs semiautomatic suturing d.
tiered-therapy antiarrhythmic d.
tinnitus relief d. (TRD)
tissue-engineered polymer d.
titanium fixation d.
Titanium Wedge electrosurgical
resection d.

device *(continued)*
tongue-locking d.
tongue-retaining d.
tooth-borne distraction d.
totally implantable lengthening d.
traction d.
Trak Back pullback d.
Tranquility Bilevel airway patency
maintenance d.
Tranquility Bilevel positive airway
pressure therapy d.
Tranquility Quest CPAP d.
transcatheter d.
transdermal fentanyl d.
transparent elastic band ligating d.
transpedicularly implanted anterior
spinal support d.
d. for transverse traction
Trapper catheter exchange d.
Trerotola thrombectomy d.
TriClip endoscopic clipping d.
TriggerWheel d.
Trimedyne Optilase d.
TriSpan aneurysm neck-bridge d.
Tru-Area Determination wound
measuring d.
TSRH corkscrew d.
TSRH mini-corkscrew d.
tube d.
tube attachment d.
Turapy d.
Ultra-Retractor d.
ultrasonic aspirating d.
UltraTLC adjustable lancing d.
Unilink anastomotic d.
Universal joint d.
urethral barrier d.
Uri-Drain male incontinence d.
urine collection d.
Urowave d.
Uterine Explora Curette endometrial
sampling d.
UV-Flash ultraviolet germicidal
exchange d.
Vacu-Aide portable suction d.
Vaculance lancing d.
vacuum-assisted closure d.
vacuum clitoral therapy d.
vacuum constriction d. (VCD)
vacuum entrapment d.
vacuum erection d. (VED)
vacuum extraction d.
vacuum fixation d.
vacuum tumescence d.
vacuum tumescence constrictor d.
Valenti arthroereisis d.
Valleylab Force 2 electrosurgical d.
Valtrac anastomosis d.
Vanguard d.

Vapr coagulation and cautery d.
variceal pressure measuring d.
VariFix spinal implant d.
VariGrip spinal implant d.
Vasceze vascular access flush d.
Vascugel d.
vascular access d. (VAD)
vascular access flush d.
vascular hemostatic d. (VHD)
vascular sealing d.
VasoSeal closure d.
VasoSeal diagnostic d.
VasoSeal ES, VHD arterial
puncture site closure d.
VasoSeal therapeutic d.
VasoSeal vascular hemostasis d.
VasoView balloon dissection d.
Vectra Genisys laser system d.
Venodyne pneumatic compressive d.
venous access d. (VAD)
Ventak Prizm AVT cardioverter d.
ventricular assist d. (VAD)
Ventritex Cadence d.
Venture demand oxygen delivery d.
Venturi aspiration vitrectomy d.
VEPTR d.
Verdict-II drug screening d.
Veriflex cardiac d.
Versalok low back fixation d.
VestaBlate system balloon d.
vest-type extrication d.
VHD closure d.
Vibrant Soundbridge implantable
middle ear hearing d.
Vidal d.
Vidal-Adrey modified Hoffmann
external fixation d.
Viking II nerve monitoring d.
Viladot arthroereisis d.
Viringe vascular access flush d.
Virtual distortion-product otoacoustic
emission d.
viscosurgical d.
Visiport d.
visor halo fixation d.
VitaCuff d.
VitaCuff infection control d.
vitallium d.
Vitrasert intraocular d.
ViziLite oral abnormality
detection d.
Volkov-Oganesian external
fixation d.
Voyager aortic IntraClusion d.
VPAP III ST bilevel d.
VTU-1 vacuum erection d.
Wagner distraction d.
Wagner external fixation d.

Wagner leg-lengthening distraction d.
Wagner-Schanz screw d.
Walk-Rite d.
Wallach Endocell d.
Wallach freezer cryosurgical d.
Wallach pencil cryosurgical d.
Wallstent delivery d.
Wanger leg-lengthening d.
WasherLoc d.
Wasserstein fixation d.
wearable cardioverter-defibrillator d.
Wedge electrosurgical resection d.
Wells Johnson transfer d.
Widex listening d.
wire-guided metal spiral retrieval d.
Wizard disposable inflation d.
woggle d.
Wolf Piezolith lithotripsy d.
Wolvek fixation d.
Wrist Pro wrist support d.
Xercise band exercise d.
Xercise tube resistive d.
Xpose 3 access d.
X-Press suture-mediated closure d.
XTB knee extension d.
Zielke distraction d.
Zimmer electrical stimulation d.
Zimmer orthopaedic d.
Zimmer Statak suturing d.
Zipper antidisconnect d.
Z sampler endometrial sampling d.
Z-Touch laser d.

DeVilbiss
    D. CPAP manometer
    D. cranial rongeur
    D. I&A unit
    D. nebulizer
    D. powder blower
    D. Pulmo-Aide LT compressor
    D. Pulmo-Aide nebulizer
    D. suction pump
    D. syringe
    D. Vacu-Aide aspirator
    D. vaginal speculum
DeVilbiss-Stacy speculum
Devine-Millard-Aufricht retractor
Devine-Millard-Frazier fiberoptic suction tube
deviometer
Dewan suprapubic urodynamics catheter
Dewar flask
DeWeese
    D. axis traction forceps
    D. vena cava clamp
DeWeese-Hunter clip
Dewey obstetrical forceps
DEXAscan bone densitometer

Dexide
    D. disposable cannula
    D. disposable trocar
Dexon
    D. absorbable synthetic polyglycolic acid suture
    D. II suture
    D. mesh
    D. Plus suture
    D. polyglycolic acid mesh
    D. surgically knitted mesh
    D. suture
DexTBrush toothbrush
dexterity
    D. pneumo sleeve
    d. protractor
dextran-70 barrier material
dextrose stick
Dextrostix reagent strip
DEY albuterol inhalation aerosol
Deyerle
    D. fixation device
    D. interlocking screw
    D. punch
Deyo device
Dey-Wash skin wound cleanser
D/Flex filter
D-Foam
DFP+/DXP+
DFS 2 mattress replacement system
DGH 2000 AP ultrasonic pachymeter
DG Softgut suture
DH pressure relief walker
DHS screw
Diab-A-Foot
    D.-A.-F. protection system
    D.-A.-F. rocker insole
Diab-A-Pad insole
Diab-A-Sheet
Diab-A-Sole
    D.-A.-S. flat insole
    D.-A.-S. molded insole
Diab-A-Thotics orthotic
diabetic
    D. Diagnostic insole
    D. D-Sole foot orthosis
    d. orthosis kit
    d. pressure relief shoe
    d. sock
Diabeticorum dressing
DiabGel hydrogel dressing
DiaB Klenz wound cleanser
diacrylate resin
Diagnodent laser device
diagnostic
    d. curette
    d. duodenoscope
    d. fiberoptic lens
    d. hysteroscope

D

diagnostic *(continued)*
>d. peritoneal lavage
>d. tube
>d. tympanometer
>d. ultrasound imaging catheter
>d. x-ray camera and imaging source

Diaket root canal cement
dial
>astigmatic d.
>d. calipers
>Mendez astigmatism d.
>Regan-Lancaster d.

dial-a-flow IV line
dialer
>angled iris hook and IOL d.
>intraocular lens d.
>IOL d.
>irrigating d.
>Spadafora MemoryLens d.
>Visitec intraocular lens d.

dial-lock orthosis
Dialock hemodialysis access system
Dialog pacemaker
dial-type ophthalmodynamometer
Dialy-Nate catheter
dialysate
>d. bag
>d. tubing

dialysis
>d. catheter
>d. shunt
>d. tubing

dialyzer
>AN69 membrane d.
>CA110 d.
>CA cellulose acetate membrane hollow-fiber d.
>capillary flow d.
>CA-series d.
>C-Dak d.
>Clirans T-series d.
>DAS single-pass d.
>Filtryzer d.
>Fresenius AG d.
>F-series d.
>Gambro d.
>Gambro Lundia coil d.
>HD Secura d.
>HF d.
>high-flux d.
>hollow-fiber capillary d.
>hollow filter d.
>parallel plate d.
>Polyflux S d.
>polysulfone d.
>Renaflo hollow-fiber d.
>Renalin d.

>Renatron d.
>Terumo d.
>Terumo-Clirans d.
>twin-coil d.

Diamatrix trapezoidal diamond knife
diamond
>d. barrel bur
>D. biomechanical table
>d. bit
>d. blade knife
>d. bur
>3-in-1 d. bur
>d. crescent blade
>d. dermabrader
>d. electrode
>d. finishing bur
>d. fraise
>d. fraise dermabrasion instrument
>d. grip needle holder
>d. high-speed air drill
>d. laser knife
>d. micrometer
>d. nail
>d. phaco knife
>d. pin cutter
>d. point needle
>d. pyramid indenter
>d. rasp
>D. stent
>d. tip wire
>D. tube
>D. valve
>D. valve flow-regulating shunt
>d. wafering blade
>d. wafering saw
>d. wound separator

Diamondback
>D. 1100 recumbent stepper
>D. 100 upright stepper

diamond-coated bur
diamond-dusted
>d.-d. bur
>d.-d. knife
>d.-d. membrane eraser
>d.-d. membrane scraper (DDMS)
>d.-d. scraper

diamond-edge Supercut scissors
Diamond-Flex trocar
Diamond-Jaw needle holder
Diamond-Lite
>D.-L. cardiovascular instrument
>D.-L. titanium instrument

Diamontek knife
diaper
>Kins prefolded flat 100% cotton flannelette d.
>reusable and washable adult pin-style d.

reusable and washable adult
snap d.
Safe & Dry d.
diaphanoscope
diaphragm
Bucky d.
d. inserter
Ortho All-Flex d.
d. pessary
Potter-Bucky d.
Ramses d.
d. of stent
wide-seal d.
Diapulse
Dia pump aspirator
diascope
DiaScreen 10 Reagent Strip
Diasensor
D. 2000 glucose monitor
D. 1000 sensor
Diasonics
D. DRF ultrasound unit
D. Therasonic lithotriptor
D. transducer
D. ultrasound
D. ultrasound scanner
Diastat vascular access graft
diastolic fluttering aortic valve
Diatek 9000 Insta-Temp
Diatest
D. diabetes breath test
D. diabetes breath test kit
diathermal
d. needle
d. snare
diathermic
d. cystenterostome
d. forceps
d. precut needle
d. retinal electrode
d. snare
diathermy
d. cord
d. electrode
d. forceps
d. knife
d. scissors
d. tip
d. unit
d. wire
Diatube-H
dichroic filter system
dichromate dosimeter
Dickinson FACS 400-series flow cytometer
Dickson paraffin bath
Dicom acquisition station

Dicon
D. CT 200 corneal topographer
D. ocular blood-flow analyzer
DIC tracheostomy tube
die
pin-deburring d.
Dieckmann intraosseous needle
Dieffenbach
D. forceps
D. serrefine
dielectric track detector
Diener forceps
Dieter-House nipper
Diethrich
D. aortic clamp
D. bulldog clamp
D. coronary artery set
Diethrich-Hegemann scissors
Diethrich-Jackson femoral graft tunneler
Dieulafoy aspirator
Difco ESP testing system
Difei glasses
differential
d. pressure valve
d. scanning colorimeter
d. stethoscope
d. temperature sensor
d. variable reluctance transducer
diffractive multifocal lens
DiffSpin slide spinner
diffuser
Aroma-Stream d.
aromatherapy d.
cylindrical d.
Ultra Scent d.
Digene cervical sampler
digestive-respiratory fistula stent
digestive tube
Digi
D. Grip traction system
D. Sleeve stockinette dressing
Digibind pneumatonometer
Digiflator digital inflation device
Digi-Flex
D.-F. exercise system
D.-F. finger exerciser
D.-F. hand exerciser
Digikit finger tourniquet
Digilab
D. FTS 40A spectrometer
D. tonometer
Digimatic calipers
Digirad
D. gamma camera
D. 2020 TC imager
D. 2020tc imager
Digiscope
Direx D.
DigiScope camera

Digi-Sound hearing aid
digit
> d. cap
> d. splint
> d. tube
> d. wrap

digital
> d. acuity card
> d. Add-On Bucky image acquisition imaging system
> d. Add-On Bucky x-ray device
> d. amorphous silicon flat-panel detector
> d. autofluoroscope
> d. calipers
> D. Cardiac Imaging system
> D. Care kit
> d. chest imaging system
> d. dermoscopy analyzer
> 3Dx d. stereo disc camera
> d. edge-detection
> d. flat-panel amorphous silicon detector-radiography system
> d. fundus imager
> d. goniometer
> d. holography system
> d. imaging spectrophotometer (DIS)
> D. Inflection Rigidometer
> d. isotope calibrator
> d. mammographic system
> d. mammography system
> D. OsteoView
> d. selenium-based chest imaging system
> d. self-retaining retractor
> d. slide scanner
> D. slit-lamp imager
> D. Strobe
> D. Traumex system
> d. voltmeter
> d. x-ray detector

digital-to-analog converter
Digit-Grip device
digitized instrument
digitizer
> Amfit d.
> Bitpad d.
> Cyberware 3030 d.
> Cyberware 3030RGB d.
> 3-dimensional sonic d.
> GP-8 sonic d.
> infrared d.
> laser d.
> Metrecom d.
> optical d.
> Pixsys FlashPoint d.
> Polhemus 3D d.
> Polhemus 3Space d.
> Scanmaster D, DX x-ray film d.

digitizing pad
Digitrace home sleep system
DigiTrak Plus Holter monitor
Digitrapper
> D. Gold MK III solid-state data logger
> D. Mark II pH monitoring system
> D. MK III
> D. Mk III portable digital recorder
> D. Mk III reflux testing device
> D. Mk III sleep monitor
> D. portable pH recorder
> Synthetics dual-channel solid-state D.

Digitron
> D. digital subtraction imaging system
> D. Koordinat angiography equipment

Dignity
> D. easy access pant
> D. Plus Briefmates beltless undergarment
> D. Plus Briefmates Guard
> D. Plus Briefmates Pad
> D. Plus Briefmates stretch mesh pant
> D. Plus liner
> D. Plus regular pant
> D. Plus underpad

digoxigenin-labeled oligonucleotide probe
Dilamezinsert
> D. device
> D. dilator
> D. penile prosthesis
> D. urologic instrument

Dilapan hygroscopic cervical dilator
Dilapan-S hygroscopic cervical dilator
dilating
> d. bougie
> d. catheter-gastrostomy tube assembly
> d. forceps
> d. pressure balloon catheter
> d. probe

dilation, dilatation
> d. balloon catheter
> Wirsung d.

dilation-tracheobronchoscope
> Edens d.-t.

dilator
> achalasia d.
> Achiever balloon d.
> AirMax external nasal d.
> Ambler d.
> American Endoscopy d.
> Amplatz d.
> Amplatz fascial d.
> anal d.

Anthony quadrisected minigraft d.
aortic d.
Backhaus d.
Bakes d.
balloon d.
Barnes common duct d.
Béniqué d.
Berens d.
biliary duct balloon d.
bisected minigraft d.
2-bladed d.
bougie d.
Breathe with EEZ nasal d.
bronchial d.
Brown-McHardy pneumatic d.
bullet-tip d.
cannula with locking d.
cardiac valve d.
cardioesophageal junction d.
cardiospasm d.
Castroviejo double-end lacrimal d.
Castroviejo lacrimal d.
d. catheter
cervical d.
circular anal d.
Clark common duct d.
Clerf d.
Cook-Amplatz d.
Cooley d.
coronary d.
cortical incision coronary d.
Councill ureteral d.
Cunningham-Cotton sleeve
 coaxial d.
DeBakey vascular d.
Delaborde tracheal d.
Delaborde-Trousseau tracheal d.
Derra valve d.
Dilamezinsert d.
Dilapan hygroscopic cervical d.
Dilapan-S hygroscopic cervical d.
disposable cervical d.
Dotter d.
double-ended d.
duct d.
Einhorn esophageal d.
Eliminator PET biliary balloon d.
ERCP d.
esophageal balloon d.
esophagospasm d.
expandable cervical d.
fascial d.
Fenton uterine d.
Ferris filiform d.
fixed cervical d.
fluoroscopy-guided balloon d.
French-Hanks uterine d.
French lacrimal d.
frontal sinus d.

Galezowski lacrimal d.
gall duct d.
gallstone d.
Garrett d.
GlideCath d.
Goodell uterine d.
graduated Garrett d.
Grüntzig balloon d.
Heath punctum d.
Hegar rectal d.
Hegar uterine d.
Henley d.
Heyner d.
high-diameter d.
Hopkins d.
Hosford double-ended lacrimal d.
Hosford lacrimal d.
House lacrimal d.
Hurst mercury-filled d.
hydrophilic d.
hydrostatic d.
hygroscopic d.
Iglesias d.
implant site d.
incision d.
infant d.
iris d.
Jackson d.
Jackson esophageal d.
Jackson triangular brass d.
Jewett uterine d.
Johnston infant d.
Jones lacrimal canaliculus d.
Jones punctum d.
Jordan wire loop d.
Kahn uterine d.
Kearns bladder d.
Kelly orifice d.
Kelly sphincter d.
Kelly uterine d.
Keuch pupil d.
KeyMed advanced d.
Kron bile duct d.
Laborde tracheal d.
lacrimal canaliculus d.
laminaria cervical d.
laminaria seaweed obstetrical
 cervical d.
Landau d.
laryngeal d.
Laufe cervical d.
LeFort d.
Mahoney d.
Maloney-Hurst d.
Maloney mercury-filled
 esophageal d.
Maloney tapered-tip d.
mandrin d.
Marritt d.

dilator *(continued)*
McCrea d.
meatal d.
Meditech fascial d.
mercury-filled d.
mercury-weighted d.
metal olive d.
micrograft d.
Microvasive CRE esophageal d.
Microvasive Rigiflex balloon d.
minigraft d.
mitral valve d.
Morcher pupil d.
Mosher d.
Muldoon lacrimal d.
nasal d.
Nettleship canaliculus d.
Nettleship-Wilder d.
Nottingham One-Step tapered d.
Nottingham ureteral d.
Nozovent nasal valve d.
Olbert balloon d.
olive-tipped plastic d.
osmotic d.
Otis bougie à boule d.
over-the-endoscope Witzel d.
pediatric rectal d.
Perfect Pupil d.
Perry exchange d.
Pharmaseal disposable cervical d.
pneumatic balloon d.
pneumostatic d.
polyurethane d.
polyvinyl d.
Porges Neoflex d.
Pratt d.
Pratt uterine d.
d. probe
probe d.
punctal d.
punctum d.
pupil d.
pyloric stenosis d.
quadrisected graft d.
quadrisected minigraft d.
Quantum TTC balloon d.
Quantum TTC biliary balloon d.
Ramstedt pyloric stenosis d.
rectal d.
Rider-Moeller cardiac d.
Rigiflex achalasia d.
Rigiflex achalasia balloon d.
Rigiflex TTS balloon d.
rocket d.
Ruedemann lacrimal d.
Russell peel-away sheath d.
Savary d.
Savary esophageal d.

Savary-Gilliard d.
Savary-Gilliard esophageal d.
Savary-Gilliard over-the-wire d.
Savary tapered thermoplastic d.
Silent Nite external nasal d.
Simpson lacrimal d.
Simpson uterine d.
Sims uterine d.
sinus d.
Sisler punctum d.
Soehendra d.
Soehendra catheter d.
sphincter d.
stapes d.
Starck d.
Stucker bile duct d.
synthetic hygroscopic cervical d.
tapered-tip d.
Teflon d.
Teflon fascial d.
telescopic aerial d.
through-the-scope d.
tissue d.
tracheal d.
tracheoesophageal puncture d.
transventricular d.
Trousseau-Jackson esophageal d.
Trousseau-Jackson tracheal d.
Trousseau tracheal d.
TTS d.
Tubbs aortic d.
Tubbs mitral valve d.
Turner d.
ureteral stone d.
urethral female d.
urethral male d.
urethral meatus d.
UroForce ureteral balloon d.
uterine d.
vaginal d.
valve d.
Van Buren d.
vascular d.
vein d.
vessel d.
Wales rectal d.
Walther urethral d.
Wilder lacrimal d.
Williams lacrimal d.
Witzel pneumatic d.
Wylie uterine d.
Young pediatric rectal d.
Ziegler lacrimal d.
dilator-sheath system
Di-Main retractor
Dimension
D. hip prosthesis

D. RxL PSA Flex reagent
cartridge
2-dimensional (2D)
2-d. linear plating system
3-dimensional (3D)
3-d. biocompatible scaffold
3-d. grid electrode
3-d. magnetic sensor
3-d. plating system
3-d. sonic digitizer
3-d. SPECT phantom
3-d. videoendoscope
Dimension-C femoral stem prosthesis
Dimitry-Bell erysiphake
Dimitry-Thomas erysiphake
Dinamap
D. Accutorr A1, A3 blood
pressure monitor
D. automated blood pressure device
D. blood pressure cuff
D. blood pressure monitor
D. monitor/Oxytrak pulse oximeter
D. Plus monitor
D. Plus multiparameter monitor
D. Plus vital signs monitor
D. pulse oximeter
D. system
D. ultrasound blood pressure
manometer
Dine
D. Digital Macro camera
D. digital scanner
Dingman
D. bone and cartilage clamp
D. bone-holding forceps
D. breast dissector
D. cartilage clamp
D. dissector
D. mouthgag
D. mouthgag frame
D. mouthgag tongue depressor
blade
D. oral retraction system
D. osteotome
D. otoplasty cartilage abrader
D. wire passer
D. zygoma elevator
D. zygoma hook retractor
Dingman-Millard mouthgag
Dingman-Pollock septal displacer
Dingman-Senn retractor
dinner pad
diode
d. detector
d. endolaser
light-emitting d. (LED)
d. microlaser
d. pumped Nd:YAG laser

**diode-pumped solid-state
photocoagulation laser**
DioLite 532 laser system
Diomed
D. EVLT laser
D. laser
D. PDT laser
D. surgical diode laser
diopsimeter
diopter
d. lens
d. prism
dioptrometer, dioptometer
dioxide
carbon d. (CO_2)
diploscope
dipstick
Chemstrip d.
Chemstrip LN d.
Kelman d.
Knolle d.
Rapid One single drug screen d.
dipyridamole thallium-201 scan
direct
d. current generator
d. gonioscopic lens
d. laryngoscope
d. ophthalmoscope
D. Optical Research Company
(DORC)
d. percutaneous jejunostomy tube
d. retainer
d. vision spectroscope
direct-beam coupler for TURP
direct-current bone growth stimulator
DirectFlow arterial catheter
Directigen Flu A + B test kit
direct-impact prosthesis
directional
d. atherectomy catheter
d. atherectomy device
Directon resin
director
grooved d.
D. Guidewire system
Kocher goiter d.
Kocher grooved d.
Koenig grooved d.
Larry rectal d.
laser fiber d.
Leksell grooved d.
ligature d.
Payr grooved d.
plain-end grooved d.
probe-ended grooved d.
probe and groove d.
Quickert grooved d.
ultrasonic flow d.

D

DirectRay
    D. direct-to-digital image capture device
    D. direct-to-digital x-ray capture device
direct-reading bilirubinometer
DirectView CR 900 imaging system
direct-vision telescope
Direx
    D. Digiscope
    D. Thermex
    D. Tripter
    D. Tripter X-1 lithotriptor
DIS
    digital imaging spectrophotometer
Disa
    D. needle electrode
    D. urograph
disarticulation chisel
disc, disk
    Acroflex artificial d.
    artificial intervertebral d.
    Charité artificial d.
    concave skull d.
    d. curette
    Eigon d.
    d. electrode
    d. endoscope
    d. forceps
    Krupin eye d.
    d. lens intraocular lens
    Lillehei-Kaster pivoting d.
    Miller ocular d.
    Molnar d.
    Moore d.
    Moran-Karaya d.
    Morcher Asti d.
    d. oxygenator
    Placido d.
    Placido da Costa d.
    planoconvex-shaped d.
    plastic-covered hydrogel d.
    Private Practice vibration reminder d.
    d. rongeur
    stroboscopic d.
    synthetic intervertebral d.
    vacuum d.
    video d.
    Z d.
discectomy, diskectomy
    d. forceps
discharge tube
DisCide disinfecting towel
discission
    d. hook
    d. knife
Discofix stopcock
discogram needle

discographic needle
disconnect wedge
discoscope
    percutaneous d.
Disc-O-Sit Jr. cushion
Discovery
    D. bone densitometer
    D. DDDR pacemaker
    D. elbow system
    D. handheld spirometer
    D. II DDD pacing system
    D. II DR pacing system
    D. II SR pacing system
    D. II SSI pacing system
    D. LS imaging system
    D. LS, ST^4 PET/CT scanner
    D. SE ultracentrifuge
DisCoVisc ophthalmic viscosurgical device
Discrene breast form
discriminator
    EMI APED amplifier d.
    gamma camera d.
    2-point d.
disengagement mechanism
Disetronic
    D. Diaport pump
    D. Dihedi 25 insulin pump
    D. D-Tron insulin pump
dish
    insemination d.
    panning d.
    petri d.
    scoop d.
    side-fire reflecting d.
    Uri-Two petri d.
Dishler
    D. Excimer Laser System for LASIK
    D. irrigation cannula
Dishler-type LASIK irrigating cannula
disimpaction forceps
disinfectant
    Vespore d.
    Wavicide d.
disinfector
    DSD-91 endoscope d.
    Kestrel d.
disintegrator
    electrohydraulic d.
DisIntek reagent strip
disk (*var. of* disc)
Diskard head halter
Disk-Criminator
    D.-C. instrument
    D.-C. nerve stimulation measuring device
diskectomy (*var. of* discectomy)

Diskhaler
    Flutide D.
    D. inhaler
    D. metered-dose inhaler
Diskus inhaler
dislocator
    Kirby lens d.
dislodger
    Councill stone d.
    Davis loop stone d.
    Dormia ureteral stone d.
    Jimmy d.
    Johnson stone d.
    spiral stone d.
    stone d.
    Storz stone d.
    Tessier d.
    ureteral basket stone d.
    Zeiss ureteral stone d.
disparometer
    Sheedy d.
Dispatch
    D. balloon
    D. infusion catheter
    D. over-the-wire catheter
dispenser
    Baxa oral d.
    Exacta-Med oral d.
    Jet Vac cement d.
    optical d.
Dispenstirs
DisperDose
dispersing
    d. electrode
    d. lens
displacement sensing device
displacer
    air uterine d.
    Dingman-Pollock septal d.
display
    virtual reality head-mouthed d.
    virtual retinol d.
disposable
    d. acupuncture needle
    d. airway
    d. aspiration needle
    d. bikini
    d. biopsy needle
    d. bottle
    d. butterfly needle
    d. cannula tip
    d. catheter
    d. cautery
    d. cervical dilator
    d. coaxial Endostat
    d. curette
    d. cystotome cannula
    d. Doppler-constant thermocouple sensor

    d. electrode pad
    d. forceps
    d. head halter
    d. injection needle
    d. intraluminal stapler
    d. iris retractor
    d. Keratoplast tip
    d. laryngoscope
    d. measuring guide
    d. microclamp
    d. muscle biopsy clamp
    d. ocutome
    d. over-the-ear earphone
    d. PD-10 column
    d. percutaneous entry thinwall needle
    d. 1-piece osteotome
    d. probe
    d. pudendal nerve electrode
    d. ReFlex wand
    d. scalpel
    d. sculptured Endostat
    d. sheathed flexible sigmoidoscope
    d. Styrofoam block
    d. surfaces EMG electrode
    d. surgical electrode
    d. suturing needle
    d. thermometer
    d. trephine
    d. trocar
    d. TUR drape
    d. vacuum curette
    d. Yankauer aspirating tube
    d. Yankauer suction tube
disposable-sheath flexible gastroscope
Disposa-Derm skin punch
Dispo-sand device
Disposa-Shield dental barrier system
Disposatrode disposable electrode
disrupter
    ultrasonic cell d.
dissect
    Endo D.
dissecting
    d. chisel
    d. clamp
    d. forceps
    d. hook
    d. microscope
    d. probe
    d. scissors
    d. tip
dissection
    d. knife
    d. scissors
dissector
    Agris-Dingman submammary d.
    aneurysm neck d.
    Angell James d.

D

dissector *(continued)*
    angled d.
    aspirating d.
    ASSI breast d.
    ball d.
    balloon d.
    Barraquer corneal d.
    batwing d.
    Beaver d.
    Berens corneal d.
    Blumenthal d.
    Blumenthal conjunctiva d.
    blunt hook d.
    bunion d.
    Castroviejo corneal d.
    Chajchir d.
    channel d.
    Cheyne d.
    corneal knife d.
    Cottle d.
    cottonoid d.
    Creed d.
    Crile gasserian ganglion knife
      and d.
    Davis dura d.
    Desmarres corneal d.
    Desmarres lamellar d.
    Dingman d.
    Dingman breast d.
    dolphin nose monopolar
      electrosurgical d.
    double-ended d.
    dura d.
    ear d.
    Emory EndoPlastic
      electrosurgical d.
    endarterectomy d.
    Endo-Assist cutting d.
    Endo Dissect d.
    endoscopic d.
    facial nerve d.
    Fisher tonsillar d.
    flap knife d.
    Freer d.
    Freer dural d.
    Freer-Sachs d.
    golf-stick d.
    Gorney d.
    Green corneal d.
    Hajek-Ballenger d.
    Hajek-Ballenger septal d.
    hand d.
    Hardy pituitary d.
    Harris d.
    Hartmann tonsillar d.
    hockey-stick d.
    Holinger d.
    Hood d.
    House d.

    Hurd d.
    hydrostatic d.
    Jackson-Pratt d.
    Jimmy d.
    joker d.
    Judet d.
    Killian d.
    King-Hurd tonsillar d.
    Kittner blunt d.
    Kleinert-Kutz d.
    knife d.
    d. knife
    Kocher goiter d.
    Kocher periosteal d.
    Kurze d.
    laminar d.
    Lane d.
    Lang d.
    laryngeal d.
    LASEK bow d.
    Lemmon intimal d.
    Lewin bunion d.
    Lewin sesamoidectomy d.
    Logan d.
    Lothrop d.
    Luetje stimulating d.
    Luikart d.
    Lynch blunt d.
    Lynch laryngeal d.
    Lynch tonsillar d.
    MacAusland d.
    Macdonald d.
    Madden d.
    Malis d.
    Manhattan Eye & Ear corneal d.
    Marino rotatable transsphenoidal
      round d.
    Marino rotatable transsphenoidal
      spatula d.
    Martinez d.
    Martinez double-ended corneal d.
    Maryland d.
    Maryland monopolar
      electrosurgical d.
    Mason tonsil suction d.
    McCabe facial nerve d.
    McCabe flap knife d.
    McDonald d.
    McDonald stone d.
    Meeker monopolar electrosurgical d.
    microsurgical d.
    Mixter d.
    Montgomery d.
    Morrison-Hurd tonsillar d.
    nasal d.
    needle d.
    neural d.
    peanut d.
    Penfield 4 d.

plasma d.
pleural d.
Polaris reusable d.
prostatic d.
Ramirez EndoFacelift d.
Ramirez EndoForehead A/M d.
Ramirez EndoForehead curved d.
Ramirez EndoForehead flap d.
Ramirez EndoForehead straight d.
Ramirez EndoForehead T d.
Rosebud d.
rotatable transsphenoidal round d.
rotatable transsphenoidal spatula d.
round d.
SAPHfinder surgical balloon d.
SAPHtrak balloon d.
septal d.
sesamoidectomy d.
Spacemaker balloon d.
Spacemaker hernia balloon d.
Spacemaker II surgical balloon d.
Spacemaker surgical balloon d.
spatula d.
sponge d.
square-tipped arterial d.
Stallard d.
straight monopolar electrosurgical d.
submammary d.
submucous d.
suction tonsillar d.
synovial d.
teardrop d.
tissue plane d.
Toennis d.
Toennis-Adson d.
Toledo d.
tonsillar d.
Touma d.
transsphenoidal d.
Troutman nonincisional lamellar d.
ultrasonic d.
ultrasonic aspirator and d.
umbrella d.
vascular d.
Wagner epiretinal membrane d.
Walker suction tonsillar d.
Wangensteen d.
West blunt d.
West hand d.
Yasargil d.
Young urological d.
Dissectron ultrasonic neurosurgical aspirator console
Dissolve-A-Way tape
Distaflo bypass graft
distal
d. catheter
d. end cutter
d. femoral cutting guide

d. locking screw
d. over-shoulder strap
d. radioulnar joint prosthesis
d. shocking coil
d. star pad
d. stimulation generator
d. targeting device
d. thigh band
distending obturator
Disten-U-Flo fluid system
distometer
Haag-Streit d.
distraction
d. bar
d. clamp
d. device
d. hook
d. instrumentation
d. pin
d. rod
d. screw
distractor
Ace OsteoGenic d.
Acufex ankle d.
Anderson d.
bidirectional telescopic d.
Bliskunov implantable femoral d.
Caspar d.
DeBastiani d.
femoral d.
femur d.
hip d.
hook d.
Ilizarov d.
intramedullary skeletal kinetic d.
Kaneda d.
Kessler metacarpal d.
Mark II distal femur d.
McCarthy hip d.
Molina mandibular d.
Monticelli-Spinelli d.
multidirectional d.
multiplanar mandibular d.
Orthofix M-100 d.
Pinto d.
plate-guided d.
Track Plus d.
turnbuckle d.
Wagner d.
distribution
vascular volume of d. (VVD)
distribution transformer
Dittel sound
Dittrich plug
Diva
D. laparoscopic morcellator
D. laparoscopic morcellator device
divergent outlet forceps
diverging collimator

D

diversion stent
diver's spectacles
diverticulectomy
Harrington esophageal d.
diverticuloscope
soft d.
divided spectacles
Dixon-Lovelace hemostatic forceps
Dixon-Thomas-Smith intestinal clamp
Dixon-Thorpe vitreous foreign body forceps
Dk IOL insertion forceps
DL
double-lumen
QuickFurl DL
DL2000 data management system
D-L internal fixator
DLP
DLP aortic root cannula
DLP cardiac sling
DLP cardioplegic catheter
DLP cardioplegic needle
DLP infant ventricular catheter
DLP left atrial pressure monitoring catheter
DLP pericardial sump
DM-400 Holter ECG cassette recorder
DME
durable medical equipment
DMI analyzer
DMP wire twister
DNA
deoxyribonucleic acid
DNA labeling kit
DNA microarray chip
DNA polymerase assay kit
DNA sequencing system
DNA template
DNA-coated stent
DNA-Prep workstation & reagent system
DNAzole cell suspension
DNAzol kit
Doane knee retractor
Dobbhoff
D. biliary stent
D. bipolar coagulation probe
D. enteral feeding bag
D. feeding tube
D. gastrectomy feeding tube
D. gastric decompression tube
D. nasogastric feeding tube
D. PEG tube
DOBI system
DOC
dynamic orthotic cranioplasty
DOC Band
Doc
D. cervical dynamic rod

D. cervical plate
D. ventral cervical stabilization system
docking needle
Docustar fundus camera
Dodd perforator
Dodick
D. laser photolysis system
D. lens-holding forceps
D. nucleus cracker
D. nucleus irrigating chopper
D. photolysis probe
D. photolysis system
Dodick-Kammann bimanual chopper
Dogbone
D. ACFS
D. anterior cervical plate fixation system
dog chain retractor
dog-leg catheter
Doherty
D. sphere
D. sphere implant
Dohlman
D. esophagoscope
D. keratoprosthesis
Dohn-Carton brain retractor
DoLi S extracorporeal shock wave lithotriptor
dolorimeter
Chatillon d.
dolphin
d. dissecting forceps
d. grasping forceps
D. hysteroscopic fluid management system
D. instrument
d. nose monopolar electrosurgical dissector
dolphin-billed grasping forceps
dolphin-type atraumatic forceps
dome
d. colpostat
d. cylinder
d. hole plug
d. plunger
Dome-Paste boot
Dome Port catheter
dome-shaped internal bumper
domino spinal instrumentation connector
Donaghy angled suture needle holder
Donaldson
D. eye patch
D. fundus camera
D. stereoviewer
D. tube
DonJoy
D. ALP brace
D. Boa Duel TLSO

D. brace
D. Drytex Wraparound Playmaker knee brace
D. Female Fource custom knee brace
D. Female Fource OTS knee brace
D. GoldPoint knee brace
D. knee splint
D. Legend ACL knee brace
D. MaxTrax diabetic walker boot
D. Opal knee brace
D. 4-point Super Sport knee brace
D. Quadrant shoulder brace
D. Ultrasling shoulder immobilizer
D. Universal ankle brace
Donnez endometrial ablation device
donor button forceps
Dontrix gauge
doobie derm patch
Dooley nail
Dopcord recorder
Doppler
Acuson color D.
Aloka color D.
D. apparatus
ATL HDI 5000 color D.
D. 4-beam laser probe
D. blood flow detector
D. blood flow monitor
color D.
color-flow D.
D. color jet
continuous-wave D.
Convergent color D.
D. coronary catheter
2D D.
D. device
D. fetal heart monitor
FetalPulse Plus fetal D.
D. fetal stethoscope
D. flow echocardiographic probe
D. FloWire
D. flowmeter
D. flow probe
D. guidewire
Hadeco ES100VX mini D.
Hadeco intraoperative D.
Hadeco MiniDop D.
Imexdop CT D.
Imex Pocket-Dop OB D.
D. IntraDop
IntraDop intraoperative D.
intravascular D.
Laserflo laser D.
D. laser velocimeter
MD2 D.
MedaSonics transcranial D.
MedaSonics Versatone perioperative D.

Mizuho surgical D.
Multi Dopplex II D.
Neuroguard transcranial D.
Nicolet Elite obstetrical D.
penile D.
power D.
D. probe
pulsed D.
D. pulsed ultrasound
pulsed wave D.
pulse wave D.
D. QAD-1
D. Quantum color-flow system
D. scope
Siemens Quantum 2000 Color D.
Smartdop D.
SonoSite pulsed wave D.
spectral D.
transcranial D. (TCD)
D. ultrasonic blood flow detector
D. ultrasonic fetal heart monitor
D. ultrasonic flowmeter
D. ultrasonic probe
D. ultrasonography
D. ultrasound
D. ultrasound monitor
D. ultrasound stethoscope
D. velocimeter
D. velocimetry
D. velocity wire
Versatone perioperative D.
Doppler-Cavin monitor
Doppler System 97
Doppler-tipped angioplasty guidewire
Dopplette
Doptone
D. fetal monitor
D. fetal pulse detector
D. fetal stethoscope
Doran pattern stimulator ophthalmoscope
DORC
Direct Optical Research Company
DORC backflush instrument
DORC fast freeze cryosurgical system
DORC handle
DORC Hexon Illumination System
DORC illuminated diamond knife
DORC microforceps and microscissors
DORC subretinal instrument set
DORC vitreous shaver
Dorian rib stripper
Doriot handpiece
Dormia
D. biliary stone basket
D. gallstone basket
D. gallstone lithotriptor

Dormia *(continued)*
>D. noose
>D. stone basket
>D. stone basket catheter
>D. ureteral stone dislodger
>D. waterbath lithotriptor

Dornhoffer Hapex implant system

Dornier
>D. compact lithotriptor
>D. HM3, HM4 electrohydraulic lithotriptor
>D. HM-series lithotriptor
>D. Medilas H holmium:YAG endourology laser
>D. MPL 9000 electrohydraulic lithotriptor ultrasound focusing system
>D. MPL 9000 gallstone lithotriptor
>D. MPL 5000 lithotriptor
>D. scanner
>D. Urotract cystoscopy table

Dorros infusion and probing catheter

dorsal
>d. angled scissors
>d. columellar implant
>d. column stimulator
>d. column stimulator implant
>d. extension splint
>d. lumbar corset
>d. plate
>d. plate extender
>d. T-plate
>d. wrist splint
>d. wrist splint with outrigger

Dorsey
>D. bayonet forceps
>D. dural separator

dorsiflexion assist ankle joint ankle-foot orthosis

dorsi stop component

Dorsiwedge night splint

Dortu phlebectomy hook

dose calibrator

dose-rate/meter

dosimeter
>criticality locket d.
>dichromate d.
>Gardray d.
>LiF thermoluminescence d.
>neutron personnel d.
>quartz fiber d.
>Rosenthal-French nebulization d.
>silicon diode d.
>silicone diode d.
>single-channel in vivo light d.
>thermoluminescence d.
>thermoluminescent d.
>Victoreen d.

dosimetrist radiation beam monitor

Dos Santos lumbar aortography needle

Doss automatic percolator irrigator

Dostent

dot-plotted probe

Dotter
>D. caged-balloon catheter
>D. catheter
>D. coaxial catheter
>D. dilator
>D. intravascular retrieval set
>D. tube

Dott-Kilner mouthgag

Dott mouthgag

Doubilet sphincterotome

Double
>D. Duty cane
>D. Duty cane reacher
>D. Play large-bore double-Y hemostasis valve

double
>d. accessory channel therapeutic endoscope
>d. approximating clamp
>d. Becker ankle brace
>d. bent Hohmann acetabular retractor
>d. breast coil
>d. bridge
>d. clamp
>d. club elevator
>d. cobra retractor
>d. concave lens
>d. convex lens
>d. crank retractor
>d. drape
>d. fishhook retractor
>d. flexible-tipped wire guide
>d. irrigating/aspirating cannula
>d. keyhole loop wire
>d. right-angle suture
>d. safe-sided chisel
>d. setup endotracheal tube
>d. skin hook
>d. spatula
>d. tantalum clip
>d. tenaculum hook
>d. towel clamp
>d. velour knitted graft
>d. Zielke instrumentation

double-action
>d.-a. ankle joint
>d.-a. bone-cutting forceps
>d.-a. cutter
>d.-a. hump forceps
>d.-a. rongeur

double-angled
>d.-a. blade
>d.-a. blade plate
>d.-a. clamp

double-armed wire suture
double-balloon
    d.-b. applicator
    d.-b. device
    d.-b. triple-lumen catheter
double-band navel appliance
double-barreled
    d.-b. injector-aspirator
    d.-b. needle
double-bubble
    d.-b. flushing reservoir
    d.-b. isolette
    d.-b. ventriculoperitoneal shunt
double-cannula tracheostomy tube
double-catheterizing fin
double-channel
    d.-c. colonoscope
    d.-c. endoscope
    d.-c. irrigating bronchoscope
    d.-c. operating sheath
    d.-c. sphincterotome
    d.-c. videoendoscope
double-chip micromanometer catheter
double-concave rat-tooth forceps
double-cuff urinary sphincter
double-cupped forceps
double-current catheter
double-cutting sharp cystotome
double-detector Vertex system
double-disc ASD closure device
double-dome reservoir
double-edged sickle knife
double-ended
    d.-e. bone curette
    d.-e. breast retractor
    d.-e. curette
    d.-e. dental curette
    d.-e. dilator
    d.-e. dissector
    d.-e. instrument
    d.-e. nail
    d.-e. root tip dental pick
    d.-e. silver probe
    d.-e. stapes curette
    d.-e. suture forceps
double-fixation forceps
double-flanged valve sewing ring
double-focus tube
double-guarded chisel
double-headed stereotactic carrier
double-hollow nail
double-hook Tyrell skin hook
double-H plate
double-hub emulsifying needle
double-insulated incubator
double-J
    d.-J catheter
    d.-J indwelling catheter
    d.-J indwelling catheter stent

    d.-J silicone stent
    d.-J stent
    d.-J stent catheter
    d.-J ureteral catheter
    d.-J ureteral stent
double-looped cerclage wire
double-loop tourniquet
double-L spinal rod
double-lumen (DL)
    d.-l. balloon catheter
    d.-l. breast implant
    d.-l. Broviac catheter
    d.-l. catheter
    d.-l. central venous catheter
    d.-l. endobronchial tube
    d.-l. endoprosthesis
    d.-l. endotracheal tube
    d.-l. gastric laryngeal mask airway
    d.-l. Hickman-Broviac catheter
    d.-l. Hickman catheter
    d.-l. implant
    d.-l. injection catheter
    d.-l. irrigation cannula
    d.-l. needle
    d.-l. silastic catheter
    d.-l. subclavian catheter
    d.-l. suction irrigation tube
    d.-l. Swan-Ganz catheter
    d.-l. tapered-tip papillotome
double-occlusal splint
double-pigtail
    d.-p. endoprosthesis
    d.-p. prosthesis
    d.-p. stent
double-plane instrument
double-plate Molteno implant
double-power injector
double-pronged
    d.-p. Cottle hook
    d.-p. forceps
    d.-p. skin hook
double-ring frame
double-rod construct
double-running penetrating keratoplasty
    suture
double-sharp forceps
double-spoon biopsy forceps
double-spring ball valve
double-stem silicone lesser MP implant
DoubleStent
    D. biliary endoprosthesis
    D. biliary endoprosthesis stent
doublet
    Wollaston d.
double-thermistor coronary sinus
    catheter
double-thickness Sheen graft
double-tipped center-threading needle
double-tooth tenaculum

D

double-umbrella device
double-vector
 d.-v. blade
 d.-v. brain spatula
double-walled incubator
double-webbed needle
Doubra lens
douche
 Massengill d.
Douek-Med ear device
Dougherty
 D. anterior chamber cannula
 D. irrigator
doughnut
 GE Signa double d.
 d. headrest
 d. magnet
 d. pessary
 stapler d.
 d. support brace
 d. transformer
doughnut-shaped balloon
Doughty tongue plate
Douglas
 D. antral trocar
 D. bag
 D. cilia forceps
 D. graft
Douvas-Barraquer speculum
Douvas rotoextractor
Dover
 D. 100% silicone Foley catheter
 D. Teflon-coated latex Foley catheter
 D. Texas Catheter Disposable Male Catheter
dovetail stress broken abutment
Dow
 D. Corning cannula
 D. Corning external breast form
 D. Corning implant
 D. hollow-fiber analyzer
Dowd II prostatic balloon dilatation catheter
dowel
 bone d.
 calf bone d.
 d. cutter
 cylindrical d.
 graft d.
 Graftech cervical d.
 Graftech structural allograft cervical d.
 d. grip
 iliac crest d.
 Thompson d.
 threaded cortical d.

Down
 D. epiphysial knife
 D. flow generator
down-angled endoscope
down-angle hook
down-biting Epstein curette
down-curved rasp
down-cutting rongeur
Downes
 D. lid clamp
 D. nasal speculum
Downing cartilage knife
Downs arthroscope
downsized circular laminar hook
down-viewing endoscope
Doyen
 D. abdominal scissors
 D. bone mallet
 D. child abdominal retractor
 D. costal rasp
 D. cylindrical bur
 D. cylindrical drill
 D. dissecting scissors
 D. elevator
 D. intestinal clamp
 D. intestinal forceps
 D. myoma screw
 D. periosteal elevator
 D. raspatory
 D. rib elevator
 D. rib rasp
 D. rib spreader
 D. spherical bur
 D. tumor screw
 D. vaginal retractor
 D. vaginal speculum
Doyen-Ferguson scissors
Doyen-Jansen mouthgag
Doyle
 D. bivalved airway splint
 D. Combo nasal airway splint
 D. ear dressing
 D. II silicone stent
 D. Shark nasal splint
Dozier radiolucent Bennett retractor
DP
 dynamic pylon
  Springlite Advantage DP
DP-1 lithotriptor
DPAP
 DPAP interactive airway management system
 DPAP Stealth device
 DPAP Stealth positive airway pressure device
DPEG
 dual percutaneous endoscopic gastrostomy

DPS

    QuickFlow DPS

DPX

    D. Bravo bone densitometer
    ER-Tracker blue-white D.

DPX-IQ densitometer

Dr.

    Dr. Grip writing device
    Dr. Joseph's diabetic foot kit
    Dr. Joseph's Original Footbrush
    Dr. Scholl's exercise sandal

Draeger

    D. forceps
    D. modified keratome
    D. tonometer

Dräger

    D. MTC transducer
    D. respirometer
    D. thermal gel mattress
    D. ventilator
    D. volumeter

dragonhead needle

dragon shaver

drain

    antral d.
    Axiom d.
    Blake silicone d.
    butterfly d.
    butterfly intravenous tube d.
    Chaffin-Pratt d.
    Charnley suction d.
    cigarette d.
    closed suction d.
    Clot Stop d.
    combination cone/tube stoma
      irrigator d.
    controlled d.
    de Pezzer d.
    dual-sump silicone d.
    DuoDERM d.
    ERCP nasobiliary d.
    external ventricular d.
    extraventricular d.
    filtered dual-sump d.
    filtered mediastinal sump d.
    fishmouth d.
    fluted d.
    fluted J-Vac d.
    fluted silicone d.
    flute-end right-angle d.
    Foley straight d.
    Freyer suprapubic d.
    glove d.
    Gomco d.
    Guibor lacrimal d.
    Hemaduct wound d.
    Hemovac d.
    Hemovac Hydrocoat d.
    Heyer-Schulte wound d.

    high-capacity silicone d.
    Hollister irrigator d.
    intercostal d.
    Jackson-Pratt d.
    Jackson-Pratt Gold wound d.
    Jackson-Pratt Hemaduct d.
    Jackson-Pratt round PVC d.
    Jackson-Pratt silicone flat d.
    Jackson-Pratt silicone round d.
    Jackson-Pratt suction d.
    Jackson-Pratt T-tube d.
    J-Vac d.
    Keith d.
    Lahey d.
    large-volume round silicone d.
    latex d.
    lumbar d.
    Malecot 2-wing d.
    Malecot 4-wing d.
    Marion d.
    mediastinal d.
    mesonephric d.
    Mikulicz d.
    Mikulicz-Radecki d.
    nasobiliary d.
    nasocystic d.
    Nélaton rubber tube d.
    occlusive d.
    Oasis dry suction chest d.
    Ocean water-seal chest d.
    papilla d.
    pencil d.
    Penrose d.
    Penrose sump d.
    Pezzer d.
    Pharmaseal closed d.
    pigtail nephrostomy d.
    polyethylene d.
    polyvinyl d.
    PVC d.
    quarantine d.
    Redivac suction d.
    Redon d.
    rubber d.
    rubber dam d.
    Salem sump d.
    seton d.
    Shirley d.
    Shirley sump wound d.
    Shirley wound d.
    silastic closed-suction d.
    silicone hubless flat d.
    silicone round d.
    silicone sump d.
    silicone thoracic d.
    Snyder d.
    soft rubber d.
    Sof-Wick d.
    Sonnenberg sump d.

D

drain *(continued)*
    spaghetti d.
    stab-wound d.
    stoma irrigator d.
    Stryker d.
    subarachnoid d.
    subgaleal d.
    suction d.
    sump d.
    suprapubic suction d.
    surgical d.
    Surgilav d.
    Surgivac d.
    T d.
    Taut capillary d.
    The MMG Golden d.
    thoracic d.
    thyroid d.
    tissue d.
    TLS suction d.
    TLS surgical d.
    transnasal pancreaticobiliary d.
    transpapillary d.
    triple-lumen sump d.
    T-tube d.
    umbilical tape d.
    U-tube d.
    Vacutainer d.
    vacuum d.
    Van Sonnenberg sump d.
    Via silicone surgical wound d.
    Vigilon d.
    Wangensteen d.
    Waterman sump d.
    waterseal d.
    watertrap d.
    2-wing Malecot d.
    4-wing Malecot d.
    wound d.
    Wound-Evac d.
    Y d.
drainable fecal collector
drainage
    d. bag
    d. catheter
    Thora-Drain III chest d.
    underwater-seal d.
    waterseal d.
drain-to-wall suction connector
Drake
    D. aneurysm clip
    D. fenestrated clip
    D. tourniquet
    D. uroflowmeter
Drake-Kees clip
Drake-Willock
    D.-W. automatic delivery system
    D.-W. delivery system
    D.-W. dialysis machine

Drapanas mesocaval shunt
drape
    3M Vi-d.
    adhesive d.
    adhesive plastic d.
    Alcon disposable d.
    barrier d.
    barrier laparoscopy d.
    d. clamp
    Convertors surgical d.
    disposable TUR d.
    double d.
    eye d.
    Eye-Pak d.
    fenestrated sterile d.
    foot d.
    Hough d.
    Incise d.
    Ioban d.
    Ioban antimicrobial incise d.
    Ioban Steri-D.
    isolation d.
    Johnson & Johnson Band-Aid
      sterile d.
    LASIK eyelid d.
    Lingeman 3-in-1 procedure d.
    Lingeman TUR d.
    lint-free d.
    MB&J hip d.
    miniophthalmic d.
    3M small aperture Steri-Drape d.
    3M Steri-Drape d.
    NeuroDrape surgical d.
    O'Connor d.
    Opmi microscopic d.
    Opraflex incise d.
    OpSite d.
    paper d.
    plastic d.
    procedure d.
    sewn-in waterproof d.
    small-aperture Steri-Drape d.
    split d.
    Steri-Drape d.
    sterile d.
    surgical d.
    Surgikos disposable d.
    towel d.
    transparent d.
    Vi-Drape d.
    Visidrape d.
    Visiflex d.
draw-over vaporizer
draw-sheet
dream
    d. pillow
    D. Ride car seat
dreamer clamp
Dremel Moto-Tool

Dressflex
    D. orthotic device
    D. shoe orthotic
Dressinet netting bandage
dressing
    Ace longitudinal strips d.
    AcryDerm border island d.
    AcryDerm Strands absorbent
      wound d.
    Acticel wound d.
    Acticoat burn d.
    Acticoat composite d.
    Acticoat foam d.
    Acticoat silver-based burn d.
    Acticoat 7 wound d.
    Actisorb Silver 220 antimicrobial
      binding d.
    Acu-Derm TPN d.
    Adaptic d.
    Adaptic gauze d.
    Adaptic nonadhering d.
    adhesive absorbent d.
    adhesive-type d.
    Aeroplast d.
    air pressure d.
    Airstrip composite d.
    AlgiDerm alginate d.
    alginate wound d.
    AlgiSite alginate wound d.
    Algisorb wound d.
    Algosteril alginate d.
    Alldress composite d.
    Alldress multilayered wound d.
    Allevyn adhesive foam d.
    Allevyn adhesive hydrocellular d.
    Allevyn cavity foam d.
    Allevyn hydrophilic polyurethane d.
    Allevyn island d.
    Allevyn island foam d.
    Allevyn Thin d.
    Allevyn tracheostomy foam d.
    Allevyn wound d.
    Amerigel topical ointment
      hydrogel d.
    AmnioGraft wound d.
    antiseptic d.
    Aquacel AG wound d.
    Aquacel Hydrofiber d.
    Aquacel Hydrofiber wound d.
    Aquacel wound packing and d.
    Aquaflo hydrogel wound d.
    Aquaphor gauze d.
    Aquaplast d.
    Aquasorb hydrogel wound d.
    Aquasorb transparent hydrogel d.
    Arglaes antimicrobial barrier
      film d.
    Arglaes film d.
    Arglaes wound d.

    ArtAssist leg compression d.
    Arthrosol d.
    Avitene flour d.
    Bactigras d.
    Band-Aid brand surgical d.
    Band-Aid composite d.
    Bard absorption d.
    Bard AlgiDERM d.
    Barnes-Hind ophthalmic d.
    Barton d.
    BGC matrix hydrocolloid d.
    bias-cut stockinette d.
    bibulous d.
    Biobrane d.
    Biobrane glove d.
    Biobrane/HF d.
    Biobrane wound d.
    Bioclusive d.
    Bioclusive MVP Select
      transparent d.
    Bioclusive transparent d.
    Biocol d.
    BioCore collagen d.
    Biolex hydrogel d.
    Biolex impregnated d.
    bioocclusive d.
    Biopatch antimicrobial foam
      wound d.
    Blenderm tape d.
    BlisterFilm transparent wound d.
    bolus d.
    Borsch d.
    BreakAway absorptive wound d.
    Breast Vest Exi-Dry 1-piece
      wound d.
    bulky d.
    bulky compressive d.
    bulky hand d.
    bulky pressure d.
    Bunnell d.
    butterfly d.
    calcium alginate d.
    calcium sodium alginate wound d.
    Calgiswab d.
    CarboFlex odor-control d.
    CarraFilm transparent film d.
    CarraFilm wound d.
    CarraSmart foam d.
    CarraSorb H calcium alginate
      wound d.
    CarraSorb hydrogel d.
    CarraSorb M freeze-dried gel
      wound d.
    Carrasyn hydrogel wound d.
    Carrasyn V viscous hydrogel
      wound d.
    Castmate plaster bandage d.
    Catrix wound d.
    cellophane d.

D

dressing *(continued)*

Centurion SorbaView composite d.
Centurion SorbaView window d.
chest d.
Chick sterile d.
Chronicure wound d.
Chux incontinent d.
Cica-Care silicone gel sheet d.
Cica-Care wound d.
CircPlus leg compression d.
Circulon d.
Circulon leg compression d.
circumferential d.
ClearSite borderless d.
ClearSite hydrogauze d.
ClearSite hydrogel absorptive
 borderline wound d.
ClearSite wound d.
Clo-Sur PAD nonwoven hydrophilic
 wound d.
Coban d.
Coban elastic d.
cocoon d.
Coe-Pak periodontal d.
Coflex d.
cohesive d.
CollaCote collagen wound d.
collagen d.
CollaPlug absorbable collagen d.
CollaPlug wound d.
collar d.
CollaTape wound d.
collodion d.
CombiDERM ACD hydrocolloid d.
CombiDERM nonadhesive
 absorbent d.
Comfeel contour d.
Comfeel hydrocolloid d.
Comfeel Plus pressure relief d.
Comfeel Plus triangle d.
Comfeel Purilon d.
Comfeel Ulcus d.
Comfeel Ulcus occlusive d.
Compeed protective d.
Compeed skin protector d.
Complex Cu3 d.
composite d.
compound d.
compression d.
conductive hydrogel wound d.
Conform d.
Conformant wound d.
contact-layer wound d.
Contreet hydrocolloid nonadhesive
 foam d.
Contura medicated d.
CoolSorb absorbent cold transfer d.
corrective soft d.
cotton-ball d.

cotton bolster d.
cotton elastic d.
cotton-wadding d.
Covaderm composite wound d.
Covaderm Plus adhesive barrier d.
Covaderm Plus V.A.D. d.
Coverlet adhesive d.
Coverlet composite d.
Coverlet O.R. adhesive surgical d.
Coverlet Strips wound d.
Cover-Roll d.
Covertell composite secondary d.
CovRSite d.
Co-Wrap d.
Cranioplastic material d.
crepe bandage d.
Cryo/Cuff ankle d.
Cryo/Cuff compression d.
Curaderm hydrocolloid d.
Curad surgical adhesive d.
Curafil gel wound d.
Curafil hydrogel d.
Curafoam foam d.
Curafoam foam wound d.
Curafoam island d.
Curafoam wound d.
Curagel hydrogel d.
Curagel hydrogel island wound d.
Curasol hydrogel d.
Curasol sterile wound d.
Curasorb calcium alginate d.
Curasorb zinc alginate d.
Curity ABD absorptive d.
Curtinova hydrocolloid d.
Cutifilm Plus composite d.
Cutifilm Plus waterproof wound d.
Cutinova alginate d.
Cutinova cavity d.
Cutinova foam d.
Cutinova Hydro d.
Cutinova hydroactive d.
Cutinova thin d.
Cutinova thin hydrocolloid d.
Cutiplast sterile wound d.
Debrisan d.
demigauntlet d.
Dermacea alginate d.
DermaCol hydrocolloid wound d.
DermaFilm d.
Dermagran-B hydrophilic wound d.
Dermagran hydrogel d.
Dermagran hydrogel wound d.
Dermagran hydrophilic gauze d.
Dermagran ointment wound d.
Dermagran zinc-saline hydrogel
 wound d.
DermaMend cavity foam d.
DermaMend foam wound d.
DermaMend hydrogel d.

DermaMend island foam d.
Dermanet contact layer wound d.
DermaSite transparent film d.
Dermasorb hydrocolloid/alginate
  wound d.
DermAssist gel/gauze d.
DermAssist glycerin hydrogel d.
DermAssist hydrocolloid d.
DermAssist transparent site d.
Dermatell hydrocolloid d.
Dermicel d.
Dermophase d.
Diabeticorum d.
DiabGel hydrogel d.
Digi Sleeve stockinette d.
Doyle ear d.
Drilac surgical d.
dry and occlusive d.
dry pressure d.
dry sterile d.
dry textile d.
DuoDERM CGF gel d.
DuoDERM CGF hydrocolloid d.
DuoDERM hydrocolloid d.
DuoDERM SCB leg
  compression d.
Dyna-Flex compression d.
Dyna-Flex leg compression d.
Eakin cohesive seal d.
Elasto d.
Elasto-Gel hydrogel wound d.
Elastomull d.
Elastoplast d.
Elastoplast elastic d.
Elta Dermal hydrogel d.
Epigard d.
Epi-Lock d.
Episeal wound d.
Esmarch roll d.
Ete low-adherent d.
ethylene oxide d.
Expo eye d.
ExuDerm hydrocolloid d.
ExuDerm RCD hydrocolloid d.
Exu-Dry absorptive d.
Exu-Dry wound d.
eye pad d.
EZ-Derm porcine biosynthetic
  wound d.
Fabco gauze d.
felt d.
Ferris PolyMem wound d.
Fibracol collagen alginate d.
Fibracol collagen alginate wound d.
figure-of-8 d.
filiform d.
film wound d.
fine mesh d.
finger cot d.

fixed d.
Flex-Aid knuckle d.
Flexderm wound d.
Flexfilm wound d.
Flex Foam d.
FlexiGel gel sheet d.
Flexigrid d.
Flexinet d.
Flexzan Extra foam adhesive d.
Flexzan foam adhesive wound d.
Flexzan foam wound d.
Flexzan topical wound d.
fluff d.
fluffed gauze d.
fluffy compression d.
foam d.
foam wound d.
Foille d.
d. forceps
FortaDerm antimicrobial wound d.
Fuller rectal d.
Furacin gauze d.
FyBron d.
FyBron calcium alginate d.
Gamgee d.
gauze stent d.
Gauztex d.
Gelfilm d.
Geliperm gel d.
Gelocast Unna boot compression d.
Gelocast Unna boot leg
  compression d.
gel wound d.
Gentell alginate wound d.
Gentell foam wound d.
Gentell hydrogel d.
Gentell isotonic saline wet d.
Gibson d.
Glasscock ear d.
GraftCyte gauze wound d.
GraftCyte moist d.
GraftCyte moist wound d.
Griffin bandage lens d.
Gypsona plaster d.
hammock d.
Handages d.
Harrison interlocked mesh d.
Hexcel cast d.
hip spica d.
hourglass d.
hyCURE collagen hemostatic
  wound d.
Hydragran absorption d.
Hydrasorb foam wound d.
hydroactive d.
Hydrocol hydrocolloid d.
hydrocolloid d.
hydrocolloid occlusive d.
Hydrocol sacral wound d.

D

dressing *(continued)*

Hydrocol wound d.
HydroDerm transparent d.
hydrofiber d.
hydrogel d.
hydrogel wound d.
HydroMed wound d.
hydrophilic polyurethane foam d.
HyFil hydrogel d.
Hypergel hydrogel wound d.
Hyperion bordered hydrocolloid d.
Hyperion hydrophilic wound gel
  hydrogel d.
Hyperion thin hydrocolloid d.
Iamin gel wound d.
Iamin hydrating gel wound d.
Iamin hydrogel d.
impermeable d.
impregnated d.
Inerpan flexible burn d.
IntraSite d.
IntraSite gel wound d.
IntraSite hydrogel d.
Iodoflex absorptive d.
Iodosorb absorptive d.
island wound d.
Ivalon d.
jacket-type chest d.
jelly d.
Jelonet d.
Jobst mammary support d.
Jobst UlcerCare d.
Johnson & Johnson d.
Jones d.
Kalginate alginate d.
Kalginate calcium alginate
  wound d.
Kalostat d.
Kaltostat d.
Kaltostat alginate d.
Kaltostat Fortex d.
Kaltostat wound packing d.
Karaya d.
Kelikian foot d.
Kerlix MD antimicrobial gauze d.
Kerlix MD antimicrobial wound d.
Kirkland cement d.
Kling adhesive d.
Kling gauze d.
Kollagen d.
Larrey d.
Lipisorb d.
Lister d.
Lukens bone wax d.
Lyofoam A, C, T foam d.
Lyofoam Extra foam d.
mammary support d.
many-tailed d.
Martin rubber d.

mastoid d.
Maxorb alginate wound d.
mechanic's waste d.
Medical Resources hydrophilic
  wound d.
Medipore Dress-it d.
Medi-Rip d.
Mediskin porcine biological
  wound d.
Medline Derma-Gel d.
Melgisorb alginate d.
Mepiform self-adherent silicone d.
Mepilex border d.
Mepilex foam d.
Mepilex Lite d.
Mepilex transfer d.
Mepitel contact layer wound d.
Mepitel nonadherent silicone d.
Mepore absorptive d.
Mepore Pro d.
MeroGel nasal d.
Mersilene mesh d.
Mesalt sodium chloride-
  impregnated d.
Mestopore continent stoma d.
Micropore d.
Mills d.
Mitraflex Plus foam d.
Mitraflex Plus wound d.
Mitraflex SC foam d.
3M Microdon d.
modified Robert Jones d.
moistened fine mesh gauze d.
moist interactive d.
moisture-retentive d.
monocular d.
Montgomery strap d.
Mother Jones d.
moustache d.
MPM composite d.
MPM hydrogel d.
3M SoftCloth adhesive wound d.
3M Tegasorb hydrocolloid d.
Multidex maltodextrin wound d.
MultiPad absorptive d.
multitrauma d.
muslin d.
mustache d.
nasal-tip d.
NeoDerm d.
neoprene d.
nonadhering d.
nonadhesive d.
nonocclusive d.
Normlgel hydrogel d.
Normlgel protective wound d.
N-Terface d.
N-Terface contact layer wound d.
N-Terface nonadherent d.

Nu-Derm foam island d.
Nu-Derm hydrocolloid d.
Nu Gauze d.
Nu-Gel clear hydrogel wound d.
Nu-Gel hydrogel wound d.
NutraCol hydrocolloid wound d.
NutraDress zinc-saline d.
NutraFill hydrophilic d.
NutraGauze hydrophilic wound d.
NutraStat calcium alginate
  wound d.
Oasis wound d.
occlusive d.
occlusive collodion d.
occlusive semipermeable d.
odor-absorbent d.
Omiderm transparent adhesive
  film d.
Omniderm d.
open d.
OpSite d.
OpSite Flexifix transparent film d.
OpSite Flexigrid d.
OpSite occlusive d.
OpSite Plus composite d.
OpSite postop composite d.
OpSite semipermeable d.
OpSite wound d.
OrCel wound d.
OsmoCyte island wound care d.
OsmoCyte PCA pillow wound d.
OsmoCyte pillow wound d.
Owens gauze d.
Owens Surgical d.
Oxycel d.
oxyquinoline d.
PanoGauze d.
Panoplex hydrogel wound d.
paraffin d.
patch d.
PEG self-adhesive elastic d.
petrolatum gauze d.
Pillo Pro d.
pink d.
plaster pants d.
plaster of Paris d.
plastic d.
Polyderm foam d.
Polyderm foam wound d.
Polyderm hydrophilic polyurethane
  foam d.
PolyMem adhesive surgical
  wound d.
PolyMem alginate d.
PolyMem foam d.
PolyMem foam wound d.
PolyMem wound care d.
Polyskin II d.
polyurethane d.

PolyWic d.
postauricular ear d.
postnasal d.
pressure-applied d. (PAD)
pressure patch d.
Priessnitz d.
Primapore tape and gauze
  wound d.
primer leg compression d.
Pro-Clude transparent wound d.
ProCyte transparent d.
ProCyte transparent adhesive
  film d.
Profore 4-layer wound d.
Profore leg compression d.
Profore wound d.
Promogran matrix wound d.
propylene d.
protective d.
pulped muscle d.
PuraPly wound d.
PVD d.
Rapid Rhino gel knit nasal d.
Red Cross adhesive d.
Release non-adhering d.
RepliCare hydrocolloid d.
RepliCare Thin hydrocolloid d.
RepliCare wound d.
Reston d.
Reston foam d.
Reston foam wound d.
Restore alginate d.
Restore alginate wound d.
Restore CalciCare d.
Restore Cx wound care d.
Restore extra-thin d.
Restore hydrocolloid d.
Restore hydrogel d.
Restore Plus wound care d.
Rhino Rocket d.
ribbon gauze d.
Robert Jones bulky soft
  compressive d.
Royl-Derm hydrogel wound d.
Royl-Derm hydrogel wound
  nonadherent d.
Saf-Gel hydrogel d.
SaliCept freeze-dried d.
saline d.
saline-saturated wool d.
Scan spray d.
scarlet red gauze d.
d. scissors
scrotal d.
scultetus binder d.
SeaSorb alginate wound d.
semicompressive d.
semiocclusive moisture-retentive d.
semipermeable d.

dressing *(continued)*
semipermeable membrane d.
Septisol soap d.
Setopress d.
Shah aural d.
sheepskin d.
SignaDress sterile hydrocolloid d.
silastic foam d.
silastic gel d.
silicone d.
Silon wound d.
Siloskin d.
silver and cadexomer iodine-based
    wound d.
Sinu-Knit dissolvable nasal d.
SiteGuard transparent d.
Skin-Prep protective d.
SkinTegrity hydrogel d.
SkinTemp biosynthetic collagen d.
SkinTemp collagen skin d.
sling d.
Snugs tapeless d.
Sof-Foam d.
Sofra-Tulle d.
Sof-Rol d.
Sofsorb absorptive d.
SoftCloth absorptive d.
Sof-Wick d.
SoloSite hydrogel d.
Sorbex hydrocolloid wound d.
Sorbex thin hydrocolloid d.
Sorbsan alginate d.
spica d.
Spray Band d.
Spyrogel hydrogel wound d.
squares of d.
starch-based copolymer d.
stent d.
sterile adhesive bubble d.
sterile compression d.
sterile dry d.
sterile gauze d.
Steri-Pad d.
d. stick
Stimson d.
stockinette d.
StrataSorb composite wound d.
Stretch Net wound d.
subclavian Tegaderm d.
super-absorptive polymer d.
SuperSkin thin film d.
SurePress leg compression d.
surgical d.
Surgilast tubular elastic d.
Surgipad Combine d.
Suture-Self d.
Sween-A-Peel wound d.
4-tailed d.
tap water wet d.

Tegaderm d.
Tegaderm occlusive d.
Tegaderm semipermeable d.
Tegaderm semipermeable
    occlusive d.
Tegaderm transparent d.
Tegagel hydrogel d.
Tegagen HG, HI alginate
    wound d.
Tegasorb d.
Tegasorb occlusive d.
Tegasorb Thin hydrocolloid d.
Tegasorb ulcer d.
Telfa Clear nonadherent wound d.
Telfa composite d.
Telfa gauze d.
Telfa island d.
Telfamax absorptive d.
Telfa plastic film d.
Telfa Plus barrier island d.
Telfa Xtra barrier island d.
Tendersorb ABD absorptive d.
Tenderwrap leg compression d.
Tensor elastic d.
Thera-Boot compression d.
Thera-Boot leg compression d.
thin film d.
THINSite d.
THINSite topical wound d.
Tielle absorptive d.
Tielle Plus hydropolymer d.
tie-over d.
tie-over bolster d.
tie-over Sellotape d.
Tierney otoplasty d.
Toe-Aid d.
Transeal transparent wound d.
TransiGel woven gauze d.
Transorbent d.
Transorbent topical wound d.
Transorb wound d.
transparent adhesive film d.
transparent film d.
Transpore surgical tape d.
Triad hydrocolloid d.
Triad hydrophilic wound d.
triangular d.
tube d.
Tubex gauze d.
Tubigrip d.
tubular d.
tulle gras d.
twill d.
ulcer d.
Ultec hydrocolloid d.
Ultec Pro alginate hydrocolloid d.
Ultec thin d.
Ultex Thin extra-thin
    hydrocolloid d.

Ultrafera wound d.
Ultrex wound d.
Uniflex d.
universal d.
Unna boot d.
Unna-Flex leg compression d.
Unna-Flex Plus d.
Unna-Pak leg compression d.
upper body d.
VAC GranuFoam heel d.
vacuum-assisted closure d.
vapor-permeable d.
Vari/Moist wound d.
Vaseline gauze d.
Velcro fastener d.
Veni-Gard stabilization d.
Ventex d.
Ventex composite d.
Viasorb d.
Viasorb composite d.
Viasorb occlusive film d.
Viasorb wound d.
Victorian collar d.
Vi-Drape d.
VigiFOAM d.
Vigilon d.
Vigilon gel d.
Vigilon primary wound d.
Vigilon semipermeable
 nonocclusive d.
Vigilon synthetic occlusive d.
VitaCuff d.
water d.
water-impermeable nonsilicone-based
 occlusive d.
Water-Jel burn d.
Watson-Jones d.
Webril d.
Weck-cel d.
wet d.
wet-to-dry d.
wick d.
wound d.
Woun'Dres hydrogel d.
Woun'Dres natural collagen
 hydrogel wound d.
wraparound d.
Xeroflo d.
Xeroform d.
Xeroform gauze d.
Y-bandage d.
Zipzoc stocking leg compression d.
Zonas porous adhesive tape d.
dressing/wrap
ArtAssist compression d./w.
Drews
D. capsule polisher
D. cataract needle
D. cilia forceps

D. ciliary forceps
D. cystotome
D. forceps
D. lens
Drews-Knolle reverse irrigating vectis
Drew-Smythe catheter
Drews-Rosenbaum iris retractor
Dreyfus prosthesis forceps
DREZ electrode
drier
Savant Speed-Vac d.
Driessen hinged plate
Dri-flo underpad
Drilac surgical dressing
drill
ACL d.
Acra-Cut wire pass d.
Acufex d.
Aesculap d.
air d.
air-powered d.
Amsco Orthairtome d.
Anspach d.
Archimedean d.
ASIF twist d.
ASSI wire pass d.
automatic cranial d.
bar d.
d. bit
Björk rib d.
Black Max high-speed d.
bone hand d.
brace d.
bur d.
Calcitek d.
Canal Master d.
cannulated d.
cannulated cortical step d.
Caspar d.
Cebotome bone cement d.
centering d.
cervical d.
d. chamber
Championnière bone d.
Charnley starting d.
Coballoy twist d.
cobra-head d.
cranial d.
Crutchfield-Raney d.
CurvTek TSR bone d.
Cushing perforator d.
dental d.
diamond high-speed air d.
Doyen cylindrical d.
Elan d.
Elan-E power d.
electric d.
extractor nail d.
fingernail d.

D

265

drill *(continued)*
Fisch d.
flat d.
Gates-Glidden d.
glenoid d.
Gray bone d.
Grosse-Kempf bone d.
d. guard
d. guide
d. guide forceps
d. guide with drill bit
Hall air d.
Hall-Dundar d.
Hall Micro-Aire d.
Hall Neurairtome d.
Hall Orthairtome d.
Hall power d.
Hall Surgairtome II d.
Hall surgical d.
Hall Versipower d.
hand d.
high-speed d.
hip fraction compaction d.
Hudson bone d.
Hudson brace d.
Hudson cranial d.
initiator d.
intramedullary d.
Jacobs chuck d.
Jordan-Day d.
Kerr electrotorque d.
Kerr hand d.
Kirschner bone d.
Kirschner wire d.
Kodex d.
Küntscher d.
lentula spiral d.
lithoclast miniature pneumatic d.
Luck bone d.
Lusskin bone d.
Macewen d.
magnetic resonance
    imaging–compatible piezoelectric
    power d.
Magnuson twist d.
Mathews hand d.
Mathews load d.
McKenzie bone d.
McKenzie cranial d.
McKenzie perforating twist d.
MedNext high-speed d.
Micro-Aire d.
MicroMax speed d.
Midas Rex d.
mini-Stryker power d.
nail d.
Neurairtome d.
nipper nail d.
ophthalmic d.

Orthairtome II d.
orthopaedic Universal d.
Osteon d.
Oto-Flex d.
Patrick d.
pencil-tip d.
penetrating d.
Penn finger d.
perforating twist d.
perforator d.
pilot d.
d. point
power d.
powered automatic-stopping d.
pronator d.
Quick Connect twist d.
Rainbow d.
rib d.
right-angle d.
Romano curved surgical d.
scissors nail d.
Skeeter otologic d.
Sklar bone d.
skull traction d.
d. sleeve
Smedberg hand d.
Smedberg twist d.
Smith automatic perforated d.
spiral d.
Spirec d.
step d.
step-down d.
d. stop cylinder
Stryker d.
Suretac d.
Surgairtome air d.
Synthes d.
tap d.
Toti trephine d.
trephine d.
Trinkle bone d.
twist d.
Uniflex calibrated step d.
union broach retention d.
Universal 2-speed hand d.
wire d.
Xomed d.
Xpress 100 disposable perforator
    bur hole d.
Zimmer Cebotome bone cement d.
Zimmer-Hall d.
Zimmer hand d.
Zimmer Micro-E fixation d.
drill-tip catheter
drill-tipped guidewire
D-Ring
D.-R. strap
D.-R. wrist support strap
Drinker tank respirator

drip
    d. chamber
    Murphy d.
driver
    automatic needle d.
    Castroviejo needle d.
    Cook endoscopic curved needle d.
    D. coronary stent
    femoral head d.
    graft d.
    Hall d.
    hand-pushed tack d.
    Haney needle d.
    Harrington hook d.
    Jewett d.
    Ken d.
    Küntscher nail d.
    K-wire d.
    laparoscopic needle d.
    Laurus ND-260 needle d.
    Linvatec d.
    Lloyd nail d.
    long vascular needle d.
    McReynolds d.
    Micro Series wire d.
    needle d.
    Orthairtome wire d.
    orthodontic band d.
    Pereyra needle d.
    plate d.
    polyethylene-faced d.
    prostatic d.
    spring-loaded automatic tack d.
    surgical pin d.
    Szabo-Berci needle d.
    Teflon-coated d.
    TLC-II portable VAD d.
    trial d.
    UAM universal fixation d.
    wire d.
    Zimmer Orthair ream d.
driver-bender-extractor
    Rush d.-b.-e.
driver-extractor
    Sage d.-e.
    Schneider d.-e.
Dromos pacemaker
drop
    sole lift/heel d.
dropfoot
    d. brace
    d. redression stocking
    d. splint
dropper
drop-piece table
drug
    d. infusion pump
    d. infusion sleeve

drug-coated stent
drug-eluting stent
drug-loaded biodegradable polymer stent
DRUJ prosthesis
drum
    d. dermatome
    d. probe
    d. scraper
Drummond
    D. hook
    D. hook holder
drum-to-footplate total ossicular reconstruction prosthesis
drum-type dermatome
dry
    d. cup
    d. eye goggles
    D. Flotation wheelchair cushion
    d. heat sterilizer and incinerator unit
    d. and occlusive dressing
    d. powder inhaler
    d. pressure dressing
    d. sterile dressing
    d. sterile fluff
    d. sterile gauze
    d. textile dressing
    d. textile gauze
dryer
    L&R X-ray film d.
Drysdale nucleus manipulator
Drystar dry imager
Drytex
    D. RocketSoc ankle brace
    D. Wraparound Playmaker knee brace
Dry-Therm sterilizer
DryView laser imaging system
drywall sanding screen
DS-60 diode laser system
DS-9 needle
DSD-91 endoscope disinfector
D-shaped implant
DSI camera
DSIS orthotic
D-Soles
    D.-S. insole
    D.-S. orthotic
D-Stat
    D.-S. clamp accessory bandage
    D.-S. 2Dry bandage
    D.-S. dry bandage
    D.-S. flowable bandage
    D.-S. flowable hemostat
    D.-S. radial bandage
DSX
    DSX automated ELISA system
    DSX Sopha camera

D

D-Tach
    D-T. removable needle
    D-T. removal needle
2D TEE system Ultra-Neb 99
D-Tron insulin pump
DTU-215 cardiac digital stimulator
DTU-one UltraSure imaging system
DTX series multimode detector
Dua antireflux stent
dual (D)
    D. AFO Boot orthotic
    d. aspiration pump
    d. aspiration pump system
    d. balloon perfusion catheter
    d. bypass connector
    d. chamber
    d. coil transvenous lead
    d. color probe
    d. distal lighted laryngoscope
    d. eye shield
    d. lateral hand positioner
    d. lateral skull block
    d. leg immobilizer
    d. lookup table
    d. mechanism lens
    d. nerve root suction retractor
    d. oblique hand positioner
    d. octapolar lead
    d. percutaneous endoscopic
      gastrostomy (DPEG)
    d. percutaneous gastrostomy tube
    d. quadrapolar lead
    D. Quattrode spinal cord
      stimulation system
    D. Range Limiter System
    d. single-crystal gamma camera
    d. square-ended Harrington rod
dual-axis confocal microscope
dual-chamber
    d.-c. AV sequential pacemaker
    d.-c. ICD
    d.-c. Medtronic Kappa 400
      pacemaker
dual-compartment gel-inflatable
  mammary implant
dual-energy
    d.-e. linear accelerator
    d.-e. x-ray absorptiometry (DXA)
    d.-e. x-ray absorptiometry
      densitometer
Dualer Plus inclinometer
dual-head
    d.-h. coincidence camera
    d.-h. coincidence detection system
    d.-h. gamma camera
Dualine digital hearing instrument
Duall 88 cement
dual-lead electrode

dual-lock
    d.-l. ankle brace
    d.-l. total hip prosthesis
    d.-l. total hip replacement system
dual-lumen
    d.-l. catheter
    d.-l. papillotome
    d.-l. silicone hemodialysis/apheresis
      catheter
    d.-l. sump nasogastric tube
DualMesh
    D. hernia mesh
    D. material
    D. Plus biomaterial
dual-mode
    dual-sensing, dual-pacing, d.-m.
      (DDD)
Dualoop
dual-pass pacemaker
dual-photon
    d.-p. densitometer
    d.-p. electrospinal orthosis
Dual-Port system
dual-probe rectilinear scanner
dual-pulse lithotriptor
dual-sensing, dual-pacing, dual-mode
  (DDD)
dual-sensor micromanometric high-
  fidelity catheter
dual-sump silicone drain
dual-switch valve
Dualtherm dual-thermistor
  thermodilution catheter
Dubois decapitation scissors
Duchenne trocar
duckbill
    d. clamp
    d. elevator
    d. forceps
    d. rongeur
    d. speculum
    d. voice prosthesis
duck-billed anodized spatula
Ducker-Hayes nerve cuff
Ducor angiographic catheter
Ducor-Cordis pigtail catheter
Ducournau fine gripping forceps
duct
    d. dilator
    d. scoop
DuctOcclud coil
Duct-Occlud system
ductus clamp
Dudley-Smith rectal speculum
Duet
    D. coronary stent
    D. glucose control monitor
    D. system

Duett
    D. arterial closure device
    D. arterial puncture site closure
      device
    D. catheter
    D. closure device
    D. diagnostic device
    D. therapeutic device
    D. vascular sealing device
Duette double-lumen ERCP instrument
Duff debridement needle
Duffield cardiovascular scissors
Dujovny microsuction dissection set
Duke
    D. boot
    D. trocar
Duke-Elder lamp
Dulaney
    D. LASIK marker
    D. lens
Dulbecco phosphate buffered saline
dull
    d. pointed forceps
    d. retractor
    d. rotation forceps
dull-pronged retractor
dull-sided diamond blade
dull-tipped horizontal chopper
Dulox suture
Dumas pessary
Dumbach
    D. mandibular reconstruction system
    D. mini mesh
    D. regular mesh
    D. titanium mesh
dumbbell
    d. needle
    d. wagon
dummy
    d. source
    d. spacer
Dumon
    D. bronchoscope
    D. endobronchial silicone stent
    D. laser bronchoscope
    D. silicone stent
    D. tracheobronchial stent
Dumon-Gilliard endoprosthesis system
Dumon-Harrell bronchoscope
Dumont
    D. jeweler's forceps
    D. Swiss dissecting forceps
    D. tweezers
Dumontpallier pessary
Duncan loop
Dundas-Grant tube
Dunhill forceps
Dunlap cold compression wrap system
Dunlop elbow traction

Dunn fracture device
Dunning elevator
DUO
    TheraPress DUO
Duo-Care combined blood glucose and wrist blood pressure monitor
Duocentric prosthesis
Duo-Cline Dual Support contoured bed wedge
Duocondylar knee prosthesis
duodecapolar catheter
duodenoscope
    diagnostic d.
    endoscopic ultrasound d.
    Fujinon DUO-XT d.
    Fujinon ED series d.
    Fujinon ED7-XT d.
    Fujinon ED-200XU d.
    Fujinon ED-310XU d.
    Fujinon EVD-XT d.
    Fujinon FD series d.
    Fujinon FD-100XU d.
    JF-200 d.
    JF-IT20 d.
    JF-1T Olympus adult d.
    JF-V10 d.
    large-channel therapeutic d.
    Machida fiber d.
    Olympus EW series fiberoptic d.
    Olympus GIF series d.
    Olympus JF series video d.
    Olympus JF1T10 fiberoptic d.
    Olympus PJF series pediatric d.
    Olympus TJF-10, -100, -200 d.
    Olympus video d.
    Pentax d.
    side-viewing d.
    standard d.
    therapeutic side-viewing d.
    TJF-100, -130 large-channel d.
duodenovideoscope
    small-caliber d.
DuoDERM
    D. CGF gel dressing
    D. CGF hydrocolloid dressing
    D. drain
    D. hydrocolloid dressing
    D. SCB leg compression dressing
    D. SCB sustained compression
      bandage
Duo-Drive cortical screw
Duo-Flow catheter
Duo-Lock
    D.-L. curved tail closure
    D.-L. hip prosthesis
Duoloid impression system
Duostat rotating hemostatic valve
Duotrak blade
Duo-Tube feeding tube

D

Duovisc viscoelastic system
Dupel
    D. blue iontophoresis electrode
    D. drug delivery system
DuPen long-term epidural catheter
Duplay
    D. nasal speculum
    D. tenaculum forceps
Duplay-Lynch nasal speculum
Du Plessis muscle hook
duplex ultrasound
duplicator
    cardiac pulse d.
    Lang denture d.
DupliCone silicone dental impression material
DuPont
    D. Cronex x-ray film
    D. distal humeral plate
    D. distal humeral plate system
    D. scanner
Dupuy-Dutemps needle
Dupuy-Weiss tonsillar needle
dura
    d. dissector
    d. hook
    Tutoplast D.
    d. twist skin hook
durable medical equipment (DME)
DuraBoot orthosis
Duracast plaster bandage
Duracell Activair hearing aid battery
Duracep biopsy forceps
Duraclose scleral clip
Duracon
    D. knee implant
    D. prosthesis
    D. PS total knee system
Durafill dental restorative material
Dura-Flex back brace
Duraflo
    Bentley D. II
DuraGen absorbable dural graft matrix
DURAglide 3 stone balloon catheter
Dura-Guard dural repair patch
Durahesive skin barrier
Durahue acrylic
Dura-II
    D.-II concealable penile implant
    D.-II positionable penile prosthesis
Dura-Kold reusable compression ice wrap
dural
    d. elevator
    d. forceps
    d. graft matrix
    d. implant
    d. microclip
    d. needle

    d. protector
    d. scissors
    d. separator
    d. substitute
    d. suction retractor
Duralay acrylic
Duraleve custom molded foot orthotic
Dura-Liner acrylic
Durallium implant
Duraloc
    D. acetabular cup
    D. acetabular cup system
    D. Option ceramic hip system
    D. prosthesis
Duralon-UV nylon membrane
Duralyn balloon
Duramer polyethylene component
Duran annuloplasty ring
Dura-Neb
    D.-N. 2000 portable nebulizer
    D.-N. portable nebulizer pump
Durapatite
    D. bone replacement material
    D. implant
Duraphase inflatable penile prosthesis
DuraPlug synthetic extended temporary punctal/canalicular plug
Durapulse pacemaker
Durascope endoscope
DuraSeal sealant
Dur-A-Sil
    D.-A.-S. ear impression material
    D.-A.-S. silicone impression system
Durasoft
    D. 2 ColorBlends lens
    D. 2 contact lens
    D. 3 Optifit Toric Colorblends contact lens
    D. 2 Optifit Toric for light eyes contact lens
Dura-Soft soft compression reusable ice or heat wrap
Durasphere injectable bulking agent
Dura-Stick adhesive electrode
Durasul
    D. head system
    D. large diameter head system
    D. polyethylene
    D. polyethylene, high wear resistant acetabular insert
    D. prosthetic component
Dura-Temp specimen transporter
Durathane cardiac device
duration
    ventricular depolarization d. (VDD)
Dura-T lens
Duraval Hook & Loop strap material
Duredge knife
Duredge-Paufique knife

Durelon dental cement
Durette
    D. dental shield
    D. external laser shield
    D. system
Durham tracheostomy tube
Durkan CTS gauge
Duromedics
    D. bileaflet mitral valve
    D. mitral valve
    D. valve prosthesis
Duros leuprolide implant
Durrani dorsal vein complex ligation
  needle
DU Series 500, DU 800 UV/Vis
  spectrophotometer
Dutchman's roll
Dutch pessary
Duval
    D. disposable dermatome
    D. elevator
    D. intestinal forceps
    D. lung clamp
    D. lung grasping forceps
    D. lung tissue forceps
Duval-Allis forceps
Duval-Collin intestinal forceps
Duval-Coryllos rib shears
Duval-Vital intestinal forceps
DuVries needle
DVI
    DVI pacemaker
    DVI Simpson AtheroCath
    DVI Simpson AtheroCath catheter
Dwyer
    D. device
    D. instrument
    D. instrumentation
Dwyer-Hall plate
DXA
    dual-energy x-ray absorptiometry
    DXA densitometer
DxI 800 immunoassay system
Dycem roll matting
Dycor
    D. Geriatric ADL single-axis foot
      prosthesis
    D. prosthetic foot
dye
    d. cuvette
    d. laser
    d. terminator cycle sequencing core
      kit
    d. yellow laser
[166]**Dy generator**
Dymedix sleep sensor
Dymer excimer delivery system
DyNA block 1000 microtiter plate
Dynabond resin

Dyna-Care pressure pad system
Dynadisc
    Exertools D.
DYNAfabric material
Dynafill
    D. graft biomedium
    D. graft biomedium mineralized
      bone matrix
DynaFix external fixation system
Dyna-Flex
    D.-F. compression dressing
    D.-F. elastic bandage
    D.-F. Layer One padding
    D.-F. Layer Three bandage
    D.-F. Layer Two bandage
    D.-F. leg compression dressing
    D.-F. multilayer compression
      system
    D.-F. wrap
Dynaflex
    D. Gyro exerciser
    D. penile implant
    D. penile prosthesis
    D. prosthesis
Dynaflo bypass graft
DynaGraft
    D. bioimplant
    D. gel
    D. granule
    D. putty
Dynagrip blade handle
DynaHeat hot pack
DynaLator ultrasound unit
Dynal CELLection system
DynaLEAP balloon material
Dynalink biliary self-expanding stent
  system
Dyna-Lok plating system
dynamic
    d. axial fixator
    d. bed
    d. bridging plate
    d. compression plate
    d. compression plate instrumentation
    d. condenser electrometer
    d. condylar screw
    d. cooling device
    D. digit extensor tube
    D. Edge rehabilitation equipment
    d. elbow orthosis
    d. EMG-assisted biomechanical
      model
    d. external fixation
    D. foot stabilizer
    d. hinge elbow fracture brace
    d. hip screw
    d. integrated stabilization chair
    D. knee orthosis

D

dynamic *(continued)*
  D. Mesh craniomaxillofacial
    preangled connecting bar
  D. Motion Foot 1D35
  d. optical breast imaging system
  d. orthotic cranioplasty (DOC)
  d. orthotic cranioplasty band
  d. orthotic cranioplasty device
  d. penile prosthesis
  d. pylon (DP)
  d. reference arc
  d. spatial reconstructor scanner
  d. spiral CT lung densitometer
  d. splint
  d. stabilization trainer
  d. transverse traction device
  D. wrist orthosis
  d. Y-stent
Dynamite mattress system
dynamometer
  back-leg-chest d.
  Baseline d.
  bicycle d.
  Biodex isokinetic d.
  bulb d.
  Chiroslide Jamar hand d.
  Collins d.
  computerized isokinetic d.
  Cybex II isokinetic d.
  Cybex isokinetic d.
  electromechanical d.
  handheld d.
  Harpenden handgrip d.
  hydraulic hand d.
  Jamar d.
  Jamar hand d.
  Jamar hydraulic hand d.
  Lido isokinetic d.
  Lido Multi Joint II isokinetic d.
  orthopaedic d.
  Padgett hydraulic hand d.
  Smedley d.
  Spark handheld d.
  squeeze d.
DynaPak electrode kit
DynaPrene splinting thermoplastic
**DynaPulse 5000A ambulatory blood
  pressure monitor**
DynaRad
  D. portable imaging system
  D. portable x-ray system

Dynaslipper night shoe
Dynasplint
  D. knee extension
  D. knee extension unit
  D. shoulder system
DynaSport athletic tape
Dynasty
  D. balloon
  D. delivery system
DynaSurg
  D. electric handpiece
  D. I, II electric irrigation system
DynaTorq wrench
Dynatrak handpiece
Dynatron
  D. 50, 125, 525 electrotherapy
  D. Mini 2000 electrotherapy
  D. 2000 muscle test
  D. TX 900 electrotherapy
  D. ultrasound
DynaVox 2 communication device
DynaWell medical compression device
Dynesys dynamic stabilization system
Dynex Immulon 1B microtiter plate
DyoCam
  D. arthroscopic videocamera
  D. arthroscopic view camera
Dyonics
  D. arthroplasty bur
  D. arthroscopic blade
  D. arthroscopic instrument
  D. basket forceps
  D. Dyosite office arthroscopy
    system
  D. 25 fluid management system
  D. full-radius resector
  D. InteliJet fluid management
    system
  D. 25 pump
  D. suction punch
  D. syringe injector
Dyopneumatic insufflator
Dyovac suction punch
dysfunction
  extrathoracic airway d.
dysplastic valve
dysprosium-holmium in vivo generator

E

E Clips computer eyewear
E Clips prescription computer lens

E-2

E-2 foot prosthesis
E-2 hydrocollator heating unit

500e

e10 electrosurgery system

E-150 Breeze ventilator

E/200 contraangle 1:5 press-button chuck

EAC catheter

eagle

E. arthroscope
e. beak bone-cutting forceps
E. FlexPlug punctum plug
E. II survey spirometer
E. inflation device
E. portable ventilation system
E. rigid anterior cervical plate system
E. spirometer

EaglePlug tapered-shaft punctum plug

EagleVision Freeman punctum plug

Eakin cohesive seal dressing

ear

e. applicator
Bionic E.
e. bougie
e. cannula
e. clip
e. cup
e. curette
e. dissector
e. dressing forceps
e.'s education and retraining system
e. fenestrometer
e. forceps with suction
e. furuncle knife
e. grasping forceps
e. hook
e. knife handle
e. loupe
e. magnet
E. Muffin disposable over-the-ear earphone
e.'s, nose, throat (ENT)
e. oximeter
e. pinna prosthesis
e. piston prosthesis
e. polyp forceps
e. polyp snare
e. probe
e. punch forceps
e. rasp
e. scissors
e. snare wire
e. snare wire carrier
e. speculum
e. spoon
e. syringe

EarCheck

E. monitor
E. Pro instrument
E. Pro otitis media detector

earclip

early

E. Fit night splint
e. opening valve

earphone

disposable over-the-ear e.
Ear Muffin disposable over-the-ear e.
Eartone e.
intrameatal e.
over-the-ear e.

EarPlanes

E. children's earplug
E. flight ear protection
E. silicone earplug

earplug

AquaNot soft silicone custom-molded e.
Children's EarPlanes e.
EarPlanes children's e.
EarPlanes silicone e.
Insta-Putty silicone e.
Mack's e.
pliable e.

earring

Brent pressure e.
compression e.
Glori pressure e.
pressure e.
pressure-producing e.

Earscope otoscope

Eartone earphone

Ear-Tronics hearing aid

EAS-1000 anterior eye segment analysis system

Easebak lumbar support cushion

Easi-Breathe inhaler

EASI catheter

Easi-Lav gastric lavage

EasiVac evacuator

EasiVent

E. valved holding chamber
E. valved holding chamber mask

Eastman
> E. cystic duct forceps
> E. dental cement
> E. Kodak scanner
> E. vaginal retractor

Easton cock-up splint
East-West soft tissue retractor
EA surgical contraangle 10:1 press-button chuck
Easy
> E. Access foot splint
> E. Air 15 compressor
> E. Cap II CO_2 detector
> E. Dial Reg oxygen regulator
> E. Introduction system
> E. Lok ankle brace
> E. Neb compressor
> E. Pivot patient lift
> E. Rider neurovascular catheter
> E. Sleeve
> E. Up cushion
> E. Wallstent stent

EasyAnchor
> GII E.

EasyBand telemetrically adjustable gastric band
Easy-Breathe
Easycath
EasyChair massage chair
EasyGuide Neuro image-guided surgery system
Easyhaler
EasyLiner
> ALPS E.

Easyloupes
> Oculus E.

Easy-On elbow brace
EasyOne spirometry system
Easy-Pull sock aide device
Easyslide sliding mat
Easyspine pedicle screw and rod system
EasyStand 6000 glider
EasyStep pressure relief walker
Easytrak coronary venous lead
EBER1 riboprobe
Eber needle-holder forceps
EBI
> EBI Array spinal system
> EBI bone healing system
> EBI external fixator
> EBI Omega21 spinal fixation system
> EBI SpF-2 implantable bone stimulator
> EBI SpF-T implantable bone stimulator
> EBI XFix DynaFix system

EBT scanner

EC-5000 excimer laser
EC50 ToxCO breath carbon monoxide monitor
E.CAM dual-head emission imaging system
ecarin clotting time test card
ECAT
> ECAT III positron tomograph
> ECAT 951/33 PET scanner
> ECAT Reveal PET/CT imaging system

E-cath catheter
eccentric
> e. drill guide
> e. dynamic compression plate
> e. dynamic compression plating
> e. monocuspid disc valve
> e. monocuspid tilting disc prosthetic valve
> E. Y adjustable finger retractor

ecchymotic mask
Eccocee
> E. CS ultrasound system
> E. ultrasound
> E. ultrasound system

Eccovision
> E. acoustic pharyngometer
> E. acoustic reflection imaging system
> E. acoustic rhinometer
> E. acoustic rhinometry system

ECD
> external cardioverter-defibrillator
> Ventak ECD

ECG
> electrocardiogram
> Cardiovit AT-series ECG
> KoKo Rhythm PC-Based ECG
> Micro-Tracer portable ECG
> Miniscope MS-3 pocket ECG
> MSC-2001 ECG
> ECG triggering unit
> Welch Allyn/Schiller AT-1 3-channel ECG
> Welch Allyn/Schiller AT-2 full-size ECG
> Welch Allyn/Schiller AT-10 hospital grade ECG
> Welch Allyn/Schiller AT-10 hospital-grade ECG
> Welch Allyn/Schiller AT-2*plus* full-size ECG
> Welch Allyn/Schiller MS-3 pocket size ECG

ECG*stat*
> PalmVue E.

Echlin
> E. bone rongeur

E. duckbill rongeur
E. rongeur forceps
Echlin-Luer rongeur
echocardiograph
Acuson e.
Siemens Sonoline SL-2 e.
Ultramark 9 e.
echocardiographic
e. probe
e. scoring system
EchoCheck
Echocheck hearing screening device
Echo-Coat ultrasound biopsy needle
echocolonoscope
CF-UM3 e.
Olympus CF-UM3 flexible e.
echodense valve
echoduodenoscope
Olympus XJF-UM20 e.
echoendoscope
CLA e.
curved-array e.
curvilinear scanning e.
electronic radial-array e.
FG-36UA curved linear-array e.
FG-36UX scanning e.
GF-UM30P linear-oriented radial
scanning e.
large-channel video curvilinear e.
linear-array e.
linear array e.
linear-type e.
mechanical longitudinal/sector
scanning e.
oblique viewing e.
oblique-viewing e.
Olympus e.
Olympus CF-UM series e.
Olympus EUM-20 e.
Olympus GF series e.
Olympus GF-UC30P e.
Olympus GF-UCT30P linear-
array e.
Olympus GF-UM30P e.
Olympus GF-UM29 radial
scanner e.
Olympus GF-UM series e.
Olympus GIF20 e.
Olympus GIF-EUM2 e.
Olympus GIF series e.
Olympus GIF-1T10 e.
Olympus JF-UM20 e.
Olympus linear-array e.
Olympus UM-20 radial e.
Olympus UM series e.
Olympus VU-M2 e.
Olympus VU series e.
Olympus XIF series e.
Olympus XIF-UM3 e.

Pentax FG-36-UX linear-array e.
Pentax FG-36UX linear scanning e.
Pentax linear-array e.
radial sector scanning e.
EchoEye
E. 3D ultrasound imaging system
E. ultrasound
E. ultrasound imaging system
EchoFlow blood velocity meter system
echogastroscope
echogenic needle
echograph
Siemens Sonoline CD e.
EchoMark
E. angiographic catheter
E. catheter
E. salpingography catheter
echoprobe
Olympus XMP-U2 catheter e.
EchoScan
Nidek E.
echoscanner
Echosight
E. Jansen-Anderson intrauterine
catheter set
E. Patton coaxial catheter set
Echospeed
E. Signa LX scanner
E. 1.5T MR machine
Echotip
E. amniocentesis needle
E. Baker amniocentesis set
E. coaxial needle biopsy set
E. Kato-Asch needle set
E. Mennuti sampling needle set
E. Norfolk aspiration needle
E. percutaneous entry needle
E. Soft-Pass embryo transfer
catheter
EchoTip Ultra endoscopic needle
Echovar Doppler system
Echowarm gel warmer
ECI automatic reprocessor
Eckardt
E. ILM microforceps
E. temporary keratoprosthesis
E. vitrectomy system
Ecker-Kazanjian forceps
Eckhoff forceps
Eclipse
E. blood collection needle
E. Gel ankle brace
E. Gel elbow strap
E. holmium laser
E. infusion system
E. MR system
E. PTMR system
E. spinal system

E

Eclipse *(continued)*
    E. TENS unit
    E. TMR laser
ECMO
    extracorporeal membrane oxygenator
    ECMO pump
EcoCheck oxygen monitor
Econo
    E. 90 lumbar home traction
    E. 90 traction unit
Econo-Cerv
    E.-C. supine cervical traction
    E.-C. traction device
Econo-Float water flotation mattress
Econolith device
economy ROM brace
EconoSoc ankle brace
Econo-Strap
Eco-Oxymax
EcstaSeat seat cushion
ECT
    ECT bone screw
    ECT internal fracture fixation
    ECT internal fracture fixation
      system
    ECT test card
    ECT time test card
Ectocor pacemaker
Ectra carpal tunnel instrument
EDAP LT.01 lithotriptor
Edelstein scissors
edema sock
Edens dilation-tracheobronchoscope
EdenTec 2000W in-home
  cardiorespiratory monitor
EdenTrace sleep system
Eder
    E. cord blood collection device
    E. gastroscope
    E. insufflator
Eder-Bernstein gastroscope
Eder-Chamberlin gastroscope
Eder-Cohn endoscope
Eder-Hufford gastroscope
Eder-Puestow
    E.-P. guidewire
    E.-P. wire
Edge
    Acufex E.
    CeeOn E.
    E. coated blade
    E. coated needle electrode
    E. III hydrogel contact lens
    E. knee brace
EdgeAhead
    E. crescent knife
    E. microsurgical knife
    E. phaco slit knife

edge-detection
    digital e.-d.
EDG system
Edison fluoroscope
Edmark mitral valve
EDM infusion catheter
Edmonton extension tongs
Edna
    E. towel clamp
    E. towel forceps
Edridge-Green lamp
EDTA-anticoagulated Vacutainer
EDTA-Vacutainer tube
Edwards
    E. AVA high-flow device
    E. catheter
    E. clamp
    E. D-L modular fixator
    E. D-L modular screw rod
    E. heart valve
    E. hook
    E. instrumentation
    E. IntroFlex introducer
    E. LifeStent LP SDS biliary stent
      system
    E. LifeStent NT self-expanding
      biliary stent system
    E. LifeStent XL SDS biliary stent
      system
    E. MC^3 annuloplasty system
    E. MC^3 ring
    E. modular system
    E. modular system compression
      construct
    E. modular system kyphoreduction
      construct
    E. modular system neutralization
      construct
    E. modular system rod crosslink
    E. modular system rod-sleeve
      construct
    E. modular system sacral fixation
      device
    E. modular system scoliosis
      construct
    E. modular system standard sleeve
      construct
    E. outflow tract fabric
    E. sacral screw
    E. seamless heart valve
    E. seamless prosthesis
    E. Teflon intracardiac implant
    E. Thrombex PMT system
    E. Universal rod
Edwards-Barbaro T-shaped syringeal
  shunt
Edwards-Carpentier aortic valve brush
Edwards-Duromedics bileaflet heart
  valve

Edwards-Levine
    E.-L. hook
    E.-L. rod
    E.-L. sleeve
Edwards-Tapp arterial graft
Edwards-Verner rasp
EDXRF
    energy dispersive x-ray fluorescence
    EDXRF spectrometer
EEA
    EEA Auto Suture
    EEA Auto Suture stapler
    EEA disposable loading unit
    EEA stapler
    EEA stapling device
EEG
    electroencephalograph
    Equinox digital EEG
    Neurotrac II EEG
EF Cutter Ergo Toothing bur
Effapoxy resin
effective lithotriptor
Effler-Groves hook
efflux pump
effusion light pipe
Efos Lite curing system
Eftekhar long-stem prosthesis
E-G alloy
eggcrate
    e. foam
    e. mattress
Eggers bone plate
Eggsercizer
    E. CTS exerciser
    E. resistive hand exerciser
Egnell
    E. breast pump
    E. vacuum
egress cannula
EGTA device
EHL probe
Ehrhardt lid forceps
Ehrlich catheter
EIA kit
Eichen irrigating cannula
EID percutaneous central venous large-bore catheter
Eigon disc
eikonometer
Eindhoven magnet
Einhorn esophageal dilator
Einthoven string galvanometer
Eisenhammer speculum
Eitest MONO P-II test
EJ bone marrow biopsy needle
ejector
    Cloward dowel e.
    Johnson & Johnson saliva e.

EKG
    electrocardiogram (*See also* ECG)
    EKG calipers
Eklund breast positioning system
E/KM surgical contraangle 40:1 press-button chuck
Ekos ultrasound catheter
El
    El Bayadi-Kajiura lens
    El Gamal cardiac device
    El Gamal coronary bypass catheter
    El Gamal guiding catheter
EL2-LS2 flexible video laparoscope
EL2-TF410 laparoscope
eLabNotebook
ELAD
    extracorporeal liver assist device
    ELAD cartridge
Elan drill
Elan-E
    E.-E electronic motor system
    E.-E power drill
Elastafit tubing kit
Elastalloy
    E. esophageal endoprosthesis
    E. esophageal stent
    E. Ultraflex Strecker nitinol stent
ElastaTrac
    E. home lumbar traction system
    E. home lumbar traction unit
    E. lumbar traction
elastic
    e. back strap
    e. bandage
    e. bougie
    e. foam bandage
    e. knee cage
    e. knee cage with medial and lateral contoured knee joints
    e. knee sleeve brace
    maxillomandibular e.
    e. O ring
    e. plastic splint
    e. rubber band
    e. silicone membrane
    e. stable intramedullary nail
    e. stocking
    e. tubing
elastic-hinge knee brace
Elastikon
    E. bandage
    E. elastic tape
Elasto dressing
Elasto-Gel
    E.-G. hot/cold wrap
    E.-G. hydrogel sheet
    E.-G. hydrogel wound dressing
elastomer
    e. catheter

E

elastomer *(continued)*
    e. shell
    silicone e.
    e. skin molding
    thermoplastic e. (TPE)
elastomeric
    e. balloon
    e. pump
Elastomull
    E. dressing
    E. elastic gauze bandage
    E. splint
Elastoplast
    E. bandage
    E. dressing
    E. elastic dressing
    E. eye occlusor
Elastorc catheter guidewire
Elastylon glove
elbow
    e. extension splint
    e. flexion splint
    e. hinge
    E. Injury Management Kit
    e. magnet
    e. orthosis
    e. sleeve
elbowed
    e. bougie
    e. catheter
Elbowlift
    E. elbow protector
    E. suspension pad
Elbow-Up Protector elbow suspension device
elbow-wrist-hand orthosis (EWHO)
Elecath electrophysiologic stimulation catheter
Elecsys
    E. 1010 analyzer
    E. 1010 and 2010 immunoanalyzer
    E. 1010, 2010 immunoanalyzer
    E. 2010 modular immunoassay analyzer
    E. total PSA test
    E. troponin T immunoassay system
Electra
    E. 1400C, 1800C coagulation system
    E. 1000C coagulation analyzer
electric
    e. bed
    e. cabinet bath
    e. cardiac pacemaker
    e. dermatome
    e. drill
    e. generator
    e. laryngofissure saw
    e. nerve stimulator

    e. probe
    e. retinoscope
    e. suction device
    e. syringe
    e. tissue morcellator
    e. vacuum aspirator
    e. wheelchair
electrical
    e. air humidifier
    e. brain stimulator
    e. grounding pad
    e. implant
    e. resistance detector
    e. stimulation device
electrically detachable coil
Electricator electrosurgical unit
electricity-driven dermatome
Electri-Cool cold therapy system
electroacupuncture device
Electro-Acuscope
    E.-A. device
    E.-A. scope
    E.-A. stimulator
electroanatomical mapping system
Electro-Blend epilator
electrocardiogram (ECG, EKG)
electrocardiograph
    bioimpedance e.
    Cambridge e.
    Cardiomatic e.
    Marquette e.
    Mingograf 62 6-channel e.
    signal-averaged e.
electrocardiographic transtelephonic monitor
electrocardioscanner
    Compuscan Hittman computerized e.
electrocautery
    AmpErase e.
    Aspen e.
    bipolar e.
    Bovie e.
    Bugbee e.
    e. cautery
    Endo Clip monopolar e.
    Fine micropoint e.
    Fox bipolar e.
    Geiger e.
    Hildreth e.
    Mentor wet-field e.
    Mira e.
    monopolar e.
    Mueller e.
    needlepoint e.
    Neomed e.
    ophthalmic e.
    Op-Temp disposable e.
    Prince e.

Rommel e.
Scheie e.
Todd e.
Valilab e.
Valleylab e.
von Graefe e.
wet-field e.
Ziegler e.
electrochemical detector
electrocoagulating biopsy forceps
electrocoagulation biterminal device
electrocoagulator
electrode
abdominal patch e.
ACMI monopolar e.
All-In-One laparoscopic e.
angled ball-end e.
angle-tip e.
anterior anodal patch e.
anterior cheek e.
antimony monocrystalline e.
antimony pH e.
ArthroCare e.
Arzbaecher pill e.
Arzco Tapsul pill e.
Aspen laparoscopy e.
atrial e.
ball e.
e. balloon
Ball reusable e.
ball-tip coagulating e.
bayonet-tip e.
Berens e.
Berkovits-Castellanos hexapolar e.
bifilar needle e.
BiLAP bipolar needle e.
BioKnit garment e.
biopotential skin e.
biopsy loop e.
bipolar e.
bipolar depth e.
bipolar glass e.
bipolar myocardial e.
bipolar needle e.
bipolar stimulating e.
Bisping e.
biterminal e.
blade e.
Bovie conization e.
Bugbee e.
Bugbee fulgurating e.
Buie fulguration e.
Burian-Allen bipolar contact lens e.
Burian-Allen contact lens e.
button e.
calomel e.
CapSure e.
e. catheter
cautery e.

Cecar e.
central terminal e.
cerebellar e.
Clarion HiFocus e.
Clark oxygen e.
Clark-type polarographic e.
closed-loop system passing e.
C-Max cutting loop e.
coagulating e.
coagulation e.
Coaguloop resection e.
coaxial needle e.
coil e.
Collings e.
Colorado MicroNeedle needle e.
combination needle e.
common pH e.
CO_2mmO_2n sensor transcutaneous
gas e.
concentric needle e.
conical-tip e.
conization e.
Copeland fetal scalp e.
corneal contact lens e.
Cortac monitoring e.
cortical e.
coudé fulgurating e.
CPI Endotak transvenous e.
Cryomedics disposable LLETZ e.
Cueva cranial nerve e.
cuff e.
cuff-type inactive e.
cup-shaped e.
curved e.
cutaneous thoracic patch e.
cutting loop e.
Cyberonics vagus nerve
stimulator e.
cyclodiathermy e.
cystoscopic fulgurating e.
Darox cutaneous thoracic patch e.
depolarizing e.
depth e.
Depthalon monitoring e.
diamond e.
diathermic retinal e.
diathermy e.
3-dimensional grid e.
Disa needle e.
disc e.
dispersing e.
disposable pudendal nerve e.
disposable surfaces EMG e.
disposable surgical e.
Disposatrode disposable e.
DREZ e.
dual-lead e.
Dupel blue iontophoresis e.
Dura-Stick adhesive e.

E

electrode *(continued)*
Edge coated needle e.
Electro-Mesh e.
EMG e.
epicardial sock e.
epidural peg e.
Eppendorf needle e.
equipotential e.
ESA acromioplasty e.
ESA hook e.
ESA meniscectomy e.
esophageal pill e.
Excel Plus e.
exploring e.
external auditory meatus e.
external canthus e.
eye diathermy e.
E-Z Clean laparoscopic e.
Fast-Patch disposable
  defibrillation/electrocardiographic e.
fetal scalp e.
fine needle e.
fine wire e.
flat spatula e.
flat-tip e.
flat-wire eye e.
flexible fulgurating e.
flexible wire e.
follicle e.
foramen ovale e.
fulgurating e.
Galloway e.
glass pH e.
e. glove
Goetz bipolar e.
gold disc Grass e.
Grass e.
Greenwald Control Tip
  cystoscopic e.
Greenwald flexible endoscopic e.
grid e.
Heatwave e.
helical e.
HiFocus e.
Hurd bipolar diathermy e.
Iglesias e.
impedance e.
implantable pronged unipolar e.
implantable unipolar endocardial e.
impregnated e.
inactive e.
indifferent e.
intracerebral depth e.
intraluminal reference e.
intrameatal e.
intravascular catheter e.
Iomed Phoresor e.
ion-selective e.
iontophoresis e.

Jewett e.
J-loop e.
Josephson quadpolar mapping e.
J-shaped pacemaker e.
Kanpolat CT e.
Karaya e.
knife e.
Kontron e.
Kronfeld surface e.
lancet-shaped e.
Lane ureteral meatotomy e.
large-loop e.
large-tip e.
Laserdish e.
LeVeen radiofrequency ablation
  needle e.
Levin thermocouple cordotomy e.
Littmann ECG e.
LLETZ-LEEP active loop e.
lobotomy e.
localizing e.
loop e.
loop ball e.
loop-tipped e.
LSI silver self-adhesive
  disposable e.
Lynch e.
mandibular notch e.
Mansfield Polaris e.
McCarthy e.
McCarthy coagulation e.
McCarthy diathermic knife e.
McCarthy fulgurating e.
McCarthy loop operating e.
McCarthy miniature loop e.
meatotomy e.
Medelec DMG 50 Teflon-coated
  monopolar e.
Medi-Trace e.
Medtronic thin flexible antimony e.
MegaDyne arthroscopic hook e.
metal surface e.
microcurrent e.
Microglass pH e.
midgastric e.
midoccipital e.
miniature loop e.
monopolar e.
monopolar needle e.
monopolar stimulating e.
monopolar temporary e.
MRI-compatible e.
multilead e.
multiple point e.
multipurpose ball e.
myocardial e.
Myowire II cardiac e.
nasopharyngeal e.
needle e.

Neil-Moore e.
Neotrode II neonatal e.
neutral e.
Nucleus 24 Contour e.
ophthalmic cautery e.
optically transparent e.
Orion e.
pacemaker e.
pacing wire e.
pad e.
e. pad
parallel-loop e.
e. paste
peg e.
pencil-tip e.
percutaneous epidural e.
periaqueductal gray e.
Pisces e.
Pisces-Quad e.
platinum-iridium e.
platinum microwire e.
platinum oxygen e.
point e.
pointed tip c.
polarographic needle e.
Polystim e.
e. positioning system
Prizm Electro-Mesh Sock e.
punctate e.
Quad e.
QuadPolar e.
quadripolar Quad e.
Ray RRE-TM thermistor e.
recording e.
reference e.
reimplanted e.
REM PolyHesive II patient
  return e.
renal sympathetic nerve activity
  recording e.
Re-Ply TENS e.
Resume e.
reusable laparoscopic e.
right-angle e.
ring e.
rod e.
roller e.
rollerbar e.
roller-barrel e.
RollerLoop vaporizing loop e.
round-loop e.
round-wire e.
saturated calomel e.
scalp e.
scalpel e.
screw-in epicardial e.
screw-in sutureless myocardial e.
semiflat tip e.
semiinvasive e.

Severinghaus e.
sew-on e.
silver bead e.
silver-silver chloride e.
Silver-Thera stocking e.
single-fiber EMG e.
single-use e.
single-wire e.
small-loop e.
Smith e.
e. sock
Somatics monitoring e.
Spencer probe depth e.
sphenoidal e.
spiral e.
Sportstim muscle stimulation e.
stab e.
stab-in epicardial e.
steroid-eluting e.
stick-on e.
stimulating e.
St. Mark pudendal e.
Storz resectoscope e.
straight-blade e.
straight-needle e.
straight-point e.
straight-tip e.
straight-wire e.
subcutaneous patch e.
subdural grid e.
subdural strip e.
surface e.
surgical e.
Surgicraft Copeland fetal scalp e.
sutured plaque e.
sutureless pacemaker e.
temporal e.
temporary percutaneous SCS e.
Teq-Trode e.
terminal e.
thermistor e.
three-quarter circle c.
tined ventricular e.
tissue desiccation needle e.
tongue plate e.
tonsillar e.
Transvene tripolar e.
transvenous e.
trigeminal e.
tripolar defibrillation coil e.
tripolar nerve cuff e.
turbinate e.
Turner cystoscopic fulgurating e.
UltrAblator e.
ultrasonic e.
Ultra Stim silver e.
underwater e.
unipolar e.
unipolar defibrillation coil e.

electrode *(continued)*
  unipolar glass e.
  ureteral meatotomy e.
  Uroloop e.
  USCI Goetz bipolar e.
  USCI NBIH bipolar e.
  USCI pacing e.
  Valleylab ball e.
  Valleylab loop e.
  VaporTome resection e.
  VaporTrode roller e.
  Vitatron catheter e.
  V-Max roller bar e.
  Walker e.
  Wilson-Cook coagulation e.
  wire e.
  Wolfram needle e.
  Ziegler cautery e.
  zinc ball e.
electrodermatome
Electrodes
  E. ball
  E. loop
  E. needle
  E. scalpel
electrodetachable balloon
electro-detachable platinum coil
electrodiaphake
Electrodyne pacemaker
electroejaculator
  G&S e.
electroencephalogram
electroencephalograph (EEG)
  biofeedback e.
  BMSI 5000 e.
  Galileo evoked potential e.
  Grass e.
  Mingograf e.
  Nihon Kohden Neurofax e.
electroencephalography
electroencephaloscope
electrogalvanometer
electrogastrograph
Electro-Gel conductivity gel
electrogoniometer
  ankle-foot e.
  6 degrees of freedom e.
electrograph
  Cardiotest portable e.
electrogustometer
electrohemostasis catheter
electrohydraulic
  e. disintegrator
  e. generator
  e. lithotripsy probe
  e. lithotriptor
  e. lithotriptor probe
  e. probe

electrokeratotome
  Castroviejo e.
electrolarynx
  Bivona OptiVox E.
Electro-Link joint wrap
electroluminescent sensitometer
electromagnet
  spring-mounted e.
  structured coil e.
electromagnetic
  e. flowmeter
  e. flow probe
  e. flow transducer
  e. focusing field probe
  e. lithotriptor
electromechanical
  e. artificial heart
  e. dynamometer
  e. impactor
  e. morcellator
Electro-Mesh
  E.-M. electrode
  E.-M. sleeve
electrometer
  dynamic condenser e.
  vibrating-reed e.
electromucotome
electromyogram (EMG)
  kinesiological e.
  e. sensor
  ulnar nerve motor/sensory e.
electromyograph (EMG)
  Counterpoint e.
  Medelec MS91 e.
  Viking II EMG system e.
Electro-Myopulse muscle stimulator
electron
  e. beam CT scanner
  e. capture detector
  e. diffraction camera
  e. gun
  e. interferometer
  e. linear accelerator
  e. microscope
  e. multiplier tube
  e. probe x-ray microanalyzer
  e. valence
  e. volt
electronic
  e. amplified stethoscope
  e. artificial larynx
  e. barostat
  e. calipers
  e. goniometer
  E. HouseCall system
  e. infusion device
  e. knife
  e. microanalyzer
  e. muscle stimulator

e. pacemaker
e. patient care reporting system
e. PCR system
e. portal imaging device
e. radial-array echoendoscope
e. radial-array endoscope
e. scale
e. stethoscope
e. stimulator
e. thermometer
e. vitreous cutter
e. voltmeter

Electronics electrical stimulation device
electronystagmogram (ENG)
electronystagmograph (ENG)
Elmed-Toennis system e.
TAR-200 dual-channel e.
electrooculogram apparatus
electrooculograph
electroperimeter
ElectrophoresisTUTOR
electropneumatic endoscopic lithotriptor
electropolished stent
electroretinograph
Ganzfeld e.
electroscope
Electroscope disposable scissors
Electroshield monitoring system
electrostatic generator
electrosurgery
e. forceps
e. snare
electro-surgical
electrosurgical
e. biopsy forceps
e. blade
e. curved scissors
e. filter
e. generator
e. instrument
e. monopolar spatula probe
e. needle
e. pencil
e. scalpel
e. spatula
e. unit (ESU)
electrotherapy
Dynatron 50, 125, 525 e.
Dynatron Mini 2000 e.
Dynatron TX 900 e.
Mettler e.
e. system
ultrasound e.
electrothermal catheter
electrotome
McCarthy infant e.
McCarthy miniature e.
McCarthy punctate e.

Elekta
E. robotic surgical microscope
E. stereotactic head frame
E. viewing wand
Elema pacemaker
Elema-Schonander pacemaker
Elema-Siemens AB pressure transducer
element
3D hexahedral e.
8000-e. linear array CCD scanner
Mira encircling e.
4-e. phased array coil
resolution e.
truss e.
2-element phased-array coil
element-specific detector
elephant cuff
Eletrohome Marquee 8500 Ultra graphics projector
elevated
e. leg support
e. rim acetabular liner
elevating forceps
elevator
Adson periosteal e.
Alexander e.
amalgam plugger e.
angular e.
APC proximal femoral e.
Apexo e.
Aufricht e.
ball-end e.
Bennett bone e.
biceps e.
Blair cleft palate e.
blunt e.
Boies nasal fracture e.
bone e.
Boyle uterine e.
Buck periosteal e.
Cameron e.
Cameron-Haight e.
Campbell periosteal e.
Carmody-Batson e.
Chandler bone e.
Cheyne periosteal e.
chisel e.
cleft palate e.
clinic exolever e.
Cloward osteophyte e.
Cloward periosteal e.
Cobb periosteal e.
Cobb spinal e.
Cohen periosteal e.
combined wire guide bone e.
Converse-MacKenty e.
Converse periosteal e.
Cottle-MacKenty e.
Cottle periosteal e.

elevator *(continued)*
    Cottle septal e.
    Cottle skin e.
    Coupland e.
    Crane e.
    Crego e.
    Crego periosteal e.
    Cronin palate e.
    Cryer dental e.
    Cryer root e.
    Cushing Little Joker e.
    Cushing periosteal e.
    Davidson-Mathieu-Alexander periosteal e.
    Davidson-Sauerbruch-Doyen periosteal e.
    Davis periosteal e.
    Dawson-Yuhl-Key e.
    Dawson-Yuhl periosteal e.
    Dean periosteal e.
    dermal e.
    Desmarres lid e.
    Dingman zygoma e.
    double club e.
    Doyen e.
    Doyen periosteal e.
    Doyen rib e.
    duckbill e.
    Dunning e.
    dural e.
    Duval e.
    Ellik kidney stone e.
    Endotrac e.
    ESI lighted suction e.
    Farabeuf periosteal e.
    Farrior-Shambaugh e.
    femoral e.
    Fibre-Lite septal e.
    file e.
    Fiske periosteal e.
    Fomon nostril e.
    Fomon periosteal e.
    footplate e.
    fracture reducing e.
    Frazier e.
    Frazier dural e.
    Frazier suction e.
    Freer e.
    Freer double-end e.
    Freer periosteal e.
    Freer septal e.
    Freer septum e.
    Friedman e.
    Gillies zygoma e.
    Goldman septal e.
    Graham scalene e.
    Haberman suction e.
    Hajek e.
    Hajek-Ballenger septal e.

    Halle nasal e.
    Halle septal e.
    hand e.
    Heel Minder foot e.
    Herczel rib e.
    Hibbs chisel e.
    Hibbs costal e.
    Hibbs periosteal e.
    Hoen periosteal e.
    Horsley e.
    Hough spatula e.
    House ear e.
    House endaural e.
    House stapes e.
    Howarth e.
    Howorth e.
    Hu-Friedy e.
    Hurd septal e.
    Iowa University periosteal e.
    Jannetta duckbill e.
    Jarit periosteal e.
    joker e.
    Jordan canal e.
    Jordan-Rosen e.
    Joseph nasal e.
    Joseph periosteal e.
    J periosteal e.
    Kartush stimulus dissection e.
    Kennerdell-Maroon e.
    Key e.
    Key periosteal e.
    Killian septal e.
    Kilner e.
    Kleinert-Kutz e.
    Kocher e.
    Kocher periosteal e.
    Koenig e.
    Ladd e.
    Lambotte e.
    laminar e.
    Lane periosteal e.
    Lange bone e.
    Langenbeck periosteal e.
    Lee-Cohen septal e.
    Lemmon sternal e.
    lemon-squeezer obstetrical e.
    Lempert heavy e.
    Lempert narrow e.
    Lempert periosteal e.
    Lewin e.
    Lewis periosteal e.
    liberator e.
    Logan periosteal e.
    Love-Adson periosteal e.
    L-shaped e.
    lumbosacral fusion e.
    Macdonald periosteal e.
    MacKenty septal e.
    Malis e.

Matson-Alexander rib e.
Matson rib e.
McCollough e.
McGee canal e.
McGlamry e.
McIndoe e.
Mead periosteal e.
Miller dental e.
modified Darrach-type e.
Molt No. 4 e.
Molt periosteal e.
Moore bone e.
mucosal e.
e. muscle
narrow proximal femoral e.
Obwegeser periosteal e.
Ohl periosteal e.
orthopaedic e.
OSI extremity e.
osteophyte e.
Overholt periosteal e.
palatorrhaphy e.
Pennington septal e.
periosteal e.
e. periosteotome
Phemister e.
Pierce e.
Pollock-Dingman e.
posterior glenoid e.
Potts e.
Potts dental e.
Pritchard e.
Ramirez EndoFacelift e.
Ramirez EndoForehead parietal e.
Ramirez periosteal e.
Rhoton e.
rib e.
Ries suction e.
right-angle e.
Rochester lamina e.
Rochester spinal e.
Roger septal e.
Rolyan arm e.
Rosen e.
round-tipped periosteal e.
Sauerbruch rib e.
Sayre e.
Sayre double-end periosteal e.
Sebileau periosteal e.
Sédillot periosteal e.
Seldin e.
septal e.
sharp e.
Sisson fracture reducing e.
skin e.
skull e.
soft tissue e.
Somer uterine e.
spiked Darrach-type e.

stapes e.
staphylorrhaphy e.
straight inclined plane e.
straight periosteal e.
suction e.
Sunday staphylorrhaphy e.
Suraci zygoma hook e.
Swanson e.
Tenzel e.
Tessier e.
T-handle e.
Traquair periosteal e.
Tronzo e.
uterine e.
Veau e.
Wadia e.
Walker submucous e.
Ward periosteal e.
Warwick James e.
Wiberg periosteal e.
wide periosteal e.
Williger periosteal e.
Winter e.
Woodson e.
Woodson dental periosteal e.
Yankauer periosteal e.
Yasargil e.
zygoma e.

elevator-periosteotome
Elgiloy
    E. clip
    E. clip material
    E. metal alloy
Elgiloy-Heifitz aneurysm clip
Elias lid retractor
Eliasoph lid retractor
Eliminator
    E. ArthroWand
    E. balloon catheter
    E. biliary stent
    E. dilatation balloon
    E. nasobiliary catheter set
    E. pancreatic stent
    E. PET biliary balloon dilator
    E. stone extraction basket
ELISA Kit Alfa-gliatest
ELISA-Light Chemiluminescent Detection system
Elite
    E. dual-chamber rate-responsive pacemaker
    E. Farley retractor
    E. hip system
    E. knee brace
    E. Plus motion analyzer
    E. posterior adjustable stop
    E. posterior spring assist
    E. Power Station gym

Elite *(continued)*
    E. System rotating resectoscope
    VasoSeal E.
Ellik
    E. bladder evacuator
    E. kidney stone basket
    E. kidney stone elevator
Ellik-Shaw obturator
Elliot
    E. corneal trephine
    E. trephine handle
Elliott obstetrical forceps
Ellipse compact spacer
ellipsometer
    retinal e.
elliptical end-capped quadrature
  radiofrequency coil
Ellis
    E. astigmatism marker
    E. foreign body needle
    E. foreign body spud
    E. foreign body spud needle probe
    E. needle holder
Ellman
    E. pressform system
    E. Surgitron
Ellsner gastroscope
Elmed
    E. BC 50 M/M digital bipolar
      coagulator
    E. diagnostic laparoscope
    E. operating laparoscope
    E. peristaltic irrigation pump
Elmed-Toennis system
  electronystagmograph
Elmiskop 101 electron microscope
Elmslie triple arthrodesis
Elsberg brain-exploring cannula
Elschnig
    E. capsule forceps
    E. cataract knife
    E. corneal knife
    E. cyclodialysis spatula
    E. extrusion needle
    E. fixation forceps
    E. pterygium knife
    E. refractor
    E. retractor
    E. spoon
    E. trephine
Elschnig-O'Brien forceps
Elschnig-O'Connor fixation forceps
Elschnig-Weber loupe
Elscint
    E. Apex 409-AG ECT camera
    E. Apex 009 Precursor camera
    E. dual-detector cardiac camera
    E. dual-head helix camera
    E. Excel 905 scanner

    E. MR scanner
    E. Prestige MRI system
    E. Twin CT scanner
    E. ultrasound
Elset long stretch bandage
Elta
    E. dermal gel
    E. Dermal hydrogel dressing
    E. Dermal impregnated gauze
    E. Dermal wound cleanser
eluting stent
Elvarex
    E. compression garment
    E. support garment
Elwrite pediatric lead
Elypse control unit
EMA appliance
E-Mac laryngoscope blade
Embarc bone repair material
EmboGold microsphere
embolectomy
    e. catheter
    Fogarty arterial e.
embolization coil
embolus, pl. **emboli**
    polyurethane foam e.
Embol-X arterial cannula and filter
  system
Emboshield
    E. bare wire filter
    E. embolic protection system
Embosphere microsphere
Embrace heart stabilizer
Embryon
    E. GIFT catheter
    E. GIFT transfer catheter set
    E. HSG catheter
embryotome
Emcee lens
Emdogain gel
EMED
    EMED insole
    EMED scanner
EMED-SF
    EMED-SF pedobarograph
    EMED-SF sensor mat
Emerald
    E. diagnostic guidewire
    E. implantation system
Emerge biomaterial
E-Merge Contour Grid eruption
  appliance
Emergence Profile implant system
emergency
    e. infusion device
    e. life support system
Emerson
    E. cuirass respirator
    E. postoperative ventilator

E. pump
E. respirator
Emerson-Segal Medimizer demand nebulizer
Emery lens
Emesco dental drill and handpiece
emesis basin
EMG
electromyogram
electromyograph
EMG biofeedback system
EMG electrode
MyoTrac EMG
Neuropack 4, 8 EMG
Nomad-LE EMG
EMG retrainer biofeedback unit
EMG stimulator
EMI
EMI APED amplifier discriminator
EMI 9813B photomultiplier
EMI brain scanner
EMI CT 500 scanner
EMI digital imaging system
EMI 7070 scanner
EMI unit
emission spectrometric detector
emitter
alpha-particle e.
Auger-electron e.
gamma e.
light e.
positron e.
Emmet
E. needle
E. tenaculum hook
Emmet-Murphy needle
Emmett-Gellhorn pessary
Emory
E. EndoPlastic electrosurgical dissector
E. EndoPlastic retractor
Empac-Cavitron I&A unit
Empire needle
EMS
EMS Immobile-VAC pediatric universal mattress
EMS 2000 neuromuscular stimulator
emulsifier
Pulsatome cataract e.
emulsion
Biafine wound dressing e.
EnAbl thermal ablation system
ENAC ultrasonic instrument system
enamel rod
Encapsulon epidural catheter
encased screw
encephaloscope
en chemise catheter

encircling
e. band
e. clip
enclavation needle
Enclose
E. anastomosis assist device
E. II anastomosis assist device
E. proximal anastomotic assist device
enclosure
air-flow e.
Encode restorative system
Encore
E. ceramic hip and knee joint replacement systems
E. monthly disposable contact lens
E. Orthopedics device
Encor pacemaker
encrusted ureteral stent
endarterectomy
e. dissector
e. scissors
c. spatula
endaural
e. curette
e. retractor
e. speculum
end-biting
e.-b. blunt-nosed rongeur
e.-b. forceps
end-cutting
e.-c. fissure bur
e.-c. reamer
Endeavor
E. drug-eluting stent
E. nondetachable silicone balloon catheter
end-end stapler
Endermologie
E. adipose destruction system
F. LPG system
E. noninvasive body contouring device
Ender nail
Endex
E. apex locator
E. apex sensor
end-expiratory film
end-fire
e.-f. transducer
e.-f. transrectal probe
end-gripping forceps with standard jaw
end-hole
e.-h. balloon-tipped catheter
e.-h. catheter
e.-h. fluid-filled catheter
e.-h. introducer
e.-h. pigtail catheter

E

end-hole *(continued)*
 e.-h. Tracker microcatheter
 e.-h. ureteral catheter
end-inspiratory film
Endius
 E. bipolar sheath
 E. endoscopic access system
 E. spinal endoscope/camera
 E. TriFix thoracolumbar pedicle
 screw system
Endless Pool physical therapy pool
Endo
 E. Babcock grasper
 E. Babcock stapler
 E. Babcock surgical grasping
 device
 E. button
 E. Catch bag
 E. Catch II device
 E. Clip applier
 E. Clip monopolar electrocautery
 E. Close suture carrier
 E. Dissect
 E. Dissect dissector
 E. GIA 30, 60 stapler
 E. GIA stapler
 E. GIA stapling device
 E. GIA surgical clip
 E. GIA 30 suture stapler
 E. GIA suture stapler
 E. Grasp device
 E. Hernia stapler
 E. Irrigator pump
 E. Multi-Mode stimulator
 E. pants
 E. Retract retractor
 E. Shears
 E. sled prosthesis
 E. Stitch instrument
 E. Stitch laparoscopic suturing
 device
 E. stop
endoanal
 e. coil
 e. ultrasound
EndoAnchor
endoaortic clamp
Endo-Assist
 E.-A. cutting dissector
 E.-A. disposable atraumatic
 grasping forceps
 E.-A. disposable hemostat
 E.-A. disposable ligature carrier
 E.-A. disposable needle holder
 E.-A. endoscopic forceps
 E.-A. endoscopic knot pusher
 E.-A. endoscopic ligature carrier
 E.-A. endoscopic needle holder
 E.-A. retractable blade

 E.-A. retractable scalpel
 E.-A. reusable knot pusher
 E.-A. sponge aspirator
Endo-Avitene
 E.-A. collagen hemostatic material
 E.-A. microfibrillar collagen
 hemostat
Endo-Babcock stapler
Endobag
 E. laparoscopic specimen retrieval
 system
 E. specimen bag
Endo-Bender bending device
endobiliary stent
EndoBlade
 LaserSonics E.
endobrachial double-lumen tube
endobronchial
 e. stent
 e. tube
EndoButton
 E. CL BTB fixation system
 closed-loop E.
 E. FM
Endocam digital camera
endocamera
 Olympus e.
 Polaroid instant e.
endocapsular
 e. artificial lens intraocular lens
 e. balloon
 e. equator ring
endocardial
 e. bipolar pacemaker
 e. cardiac lead
 e. screw
 e. wire
endocardiographic amplifier
Endocare nitinol stent
endocavitary
 e. applicator system
 e. probe
Endocell
 E. endometrial cell collector
 E. endometrial cell sampler
endocervical
 e. aspirator
 e. biopsy curette
 e. probe
endochondral bone
EndoCinch suturing system
EndoClamp-ST II aortic catheter
endocoagulator
EndoCoil
 E. biliary stent
 E. esophageal stent
EndoCPB catheter
Endocut

endocutter
    Long45 e.
endodiathermy
Endodirect system
endodontic
    e. broach
    e. bur
    e. curette
    e. endosteal implant
    E. Meter SII
    e. plugger
    e. reamer
Endo-Dop transendoscopic Doppler catheter probe system
Endodynamics suction polyp trap
EndoENT probe
endoesophageal
    e. MRI coil
    e. stent
    e. tube
Endofix
    E. absorbable interference screw
    E. bioabsorbable interference screw
Endo-FixL screw
EndoFlex endotracheal tube
Endo-Flo
    E.-F. irrigation system
    E.-F. irrigator
EndoForehead cannula
Endo-Gauge
endograft
    AneuRx e.
    Prograft bifurcated e.
    Talent bifurcated e.
    Vanguard e.
Endo-Grasper
    Babcock E.-G.
endograsper
    roticulating e.
EndoGrip endotracheal tube holder
Endo-Gripper endodontic handpiece
endoilluminator
    Grieshaber e.
Endoknot suture
EndoLase C0$_2$ laser
endolaser
    diode e.
    e. probe
Endolav
    Meditron EL-100 E.
EndoLift device
Endolite transtibial system
EndoLive 3D stereo video endoscope
Endoloop
    E. chromic ligature suture instrument
    E. ligature
    E. suture

EndoLumina
    E. bougie
    E. II transillumination system
    E. illuminated bougie
endoluminal
    e. stent
    e. stent graft
endolymphatic shunt tube introducer
endolymphatic-subarachnoid shunt
EndoMate grab bag
EndoMax endoscopic instrumentation
endometrial
    e. ablator
    e. aspirator
    e. brush
    e. cannula
    e. curette
    e. polyp forceps
Endo-Model
    E.-M. hinged knee prosthesis
    E.-M. rotating knee joint prosthesis
    E.-M. sled prosthesis
endonerve stripper
EndoNet
    Pentax E.
EndoOctopus
endoootoprobe
    Horn e.
    Maloney e.
Endopap endometrial sampler
Endopath
    E. bladeless trocar
    E. dilating tip trocar
    E. EMS hernia stapler
    E. endoscopic articulating stapler
    E. ETS-Flex endoscopic articulating linear cutter
    E. EZ35 endoscopic linear cutter
    E. needle-tip electrosurgery probe
    E. Optiview laparoscopic obturator
    E. Optiview optical surgical obturator
    E. Pneumoneedle insufflation needle
    E. 30, 60 stapler
    E. TriStar trocar
    E. Ultra Veress needle
    E. Xcel bladeless trocar
    E. Xcel blunt-tip trocar
EndoPearl
    E. bioabsorbable device
    E. fixation device
EndoPlastic retractor
Endopledge sinus catheter
Endo-Pool suction cannula
Endopore
    E. dental implant system
    E. implant
Endo-Port

E

Endopost
  Kerr E.
Endopouch
  E. Pro specimen-retrieval bag
  E. retriever
Endo-P-Probe
endoprobe
  rotating e.
  single-crystal e.
endoprosthesis
  acetabular e.
  biliary e.
  Bio-Moore e.
  Carey-Coons soft stent biliary e.
  Celestin e.
  constrained Wallgraft e.
  Coons/Carey e.
  crutched stick-type polyurethane e.
  cuffed esophageal e.
  double-lumen e.
  double-pigtail e.
  DoubleStent biliary e.
  Elastalloy esophageal e.
  endoscopic biliary e.
  expandable biliary e.
  expandable metal mesh e.
  femoral e.
  Gore Tag thoracic e.
  Gore Viabil biliary e.
  Hemobahn e.
  IntraCoil e.
  IntraStent DoubleStent biliary e.
  IntraStent DoubleStrut biliary e.
  large-bore bile duct e.
  large-bore biliary e.
  Leinbach head and neck e.
  Medoc-Celestin e.
  metallic biliary e.
  metatarsophalangeal e.
  nonporous-coated e.
  pancreatic e.
  peroral e.
  pigtail e.
  plastic e.
  polyethylene e.
  Proctor-Livingston e.
  Schneider Wallstent biliary e.
  self-expandable stainless steel
    braided e.
  self-expanding metallic e.
  self-expanding Wallstent e.
  smooth e.
  straight e.
  Thompson e.
  three-quarter pigtail plastic e.
  tibial e.
  Titan e.
  TPP hip e.
  transpapillary endoscopic e.

  tumor replacement e.
  UroLume e.
  Viabahn e.
  Viabil biliary e.
  Viatorr e.
  Wallgraft e.
  Wallgraft tracheobronchial e.
  Wallstent e.
  Wallstent biliary e.
  Wilson-Cook e.
endoprosthetic flange
**Endoprothetik CSL-Plus cemented-hip
  system**
endopyelotomy
  Acucise e.
endorectal coil
endorectal-pelvic phased-array coil
Endosac specimen bag
**Endosampler disposable endometrial
  biopsy curette**
Endosaph vein harvest system
endoscissors
  rotating e.
endoscope
  AccuSharp e.
  activated capsule e.
  Agee e.
  angled-lens e.
  angled-shaft e.
  battery-powered e.
  cap-fitted e.
  charge-coupled device e.
  Cho/Dyonics 2-portal e.
  Cho 2-portal Dyonics e.
  Circon-ACMI e.
  disc e.
  double accessory channel
    therapeutic e.
  double-channel e.
  down-angled e.
  down-viewing e.
  Durascope e.
  Eder-Cohn e.
  electronic radial-array e.
  EndoLive 3D stereo video e.
  end-viewing e.
  EUM-series e.
  Evis Exera e.
  Evis 140 Q series e.
  Evis "Q" series e.
  Evis 140 S wide-screen e.
  FG-series 2-channel e.
  fiberoptic e.
  flexible e.
  flexible fallopian tube e.
  foroblique e.
  forward-viewing e.
  French-McCarthy e.
  Fujinon EG-FP series e.

Fujinon EG series e.
Fujinon EVE series e.
Fujinon EVG-CT e.
Fujinon EVG-CT series e.
Fujinon EVG-FP series e.
Fujinon EVG-F series e.
Fujinon EVG series e.
Fujinon FP series e.
Fujinon UGI-FP series video e.
Gaab e.
GIF-HM e.
GIF-N30 fiberoptic pediatric e.
GIF-Q240 upper digestive tract e.
GIF-XP20 e.
GIF-XP series e.
GIF-XQ series e.
Hamou e.
Hopkins II e.
Hopkins rod e.
Image 1 Pendulum e.
intraductal e.
JFB III e.
JF-20 side-viewing fiberoptic e.
J-shaped e.
Karl Storz e.
Karl Storz Calcutript e.
Karl Storz flexible e.
Kelly e.
Kuda e.
large-channel e.
lateral-viewing e.
Lowsley-Peterson e.
lung imaging fluorescence e.
Machida flexible e.
magnetic resonance e.
McCarthy e.
Messerklinger e.
MicroLap e.
Microprobe integrated laser e.
mother-baby e.
mother-daughter e.
Navigator flexible e.
near infrared electronic e.
nonferromagnetic MR e.
oblique viewing e.
Olympus CF-2301 e.
Olympus CF-UM20 ultrasonic e.
Olympus CF-UM20 ultrasound e.
Olympus CF-200Z e.
Olympus CV series e.
Olympus EUM-20 e.
Olympus EUS series e.
Olympus EVIS Q series e.
Olympus EVIS Q-200V e.
Olympus EVIS series e.
Olympus forward-viewing e.
Olympus GF-UM30P e.
Olympus GF-UM20 radial
  scanning e.

Olympus GF-UM3 ultrasonic e.
Olympus GF-UM20 ultrasound e.
Olympus GIF-D2 e.
Olympus GIF-HM-series e.
Olympus GIF-HM series e.
Olympus GIF-J series e.
Olympus GIF-P e.
Olympus GIF-Q200 e.
Olympus GIF-2T10 e.
Olympus GIF-2T200 e.
Olympus GIF-2T20 end-viewing e.
Olympus GIF-XP series e.
Olympus GIF-XP10 video e.
Olympus GIF-XQ240 e.
Olympus GIF-XV series e.
Olympus JF1T e.
Olympus JF-T series e.
Olympus JF-TV series e.
Olympus JF-V series e.
Olympus N series ultrathin e.
Olympus PJF e.
Olympus PJF series pediatric e.
Olympus P series e.
Olympus side-viewing e.
Olympus SIF-SW fiberoptic e.
Olympus SIF-100 video push e.
Olympus 2T100 e.
Olympus TJF-100 e.
Olympus UM series e.
Olympus V series e.
Olympus VU-M2 e.
Olympus XCF series e.
Olympus XCF-XK series e.
Olympus XGF-UCT30 e.
Olympus XK-10 e.
Olympus XP series e.
Olympus XQ series e.
Olympus XQ-200, XQ-230
  video e.
Olympus Zoom e.
ophthalmic e.
oral e.
OtoView rod lens e.
Padgett e.
pediatric e.
Pentax EC series video e.
Pentax EG-2901, -2940, -3800 e.
Pentax EndoNet digital e.
Pentax ESI-2000 fiberoptic e.
Pentax FG-38X e.
Pentax flexible e.
Pentax side-viewing e.
Pentax VSB-2000 fiberoptic e.
percutaneous spinal e.
Perneczky-designed microscope-
  assisting e.
rigid intranasal e.
rigid open-tube e.
rigid rod-lens e.

E

endoscope *(continued)*
    ROAM right-angled e.
    semiflexible e.
    semirigid e.
    Sensatec e.
    side-viewing e.
    Simpson e.
    Storz e.
    Storz Sine-U-View e.
    stylet-scope e.
    Surgenomic e.
    therapeutic e.
    transpapillary e.
    UGI e.
    ultrasonic e.
    ultrathin e.
    variable-stiffness e.
    velolaryngeal e.
    e. videocamera
    Visicath e.
    Weerda e.
    wireless capsule e.
    Wolf e.
    Zeiss EndoLive e.
endoscope/camera
    Endius spinal e./c.
endoscopic
    e. access port
    e. Babcock grasper
    e. band ligator
    e. biliary endoprosthesis
    e. biopsy forceps
    e. carpal tunnel release system
    e. color Doppler ultrasonography
    e. dissector
    e. flowprobe
    e. forceps
    e. heat probe
    e. hemoclip device
    e. in-line needle holder
    e. knot pusher
    e. laser
    e. linear cutter
    e. quadrature radiofrequency coil
    e. retractor
    e. retrograde
    cholangiopancreatogram (ERCP)
    e. retrograde
    cholangiopancreatography catheter
    e. rotating clip applier (ERCA)
    e. scissors
    e. sewing machine
    e. Splash-Shield
    e. suction cap
    e. suture punch
    e. telescope
    e. thermodisinfector
    e. threaded imaging port
    e. ultrasound duodenoscope

    e. ultrasound probe
    e. washing pipe
endoscopically deliverable tissue-transfixing device
endoscopy
    UGI e.
Endoscrub device
Endo-Set
    Haag-Streit E.-S.
Endoshears
EndoSheath
    E. endoscopy system
    Slide-On E.
    E. system
    Vision System E.
endoskeletal socket
endoskeleton
    stationary ankle flexible e.
    E. TA structural device
Endo-Sock specimen retrieval bag
Endosoft reinforced cuffed tube
EndoSonics
    E. balloon dilatation catheter
    E. IVUS/balloon dilation catheter
endosonography instrument
Endosound
    E. endoscopic ultrasound
    E. endoscopic ultrasound catheter
    E. ultrasound probe
endospeculum
    Kogan e.
endosseous
    e. dental implant
    e. HA implant
    e. hydroxyapatite implant
Endostaple device
Endostapler
EndoStasis probe
Endostat
    Coaxial E.
    disposable coaxial E.
    disposable sculptured E.
    E. II bipolar/monopolar
    electrosurgical generator
    Sculptured E.
endostethoscope
Endotak
    E. C lead catheter
    E. C tripolar transvenous lead
    E. DSP lead
    E. lead defibrillator
    E. lead system
    E. nonthoracotomy implantable
    cardioverter-defibrillator
    E. pacemaker
    E. Picotip
    E. Picotip defibrillation lead
    E. Reliance lead
Endotec spreader

Endotek
   E. machine
   E. OM-3 Urodata monitor
   E. UDS-1000 monitor
   E. urodynamics system
endothelial specular microscope
endothelin-1
   e.-1 platinum Dacron microcoil
   e.-1 platinum Dacron microcoil endotracheal tube
Endo-therapy disposable biopsy forceps
Endotine TransBleph implant
EndoTIP
   EndoTIP imaging port
Endotorque
   Greenen E.
Endotrac
   E. blade system
   E. cannula
   E. carpal tunnel release system
   E. elevator
   E. endoscopic carpal tunnel release system
   E. obturator
   E. probe
   E. rasp
   E. retractor
endotracheal (ET)
   e. cardiac output monitor
   e. catheter
   e. catheter forceps
   e. stylet
   e. tube
   e. tube cuff
Endotrol
   E. endotracheal tube
   E. tracheal tube
Endotron-Lipectron ultrasonic scalpel
Endo-Tube nasojejunal feeding tube
endovaginal
   e. coil
   multiplanc c.
   e. transducer
endovascular
   e. aortic graft
   e. coil
   e. stent
EndoVasix EPAR laser system
Endovations disposable cytology brush
Endovent pulmonary catheter
EndoView
   E. camera
   E. sapphire lens
EndoWrist instrument
Endozime sponge
endplate
   artificial e.
   metallic e.

ends
   esophageal Z-stent with fully coated flange e.
end-to-end
   e.-t.-e. anastomosis stapling device
   e.-t.-e. suture
end-to-side suture
Endura dressing forceps
EnduraFIX tape
Endurance
   E. all-polyethylene acetabular cup system
   E. bone cement
EnduraSPORTS tape
EnduraTape tape
Enduron acetabular liner
Endur resin
end-viewing
   e.-v. endoscope
   e.-v. gastroscope
end-Z file
energometer
energy
   e. dispersive spectrometer
   e. dispersive x-ray fluorescence (EDXRF)
   E. Plus shoe insert
energy-storing foot prosthesis
Enertrax
   E. 7100 pacemaker
   E. pacemaker
e-Net headpiece
Enfant pediatric vision testing system
enforcer
   E. balloon dilation catheter
   Cook e.
   E. SDS coronary stent
ENG
   electronystagmogram
   electronystagmograph
   Nystar Plus ENG
Engelmann thigh splint
Engel-May nail
Engel plaster saw
Engen
   E. palmar finger orthosis
   E. palmar wrist splint
Engh porous metal hip prosthesis
engine
   Acrotorque hand e.
   e. H-file
   Kodak Mammography CAD e.
   Robbins Acrotorque hand e.
   e. S-file
   e. T-file
Englehardt femoral prosthesis
Englert forceps
English
   E. anvil nail nipper

E

English *(continued)*
    E. brace
    E. cane
    E. cane board
English-McNab shoulder prosthesis
Engstrom respirator
enhanced
    e. external counterpulsation unit
    E. Torque guiding catheter
enhancement
    bioelectric field e.
    e. gun
    V-Lace real-time digital video e.
enhancer
    Ace aerosol cloud e.
    aerosol cloud e.
    Avance hearing e.
    e. cushion
    ResQPOD circulatory e.
    universal aerosol cloud e.
enlarging bur
Enneking rod
EnPulse pacing system
EnRhythm
    E. pacemaker
    E. pacing system
ensheathing trocar
EnSite
    E. 3000 imaging system
    E. multielectrode array transvenous
      catheter
    E. NavX intracardiac
      nonfluoroscopic navigation system
    E. 3000 system
Ensolite padded transfer bench
ENT
    ears, nose, throat
    ENT scope
    ENT wash
ENTec
    E. Coblator plasma system
    E. Plasma Wand
    E. surgery system
Entegra prosthesis
EnteraFlo feeding tube
enteral
    VTR-300 e. feeding pump
enteroclysis tube
Enteroport feeding pump
enteroscope
    dedicated push e.
    Olympus 215-cm e.
    Olympus SIF-10 e.
    Olympus SIF-M series video e.
    Olympus SIF-Q240 e.
    Olympus SIF-SW series video e.
    Olympus SIF-100 video e.
    Olympus SIF-100 video push e.
    Pentax VSB-P series e.

    push e.
    Sonde e.
    variable-stiffness e.
    video push e.
enteroscopy
    push-type e.
enterostomy clamp
enterotomy scissors
Enterra
    E. gastrointestinal pacemaker
    E. Therapy implantable
      neurostimulation system
Enteryx GERD procedure kit
Entity pacemaker
ENTrak Plus
entrapment
    e. sac
    e. sack
    e. sack introducer
Entree
    E. disposable CO_2 insufflation
      needle
    E. II trocar
    E. II trocar and cannula system
    E. Plus trocar and cannula system
    E. thoracoscopy cannula
    E. thoracoscopy trocar
Entrex small joint arthroscopy
    instrument set
Entri-Pak enteral feeding bag
EntriStar
    E. feeding tube
    E. gastrostomy system
    E. polyurethane PEG tube
entropion forceps
ENTsol
    E. adaptor
    E. refillable bottle
enucleation
    e. compressor
    e. scissors
    e. scoop
    e. spoon
    e. wire snare
enucleator
    Banner snare e.
    Castroviejo snare e.
    Foster snare e.
    Hardy bayonet e.
    Hardy microsurgical e.
    Marino rotatable transsphenoidal e.
    rotatable transsphenoidal e.
    snare e.
    transsphenoidal e.
    Young e.
enuresis alarm
envelope arm sling
Envisan dextranomer pad

Envision
 E. anterior cervical plate system
 E. CT power injector
 E. endocavity probe
 E. TD implant
 E. TD intravitreal implant
 E. TD ophthalmic drug delivery device
Envision² anterior cervical plate
EnVision non-avidin-biotin detection system
Envoy
 E. guide catheter
 E. middle ear implantable system
 E. totally implantable hearing restoration system
Envy catheter
Enzact
 Pro-PredictRx E.
enzymatic débriding agent
EOA device
EOC goniometer
Eon femoral stem
EP
 Heartwave EP
EP2000 electrophysiology imaging system
EPAR laser system
Epi
 E. E-Z Pen
 E. E-Z Pen-Jr
Epic
 E. ophthalmic 3-in-1 laser
 E. valve
 E. wheelchair
epicardial
 e. defibrillator patch
 e. Doppler flow sector transducer
 e. lead
 e. pacemaker
 e. retractor
 e. sock electrode
Epicel
 E. cultured epidermal autograft
 E. skin graft material
Epics
 E. Altra cell sorting system
 E. C flow cytometer
 E. Elite flow cytometer
 E. Profile flow cytometer
 E. 700-series flow cytometer
 E. V flow cytometer
 E. XL flow cytometer
 E. XL, XLMCL flow cytometer system
Epi-Derm silicone gel sheeting
epidiascope

epidural
 e. electrode array
 e. peg electrode
EpiFlex heel and elbow protector
EpiFLO SD transdermal sustained oxygen delivery system
Epigard
 E. dressing
 E. synthetic skin
epiglottis retractor
Epi-Guide bioresorbable barrier matrix
epi-illuminated microscope
epikeratome
 Amadeus e.
 Norwood EyeCare e.
Epi-K microkeratome
EpiLaser
 E. hair removal laser
 E. laser-based hair removal system
 Palomar E.
 E. system
epilation
 e. forceps
 e. needle
epilator
 Electro-Blend e.
 high-frequency tweezer-type e.
 Removatron e.
epilepsy implant
EpiLift epikeratome system
EpiLight
 E. flashlamp
 E. hair removal system
Epi-Lock
 E.-L. dressing
 E.-L. elbow support
epiluminescent skin surface microscope
Epi-Peeler
 Sloane E.-P.
EpiPen
 E. injection device
 E. Jr.
EpiPen-Jr injection device
Epipoint elbow support
Epiquick
epiretinal delamination diamond knife
episcleral
 e. forceps
 e. sponge
Episeal wound dressing
episiotomy scissors
Epi-Sport epicondylitis clasp
EpiStar diode laser system
Epistat
 E. balloon
 E. double balloon catheter
 E. II nasal catheter
 E. nasal catheter
epistaxis balloon

E

Epi-Stay device
epithelial
  e. rete peg
  e. scraper
  e. trephine
epithelium-derived orthotopic corneal
  allograft
Epitome scalpel
EpiTouch
  E. Alex laser hair removal system
  E. laser
  E. Ruby SilkLaser
  E. Ruby SilkLaser hair removal
    system
Epitrain
  E. active elbow support
  E. elastic elbow support
  E. elbow splint
  E. knitted elbow support
  E. Viscoped support
EpiVision blade
EPL
  Piezolith E.
E-Plate
  ABC E.-P.
Epoca RH humeral resurfacing head
  implant
Epoch hip prosthesis
Epos Ultra extracorporeal shock wave
  therapy device
epoxy
  E. Die material
  e. resin sealer
epoxy-mounted preamplifier
Eppendorf
  E. catheter
  E. 5702 centrifuge
  E. filtertip
  E. microdissector
  E. needle electrode
  E. pO$_2$ microelectrode
  E. Repeater Pro pipette
  E. tube
Eppendorfer
  E. biopsy forceps
  E. biopsy punch
Epson 3200 Perfect Scanner
Epstein
  E. bone rasp
  E. collar stud acrylic implant
  E. collar stud acrylic lens
  E. curette
  E. intraocular lens
  E. neurological hammer
  E. posterior chamber lens
Epstein-Copeland lens
EPT-1000 XP cardiac ablation system
EPT-Dx steerable diagnostic catheter

EPTFE
  expanded polytetrafluoroethylene
    EPTFE augmentation membrane
    EPTFE graft prosthesis
    EPTFE implant
    EPTFE vascular suture
    EPTFE ventricular shunt catheter
epX suspension sleeve
EP-XT steerable catheter
Equalizer
  E. air walker
  E. Pro massager
  E. short leg walking cast
Equation spinal system
Equi-Flow valve
Equinox
  E. balloon microcatheter
  E. digital EEG
  E. digital EEG system
  E. EEG acquisition device
  E. EEG neuromonitoring system
  E. occlusion balloon catheter
  E. occlusion balloon system
Equinoxe shoulder system
equipment
  Acuson echocardiographic e.
  American Medical Source
    laparoscopic e.
  Angiostar Plus vascular imaging e.
  AquaMED dry hydrotherapy e.
  Body-Solid exercise e.
  Cell Saver 4 cardiopulmonary
    bypass blood centrifuge and
    washing e.
  chemical detection e.
  Cybex back rehabilitation e.
  Digitron Koordinat angiography e.
  durable medical e. (DME)
  Dynamic Edge rehabilitation e.
  ERCP e.
  Heart Aide Ezd noninvasive
    monitoring e.
  individual protective e.
  Invertrac e.
  Luxar Silhouette noninvasive body
    appearance e.
  OsseoCare drilling e.
  OsteoStat single-use power
    surgical e.
  personal protective e.
  Polytron DSA e.
  RapidScreen RS-2000 x-ray e.
  Reflex exercise and
    rehabilitation e.
  reflex exercise and rehabilitation e.
  Response rehabilitation and
    fitness e.
  static gray scale ultrasound e.
  StereoGuide breast biopsy e.

equipotential electrode
EquiTest
    E. motor coordination test
    E. sensory organization test
ERA
    ERA 300 dual-chamber pacing system analyzer
    ERA resectoscope sheath
eraser
    e. cautery
    diamond-dusted membrane e.
    hemostatic e.
    Mentor curved e.
    Mentor wet-field e.
    PeaceKeeper extrusion aspiration cannula e.
    Tano e.
eraser-tip cautery
Erbe
    E. cryoprobe
    E. electrical coagulation instrument
    E. electrical coagulation instrument
    E. electrical cutting instrument
    E. electrical cutting instrument
    E. electrocautery unit
    E. ICC electrosurgical generator
    E. Unit argon plasma coagulator
    E. Unit argon plasma coagulator
erbium
    e. CrystaLase laser
    e. laser
    e. resurfacing laser
    2040 e. SilkLaser
erbium:YAG
    e:YAG infrared laser
    e:YAG laser
    e:YAG laser system
ERCA
    endoscopic rotating clip applier
ERCP
    endoscopic retrograde cholangiopancreatogram
    ERCP balloon extractor
    ERCP cannula
    ERCP catheter
    ERCP conventional prosthesis
    ERCP dilator
    ERCP equipment
    ERCP guidewire
    ERCP nasobiliary drain
    ERCP sphincterotome
ErCr:YAG laser
ErecAid
    E. vacuum
    E. vacuum erection device
    E. vacuum system
Erection
    Medicated Urethral System for E.
erector spinae retractor

ERG-Jet disposable contact lens
Ergo
    E. Cush back support
    E. style flexion table
Ergociser
    Cateye E.
    E. exercise cycle
Ergoflex Premiere back support
ergograph
    Mosso e.
Ergolift device
Ergoline bicycle ergometer
ErgoLogic keyboard
ergometer
    bicycle e.
    Biodex cycle e.
    Bosch ERG 500 e.
    Concept II rowing e.
    Corival 400 e.
    Cybex e.
    Cybex cycle e.
    Ergoline bicycle e.
    Lode BV Excalibur braked cycle e.
    Monark bicycle e.
    pedal-mode e.
    Siemens-Elema AG bicycle e.
    Tunturi bicycle e.
    upper body e.
ergonomically correct chair
ergonomic vascular access needle (EVAN)
Ergos
    E. O_2 dual-chamber rate-responsive pacemaker
    E. work simulator
ErgoTec vitreoretinal instrument system
Erhardt
    E. ear speculum
    E. lid clamp
    E. lid forceps
Erich
    E. dental arch bar
    E. facial fracture appliance
    E. malleable arch bar
    E. maxillary splint
    E. nasal splint
Erich-Winter arch bar
Eriksson
    E. knee prosthesis
    E. muscle biopsy cannula
Eriksson-Paparella holder
erisophake (*var. of* erysiphake)
Erkoflex plastic
Erlangen papillotome
Erlanger sphygmomanometer
Erlenmeyer flask
Ernest-McDonald
    E.-M. soft intraocular lens

E

Ernest-McDonald (*continued*)
    E.-M. soft intraocular lens-folding forceps
    E.-M. soft IOL folding forceps
Ernest nucleus cracker
Ernst radium applicator
Eros-CTD
    E.-CTD eroscillator device
    E.-CTD female sexual therapy device
ER-Tracker blue-white DPX
ERx avulsed tooth kit
ERxin multicomponent penile injection
Er:YAG
    Er:YAG laser
    Er:YAG phacolase
erysiphake, erisophake
    corneal e.
    Dimitry-Bell e.
    Dimitry-Thomas e.
    Esposito e.
    Floyd-Grant e.
    Johnson e.
    Maumenee e.
    oval cup e.
    right-angle e.
    Simcoe nucleus e.
Erythroflex hydromer-coated central venous catheter
erythrolabe
ESA
    ESA acromioplasty electrode
    ESA Coulochem multi-electrode
    ESA hook electrode
    ESA meniscectomy electrode
    ESA system
Esaote extremity scanner
escape
    E. nitinol stone retrieval basket
    e. pacemaker
Eschenbach
    E. highlighter
    E. low-vision rehabilitation guide
    E. monocular telescope
    E. Optik lens
Eschmann endotracheal tube introducer
E-Scope electronic stethoscope
ESI
    ESI fiberoptic light source
    ESI fiberoptic sigmoidoscope
    ESI lighted suction elevator
    ESI light-weight narrow mammaplasty retractor
    ESI Lite-Pipe fiberoptic cable
    ESI Lite-Pipe fiberoptic instrument
    ESI Lite-Pipe plastic surgery instrument
    ESI long narrow mammaplasty retractor
    ESI mammary retractor
Eska modular hip system
Esmarch
    E. ball
    E. bandage
    E. bandage scissors
    E. plaster knife
    E. plaster shears
    E. probe with Myrtle leaf end
    E. roll dressing
    E. tourniquet
    E. tube
EsophaCoil
    E. biliary stent
    E. prosthesis
    E. self-expanding esophageal stent
    E. stent
esophageal
    e. balloon
    e. balloon catheter
    e. balloon dilator
    e. balloon tamponade
    e. detection device
    e. detector device
    e. forceps
    e. I stent
    e. manometry catheter
    e. mercury-filled bougie
    e. obturator
    e. obturator airway
    e. perfusion catheter
    e. pill electrode
    e. prosthesis
    e. retractor
    e. scissors
    e. stent
    e. stethoscope
    e. Strecker stent
    e. tracheal Combitube
    e. Z stent with anchors
    e. Z stent with Dua antireflux stent
    e. Z stent with Dua antireflux valve
    e. Z-stent with fully coated flange ends
    e. Z-stent with uncoated flange
esophagofiberscope
    Olympus e.
esophagoprobe
    Olympus ultrasonic e.
esophagoscope
    ACMI fiberoptic e.
    ballooning e.
    Blom-Singer e.
    Boros e.
    Broyle e.

Bruening e.
Chevalier Jackson e.
child e.
Denck e.
Dohlman e.
fiberoptic e.
Foregger rigid e.
foroblique fiberoptic e.
full-lumen e.
Haslinger e.
Holinger infant e.
infant e.
Jackson e.
Jesberg e.
J-scope e.
Lell e.
LoPresti fiberoptic e.
Moersch e.
Mosher e.
Moure e.
Olympus e.
optical e.
oval e.
oval open e.
pediatric e.
Roberts folding e.
Roberts oval e.
Sam Roberts e.
Schindler e.
standard full-lumen e.
Storz e.
Tesberg e.
Tucker e.
Universal e.
upper e.
Yankauer e.

esophagospasm dilator
esophagotome
esophagotracheal combination tube
ESP
ESP II system
ESP radiation reduction examination
gloves
Espaillat-Deblasio nucleus rotator
Espe
E. Ketac-Bond Aplicap
E. Photac-Bond Aplicap
E-speed intraoral film
Espocan combined spinal/epidural needle
Esposito erysiphake
ESPrit ear level speech processor
Esprit ventilator
Esquire dental sterilizer
ESRA-10 erythrocyte sedimentation rate
analyzer
ESR-Auto Plus sedimentation rate
analyzer

Essential
E. Energy cup
E. Energy whole house wand
ESSential shaver system
Esser graft
Essig arch bar
Esteem
E. advanced vacuum therapy for
impotence
E. synergy
EsteLux
Palomar E.
E. system
esthesiometer
manual e.
monofilament pressure e.
noncontact corneal e.
noncontact pneumatic e.
esthetic
e. CO_2 laser
e. laser system
e. Taylor mandibular angle implant
estimator
bone e.
Vilex bone e.
Estrace VR intravaginal ring
Estring
E. estradiol vaginal ring
E. silicone vaginal ring
ESU
electrosurgical unit
Aspen Excalibur ESU
ESU dispersive pad
ET
endotracheal
ET tube
etafilcon A disposable contact lens
etch system
ETDRS acuity chart
Ete low-adherent dressing
Ethalloy needle
ether
e. guard
e. screen
Ethibond polybutilate-coated polyester
suture
Ethicon
E. BV-75-3 needle
E. CDH29 stapler
E. circular stapler
E. clip
E. disposable cannula
E. disposable trocar
E. Endopath EZ45 stapler
E. Ligaclip
E. mesh
E. micropoint suture
E. Sabreloc suture
E. SAS

Ethicon *(continued)*
  E. silk suture
  E. ST-4 straight taper-point needle
  E. suture
  E. TLH30 stapler
  E. trocar
Ethicon-Atraloc suture
Ethiflex
  E. retention suture
  E. suture
Ethiguard needle
Ethilon
  E. nylon suture
  E. suture
ethiodized oil
Ethi-pack suture
ethmoid
  e. Blakesley forceps
  e. cutting forceps
  e. forceps
  e. punch forceps
ethmoidal
  e. chisel
  e. curette
  e. punch
Ethox
  E. bite block
  E. cuff
  E. feeding tube
ethyl cyanoacrylate glue
ethylene oxide dressing
ETO
  ETO Sleuth
  ETO Sleuth monitor
E-to-A adapter
e-TRAIN 110 AngioJet catheter
Etude cystometer uroflowmeter
ETView endotracheal tube
E-type dental implant
EUB-405
  EUB-405 ultrasound scanner
  EUB-405 ultrasound system
Eudermic surgical glove
EUM-series endoscope
Eureka collimator
Euro-Collins multiorgan perfusion kit
EuroCuff forearm crutch
Euroglide MKII slide board
Euro-Med
  E.-M. biopsy punch
  E.-M. FNA-21 aspiration needle
European/German bipolar cable
European in-the-bag lens
EuroPeel system
Euro Precision Technology submicron lathe machine
Eurotaper 12/14 taper
Eurotech
  E. Diamond table

  E. Emerald table
  E. Platinum table
  E. Sapphire table
EUSN-1 EchoTip needle
eustachian
  e. catheter
  e. tube
euthyscope
ev3
  ev3 premounted balloon-expandable stent
  ev3 self-expanding stent
  ev3 unmounted balloon-expandable stent
EVac
  E. 70 suction wand
  E. T&A suction wand
evacuation device
evacuator
  AspenVac smoke e.
  Bard e.
  bladder e.
  EasiVac e.
  Ellik bladder e.
  high-volume e.
  ice clot e.
  Iglesias e.
  Laparofan smoke e.
  Laufe portable uterine e.
  McCarthy e.
  McCarthy bladder e.
  smoke e.
  Toomey e.
  e. tubing
  Urovac bladder e.
  uterine e.
evaluator
  computer-aided sensory e.
  Touch-Test sensory e.
EVAN
  ergonomic vascular access needle
Evans articulator
Evans-Vital tissue forceps
Evazote
  E. cushioning material
  E. foam
EVE Fujinon videocolonoscope
Eve-Neivert tonsillar wire
event
  e. monitor
  e. recorder
  e. recorder monitor
event/episode counter
eVent Inspiration ventilator system
Everest
  E. alloy
  E. disposable inflation device
Everett pile forceps
Ever-Flex insole

EverGrip clamp insert
Evershears
- E. bipolar curved scissors
- E. bipolar laparoscopic forceps
- E. bipolar laparoscopic scissors
- E. surgical instrument device

everter
- Berens lid e.
- Berke double-end lid e.
- lid e.
- Roveda lid e.
- Schachne-Desmarres lid e.
- Struble lid e.
- Walker lid e.

everting mattress suture
Evert-O-Cath drug delivery catheter
Everyday Objects ColorCards
Eves-Neivert tonsillar snare
Eves tonsillar snare
Evis
- E. 140 endoscope reprocessing system
- E. Exera
- E. Exera endoscope
- E. Exera video system
- E. 200I colonoscope
- E. 140 Q series endoscope
- E. "Q" series endoscope
- E. 140 S wide-screen endoscope

evisceration spoon
EVLT laser
Evolis femoral cutting guide
Evolution
- E. CT scanner
- E. hip prosthesis
- E. 1 precision robot
- R-Test E.
- E. scanner
- E. XP scanner

EVS
- expanding vascular stapling
- EVS mechanical closure device
- EVS vascular closure system

Ewald
- E. gastroscope
- E. tissue forceps
- E. tube

Ewald-Walker knee implant
EWIIO
- elbow-wrist-hand orthosis

Ewing lid clamp
EX
- Filter Wire E.

EX-2000 DeVilbiss conserver
ExAblate 2000 ultrasound system
Exacta-Med oral dispenser
ExacTech
- E. blood glucose meter
- E. blood glucose meter test

- E. glucose measuring device
- E. RSG glucose meter

Exactech
- E. Equinoxe shoulder system
- E. hip system

Exact-Fit broaching system
Exact-Touch Saccomanno Pap smear collection system
Exakt
- E. cutting/grinding system
- E. cutting/grinding unit

Exami-Gown MRI gown
examination retractor
examining
- e. lamp
- e. spotlight
- e. telescope

Ex-Balls medicine ball
Excalibur
- E. handpiece
- E. introducer

excavating bur
excavator
- Clev-Dent e.
- dental e.
- fenestration e.
- Henry Schein e.
- Lempert e.
- middle ear e.
- sinus tympani e.
- stapes e.

Excel
- E. disposable biopsy forceps
- E. double-tipped microcatheter
- E. fracture system
- E. GE
- E. GE electrochemical glucose monitoring test strip
- E. Plus electrode
- E. Plus underpad
- E. quilted underpad

Excel-14 microcatheter
eXcel-DR
- e.-DR disposable/reusable Glasser laparoscopic needle
- e.-DR disposable/reusable instrument
- e.-DR Glasser laparoscopic needle

Excell DXA bone densitometry system
Excelsior 1018 microcatheter
exchange
- e. guidewire
- rapid e. (RX)
- e. tip deflecting wire guide handle

exchanger
- countercurrent heat e.
- head/moisture e.
- heat e.
- heat and moisture e. (HME)
- HumidFilter heat and moisture e.

E

exchanger *(continued)*
> hygroscopic heat and moisture e.
> moisture e.
> Portex Thermovent heat and
>   moisture e.
> Thermovent heat and moisture e.

exchange-tip deflecting wire guide
handle

Excilon
> E. drain sponge
> E. dressing sponge
> E. IV sponge

ExciMed
> E. UV200 excimer laser
> E. UV200LA laser

excimer
> e. cool laser
> e. gas laser
> e. laser
> e. laser system
> e. sheath
> e. ultraviolet laser

excitatory amino acid neurotransmitter
Excluder stent-graft
exclusion clamp
excretory urography
excursion amplifier sleeve
exdwelling ureteral occlusion balloon
catheter

executive
> e. bifocal
> e. trifocal

Exera
> Evis E.

Exerball kit
Exerband
> E. Pak bilateral tube
> E. Pak unilateral tube
> E. therapy band
> E. tubing

Exerboard
> Velcro Hand E.

exercise
> Back Revolution Stick e.
> e. band
> Cardiac Assessment System for E.
>   (CASE)
> cardiopulmonary e.
> e. grab bar
> E. Sandal
> Thera-Band Max resistive e.
> e. treadmill

exerciser
> AccessTrainer e.
> animal beanbag e.
> Ankle Isolator foot and ankle e.
> axial resistance e.
> Böhler e.
> Builder Grip hand e.

Carpal Care carpal tunnel e.
Carpal Tunnel Stretch e.
Cat's Paw e.
ChairCiser adjustable e.
Cybex II, II+ isokinetic e.
Danniflex CPM e.
Digi-Flex finger e.
Digi-Flex hand e.
Dynaflex Gyro e.
Eggsercizer CTS e.
Eggsercizer resistive hand e.
Exer-Cor e.
ExtendaFLEX e.
finger e.
Finger Helper hand e.
Finger Platter hand e.
Flextender Plus hand e.
Grahamizer I e.
Gripp squeeze ball hand e.
Gyro-Flex upper extremity e.
hand e.
Hand Helper hand e.
isokinetic Unex III e.
Iso-Quadron e.
Jace shoulder e.
jaw e.
Jux-A-Cisor e.
Kinetec clubfoot CPM e.
Knead-A-Ball e.
microcomputer upper limb e.
MiniMedBall hand e.
Morpho E.
Motivator FTR2000 e.
Mule upper limb e.
NordiCare Enabler e.
NordiCare Strider e.
NordicTrack ski e.
NuStep e.
Omni-Flexor wrist e.
Oppociser hand e.
Orthotron e.
pedal e.
Plyo-Sled e.
Powerflex CMP e.
Power Pogo stationary e.
Power Web hand e.
Power Web Jr. e.
Preston Traveler CPM e.
ProStretch e.
Pul-Ez e.
resistive e.
rickshaw rehab e.
rickshaw rehabilitation e.
rocky boat e.
Rotaflex e.
Roylan ergonomic hand e.
Seated Cable Row e.
Soft Touch hand e.
squeeze e.

strengthening e.
Stronghands hand e.
Stryker CPM e.
Stryker leg e.
Swanson Grip-X hand e.
Thera-Band Assist e.
Thera-Band hand e.
Thera-Band resistive e.
TheraBite jaw e.
Thera Cane shoulder e.
Theraflex wrist e.
Ther-A-Hoop e.
Thera-Loop e.
Thera-Putty CTS e.
Toronto Medical CPM e.
Tuf Nex neck e.
Tunturi hand e.
Versa-Trainer e.
Walk-'n-Tone e.
Wilco ankle e.
Wristiciser e.
Zimmer continuous anatomical
   passive e.
Exer-Cor exerciser
ExerFlex ball
Exer-Pedic cycle
Exerstrider
   E. machine
   E. walking pole
Exertools
   E. Dynadisc
   E. gymball
Exeter
   E. intramedullary bone plug
   E. intramedullary bone plug device
   E. ophthalmoscope
   E. stem
Exeter-Femora press-fit prosthesis
EX-FI-RE
   EX-FI-RE external fixation device
   EX-FI-RE external fixation system
eXit disposable puncture closure device
exit tip
Exmoor aural grommet
Exo-Bed
   E.-B. traction unit
   E.-B. tractor
Exogen
   E. 2000+ low-intensity ultrasound
      fracture healing system
   E. 2000 noninvasive low-intensity
      pulsed ultrasound device
   E. noninvasive ultrasound
   E. 2000 sonic accelerated fracture
      healing system
exolever forceps
Exonix ultrasonic surgical system
Exo-Overhead traction unit

exophthalmometer
   Hertel e.
   Luedde e.
   Marco prism e.
   Naugle e.
exophthalmometry
   Krahn e.
exoplant
   Miragel e.
EX-OP operating table
Exo-Static cervical collar
Exotec brace
Expand212 helical stone basket
expandable
   e. access catheter
   e. biliary endoprosthesis
   e. blade
   e. breast implant
   e. cervical dilator
   e. esophageal stent
   e. Gianturco metallic stent
   e. intrahepatic portacaval shunt
      stent
   e. LeMaitre valvulotome
   e. metallic stent
   e. metal mesh endoprosthesis
   e. prosthesis
Expandacell sponge
expanded
   e. foam immobilization device
   e. polytetrafluoroethylene (EPTFE)
   e. polytetrafluoroethylene-covered
      nitinol TIPS stent graft
   e. polytetrafluoroethylene implant
   e. polytetrafluoroethylene SoftForm
      facial implant
   e. polytetrafluoroethylene vascular
      graft
expander
   AccuSpan tissue e.
   anatomic e.
   Becker tissue e.
   Beehler irrigating pupil e.
   Biospan anatomical tissue e.
   Biospan breast tissue e.
   croissant tissue e.
   field e.
   Graether pupil e.
   Heyer-Schulte subcutaneous
      tissue e.
   Integra tissue e.
   irrigating pupil e.
   e. mammary implant material
   McGhan tissue e.
   Mentor tissue e.
   Miami Star tissue e.
   PMT AccuSpan tissue e.
   Radovan subcutaneous tissue e.
   rectal e.

E

expander *(continued)*
    saline-filled e.
    self-inflating tissue e.
    silastic HP tissue e.
    slow palatal e.
    soft tissue e.
    e. stent
    subperiosteal tissue e.
    surgical skin graft e.
    Surgitek T-Span tissue e.
    tissue e.
    T-Span tissue e.
    Versafil tissue e.

expanding
    e. reamer
    e. vascular stapling (EVS)

Expand-O-Graft cutter

expansible infrastructure endosteal implant

expansile forceps

expansion
    controlled radial e.
    E. control Waffle mattress pad
    e. screw

Expedium anterior spine system

experimental apparatus

Expert bone densitometer

Expert-XL densitometer

expiratory valve

explorer
    E. common bile duct exploration system
    cowhorn e.
    curved e.
    E. 360-degree rotational diagnostic catheter
    E. 360-degree rotational diagnostic EP catheter
    dental e.
    operative e.
    Orban-type e.
    pigtail e.
    E. pre-curved diagnostic EP catheter
    shepherd's hook e.
    sickle e.
    E. ST fixed curve diagnostic catheter
    straight e.
    subgingival e.
    E. X70 intraoral radiography system

exploring
    e. cannula
    e. electrode
    e. needle

Expo
    E. angiographic catheter
    E. diagnostic catheter
    E. eye dressing

Export catheter

expoSURE

exposure meter

Express
    E. balloon
    E. balloon-expanded stent
    E. biliary LD stent
    E. PTCA catheter
    E. seeding cartridge system

ExpresSew suture passer

Ex-PRESS mini glaucoma shunt

expressor
    Arruga e.
    Berens e.
    Berens lens e.
    follicle e.
    Heilen e.
    e. hook
    hook e.
    intracapsular lens e.
    iris e.
    Kirby hook e.
    Kirby intracapsular lens e.
    lens e.
    lid e.
    McDonald e.
    Medallion lens e.
    meibomian gland e.
    nucleus e.
    ring lens e.
    Saalfield e.
    Schamberg e.
    Smith lens e.
    tonsillar e.
    Unna e.
    Verhoeff lens e.
    Walton e.
    Zimmerman-Walton e.

Exprin DQ1 biopsy instrument

expulsion stent

Extend
    E. absorbable synthetic punctal implant
    E. punctal plug
    E. stem
    E. total hip system

ExtendaFLEX exerciser

extended
    e. anatomical chin
    e. anatomical high-profile malar implant
    e. collection device
    e. round needle
    e. sector ultrasonic probe
    e. shank Gracey curette
    e. steel-shank shoe

e. wear self-adhering urinary external catheter

e. wear self-adhering urinary external catheter starter kit

e. wear self-adhering urinary external catheter with removable tip

e. wear soft contact lens

extended-curve thermistor catheter
extender

dorsal plate e.

Frechet e.

Küntscher nail e.

rear-tip e.

Rousek e.

Superstabilizer cemented stem e.

Superstabilizer press-fit stem e.

Taq e.

Extend-It finger splint
extension

e. aid

e. apparatus

bifurcated drain e.

e. bone clamp

e. bow

brake lever e.

Buck e.

Centurion needleless catheter e.

Codivilla e.

Dynasplint knee e.

Hudson cerebellar e.

Jackson-Pratt bifurcated drain e.

Linx guidewire e.

LOC guidewire e.

e. nail

NexGen offset stem e.

Orascoptic loupe e.

PSG LOC guidewire e.

radiolucent operating room table e.

e. tube

e. tubing with connector

Extensometer

Laser E.

extensor hood
exterior pelvic device
external

e. abdominal ring

e. alignment compression jig

e. asynchronous pacemaker

e. auditory meatus electrode

e. biliary drainage catheter

e. canthus electrode

e. cardioverter-defibrillator (ECD)

e. collimator

e. counterpressure device

e. demand pacemaker

e. fixator

e. functional neuromuscular stimulator

e. immobilizer

e. inflatable compressor

e. monitor

e. orthosis

e. pacemaker

e. pacemaker battery

e. pressure transducer

e. retractor

e. sequential pneumatic compression boot

e. spinal skeletal fixator

e. straightener

e. tachyarrhythmia control device

e. transthoracic pacemaker

e. ureteral catheter

e. urethral barrier

e. vascular compression device

e. vein stripper

e. ventricular drain

external-alignment compression jig
external-internal pacemaker
externally

e. controlled noninvasive programmed stimulation pacemaker

e. powered tenodesis orthosis

e. supported Dacron graft

Extra

E. Back-up guiding catheter

Precision E.

E. Sport coronary guidewire

extracapsular forceps
extracardiac right-to-left shunt
extracellular matrix protein
extrachromic suture
extracoronal retainer
extracorporeal

e. assist device

e. bypass pump

e. life support

e. liver assist device (ELAD)

e. membrane oxygenation system

e. membrane oxygenator (ECMO)

e. organ bioartificial liver device

e. piezoelectric lithotriptor

e. pump oxygenator

e. shock wave lithotriptor

extracranial shunt
extracting forceps
extraction

e. atherectomy device

e. balloon

e. forceps

e. generator

e. hook

e. pliers

e. trap

Extract-N-Amp Blood PCR kit
extractor

acetabular cup e.

E

extractor *(continued)*
Amico e.
Applied Biosystems 340A nucleic acid e.
Atlas Wire stone e.
Austin Moore e.
Bird vacuum e.
bone e.
bone plug e.
broach e.
buccal fat e.
Captura helical stone e.
cloverleaf pin e.
CMI vacuum e.
comedo e.
cortex e.
Councill ureteral stone e.
ERCP balloon e.
femoral trial e.
fetal head e.
fetal vacuum e.
food e.
head e.
e. injector
intramedullary nail e.
irrigating C-hook e.
irrigating cortex e.
Jewett e.
Jewett bone e.
Kalish Duredge wire e.
Kobayashi vacuum e.
Krwawicz cataract e.
Küntscher e.
Lewicky cortex e.
Lloyd nail e.
Look cortex e.
E. 3-lumen retrieval balloon
E. 3-lumen retrieval balloon catheter
Luxator e.
magnetic e.
Malmstrom vacuum e.
Malström vacuum e.
Mark II femoral component e.
Mark II tibial component e.
McDermott e.
McReynolds e.
metatarsal head e.
Mityvac vacuum e.
M-type e.
mucus e.
Murless vacuum e.
e. nail drill
NCircle nitinol tipless stone e.
NCompass nitinol stone e.
NForce nitinol helical stone e.
O'Neil vacuum e.
Perc NCircle rapid atraumatic PCNL stone e.

RNAzol Reagent E.
Rousek e.
Rutner stone e.
Sawyer e.
Schamberg comedo e.
Silc e.
Simcoe cortex e.
Snap Lock wire/pin e.
Soehendra stent e.
soft-cup e.
stem e.
Sven-Johansson e.
Take-Out E.
T-C ring-handle pin and wire e.
Tender Touch e.
TRIzol RNA e.
Universal modular femoral hip component e.
Unna comedo e.
ureteral stone e.
vacuum e.
Visitec cortex e.
Walton e.
Walton comedo e.
Welsh cortex e.
Wilson-Cook 8-wire basket stone e.
E. XL triple-lumen retrieval balloon
extractor-driver
Schneider e.-d.
extractor/injector cannula
eXtract specimen bag
extracutaneous vas fixation clamp
extra-depth
e.-d. posterior acetabular retractor
e.-d. shoe
extraflexible wire
extrahepatic shunt
extra large (XL)
extra-large hip retractor
extramedullary
e. alignment arch
e. alignment guide
e. tibial alignment jig
extraoral
e. bone-anchored implant
e. fracture appliance
e. prosthesis
e. sigmoid notch retractor
extra-stiff
e.-s. Amplatz wire
e.-s. guidewire
extra-support guidewire
extrathoracic airway dysfunction
extravasation detection accessory
extraventricular drain
Extreme
E. foot orthotic

E. II peripheral excimer laser catheter
E. Select ligament brace
E³xtreme Access
extremity, pl. extremities
    e. coil
    e. mobilization strap
    e. pump
ExtreSafe phlebotomy device
extrication device
extruded bar polyethylene
extrusion
    Kensey rotation atherectomy e.
    e. needle
exudate disposal bag
ExuDerm
    E. hydrocolloid
    E. hydrocolloid dressing
    E. hydrocolloid dressing material
    E. RCD hydrocolloid dressing
Exu-Dry
    E.-D. absorptive dressing
    E.-D. wound dressing
eye
    artificial e.
    e. bandage
    e. blade
    e. calipers
    4-e. catheter
    6-e. catheter
    e. cup
    e. curette
    e. diathermy electrode
    e. drape
    e. dressing forceps
    e. fixation forceps
    e. holder
    e. knife
    e. knife guard
    e. lens
    e. magnet
    e. movement measuring apparatus
    e. needle holder
    e. occluder
    e. pad
    e. pad dressing
    e. patch
    e. probe
    e. protector
    E. Scan corneal analyzer
    e. shield
    Snellen reform e.
    e. spear
    e. speculum
    e. spherical implant
    e. stitch scissors
    e. suture scissors
    e. swab
EyeArmor safety glasses

EyeCap ophthalmic image capture system
EyeClose
    E. adhesive strip
    E. external eyelid weight
Eyecor camera
Eyecuity wireless visual acuity test
eyed suture needle
eyeFix speculum system
eyeglass
    e. case
    e. frame
    e. hearing aid
    e. retainer
eyeless atraumatic suture needle
eyelet clasp
eyelid
    e. crease suture
    e. forceps
    e. retractor
    e. spacer
EyeLite photocoagulator
EyeMap EH-290 corneal topography system
Eye-Pak drape
eyepiece
    comparison e.
    compensating e.
    demonstration e.
    Huygenian e.
    Huygens e.
    negative e.
    positive e.
    Ramsden e.
    wide-field e.
eyestone
EyeSys
    E. corneal analysis system
    E. 2000 corneal topographic mapping system
    E. surface topography system
    E. videokeratograph
    E. videokeratoscope
EyeSys System 2000
eye-tracking system
eyewear
    E Clips computer e.
    polycarbonate ballistic protective e.
    Timex TMX optical e.
EZ
    EZ Bend sponge
    EZ Detect colorectal screening test kit
    FilterWire EZ
    EZ hand pump
    EZ Hold manual compression device
    EZ Lift table
    Octopus 500 EZ

E

EZ *(continued)*
  EZ Rider support chair
  EZ ROM postoperative knee brace
  EZ "T" orthopaedic shirt
E-Z
  E-Z arm abduction orthosis
  E-Z Cath catheter
  E-Z Clean cautery tip
  E-Z Clean laparoscopic electrode
  E-Z Flap
  E-Z Flap bur hole cover
  E-Z Flap cranial flap fixation
  system
  E-Z Flap titanium miniplate system
  E-Z Flex jaw exercising device
  E-Z guide
  E-Z Heat hot pack
  E-Z hold adhesive catheter tube
  holder pad
  E-Z hold adhesive/stretchable strap
  catheter tube holder
  E-Z Lets II lancing device
  E-Z mount disinfectant kit
  E-Z Reacher
  E-Z ROC anchor
  E-Z syringe
  E-Z Tac soft-tissue reattachment
  system

EZ.1 multifocal contact lens
EZ45 thoracic linear cutter
EZBrace orthosis
EZ-Derm porcine biosynthetic wound
  dressing
EZ-Dish pressure relief cushion
Ezeform splint
EZ-EM
  EZ-EM Bio-Gun automated biopsy
    system
  EZ-EM cut biopsy needle
  EZ-EM PercuSet amniocentesis tray
E-Z-Guard mouthpiece
EZ-HP *Helicobacter pylori* **test**
EZ-Ject injector
EZLoc femoral fixation device
Ezo denture cushion
EZ-On traction belt system
E-Z-On vest
EZ-Pro R4 ambulance cot
EZ-Trac orthopaedic suspension device
EZ-Up inversion table
EZVue violet haptic intraocular lens
Ezy
  E. Wrap lumbosacral support
  E. Wrap shoulder immobilizer

F-1200, -2000 -4500
F2L Multineck femoral stem
Fabco
    F. gauze bandage
    F. gauze dressing
    F. wrap
Fab fragment
Fabian
    F. screw
    F. stent
fabric
    f. baffle
    Bard Edwards outflow tract f.
    Edwards outflow tract f.
    f. leg bag strap
    neoprene f.
    Solumbra 30+ SPF f.
    Staph-Chek Synergy f.
Fabry coagulator
face
    f. mask
    f. rest
    f. shield
facebow, face-bow
    Asher high-pull f.
    Kinematic f.
    Kloehn f.
    Rampton f.
    root high-pull f.
Face-It protective shield
facelift, face-lift
    f. D'Assumpcão marker
    f. flap marker
    f. retractor
    f. scissors
face-out whole-body plethysmograph
faceplate
    Coloplast irrigation f.
    Sur-Fit irrigation adapter f.
facet
    f. rasp
    f. screw system
facial
    f. compression finger closure
    f. compression skullcap closure
    f. fracture appliance
    f. fracture appliance dental arch bar
    f. implant
    f. nerve dissector
    f. nerve knife
    f. nerve stimulator
    f. plastics garment
    f. plastic surgery scissors

    f. prosthesis
    f. support
Facit uterine polyp forceps
FACSCalibur flow cytometer
FACScan flow cytometer
FACSort flow cytometer
FACStar Plus flow cytometer
FACSVantage
    F. cell sorter
    F. flow cytometer
factor
    insulin-like growth f.
    platelet-derived growth f.
    Stuart-Prower f.
Faden suture
Fader Tip ureteral stent
Fahey-Compere pin
Fahey pin
Fahrenheit flat bath thermometer
fail-safe device
failure
Fairdale orthodontic appliance
Fair urethral stent
Falcon
    F. coronary catheter
    F. filter
    F. lens
    F. Omniflex balloon
    F. plastic flask
    F. single-operator exchange balloon catheter
Falconer rongeur
Falk appendectomy spoon
fallopian
    f. cannula
    f. catheter
    f. tube forceps
falloposcope endoscopic instrument
Falope
    F. ring
    F. ring applicator
    F. ring tubal occlusion band
false neurochemical transmitter
fan
    f. elevator retractor
    Schmitt f.
Fanal Finder system
fan-beam collimator
Fanta speculum
Fantastic Burr nail bur
fan-type laparoscopic retractor
Farabeuf
    F. bone-holding forceps
    F. bone rasp
    F. double-ended retractor

F

Farabeuf *(continued)*
  F. periosteal elevator
  F. saw
Farabeuf-Collin rasp
Farabeuf-Lambotte
  F.-L. bone-holding clamp
  F.-L. bone-holding forceps
  F.-L. rasp
Faraday
  F. cage
  F. shield
  F. shielded resonator
Farkas-Bracken fixation forceps
Farley Elite spinal retractor
Farnham nasal-cutting forceps
Farr
  F. self-retaining retractor
  F. spring retractor
  F. wire retractor
Farrior
  F. ear curette
  F. ear speculum
  F. otoplasty knife
  F. oval speculum
  F. septal cartilage stripper knife
  F. wire-crimping forceps
Farrior-Derlacki chisel
Farrior-Joseph
  F.-J. bayonet saw
  F.-J. nasal saw
Farrior-McHugh ear knife
Farrior-Shambaugh elevator
Farris tissue forceps
Fasanella
  F. double-ended iris retractor
  F. lacrimal cannula
fascia
  f. lata heart valve
  f. lata implant
  f. lata prosthesis
  f. lata stripper
fascial
  f. cutter
  f. dilator
  f. needle
  f. zipper
fasciotome
  Masson f.
  Moseley f.
Fasguide catheter
FasLata allograft tissue
Fasplint vacuum splint
FAST
  flow-assisted short-term
    FAST 1 intraosseous infusion
    system
fast
  F. Dasher 14 wire

  f. Fourier transform
  f. Fourier transformation spectrum
    analyzer
  F. Lanex rare earth screen
  f. motor unit
FASTak
  F. suture anchor
  F. suture anchor system
fast-breeder reactor
Fastcard
Fast-Cath
  F.-C. Duo introducer
  F.-C. hemostasis introducer catheter
  F.-C. introducer catheter
fastener
  Brown-Mueller T-bar f.
  Cath-Strip catheter f.
  Intrafix ACL tibial f.
  NG strip nasal tube f.
  Percu-Stay catheter f.
  ROC XS suture f.
FastFill brachytherapy needle
Fast-Fit vascular stocking
Fast-Flap cranial flap fixation system
FastGrind lens system
Fastin
  F. RC threaded anchor
  F. suture anchor
  F. threaded anchor
Fastlok implantable staple
FastOut device
FastPack blood analyzer system
Fast-Pass lead pacemaker
**Fast-Patch disposable
  defibrillation/electrocardiographic
  electrode**
FastPrep DNA kit
Fastrac
  F. hydrophilic-coated guidewire
  F. introducer
Fastrach laryngeal mask airway
FasTracker
  F. catheter
  F. 325 coaxial microcatheter
FasTracker-18 infusion catheter
fast-setting acrylic
FastStart
  F. EMS neuromuscular stimulator
  F. HVPC pulsed stimulator
**FastTake blood glucose monitoring
  system**
fat
  f. pad retractor
  f. towel
Fathom steerable guidewire
fat-injection needle
Fat-O-Meter skinfold calipers
fat-suppressed body coil

FatTrack
> F. Digital body fat calipers
> F. skinfold calipers

faucet aspirator
faucial eustachian catheter
Faught sphygmomanometer
Faulkner
> F. curette
> F. ethmoidal curette
> F. folder
> F. lens-holding forceps

Faulkner-Browne chisel
Faure
> F. peritoneal forceps
> F. uterine biopsy forceps

Fauvel laryngeal forceps
Favaloro-Morse rib spreader
Favaloro proximal anastomosis clamp
Favaloro-Semb ligature carrier
Favorite clamp
Faxitron x-ray machine
Fazio-Montgomery cannula
FB-25K jumbo biopsy forceps
FCD
> fecal containment device

FCI Ready-Set punctal plug
Feaster
> F. adjustable eyelid speculum
> F. Dualens lens
> F. K7-5460 hydrodissecting cannula
> F. radial keratotomy knife

Feather
> F. carbon breakable blade
> F. clear cornea knife
> F. knife
> F. scalpel

feathered extended malar implant
Feather-Lite Pouching System
FeatherTouch
> F. automated rasp
> F. CO_2 laser
> F. SilkLaser
> F. SilkLaser system

fecal
> f. containment device (FCD)
> f. containment system
> f. marker

Fechtner
> F. conjunctiva forceps
> F. ring forceps
> F. trabeculectomy marker

Federov 4-loop iris clip
feedback system
feeder
> Brecht f.
> Haberman f.
> offset suspension f.
> suspension f.
> Tumble Forms f.

feeding
> f. button
> f. tube
> f. tube attachment device

Feeln' Sure pant
Fe-Ex orogastric tube magnet
Fehland
> F. intestinal clamp
> F. intestinal forceps
> F. right-angled colon clamp

Fehling TOP ejector punch
Feilchenfeld splinter forceps
Feldenkrais cylinder
Feldman
> F. adaptometer
> F. aortic stenosis catheter
> F. bur
> F. RK optical center marker

Feldstein blepharoplasty clip
Felig insulin pump
Fell-O'Dwyer apparatus
Fell sucker tip
felt
> f. brace
> f. dressing
> f. patch
> F. shears
> f. strip
> Teflon f.

female
> f. catheter
> f. condom
> F. Fource custom knee brace
> F. Fource OTS knee brace
> f. sound
> f. urinary pouch
> f. washer

FemCap barrier contraceptive device
Femcept device
Fem-Flex II femoral cannulae
Feminal urinal
Femina vaginal weight
femoral
> f. aligner
> f. artery cannula
> f. broach
> f. canal restrictor
> f. cerebral catheter
> f. clamp
> f. distractor
> f. elevator
> f. endoprosthesis
> f. guide pin
> f. guiding catheter
> f. head bone removal reamer
> f. head driver
> f. head implant component
> f. hemodialysis catheter
> f. impactor

F

femoral *(continued)*
    f. intramedullary guide
    f. introducer sheath
    f. neck nail
    f. neck retractor
    f. notch guide
    f. perfusion cannula
    f. plug
    f. rasp
    f. resector
    f. shaft reamer
    f. stem
    f. trial extractor
femorofemoral crossover prosthesis
FemoStop
    F. femoral artery compression arch
    F. femoral compression system
    F. inflatable pneumatic compression
      device
FemSoft
    F. continence insert
    F. insert
    F. urethral insert
FemTone vaginal weight
femtosecond
    f. laser
    f. laser keratome
    f. laser system
femur
    f. distractor
    F. Finder instrument
fence
    Kirklin f.
    f. splint
fenestra implant
fenestrated
    f. aneurysm clip
    f. blade forceps
    f. catheter
    f. compression plate
    f. cup biopsy forceps
    f. ellipsoid spiked open-span
      biopsy forceps
    f. forceps
    f. Moore-type femoral stem
    f. spiked open-span jumbo biopsy
      forceps
    f. sterile drape
    f. tracheostomy tube
    f. tube
fenestration
    f. bur
    f. curette
    f. excavator
    f. hook
fenestrator
    Montgomery tracheal f.
    tracheal f.

fenestrometer
    ear f.
Fenger gall duct probe
Fenlin total shoulder system
Fenton uterine dilator
Fenwal CS 3000 Plus cell separator
Fenzel angled manipulating hook
FEP-ringed Gore-Tex vascular graft
Ferciot wire guide
Fergie needle
Ferguson
    F. abdominal scissors
    F. anal retractor
    F. angiotribe
    F. angiotribe forceps
    F. anoscope
    F. bone holder
    F. bone-holding forceps
    F. gallstone scoop
    F. implant
    F. mouthgag
    F. needle
    F. suction
    F. suture needle
    F. tenaculum forceps
Ferguson-Brophy mouthgag
Ferguson-Frazier suction tube
Ferguson-Gwathmey mouthgag
Ferguson-Metzenbaum scissors
Ferguson-Moon rectal retractor
Fergus percutaneous introducer kit
Fergusson
    F. forceps
    F. knife
    F. tubular vaginal speculum
Fergusson-Ackland mouthgag
Ferkel C guide
fermentation tube
Fermit-N occlusal hole blockage
    material
Ferno
    F. AquaCiser underwater treadmill
      system
    F. custom therapy pool
Ferran awl
Ferree-Rand perimeter
ferric hyaluronate adhesion barrier
Ferrier
    F. coupler
    F. 212 gingival clamp
    F. separator
Ferris
    F. chart
    F. common duct scoop
    F. disposable bone marrow
      aspiration needle
    F. filiform dilator
    F. PolyMem wound dressing

Ferris-Smith
    F.-S. bone-biting forceps
    F.-S. fragment forceps
    F.-S. intervertebral disc rongeur
    F.-S. needle holder
    F.-S. orbital retractor
    F.-S. pituitary rongeur
    F.-S. punch
    F.-S. retractor
    F.-S. rongeur forceps
    F.-S. tissue forceps
Ferris-Smith-Gruenwald rongeur
Ferris-Smith-Halle sinus bur
Ferris-Smith-Kerrison
    F.-S.-K. disc rongeur
    F.-S.-K. forceps
    F.-S.-K. forceps
    F.-S.-K. laminectomy rongeur
    F.-S.-K. laminectomy rongeur
    F.-S.-K. punch
Ferris-Smith-Lyman periosteotome
Ferris-Smith-Sewall orbital retractor
Ferris-Smith-Spurling disc rongeur
Ferris-Smith-Takahashi
    F.-S.-T. forceps
    F.-S.-T. rongeur
Ferritin IRMA kit
ferromagnetic
    f. intracerebral aneurysm clip
    f. monitoring device
    f. rod
ferrule clamp
FertilMARQ
    F. fertility screening test
    F. home diagnostic screening test
     kit
    F. male fertility screening test kit
fetal
    f. Dopplex monitor
    f. head extractor
    f. heart rate monitor
    f. incontinence collector
    f. scalp electrode
    f. stethoscope
    f. vacuum extractor
FetalPulse
    F. Plus fetal Doppler
    F. Plus monitor
Fetasonde fetal monitor
Feth-R-Kath epidural catheter
fetoscope
    Hillis-DeLee f.
    Pinard f.
Fett carpal prosthesis
Feuerstein split ventilation tube
F&F
    filiform and follower
F-1200, -2000, -4500 fluorescence
  spectrophotometer

FG-36UX scanning echoendoscope
FG diamond bur
FG-series 2-channel endoscope
FG-36UA curved linear-array
  echoendoscope
fiber
    braided polyester f.
    f. cleaver
    Dacron f.
    FiberLase flexible f.
    Indigo diffuse f.
    laser f.
    Laserscope disposable Endostat f.
    f. mallet
    f. metal taper
    Micro Link endoscope f.
    micro-thin plastic f.
    nonmedullated nerve f.
    Pinnacle contact Nd:YAG f.
    Prolase f.
    Trimedyne Flex MAX f.
    UltraLine f.
    UltraLine Nd:YAG laser f.
    Urolase neodymium:YAG laser f.
    X-Static silver fiber shoe lining f.
fibercolonoscope
    Olympus CF-20 f.
fiberduodenoscope
fiberendoscope
fibergastroscope
    fluorescence f.
fiberglass
    f. bandage
    f. graft
    f. splint
    f. staff
fiberglass-free cast tape
FiberLase
    F. beam delivery system
    F. flexible fiber
    F. flexible fiberoptic delivery
     system
    F. laser
Fiberlite microscope
fiber-metal peg
fiberoptic
    f. absorbable plate
    f. anoscope
    f. arthroscope
    f. bronchoscope
    f. catheter
    f. catheter delivery system
    f. choledochoscope
    f. delivery device
    f. digital fundus camera
    f. endoscope
    f. esophagoscope
    f. gastroscope
    f. headband

F

fiberoptic *(continued)*
    f. headlight
    f. hysteroscope
    f. illuminator
    f. laryngoscope
    f. laryngoscope blade
    f. light cable
    f. light carrier
    f. lighted mirror
    f. light pipe
    f. light projector
    f. light source
    f. loupe
    f. microscope
    f. otoscope
    f. oximeter catheter
    f. PCO_2 sensor
    f. pick
    f. pressure catheter
    f. probe
    f. proctosigmoidoscope
    f. right-angle telescope
    f. sensor
    f. sheath
    f. sigmoidoscope
    f. slide laryngoscope
    f. smoke evaluating retractor
    f. suction tube
    f. surgical field illuminator
    f. tip
    f. vaginal speculum
    f. videoendoscope
    f. video glasses
fiberscope
    gastrointestinal f.
    Hirschowitz gastroduodenal f.
    nasopharyngeal f.
    Olympus GF-EU1 gastrointestinal f.
    Olympus GIF-Q30 f.
    Olympus OES f.
    Olympus XK series oblique-viewing
      flexible f.
    pediatric f.
    Pentax f.
    side-viewing f.
    superfine f.
FiberWire suture
Fibracol
    F. collagen
    F. collagen alginate dressing
    F. collagen alginate wound
      dressing
Fibra Sonics phaco aspirator
FibreKor post
Fibrel gelatin matrix implant
Fibre-Lite septal elevator
fibrillar collagen strip
fibrillation
    atrial f. (AF)

Fibrimage diagnostic imaging agent
fibrin
    f. adhesive sealant
    Cell-Tak autologous f.
    f. film stent
    f. gel
    f. glue
    f. glue adhesive
    f. glue-soaked Gelfoam
    f. sealant
    f. sealant adhesive
fibroid hook
FIBROSpec test
fibrotome
fibrous shell
Ficoll cushion
Ficoll-Hypaque density gradient
    centrifuge
fiducial skin marker
field
    automated visual f.
    F. blade
    f. emission tube
    f. expander
    f. lens
    F. tourniquet
field-effect transistor
Field-Lee biopsy needle
field-of-view camera
figure
    Allen f.
figure-of-8
    f.-o.-8 bandage
    f.-o.-8 brace
    f.-o.-8 clavicle strap
    f.-o.-8 coil
    f.-o.-8 dressing
    f.-o.-8 harness
    f.-o.-8 suture
filament
    Charcot-Bottcher f.
    cytokeratin f.
    desmin f.
    Semmes-Weinstein pressure
      aesthesiometer f.
    f. suture
    f. transformer
    vimentin f.
filamentary keratome
Filcard temporary removable vena cava
    filter
file
    Aagesen f.
    bone f.
    f. elevator
    end-Z f.
    Flexicut f.
    Flex-R-File f.
    Hedstrom f.

Kerr K-Flex f.
Kleinert-Kutz bone f.
K root canal f.
McXIM f.
Miller bone f.
Mity Hedström f.
Mity Turbo f.
nickel-titanium f.
Nordent bone f.
orthopaedic bone f.
precurving endosonic f.
ProFile f.
pulp canal f.
Putti bone f.
root canal f.
SureFlex nickel-titanium hand f.
surgical f.
taper hand f.
turbo f.

filiform

f. bougie
f. bougie probe
f. catheter
f. dressing
f. and follower (F&F)
f. guide
LeFort f.
f. steel needle

filiform-tipped catheter

Fillauer

F. bar
F. dorsiflexion assist ankle joint
F. endoskeletal alignment system
F. modular shuttle lock system
F. night splint
F. PDC ankle joint
F. prosthesis liner
F. Scottish Rite orthosis kit
F. silicone suction liner
F. silicone suspension liner

filler

AcryDerm Strands f.
BF+ bone void f.
Bio-Oss maxillofacial bone f.
BonePlast bone void f.
calcium sulfate bone void f.
cellular wrinkle f.
Cerasorb resorbable synthetic bone
void f.
Cortoss bone void f.
Cutinova cavity wound f.
DBX bone void f.
DermAssist f.
Humatrix Microclysmic Gel f.
Multidex f.
OsteoSet bone f.
paste f.
PolyWic f.

ProOsteon implant 500 coralline
hydroxyapatite bone void f.
spiral f.
Springlite toe f.
synthetic cancellous bone void f.
synthetic cortical bone void f.
TheriLok bone void f.
TricOs T bone void f.
Vitoss Scaffold foam bone void f.
Vitoss Scaffold synthetic cancellous
bone void f.
wrinkle f.

filling

muscle f.
Retroplast f.

film

absorbable gelatin f.
AccuFilm articulating f.
Agfa Dentus M2 comfort intraoral
radiograph f.
Agfa Dentus RP 6 blue-sensitive
extraoral radiograph f.
Agfa Dentus ST8 G green-sensitive
extraoral radiograph f.
f. alternator
autoradiographic f.
f. badge
Bard protective barrier f.
Bioclusive MVP transparent f.
BlisterFilm transparent f.
Bucky f.
CarraFilm transparent f.
Centurion SiteGuard MVP
transparent f.
f. changer
contraceptive f.
Curix Ultra UV-L f.
Dentus x-ray f.
DermAssist transparent f.
DuPont Cronex x-ray f.
end-expiratory f.
end-inspiratory f.
E-speed intraoral f.
Gelfilm ophthalmic f.
f. hanger
in-department f.
intraoperative f.
Knuttsen bending f.
Kodak Min-R f.
Kodak XAR-5 x-ray f.
Kodak XRP-1 x-ray f.
lateral cervical spine f.
3M No Sting barrier f.
mobility f.
No Sting barrier f.
NUVO barrier f.
Omniderm transparent f.
OpSite f.
OpSite Flexigrid transparent f.

F

film *(continued)*

Polyskin II transparent f.
Polyskin M.R. transparent f.
Pro-Clude transparent f.
ProCyte transparent f.
Repel bioresorbable barrier f.
Repel-CV bioresorbable adhesion-barrier f.
runoff f.
Scopix Laser f.
f. screen cassette
screenless mammography f.
semierect f.
Softopac intraoral f.
soft x-ray f.
SureSite transparent f.
Tegaderm HP transparent f.
Transeal transparent f.
UP7 f.
upright compression spot f.
vaginal contraceptive f.
f. wound dressing
X-Omat AR f.
x-ray f.

FilmFax teleradiology system
film-screen combination
Filshie

F. clip
F. clip applicator
F. clip minilaparotomy applicator
F. female sterilization clip

filter

Ace Autografter bone f.
Amicon D-20 f.
ARI Group I–IV f.
arterial f.
autoadhesive cellulose nitrate f.
bacterial f.
bandpass f.
Baxter CA-210 f.
Berkefeld f.
bidirectional 4-pole Butterworth high-pass digital f.
bird's nest f.
bird's nest IVC f.
BTF-37 arterial blood f.
Butterworth bidirectional 4-pole high-pass digital f.
Celect vena cava f.
Centricon-10 f.
charcoal f.
Clear Advantage spirometry f.
Coloplast 1-piece closed pouch with f.
Coloplast 2-piece stoma cap with f.
Cook Celect vena cava f.
D/Flex f.
electrosurgical f.

Emboshield bare wire f.
Falcon f.
Filcard temporary removable vena cava f.
flattening f.
fluorescence excitation f.
Fresenius F-40 f.
Gambro FH88H f.
Gene Screen nylon membrane f.
Gianturco-Roehm bird's nest vena cava f.
f. glasses for color testing
Greenfield f.
Greenfield IVC f.
Greenfield titanium IVC f.
Greenfield vena cava f.
Günther Tulip vena cava MReye f.
Haag-Streit 900 cobalt blue f.
Hann f.
HEPA f.
heparin arterial f.
high-efficiency particulate air f.
high-pass f.
Holter in-line shunt f.
Hospal Biospal f.
Hybond N f.
inferior vena cava umbrella f.
InsuFilter f.
Interface arterial blood f.
interference f.
interference barrier f.
IVC f.
Jostra arterial blood f.
Kalman f.
K-edge f.
Keeper vena cava f.
Kim-Ray Greenfield vena cava f.
KoKo Moe pulmonary function f.
K-37 pediatric arterial blood f.
leukocyte depletion f.
leukocyte removal f.
leukodepletion f.
LeukoNet F.
LGM f.
Liposorber cholesterol f.
low-pass f.
f. maintainer
mediastinal sump f.
Meditech IVC f.
Metz spatially varying f.
Millex f.
Millex-GS pore-size f.
Millex-GV f.
Millipore f.
Millipore ultrafree-CL centrifugal f.
Mobin-Uddin f.
Mobin-Uddin umbrella vena cava f.
Mobin-Uddin vena cava f.
f. mold

MultiSPIRO Clear Advantage
  pulmonary function f.
muscle f.
Nalgene capsule f.
f. needle
neutral density f.
notch f.
Nucleopore f.
OptEase permanent vena cava f.
over-the-wire Greenfield f.
Pall ELD-96 Set Saver f.
Pall leukocyte removal f.
Pall Leukogard-6 leukocyte
  reduction arterial blood f.
Pall PL100 f.
Pall RC100 f.
Pall RC50 f.
Pall transfusion f.
f. paper
Percoll f.
pocket red f.
power peak f.
prophylactic IVC f.
Recovery f.
Recovery nitinol f.
Recovery vena cava f.
red-free f.
Re/Flex f.
Renal System HF250 f.
retrievable IVC f.
rhodium f.
SafeFlo IVC f.
F. Security closed minipouch
shunt f.
Simon nitinol inferior vena cava f.
Simon nitinol IVC f.
software-controlled internal
  hardware f.
stainless-steel Greenfield f.
suprarenal Greenfield f.
Sur-Fit auto-lock closed-end pouch
  with f.
Sur-Fit Natura opaque closed-end
  pouch with f.
Tempofilter vena cava f.
Tetko nylon mesh f.
third-order Butterworth f.
Thoreau f.
titanium Greenfield f.
TrapEase inferior vena cava f.
TrapEase permanent IVC f.
TrapEase permanent vena cava f.
TrapEase vena cava f.
tunable notch f.
umbrella f.
UV blocking f.
vena cava f.
Vena Tech f.
Vena Tech dual vena cava f.

Vena Tech LGM f.
Vena Tech LGM vena cava f.
Vena Tech low-profile f.
Vena Tech LP vena cava f.
Vitalograph bacterial/viral f.
wedge f.
Weiner spatially varying f.
Wiener f.
Wiener MRI f.
William Harvey arterial blood f.
F. Wire EX
Wratten f.
Zeta probe nylon f.

filtered
  f. dual-sump drain
  f. mediastinal sump drain
  f. specimen trap
FilterLine circuit
filtertip
  Eppendorf f.
FilterWatch sensor
FilterWire
  F. distal embolic protection device
  F. distal protection device
  F. EX embolic protection system
  F. EZ
FiltraCheck-UTI
  F.-U. colorimetric filtration system
  F.-U. disposable colorimetric
    bacteriuria detection system
filtration
  Millipore f.
  f. system
  Van Herick f.
Filtryzer dialyzer
fin
  convertible f.
  DePuy Global shoulder glenoid
    component with f.
  double-catheterizing f.
  prosthesis f.
final-cut acetabular reamer
Finapres
  F. blood pressure monitor
  F. Dinamap blood pressure
    machine
  F. finger cuff
finder
  angle f.
  Dasco Pro angle f.
  gravity-driven angle f.
  hamate f.
  lumen f.
  pedicle f.
  Tucker vertebrated lumen f.
Findley folding pessary
fine
  f. angled curette
  f. arterial forceps

F

fine *(continued)*
  F. bimanual handpiece set
  f. blade
  f. bone curette
  f. chromic suture
  F. crescent fixation ring
  f. cup forceps
  f. curette
  F. dissecting forceps
  F. folding block
  F. gripping forceps
  F. III inserter
  f. intestinal needle
  F. irrigating capsulorrhexis forceps
  F. irrigating reverse actuating
    splitting chopper
  F. magnetic implant
  f. mesh dressing
  f. micropoint cautery
  F. micropoint electrocautery
  f. needle electrode
  f. olive bur
  F. sideport actuating quick chopper
  F. sideport capsulorrhexis forceps
  f. silk suture
  F. suture scissors
  F. suture-tying forceps
  F. tissue forceps
  f. wire electrode
fine-bore catheter
Fine-Castroviejo suturing forceps
Fine-Gill corneal knife
Fine-Ikeda capsulorrhexis forceps
Fineline II Sterox lead
fine-line tissue marker
Fine-Nagahara phaco chopper
Finesse
  F. cardiac device
  F. guiding catheter
  F. large-lumen guiding catheter
Fine-Thornton scleral fixation ring
fine-tipped
  f.-t. mosquito hemostat
  f.-t. up-angled and down-angled
    bipolar forceps
fine-tooth
  f.-t. clamp
  f.-t. electric saw
fine-toothed
  f.-t. clamp
  f.-t. forceps
fine-wire speculum
finger
  f. blocking tree
  f. circumference gauge
  f. clip sensor
  f. cot
  f. cot dressing
  f. cot splint

  f. cuff
  f. exerciser
  F. Fitness Spring Ball
  f. flexion glove
  f. flexion splint
  f. gauge
  f. gauze
  f. goniometer
  F. Helper hand exerciser
  f. hook
  HP-100 prosthetic f.
  f. indicator
  f. joint implant
  f. ladder
  f. loop
  mechanical f.
  f. oximeter
  F. Phantom pulse oximeter testing
    system
  f. photoplethysmographic device
  f. plate
  F. Platter hand exerciser
  f. rake retractor
  f. ring cutter
  f. ring saw
  f. separator
  f. sled splint
  f. sling
  f. splint
Finger-Hugger splint
fingernail drill
FingerPrint handheld pulse oximeter
fingertip unit
fingertrap suture
finish bur
finisher
  Küntscher f.
finishing bur
Finite dental glazing compound
Fink-Jameson oblique muscle forceps
Fink-Rowland keratome
Fink valve
Fink-Weinstein 2-way syringe
Finn
  F. chamber
  F. chamber patch test device
  F. hinged knee prosthesis
  F. knee revision prosthesis
  F. knee revision system
  F. knee system
finned pacemaker lead
finned stem punch
Finney
  F. Flexirod penile prosthesis
  F. penile implant
Finnoff
  F. sinus transilluminator
  F. transilluminator

Finochietto
F. arterial clamp
F. bronchial clamp
F. clamp carrier
F. forceps
F. hand retractor
F. infant rib contractor
F. infant rib retractor
F. needle holder
F. retractor
F. rib spreader
F. stirrup
F. thoracic forceps
F. thoracic scissors
Finochietto-Burford
F.-B. rib contractor
F.-B. rib spreader
Finochietto-Geissendorfer rib retractor
Finochietto-Stille rib spreader
Fino DVT catheter
Finsen
F. bath
F. lamp
F. retractor
Finsterer suction tube
Firlit-Kluge urethral stent
firm D-ring wrist support
FirmFlex
F. custom orthosis
F. custom orthotic
first
F. Aid triple-antibiotic bandage
F. Beat ultrasound stethoscope
F. Check Ecstasy test kit
F. Quality belted undergarment
F. Quality full-fit brief
F. Quality high-performance and
nighttime underpad
F. Quality pad insert and pant
F. Response manual resuscitator
f. rib shears
F. Step select low-air overlay
F. Teeth Infa-dent Combo Pack
F. Temp Genius tympanic
thermometer
FirstChoice
F. closed pouch
F. drainable pouch
F. postoperative drainable pouch
F. urostomy pouch
FirstCyte
F. Aspirator
F. microcatheter
FirstQ departure alert system
**FirstSave automated external
defibrillator**
FirstStep
F. mattress
F. tibial osteotomy instrument

**FirstTemp Genius tympanic
thermometer**
Fisch
F. bone rongeur
F. cutting bur
F. drill
F. dural hook
F. dural retractor
Fischer
F. burner
F. compliance meter
F. modular stereotaxic system
F. nasal rasp
F. & Paykel HC100 heated
humidifier
F. pneumothoracic needle
F. stripper
F. tendon stripper
**Fischer-Leibinger bur hole-mounted
fixation device**
Fisher
F. Accumet pH meter
F. advancement forceps
F. bed
F. brace
F. capsular forceps
F. double-ended retractor
F. eye needle
F. eye spoon
F. fenestrated lid retractor
F. half pin
F. iris forceps
F. lid retractor
F. microcapillary tube reader
F. and Paykel RD1000 resuscitator
F. Scientific Histo-freeze 2000
freezing spray
F. spoon
F. spud
F. tonsillar dissector
F. tonsillar knife
F. tonsillar retractor
F. ventricular cannula
Fisher-Arlt iris forceps
fisherman's pliers
Fisher-Nugent retractor
Fisher-Paykel
F.-P. heated humidifier
F.-P. MR290 water-feed chamber
F.-P. RD1000 resuscitator
Fisher-plus slide
Fisher-Price polycarbonate lens
Fisher-Smith spatula
fishhook
f. lead
f. needle
Fishkind eye speculum
fishmouth drain
Fish sinus probe

F

fishtail
    f. burnisher
    f. chisel
    f. spatula
Fiskars scissors
Fiske periosteal elevator
Fisk tractor
Fisoneb ultrasonic nebulizer
Fison indirect binocular ophthalmoscope
Fisons nebulizer
fissure
    f. bur
    f. burnisher
    f. sealant
fistula
    Cimino f.
    Cimino-Brescia arteriovenous f.
    Gore-Tex AF f.
    Gore-Tex aortofemoral f.
    f. hook
    f. needle
    f. probe
    f. scissors
fistulotome
    needle-knife f.
Fitch obturator
Fit-Lastic
    F.-L. therapy band
    F.-L. therapy tubing
Fitness Ball
Fitnet joint testing system
Fits-All
    F.-A. sling
    F.-A. support
Fitstep II stair climber
fitting
    Luer-Lok f.
Fitz-all fabric leg strap
Fitzgerald
    F. aortic aneurysm clamp
    F. aortic aneurysm forceps
    F. forceps
Fitzpatrick suction tube
Fix
    B-plus F.
    F. and Perm permeabilizing kit
Fixateur
    F. Interne fixation system
    F. Interne rod
    F. Interne screw
fixation
    Ace-Colles f.
    AO rigid f.
    f. apparatus
    Association for
      Osteosynthesis/American Society
      of Internal F. (AO/ASIF)
    f. bandage
    f. base

    f. binocular forceps
    f. button
    DeBastiani f.
    f. device
    dynamic external f.
    ECT internal fracture f.
    f. forceps
    Ganz f.
    f. hook
    hook-plate f.
    Hughes f.
    Ikuta f.
    f. jig
    Kempf internal screw f.
    Kirschner pin f.
    Kirschner wire f.
    Kronner ring f.
    K-wire f.
    LactoSorb resorbable
      craniomaxillofacial f.
    Luque rod f.
    MacroPore mesh f.
    Magerl transarticular screw f.
    f. mechanism
    Meniscus Arrow f.
    Modulock posterior spinal f.
    Murray f.
    Obwegeser-Dalpont internal screw f.
    Orthofix large-pin f.
    OrthoFrame external f.
    OrthoSorb pin f.
    f. pick
    f. pin
    ReUnite hand f.
    f. ring
    Roger Anderson f.
    f. screw
    screw-and-keel f.
    Searcy f.
    Seidel intramedullary f.
    Shepherd internal screw f.
    Slatis f.
    SmartTack f.
    Sof'Wire spinal f.
    Stableloc II external f.
    Sukhtian-Hughes f.
    TransFix ACL system f.
    True-Lok external f.
    f. twist hook
    Wagner f.
    Wasserstein f.
    Zickel nail f.
    Zickel subtrochanteric fracture f.
fixation/anchor forceps
fixator
    Ace-Fischer external f.
    articulated external f.
    1-bar external f.
    biplanar f.

Block f.
cantilever external f.
circular external f.
circular fine-wire external f.
Clyburn Colles fracture f.
Compass Hinge external f.
DeBastiani external f.
D-L internal f.
dynamic axial f.
EBI external f.
Edwards D-L modular f.
external f.
external spinal skeletal f.
Herbert screw f.
Hex-Fix monolateral external f.
hinged articulated f.
Hoffman external f.
Hoffmann C-series Colles wrist f.
Hoffmann external f.
HTO f.
Ilizarov circular external f.
Ilizarov external f.
Ilizarov external ring f.
Ilizarov hybrid f.
Kessler external f.
L-frame f.
mini-Hoffmann external f.
mini-Kessler external f.
mini-Orthofix f.
Monofixateur external f.
Olerud internal f.
Orthofix monolateral femoral
  external f.
Oxford f.
Pennig dynamic wrist f.
Rezaian spinal f.
spanning external f.
Stableloc Colles fracture external f.
thin-wire Ilizarov f.
Thomas f.
Vermont spinal f. (VSF)
Wiltse f.
fixed
f. anatomic patellar implant
f. appliance
f. arch bar
f. bearing knee implant
f. cervical dilator
f. detachable mandibular prosthesis
f. dressing
f. expansion prosthesis
f. femoral head prosthesis
f. forceps
f. mandibular implant
f. offset guide
f. ring retractor
f. suction unit
fixed-angle AO blade-plate
fixed-beam portal

fixed-focus scope
fixed-head screw
fixed-rate
f.-r. asynchronous atrial pacemaker
f.-r. asynchronous ventricular
  pacemaker
fixed-wing transport
fixed-wire
f.-w. balloon
f.-w. coronary balloon catheter
fixer
Wagner f.
Fixion intramedullary humeral nail
fixture
osseointegrated f.
zygoma f.
FK-13K-1 jumbo biopsy forceps
F. L.
F. L. Fischer microsurgical
  neurectomy bayonet scissors
F. L. Fischer modular stereotaxy
  system
**FL3095 fluorescence spectrometer
  system**
Flagg
F. blade
F. fiberglass knee brace
F. laryngoscope
F. stainless steel laryngoscope
  blade
flail implant
flame
f. bur
f. ionization detector
f. photometer
f. photometric detector
flame-tip bur
flamingo
f. antrostomy forceps
F. stent
Flanagan spinal fusion gouge
flange
adhesive f.
Assura pediatric skin barrier f.
ConQuest female continence system
  pressure pad with preattached f.
ConQuest male continence system
  condom catheter with
  preattached f.
endoprosthetic f.
esophageal Z-stent with uncoated f.
tracheostomy tube f.
flanged
4-f. nail
f. revision prosthesis
f. Teflon tube
flap
Abbe f.
Antia composite f.

flap *(continued)*
    f. demarcator
    f. dissector cannula
    E-Z F.
    f. knife
    f. knife dissector
    Leibinger E-Z f.
    muscle f.
    peg f.
    prefabricated composite f.
    Schrudde rotational f.
    f. tip
FlapMaker
    F. disposable microkeratome
    F. microkeratome system
flared
    f. ABS tip
    f. patch mesh
    f. spinal rod
flash
    F. portable spirometer
    f. pump dye laser
FlashCast
    Delta-Lite F.
flashlamp
    EpiLight f.
    f. pulsed Nd:YAG laser
    f. pumped pulsed dye laser
flashlamp-pulsed
    f.-p. dye laser
    f.-p. Nd:YAG laser
FlashPoint
    F. image-guided surgical instrument
    F. optical localizer
flashscanner-enhanced CO_2 laser
flask
    Dewar f.
    Erlenmeyer f.
    Falcon plastic f.
    Primaria tissue culture f.
    tissue culture f.
flat
    f. back curette
    f. bottom reservoir
    f. brain spatula support
    f. burnisher
    f. drill
    f. eye bandage
    F. Foot insole
    f. hook
    f. needle spud
    f. plate
    f. spatula
    f. spatula electrode
    f. spatula needle
    f. tenotomy hook
    f. tube pressure sensor
    f. wire coil stent
flat-bladed nasal speculum

flat-blade-tipped catheter
flat-bottomed Kerrison rongeur
flat-end cutter
flat-panel megavoltage imager
flat-plate detector
Flatt
    F. finger prosthesis
    F. implant
flattened irrigating cannula
flattening filter
F&L attenuating glove
flat-tip electrode
flat-wire eye electrode
flavine wool mold
Flaxedil suture
Fleischer ring
Fleisch pneumotachograph
Fleming ovoid
Flents breast comfort pack
Fletcher
    F. afterloader
    F. sponge forceps
Fletcher-Delclos dome cylinder
Fletcher-Pierce cannula
Fletcher-Suit
    F.-S. afterloading tandem
    F.-S. applicator
    F.-S. polyp forceps
    F.-S. tandem and ovoid
Fletcher-Suit-Delclos
    F.-S.-D. system
    F.-S.-D. tandem
Fletching femoral hernia implant
    material
Flex
    F. DIC tracheostomy tube
    F. Foam brace
    F. Foam dressing
    F. Foam orthosis
    F. H/A total ossicular prosthesis
    F. 4 microwave surgical ablation
        system
    F. 10 microwave surgical ablation
        system
    F. Ranger stretch cable with
        pulley
    F. stent
    F. Tip guidewire
Flex-Aid knuckle dressing
Flexall gel
Flexart MRI scanner
Flexblock temporal fossa implant
Flex-Cath double-lumen intraaortic
    balloon catheter
Flexderm
    F. hydrogel sheet
    F. wound dressing
Flexercell strain unit
Flex-E-Z wax

Flexfilm wound dressing
Flex-Foot Modular III prosthesis
Flexguide intubation guide
Flexiblade laryngoscope
flexible
- f. angioscope
- f. aortic clamp
- f. arm
- f. arm microretractor
- f. aspiration needle
- f. balloon-tipped catheter
- f. bandage
- f. biopsy needle
- f. blade osteotome
- f. bronchoscopy simulator
- f. cardiac valve
- f. coil stent
- f. contact lens
- f. delivery device
- f. digital implant
- f. Dualens implant
- f. endoscope
- f. endoscopic overtube
- f. endoscopic suturing device
- f. endosonography probe
- f. fallopian tube endoscope
- f. fiberoptic bronchoscope
- f. fluoropolymer
- f. fluoropolymer contact lens
- f. foreign body forceps
- f. forward-viewing panendoscope
- f. fulgurating electrode
- f. gastroscope
- f. guidewire
- f. hysteroscope
- f. injection needle
- f. intramedullary nail
- f. laminar bone strip
- f. metal catheter
- f. myocardial biopsy forceps
- f. nasopharyngoscope
- f. Olympus GF-eUM3 device
- f. optical biopsy forceps
- f. orthosis
- f. over-wire system
- f. plastic catheter
- f. plastic suction catheter
- f. pump
- f. radiofrequency coil
- f. reamer
- f. retinal brush
- f. retractor pressure clamp
- f. retractor sliding clamp
- f. rod penile implant
- f. scope
- F. Sew-Right device
- f. sigmoidoscope
- f. silicone implant
- f. socket
- f. sound
- f. spiral wire
- f. stretcher
- f. surface coil
- f. surface coil-type resonator
- f. Teflon catheter
- F. Ti-Knot device
- f. translimbal iris retractor
- f. ureteroscope
- f. vascular clamp
- f. video laparoscope
- f. videolaparoscope
- f. wand
- f. wire electrode

flexible-loop
- f.-l. anterior chamber intraocular lens
- f.-l. posterior chamber intraocular lens

flexible-tip guidewire
flexible-wire bundle reamer
Flexicair
- F. bed
- F. eclipse low-air-loss therapy unit
- F. II low-air-loss therapy unit bed
- F. MC3 low-air-loss therapy unit bed

Flexicath silicone subclavian cannula
Flexicon gauze bandage
Flexi-Cut directional debulking system
Flexicut file
Flexi-Flate
- F.-F. I, II penile prosthesis
- F.-F. penile implant

Flexiflo
- F. Companion enteral feeding pump
- F. enteral feeding tube
- F. gastrostomy tube enteral delivery system
- F. II enteral feeding pump
- F. Inverta-PEG gastrostomy kit
- F. Inverta-PEG tube
- F. Lap G laparoscopic gastrostomy kit
- F. Lap J laparoscopic jejunostomy kit
- F. over-the-guidewire gastrostomy kit
- F. Sacks-Vine tube
- F. stoma-creator tube
- F. Stomate low-profile gastrostomy tube
- F. suction feeding tube
- F. top-fill enteral nutrition system
- F. tungsten weighted feeding tube
- F. Versa-PEG tube

FlexiGard

FlexiGel
F. gel sheet dressing
F. Strands
Flexigrid dressing
Flexi-Grip exercise putty
Flexilite conforming elastic bandage
Flexima
F. biliary drainage catheter
F. biliary stent
F. ureteral catheter
Fleximatic massage/percussion unit
Flexinet dressing
flexion-distraction chiropractic table
flexion glove
Flexipath flexible surgical thoracic trocar
Flexipet micro-manipulation pipette
Flexipost
Flexi-Rod II penile implant
Flexirod penile prosthesis
Flexi-Seal
F.-S. fecal collector
F.-S. fecal collector & tail clip
Flexisensor sensor
Flexisplint flexed arm board
FlexiSport orthotic
Flexi-Stent
Freeman pancreatic F.-S.
FlexiTherm diabetic diagnostic insole
Flexi-Therm liquid crystal system
Flexitip sclerotherapy needle
Flexi-Tip ureteral catheter
Flexitone suture
Flexi-Trak skin anchoring device
Flexlens lens
FlexLite hinged knee support
Flexner-Worst iris claw lens
FlexoFiles
Dentsply F.
Flex-O-Jet aspirator
flexometer
Moeltgen f.
Flexon steel suture
flexor
F. Check-Flo introducer set
f. hinge hand splint brace
F. introducer
Flexoreamer Batt tip
FlexPosure endoscopic retractor
Flex-R-File file
Flex-Rite lumbar support
Flexseat cushion
Flexsite heart stabilizer
Flex-Sprint prosthesis
FlexStent
Cook F.
Gianturco-Roubin F.
F. stent
FlexStrand cable

FlexSure
F. HP
F. in-office rapid serology test kit
FlexTech knee brace
Flextend
F. pacing lead
F. steroid-eluting transvenous pace/sense lead
Flextender Plus hand exerciser
Flex-T guidewire
FlexTip
Arrow Blue F.
F. intervertebral rongeur
FlexVision flexible ureteroscope
Flex-Walk
F.-W. II prosthesis
F.-W. II prosthetic foot
F.-W. prosthesis
Flex-Wrap self-adherent wrap
Flexx biliary stent
Flexxicon
F. Blue dialysis catheter
F. II PC internal jugular catheter
Flexzan
F. Extra foam adhesive dressing
F. foam adhesive wound dressing
F. foam wound dressing
F. topical wound dressing
flicker photometer
Flieringa-Kayser fixation ring
Flieringa-LeGrand fixation ring
Flieringa scleral fixation ring
Flimm-Fighter percussor
Flint glass speculum
flip-flap
Mathieu-Horton-Devine f.-f.
Flip-Flop pillow
Flixene vascular graft
Floam ankle stirrup brace
floater eye model
floating
f. alveolar device
f. catheter
f. lead
f. stent
f. table
floating-disc heart valve
Flocare 500 feeding pump
Flo-Fit
F.-F. Comfortseat
F.-F. cushion
Flo-Gard pump
FloMap
F. guidewire
F. velocimeter
floor-standing surgical light
FloPoint uroflowmeter
floppy guidewire
floppy-tip guidewire

floppy-tipped guidewire
Flo-Rester
    F.-R. vascular occluder
    F.-R. vessel occluder
Florex medical compression stocking
Florida
    F. back brace
    F. cervical brace
    F. contraflexion brace
    F. extension brace
    F. hyperextension brace
    F. J-24, J-35, J-45, J-55 brace
    F. postfusion brace
    F. pouch
    F. spinal brace
    F. urinary pouch
FloSeal matrix hemostatic sealant
floss
    Glide f.
flossAwl floss holder
FlossBrite dental floss device
Floss Rite floss holder
Flo-Stat
    F.-S. fluid management system
    F.-S. fluid monitor
flotation
    f. catheter
    f. gel pad
Flo-Tech prosthetic socket
Flotem IIe fluid-warming device
Flo-Thru shunt
Flo-Trol drinking cup
flow
    f. controller
    f. cytometer
    f. meter
    f. probe
    f. regulated suction tube
    f. restricted oxygen-powered ventilation device
    F. Rider flow-directed catheter
    F. Rider microcatheter
    F. Rider neurovascular catheter
    f. wire
flow-assisted
    f.-a. short-term (FAST)
    f.-a. short-term balloon catheter
flow-based pump
flow-controlled
    f.-c. device
    f.-c. valve
flow-cycled ventilator
flow-directed
    f.-d. balloon cardiovascular catheter
    f.-d. balloon-tipped catheter
    f.-d. end-hole catheter
    f.-d. thermodilution catheter
Flowers
    F. Extended Tear Trough implant

    F. mandibular glove
    F. mandibular glove implant
    F. mandibular implant
    F. tear trough implant
FlowGel barrier material
FloWire
    Doppler F.
    F. Doppler catheter
    F. Doppler guidewire
    F. ultrasound device
flowmeter, flow meter
    AccuTrax peak f.
    AirZone peak f.
    asmaPLAN+ peak f.
    Assess peak f.
    Astech peak f.
    Asthma Check peak f.
    AsthmaMentor peak f.
    blood f.
    CLBF-100 blood f.
    clinical electromagnetic f.
    Dantec rotating disc f.
    Dantec Urodyn 1000 f.
    Doppler f.
    Doppler ultrasonic f.
    electromagnetic f.
    FM color-coded f.
    Gould electromagnetic f.
    Heidelberg retinal f.
    infrared laser Doppler f.
    laser Doppler f.
    Life-Tech f.
    Mini-Wright peak f.
    Narcomatic f.
    Parks bidirectional Doppler f.
    Parks 800 bidirectional Doppler f.
    Periflux PF 1 D blood f.
    Personal Best peak f.
    PocketPeak peak f.
    pulsed Doppler f.
    pulsed Doppler ultrasonic f.
    SensorMedics mass flow sensor heated wire f.
    Spir-O-Flow peak f.
    Statham f.
    Thorpe f.
    transit time f.
    Transonics f.
    Transonics laser Doppler f.
    TruZone peak f.
    Wright peak f.
    Youlten nasal inspiratory peak f.
flow-over vaporizer
flow-oximetry catheter
Flowplus therapeutic pneumatic compression system
flowprobe
    endoscopic f.
flow-regulated suction tube

F

flow-regulator clamp
flow-restricted oxygen-powered
ventilation device
flow-sensing
    f.-s. pneumotachograph
    f.-s. spirometer
Flow-Thru feeding tube
Flowtron
    F. DVT compression device
    F. DVT external pneumatic
      compression system
    F. DVT prophylactic deep venous
      thrombosis unit
    F. DVT pump
    F. DVT pump system
    F. Excel DVI prophylaxis system
    F. pneumatic compression system
      BioCryo system
    F. thigh-high device
Floxite mirror light
Floyd-Barraquer wire speculum
Floyd-Grant erysiphake
Fluency tracheobronchial stent graft
fluff
    f. dressing
    dry sterile f.
fluffed gauze dressing
fluffy compression dressing
fluffy-cuffed tube
Fluftex
    F. gauze roll
    F. gauze rolls and sponge
Flu-Glow strip
Fluhrer
    F. bullet probe
    F. rectal probe
fluid
    f. barrier boot
    f. control trauma pad
    f. prosthesis
    f. warmer
Fluid-Air Plus bed
fluid-filled
    f.-f. balloon
    f.-f. balloon cardiovascular catheter
    f.-f. balloon-tipped flow-directed
      catheter
    f.-f. catheter
    f.-f. pigtail catheter
    f.-f. pressure monitoring guidewire
    f.-f. pressure transducer
Fluidics
    Concentrix F.
Fluidotherapy sterile dry heat modality
fluid-ventilated lens
FluidVision implant
fluorescein angiographer
fluorescence
    f. detector

energy dispersive x-ray f.
    (EDXRF)
    f. excitation filter
    f. fibergastroscope
    f. microscope
fluorescence-activated
    f.-a. cell sorter
    f.-a. cell sorter scan
fluorescence-guided smart laser
fluorescent
    f. lamp
    f. probe
    f. sun lamp
Fluorescite syringe
Fluorets
    F. fluorescein sodium strip
    F. fluorescein sodium strips
Fluorex 300, 500 contact lens
fluoride
    argon f. (ArF)
fluorinated ethylene propylene
Fluor-i-Strip
Fluoro-4 silicone ureteral stent
FluoroCatcher
Fluoro-Free
Fluorognost HIV-1 IFA assay kit
fluorometer
    CytoFluor II f.
    scanning f.
    96-well scanning f.
FluoroNav virtual fluoroscopy system
Fluoropassiv thin-wall carotid patch
fluorophotometer
    Fluorotron master f.
    slit-lamp f.
FluoroPlus
    F. Cardiac
    F. Cardiac digital imaging system
    F. real-time digital imaging system
    F. Roadmapper
    F. Roadmapper digital fluoroscopy
      system
fluoropolymer
    flexible f.
fluoroptic
    f. thermometry probe
    f. thermometry system
FluoroScan
    F. C-arm fluoroscope
    F. imaging system
fluoroscope
    C-arm f.
    Edison f.
    FluoroScan C-arm f.
    XiScan f.
fluoroscopic
    f. foreign body forceps
    f. gantry
    f. imaging chair

fluoroscopy-guided balloon dilator
Fluorospheres
    Immuno-Brite F.
Fluoro Tip ERCP cannula
Fluorotome double-lumen sphincterotome
FluoroTrak fluoroscopy-based surgical navigation system
Fluorotron
    Coherent radiation F.
    F. master fluorophotometer
FluoroVision
Fluotec vaporizer
flush chamber
flushing
    f. device
    f. reservoir
    f. valve
flute
    f. cannula
    f. needle
    f. pipe
fluted
    f. drain
    f. finishing bur
    f. J-Vac drain
    f. reamer
    f. Sampson nail
    f. silicone drain
    f. spiral tubing
    f. stem punch
    f. titanium nail
flute-end right-angle drain
Flutide Diskhaler
Flutter
    F. mucus clearance device
    F. therapeutic device
FLX flexible treatment coilette
FLx/TDx immunoassay analyzer
flying
    f. spot excimer laser system
    f. spot microscope
Flynn
    F. extrusion needle
    F. lens loop
    F. lens loupe
    F. scleral depressor
FM
    F. color-coded flowmeter
    EndoButton F.
    F. wireless assistive listening device
F-MAT screening system
F/M base curve contact lens
FMP acetabular system
FMS Intracell stick
FNA-21
    FNA-21 fine-needle aspiration device

FNA-21 needle
FNA-21 syringe
foam
    Allevyn f.
    CarraSmart f.
    CIDA f.
    f. collar
    copolymer f.
    crosslinked EVA copolymer f.
    f. cube
    f. cube mattress
    f. cushion
    DermaMend f.
    f. dressing
    eggcrate f.
    Evazote f.
    foam compression molded ethylene vinyl acetate f.
    high-density f.
    Ivalon f.
    Neoplush f.
    nonadherent f.
    Oleeva f.
    open-celled f.
    f. pad
    Pedilen polyurethane f.
    Plastazote f.
    polyethylene f.
    polyvinyl alcohol f.
    prosthetic f.
    PV f.
    Reston polyurethane f.
    f. ring
    f. rubber vaginal stent
    f. slant
    soft copolymer f.
    Synthaderm f.
    f. tape
    tube f.
    f. tubing
    f. vacuum pillow
    f. wedge wheelchair cushion
    f. wound dressing
Foamart foot impression system
FoamCare
    F. cleansing system
    F. double scrub brush
foam-padded Velcro restraint
FoamTrac traction bandage
FoamWrap
    F. BuddyWrap
    F. Final Flexion wrap
    F. finger sling
    F. finger trapper
    F. ThumDuction strap
    F. ThumWrap
Fobi pouch
FocalSeal-L surgical sealant
FocalSeal-R neurosurgical stent

F

FocalSeal-S surgical sealant
focimeter
Focus
    F. Dailies toric contact lens
    F. glucose monitoring system
    F. Night & Day contact lens
    F. Night & Day lens
    F. PV catheter
    F. test strip
focused
    f. rigidity casting (FRC)
    f. segmented ultrasound machine
focusing collimator
Foerger airway
Foerster
    F. capsulotomy knife
    F. forceps
    F. iris forceps
    F. sponge-holding forceps
    F. tissue forceps
Foerster-Ballenger forceps
Foerster-Bauer sponge-holding forceps
Foerster-Mueller forceps
Fogarty
    F. adherent clot catheter
    F. arterial embolectomy
    F. arterial embolectomy catheter
    F. arterial irrigation catheter
    F. atrioseptostomy catheter
    F. balloon
    F. balloon biliary catheter
    F. balloon catheter
    F. balloon embolectomy catheter
    F. biliary balloon probe
    F. clamp
    F. dilation catheter
    F. embolectomy catheter
    F. embolus catheter
    F. forceps
    F. graft thrombectomy catheter
    F. Hydragrip clamp
    F. insert
    F. occlusion catheter
    F. spring clip
    F. Thru-Lumen catheter
    F. vascular catheter
    F. venous irrigation catheter
    F. venous thrombectomy catheter
fog reduction/elimination device
FOII powder inhaler
foil
    f. carrier
    scattering f.
    f. sheet
    Shimstock occlusion f.
    titanium f.
Foille dressing
Folatex catheter

foldable
    f. acrylic lens
    f. intraocular lens
    f. iris-claw phakic IOL
    f. 3-piece silicone IOL
    f. plate-haptic silicone intraocular
    lens
    f. silicone implant
    f. silicone IOL
folded aluminum ear splint
folder
    Faulkner f.
    intraocular lens f.
fold forceps
folding
    f. blade
    f. forceps
    f. laryngoscope
    f. lens
folding-frame wheelchair
fold-over finger splint
Foley
    F. balloon
    F. balloon catheter
    F. catheter
    F. cone-tip catheter
    F. Cordostat
    F. hemostatic bag
    F. plate
    F. straight drain
    F. tube
    F. 3-way catheter
Foley-Tractor
    Rutner F.-T.
follicle
    f. aspiration tube
    f. electrode
    f. expressor
follower
    Atala-Shepard coaxial balloon f.
    filiform and f. (F&F)
    Le Fort f.
Foltz
    F. catheter
    F. flushing reservoir
    F. needle
Foltz-Overton cardiac catheter
Fome-Cuf
    F.-C. endotracheal tube
    F.-C. laser kit
    F.-C. pediatric tracheostomy tube
    F.-C. tracheostomy tube
Fomon
    F. angular scissors
    F. chisel
    F. double-edge knife
    F. facelift scissors
    F. hook retractor
    F. lower lateral scissors

F. nasal chisel
F. nasal hook
F. nasal rasp
F. nasal retractor
F. nostril elevator
F. nostril retractor
F. osteotome
F. periosteal elevator
F. periosteotome
F. rasp
F. saber-back scissors
F. upper lateral scissors

Fonar

F. Quad MRI scanner
F. Standing Ovation MRI system
F. Stand-Up MRI scanner

Fonar-360 MRI scanner
Fonix

F. 6500-CX hearing aid test
system
F. hearing aid

food

f. extractor
NutraPrep f.

foot

Carbon Copy II Light f.
Cirrus composite prosthetic f.
College Park TruStep f.
ComfortWalk prosthetic f.
ComfortWalk$_2$ prosthetic f.
f. cradle
f. cushion
C-Walk foot 1C40 prosthetic f.
f. drape
Dycor prosthetic f.
Dynamic Motion F. 1D35
Flex-Walk II prosthetic f.
f. holder
F. Hugger foot support
f. imprinter
Kingsley Steplite f.
F. Levelers custom orthotic
F. Levelers orthosis
F. Levelers Sandalthotics
Lo Rider prosthetic f.
f. magnet
f. model
multiaxis f.
f. orthosis
f. orthotic device
Otto Bock 1A30 Greissinger
Plus f.
Otto Bock 1D25 Dynamic Plus f.
Pathfinder prosthetic f.
f. pillow
QuickFlow DPS f.
f. rest
SACH f.
Silhouette prosthetic f.

single-axis Syme DYCOR f.
f. sling
f. stabilizer
f. stool
Sure-Flex III prosthetic f.
Syme Dycor prosthetic f.
The Beachcomber prosthetic f.
Trowbridge TerraRound f.
Vari-Flex prosthetic f.
f. volumeter
F. Waffle positioner

foot-ankle brace
Footbrush

Dr. Joseph's Original F.

Footdeck Sport exercising footrest
footdrop

f. brace
f. night splint
f. stop
f. strap

footed

3-f. intraocular lens
4-f. lens

Foot-Fitter
FootFlex performance stretching device
footgear

Comed f.
Comed postsurgical f.

Footmaster orthotic
footplate, foot plate

f. elevator
f. hook
f. pick

footrest

Footdeck Sport exercising f.

footwear

Ambulator biomechanical f.
Ambulator conform f.
AquaRunners resistance f.
Comfort Rite f.
Milano Shoethotic f.
Mobils Professionals Pedorthic f.

foramen ovale electrode
foramen-plugging forceps
force

F. balloon
F. balloon dilatation catheter
F. 2 CEM generator
f. fulcrum retractor
F. FX generator
F. GSU argon-enhanced
electrosurgery system
F. GSU laparoscopic handset
f. transducer
F. wire

forced

f. air active cooling device
f. air blanket

forced (*continued*)
f. displacement transducer
f. generation

forceps
abscess f.
Acland clamp-applying f.
Acufex curved basket f.
Adair-Allis tissue f.
Adair uterine f.
adenoid f.
adnexal f.
Adson f.
Adson bayonet dressing f.
Adson bipolar f.
Adson-Brown f.
Adson-Brown tissue f.
Adson clip-introducing f.
Adson dressing f.
Adson hemostatic f.
Adson hypophysial f.
Adson monopolar f.
Adson thumb f.
Adson tissue f.
Adson toothed f.
advancement f.
adventitial f.
Aesculap bipolar cautery f.
air-powered f.
Akahoshi acrylic intraocular lens f.
Akahoshi acrylic IOL loading f.
Akahoshi implantation f.
Akahoshi prechopper f.
Alabama tying f.
Alabama University utility f.
Alexander-Farabeuf f.
Alfonso nucleus f.
Alio capsulorrhexis f.
Alio enclavation f.
Alio iridectomy f.
Alio MICS capsulorrhexis f.
alligator f.
alligator bone-reduction f.
alligator cup f.
alligator ear f.
alligator grasping f.
alligator jaws Olympus FG 6L
  grasping f.
Allis f.
Allis-Abramson breast biopsy f.
Allis-Adair tissue f.
Allis delicate tissue f.
Allis-Duval f.
Allis intestinal f.
Allis tissue f.
Alvis fixation f.
American Catheter Corp. biopsy f.
anastomosis f.
aneurysm f.
Angell James hypophysectomy f.

angiotribe f.
angled capsular f.
angled capsule f.
angled-down f.
angled stone f.
angled-up f.
Anis corneal f.
Anis lens-holding f.
Anis tying f.
anterior f.
anterior capsule f.
antrum punch f.
AO reduction f.
aortic aneurysm f.
Apfelbaum bipolar f.
Apple Medical bipolar f.
applicator f.
apposition f.
approximation f.
Archer splinter f.
Arroyo f.
Arruga f.
Arruga capsule f.
Arruga-Nicetic ophthalmology f.
arterial f.
Arthroforce basket cutting f.
Arthur splinter f.
articulating paper f.
Asch septal f.
Ash septum-straightening f.
Asico capsulorrhexis f.
ASSI bipolar coagulating f.
ASSI capsulorrhexis f.
ASSI IOL inserter f.
ASSI tubing introducer f.
ASSI universal lens folding f.
atraumatic f.
atraumatic locking/grasping f.
atraumatic tissue f.
aural f.
axis traction f.
Azar utility f.
Babcock f.
Babcock intestinal f.
Babcock thoracic tissue f.
Babcock-Vital atraumatic f.
Babcock-Vital tissue f.
baby Adson f.
baby Crile f.
baby Lane f.
baby Mixter f.
baby mosquito f.
baby Overholt f.
backbiting f.
Backhaus f.
Backhaus-Roeder f.
Baer bone-cutting f.
Bahnson-Brown f.
Bailey chalazion f.

Bailey-Williamson obstetrical f.
Bainbridge intestinal f.
Bainbridge thyroid f.
Baird chalazion f.
ball f.
Ballenger sponge f.
Bane rongeur f.
Bangerter muscle f.
Banner f.
Bansal LASIK f.
Bardeleben bone-holding f.
Bard-Parker f.
Bard Precisor direct bite f.
Barnes-Crile hemostatic f.
Barracuda flexible cystoscopic hot
 biopsy f.
Barraquer f.
Barraquer cilia f.
Barraquer-Colibri f.
Barraquer conjunctival f.
Barraquer hemostatic mosquito f.
Barraquer-Katzin f.
Barraquer-von Mandach capsule f.
Barraya tissue f.
Barron alligator f.
Barton f.
Barton obstetrical f.
basket f.
basket cutting f.
basket punch f.
basket-type crushing f.
Bauer sponge f.
Baum-Hecht tarsorrhaphy f.
bayonet f.
bayonet bipolar f.
bayonet monopolar f.
bayonet root tip f.
beaked f.
bean f.
Beardsley intestinal f.
Beasley-Babcock tissue f.
Beaupre cilia f.
Bechert lens-holding f.
Bechert-McPherson tying f.
Beck aorta f.
Beebe hemostatic f.
Bellucci ear f.
Bengolea arterial f.
Bennett cilia f.
Berens corneal transplant f.
Berens muscle f.
Berens ptosis f.
Berens suturing f.
Bergh ciliary f.
Berke cilia f.
Berkeley Bioengineering ptosis f.
Berke ptosis f.
B-H f.
biarticular bone-cutting f.

BiCoag f.
Bierer ovum f.
Billroth uterine tumor f.
binocular fixation f.
biopsy f.
biopsy punch f.
biopsy specimen f.
bipolar f.
bipolar bayonet f.
bipolar coagulating f.
bipolar coaptation f.
bipolar cutting f.
bipolar electrocautery f.
bipolar irrigating f.
bipolar laparoscopic f.
bipolar long-shaft f.
bipolar suction f.
Bircher-Ganske meniscal cartilage f.
Birkett hemostatic f.
Bishop-Harmon crisscross f.
Bishop-Harmon iris f.
Bishop-Harmon ophthalmic f.
Bishop tissue f.
Bissinger detachable bipolar
 coagulation f.
bite biopsy f.
biting f.
Björk diathermy f.
Björk-Stille diathermy f.
Blake dressing f.
Blake ear f.
Blake gallstone f.
Blakesley ethmoid f.
Blakesley-Weil upturned ethmoid f.
Blalock pulmonary artery f.
Blanchard hemorrhoid f.
Blaydes corneal f.
Blaydes lens-holding f.
blepharochalasis f.
Bloodwell f.
Bloodwell-Brown f.
blunt f.
Boer craniotomy f.
Boerma obstetrical f.
Boettcher f.
Boies cutting f.
Bolton f.
Bonaccolto cup jaws f.
Bonaccolto fragment f.
Bonaccolto jeweler's f.
Bonaccolto magnet tip f.
Bonaccolto utility and splinter f.
bone f.
bone-biting f.
bone-cutting f.
bone-holding f.
bone punch f.
bone-reduction f.
bone-splitting f.

F

forceps *(continued)*

Bonn iris f.
Bonn suturing f.
Bores corneal fixation f.
Bores U-shaped f.
Botvin iris f.
Bovie coagulating f.
bowel f.
box-joint f.
Boys-Allis tissue f.
Bozeman f.
Bozeman-Douglas dressing f.
Bozeman LR dressing f.
Bozeman uterine f.
Bozeman uterine dressing f.
Bozeman uterine packing f.
Bracken fixation f.
Bracken iris f.
brain clip f.
brain dressing f.
brain spatula f.
brain tissue f.
brain tumor f.
Brand tendon-holding f.
Brand tendon-passing f.
Bridge deep surgery f.
Bridge hemostatic f.
Brigham thumb tissue f.
bronchial-grasping f.
Broncho pulmonary disposable biopsy f.
bronchus-grasping f.
Brophy dressing f.
Brophy tissue f.
Brown-Adson f.
Brown-Adson side-grasping f.
Brown-Adson tissue f.
Brown-Buerger f.
Brown-Cushing f.
Brown-Grabow capsulorrhexis cystotome f.
Brown insertion f.
Brown side-grasping f.
Brown tissue f.
Bruening f.
Bruening septal f.
Brunner intestinal f.
Brunner tissue f.
Buie biopsy f.
bulldog clamp-applying f.
bullet f.
Buratto f.
Buratto flap f.
Buratto III acrylic implantation f.
Buratto LASIK f.
Buratto ophthalmic f.
Cairns hemostatic f.
Callahan fixation f.
Cameron-Miller type monopolar f.

cannulated bronchoscopic f.
capsular f.
capsule f.
capsule fragment f.
capsule-grasping f.
capsulorrhexis f.
capsulotomy f.
carbide-jaw f.
Cardona threading f.
Carmalt f.
Carmalt splinter f.
Carmody-Brophy f.
Carrel mosquito f.
Carroll bone-holding f.
Carroll dressing f.
Carroll tendon-pulling f.
Carroll tissue f.
cartilage f.
cartilage-holding f.
Cartman lens insertion f.
Casebeer capsulorrhexis f.
Caspar alligator f.
Castroviejo f.
Castroviejo-Arruga capsular f.
Castroviejo capsule f.
Castroviejo clip-applying f.
Castroviejo-Colibri corneal f.
Castroviejo corneal-holding f.
Castroviejo eye suture f.
Castroviejo fixation f.
Castroviejo lid f.
Castroviejo scleral fold f.
Castroviejo suture f.
Castroviejo suturing f.
Castroviejo transplant-grafting f.
Castroviejo tying f.
Castroviejo wide-grip handle f.
catheter-introducing f.
Cauer chalazion f.
Cavanaugh-Wells tonsillar f.
center-action f.
cervical biopsy f.
cervical punch f.
cesarean f.
chalazion f.
Chamberlen obstetrical f.
Championnière f.
Chandler iris f.
Chandler spinal perforating f.
Chaput tissue f.
Charnley suture f.
Charnley wire-holding f.
Cheatle sterilizing f.
Cheron uterine dressing f.
chicken-bill rongeur f.
Child intestinal f.
Children's Hospital intestinal f.
Choyce lens-inserting f.
cilia suture f.

circular cup bronchoscopic
  biopsy f.
Citelli punch f.
Civiale f.
clamp f.
Clark capsule fragment f.
Clarke ligator scissor f.
claw f.
Clayman lens-holding f.
Clayman lens implant f.
Clayman lens-inserting f.
cleft palate f.
Clemetson uterine f.
Clerf f.
Cleveland bone-cutting f.
clip f.
clip-applying aneurysm f.
clip-bending f.
clip-cutting f.
clip-introducing f.
clip-removing f.
closer f.
closing f.
clot f.
coagulating f.
coagulation f.
coaptation bipolar f.
coarctation f.
coated biopsy f.
Codman ovary f.
Cohen corneal f.
cold biopsy f.
cold cup biopsy f.
Colibri f.
College f.
Collier-Crile hemostatic f.
Collin-Duval intestinal thumb f.
Collin intestinal f.
Collin lung-grasping f.
Collin-Pozzi uterine f.
Collin tissue f.
Collin tongue f.
Collin tongue-seizing f.
Collin uterine-elevating f.
Colver tonsil-seizing f.
common duct-holding f.
compression f.
conjunctival fixation f.
connector f.
Connor capsulorrhexis peeler f.
contact compressive f.
continuous clip f.
Cook flexible biopsy f.
Cooley f.
Cooley aortic f.
Cooley coarctation f.
Cooley vascular tissue f.
Corey ovum f.
cornea-holding f.

corneal fixation f.
corneal prosthesis f.
corneal splinter f.
corneal utility f.
corneoscleral f.
Cornet f.
coronary artery f.
Corson myoma grasping f.
Cottle-Arruga cartilage f.
Cottle biting f.
Cottle-Jansen rongeur f.
Cottle-Kazanjian bone-cutting f.
Cottle-Kazanjian nasal f.
Cottle-Kazanjian nasal-cutting f.
Cottle lower lateral f.
Crafoord arterial f.
Craoord-Sellors hemostatic f.
Craig septal f.
Craig septum bone-cutting f.
cranial f.
cranium clip-applying f.
Crawford f.
Crile f.
Crile arterial f.
Crile gall duct f.
Crile hemostatic f.
Crile-Rankin f.
crimper f.
crimping f.
crocodile biopsy f.
cross-action capsule f.
Cryer Universal f.
Culler fixation f.
Cummings folding f.
cup f.
cup biopsy f.
cupped f.
cup-shaped curette f.
curette f.
curved dissecting f.
curved iris f.
curved knot-tying f.
curved Maryland f.
curved microbipolar f.
curved tip jeweler's bipolar f.
curved tying f.
Cushing f.
Cushing bayonet f.
Cushing bipolar neurosurgical f.
Cushing brain f.
Cushing-Brown tissue f.
Cushing dressing f.
Cushing-Taylor carbide-jaw f.
Cushing thumb f.
Cushing tissue f.
cutting f.
cystic duct f.
cystoscopic f.
Dale femoropopliteal anastomosis f.

F

forceps *(continued)*

Dallas lens-inserting f.
Dan chalazion f.
Dandy hemostatic f.
Dandy scalp hemostatic f.
Dardenne nucleus f.
Davis f.
Davis diathermy f.
Davis sterilizing f.
Davis thoracic tissue f.
Dawson-Yuhl-Kerrison rongeur f.
Dawson-Yuhl-Leksell rongeur f.
Dawson-Yuhl rongeur f.
De Alvarez f.
Dean-Shallcross tonsil-seizing f.
Dean tonsillar f.
DeBakey f.
DeBakey arterial f.
DeBakey Atraugrip f.
DeBakey-Colovira-Rumel thoracic f.
DeBakey-Derra anastomosis f.
DeBakey-Diethrich coronary
 artery f.
DeBakey-Diethrich vascular f.
DeBakey dissecting f.
DeBakey-Kelly hemostatic f.
DeBakey-Mixter thoracic f.
DeBakey-Péan cardiovascular f.
DeBakey-Rankin hemostatic f.
DeBakey-Reynolds anastomosis f.
DeBakey-Rumel thoracic f.
DeBakey thoracic f.
DeBakey tissue f.
DeBakey vascular f.
deep surgery f.
deep vessel f.
DeJuan ophthalmic pick f.
DeLee cervical f.
DeLee obstetrical f.
DeLee-Simpson f.
delicate grasping f.
Demel wire-tightening f.
Demel wire-twisting f.
Denis f.
Denis Browne tonsil f.
Dennen f.
dental dressing f.
depilatory dermal f.
Derra-Cooley f.
D'Errico dressing f.
D'Errico hypophysial f.
D'Errico tissue f.
Desjardins f.
Desjardins gallstone f.
Desmarres chalazion f.
DeWeese axis traction f.
Dewey obstetrical f.
diathermic f.
diathermy f.

Dieffenbach f.
Diener f.
dilating f.
Dingman bone-holding f.
disc f.
discectomy f.
disimpaction f.
disposable f.
dissecting f.
divergent outlet f.
Dixon-Lovelace hemostatic f.
Dixon-Thorpe vitreous foreign
 body f.
Dk IOL insertion f.
Dodick lens-holding f.
dolphin-billed grasping f.
dolphin dissecting f.
dolphin grasping f.
dolphin-type atraumatic f.
donor button f.
Dorsey bayonet f.
double-action bone-cutting f.
double-action hump f.
double-concave rat-tooth f.
double-cupped f.
double-ended suture f.
double-fixation f.
double-pronged f.
double-sharp f.
double-spoon biopsy f.
Douglas cilia f.
Doyen intestinal f.
Draeger f.
dressing f.
Drews f.
Drews cilia f.
Drews ciliary f.
Dreyfus prosthesis f.
drill guide f.
duckbill f.
Ducournau fine gripping f.
dull pointed f.
dull rotation f.
Dumont jeweler's f.
Dumont Swiss dissecting f.
Dunhill f.
Duplay tenaculum f.
Duracep biopsy f.
dural f.
Duval-Allis f.
Duval-Collin intestinal f.
Duval intestinal f.
Duval lung grasping f.
Duval lung tissue f.
Duval-Vital intestinal f.
Dyonics basket f.
eagle beak bone-cutting f.
ear dressing f.
ear grasping f.

ear polyp f.
ear punch f.
Eastman cystic duct f.
Eber needle-holder f.
Echlin rongeur f.
Ecker-Kazanjian f.
Eckhoff f.
Edna towel f.
Ehrhardt lid f.
electrocoagulating biopsy f.
electrosurgery f.
electrosurgical biopsy f.
elevating f.
Elliott obstetrical f.
Elschnig capsule f.
Elschnig fixation f.
Elschnig-O'Brien f.
Elschnig-O'Connor fixation f.
end-biting f.
Endo-Assist disposable atraumatic
  grasping f.
Endo-Assist endoscopic f.
endometrial polyp f.
endoscopic f.
endoscopic biopsy f.
Endo-therapy disposable biopsy f.
endotracheal catheter f.
Endura dressing f.
Englert f.
entropion f.
epilation f.
episcleral f.
Eppendorfer biopsy f.
Erhardt lid f.
Ernest-McDonald soft intraocular
  lens-folding f.
Ernest-McDonald soft IOL
  folding f.
esophageal f.
ethmoid f.
ethmoid Blakesley f.
ethmoid cutting f.
ethmoid punch f.
Evans-Vital tissue f.
Everett pile f.
Evershears bipolar laparoscopic f.
Ewald tissue f.
Excel disposable biopsy f.
exolever f.
expansile f.
extracapsular f.
extracting f.
extraction f.
eye dressing f.
eye fixation f.
eyelid f.
Facit uterine polyp f.
fallopian tube f.
Farabeuf bone-holding f.

Farabeuf-Lambotte bone-holding f.
Farkas-Bracken fixation f.
Farnham nasal-cutting f.
Farrior wire-crimping f.
Farris tissue f.
Faulkner lens-holding f.
Faure peritoneal f.
Faure uterine biopsy f.
Fauvel laryngeal f.
FB-25K jumbo biopsy f.
Fechtner conjunctiva f.
Fechtner ring f.
Fehland intestinal f.
Feilchenfeld splinter f.
fenestrated f.
fenestrated blade f.
fenestrated cup biopsy f.
fenestrated ellipsoid spiked open-
  span biopsy f.
fenestrated spiked open-span jumbo
  biopsy f.
Ferguson angiotribe f.
Ferguson bone-holding f.
Ferguson tenaculum f.
Fergusson f.
Ferris-Smith bone-biting f.
Ferris-Smith fragment f.
Ferris-Smith-Kerrison f.
Ferris-Smith-Kerrison f.
Ferris-Smith rongeur f.
Ferris-Smith-Takahashi f.
Ferris-Smith tissue f.
fine arterial f.
Fine-Castroviejo suturing f.
fine cup f.
Fine dissecting f.
Fine gripping f.
Fine-Ikeda capsulorrhexis f.
Fine irrigating capsulorrhexis f.
Fine sideport capsulorrhexis f.
Fine suture-tying f.
fine-tipped up-angled and down-
  angled bipolar f.
Fine tissue f.
fine-toothed f.
Fink-Jameson oblique muscle f.
Finochietto f.
Finochietto thoracic f.
Fisher advancement f.
Fisher-Arlt iris f.
Fisher capsular f.
Fisher iris f.
Fitzgerald f.
Fitzgerald aortic aneurysm f.
fixation f.
fixation/anchor f.
fixation binocular f.
fixed f.
FK-13K-1 jumbo biopsy f.

F

forceps (*continued*)
flamingo antrostomy f.
Fletcher sponge f.
Fletcher-Suit polyp f.
flexible foreign body f.
flexible myocardial biopsy f.
flexible optical biopsy f.
fluoroscopic foreign body f.
Foerster f.
Foerster-Ballenger f.
Foerster-Bauer sponge-holding f.
Foerster iris f.
Foerster-Mueller f.
Foerster sponge-holding f.
Foerster tissue f.
Fogarty f.
fold f.
folding f.
foramen-plugging f.
foreign body f.
foreign body cystoscopy f.
foreign body eye f.
foreign body retrieving f.
Förster iris f.
forward-grasping f.
Foss clamp f.
Foster-Ballenger f.
Fox cartilage f.
Fox tissue f.
Fraenkel f.
fragment f.
Francis spud chalazion f.
Fränkel cutting tip f.
Fränkel esophagoscopy f.
Fränkel laryngeal f.
Fränkel tampon f.
Frankfeldt grasping f.
Freer septal f.
French-pattern f.
Friedman rongeur f.
Fry nasal f.
Fuchs capsular f.
Fuchs capsule f.
Fuchs capsulotomy f.
Fuchs extracapsular f.
Fuchs iris f.
Fujinon biopsy f.
galea f.
gallbladder f.
gall duct f.
gallstone f.
Gardner bone f.
Garland hysterectomy f.
Garrison f.
Gaskin fragment f.
gastrointestinal f.
Gauss hemostatic f.
Gaylor uterine biopsy f.
Gelfilm f.

Gelfoam pressure f.
Gellhorn uterine biopsy f.
Gelpi hysterectomy f.
Gemini gall duct f.
Gemini hemostatic f.
Gemini Mixter f.
general tissue f.
general wire f.
Gerald f.
Gerald bayonet microbipolar neurosurgical f.
Gerald bipolar f.
Gerald dressing f.
Gerald tissue f.
Gerbode f.
GI f.
GIA f.
Gifford fixation f.
Gifford iris f.
Gill-Arruga capsular f.
Gill-Chandler iris f.
Gill-Colibri f.
Gill curved iris f.
Gillespie obstetrical f.
Gill-Fuchs capsular f.
Gill-Hess iris f.
Gillies dissecting f.
Gillies tissue f.
Gill iris f.
Gill-Safar f.
Ginsberg tissue f.
giraffe biopsy f.
Girard corneoscleral f.
Glassman-Allis noncrushing tissue-holding f.
Glassman-Babcock f.
Glassman noncrushing pickup f.
Glassman pickup f.
glenoid reaming f.
globular object f.
Glover coarctation f.
Glover curved f.
Glover patent ductus f.
Glover spoon-shaped f.
Gold deep surgery f.
Gold hemostatic f.
Goldman capsulorrhexis f.
Goldman-Kazanjian nasal f.
Gomco f.
Gordon bead f.
Gordon ciliary f.
Gordon uterine f.
Gordon vulsellum f.
Grabow f.
Gradle cilia f.
Gradle ciliary f.
Graefe f.
Graefe curved iris f.
Graefe dressing f.

Graefe eye fixation f.
Graefe fixation f.
Graefe iris f.
Graefe straight iris f.
Graefe tissue f.
Graefe tissue-grasping f.
Grafco-Halsted f.
grasping f.
grasping biopsy f.
grasping tripod f.
Gray arterial f.
Gray cystic duct f.
Grayson corneal f.
Grazer blepharoplasty f.
Green-Armytage hemostatic f.
Green cystic duct f.
Greene f.
Green fixation f.
Green tissue grasping f.
Greenwood bayonet f.
Greenwood bipolar coagulation-
 suction f.
Gregory f.
Greven alligator f.
Grey Turner f.
Grieshaber diamond-coated f.
Grieshaber internal limiting
 membrane f.
Grieshaber iris f.
Grieshaber manipulator f.
Griffiths-Brown f.
grooved tying f.
Gross dressing f.
Gross sponge f.
f. guard
guide f.
guillotine f.
Guist fixation f.
Gunderson bone f.
Gunderson muscle f.
Gunderson muscle recession f.
Guyton-Clark f.
Guyton-Noyes fixation f.
Hajek antral punch f.
Hajek-Koffler bone punch f.
Hajek-Koffler sphenoidal f.
Hajek sphenoid punch f.
Halberg contact lens f.
Hale obstetrical f.
hallux f.
Halsted f.
Halsted arterial f.
Halsted curved mosquito f.
Halsted hemostatic mosquito f.
Hamilton deep surgery f.
Hardy bayonet dressing f.
Hardy bayonet neurosurgical
 bipolar f.

Hardy microsurgical bayonet
 bipolar f.
harelip f.
Harken f.
Harman fixation f.
Harms-Colibri f.
Harms corneal f.
Harms microtying f.
Harms suture-tying f.
Harms-Tubingen tying f.
Harms tying f.
Harrington f.
Harrington lung-grasping f.
Harrington-Mayo tissue f.
Harrington-Mixter thoracic f.
Harrington thoracic f.
Harrison bone-holding f.
Harris suture-carrying f.
Hartmann alligator f.
Hartmann ear f.
Hartmann ear dressing f.
Hartmann ear polyp f.
Hartmann hemostatic mosquito f.
Hartmann mosquito f.
Hartmann mosquito hemostatic f.
Hartmann nasal-cutting f.
Hartmann nasal-dressing f.
Hartmann nasal polyp f.
Hartmann-Noyes nasal-dressing f.
Hartmann tonsillar punch f.
Hartmann uterine biopsy f.
Hartmann-Weingärtner ear f.
Haslinger tip f.
Hasner lid f.
Hasson bullet-tip f.
Hasson grasping f.
Hasson needle-nose f.
Hasson ring f.
Hasson spike-tooth f.
Hawkins cervical biopsy f.
Hawks-Dennen obstetrical f.
Hayes anterior resection f.
Hayton-Williams f.
Healy gastrointestinal f.
Healy intestinal f.
Healy suture removing f.
Healy uterine biopsy f.
Heaney hysterectomy f.
Heaney-Simon hysterectomy f.
Heaney tissue f.
Heath chalazion f.
Heath clip-removing f.
Heath nasal f.
Heermann alligator f.
Heermann ear f.
Hegenbarth clip-applying f.
Heiss arterial f.
Heiss hemostatic f.
Heller biopsy f.

F

forceps *(continued)*

hemorrhoidal f.
hemostatic f.
hemostatic cervical f.
hemostatic clip-applying f.
hemostatic neurosurgical f.
hemostatic tissue f.
hemostatic tonsillar f.
hemostatic tracheal f.
Henrotin vulsellum f.
Henry cilia f.
Henry ciliary f.
Herrick kidney f.
Hersh LASIK retreatment f.
Hertel kidney stone f.
Hertel stone f.
Hess f.
Hess capsular f.
Hess iris f.
Heyman nasal f.
Heyner f.
Heywood-Smith dressing f.
Hibbs bone-cutting f.
Hibbs bone-holding f.
high f.
high-frequency hemostatic f.
Hildebrandt uterine hemostatic f.
Hinderer cartilage f.
Hirsch hypophysis punch f.
Hirschman lens f.
Hirst placental f.
Hodge obstetrical f.
Hoffmann ear punch f.
holding f.
hollow-object f.
Holmes fixation f.
Holth f.
Holth punch f.
hook f.
Hopkins f.
Hopkins aortic f.
Horsley bone-cutting f.
Horsley-Stille bone-cutting f.
Horsley-Stille rib shears f.
Hoskins beaked Colibri f.
Hoskins fine straight f.
Hoskins fixation f.
Hoskins miniaturized micro straight f.
Hoskins straight microiris f.
Hoskins suture f.
host tissue f.
hot biopsy f.
hot flexible f.
Hot Sampler disposable hot biopsy f.
House alligator crimper f.
House alligator grasping f.
House alligator strut f.
House cup f.
House-Dieter eye f.
House ear f.
House Gelfoam pressure f.
House grasping f.
House miniature f.
House oval-cup f.
House pressure f.
House strut f.
Howmedica Microfixation System f.
Hubbard corneoscleral f.
Hudson f.
Hudson brain f.
Hudson cranial f.
Hudson dressing f.
Hudson rongeur f.
Hudson tissue f.
Hufnagel mitral valve f.
Hulka clip f.
Hulka tenaculum f.
hump f.
Hunt f.
Hunt angled serrated ring f.
Hunt angled tip f.
Hunt bipolar f.
Hunt chalazion f.
Hunter splinter f.
Hunt grasping f.
Hurd bone f.
Hurd bone-cutting f.
Hurd septal bone-cutting f.
Hurd septum-cutting f.
Hyde double-curved f.
hyoid cutting f.
hypogastric artery f.
hypophysial f.
hysterectomy f.
Ikeda microcapsulorrhexis f.
Ilg curved micro tying f.
iliac f.
IM Jaws alligator f.
implant f.
implantation f.
Inamura small incision capsulorrhexis f.
infant biopsy f.
infundibular f.
inlet f.
insertion f.
instrument grasping f.
insulated f.
insulated bayonet f.
insulated monopolar f.
insulated tissue f.
intervertebral disc f.
intestinal anastomosis f.
intestinal closing f.
intestinal holding f.
intestinal tissue f.

intracapsular lens f.
intraocular f.
intraocular irrigating f.
intraocular lens f.
intrathoracic f.
introducing f.
Iowa membrane f.
Iowa State fixation f.
iris f.
iris bipolar f.
iris tissue f.
Iselin f.
isolation f.
Jackson alligator grasping f.
Jackson approximation f.
Jackson biopsy f.
Jackson broad staple f.
Jackson button f.
Jackson conventional foreign
  body f.
Jackson cross-action f.
Jackson cylindrical object f.
Jackson double-prong f.
Jackson dressing f.
Jackson dull rotation f.
Jackson endoscopic f.
Jackson flexible upper lobe
  bronchus f.
Jackson forward grasping f.
Jackson hollow object f.
Jackson laryngeal applicator f.
Jackson laryngeal basket f.
Jackson laryngeal punch f.
Jackson laryngeal ring-rotation f.
Jackson laryngofissure f.
Jackson papilloma f.
Jackson ring jaw globular object f.
Jackson ring rotation f.
Jackson sharp-pointed rotation f.
Jackson tendon-seizing f.
Jacob capsule fragment f.
Jacobs biopsy f.
Jacobson f.
Jacobson hemostatic f.
Jacobson mosquito f.
Jacobs vulsellum f.
Jaffe capsulorrhexis f.
Jako laryngeal f.
Jako microlaryngeal cup f.
Jako microlaryngeal grasping f.
Jameson muscle f.
Jameson muscle recession f.
Jameson strabismus f.
James wound f.
Jansen bayonet dressing f.
Jansen dissecting f.
Jansen dressing f.
Jansen-Middleton nasal cutting f.
Jansen-Middleton punch f.

Jansen-Middleton septal f.
Jansen-Middleton septotomy f.
Jansen-Middleton septum cutting f.
Jansen monopolar f.
Jansen nasal dressing f.
Jansen thumb f.
Jarcho tenaculum f.
Jarell f.
Jarit microsuture tying f.
Jarit mosquito f.
Jarit tendon-pulling f.
Jarit tube-occluding f.
Jawz disposable biopsy f.
Jensen intraocular lens f.
Jerald f.
Jervey capsule fragment f.
Jervey iris f.
jeweler's f.
jeweler's bipolar f.
jeweler's pickup f.
Johns Hopkins gallbladder f.
Johns Hopkins gall duct f.
Johns Hopkins hemostatic f.
Johns Hopkins occluding f.
Johns Hopkins serrefine f.
Johnson brain tumor f.
Johnson ptosis f.
Johnson thoracic f.
Jones f.
Jones hemostatic f.
Jones IMA f.
Jones towel f.
Jordan strut f.
Judd f.
Judd-Allis intestinal f.
Judd-Allis tissue f.
Judd strabismus f.
Judd suture f.
Juers crimper f.
Juers-Lempert rongeur f.
Juers lingual f.
Julian splenorenal f.
Julian thoracic f.
Julian thoracic artery f.
jumbo f.
jumbo biopsy f.
Kahler f.
Kahler bronchial biopsy f.
Kahler bronchoscopic f.
Kahler bronchus grasping f.
Kahler laryngeal biopsy f.
Kahler polyp f.
Kahn tenaculum f.
Kalman occluding f.
Kalman tube-occluding f.
Kalt f.
Kalt capsular f.
Kansas fragment lens f.
Kansas University corneal f.

F

forceps *(continued)*

Kantor f.
Kantrowitz dressing f.
Kantrowitz thoracic f.
Kantrowitz tissue f.
Kapp f.
Kapp-Beck f.
Karl Storz reusable multifunction
  valve trocar take-apart scissors f.
Katena capsulorrhexis f.
Katzin-Barraquer f.
Kaufman ENT f.
Kawai capsulorrhexis f.
Kazanjian bone-cutting f.
Kazanjian cutting f.
Kazanjian nasal hump f.
Keeler extended round tip f.
Keeler intraocular foreign body
  grasping f.
Keen Edge disposable biopsy f.
Kelly f.
Kelly arterial f.
Kelly dressing f.
Kelly-Gray uterine f.
Kelly hemostatic f.
Kelly-Murphy f.
Kelly ovum f.
Kelly placental f.
Kelly polypus f.
Kelly-Rankin f.
Kelly tissue f.
Kelly urethral f.
Kelly vulsellum f.
Kelman implantation f.
Kelman intraocular f.
Kelman irrigator f.
Kelman-McPherson corneal f.
Kelman-McPherson lens-holding f.
Kelman-McPherson microtying f.
Kelman-McPherson suture f.
Kelman-McPherson suturing f.
Kelman-McPherson tissue f.
Kelman-McPherson tying f.
Kennedy vulsellum f.
Kennerdell bayonet f.
Kent deep surgery f.
Kern bone-holding f.
Kern-Lane bone f.
Kerrison f.
Kershner butterfly capsulorrhexis f.
Kershner LASIK flap f.
Kershner 1-step micro
  capsulorhexis f.
Kevorkian uterine biopsy f.
Kevorkian-Younge cervical
  biopsy f.
Kevorkian-Younge uterine biopsy f.
Khodadad microclip f.
kidney elevating f.

kidney pedicle f.
kidney stone f.
Kielland f.
Killian septal compression f.
Kinder Design pedo f.
King-Prince muscle f.
King-Prince recession f.
Kingsley grasping f.
King tissue f.
King wound f.
Kirby capsular f.
Kirby capsule f.
Kirby corneoscleral f.
Kirby eye tissue f.
Kirby fixation f.
Kirby intracapsular lens f.
Kirby iris f.
Kirby tissue f.
Kjelland f.
Kjelland obstetrical f.
KleenSpec f.
Kleinert-Kutz bone-cutting f.
Kleinert-Kutz rongeur f.
Kleinert-Kutz tendon f.
Kleinert-Kutz tendon-passing f.
Kleinert-Kutz tendon-retrieving f.
Kleppinger bipolar f.
Knapp f.
Knapp trachoma f.
Knight bone-cutting f.
Knight nasal-cutting f.
Knight nasal septum-cutting f.
Knight polyp f.
Knight septal f.
Knight septum-cutting f.
Knight turbinate f.
Knolle lens implantation f.
Knolle-Shepard lens f.
Knolle-Shepard lens-holding f.
knot-holding f.
knotting f.
Kocher f.
Kocher arterial f.
Kocher artery f.
Kocher hemostatic f.
Kocher kidney elevating f.
Koeberlé f.
Koenig vascular f.
Koerte gallstone f.
Kogan endospeculum f.
Kolodny f.
Kraff fixation f.
Kraff intraocular utility f.
Kraff lens-holding f.
Kraff lens-inserting f.
Kraff suturing f.
Kraff tying f.
Kraff-Utrata capsulorrhexis f.
Kraff-Utrata intraocular utility f.

Kraff-Utrata tear capsulotomy f.
Kraft f.
Kramer f.
Kratz lens-inserting f.
Krause biopsy f.
Krause esophagoscopy f.
Krause punch f.
Krause universal f.
Kremer corneal fixation f.
Kremer 2-point fixation f.
Kronfeld micropin f.
Kronfeld suturing f.
Krönlein hemostatic f.
Krukenberg pigment spindle f.
Kuehne coverglass f.
Kuhnt capsular f.
Kuhnt fixation f.
Kulvin-Kalt iris f.
Kurstin flap-stretching f.
Kurze pickup f.
Küstner uterine tenaculum f.
Laborde f.
Lahey arterial f.
Lahey-Babcock f.
Lahey dissecting f.
Lahey gall duct f.
Lahey goiter seizing f.
Lahey goiter vulsellum f.
Lahey hemostatic f.
Lahey lock arterial f.
Lahey-Péan f.
Lahey thoracic f.
Lahey thyroid tenaculum f.
Lahey thyroid tissue traction f.
Lahey thyroid traction vulsellum f.
Lalonde delicate hook f.
Lalonde extra-fine skin hook f.
Lalonde hook f.
Lambert chalazion f.
Lambert hook f.
Lambert-Kay anastomosis f.
Lambotte bone-holding f.
Lambotte fibular f.
Lancaster-O'Connor f.
lancet-shaped biopsy f.
Landers vitrectomy lens f.
Landolt spreading f.
Lane bone-holding f.
Lane gastrointestinal f.
Lane intestinal f.
Lane screw-holding f.
Lane tissue f.
Lange approximation f.
Langenbeck bone-holding f.
Lang iris f.
laparoscopic plasma f.
Laplace f.
large angled f.
large cup f.

LaRoe undermining f.
Larsen tendon f.
Larsen tendon-holding f.
laryngeal applicator f.
laryngeal basket f.
laryngeal biopsy f.
laryngeal bronchial grasping f.
laryngeal curette f.
laryngeal grasping f.
laryngeal punch f.
laryngeal rotation f.
laryngeal sponging f.
laryngofissure f.
laser microlaryngeal cup f.
laser microlaryngeal grasping f.
laser ovary f.
Laufe divergent outlet f.
Laufe obstetrical f.
Laufe-Piper f.
Laufe-Piper obstetrical f.
Laufe-Piper uterine polyp f.
Laufe uterine polyp f.
Laurer f.
Lawrence deep surgery f.
Lawrence hemostatic f.
Lawton f.
Leahey chalazion f.
Lebsche f.
Lees arterial f.
Lees nontraumatic f.
Leff f.
Lefferts bone-cutting f.
Lehner-Utrata capsulorrhexis f.
Leibinger Micro System plate-holding f.
Leigh capsule f.
Lejeune thoracic f.
Leksell rongeur f.
Leland-Jones f.
Lemoine f.
Lempert rongeur f.
lens implantation f.
lens loop f.
lens threading f.
Leonard f.
Leo Schwartz sponge-holding f.
Leriche hemostatic f.
Leriche tissue f.
LeRoy clip-applying f.
Lester fixation f.
Lester muscle f.
Levret f.
Lewin f.
Lewin bone-holding f.
Lewin spinal perforating f.
Lewis septal f.
Lewis tonsillar hemostatic f.
Lewis ureteral stone isolation f.
Lewkowitz lithotomy f.

F

forceps *(continued)*

Lewkowitz ovum f.
Lewkowitz placental f.
Lexer tissue f.
lid f.
Lieberman lens-holding f.
Lieberman micro-ring lens f.
Lieberman suturing f.
Lieberman tying f.
Lieb-Guerry f.
ligament grasping f.
ligamentum flavum f.
ligature f.
ligature carrying f.
Lillie intestinal f.
Lillie tissue-holding f.
Lindstrom lens-insertion f.
lingual f.
Linnartz f.
lion f.
lion-jaw f.
lion-jaw bone-holding f.
Lister f.
Lister conjunctival f.
Liston bone-cutting f.
Liston-Key bone-cutting f.
Liston-Key-Horsley f.
Liston-Littauer bone-cutting f.
Liston-Stille bone-cutting f.
lithotomy f.
Littauer bone-cutting f.
Littauer cilia f.
Littauer ear dressing f.
Littauer ear polyp f.
Littauer-Liston bone-cutting f.
Littauer nasal dressing f.
Littauer-West cutting f.
Littlewood tissue f.
Livernois lens-holding f.
Livernois pickup and folding f.
Livingston f.
Llorente dissecting f.
Lloyd-Davies occlusion f.
lobectomy f.
lobe grasping f.
lobe holding f.
lobster bone-reduction f.
Lockwood-Allis intestinal f.
Lockwood-Allis tissue f.
Lockwood intestinal f.
Lockwood tissue f.
Lombard-Beyer f.
London tissue f.
Long Island College Hospital placental f.
long-jaw basket f.
long-jaw disposable f.
long tissue f.
loop-type snare f.

loop-type stone-crushing f.
loose body suction f.
Lordan chalazion f.
Lore subglottic f.
Lore suction tube-holding f.
Lore suction tube and tip-holding f.
Lothrop ligature f.
Love-Gruenwald alligator f.
Love-Gruenwald pituitary f.
Love-Kerrison rongeur f.
Lovelace bladder f.
Lovelace gallbladder traction f.
Lovelace hemostatic f.
Lovelace lung grasping f.
Lovelace thyroid traction vulsellum f.
Lovelace tissue f.
Lovelace traction lung f.
Lovelace traction tissue f.
low f.
Löw-Beer f.
Löwenberg f.
lower gall duct f.
lower lateral f.
Lowman bone-holding f.
low outlet f.
Lowsley grasping f.
Lowsley prostatic f.
Luc f.
Lucae bayonet dressing f.
Lucae bayonet ear f.
Lucae bayonet tissue f.
Lucae dissecting f.
Lucae dressing f.
Luc ethmoidal f.
Luc nasal cutting f.
Luc septal f.
Luc septum cutting f.
Luer curette f.
Luer hemorrhoidal f.
Luer rongeur f.
Luer-Whiting rongeur f.
Luhr microfixation system plate-holding f.
Luikart f.
Luikart-Bill f.
Luikart-Kjelland obstetrical f.
Luikart-Simpson obstetrical f.
lung grasping f.
lung tissue f.
Lusk f.
Lutz septal f.
Lynch cup-shaped curette f.
Lynch laryngeal f.
Lyon f.
MacCarty f.
Machemer diamond dust-coated foreign body f.

Machemer diamond-dusted f.
Madden f.
Madden-Potts intestinal f.
Madden-Potts tissue f.
Magill f.
Magill catheter f.
Magill endotracheal f.
Maier dressing f.
Maier polyp f.
Maier sponge f.
Maier uterine f.
Maingot hysterectomy f.
Malis angled bayonet f.
Malis bipolar coagulation f.
Malis bipolar cutting f.
Malis bipolar irrigating f.
Malis cup f.
Malis-Jensen bipolar f.
Malis-Jensen microbipolar f.
Malis jeweler's bipolar f.
Malis titanium microsurgical f.
malleus f.
mammary-coronary tissue f.
Manche LASIK f.
Manhattan Eye & Ear suturing f.
Manning f.
Mansfield f.
Mantis retrograde f.
marginal chalazion f.
Markwalder rib f.
Martin bipolar coagulation f.
Martin cartilage f.
Martin meniscal f.
Martin nasopharyngeal biopsy f.
Martin thumb f.
Martin uterine tenaculum f.
Maryland tissue-grasping f.
Masket capsulorrhexis f.
Masterson hysterectomy f.
Mastin goiter f.
Mastin muscle f.
Mathieu foreign body f.
Mathieu tongue f.
Mathieu urethral f.
matte black f.
Matthew f.
Maumenee f.
Maumenee capsular f.
Maumenee capsule f.
Maumenee-Colibri corneal f.
Maumenee corneal f.
Maumenee cross-action capsular f.
Maumenee straight-action
  capsular f.
Maumenee tissue f.
Max Fine f.
Max Fine tying f.
maxillary disimpaction f.
maxillary fracture f.

Maxum Carr-Locke angled f.
Maxum reusable f.
Maxum reusable endoscopic f.
Mayer f.
Mayfield f.
Mayfield aneurysm f.
Mayo bone-cutting f.
Mayo-Harrington f.
Mayo kidney pedicle f.
Mayo-Ochsner f.
Mayo-Robson gastrointestinal f.
Mayo tissue f.
Mayo ureter isolation f.
Mazzariello-Caprini f.
McCain TMJ f.
McCarthy visual hemostatic f.
McClintock placental f.
McClintock uterine f.
McCollough tying f.
McCoy septal f.
McCoy septum cutting f.
McCullough strabismus f.
McCullough suture-tying f.
McCullough suturing f.
McDonald lens-folding f.
McDonald soft IOL folding f.
McGannon lens f.
McGee-Priest wire f.
McGee wire closure f.
McGee wire-crimping f.
McGill f.
McGivney f.
McGivney hemorrhoidal f.
McGregor conjunctival f.
McGuire marginal chalazion f.
McIndoe bone-cutting f.
McIndoe dissecting f.
McIndoe dressing f.
McIndoe rongeur f.
McIntosh suture-holding f.
McKenzie clip applying f.
McKernan-Adson f.
McKernan Potts f.
McLane f.
McLane obstetrical f.
McLane pile f.
McLane-Tucker obstetrical f.
McLean capsular f.
McLean muscle-recession f.
McLean ophthalmic f.
McNealey-Glassman-Mixter f.
McPherson f.
McPherson angled f.
McPherson bent f.
McPherson-Castroviejo f.
McPherson corneal f.
McPherson irrigating f.
McPherson lens f.
McPherson microbipolar f.

F

forceps *(continued)*

McPherson microcorneal f.
McPherson microiris f.
McPherson microsuture f.
McPherson-Pierse microcorneal f.
McPherson-Pierse microsuturing f.
McPherson straight bipolar f.
McPherson suture-tying f.
McPherson suturing f.
McPherson tying iris f.
McQuigg f.
McWhorter tonsillar f.
mechanical finger f.
Medicon wire twister f.
medium f.
Meeker deep surgery f.
Meeker gallbladder f.
Meeker hemostatic f.
Meeker intestinal f.
meibomian expressor f.
membrane f.
membrane peeling f.
membrane puncturing f.
Mendez multipurpose LASIK f.
meniscal basket f.
meniscus f.
Mermoud nonpenetrating
  glaucoma f.
Michel clip-applying f.
Michel clip-removing f.
Michigan intestinal f.
micro-Allis f.
microarterial f.
microbayonet f.
microbiopsy f.
microbipolar f.
MicroBite f.
microbronchoscopic tissue f.
microclamp f.
microclip f.
micro Colibri f.
microcorneal f.
microcup pituitary f.
microdissecting f.
microdressing f.
micro Halstead arterial f.
microneedle holder f.
microneurosurgical f.
Micro-One dissecting f.
micropin f.
microserrated Tano asymmetrical
  peeling f.
microsurgical biopsy f.
microsurgical grasping f.
microsurgical tying f.
microtip bipolar jeweler's f.
microtissue f.
Micro-Two f.
microtying f.

microvascular clamp-applying f.
microvascular tying f.
Microvasive disposable alligator-
  shaped f.
Microvasive radial-jaw biopsy f.
middle ear strut f.
Mighty Bite Zimmon lateral biopsy
  cup f.
Mikulicz peritoneal f.
Miles punch biopsy f.
Miller articulating f.
Millin f.
Millin capsular f.
Millin prostatectomy f.
Mill-Rose RiteBite biopsy f.
miniature f.
miniature intestinal f.
mitral valve-holding f.
Mixter f.
Mixter baby hemostatic f.
Mixter mosquito f.
Mixter thoracic f.
monopolar coagulating f.
monopolar insulated f.
Moody fixation f.
mosquito f.
mosquito hemostatic f.
Mount intervertebral disc f.
Mount-Mayfield aneurysm f.
mouse-tooth f.
Moynihan artery f.
Moynihan towel f.
Multibite multiple sample biopsy f.
multipurpose f.
multitooth f.
Murphy-Péan hemostatic f.
muscle f.
Museau uterine f.
Museau vulsellum f.
Myerson laryngeal f.
Myles hemorrhoidal f.
Myles nasal f.
Nadler bipolar coaptation f.
Naegele obstetrical f.
nail-cutting f.
nail-extracting f.
nail-pulling f.
Nakao Ejector biopsy f.
nasal alligator f.
nasal bone f.
nasal cartilage-holding f.
nasal cutting f.
nasal dressing f.
nasal hump-cutting f.
nasal insertion f.
nasal lower lateral f.
nasal needle holder f.
nasal polyp f.
nasal septal f.

nasopharyngeal biopsy f.
National Institutes of Health mitral
  valve grasping f.
needle f.
needle holder f.
Nelson tissue f.
neonatal vascular f.
nephrolithotomy f.
Neville-Barnes f.
Newman collagen plug inserter f.
New Orleans Eye & Ear
  fixation f.
New tissue f.
Nicola f.
Niro bone-cutting f.
Niro wire-twisting f.
Noble f.
noncrushing intestinal f.
nonfenestrated f.
nonperforating towel f.
nontoothed f.
no-scalpel vasectomy fixator ring
  clamp f.
Noto polypus f.
Noto sponge f.
Noyes f.
Noyes ear f.
Noyes nasal f.
Nugent utility f.
Nussbaum intestinal f.
O'Brien fixation f.
O'Brien tissue f.
obstetric f.
obstetrical f.
occluding f.
Ochsner arterial f.
Ochsner hemostatic f.
Ochsner tissue/cartilage f.
O'Connor iris f.
O'Connor sponge f.
O'Gawa tying f.
Ogura tissue/cartilage f.
O'Hara f.
Oldberg intervertebral disc f.
Olivecrona clip-applying and
  removing f.
Olivecrona-Toennis clip-applying f.
Olympus Endo-Therapy disposable
  biopsy f.
Olympus FB-20C endoscopic f.
Olympus FBK-13 f.
Olympus FB-25K endoscopic f.
Olympus FB series biopsy f.
Olympus FB-24U biopsy f.
Olympus FG-12U wide-mouth f.
Olympus FK-13-1 biopsy f.
Olympus FS-K series endoscopic
  suture-cutting f.
Olympus grasping rat-tooth f.

Olympus hot biopsy f.
Olympus reusable oval cup f.
Olympus tripod-type endoscopic f.
Ombrédanne f.
optical biopsy f.
oral rongeur f.
orthopaedic f.
Osher foreign body f.
Osher superior rectus f.
ossicle-holding f.
outlet f.
oval f.
oval cup f.
ovary f.
Overholt clip-applying f.
Overholt-Geissendörfer arterial f.
Overholt-Mixter dissecting f.
ovum f.
Packer mosquito f.
packing f.
Palmer ovarian biopsy f.
papilloma f.
parametrium f.
partial occlusion f.
Passarelli 1-pass capsulorrhexis f.
passing f.
patent ductus f.
Paton anterior chamber lens
  implant f.
Paton capsule f.
Paton corneal transplant f.
Paton suturing f.
Paton tying/stitch removal f.
Paufique suturing f.
Payne-Péan arterial f.
Payr pylorus f.
Péan arterial f.
Péan hemostatic f.
Péan hysterectomy f.
Péan intestinal f.
Péan sponge f.
peanut grasping f.
peanut sponge-holding f.
peapod bead-type f.
peapod intervertebral disc f.
pediatric f.
pedicle f.
Peet f.
Peet splinter f.
pelican biopsy f.
pelvic reduction f.
pelvic tissue f.
Pennington hemostatic f.
Pennington tissue f.
Pennington tissue grasping f.
Percy intestinal f.
Percy tissue f.
Perez-Castro f.
perforating f.

F

forceps *(continued)*

peripheral blood vessel f.
peripheral iridectomy f.
peripheral vascular f.
peritoneal f.
Perman cartilage f.
Perone LASIK flap f.
Peyman-Green vitreous f.
phalangeal f.
Phaneuf hysterectomy f.
Phaneuf peritoneal f.
Phaneuf uterine artery f.
Phillips fixation f.
phimosis f.
phrenicectomy f.
pickup f.
pickup noncrushing f.
Pierse-Colibri corneal utility f.
Pierse corneal Colibri-type f.
Pierse fixation f.
Pierse tip f.
pillar grasping f.
Pilling Weck Y-stent f.
pin-bending f.
pinch f.
pin-seating f.
Piper obstetrical f.
Pistofidis cervical biopsy f.
pituitary f.
placement f.
placenta previa f.
plain f.
plastic f.
plate-holding f.
platform f.
pleurectomy f.
Pley capsular f.
Pley extracapsular f.
point f.
Polaris reusable f.
Pollock f.
polyp f.
polypus f.
Poppen f.
Poppen intervertebral disc f.
Positrap 3-prong nonretracting grasping f.
Post f.
posterior f.
postnasal sponge f.
Potts f.
Potts bronchial f.
Potts bulldog f.
Potts-Smith bipolar f.
Potts-Smith dressing f.
Potts-Smith monopolar f.
Potts-Smith tissue f.
Potts thumb f.
Pozzi tenaculum f.

pre-chopping f.
Precisor Broncho pulmonary disposable biopsy f.
Precisor Direct Bite biopsy f.
Precisor disposable biopsy f.
prepuce f.
pressure f.
Preston ligamentum flavum f.
Primbs suturing f.
Prince advancement f.
Prince muscle f.
Prince trachoma f.
3-prong grasping f.
prostatectomy f.
prostatic lobe f.
Providence Hospital arterial f.
ptosis f.
pulmonary arterial f.
pulmonary vessel f.
punch f.
Puntenney f.
pupil spreader/retractor f.
quadripolar cutting f.
Quevedo fixation f.
Quinones-Neubüser uterine-grasping f.
Quinones uterine-grasping f.
Quire foreign body f.
Quire mechanical finger f.
Raaf-Oldberg intervertebral disc f.
Radial Jaw biopsy f.
Radial Jaw bladder biopsy f.
Radial Jaw hot biopsy f.
Radial Jaw III Max Capacity 1589 biopsy f.
Radial Jaw III Max Capacity with needle biopsy f.
Radial Jaw III single-use biopsy f.
Raimondi hemostatic f.
Raimondi scalp hemostatic f.
Ramirez EndoForehead f.
Rampley sponge f.
Rampley sponge-holding f.
Randall stone f.
Raney scalp clip-applying f.
Rankin-Crile f.
Rappazzo intraocular foreign body f.
rat-tooth f.
rat-tooth Olympus FG 8L grasping f.
reach-and-pin f.
recession f.
rectal f.
Reese muscle f.
Reich-Nechtow hysterectomy f.
Reiner-Knight f.
Reisinger lens-extracting f.
renal artery f.

resection intestinal f.
retrieval f.
reverse-action hypophysectomy f.
Rhein Artisan lens-holding f.
Rhein capsulorrhexis cystotome f.
Rhein fine foldable lens-insertion f.
Rhein LASIK flap f.
rib f.
rib rongeur f.
Rica clip-applying f.
Riches artery f.
Riches diathermy f.
Richter-Heath clip-removing f.
ridge f.
right-angle f.
rigid biopsy f.
rigid kidney stone f.
ring f.
ring rotation f.
ring tip f.
RiteBite biopsy f.
Rizzuti rectus f.
Roberts arterial f.
Robson intestinal f.
Rochester-Carmalt f.
Rochester-Ochsner f.
Rochester oral tissue f.
Rochester-Péan f.
Rochester-Péan hysterectomy f.
Rochester Russian tissue f.
Roeder f.
Roger f.
Rolf f.
roller f.
rongeur f.
rotating f.
round f.
round-handled f.
round punch f.
Rowe disimpaction f.
Rowe glenoid reaming f.
Rowe-Harrison bone-holding f.
Rowe-Killey f.
Rowe maxillary f.
Rowe modified Harrison f.
Rowland double-action f.
rubber-shod f.
Rudd Clinic hemorrhoidal f.
Ruel f.
Ruskin bone-cutting f.
Ruskin-Liston bone-cutting f.
Ruskin rongeur f.
Ruskin-Rowland bone-cutting f.
Russian Péan f.
Rycroft tying f.
Sachs tissue f.
Saenger ovum f.
Samuels f.
Samuels hemoclip-applying f.

Sanders-Castroviejo suturing f.
Sandt f.
Sarot arterial f.
Satinsky f.
Sattler advancement f.
Sauerbruch rib f.
Sauer suture f.
Sauer suturing f.
Saupe cilia f.
Sawtell artery f.
scalp clip-applying f.
Scanzoni f.
Schaaf foreign body f.
Schepens f.
Schlesinger cervical punch f.
Schlesinger intervertebral disc f.
Schlesinger rongeur f.
Schnidt thoracic f.
Scholten biopsy f.
Scholten endomyocardial biopsy f.
Schroeder-Braun uterine f.
Schroeder uterine vulsellum f.
Schubert cervical biopsy f.
Schubert uterine biopsy f.
Schumacher biopsy f.
Schwartz clip-applying f.
Schwartz temporary clamp-
  applying f.
Schweigger capsule f.
scissors f.
scleral twist-grip f.
Scott lens-insertion f.
Scoville clip-applying f.
Scoville-Greenwood bayonet
  neurosurgical bipolar f.
screw-holding f.
Scudder intestinal f.
Segond hysterectomy f.
Segond-Landau hysterectomy f.
Seitzinger tripolar cutting f.
seizing f.
self-centering bone-holding f.
self-opening f.
self-retaining bone f.
Selman tissue f.
Selverstone intervertebral disc f.
Selverstone rongeur f.
Semb bone f.
Semb bone-cutting f.
Semb bone-holding f.
Semb ligature f.
Semb rib f.
Semken f.
Semken dressing f.
Semken thumb f.
Semken tissue f.
septal f.
septal bone f.
septal compression f.

F

forceps *(continued)*
    septal ridge f.
    septum cutting f.
    septum-straightening f.
    sequestrum f.
    series 5 f.
    serrated f.
    serrated conjunctival f.
    serrefine f.
    Shaaf cilia foreign body f.
    Shallcross cystic duct f.
    Shark disposable biopsy f.
    sharp-pointed f.
    Shea f.
    Shearer f.
    Shearer chicken-bill f.
    Sheets-McPherson angled f.
    Sheets-McPherson tying f.
    Shepard intraocular lens f.
    Shepard intraocular lens-holding f.
    Shepard-Reinstein f.
    Shepard tying f.
    Shields f.
    Shoemaker intraocular lens f.
    short tooth f.
    Shutt Aggressor f.
    Shutt alligator f.
    Shutt basket f.
    Shutt B-scoop f.
    Shutt grasping f.
    Shutt Mantis retrograde f.
    Shutt Mini-Aggressor f.
    Shutt retrograde f.
    Shutt shovel-nosed f.
    Shutt suction f.
    side-biting Stammberger punch f.
    side-curved f.
    side-cutting basket f.
    side-grasping f.
    side-lip f.
    silicone rod and sleeve f.
    silicone sponge f.
    Simcoe lens-inserting f.
    Simcoe nucleus f.
    Simcoe posterior chamber f.
    Simcoe superior rectus f.
    Simpson f.
    Simpson-Braun obstetrical f.
    Simpson-Luikart obstetrical f.
    Simpson obstetrical f.
    Sims-Maier sponge and dressing f.
    single-tooth f.
    Singley tissue f.
    Singley-Tuttle dressing f.
    Singley-Tuttle intestinal f.
    Singley-Tuttle tissue f.
    Sinskey lens-holding f.
    sinus biopsy f.
    sister-hook f.

    skeleton fine f.
    Skene tenaculum f.
    Skene vulsellum f.
    Skillman mosquito f.
    skin f.
    sleeve-spreading f.
    Sluder-Ballenger tonsillar punch f.
    small cup biopsy f.
    small plate f.
    Smart f.
    Smart chalazion f.
    Smellie obstetrical f.
    Smith-Leiske cross-action intraocular
     lens f.
    Smith & Nephew Richards
     bipolar f.
    Smithwick clip-applying f.
    smooth dressing f.
    smooth grasping f.
    smooth-tipped jeweler's f.
    smooth tissue f.
    Snellen f.
    Snellen entropion f.
    Snyder corneal spring f.
    Snyder deep surgery f.
    Sopher ovum f.
    Spaleck f.
    Sparta micro-iris f.
    spatula f.
    specimen f.
    speculum f.
    Spencer biopsy f.
    Spencer chalazion f.
    Spence rongeur f.
    Spencer plication f.
    Spencer-Wells arterial f.
    Spero f.
    sphenoidal punch f.
    spicule f.
    spinal perforating f.
    spiral f.
    spiral gallstone f.
    splaytooth f.
    splinter f.
    splitting f.
    sponge f.
    sponge-holding f.
    spoon f.
    spoon-shaped f.
    spreading f.
    spring-handled f.
    Spurling intervertebral disc f.
    Spurling-Kerrison rongeur f.
    Spurling rongeur f.
    square specimen f.
    squeeze-handle f.
    Stammberger punch f.
    Stamm bone-cutting f.
    standard arterial f.

stapedectomy f.
stapes f.
staple f.
Starr fixation f.
Steinmann tendon f.
Stephens soft IOL-inserting f.
sterilizing f.
sternal punch f.
Stern-Castroviejo locking f.
Stevens iris f.
Stevenson cupped-jaw f.
Stevenson microsurgical f.
Stieglitz splinter f.
Stille-Björk f.
Stille-Horsley bone f.
Stille-Horsley bone-cutting f.
Stille-Horsley rib f.
Stille-Liston bone f.
Stille-Liston bone-cutting f.
Stille-Liston rib-cutting f.
Stille-Luer rongeur f.
Stiwer bone-holding f.
S&T Lalonde hook f.
St. Martin eye f.
St. Martin suturing f.
Stolte capsulorrhexis f.
stone crushing f.
stone extraction f.
stone grasping f.
Stone intestinal f.
Stone tissue f.
Storz biopsy f.
Storz-Bonn suturing f.
Storz capsule f.
Storz cilia f.
Storz corneal f.
Storz curved f.
Storz esophagoscopic f.
Storz kidney stone f.
Storz Microsystems plate-holding f.
Storz nasopharyngeal biopsy f.
Storz stone crushing f.
strabismus f.
straight f.
straight coagulating f.
straight-end cup f.
straight knot-tying f.
straight-line bayonet f.
straight line bayonet f.
straight Maryland f.
straight microbipolar f.
straight single tenaculum f.
straight-tip bipolar f.
straight-tip jeweler's bipolar f.
straight tying f.
2-stream irrigating f.
Strow corneal f.
strut f.
Struycken turbinate f.

St. Vincent tube-occluding f.
subglottic f.
suction f.
superior rectus f.
SureBite biopsy f.
suture clip f.
suture tag f.
suture tying platform f.
suturing f.
Sweet clip-applying f.
synovium biopsy f.
Synthes Microsystems plate-holding f.
Tabb crura tissue f.
tack-and-pin f.
Takahashi cutting f.
Takahashi ethmoidal f.
Takahashi iris retractor f.
Takahashi nasal f.
take-apart f.
tampon f.
tangential f.
Tano microserrated f.
taper-jaw f.
Tarnier axis traction f.
Tarnier obstetrical f.
Taylor dissecting f.
Taylor tissue f.
Teale tenaculum f.
Teale uterine f.
Teale vulsellum f.
tenaculum f.
tenaculum reducing f.
tendon f.
tendon-holding f.
tendon-passing f.
tendon-pulling f.
tendon-retrieving f.
tendon-seizing f.
Tennant-Colibri corneal f.
Tennant intraocular lens f.
Tennant lens f.
Tennant titanium suturing f.
Tennant-Troutman superior rectus f.
Tennant tying f.
Tenzel bipolar f.
Terson capsular f.
Terson capsule f.
Terson extracapsular f.
Tessier disimpaction device f.
Tessier rib-contouring f.
Therma Jaw disposable hot biopsy f.
Therma Jaw hot urologic f.
Thomas fixation f.
Thoms-Allis tissue f.
Thoms-Gaylor uterine f.
Thoms tissue f.
thoracic artery f.

F

349

forceps *(continued)*

thoracic tissue f.
Thorpe-Castroviejo vitreous foreign body f.
Thorpe conjunctival f.
Thorpe corneal f.
Thrasher lens implant f.
throat f.
through-cutting sinus surgery f.
thumb f.
thumb tissue f.
thyroid f.
Tiemann bullet f.
Tilley-Henckel f.
Tilley nasal dressing f.
Tischler cervical biopsy f.
Tischler cervical biopsy punch f.
Tischler-Morgan uterine biopsy f.
tissue f.
tissue grasping f.
tissue holding f.
tissue spreading f.
titanium microsurgical bipolar f.
Tobey ear f.
Tobold laryngeal f.
Toennis-Adson f.
Toennis tumor f.
tongue f.
tonsil f.
tonsillar abscess f.
tonsillar artery f.
tonsillar hemostatic f.
tonsillar pillar grasping f.
tonsillar punch f.
toothed f.
2-toothed f.
toothed thumb f.
toothed tissue f.
tooth-extracting f.
toothless f.
torsion f.
tracheal f.
trachoma f.
traction f.
transfer f.
transsphenoidal bipolar f.
traumatic grasping f.
triangular punch f.
tripod grasping f.
Troeltsch dressing f.
Troeltsch ear f.
Trousseau dilating f.
Troutman-Barraquer-Colibri f.
Troutman-Barraquer corneal fixation f.
Troutman-Barraquer iris f.
Troutman corneal f.
Troutman-Llobera fixation f.
Troutman microsurgery f.

Troutman rectus f.
Troutman superior rectus f.
Troutman tying f.
TruLine f.
T-shaped f.
tube-occluding f.
tubing introducer f.
tubular f.
Tucker hallux f.
Tucker-McLane f.
Tucker-McLane axis traction f.
Tucker-McLane-Luikart f.
Tucker-McLane obstetrical f.
Tucker staple f.
Tucker tack-and-pin f.
Tudor-Edwards bone-cutting f.
Tuffier arterial f.
tumor f.
tumor-grasping f.
turbinate f.
Turner-Warwick stone f.
Turrell rectal biopsy f.
Tuttle thoracic f.
Tuttle thumb f.
Tuttle tissue f.
Tydings tonsillar f.
tying f.
tying/stitch removal f.
tympanoplasty f.
Ulrich bone-holding f.
Ulrich-St. Gallen f.
Ultrata capsulorrhexis f.
unipolar hand-switching needlepoint electrocautery f.
Universal bone grafting/impacting f.
Universal II f.
Universal lens-folding f.
upbiting f.
upbiting biopsy f.
upbiting cup f.
up-cupped f.
upcurved basket f.
upturned f.
ureteral catheter f.
ureteral isolation f.
ureteral stone f.
U-shaped f.
uterine artery f.
uterine biopsy punch f.
uterine dressing f.
uterine elevating f.
uterine grasping f.
uterine holding f.
uterine manipulating f.
uterine packing f.
uterine polyp f.
uterine specimen f.
uterine tenaculum f.
uterine vulsellum f.

utility f.
Utrata f.
Utrata capsulorrhexis f.
Utrata-Kershner capsulorrhexis
  cystotome f.
vaginal hysterectomy f.
Van Buren bone-holding f.
Van Buren sequestrum f.
Vantage tube-occluding f.
Varco thoracic f.
vascular tissue f.
vasectomy f.
vena cava f.
Verbrugge bone-holding f.
Verhoeff capsule f.
vertical f.
vessel f.
Vickers f.
Vickers ring-tip f.
Virtus splinter f.
viscera-holding f.
visceral f.
visual hemostatic f.
vitreous foreign body f.
vitreous grasping f.
vomer septal f.
von Graefe fixation f.
von Graefe iris f.
von Graefe tissue f.
von Petz f.
vulsellum f.
Wachenfeldt clip-applying f.
Waldeau fixation f.
Walker f.
Walsham f.
Walsham nasal f.
Walsham septal f.
Walsham septum-straightening f.
Walter-Liston f.
Walter splinter f.
Walton-Ruskin f.
Walton wire-pulling f.
Wangensteen tissue f.
watchmaker f.
Watson duckbill f.
Watson-Williams nasal f.
Watson-Williams polyp f.
Watzke f.
Waugh dissection f.
Waugh dressing f.
Waugh tissue f.
wave-tooth f.
Weaver chalazion f.
Weck hysterectomy f.
Weck uterine biopsy f.
wedge and post f.
Weil-Blakesley ethmoidal f.
Weil ear f.
Weingartner alligator ear f.

Weiss f.
Welch Allyn anal biopsy f.
Weller cartilage f.
Weller meniscal f.
Wells f.
Welsh pupil-spreader f.
Wertheim-Cullen compression f.
Wertheim-Cullen hysterectomy f.
Wertheim-Cullen kidney pedicle f.
Wertheim hysterectomy f.
Wertheim uterine f.
Wertheim vaginal f.
West nasal dressing f.
White tonsillar f.
Whitney superior rectus f.
Wiener hysterectomy f.
Wies chalazion f.
Wiet cup f.
Wikström arterial f.
Wilde f.
Wilde-Blakesley ethmoidal f.
Wilde ear f.
Wilde ethmoid f.
Wilde ethmoidal exenteration f.
Wilde intervertebral disc f.
Wilde nasal dressing f.
Wilder dilating f.
Wilde rongeur f.
Wilde septal f.
Wilkerson intraocular lens
  insertion f.
Willauer-Allis thoracic f.
Willauer-Allis tissue f.
Willauer intrathoracic f.
Willett placenta previa f.
Willett scalp flap f.
Williams discectomy f.
Williams intestinal f.
Williams splinter f.
Williams tissue f.
Wills Hospital ophthalmic f.
Wills utility f.
Wilmer iris f.
Wilson-Cook bronchoscope
  biopsy f.
Wilson-Cook colonoscope biopsy f.
Wilson-Cook gastroscope biopsy f.
Wilson-Cook grasping f.
Wilson-Cook hot biopsy f.
Wilson-Cook retrieval f.
Wilson-Cook tripod retrieval f.
Wilson vitreous foreign body f.
Winter ovum f.
Winter placental f.
wire closure f.
wire crimping f.
wire-cutting f.
wire-extracting f.
wire-holding f.

F

forceps *(continued)*
- wire prosthesis crimping f.
- wire-pulling f.
- wire-tightening f.
- wire-twisting f.
- Wittner uterine biopsy f.
- Wolf biopsy f.
- Wolf curved basket f.
- Wolfe f.
- Wolfe eye f.
- Wolfson f.
- Woodward f.
- Worst implantation f.
- Worth advancement f.
- Worth strabismus f.
- wound f.
- wound clip f.
- Wrigley f.
- W-shape f.
- Wullstein ear f.
- Wullstein tympanoplasty f.
- Wylie uterine f.
- Yankauer ethmoid-cutting f.
- Yasargil angled f.
- Yasargil applying f.
- Yasargil bipolar f.
- Yasargil flat serrated ring f.
- Yasargil microvessel clip-applying f.
- Yasargil neurosurgical bipolar f.
- Yasargil straight f.
- Yeoman f.
- Young lobe f.
- Young prostatectomy f.
- Young prostatic f.
- Young tongue f.
- Zaldivar iridectomy f.
- Zaldivar microacrylic lens implantation f.
- Zaldivar reverse capsulorrhexis f.
- Z-clamp hysterectomy f.
- Zenker f.
- Ziegler cilia f.
- Zurich suturing f.

Ford-Deaver retractor
Forder retractor
forearm
- f. flexion control strap
- f. lift assist adjustable spring-loaded device
- f. tourniquet

forefoot compression sleeve
Foregger
- F. bronchoscope
- F. laryngoscope
- F. rigid esophagoscope

Foregger-Racine adapter
foreign
- f. body bur
- f. body curette
- f. body cystoscopy forceps
- f. body eye forceps
- f. body forceps
- f. body locator
- f. body loop
- f. body magnet
- f. body needle
- f. body probe
- f. body remover
- f. body retrieval system
- f. body retrieving forceps
- f. body screw
- f. body spud

ForeRunner
- F. automatic external defibrillator device
- F. coronary sinus guiding catheter
- F. defibrillator

forged cobalt-chromium alloy prosthesis
forged femoral head
fork
- Gardiner-Brown neurological tuning f.
- f. hammer
- Hardy 3-prong f.
- Hartmann tuning f.
- knife and f.
- magnesium tuning f.
- McCabe crus guide f.
- neurological tuning f.
- 3-prong f.
- Riverbank Laboratories tuning f.
- f. stent
- f. strap
- Sugita f.
- tuning f.

Forker retractor
form
- Amoena breast f.
- breast-mound f.
- Discrene breast f.
- Dow Corning external breast f.
- F. Fit intracanalicular plug
- Jettmobile Tumble F.'s
- Lucite f.
- mastopexy f.
- Nearly Me breast f.
- Spenco external breast f.
- Trulife silicone breast f.
- Vestibulator positioning tumble f.

formaldehyde catgut suture
Forman diamond rasp
Formatray mandibular splint
Forma water-jacketed incubator
formboard
- Séguin f.

formed nonirrigating cystotome
Formfit thumb spica

FormFlex lens
formula, pl. **formulas, formulae**
    Attain tube feeding f.
    Ostofresh f.
foroblique
    f. bronchoscope
    f. bronchoscopic telescope
    f. endoscope
    f. fiberoptic esophagoscope
    f. lens
    f. microlens resectoscope
    f. resectoscope
Forrester clamp
ForSite pupillometer
Förster
    F. enucleation snare
    F. iris forceps
    F. photometer
    F. photoptometer
FortaDerm antimicrobial wound dressing
FortaPerm surgical sling
Forte ES instrument
Fortitude
    F. Ti titanium spinal fixation product
    F. Vue titanium spinal fixation product
Fortuna syringe
Fort urethral bougie
forward-cutting knife
forward fluorescence detector
forward-grasping forceps
forward-viewing endoscope
Foss
    F. anterior resection clamp
    F. clamp forceps
    F. intestinal clamp
fossa
    f. curette
    f. eminence prosthesis
    f. of Rosenmüller
Fossfill health pillow
Foster
    F. bed
    F. enucleation snare
    F. frame
    F. needle holder
    F. snare enucleator
    F. suture
Foster-Ballenger forceps
Fothergill suture
Fotofil
    F. activator light
    F. dental restorative material
FotoFinder Derma
Foundation
    F. total hip system

    F. total knee and hip system
    F. total knee system
fountain
    F. infusion system and catheter
    xenon cold-light f.
Fourier transformation spectrum analyzer
Fournier tip
Fowler-Zollner knife
Fox
    F. aluminum eye shield
    F. aluminum shield
    F. bipolar electrocautery
    F. cartilage forceps
    F. curette
    F. dermal curette
    F. eye shield
    F. impactor-extractor
    F. internal fixation device
    F. irrigating/aspirating unit
    F. irrigator
    F. LASIK spatula
    F. postnasal balloon
    F. prosthesis
    F. PTA catheter
    F. speculum
    F. sphere implant
    F. tissue forceps
Fox-Blazina prosthesis
FP5000 pump system
FPS system
FracSure appliance
Fractomed splint
fracture
    f. band
    f. bar
    f. bed
    f. boot
    f. chisel
    f. computer-aided surgery system
    f. fixation device
    f. frame
    f. reducing elevator
    f. splint
    f. table
fracture-banding apparatus
Fraenkel forceps
fragmatome
    CooperVision f.
    Girard f.
    f. tip
fragment
    Fab f.
    f. forceps
fragmentation/aspiration handpiece
fragmentation probe
fragmentor
    Lieberman f.

F

fraise
diamond f.

frame
Alexian Brothers overhead f.
Andrews spinal surgery f.
anterior quadrilateral triplane f.
Assistant Free hip surgery square f.
Assistant Free hip surgery standard f.
Balkan fracture f.
basic f. (type IV)
Böhler-Braun fracture f.
Böhler reducing fracture f.
Bookwalter Wishbook adjustable f.
Braun f.
Brown-Roberts-Wells f.
Brown-Roberts-Wells head f.
Brown-Roberts-Wells stereotactic f.
Chick CLT operating f.
CHOP f.
Colles external fixation f.
Compass stereotactic f.
Cosman-Roberts-Wells stereotactic head f.
couch-mounted head f.
CT/MRI-compatible stereotactic head f.
detachable stretcher f.
Dingman mouthgag f.
double-ring f.
Elekta stereotactic head f.
eyeglass f.
Foster f.
fracture f.
fusion f.
GaitMaster low-profile f.
Gardner-Wells fixation f.
Gill-Thomas-Cosman f.
Goldthwait fracture f.
Greenberg retractor f.
halo fracture f.
halo head f.
head f.
Hibbs fracture f.
Hitchcock stereotactic immobilization f.
Horsley-Clarke stereotactic f.
hyperextension fracture f.
Ilizarov f.
imaging compatible stereotactic coordinate f.
Jewett f.
Jones abduction f.
Joseph septal f.
Kessler traction f.
Komai stereotactic head f.
Laitinen stereotactic head f.
laminectomy f.

Leksell D-shaped stereotactic f.
Leksell-Elekta stereotactic f.
Leksell G stereotactic head f.
Leksell stereotaxic f.
Maddacrawler f.
Malcolm-Lynn C-RXF cervical retractor f.
Malcolm-Rand cranial x-ray f.
Mayfield fixation f.
Monticelli-Spinelli f.
mouthgag f.
mouth gag f.
MTL trial f.
nitinol mesh-covered f.
nonferromagnetic MR-compatible f.
Oculus trial f.
Olivier-Bertrand-Tipal f.
Ostby dam f.
OSU f.
Otsby dam f.
Pelorus stereotactic f.
phantom f.
Pittsburgh triangular f.
3-point fixation f.
4-poster f.
quadriplegic standing f.
radiolucent spine f.
Radionics CRW stereotactic head f.
reducing fracture f.
Reichert-Mundinger-Fischer stereotactic f.
Reichert-Mundinger stereotactic head f.
retractor oval sprocket f.
Risser f.
robotics-controlled stereotactic f.
Scappa f.
servohydraulic test f.
sling f.
spinal turning f.
static testing f.
Stealth f.
stereotactic head f.
stereotactic localization f.
Stryker f.
Stryker turning fracture f.
Sugita multipurpose head f.
Talairach stereotactic f.
Tarbell-Loeffler-Cosman f.
Taylor spinal f.
Thomas fracture f.
Thomas hyperextension f.
Todd-Wells stereotactic f.
trial f.
trial fracture f.
triangular ankle fusion f.
Watson-Jones f.
Whitman f.
Whitman fracture f.

Wilson convex f.
Wilson spinal f.
Wishbook adjustable f.
Wolfson f.
Young rubber dam fracture f.
Zimmer fracture f.

frame-based radiosurgical system
frameless
    f. air support therapy system
    f. stereotactic device
    f. stereotaxy system
FrameLock reference-arc fixation device
frame-mounted pump
framer
    F. finger extension bow
    GTC repeated stereotactic
      localizer f.
    F. splint
    F. tendon passer
    F. tendon-passing needle
Franceschetti corneal trephine
Francis
    F. spud
    F. spud chalazion forceps
Francis-Gray wire crimper
Francke needle
Franco triflange ventilation tube
Frank
    F. ECG lead placement system
    F. EKG lead placement system
    F. XYZ orthogonal lead
    F. XYZ orthogonal lead system
Fränkel
    F. appliance
    F. cutting tip forceps
    F. esophagoscopy forceps
    F. head band
    F. laryngeal forceps
    F. sinus probe
    F. speculum
    F. tampon forceps
Frankfeldt
    F. diathermy snare
    F. grasping forceps
    F. hemorrhoidal needle
    F. rectal snare
Franklin
    F. glasses
    F. liver puncture needle
    F. malleable retractor
    F. spectacles
Franklin-Silverman
    F.-S. biopsy cannula
    F.-S. prostatic biopsy needle
Franseen
    F. liver biopsy needle
    F. lung biopsy needle
    F. needle

Franz
    F. abdominal retractor
    F. monophasic action potential
      catheter
Franzen needle guide
Fraser Harlake respirometer
Frazer wrist brace
Frazier
    F. aspirating tube
    F. brain suction tube
    F. Britetrac nasal suction tube
    F. dura hook
    F. dural elevator
    F. dural guide
    F. dural scissors
    F. elevator
    F. fiberoptic suction tube
    F. laminectomy retractor
    F. nasal suction tube
    F. nerve hook
    F. skin hook
    F. stylet
    F. suction
    F. suction cannula
    F. suction elevator
    F. suction tip
    F. suction-tip aspirator
    F. suction tube
    F. suction tube obturator
    F. ventricular needle
Frazier-Adson osteoplastic flap clamp
Frazier-Fay retractor
Frazier-Ferguson
    F.-F. aspirating tube
    F.-F. ear suction tube
Frazier-Paparella mastoid suction tube
Frazier-Sachs clamp
Frazier-Shepherd skin hook
FRC
    focused rigidity casting
    FRC system
Frechet extender
Frederick
    F. pneumothoracic needle
    F. sleeve spreader
Frederick-Miller tube
Fredricks mammary prosthesis
free
    F. & Active incontinence pant
    f. fibered coil
    f. implant
Freedom
    F. accommodator arch support
    Accu-Chek II F.
    F. arthritis support
    F. back support
    F. Cath
    F. Clear long-seal male external
      catheter line

F

Freedom *(continued)*
  F. Clear LS male external catheter line
  F. Clear sport-sheath male external catheter line
  F. Clear SS male external catheter line
  F. dental unit
  F. elastic long wrist support
  F. external catheter
  F. knife
  F. leg bag collection system
  F. Micro Pro stimulator
  F. neutral position splint
  F. omni progressive splint
  F. palm guard
  F. Progressive Resting splint
  F. SportsFit splint
  F. stent
  F. thumbkeeper
  F. thumb spica
  F. thumb stabilizer
  F. T-tap leg bag
  F. T-tap leg bag kit
  F. ultimate grip splint
  F. USA wristlet
FreeDop
  F. Doppler monitor
  F. portable Doppler unit
FreeFlo
  F. proximal nitinol stent
  F. stent-graft
Free-Flow system prosthesis
Freegenol cement
freehand
  F. neuroprosthetic system
  f. probe
  F. prosthesis system
Free-Lock femoral fixation system
Freeman
  F. capsule polisher
  F. cookie cutter areola marker
  F. femoral component
  F. high-neck press-fit prosthesis
  F. modular total hip prosthesis
  F. pancreatic Flexi-Stent
  F. positioning cannula
  F. punctum plug
  F. rhytidectomy scissors
  F. surgical headrest
  F. transorbital leukotome
Freeman-Samuelson knee prosthesis
Freeman-Schepens scissors
Freeman-Swanson knee prosthesis
Freer
  F. bone chisel
  F. chisel
  F. dissector
  F. double-end elevator

  F. dural dissector
  F. elevator
  F. lacrimal chisel
  F. nasal chisel
  F. nasal gouge
  F. nasal knife
  F. nasal spatula
  F. nasal submucous knife
  F. periosteal elevator
  F. periosteotome
  F. septal elevator
  F. septal forceps
  F. septal knife
  F. septum elevator
  F. skin hook
  F. skin retractor
  F. submucous chisel
  F. submucous retractor
Freer-Sachs dissector
free-spinning probe
freestanding
  f. implant
  f. single crown
  f. stent
  f. tissue retraction bridge system
Freestyle
  F. aortic root bioprosthesis
  F. bioprosthetic heart valve
  F. CAPD catheter adapter
  F. stentless aortic heart valve
  F. stentless bioprosthesis
FreeStyle
  F. blood glucose monitoring system
  F. Flash blood glucose meter
  F. test strip
  Therasense F.
  F. Tracker glucose meter
Freeway Lite portable aerosol compressor
freeze-dried bone pin
freezer
  CryoMed 1010A f.
  Gentle Jane Snap f.
  Wallach cryosurgery f.
freeze-thaw cryotherapy
freezing point osmometer
Freezor
  F. CryoAblation system
  F. cryocatheter
Freiberg cartilage knife
Freiburg mediastinoscope
Freitag stent
Frejka
  F. cast
  F. hip pillow
  F. jacket
  F. orthosis
  F. pillow

F. pillow splint
F. traction
French
F. angiographic catheter
F. catheter
F. catheter gauge
F. chisel
F. Cope loop nephrostomy catheter
F. curve out-of-plane catheter
F. cystoscope
F. double-lumen catheter
F. Foley catheter
F. Gesco catheter
F. hook spatula
F. hysteroscope
F. lacrimal dilator
F. lacrimal probe
F. lacrimal spatula
F. nasogastric tube
F. needle holder
F. pattern spatula
F. Pharmacovigilance system
F. rod bender
F. rod bender frontal
F. SAL catheter
F. scoop
F. shaft catheter
F. sizing of catheter
F. spring-eye needle
F. steel sound
F. stent
F. Swan-Ganz balloon
F. Teflon pyeloureteral catheter
F. tip catheter
F. T tube
French-eye needle
French-Hanks uterine dilator
French-McCarthy endoscope
French-pattern
F.-p. forceps
F.-p. osteotome
French-Stern-McCarthy retractor
Frenta
F. enteral feeding bag
F. Mat feeding pump
F. System II feeding pump
Frenzel
F. goggles
F. lens
frequency, pl. frequencies
f. doubled double pulse ND:YAG laser
f. doubled nd:YAG laser
f. doubled neodymium:yttrium-aluminum-garnet laser
F. 38 monthly disposable contact lens
f. shifter
f. tracer

Fresenius
F. AG dialyzer
F. Euro-Collins kit
F. F-40 filter
F. 2008H hemodialysis machine
F. volumetric dialysate balancing system
fresh-frozen nonirradiated bone-patellar tendon-bone allograft
FreshLook contact lens
FreshStart mammary support garment
Fresnel
F. goggles
F. lens
F. lens pusher
F. prism
F. zone plate
Freyer suprapubic drain
Frey-Freer bur
Frey-Sauerbruch rib shears
Frey tunneled eye implant
Frialit-2 dental implant system
Frialoc transgingival threaded dental implant
Friatec
F. implant
F. manual arthroscopy instrument
Fricke gel
friction-fit adapter
friction lock pin
friction-reduced
f.-r. examination table
f.-r. segmented table
Friedenwald
F. funduscope
F. ophthalmoscope
Friedländer incision marker
Friedman
F. bone rongeur
F. elevator
F. handheld Hruby lens
F. phaco/IOL manipulator
F. rongeur forceps
F. splint
F. splint brace
F. tantalum clip
F. vaginal retractor
Friedmann visual field analyzer
Friedman-Otis bougie à boule
Friend catheter
Friend-Hebert catheter
Friesner ear knife
Frigitronics
F. colposcope
F. cryoprobe
F. cryosurgical unit
F. freeze-thaw cryopexy probe

F

Frigitronics *(continued)*
F. nitrous oxide cryosurgery
apparatus
F. vitrector
**Frimberger-Karpiel 12 o'clock
papillotome**
Fritsch
F. abdominal retractor
F. catheter
F. retractor
Fritz vitreous transplant needle
frog-leg splint
frog splint
Froimson splint
Fromm triangle orthopaedic device
front
f. build-up implant
corset f.
f. support strap
f. surface dental mirror
frontal
French rod bender f.
f. plate
f. sinus cannula
f. sinus chisel
f. sinus curette
f. sinus dilator
f. sinus probe
f. sinus rasp
f. sinus wash tube
frontalis snare
front-entry guide
front-wheeled walker
Frost
F. scissors
F. suture
Frosted Flex earmold material
FRS
fusion and reconstruction system
FRS standard staple
FRS twist-off screw
Fruehevald splint
Frumin valve
Frye aspirator
Frykholm bone rongeur
Fry nasal forceps
F-Scan
F.-S. foot force and gait analysis
system
F.-S. in-shoe system
F.-S. pressure measurement system
FSD colpostat
F-series
F-s. dialyzer
F-s. fluorescence spectrophotometer
FS30 femtosecond laser
Fuchs
F. capsular forceps
F. capsule forceps

F. capsulotomy forceps
F. extracapsular forceps
F. iris forceps
F. lancet-type keratome
F. retinal detachment syringe
F. 2-way eye syringe
F. 2-way syringe
Fuchs-Rosenthal chamber
Fugo
F. blade
F. plasma knife
Fuhrman pleural drainage set
**Fuji AC2 storage phosphor computed
radiology system**
Fuji Dentacam EDC 2
Fujinon
F. biopsy forceps
F. diagnostic laparoscope
F. DUO-XT duodenoscope
F. EB-410S bronchoscope
F. EC-130LT colonoscope
F. EC-200LT colonoscope
F. EC-410MP colonoscope
F. EC-300MS colonoscope
F. EC series video colonoscope
F. ED series duodenoscope
F. ED7-XT duodenoscope
F. ED-200XU duodenoscope
F. ED-310XU duodenoscope
F. EG-310D gastroscope
F. EG-200FP gastroscope
F. EG-FP series endoscope
F. EG-410HR gastroscope
F. EG series endoscope
F. EG series gastroscope
F. ES-200ER sigmoidoscope
F. EVD-XT duodenoscope
F. EVE series endoscope
F. EVG-CT endoscope
F. EVG-CT series endoscope
F. EVG-FP series endoscope
F. EVG-F series endoscope
F. EVG series endoscope
F. FD series duodenoscope
F. FD-100XU duodenoscope
F. FE-100LR colonoscope
F. flexible bronchoscope
F. flexible hysteroscope
F. flexible sigmoidoscope
F. FP series endoscope
F. FS-100ER sigmoidoscope
F. GF-100PE gastroscope
F. 400-series super image video
gastroscope
F. SIG-E2 fiberoptic sigmoidoscope
F. SP-501 sonoprobe system
F. super-image videogastroscope
F. UGI-FP series video endoscope
F. videocolonoscope

F. videoduodenoscope
F. videoelectroscope
F. videoendoscope
Fukasaku
F. anesthesia cannula
F. small pupil snapper hook
F. snap & split-tip irrigating chopper
F. spatula
Fukasaku-Lieberman phacoemulsification spatula
Fukuda humeral head retractor
Fukusaku spatula
Fukushima
F. C-clamp
F. malleable brain spatula
F. monopolar malleable coagulator
F. retractor
F. ring curette
F. rongeur
Ful-Glo fluorescein strip
fulgurating electrode
full
f. denture prosthetics
f. hand splint
f. lower denture
f. occlusal splint
f. ring scanner
f. spine board
f. upper denture
full-circle goniometer
full-curved clamp
full-dimpled Lucite implant
Fuller
F. rectal dressing
F. shield
full-field digital mammography system
full-intensity needle
full-lumen esophagoscope
full-radius
f.-r. cutter
f.-r. resector
full-thickness implant
full-time occlusion eye patch
full-wave rectifier
fully
f. automated defibrillator
f. automatic atrioventricular Universal dual-channel pacemaker
f. constrained tricompartmental knee prosthesis
Fulton
F. laminectomy rongeur
F. mouthgag
F. retractor
Ful-Vue
F.-V. ophthalmoscope
F.-V. spot retinoscope
F.-V. streak retinoscope

function
Cineloop memory f.
Shepp-Logan filter f.
functional
f. electronic peroneal brace
f. fracture brace
f. funnel
f. grip pushup block
f. orthotic
f. resting position splint
f. splint
f. visual acuity meter
fundamental frequency indicator
fundus, pl. **fundi**
f. camera
f. contact lens
f. focalizing lens
funduscope
Friedenwald f.
funnel
functional f.
stent f.
funnelform taper
Funsten supination splint
Furacin gauze dressing
furcation slim-diameter tip
Furlong tendon stripper
Furlow
F. cylinder passer
F. introducer
Furniss-Clute duodenal clamp
furniture brace
fused bifocal lens
fused-tip catheter
fusiform bougie
fusion
Albee lumbar spinal f.
anterior lumbar interbody f. (ALIF)
f. bed
f. cage
f. frame
f. plate
posterior lumbar interbody f. (PLIF)
f. and reconstruction system (FRS)
Zielke instrumentation for scoliosis spinal f.
Futrex analyzer
Futura
F. conical subtalar implant
F. flexible digital implant
F. metal hemi-toe implant
F. resectoscope sheath
Future implant
Futuro
F. splint
F. wrist brace
F. wrist support
FX miniRAIL RX PTCA catheter

F

FX-wire
    Cragg FX-w.
FyBron
    F. alginate wound cover

F. calcium alginate dressing
F. dressing

G5

G5 Fleximatic massager/percussor massager
G5 Flimm-Fighter percussor
G5 massage and percussion machine
G5 Neocussor percussor
G5 Porta-Plus muscle stimulator
G5 Vibracare massager/percussor

G3PDH CDNA probe

G91-9215 monocrystant antimony pH catheter

Gaab endoscope

Gabbay-Frater suture guide

Gabriel

G. proctoscope
G. syringe

gadolinium scan

Gaeltec catheter-tip pressure transducer

Gaenslen spike

gaff

Gaffee speculum

Gaffney

G. ankle prosthesis
G. joint

gag (*See* mouthgag)

Gaillard-Arlt suture

gait

g. belt
g. lock splint
g. lock splint brace
g. plate

gaiter brace

GaitKeeper cast shoe

GaitMaster low-profile frame

GAITRite mat

GAIT spacer

galactometer

Galand-Knolle modified J-loop intraocular lens

Galante

G. hip guide
G. hip prosthesis

Galaxy

G. 900HS adjusting table
G. IVUS imaging system
G. McManis hylo table

galea forceps

Galen

G. Scan scanner
G. teleradiology system

Galetti articulator

Galezowski lacrimal dilator

Galilean

G. loupe
G. microscope

Galilei dual Scheimpflug analyzer

Galileo

G. evoked potential electroencephalograph
G. intravascular radiotherapy system
G. rigid hysteroscope
G. ventilator

Galin

G. bleb cup
G. intraocular implant lens
G. lens spatula

gall

g. duct dilator
g. duct forceps
g. duct probe
g. duct scoop

Gall-Addison uterine manipulator

Gallagher rasp

Gallannaugh bone plate

gallbladder

g. cannula
g. forceps
g. retractor
g. scissors

Gallie

G. fascial needle
G. fusion-using cable

Gallini bone marrow aspiration needle

gallium-aluminum-arsenide 904-nm laser

gallium-arsenide laser

Galloway electrode

Gallows splint

gallows-type retractor

gallstone

g. basket
g. dilator
g. forceps
g. probe
g. scoop

Galtac device

Galton

G. ear whistle
G. galvanometer

Galt skull trephine

galvanic

g. electrode stimulator
g. probe
g. skin response device
g. skin response meter

galvanogustometer

galvanometer

d'Arsonval g.

G

galvanometer *(continued)*
    Einthoven string g.
    Galton g.
Galveston
    G. fixation with TSRH
    G. fixation with TSRH crosslink
    G. metacarpal brace
    G. plate
    G. splint
Gambee suture
Gamboscope
Gambro
    G. AK10 machine
    G. catheter
    G. dialyzer
    G. dialyzer holder
    G. FH88H filter
    G. freezing bag
    G. hemodialyzer
    G. hemofiltration system
    G. Lundia coil dialyzer
    G. Lundia Minor artificial kidney
    G. Lundia Minor hemodialyzer
    G. oxygenator
game
    Boloxie OT Prehension G.
    Cone checkers g.
Gamgee dressing
gamma
    g. camera
    g. camera discriminator
    crosslink g.
    g. detection probe
    g. emitter
    G. Knife
    g. locking nail
    g. probe
    g. probe radiation detector
    g. radiation therapy system
    g. ray counter
    g. ray level indicator
    g. ray scanner
    g. ray spectrometer
    g. scintillation camera
    G. trochanteric locking nail
    g. well counter
gamma-detecting probe
gamma-irradiated plug
Gammatone II gamma camera
Gammex
    G. RMI DAP meter
    G. RMI scanner
Gamow bag
GAN-19 needle
ganciclovir implant
Gandhi knife
Gandy clamp

ganglion
    g. hook
    g. scissors
Ganley splint
Gans cyclodialysis cannula
Gant clamp
gantry
    CT scan g.
    fluoroscopic g.
    LINAC g.
gantry-free gamma camera
Ganz
    G. cup
    G. fixation
Ganz-Edwards coronary infusion catheter
Ganzfeld
    G. bowl
    G. electroretinograph
    G. stimulator
Gap cup
Garceau ureteral catheter
Garcia aortic clamp
Garcia-Ibanez M picture camera
Garcia-Novito eye implant
Garcia-Rock endometrial biopsy curette
Gard-all boot shoe
Garden screw
Gardiner-Brown neurological tuning fork
Gardner
    G. bone chisel
    G. bone forceps
    G. chair
    G. headholder
    G. needle
    G. needle holder
Gardner-Wells
    G.-W. fixation frame
    G.-W. tongs
    G.-W. traction tongs
Gardray dosimeter
Garfield-Holinger laryngoscope
Gariel pessary
Gariot articulator
Garland hysterectomy forceps
garment
    Canfield facial plastics g.
    compression g.
    console compression g.
    crotchless compression g.
    Elvarex compression g.
    Elvarex support g.
    facial plastics g.
    FreshStart mammary support g.
    Jobst pressure g.
    Marena compression g.
    Medical Z post-surgery g.
    pneumatic g.

pneumatic antishock g.
PresSsion pneumatic g.
second-stage g.
surgical compression g.
V-brace support g.
Garren-Edwards gastric balloon
Garrett
G. dilator
G. peripheral vascular retractor
Garrigue weighted vaginal speculum
Garrison forceps
garter
Goffman eye g.
Gärtner tonometer
gas
g. chromatograph
g. cylinder
g. discharge lamp
g. insufflator
g. isotope ratio mass spectrometer
g. laser
g. permeable contact lens
GaSampler collection system
GasBGon filter seat cushion
Gaskell clamp
gasket
Gaskin fragment forceps
gasless laparoscopic system
Gas-Lyte ABG syringe
Gasparotti bevel tip
Gass
G. cataract aspirating cannula
G. corneoscleral punch
G. dye applicator
G. irrigating/aspirating unit
G. muscle hook
G. retinal detachment cannula
G. retinal detachment hook
G. scleral marker
G. scleral punch
G. sclerotomy punch
G. vitreous aspirating cannula
gasserian ganglion hook
gastric
g. balloon
g. bubble
g. clamp
g. lavage tube
g. resection retractor
g. shield
g. tube
g. volvulus
Gastrin RIA kit II
gastrocamera
Olympus g.
gastroenterostomy
g. catheter
g. clamp
gastroesophageal antireflux device

gastrofiberscope
GastrographH
G. ambulatory pH monitoring system
G. Mark III pH analyzer
gastrointestinal (GI)
g. clamp
g. fiberscope
g. forceps
g. needle
g. surgical gut suture
g. surgical linen suture
g. surgical silk suture
g. therapeutic system
upper g. (UGI)
gastrojejunostomy
g. catheter
g. tube
GastroPanel assay kit
gastroplasty stapler
Gastro-Port
G.-P. II feeding device
G.-P. II feeding tube
Gastroreflex
G. ambulatory pH monitor
G. ambulatory pH monitor/recorder
gastroscope
ACMI g.
Benedict operating g.
Bernstein g.
Cameron omniangle g.
Chevalier Jackson g.
disposable-sheath flexible g.
Eder g.
Eder-Bernstein g.
Eder-Chamberlin g.
Eder-Hufford g.
Ellsner g.
end-viewing g.
Ewald g.
fiberoptic g.
flexible g.
Fujinon EG-310D g.
Fujinon EG-200FP g.
Fujinon EG-410HR g.
Fujinon EG series g.
Fujinon GF-100PE g.
Fujinon 400-series super image video g.
GFC g.
GFT Olympus g.
Herman-Taylor g.
Hirschowitz g.
Housset-Debray g.
Janeway g.
Jenning-Streifeneder g.
Kelling g.
Krentz g.
Mancke flex-rigid g.

G

gastroscope *(continued)*
    Olympus GIF-K series g.
    Olympus GIFxP10 g.
    Olympus GIF-XQ30 flexible g.
    Olympus 2T-2000 twin-channel
      therapeutic g.
    Olympus XQ230 g.
    pediatric g.
    Pentax ELLB 6000, 6500
      ultrasound g.
    Pentax EUP-EC series
      ultrasound g.
    Pentax EUP-EC124 ultrasound g.
    peroral g.
    Q200 g.
    Sielaff g.
    Taylor g.
    Tomenius g.
    Universal g.
    Wolf-Henning g.
    Wolf-Knittlingen g.
    Wolf-Schindler g.
gastrostomy
    g. button
    g. catheter
    dual percutaneous endoscopic g.
      (DPEG)
    g. feeding tube
    percutaneous endoscopic g. (PEG)
    g. plug
    g. tube
Gatch bed
gate clip
gated CT scanner
Gatekeeper reflux repair system
Gates-Glidden
    G.-G. bur
    G.-G. drill
gator
    G. meniscal cutter
    g. plastic orthosis
    G. resector
    G. shaver
Gauderer-Ponsky PEG
Gauder Silicon PEG catheter
Gau gastric balloon
gauge
    Arnett-TMP depth g.
    B&L pinch g.
    Boley g.
    bone screw depth g.
    Bourdon g.
    Bourdon tube pressure g.
    calibrated depth g.
    Charnley femoral condyle radius g.
    Charnley socket g.
    Chatillon digital force g.
    clip g.
    Cloward depth g.

CTS g.
Dacomed snap g.
Deitz incision depth g.
Deitz ophthalmic g.
depth g.
Dontrix g.
Durkan CTS g.
finger g.
finger circumference g.
French catheter g.
Harris femoral head g.
isometric strain g.
Jamar hydraulic pinch g.
Katena depth g.
Knolle lens g.
leaf g.
LeVeen inflator with pressure g.
manual dermatome thickness g.
Marco radius g.
measuring g.
Mendez degree g.
mercury-in-silastic strain g.
orthopaedic depth g.
oval piston g.
pain threshold g.
Philips toe force g.
pinch g.
pinwheel sensation g.
pressure g.
Preston pinch g.
Reichert radius g.
Rocabado posture g.
Rosette strain g.
Rowen white-to-white corneal g.
screw depth g.
Shepard incision depth g.
silastic strain g.
snap g.
Snap-Gauge g.
spanner g.
standard wire g.
Steinert-Deacon incision g.
strain g.
Synthes mini-depth g.
Tycos g.
uniaxial strain g.
Vernier caliber g.
water g.
Zaldivar degree g.
Gaulian knife guide
gauntlet
    ankle/foot g. (AFG)
    g. bandage
    leather lacer g.
Gauss hemostatic forceps
Gauthier retractor
Gautier ureteroscope
gauze
    Adaptic g.

Aquaphor g.
Avant Gauze nonwoven g.
Bactigras g.
g. bandage
Biolex impregnated g.
BIPP ribbon g.
BloodSTOP EX hemostatic g.
CarraGauze impregnated g.
ClearSite impregnated g.
Cover-Roll g.
Cover-Roll adhesive g.
Curafil hydrogel-impregnated g.
Curafil impregnated g.
Curasol impregnated g.
Dermagran impregnated g.
DermAssist impregnated g.
g. dissector sponge
dry sterile g.
dry textile g.
Elta Dermal impregnated g.
finger g.
Gentell impregnated g.
GraftCyte g.
Intersorb fine mesh g.
Intersorb 6-ply absorbent roll
  stretch g.
Intersorb wide mesh g.
iodoform g.
Kling g.
MPM GelPad impregnated g.
N-Terface g.
Oxycel g.
g. pack
g. packer
g. pad
g. pad carrier
PanoGauze hydrogel-impregnated g.
PanoGauze impregnated g.
paraffin g.
petrolatum g.
plain g.
Restore impregnated g.
g. roll
g. rosebud sponge
Safe-Wrap g.
g. scissors
SkinTegrity impregnated g.
sodium chloride-impregnated g.
Sof-Form conforming g.
Sta-Tite 2-ply elastic roll g.
g. stent
g. stent dressing
surgical steel g.
Surgicel g.
Surgitube tubular g.
tantalum g.
Telfa g.
g. tissue bag
Topper nonadherent g.

TransiGel hydrogel-impregnated g.
TransiGel impregnated g.
Vaseline-coated g.
Vaseline-impregnated g.
g. wick
woven cotton g.
Xeroform g.

Gauztape bandage
Gauztex
  G. bandage
  G. dressing
Gaylor uterine biopsy forceps
Gaymar
  G. Thermacare warming unit
  G. water-circulating blanket
Gazayerli
  G. endoscopic retractor
  G. knot pusher
Gazayerli-Mediflex retractor
Gazelle balloon dilatation catheter
G-bevel cannula
G-C
  G-C filling instrument
  G-C polishing strip
  G-C syringe
  G-C Vest investment material
  G-C wax carver
GC-16
  Surgitek graduated cystocope G.
GDC
  Guglielmi detachable coil
  GDC 360-degree detachable coil
  GDC SynerG detachment device
  UltraSoft GDC
GDC-10 soft coil
GD-LD-208C minicamera
GDLH posterior spinal system
GDS
  graft delivery system
Gd-Tex radiation sensitizer
GDx
  G. Access scanning laser
    polarimeter
  G. nerve fiber analyzer
  G. scanning laser polarimeter
  G. VCC scanning laser polarimeter
GDx-variable corneal compensator
GE
  GE 400AC/T; STAR II camera
  GE Advance PET scanner
  GE Advantage II ultrasound
  GE Advantage imager
  GE Advantx system
  GE CT Advantage high-speed CT
    system
  GE CT Advantage scanner
  GE CT HiSpeed Advantage CT
    system
  GE CTI 9800 scanner

G

GE *(continued)*
GE CTI single detector scanner
GE CT Max scanner
GE CT Pace scanner
GE 9800 CT scanner
GE 9800 CT system
GE CT/T 8800 scanner
GE CT/T7 scanner
GE 8800 CT/T scanner
GE EchoSpeed whole-body MR imager
GE Electric Advantx system
Excel GE
GE gamma camera
GE Genesis CT scanner
GE GN 500-MHz scanner
GE GN300 7.05-T/89-mm bore multinuclear spectrometer
GE 9800 high-resolution CT scanner
GE HiSpeed Advantage helical CT scanner
GE HiSpeed single detector scanner
GE Lightspeed CT scanner
GE Maxicamera gamma camera
GE MR Max scanner
GE MR Signa scanner
GE MR Vectra scanner
GE Neurocam camera
GE NMR spectrometer
GE Omega 500-MHz scanner
GE Pace CT scanner
GE pacemaker
GE proton head coil probe
GE QE 300-MHz scanner
GE Quest 300-H scanner
GE RT 3200 Advantage II
GE Senographe 2000D digital mammography system
GE Signa double doughnut
GE Signa Genesis MR imager
GE Signa 5.4 Genesis MR imager
GE Signa Horizon EchoSpeed MR imager
GE Signa 5.5 Horizon EchoSpeed MR imager
GE Signa Horizon SR 120 whole-body scanner
GE Signa magnet
GE Signa 4.7 MRI scanner
GE Signa MRI system
GE Signa MR system
GE Signa scanner
GE Signa 5.2 with SR-230 3-axis EPI gradient upgrade scanner
GE single-axis SR-230 echoplanar system
GE single-detector SPECT-capable camera
GE SPECT imager
GE Spiral CT scanner
GE Starcam single-crystal tomographic scintillation camera
GE Vectra MR scanner
GE Voluson 730 4D ultrasound system

gear
g. shift pedicle probe
turnout g.

Geenan Endotorque guidewire
Geggel corneal transplant marker
Gehrung pessary
Geiger
G. cautery
G. counter
G. electrocautery
G. electrocautery unit

Geiger-Müller
G.-M. counter
G.-M. detector
G.-M. survey meter
G.-M. tube

gel
Adcon adhesive control g.
Adcon-L anti-adhesion barrier g.
Aquagel lubricating g.
Aquasonic 100 ultrasound transmission g.
Avosil scar g.
CarraSmart g.
Carrington Dermal wound g.
g. cast
Cica-Care adhesive silicone g.
Crystal polymer g.
g. cushion
DynaGraft g.
Electro-Gel conductivity g.
Elta dermal g.
Emdogain g.
g. eye mask
fibrin g.
Flexall g.
Fricke g.
GenTeal lubricant eye g.
Grafton DBM demineralized bone graft g.
Hylaform viscoelastic g.
IntraSite g.
IPM wound g.
LAM IPM wound g.
Nasal Moist g.
osteoinductive enhanced graft g.
Oxiplex/SP g.
g. pack
g. pad
poloxamer-based g.

PRO/Gel ultrasound transmission g.
Scan ultrasound g.
g. sheeting
silicone g.
Silipos g.
Silosheath g.
sodium dodecyl sulfate-
  polyacrylamide gradient slab g.
sodium hyaluronate wound g.
SoloSite wound g.
g. stump sock
g. suspension sleeve
g. tubing
ultrasound g.
g. warmer
g. wound dressing
g. wrap
Gelastic bed
gelatin
g. compression boot
g. sponge
g. sponge packing
g. sponge pad
g. sponge pledget
gelatin-covered mesh stent
gelatin-resorcin-formalin
g.-r.-f. glue
g.-r.-f. tissue glue adhesive
gelatin-subbed slide
GelBand arm band
Gel-Bank patellar strap
Gelbfish-Endovasc device
gel-filled
g.-f. bladder
g.-f. implant
g.-f. prosthesis
Gelfilm
G. cap
G. dressing
G. forceps
G. ophthalmic film
G. plate
G. retinal implant
Gelfoam
G. cookie
G. cube
fibrin glue-soaked G.
G. pack
G. packing
G. pad
G. pledget
G. pressure forceps
G. punch
G. sponge
thrombin-soaked G.
TobraDex-soaked G.
G. torpedo
Geliperm gel dressing

Gellhorn
G. pessary
G. uterine biopsy forceps
Gellman instrumentation
Gelocast
G. bandage
G. Unna boot
G. Unna boot compression dressing
G. Unna boot compression wrap
G. Unna boot leg compression
  dressing
Gelpi
G. abdominal retractor
G. hysterectomy forceps
G. perineal retractor
G. retractor
G. self-retaining retractor
G. vaginal retractor
gel-saline Surgitek mammary prosthesis
Gel-Sole shoe insert
Gély suture
gem
Ampliwax PCR g.
G. DR implantable defibrillator
G. II DR dual-chamber defibrillator
G. III AT implantable cardioverter-
  defibrillator
G. II VR implantable cardioverter-
  defibrillator
G. Premier Plus blood
  gas/electrolyte analyzer
G. 21S enhanced tissue
  regeneration system
G. SensiCath blood gas monitoring
  system
G. total knee system
Gemini
G. automated centrifugal analyzer
G. chiropractic table
G. clamp
G. cup
G. gall duct forceps
G. hemostatic forceps
G. hip
G. hip system prosthesis
G. laser system
G. Mixter forceps
G. MKII mobile bearing knee
  implant
G. paired wire helical basket
G. syringe
GEM nonlatex medical bag
**GEM-Premier point-of-care blood
  analyzer**
GemStar infusion system
Gendron bariatric wheelchair
Gene
G. Clean II kit

Gene *(continued)*
    G. scissors
    G. Screen nylon membrane filter
GeneAmp PCR System 9600
  thermocycler
GeneChip
GenePhor
    G. DNA fragment analyzer
    G. DNA silver staining kit
general
    g. closure needle
    g. closure suture
    G. Electric Advantx system
    G. Electric pacemaker
    G. Electric Signa scanner
    g. probe
    g. retractor
    g. tissue forceps
    g. utility scissors
    g. wire forceps
General Aspirator Q
generation
    Chiron RIBA HCV test system
      second g.
    forced g.
    G. II 3DX brace
    G. II KAFO
    G. II knee brace
    G. II Unloader ADJ knee brace
    G. II Unloader Select knee brace
    G. 6 integrated radiotherapy system
    Ortho HCV ELISA test system
      second g.
    Zest Anchor Advanced G. (ZAAG)
generator
    aerosol g.
    Angeion 2000 ICD g.
    Atakr g.
    ballistic energy g.
    banana plug dipolar g.
    bipolar g.
    carbon dioxide g.
    Cardioblate RF g.
    CardioRhythm g.
    Chardack-Greatbatch implantable
      cardiac pulse g.
    Closure catheter/radiofrequency g.
    CO_2 g.
    computerized pattern g.
    Cosmos II multiprogrammable dual-
      chamber cardiac pulse g.
    Cosmos II pulse g.
    CPI-PRx pulse g.
    deuterium-tritium g.
    direct current g.
    distal stimulation g.
    Down flow g.
    ^{166}Dy g.
    dysprosium-holmium in vivo g.

electric g.
electrohydraulic g.
electrostatic g.
electrosurgical g.
Endostat II bipolar/monopolar
  electrosurgical g.
Erbe ICC electrosurgical g.
extraction g.
Force 2 CEM g.
Force FX g.
Grass visual pattern g.
high-voltage g.
^{166}Ho in vivo g.
implantable pulse g.
Instant Response technology g.
Intec AID cardioverter-
  defibrillator g.
Itrel I unipolar pulse g.
Itrel II quadripolar pulse g.
Itrel pulse g.
light beam g.
Lithoclast ballistic energy g.
Little Black Box frequency g.
magnet application over pulse g.
Maxilith pacemaker pulse g.
Medstone STS shock wave g.
Medtronic pulse g.
Medtronic 3470 pulse g.
microexplosive g.
Microlith pacemaker pulse g.
Microny II SR+ pulse g.
Microny SR+ single-chamber rate-
  responsive pulse g.
Minilith pacemaker pulse g.
molybdenum-99 g.
molybdenum-technetium g.
multiprogrammable pulse g.
Northgate SD-100 EHL g.
Pacesetter Affinity SR g.
Pacesetter Synchrony III pulse g.
Pacesetter Trilogy DR+ pulse g.
PCD ICD g.
3-phase g.
piezoelectric g.
polyphase g.
Programalith III pulse g.
programmable pulse g.
pulse g.
6-pulse 3-phase g.
12-pulse 3-phase g.
quadripolar Itrel 2 pulse g.
radiofrequency g.
Radionics radiofrequency g.
Radionics radiofrequency lesion g.
radionuclide g.
rate-responsive pulse g.
Regency SR, SR+ pulse g.
resonance g.
RF2000 Radiofrequency G.

Scan Pattern g.
SensorMedics g.
single-chamber pulse g.
small-particle aerosol g.
spark-gap shock wave g.
Super 50 CP high-voltage g.
supervoltage g.
Symmetry endobipolar g.
Synchrony II, III DDDR pulse g.
g. system
tantalum-178 g.
technetium-99m g.
Trilogy DC, DR, SR pulse g.
Triphasix g.
ultrasound g.
Valleylab g.
Valleylab Force IC
  electrosurgical g.
Valleylab II g.
Van de Graaf g.
ventricular demand pulse g.
Ventritex g.
VNUS Closure
  catheter/radiofrequency g.
VNUS radiofrequency g.
VPAP II ST-A bilevel flow g.
waveform g.
x-ray g.
GenESA
G. closed-loop delivery system
G. system
G. system for radionuclide imaging
  stress test
Genesis
G. arthroplasty hardware
G. 2000 carbon dioxide laser
G. diamond blade
G. II foot/ankle system
G. II foot system
G. II mobile-bearing knee implant
G. II total knee system
G. knee prosthesis
G. lens
G. neurostimulation system
G. stent
G. unicompartmental knee
**Genesys Vertex variable-angle gamma
  camera**
**Genetics Systems microplate reader
  spectrophotometer**
genial advancement plate
Genic coronary stent delivery system
Genie
G. lancet
G. resin
Genisis dual-chamber pacemaker
**Genitor mini-intrauterine insemination
  cannula**
Gennari band

**GenomeLab SNPstream genotyping
  system**
genomic probe
Genotropin
G. 2-chamber cartridge
G. mixer
G. Pen 5
G. pen
G. Pen 5 growth hormone delivery
  device
G. system
Genous bioengineered R stent
Gen-Probe hybridization kit
Gen-S
G.-S automated cell-counting
  instrument
G.-S hematology analyzer
Gensini
G. cardiac device
G. coronary arteriography catheter
G. Teflon catheter
GenSpin gDNA purification kit
gentamicin
g. high viscosity (G-HV)
g. implant
Genta slide
GenTeal lubricant eye gel
Gentell
G. alginate wound cover
G. alginate wound dressing
G. foam wound dressing
G. hydrogel dressing
G. impregnated gauze
G. isotonic saline wet dressing
G. wound cleanser
Gentex PDQ polycarbonate lens
gentian violet marking pen
Gentle
G. Jane Snap freezer
G. Threads interference screw
G. Touch colostomy appliance
G. Touch loop ostomy system
Gentle-Flo suction catheter
Gentle-Lance lancet device
GentleLASE
G. laser
G. Plus
G. Plus laser system
GentlePeel skin exfoliation system
GentleStep shoe
**Gentra Systems Puregene DNA isolation
  kit**
Genucentric knee hinge
Genucom
G. ACL laxity analysis system
G. arthrometer
G. knee flexion analysis system
genuine
g. sheepskin crutches accessory kit

G

genuine *(continued)*
  g. sheepskin elbow protector
  g. sheepskin heel protector
Genus stent
Genutrain
  G. knee brace
  G. P3 active knee support
  G. P3 knee support
GeoFlex
  G. knee
  G. knee prosthesis
Geo-Matt
  G.-M. contour cushion
  G.-M. 30-degree body aligner
  G.-M. gel cushion
  G.-M. PRT cushion
  G.-M. therapeutic foam overlay
  G.-M. wheelchair cushion
Geo-Mattress bariatric mattress
geometric
  g. device
  G. total knee prosthesis
Geo Rectangles spinal implant
George Washington strut
Georgiade
  G. breast prosthesis
  G. fixation device
  G. rasp
  G. visor
  G. visor cervical collar
  G. visor cervical traction
  G. visor halo fixation apparatus
Georgia valve
Gerald
  G. bayonet microbipolar
    neurosurgical forceps
  G. bipolar forceps
  G. dressing forceps
  G. forceps
  G. tissue forceps
Gerber space maintainer
Gerbode forceps
**GERDcheck ambulatory esophageal pH
  monitoring system**
Gerdy intraauricular loop
Gerhardt table
geriatric
  g. chair
  g. chair trunk support
Geristore dental implant
German lock
**Gerow-Harrington heart-shaped distal
  end retractor**
Gerster
  G. bone clamp
  G. traction bar
  G. traction device

Gertie
  G. ball
  G. Marx spinal needle
Gerzog
  G. bone hammer
  G. bone mallet
  G. ear knife
Gerzog-Ralks knife
Gesco
  G. aspirator
  G. cannula
  G. catheter
Gess I/A cannula
Get-A-Grip grip
Geuder injector
GFC gastroscope
**GFS Mark II inflatable penile
  prosthesis**
GFT Olympus gastroscope
**GF-UM30P linear-oriented radial
  scanning echoendoscope**
GF-UM3 scanner
GFX
  GFX 2 coronary stent system
  GFX Micro stent III
  GFX over-the-wire coronary stent
**GFXTM Genomic blood DNA
  purification kit**
Ghajar guide
G-HV
  gentamicin high viscosity
GI
  gastrointestinal
  GI clamp
  GI forceps
  Innerview GI
  GI pop-off silk suture
GIA
  GIA forceps
  GIA II loading unit
  GIA staple
  GIA stapler
  GIA 60, 80 stapler
  GIA stapling device
Giannestras turnbuckle
Gianturco
  G. biliary Z-stent
  G. coil
  G. expandable self-expanding
    metallic biliary prosthesis
  G. expandable self-expanding
    metallic biliary stent
  G. expanding metallic stent
  G. metal urethral stent
  G. occlusion coil
  G. prosthesis
  G. steel coil
  G. stent
  G. wool-tufted wire coil

G. zigzag stent
G. Z-stent
Gianturco-Grifka vascular occlusion device
Gianturco-Roehm bird's nest vena cava filter
Gianturco-Rosch
    G.-R. biliary stent
    G.-R. biliary Z-stent
    G.-R. self-expandable biliary Z-stent
    G.-R. self-expandable Z-stent
Gianturco-Roubin
    G.-R. flexible coil stent
    G.R. Flex II stent
    G.-R. FlexStent
    G.-R. FlexStent coronary stent
    G.-R. II stent
Gianturco-Wallace-Anderson coil
Gibbon
    G. indwelling ureteral stent
    G. urethral catheter
Gibbs eye punch
Gibbs-Gradle scissors
Gibney
    G. boot
    G. fixation bandage
Gibson
    G. bandage
    G. dressing
    G. inner ear shunt
    G. irrigating/aspirating unit
    G. irrigator
Gibson-Balfour abdominal retractor
Gibson-Cooke sweat test apparatus
Gibson-Ross board
Giebel blade-plate
Giertz rib shears
Giertz-Shoemaker rib shears
Giertz-Stille
    G.-S. rib shears
    G.-S. scissors
Gifford
    G. fixation forceps
    G. iris forceps
    G. mastoid retractor
    G. needle holder
    G. retractor
Gifford-Jansen mastoid retractor
GIF-HM endoscope
GIF-N30 fiberoptic pediatric endoscope
GIF-Q240 upper digestive tract endoscope
GIF-XP20 endoscope
GIF-XP series endoscope
GIF-XQ series endoscope
Gigli
    G. saw
    G. saw blade
    G. saw conductor

G. saw guide
G. saw handle
G. solid-handle saw
G. wire saw
Gigli-Strully saw
GII
    GII EasyAnchor
    GII KAFO
    GII Snap-Pak anchor
    GII Unloader ADJ knee brace
    GII Unloader OA brace
Gilbert-Graves speculum
Gilbert-type Bardex Foley catheter
Gilfillan humeral prosthesis
Giliberty
    G. acetabular prosthesis
    G. device
Gill
    G. biopsy brush
    G. blade
    G. corneal knife
    G. curved iris forceps
    G. double I&A cannula
    G. intraocular implant lens
    G. iris forceps
    G. needle
    G. renal tourniquet
    G. respirator
    G. scissors
Gill-Arruga capsular forceps
Gill-Chandler iris forceps
Gill-Colibri forceps
Gillespie obstetrical forceps
Gillette
    G. Blue Blade
    G. brace
    G. double-flexure ankle joint
    G. double-flexure ankle joint system
    G. joint
    G. joint orthosis
    G. joint prosthesis
    G. modification of ankle-foot orthosis
Gill-Fine corneal knife
Gill-Fuchs capsular forceps
Gill-Hess iris forceps
Gillies
    G. bone hook
    G. dissecting forceps
    G. dural hook
    G. horizontal dermal suture
    G. nasal hook
    G. needle holder
    G. scissors
    G. single-hook skin retractor
    G. skin hook
    G. suture scissors
    G. tissue forceps

G

Gillies *(continued)*
G. zygoma elevator
G. zygoma hook
Gillies-Converse skin hook
Gillies-Dingman tenaculum hook
Gillmore needle
Gillquist-Stille arthroplasty suction tube
Gills
G. double Luer-Lok cannula
G. pop-up arcuate diamond knife
Gill-Safar forceps
Gills-Welsh
G.-W. aspirating cannula
G.-W. curette
G.-W. guillotine port
G.-W. irrigating cannula
G.-W. knife
G.-W. scissors
G.-W. spatula
Gill-Thomas-Cosman frame
Gill-Thomas locator
Gill-Welsh-Morrison lens loupe
Gilman-Abrams gastric tube
Gilmer
G. dental splint
G. tooth splint
G. wire
Gilmore probe
Gil-Vernet renal sinus retractor
Gimbel
G. fountain cannula
G. glove
G. stabilization ring
G. stabilizing ring
gingival clamp
gingivectomy knife
Ginsberg
G. eye speculum
G. tissue forceps
GIP/Medi-Globe prototype needle
giraffe biopsy forceps
Girard
G. anterior chamber needle
G. cataract-aspirating needle
G. corneoscleral forceps
G. corneoscleral scissors
G. fragmatome
G. irrigating cannula
G. irrigating tip
G. keratoprosthesis prosthesis
G. phacofragmatome needle
G. phakofragmatome
G. scleral expander ring
G. synechia spatula
G. ultrasonic unit
Girard-Swan
G.-S. knife
G.-S. needle

girdle
Ace halo pelvic g.
compression g.
Lipo-Medi g.
male compression g.
Girdner probe
girth hitch
Gissane spike
Gittes needle
Given
G. diagnostic imaging system
G. M2A endoscopic videocapsule
G. videocapsule system
Givmohr upper extremity sling
Gizmo catheter
glabellar rasp
Glacier
G. ceramic 4-in-1 cutting guide
G. ceramic knee cutting guide
G. ceramic 4-in-1 knee cutting
guide
G. Pack
Gladiator shock suit
Gladstone-Putterman transmarginal
rotation entropion clamp
glarometer
Glaser laminectomy retractor
Glasgold Wafer chin implant
glass
g. bead
g. bead sterilizer
g. ionomer cement
g. penile prosthesis
g. pH electrode
g. sphere eye implant
g. sphere implant
g. thermometer
g. tract detector
g. vaginal plug
Glasscock ear dressing
Glasscock-House knife
Glaser fixation screw
glasses
bifocal g.
contact g.
Crookes g.
crutch g.
Difei g.
EyeArmor safety g.
fiberoptic video g.
Franklin g.
Hallauer g.
hyperbolic g.
liquid crystal g.
magnifying g.
Masselon g.
nystagmus g.
presbyopia g.
protective g.

safety g.
self-adjusted g.
trifocal g.
Wood g.

Glassman
G. basket
G. bowel atraumatic clamp
G. brush
G. clamp
G. intestinal clamp
G. noncrushing gastroenterostomy clamp
G. noncrushing gastrointestinal clamp
G. noncrushing pickup forceps
G. pickup forceps

Glassman-Allis noncrushing tissue-holding forceps
Glassman-Babcock forceps
Glattelast compression pantyhose
glaucoma
g. drainage device
g. pencil
g. wick

Glaucoma-Scope
Gleason guide
Glenn shunt
glenoid
g. alignment peg
g. drill
g. drill guide
g. fin broach
g. fixation screw
g. reaming forceps

Gliadel
G. implant
G. wafer

GliaSite
G. radiation therapy RTS system
G. radiation therapy system
G. radiotherapy system
G. RTS system

Glick
G. hip kit
G. instrument

glide
G. Cobra catheter
G. floss
Hessburg intraocular lens g.
g. hook
intraocular lens g.
mushroom walker g.
Sheets lens g.

Glidecath
G. hydrophilic coated catheter
G. XP catheter

GlideCath
G. dilator
G. entry needle

G. guidewire
G. hydrophilic coated catheter
G. sheath
G. syringe
G. torque device

Glidecatheter
glider
G. articular cartilage probe
g. cane
g. cane board
EasyStand 6000 g.
G. II patient transfer system

Glidesheath introducer sheath
Glidewire (*See also* guidewire)
angled G.
angle-tip G.
G. catheter
G. Gold surgical guidewire
long taper stiff shaft G.
Microvasive G.
Radifocus G.
Terumo G.
Terumo Radifocus G.

Glidex coated Percuflex catheter
gliding hinge joint
Glisson snare
global
G. Advantage CTA humeral head
G. conservative anatomic prosthesis
g. force applicator
G. Fx shoulder fracture system
G. Therapeutics Freedom stent
G. Therapeutics V-Flex stent
G. total shoulder arthroplasty
G. total shoulder arthroplasty system
G. total shoulder implant

globe prolapsus pessary
globular object forceps
Glori pressure earring
Glo-tip biliary catheter
glottic prosthesis
glove, pl. **gloves**
antivibration g.
Biobrane g.
Bio-Form g.
Biogel Diagnostic surgical g.
Biogel M surgical g.
Biogel Neotech surgical g.
Biogel orthopaedic surgical g.
Biogel Reveal g.
Biogel Reveal/Indicator surgical g.
Biogel Sensor surgical g.
Biogel Super-Sensitive surgical g.
Biogel surgeons' g.
carpal tunnel g.
compression g.
cotton g.
Dermapor g.

glove *(continued)*
   g. drain
   Elastylon g.
   electrode g.
   ESP radiation reduction
    examination g.
   Eudermic surgical g.
   finger flexion g.
   F&L attenuating g.
   flexion g.
   Flowers mandibular g.
   Gimbel g.
   Handeze fingerless g.
   impact g.
   Isotoner g.
   Jobst g.
   Kevlar g.
   Kid G.
   Life Liner stick and cut-
    resistant g.
   Maxxus orthopaedic latex
    surgical g.
   Medak g.
   Medarmor puncture-resistant g.
   mesh g.
   Micro-Touch Platex medical g.
   N-DEX non-latex g.
   Necelon surgical g.
   Neolon surgical g.
   nitrile g.
   Nouvisage Deep Hydration g.
   peripheral nerve g.
   pressure g.
   puncture-proof g.
   Push-Ease wheelchair g.
   radial nerve g.
   SensiCare synthetic powder-free
    surgical g.
   Skinsense g.
   SoftFlex computer g.
   Sorbothane antivibration g.
   Tactyl 1 g.
   TheraKnit electrode g.
   Tubigrip g.
   vibration g.
   vinyl g.
   weighted g.
Glove-n-Gel amniotomy kit
Glover
   G. auricular clamp
   G. bulldog clamp
   G. coarctation forceps
   G. curved clamp
   G. curved forceps
   G. patent ductus clamp
   G. patent ductus forceps
   G. spoon-shaped anastomosis clamp
   G. spoon-shaped forceps
   G. vascular clamp

Glover-DeBakey clamp
Glover-Stille clamp
gloves *(pl. of* glove)
glow modular tube
GLS
   GLS brace
   GLS suture anchor
Glucatell beta-glucagon blood test kit
Gluck rib shears
Glucoband electronic scanning device
Glucolet
   G. Automatic lancing device
   G. lancet device
glucometer
   Accu-Chek II g.
   Advantage g.
   Ascensia Breeze g.
   Bayer g.
   G. DEX blood glucose monitor
   G. DEX diabetes care system
   G. Elite R meter
   Glucostat II g.
   GlucoWatch g.
   G. II home glucose monitoring
    system
   OneTouch basic g.
GlucoNIR glucose sensor
Gluco-Protein OTC self-test
Glucoscan monitor
glucose
   blood g. (bG)
   g. meter
Glucostat II glucometer
GlucoWatch
   G. Biographer
   G. Biographer meter
   G. Biographer transdermal sensor
   G. bloodless glucose monitor
   G. G2 Biographer diabetes
    monitoring system
   G. glucometer
   G. glucose monitor
   G. glucose monitoring device
glue
   BioGlue g.
   Biolex wound g.
   butyl cyanoacrylate g.
   CoSeal fibrin g.
   cyanoacrylate g.
   cyanoacrylate tissue g.
   ethyl cyanoacrylate g.
   fibrin g.
   gelatin-resorcin-formalin g.
   Histoacryl g.
   Loctite 15494 ethyl
    cyanoacrylate g.
   methyl cyanoacrylate g.
   N-butyl-2-cyanoacrylate g.
   g. patch

self-gelling g.
surgical g.
Technovit 7210 VLC contact g.
Tisseel fibrin g.
Tisseel surgical g.
tissue g.
TruFill n-BCA surgical g.
glued-on hard contact lens
glue-in suture
glutameter
glutaraldehyde alarm
glutaraldehyde-tanned
g.-t. bovine collagen tube
g.-t. bovine graft
g.-t. bovine heart valve
g.-t. porcine heart valve
glycerine syringe
glycerin-preserved graft
glycolide trimethylene carbonate material
GlyMed Camouflage system
GM
GM alloy
GM instrument
Gnatholator
gnathologic instrument
Gobble Plus removal instrument
Gobi dehumidifier
Goddio disposable cannula
Goelet double-ended retractor
Goeltec catheter
Goetz
G. bipolar electrode
G. cardiac device
Goffman eye garter
goggles
Avotec MR-compatible liquid crystal display g.
dry eye g.
Frenzel g.
Fresnel g.
moisture g.
sports g.
swimmer's g.
Zoom and Sniper sports g.
goiter
g. clamp
g. hook
g. retractor
g. scissors
Golaski knitted Dacron graft
Golaski-UMI vascular prosthesis
Golay gradient coil
gold
g. biocompatible implant
g. bur
g. burnisher
G. deep surgery forceps

g. disc Grass electrode
g. ear marker
g. eyelid implant
g. eyelid load implant
G. hemostatic forceps
G. Medal foot prosthesis
Medtronic MiniMed CGMS system g.
g. needle
25 G. portable CO_2 laser
G. Probe
G. Probe bipolar hemostasis catheter
G. Probe Direct bipolar hemostasis catheter
G. Probe electrohemostasis catheter
g. ring
g. saw
G. Series bone drilling system
g. weight
g. weight and wire spring implant material
Goldberg-MPC mediastinoscope
Goldberg side port splitter
Goldblatt
G. clamp
G. kidney
gold-coated
g.-c. Inflow coronary stent
g.-c. inflow coronary stent
Golden
G. Comfort orthotic
G. Fitness orthotic
G. Retriever
Goldenberg
G. footplate shoe
G. hydroxylapatite implant
G. implant system
G. Snarecoil bone marrow biopsy needle
GoldenEye arthroscope
gold-handled chuck
Goldman
G. applanation tonometer
G. capsulorrhexis forceps
G. curette
G. guarded chisel
G. saw
G. scleral fixation ring and blepharostat
G. septal elevator
G. tonometer
G. vaporizer
Goldman-Fox
G.-F. gum scissors
G.-F. knife
G.-F. probe
G.-F. wound debridement scissors

G

Goldman-Kazanjian
- G.-K. nasal forceps
- G.-K. rongeur

Goldmann
- G. contact lens prism
- G. goniolens
- G. macular contact lens
- G. 3-mirror contact diagnostic lens
- G. 3-mirror gonioscopy lens
- G. multi-mirror lens
- G. perimeter
- G. serrated knife

Goldmann-Weekers adaptometer
gold-marked stent
Gold-Mules eye implant
gold-paneled chisel
GoldPoint
- G. ACL functional knee brace
- G. hinged knee brace
- G. PCL functional knee brace

GoldSeal nasal mask
Goldstein
- G. anterior chamber syringe
- G. cannula
- G. golf-club spud
- G. Grasp atraumatic cervical stabilizer
- G. irrigating cannula
- G. lacrimal cannula
- G. lacrimal sac retractor
- G. lacrimal syringe
- G. Microspike approximator clamp
- G. Microspike approximator clamp for vasoepididymostomy
- G. Microspike approximator clamp for vasovasostomy
- G. refractor
- G. retractor
- G. sonohysterography catheter

Goldthwait
- G. brace
- G. fracture appliance
- G. fracture frame

Gold-tip micro guidewire
Goldwasser suture carrier
golf
- g. club spud
- G. exercise system
- g. tee hollow titanium cannula
- g. tee-shaped polyvinyl prosthesis
- g. tee UAL cannula

golf-stick dissector
Golgi
- G. apparatus
- G. device

Goligher
- G. modification of Berkeley-Bonney retractor
- G. retractor

- G. speculum
- G. sternal-lifting retractor

Gomco
- G. bell
- G. bell clamp
- G. bloodless circumcision clamp
- G. circumcision bell
- G. circumcision clamp
- G. clamp
- G. drain
- G. forceps
- G. pump
- G. suction tube
- G. thoracic drainage pump
- G. umbilical clamp
- G. uterine aspirator

Gomez gastric retractor
gonad shield
Gonin
- G. cautery
- G. marker

Gonin-Amsler scleral marker
goniofocalizing lens
goniogram
- Becker g.

goniolaser
- Thorpe 4-mirror g.

goniolens
- Allen-Thorpe g.
- Barkan g.
- Goldmann g.
- Koeppe g.
- 4-mirror g.
- single-mirror g.
- Thorpe-Castroviejo g.
- Thorpe 4-mirror g.
- Zeiss g.

goniometer
- 2-arm g.
- Bailliart g.
- Conzett g.
- digital g.
- electronic g.
- EOC g.
- finger g.
- full-circle g.
- International standard g.
- orthopaedic g.
- Polk finger g.
- Sammons biplane g.
- Sedan g.
- Universal g.
- Zimmer g.

gonion gradient coil
goniophotography
gonioprism
- Posner diagnostic g.
- Posner surgical g.

goniopuncture knife

gonioscope
  Heine g.
  Sussman 4-mirror g.
  Thorpe surgical g.
  Troncoso g.
  Zeiss g.
gonioscopic
  g. implant
  g. lens
  g. prism
goniotomy
  g. knife
  g. knife cannula
  g. needle holder
Gonzalez specialized dissecting cannula
Gooch retractor
Good
  G. Grips utensil
  G. 'N Bed wedge
  G. rasp
  G. retractor
Goodale-Lubin
  G.-L. cardiac catheter
  G.-L. cardiac device
  G.-L. catheter
Goode
  G. nasal splint
  G. T tube
  G. T-tube ventilating tube
  G. wrap
Goodell uterine dilator
Goodhill-Pynchon tonsillar suction tube
GoodKnight 418A, 418G, 418P CPAP system
Good-Reiner scissors
Goodwin bone clamp
gooseneck
  g. chisel
  g. rongeur
  g. snare
Goosen vascular punch
Gordon
  G. bead forceps
  G. ciliary forceps
  G. splint
  G. uterine forceps
  G. vulsellum forceps
Gordon-Broström single-contrast arthrogram
Gore
  G. cast liner
  G. cast liner material
  G. covered biliary stent-graft
  G. HemaCarotid vascular patch
  G. HemaPatch vascular graft
  G. Preclude MVP dura substitute
  G. Preclude PDX dura substitute
  G. Resolut Adapt bioresorbable
    regenerative membrane

  G. Resolut Adapt LT regenerative
    membrane
  G. S.A.M. patch material
  G. subcutaneous augmentation
    material
  G. suture passer
  G. Tag endoprosthesis system
  G. Tag thoracic endoprosthesis
  G. thyroplasty device
  G. torso array MRI surface coil
  G. Viabil biliary endoprosthesis
Gore-Tex
  G.-T. Acuseal cardiovascular patch
  G.-T. AF fistula
  G.-T. alloplastic material
  G.-T. aortofemoral fistula
  G.-T. baffle
  G.-T. bifurcated vascular graft
  G.-T. cardiovascular patch
  G.-T. catheter
  G.-T. DualMesh biomaterial
  G.-T. DualMesh Plus biomaterial
  G.-T. FEP-ringed vascular graft
  G.-T. graft
  G.-T. Intering vascular graft
  G.-T. jump graft
  G.-T. knee prosthesis
  G.-T. membrane
  G.-T. Mycromesh biomaterial
  G.-T. Mycromesh Plus biomaterial
  G.-T. nasal implant
  G.-T. periodontal material
  G.-T. peritoneal catheter
  G.-T. regenerative material
  G.-T. SAM facial implant
  G.-T. shunt
  G.-T. sling reinforcement
  G.-T. soft tissue patch
  G.-T. stretch vascular graft
  G.-T. strip
  G.-T. surgical membrane
  G.-T. suture
  G.-T. tag
  G.-T. tapered vascular graft
  G.-T. tube
  G.-T. vascular implant
  G.-T. waterproof cast liner
Gorlin pacing catheter
Gorney
  G. dissector
  G. facelift scissors
  G. rhytidectomy scissors
  G. septal scissors
  G. straight facelift scissors
  G. turbinate scissors
Gorney-Freeman straight facelift scissors
gossamer silk suture
Gosset
  G. abdominal retractor

G

Gosset *(continued)*
    G. appendectomy retractor
    G. self-retaining retractor
Gotfried percutaneous compression plating
Gothic arch tracer
Gott
    G. butterfly heart valve
    G. cannula
    G. implant
    G. low-profile prosthesis
    G. malleable retractor
    G. shunt
    G. tube
Gott-Balfour blade
Gott-Daggett heart valve prosthesis
Gott-Harrington blade
Gottschalk
    G. nasostat
    G. transverse saw
Gouffon hip pin
gouge
    Acufex g.
    Alexander mastoid bone g.
    anular g.
    AO g.
    Ballenger g.
    Bishop mastoid g.
    bone g.
    Buck-Gramcko g.
    Capener g.
    Chermel bone g.
    Cobb spinal g.
    concave g.
    curved g.
    Flanagan spinal fusion g.
    Freer nasal g.
    Guy g.
    Hibbs bone g.
    Hibbs spinal fusion g.
    hip arthroplasty g.
    Hoen g.
    Hough g.
    hump g.
    Jewett g.
    Killian g.
    Kuhnt g.
    lacrimal sac g.
    Lahey Clinic spinal fusion g.
    Lexer g.
    Lillie g.
    long-handle offset g.
    Lucas g.
    Mannerfelt g.
    Martin hip g.
    mastoid g.
    Metzenbaum g.
    Moe g.
    Murphy g.

    nasal g.
    orthopaedic g.
    Partsch g.
    Read g.
    Rubin g.
    semicircular g.
    Sheehan g.
    Smith-Petersen gooseneck g.
    spinal fusion g.
    g. spud
    Stagnara g.
    Stille bone g.
    surgical g.
    tendon g.
    Todd g.
    Turner spinal g.
    U.S. Army g.
    U X-Acto g.
    vomerine g.
    Walton foreign body g.
    Watson-Jones bone g.
    West g.
    West bone g.
    West nasal g.
    X-Acto g.
    Zielke g.
    Zimmer g.
Gould
    G. electromagnetic flowmeter
    G. ES 1000 recorder
    G. Instrument Systems spirometer
    G. intraocular implant lens
    G. PentaCath 5-lumen thermodilution catheter
    G. polygraph
    G. polygraph gastric motility measuring device
    G. pressure monitor
    G. pressure transducer
    G. suture
Gould-Brush 481 8-channel recorder
Gould-Statham pressure transducer
Goulian
    G. blade
    G. dermatome
    G. knife
Goulter device
Gowen decompression tube
gown
    barrier g.
    Exami-Gown MRI g.
GP-8 sonic digitizer
GPI
    Vitek GPI
GPX rotary instrument
grab bar
grabber
    arthroscopic g.
    meniscal suture g.

Tab G.
   tendon g.
Grabow forceps
Grace plate 4-hole adapter
Gracey Deep Pocket curette
Gradal individual customized
  progressive lens
gradient
   g. amplifier
   g. coil
   g. index lens
   Power Trak 6000 g.
   g. sheet coil
gradiometer
   axial g.
Gradle
   G. cilia forceps
   G. ciliary forceps
   G. corneal trephine
   G. eyelid retractor
   G. scissors
   G. stitch scissors
graduated
   g. catheter
   g. compression stocking
   g. electronic decelerator
   g. Garrett dilator
Graduate measuring wire guide
Graefe
   G. cataract knife
   G. cataract spoon
   G. curved iris forceps
   G. cystitome knife
   G. cystotome
   G. dressing forceps
   G. eye fixation forceps
   G. eye speculum
   G. fixation forceps
   G. flexible cystotome
   G. forceps
   G. instrument
   G. iris forceps
   G. iris hook
   G. iris knife
   G. iris needle
   G. knife
   G. scarifier
   G. strabismus hook
   G. straight iris forceps
   G. tissue forceps
   G. tissue-grasping forceps
Graether
   G. button hook
   G. collar button
   G. mushroom hook
   G. pupil expander
   G. refractor
   G. retractor

Grafaster
   Jostent G.
Grafco
   G. breast pump
   G. cannula
   G. colostomy bag
   G. cotton-tip applicator
   G. eye shield
   G. incontinence clamp
   G. laryngeal mirror
   G. magnet
   G. ophthalmoscope
   G. otoscope
   G. percussion hammer
   G. seizure stick
   G. tourniquet
   G. umbilical cord clamp
Grafco-Halsted forceps
Graflex material
Graf stabilization system
graft
   accordion g.
   G. ACE fixed-wire balloon catheter
   acellular human dermal g.
   acrylic g.
   Advanta PTFE vascular g.
   Albee bone g.
   albumin-coated vascular g.
   aldehyde-tanned bovine carotid
    artery g.
   AlloDerm acellular dermal g.
   AlloDerm onlay g.
   AlloDerm processed tissue g.
   AlloDerm spacer g.
   AlloDerm universal dermal
    tissue g.
   Ancure tube g.
   aortic tube g.
   Apligraf g.
   Aria coronary artery bypass g.
   Artegraft natural collagen
    vascular g.
   autogenic g.
   autogenous quadrupled hamstring
    tendon g.
   batten g.
   BCP bone g.
   bifurcated vascular g.
   Biobrane glove g.
   Biocoral g.
   Biograft g.
   Biogran resorbable synthetic
    bone g.
   biopolymeric vascular g.
   Björk-Shiley g.
   Blair-Brown g.
   g. board
   Bonfiglio bone g.
   Boplant g.

G

graft *(continued)*
  bovine pericardium dural g.
  Braun-Wangensteen g.
  brephoplastic g.
  buttress g.
  cable g.
  Calcitite bone g.
  CardioPass coronary artery
    bypass g.
  CardioPass layered microporous
    small-bore vascular g.
  g. carrier spoon
  CenterFlex g.
  chemosterilized g.
  g. clamp
  clip g.
  Codivilla g.
  compressed Ivalon patch g.
  g. containment system
  Corvita endoluminal g.
  Corvita endoprosthesis stent g.
  Corvita endovascular g.
  Cragg endoluminal g.
  CryoLife valvular g.
  Dacron-covered stent g.
  Dacron knitted g.
  Dacron preclotted g.
  Dacron tube g.
  Dacron tubular g.
  Dacron velour g.
  Dardik umbilical g.
  Davis g.
  DeBakey g.
  g. delivery system (GDS)
  Dembone g.
  Dermagraft g.
  Diastat vascular access g.
  Distaflo bypass g.
  double-thickness Sheen g.
  double velour knitted g.
  Douglas g.
  g. dowel
  g. driver
  Dynaflo bypass g.
  Edwards-Tapp arterial g.
  endoluminal stent g.
  endovascular aortic g.
  Esser g.
  expanded polytetrafluoroethylene-
    covered nitinol TIPS stent g.
  expanded polytetrafluoroethylene
    vascular g.
  externally supported Dacron g.
  FEP-ringed Gore-Tex vascular g.
  fiberglass g.
  Flixene vascular g.
  Fluency tracheobronchial stent g.
  glutaraldehyde-tanned bovine g.
  glycerin-preserved g.

  Golaski knitted Dacron g.
  Gore HemaPatch vascular g.
  Gore-Tex g.
  Gore-Tex bifurcated vascular g.
  Gore-Tex FEP-ringed vascular g.
  Gore-Tex Intering vascular g.
  Gore-Tex jump g.
  Gore-Tex stretch vascular g.
  Gore-Tex tapered vascular g.
  Grafton DBM crunch demineralized
    bone g.
  Grafton DBM flex g.
  Grafton DBM flex demineralized
    bone g.
  Grafton DBM matrix PLE
    demineralized bone g.
  Graftpatch g.
  Hancock pericardial valve g.
  Hancock vascular g.
  HemaPatch vascular g.
  Hemashield Gold 1, 4 branch
    AAA g.
  Hemashield Gold Microvel knitted
    double velour g.
  Hemashield Vantage vascular g.
  Hybrid g.
  IMA g.
  Impra g.
  Impra Carboflo ePTFE vascular g.
  Impra CenterFlex g.
  Impra Distaflo bypass g.
  Impra Flex vascular g.
  Impra microporous PTFE
    vascular g.
  Impra Venaflo vascular g.
  InFuse bone g.
  InterGard heparin g.
  InterGard Silver vascular g.
  InterGard vascular g.
  Intering vascular g.
  Ionescu-Shiley pericardial valve g.
  Ionescu-Shiley vascular g.
  irradiation sterilized g.
  Ivalon compressed patch g.
  Kimura cartilage g.
  knitted g.
  Koenig g.
  Krause-Wolfe g.
  LAD composite g.
  latex sponge g.
  Lee g.
  LifeCell AlloDerm acellular
    dermal g.
  ligamentous anterior dislocation
    composite g.
  Lo-Por vascular g.
  mandrel g.
  Marlex g.
  Marlex mesh g.

Meadox g.
Meadox Microvel arterial g.
Meadox Microvel double velour
  Dacron g.
Meadox vascular g.
g. measuring instrument
Mersilene g.
mesh g.
methyl methacrylate g.
Microknit patch g.
Microvel double velour g.
Millesi interfascicular g.
modified human graft umbilical
  vein g.
modular stent g.
Mules g.
Mystique resorbable g.
nonvalved g.
Ollier g.
Ollier-Thiersch g.
OP-1 bone g.
OP-1 implant/bone g.
Opteform 100HT bone g.
OsSatura BCP bone g.
OsSatura TCP bone g.
OsteoGen bone g.
osteogenic protein-1 bone g.
Padgett mesh skin g.
Papineau bone g.
patch g.
PepGen P-15 bone g.
Peri-Guard vascular g.
PerioGlas synthetic bone g.
Perma-Flow coronary bypass g.
Perma-Seal dialysis access g.
pigskin g.
polyethylene g.
polytetrafluoroethylene stent g.
polyurethane g.
polyvinyl g.
porcine g.
portacaval H g.
ProKera amniotic membrane g.
Pro-Osteon 500 bone implant g.
Proplast g.
prosthetic g.
PTFE Gore-Tex g.
PTFE stent g.
Rastelli g.
Reverdin g.
Sauvage filamentous velour g.
seamless g.
Sheen g.
Sheen tip g.
sieve g.
silastic g.
Siloxane g.
in situ tricortical iliac crest block
  bone g.

sponge g.
spongiosa bone g.
spreader g.
St. Jude composite valve g.
strut g.
g. suction tube
Supramid g.
Talent bifurcated abdominal aortic
  stent g.
Talent stent g.
tarsoconjunctival composite g.
Teflon g.
Thiersch g.
TransCyte skin substitute g.
tube g.
tunnel g.
Ulramax knitted double velour
  vascular g.
Vanguard III endovascular aortic g.
Varivas loop g.
Varivas R vein g.
VascuLink vascular access g.
Vascutek Gelseal vascular g.
Vascutek knitted vascular g.
Vascutek woven vascular g.
velour collar g.
Venaflo vascular g.
VertiGraft textured allograft
  bone g.
Vitagraft vascular g.
Weavenit patch g.
Wolf g.
Wölfe-Krause g.
woven Dacron fabric g.
woven Dacron tube g.
XenoDerm g.
xenogeneic g.
Zenith AAA endovascular g.

Graftac absorbable skin tack
Graftac-S skin stapler
GraftAssist
  G. vein and graft holder
  G. vein-graft holder
GraftCyte
  G. gauze
  G. gauze wound dressing
  G. moist dressing
  G. moist wound dressing
Graftech
  G. anterior ramp
  G. cervical dowel
  G. cervical spacer
  G. posterior ramp
  G. structural allograft anterior ramp
  G. structural allograft cervical
    dowel
  G. structural allograft cervical
    spacer

G

Graftech (*continued*)
  G. structural allograft posterior
    ramp
Graftjacket
  G. acellular periosteum replacement
    scaffold
  G. regenerative tissue matrix
  G. rotator cuff tendon
    reinforcement scaffold
  G. ulcer repair matrix
Graftmaster device
Grafton
  G. bone grafting material
  G. bone matrix/marrow combination
  G. DBM crunch demineralized
    bone graft
  G. DBM demineralized bone graft
    gel
  G. DBM flex demineralized bone
    graft
  G. DBM flex graft
  G. DBM matrix demineralized
    bone graft plug
  G. DBM matrix PLE demineralized
    bone graft
  G. DBM matrix strip
  G. DBM Orthoblend
  G. DBM putty
  G. demineralized bone matrix putty
    material
  G. flexible sheet
  G. moldable putty
  G. Plus DBM demineralized bone
    graft paste
  G. Plus DBM paste
Graftpatch graft
graft-seeking catheter
Graftskin
  Apligraf G.
Graham
  G. blunt hook
  G. catheter
  G. deep surgery scissors
  G. dural hook
  G. muscle hook
  G. nerve hook
  G. pediatric scissors
  G. scalene elevator
Grahamizer I exerciser
Graham-Kerrison punch
Gram cannula
Granberg cervical traction system
Grand
  G. Sahara dehumidifier
  G. Stand support stand
Grandon
  G. cortex extractor set
  G. T-incision marker
GraNee needle

Granger articulator
Grant abdominal aortic aneurysmal
  clamp
granule
  Conduit TCP g.
  Dembone demineralized cortical g.
  DynaGraft g.
  ProOsteon Implant 500 g.
  TruGraft BGS g.
graphic level recorder
Graseby anesthesia pump
grasper
  Acufex g.
  Blakesley g.
  bowel g.
  Captura 3-prong g.
  Daniel g.
  Delta wire g.
  Endo Babcock g.
  endoscopic Babcock g.
  Hasson g.
  laparoscopic g.
  Lion's Claw g.
  Lion's Paw g.
  loose body g.
  MetraGrasp ligament g.
  Polaris g.
  Polaris reusable g.
  polyp g.
  3-pronged g.
  Ramirez EndoForehead g.
  tripod g.
grasping
  g. biopsy forceps
  g. clamp
  g. forceps
  g. forceps tip
  g. instrument
  g. tripod forceps
Grass
  G. electrode
  G. electroencephalograph
  G. force displacement fluid
    collector
  G. model S9 stimulator
  G. neurostimulator
  G. pressure-recording device
  G. S88 muscle stimulator
  G. stimulation isolation unit
  G. visual pattern generator
Grasshopper positioner
GRASS system
grater
  acetabular g.
grater-type reamer
grating monochromator
Graves
  G. bivalve speculum
  G. open-side vaginal speculum

gravimetric device
gravitational device
gravity
  g. equinus cast
  g. extension locking system
  g. infusion cannula
gravity-driven angle finder
Gravlee jet washer
Gray
  G. arterial forceps
  G. bone drill
  G. clamp
  G. cystic duct forceps
  G. flexible intramedullary reamer
  G. photochromic lens
  G. reamer
  G. revision instrument system
  G. surgical retractor
gray-level histogram
gray-scale
  g.-s. monitor
  g.-s. ultrasonogram
Grayson corneal forceps
Grazer blepharoplasty forceps
great
  g. big Barbie retractor
  G. Ormond Street pediatric
    tracheostomy tube
  G. Smokies Diagnostic Laboratories
    intestinal permeability test kit
  g. toe implant
Greco cutting block
green
  g. braided suture
  G. bulldog clamp
  G. cataract knife
  G. corneal dissector
  G. cystic duct forceps
  G. Endo-Ice pulp tester
  G. eye shield
  G. fixation forceps
  g. laser light photocoagulator
  G. lens spatula
  G. lid clamp
  g. Mersilene suture
  g. monofilament polyglyconate
    suture
  G. mouthgag
  G. muscle hook
  g. needle holder
  g. pulsed dye laser
  G. refractor
  G. Sleeve compression device
  G. strabismus hook
  G. strabismus tucker
  G. thyroid retractor
  G. tissue grasping forceps
Green-Armytage hemostatic forceps

Greenberg
  G. bar
  G. clamp
  G. instrument holder
  G. retracting system
  G. retractor frame
  G. retractor mounting system
  G. retractor set
  G. Universal retractor
Greenberg-Sugita
  G.-S. retractor
  G.-S. retractor grid
Greene
  G. endocervical curette
  G. forceps
  G. needle
  G. renal transplant stent
  G. uterine curette
Greenen
  G. Endotorque
  G. pancreatic stent
Greenfield
  G. catheter
  G. caval catheter
  G. filter
  G. IVC filter
  G. needle
  G. titanium IVC filter
  G. vena cava filter
  G. vena cava filter system
Green-Gould needle
Green-Kenyon corneal marker
GreenLight PV laser system
Green-Seligson-Henry nail
Green-Sewall mouthgag
Greenwald
  G. Control Tip cystoscopic
    electrode
  G. flexible endoscopic electrode
  G. needle
  G. retractor
  G. Roth Grip-Tip suture guide
  G. sound
Greenwood
  G. bayonet forceps
  G. bipolar coagulation-suction
    forceps
Gregg cannula
Gregory
  G. carotid bulldog clamp
  G. external clamp
  G. forceps
  G. stay suture clamp
  G. vascular miniature clamp
Greifer prosthesis
Greiling gastroduodenal tube
Greiner Vacuette coagulation plastic
  tube
Greishaber self-retaining retractor

Greissinger foot prosthesis
Greven alligator forceps
Grey-Hess screen
Greyhound adjustable spring clip
Grey Turner forceps
Grice suture needle
grid
  Amsler g.
  Bucky g.
  g. cabinet
  copper g.
  g. electrode
  Greenberg-Sugita retractor g.
  g. maze board
  g. maze set
  nickel g.
  ocular g.
  oscillating g.
  radiographic g.
  scatter g.
  Shar-Tek foot positioning g.
Gridley intraocular lens
Grierson meniscal shaver
Grieshaber
  G. blade
  G. calibrated trephine
  G. corneal needle
  G. corneal trephine
  G. diamond-coated forceps
  G. endo-illuminator
  G. flexible iris retractor
  G. 2-function manipulator
  G. 3-function manipulator
  G. internal limiting membrane
    forceps
  G. iris forceps
  G. iris needle
  G. keratome
  G. manipulator forceps
  G. microbipolar coagulator
  G. needle holder
  G. ophthalmic needle
  G. power injector system
  G. ruby knife
  G. self-retaining retractor
  G. ultrasharp knife
  G. vertical cutting scissors
  G. vitreous scissors
Grieshaber-Balfour retractor
Griffin bandage lens dressing
Griffiths-Brown forceps
grinder
  Kontes Pellet Pestle disposable
    microtissue g.
  Potter-Elvehjem handheld tissue g.
GRIN lens
grip
  dowel g.
  Get-A-Grip g.

Neo-Fit neonatal endotracheal
  tube g.
Polly power g.
Posey g.
screw g.
Skil-Care cushion g.
g. torque device
Grip-Ease device
Gripp
  G. squeeze ball
  G. squeeze ball hand exerciser
gripper
  g. needle
  Steeper powered G.
Grip-Tip suture guide
GripTrack Commander strength tester
grit-blasted prosthesis
Grizzard subretinal fluid cannula
Grollman
  G. pigtail catheter
  G. pulmonary artery-seeking
    catheter
grommet
  g. bone liner
  g. drain tube
  Exmoor aural g.
  g. myringotomy tube
  Shah g.
  Shepard g.
  silastic g.
  g. tube
  g. ventilating tube
Groningen
  G. button
  G. valve
  G. voice prosthesis
grooved
  g. director
  g. silicone implant
  g. silicone sponge
  g. tying forceps
groover
groove suture
grooving reamer
Groshong
  G. catheter
  G. distal-valve catheter
  G. double-lumen catheter
  G. NXT PICC
Gross
  G. dressing forceps
  G. ear curette
  G. ear hook
  G. ear spoon
  G. sponge forceps
Grossan
  G. nasal irrigator tip with Water
    Pik

G. nasal irrigator tip with Water Pik and saline

Grosse-Kempf

G.-K. bone drill
G.-K. femoral nail
G.-K. locking nail
G.-K. tibial nail

Gross-Pomeranz-Watkins retractor

Grote 2000 ossicular replacement system

grounding pad

Grover

G. clamp
G. meniscotome
G. meniscus knife

GrowTrak Plus

Gruber

G. bougie
G. ear speculum

Gruca-Weiss spring

Gruening eye magnet

Grüning magnet

Grüntzig

G. arterial balloon catheter
G. balloon
G. balloon angiography catheter
G. balloon catheter
G. balloon catheter angioplasty
G. balloon dilatation catheter
G. balloon dilator
G. Dilaca catheter
G. femoral stiffening cannula
G. G, S dilating catheter
G. steerable catheter

Grüntzig-Dilaca catheter

GS-9

GS-9 blade
GS-9 needle

GSA-9 blade

GSB

GSB elbow prosthesis
GSB knee prosthesis

G&S electroejaculator

GSH nail

GSI

GSI 16 audiometer
GSI balloon dissector system
GSI 60 distortion product otoacoustic emission device

GS Modular pulmonary testing system

G-suit device

GT

Cytobrush Plus GT

GTC repeated stereotactic localizer framer

GTR

guided tissue regeneration

GTS

guided trephine system

GTS great toe system
GTS 2-piece implant system
TMS-1 videokeratoscope GTS

Guangzhou GD-1 prosthetic valve

guard

Albany eye g.
ankle g.
Attends pad and g.
Breast Biopsy G.
cannula g.
CastGuard g.
cataract knife g.
Cloward cervical drill g.
Combiguard II irrigation splash g.
Dignity Plus Briefmates G.
drill g.
ether g.
eye knife g.
forceps g.
Freedom palm g.
Horsley g.
intracardiac sucker g.
Joseph g.
keratome g.
Kneed-It knee g.
laser-assisted intrastromal keratomileusis cannula eye g.
LASIK eye g.
McDavid ankle g.
McDavid hinged knee g.
Midas Rex bur g.
mouth g.
Omed vented instrument g.
PAL-Guard postamputation limb g.
palm g.
Peri-Guard vascular graft g.
pin g.
plastic mouth g.
Pro-Designed wrist g.
Progressive palm g.
scalpel g.
snore g.
Somatics mouth g.
Storz Teflon forceps g.
tip g.
tooth g.
Twist-Lock drill g.
Ullrich drill g.
UltraPower bur g.

guarded

g. bur
g. chisel
g. irrigating cystotome
g. osteotome

Guardian

G. AICD
G. catheter
G. DNA system
G. ICD

G

Guardian *(continued)*
    G. limb salvage system
    G. pacemaker
    G. 2-piece ostomy system
    G. 1-piece ostomy system sterile
      drainage OR set
    G. Red Dot walker
    G. vaginal retractor
guard-ring tocodynamometer
Guardsman femoral interference screw
Guardwire
    G. angioplasty system
    G. embolus containment system
GuardWire
    G. distal balloon
    PercuSurge G.
    G. Plus
    G. Plus system
    G. temporary occlusion and
      aspiration system
Guedel
    G. airway
    G. laryngoscope
    G. laryngoscope blade
Guedel-Negus laryngoscope
Guell
    G. irrigation cannula
    G. LASIK cannula
    G. LASIK irrigating cannula
    G. LASIK speculum
Guell-type LASIK speculum
Guepar II hinged knee prosthesis
Guest needle
Guggenheim-Schuknecht scissors
Guglielmi
    G. detachable coil (GDC)
    G. detachable coil system
Guibor
    G. canaliculus intubation set
    G. Expo eye bubble
    G. lacrimal drain
    G. shield
    G. silastic tube
Guidant
    G. balloon
    G. CRM pacemaker
    G. defibrillator
    G. guidewire
    G. guiding catheter
    G. Heart Rhythm Technologies
      Linear Ablation system
    G. Megalink peripheral stent
    G. Multi-Link Tetra coronary stent
      system
    G. Triad 3-electrode energy
      defibrillation system
    G. TRIAD three-electrode energy
      defibrillation system
Guidant-CPI device

guide
Accu-Cut osteotomy g.
Accu-Line g.
Accu-Line chamfer resection g.
acetabular angle g.
acetabular shell g.
Achillon instrument g.
ACL drill g.
Acufex alignment g.
Acufex drill g.
Adapteur multifunctional drill g.
adjustable-angle g.
Adson drill g.
aiming g.
Amplatz tapered extra-stiff wire g.
Amplatz tube g.
Amplatz ultra-stiff wire g.
angel wing g.
anterior cruciate ligament drill g.
antirotation g.
AO stopped drill g.
apical axis g.
Arthrex femoral g.
Arthrex tibial tunnel g.
Ascension Neurolac nerve g.
Bailey Gigli saw g.
Bailey saw g.
g. barrel
barrel g.
Bentson Plus cerebral wire g.
bone wire g.
Bow & Arrow cannulated drill g.
Brown limbal relaxing incision g.
Brown-Roberts-Wells CT
    stereotactic g.
BRW CT stereotaxic g.
Bullseye femoral g.
catheter g.
CCK femoral stem provisional g.
chamfer g.
Cloward drill g.
contoured anterior spinal plate
    drill g.
Cook stereotactic g.
Cooper nasal ganglia g.
Cope nitinol mandril wire g.
Cor-Flex wire g.
Cottle knife g.
cruciate ligament g.
curved tapered Tefcor movable
    core wire g.
Cushing saw g.
custom drill g.
Davis saw g.
Delta Recon proximal drill g.
disposable measuring g.
distal femoral cutting g.
double flexible-tipped wire g.
drill g.

eccentric drill g.
Eschenbach low-vision
  rehabilitation g.
Evolis femoral cutting g.
extramedullary alignment g.
E-Z g.
femoral intramedullary g.
femoral notch g.
Ferciot wire g.
Ferkel C g.
filiform g.
fixed offset g.
Flexguide intubation g.
g. forceps
Franzen needle g.
Frazier dural g.
front-entry g.
Gabbay-Frater suture g.
Galante hip g.
Gaulian knife g.
Ghajar g.
Gigli saw g.
Glacier ceramic 4-in-1 cutting g.
Glacier ceramic knee cutting g.
Glacier ceramic 4-in-1 knee
  cutting g.
Gleason g.
glenoid drill g.
Graduate measuring wire g.
Greenwald Roth Grip-Tip suture g.
Grip-Tip suture g.
guidepin g.
gutter g.
Guyon curved catheter g.
handheld drill g.
Harris precoat neck osteotomy g.
Hewson ligament drill g.
HiWire highly elastic nitinol core
  wire g.
hollow needle g.
House strut g.
Howell tibial g.
humeral cutting g.
hydrophilic g.
intramedullary g.
Iowa pudendal needle g.
Iowa trumpet needle g.
Joseph saw g.
Kazanjian g.
Lebsche saw g.
LeFort filiform g.
Levin drill g.
ligature g.
long nail-mounted drill g.
L-resection g.
Lu-Mendez LRI g.
Lunderquist extra-stiff wire g.
Lunderquist-Ring torque g.
Maggi disposable biopsy needle g.

McGuire suture g.
McNamara renal exchange wire g.
measuring g.
microdrilling g.
Müller catheter g.
Navigus trajectory g.
needle-point suture passer/incision
  closure g.
Neivert knife g.
NeuraGen nerve g.
Neurolac nerve g.
New York catheter exchange
  wire g.
nut alignment g.
patellar drill g.
patellar reamer g.
patellar resection g.
Pilot suturing g.
g. pin
pin g.
Poppen Gigli saw g.
ProTrac ACL tibial g.
Puddu drill g.
pudendal needle g.
punch g.
Raney saw g.
rear-entry ACL drill g.
Reece osteotomy g.
Reuter tip deflecting wire g.
Richards angle g.
Roadrunner extra-support wire g.
Roth Grip-Tip suture g.
SAM OnScene patient
  assessment g.
Savary-Gilliard wire g.
scaphoid screw g.
Scott-RCE osteotomy g.
side-exiting g.
Slick stylette endotracheal tube g.
stationary angle g.
Stewart cruciate ligament g.
stoma-centering g.
straight catheter g.
surgical instrument g.
suture g.
targeting drill g.
telescopic view g.
telescoping g.
TFE-coated wire g.
The Asta-Cath female catheter g.
tibial cutter g.
tibial drill g.
tissue anchor g. (TAG)
Todd-Wells g.
Torq-Flex wire g.
Tracer hybrid wire g.
Trailblazer screw g.
transpedicular drill g.
TrueTorque wire g.

G

guide *(continued)*
    trumpet needle g.
    Tucker vertebrated g.
    tunnel drill g.
    Uslenghi drill g.
    vacuum centering g.
    Van Buren catheter g.
    variable-stiffness wire g.
    Vista Brite Tip IG introducer g.
    Wilson-Cook standard wire g.
    wire g.
    wound measuring g.
    Yasargil ligature g.
guide-catheter
guided
    g. tissue regeneration (GTR)
    g. trephine system (GTS)
guidepin, guide pin
    g. guide
guider
GuideRight guidewire
guidewire, guide wire *(See also* wire, Glidewire)
    ACS Amplatz g.
    ACS extra-support g.
    ACS Hi-Torque Balance middleweight g.
    ACS LIMA g.
    Amplatz Super Stiff g.
    Amplex g.
    angled g.
    angle-tip g.
    AQUALiner hydrophilic Ni-Ti alloy g.
    argon g.
    Asahi Prowater g.
    Athlete GT coronary g.
    ATW steerable g.
    Bard Commander PTCA g.
    Bard Director g.
    beaded g.
    Becton-Dickinson g.
    Bentson exchange straight g.
    Bentson floppy-tip g.
    Bentson floppy-tipped g.
    Bentson-style g.
    Bentson-type Glidewire g.
    Cannu-Flex g.
    cannula with preloaded g.
    Cardiometrics FloWire g.
    catheter g.
    catheter g.
    Choice PT g.
    color-coded g.
    Commander angioplasty g.
    Conceptus Robust g.
    ControlWire g.
    Control Wire g.
    Cook straight g.

Coons Super Stiff long tip g.
Cope mandrel g.
Critikon g.
Crosswire nitinol hydrophilic g.
Crosswire PTCA g.
Dasher g.
delivery g.
Doppler g.
Doppler-tipped angioplasty g.
drill-tipped g.
Eder-Puestow g.
Elastorc catheter g.
Emerald diagnostic g.
ERCP g.
exchange g.
Extra Sport coronary g.
extra-stiff g.
extra-support g.
Fastrac hydrophilic-coated g.
Fathom steerable g.
flexible g.
flexible-tip g.
Flex-T g.
Flex Tip g.
FloMap g.
floppy g.
floppy-tip g.
floppy-tipped g.
FloWire Doppler g.
fluid-filled pressure monitoring g.
Geenan Endotorque g.
GlideCath g.
Glidewire Gold surgical g.
Gold-tip micro g.
Guidant g.
GuideRight g.
Headliner g.
Hi-Torque balance middleweight universal g.
Hi-Torque Floppy g.
Hi-Torque Floppy exchange g.
Hi-Torque Floppy II g.
Hi-Torque Floppy intermediate g.
Hi-Torque Modified J-GW g.
Hi-Torque Spartacore 14 g.
Hi-Torque Standard g.
Hi-Torque Steelcore 18 g.
Hi-Torque steerable g.
Hi-Torque Supracore 35 g.
HydroGlide g.
hydromer-coated micro g.
hydrophilic g.
hydrophilic angulated g.
hydrophilic-coated g.
hydrophilic polymer-coated steerable g.
Hydro Plus coated g.
HydroSteer hydrophilic g.
InQwire g.

intracoronary Doppler flow g.
intravascular Doppler-tipped g.
J g.
Jagwire g.
Jindo tapered peripheral g.
J-tip g.
J-tipped g.
Katzen infusion g.
Kayak hydrophilic g.
Linx exchange g.
Linx extension g.
Lubriglide-coated g.
Lumina g.
Lunderquist g.
Lunderquist exchange g.
Lunderquist-Ring g.
Magic Torque g.
Magnum g.
micro g.
micropuncture g.
Microvasive angled hydrophilic g.
Microvasive Geenen Endotorque g.
Microvasive Glidewire g.
Microvasive stiff piano wire g.
Mirage hydrophilic g.
Monorail g.
movable core g.
Mustang steerable g.
nail-driving g.
Newton g.
nitinol g.
Nitrex ev3 g.
Nitrex nitinol g.
nonconductive g.
Pathfinder exchange g.
Patriot moderate support g.
Placer g.
Platinum Plus g.
platinum tip g.
PressureWire g.
Prima laser g.
Prowater g.
Puestow g.
QuickSilver hydrophilic-coated g.
Radifocus g.
Radifocus catheter g.
Radifocus hydrophilic coated g.
Reflex steerable g.
Ring g.
Roadrunner NaviGuide g.
Rosen g.
Rosen curved g.
RotaWire Floppy Gold g.
Safe-Steer g.
safety g.
Schwarten LP g.
Seeker g.
Shinobi radiolucent steerable g.
silk g.

Silver Speed hydrophilic g.
slipper-tipped g.
Sniper Elite hydrophilic g.
Sniper Elite hydrophilic Ni-Ti
  alloy g.
Sniper hydrophilic nitinol g.
SOS g.
Spartacore 14 g.
Spectranetics Prima laser g.
spring-tipped g.
Stabilizer balanced performance g.
Stabilizer marker wire steerable g.
Stabilizer Plus steerable g.
Stabilizer XS extra-support
  steerable g.
Stabilizer XS steerable g.
stainless steel g.
standard fixed core g.
steerable angioplastic g.
stiff g.
straight g.
super-stiff g.
Supracore 35 g.
Suretac g.
SV g.
Synchro microfabricated nitinol g.
Synchro neurovascular g.
tapered core g.
tapered-tip g.
Tapered Torque g.
Teflon-coated g.
Terumo g.
Terumo Crosswire PTCA g.
Terumo hydrophilic g.
Terumo/Meditech g.
Terumo-Radiofocus hydrophilic
  polymer-coated g.
TherOx infusion g.
tip-deflecting g.
Tomcat PTCA g.
torqueable g.
Transend steerable g.
Ultra-Select nitinol PTCA g.
variable-stiffness g.
WaveWire angioplasty g.
Wholey Hi-Torque Floppy g.
Wholey Hi-Torque modified J g.
Wholey Hi-Torque standard g.
Wilson-Cook Protector g.
Wilson-Cook THSF-series g.
Wilson-Cook Tracer g.
Wizdom ST steerable g.
x-shaped g.
XWire biliary g.
Zebra exchange g.
guidewire/basket lasso
guiding
  g. cannula
  g. catheter

G

Guidor
 G. matrix barrier
 G. membrane
Guild-Pratt rectal speculum
Guilford
 G. cervical brace
 G. scissors
Guilford-Schuknecht wire-cutting scissors
Guilford-Wright
 G.-W. bur saw
 G.-W. footplate pick
 G.-W. suction tube
 G.-W. wire cutter
Guilford-Wullstein bur saw
guillotine
 g. adenotome
 Charnley femoral inlay g.
 g. cutting tip
 g. forceps
 Lilienthal rib g.
 Myles g.
 rib g.
 g. scissors
 Sluder tonsillar g.
 tonsil g.
 tonsillar g.
 g. vitrectomy instrument
 g. vitrector
guillotine-type cutter
Guimaraes
 G. flap spatula
 G. implantable contact lens manipulator
 G. ophthalmic flap spatula
 G. ophthalmic spatula
Guist
 G. fixation forceps
 G. speculum
Gulani
 G. globe stabilizer and flap restrainer
 G. triple function LASIK cannula
Guleke bone rongeur
Gulick II tape
Gullstrand
 G. lens
 G. lens loupe
 G. ophthalmoscope
 G. slit-lamp
 G. 6-surface eye model
gum elastic bougie introducer
gun
 Arthrex meniscal dart g.
 automated biopsy g.
 Bard Biopty g.
 Biofix arrow g.
 biopsy g.
 Biopty g.
 Biopty biopsy g.

 bone injection g.
 caulking g.
 CMW cement g.
 Cobe staple g.
 Cook biopsy g.
 coring biopsy g.
 electron g.
 enhancement g.
 Heaf g.
 heat g.
 introducer g.
 Mentor g.
 Mentor injector g.
 Messing root canal g.
 modified caulking g.
 Moss T-anchor introducer g.
 Moss T-anchor needle introducer g.
 reflex g.
 rivet g.
 seam-sealer g.
 spring-loaded biopsy g.
 Sterivap cement g.
 surgical stapling g.
Gunderson
 G. bone forceps
 G. muscle forceps
 G. muscle recession forceps
GunSlinger shoulder orthosis
Günther Tulip vena cava MReye filter
gurney
 SafetySure transfer g.
Gusberg
 G. cervical biopsy curette
 G. cervical cone curette
Gussenbauer suture
Gustilo
 G. knee prosthesis
 G. unconstrained prosthesis
Gustilo-Kyle
 G.-K. cementless total hip arthroplasty
 G.-K. total hip
 G.-K. total knee
gut
 g. clamp
 g. suture
Guthrie
 G. card
 G. eye fixation hook
 G. iris hook
 G. retractor
 G. skin hook
Guthrie-Smith apparatus
gutta-percha
 g.-p. point
 g.-p. spreader
gutter
 g. guide
 g. splint

Guttmann
G. obstetrical retractor
G. vaginal retractor
G. vaginal speculum
guy
G. gouge
g. suture
Guyon
G. curved catheter guide
G. kidney clamp
G. sound
G. ureteral catheter
G. urethral sound
G. vessel clamp
Guyon-Péan vessel clamp
guy-steading suture
Guyton-Clark forceps
Guyton corneal transplant trephine
Guyton-Lundsgaard
G.-L. cataract knife
G.-L. keratome
Guyton-Minkowski potential acuity meter
Guyton-Noyes fixation forceps
Guyton-Park eye speculum
Guyuron endoscopic access device
G/W Heel Lift, Inc. orthosis
gym
g. ball
Elite Power Station g.
hand g.
limb g.
Total G.
Zuni g.
gymball
Exertools g.
Gymmy exercise unit
Gymnastik ball
Gymnic Plus exercise ball
Gynecare
G. Monitorr urodynamic measurement system

G. Monitorr urodynamic measuring system
G. Thermachoice uterine balloon therapy system
G. TVT obturator system
G. TVT support system
G. Veristat fluid management system
G. Versascope hysteroscope
G. Versascope hysteroscopy system
G. X-Tract tissue morcellator
Gynemesh
G. PS
G. PS polypropylene mesh support
Gynkotek pump
GynoSampler
G. endometrial aspirator
G. endometrial sampling device
Gynoscann
Gypsona
G. cast
G. plaster dressing
Gyratome
Gyro-Flex upper extremity exerciser
gyrometer
Gyroscan
ACS G.
G. ACS-NT
G. ACS-NT MRI scanner
G. ACS-NT MR scanner
G. ACS-NT MR unit
G. HP Philips 15S whole-body system
G. Interna scanner
G. NT 10 magnet
Philips G.
G. S15 scanner
G. superconducting magnet
GyroTwister
Gyrus endourology system
Gysi articulator

G

H1 catheter
H2 Score office-based diagnostic device
HA
hydroxyapatite
HA adhesive
HA membrane
Proplast HA
Haab
H. eye knife
H. eye magnet
H. knife needle
H. scleral resection knife
Haag-Streit
H.-S. Biomicroscope 900 slit-lamp
H.-S. 900 cobalt blue filter
H.-S. distometer
H.-S. Endo-Set
H.-S. keratometer
H.-S. ophthalmometer
H.-S. slit-lamp
H.-S. slit-lamp biomicroscope
Haake rheometer
Haas intrauterine insemination catheter
Haberer intestinal clamp
Haberman
H. feeder
H. suction elevator
Haci needle
Hackett
H. sacral belt
H. sacroiliac cinch belt
HA-coated
HA-c. hip implant
HA-c. Micro-Vent implant
HA-c. root-form dental implant
Hadeco
H. ES100VX mini Doppler
H. intraoperative Doppler
H. MiniDop Doppler
Hader
H. aneroid sphygmomanometer
H. bar clip
H. dental attachment
H. implant bar
Hadfield hand board
Haefliger cleaver
Haelan tape
Haemogram blood loss monitor
Haemolance
H. lancet
H. Plus lancet device
Haemolite
H. autologous blood recovery
system
Cell Saver H.

Haemonetics
H. Cell Saver
H. Cell Saver system
Hagedorn
H. needle
H. needle holder
H. suture needle
Hagie
H. pin
H. pin nail
H. wrench
Haglund spreader
Haglund-Stille plaster spreader
Hagner
H. bag catheter
H. hemostatic bag
H. urethral bag
Hague cataract lamp
Hahn
H. bone nail
H. screw
Hahnenkratt
H. backing
H. lingual bar
H. matrix band
H. root canal pin
H. root canal post
Haid
H. cervical plate
H. UBP system
H. Universal bone plate
H. Universal bone plate system
Haidinger
H. brush
H. brush test
Haifa camera
Haight
H. baby retractor
H. pediatric rib spreader
hair
h. densitometer
h. transplant punch
hairpin splint
Hajek
H. antral punch forceps
H. antral retractor
H. antral rongeur
H. chisel
H. elevator
H. lip retractor
H. mallet
H. septal chisel
H. sphenoid punch forceps
Hajek-Ballenger
H.-B. dissector

Hajek-Ballenger *(continued)*
    H.-B. septal dissector
    H.-B. septal elevator
Hajek-Koffler
    H.-K. bone punch forceps
    H.-K. sphenoidal forceps
Hakim
    H. catheter
    H. high-pressure valve
    H. precision valve
    H. programmable valve system
    H. shunt
Halberg
    H. clip
    H. contact lens forceps
    H. trial clip occluder
Haldane
    H. apparatus
    H. tube
Haldane-Priestley tube
Hale obstetrical forceps
Hales piesimeter
half
    h. backboard
    h. pin
    h. ring
half-and-half nail
half-circle plate
half-eye spectacles
half-glass spectacles
half-intensity needle
half-ring leg splint
Halifax
    H. fine adjustment instrument
    H. interlaminar clamp
    H. interlaminar clamp system
Hall
    H. air drill
    H. arthrotome
    H. bone bur
    H. dermatome
    H. driver
    H. large bone instrument
    H. mandibular implant system
    H. Micro-Aire drill
    H. Micro E power instrument
    H. modular acetabular reamer
      system
    H. Neurairtome drill
    H. Orthairtome drill
    H. Osteon drill system kit
    H. Osteon irrigation kit
    H. power drill
    H. prosthetic heart valve
    H. sagittal saw
    H. screwdriver
    H. self-holding introducer
    H. series 4 large bone instrument
    H. Surgairtome II drill

    H. surgical drill
    H. valvulotome
    H. Versipower drill
    H. Versipower oscillating saw
    H. Versipower reamer
    H. Versipower reciprocating saw
Hallauer
    H. glasses
    H. spectacles
Hall-Dundar drill
Halle
    H. bone curette
    H. chisel
    H. dural knife
    H. ethmoidal curette
    H. infant nasal speculum
    H. nasal elevator
    H. septal elevator
    H. sinus curette
Hall-effect strain transducer
Halle-Tieck nasal speculum
Hall-Kaster
    H.-K. heart valve
    H.-K. tilting disc valve prosthesis
Hall-Morris biphase
Hallu Fix MTP fusion system
hallux
    h. forceps
    h. valgus orthosis
Hall-Zimmer power instrument
halo
    Ace Mark III h.
    h. apparatus
    h. brace
    Bremer h.
    BRW head ring h.
    h. cervical orthosis
    h. cervical traction system
    h. craniomaxillofacial fixation
      device
    h. femoral traction device
    h. fracture frame
    h. gravity traction device
    h. head frame
    h. hoop device
    Lerman noninvasive h.
    h. retractor
    h. retractor system
    h. ring
    H. Sleep System
    Surgairtome II drill h.
    h. tractor
    h. vest
    h. vest orthosis
    H. XP electrophysiology catheter
halogen
    h. coaxial ophthalmoscope
    h. dual lightsource
    h. dual light source

h. lamp
h. light source
h. ophthalmoscope
h. otoscope
halo-Ilizarov distraction instrumentation
Haloscale respirometer
haloscope
phase difference h.
halothane hepatotoxicity
Halsey
H. nail scissors
H. needle
H. needle holder
Halsted
H. arterial forceps
H. clamp
H. curved mosquito clamp
H. curved mosquito forceps
H. forceps
H. hemostat
H. hemostatic mosquito forceps
H. mattress suture
H. mosquito hemostat
H. strabismus scissors
H. straight mosquito clamp
halter
deluxe head h.
Diskard head h.
disposable head h.
head h.
neck-wrap h.
Repro head h.
standard head h.
TMJ h.
Zimfoam head h.
Zimmer head h.
**Hamamatzu high-sensitivity
photomultiplier tube**
hamate finder
Hamilton
H. bandage
H. deep surgery forceps
H. fluid warmer
H. repeating pipette dispenser
system
H. syringe
H. ventilator
Hamilton-Russell traction
Hamilton-Thorn motility analyzer
hammer
Babinski percussion h.
Berliner neurological h.
Berliner percussion h.
Buck neurological h.
Buck percussion h.
cervical/lumbar h.
Cloward h.
Davis percussion h.
Dejerine-Davis percussion h.

Dejerine percussion h.
Epstein neurological h.
fork h.
Gerzog bone h.
Grafco percussion h.
Hibbs h.
intranasal h.
Kirk bone h.
Kirk orthopaedic h.
Küntscher h.
Lucae bone h.
neurological percussion h.
orthopaedic h.
OrthoVise with slap h.
percussion h.
Quisling intranasal h.
Rabiner neurological h.
reflex h.
slide h.
sliding h.
surgical h.
tapping h.
Taylor percussion h.
Taylor reflex h.
Troemner percussion h.
Williger h.
Hammersmith
H. heart valve
H. mitral prosthesis
H. mitral valve prosthesis
hammock
h. bandage
h. dressing
Mersilene gauze h.
Hammond
H. alloy
H. orthodontic splint
H. splint
Hamou
H. contact microhysteroscope
H. endoscope
H. hysteroscope
H. microcolpomicrohysteroscope
H. Micro-Hysteroflator
Hampton electrosurgical unit
hamstring stretcher
Hanalux Oslo light
Hanau
H. 130-21 articulator
H. face bow
Hancock
H. aortic valve prosthesis
H. bioprosthetic heart valve
H. coronary perfusion catheter
H. embolectomy catheter
H. fiberoptic catheter
H. heterograft heart valve
H. hydrogen detection catheter
H. II porcine bioprosthesis

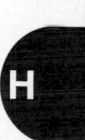

Hancock (*continued*)
    H. II tissue valve
    H. luminal electrophysiologic
      recording catheter
    H. mitral valve prosthesis
    H. modified orifice valve
    H. MO II bioprosthesis porcine
      valve
    H. M.O. II porcine bioprosthesis
    H. pericardial valve graft
    H. porcine heterograft
    H. porcine valve
    H. temporary cardiac pacing wire
    H. thermodilution catheter
    H. vascular graft
    H. wedge pressure catheter

hand
    h. block
    h. brace
    h. cock-up splint
    h. cone
    h. cuff
    h. dissector
    h. drill
    h. elevator
    h. evaluation set
    h. exercise ball
    h. exerciser
    h. gym
    H. Helper device
    H. Helper hand exerciser
    Hunstad h.
    lead h.
    Naeser laser home treatment
      program for the h.
    h. orthosis
    Otto Bock system electric h.
    pediatric retractor malleable wire h.
    h. retractor
    1-h. speculum
    h. surgery rasp
    h. trephine
    h. volumeter
    Winter Helping H.
Handages dressing
Hand-Aid arterial wrist support
Hand-E-Vent
Handeze fingerless glove
hand-glove prosthesis
handgun aspirator
handheld
    h. aerosol inhaler
    h. dermatoscope
    h. drill guide
    h. dynamometer
    h. exploring electrode probe
    h. eye magnet
    h. flutter device
    h. fundus camera

    h. Hruby lens
    h. magnifier
    h. magnifying reticle
    h. mapping probe
    h. nebulizer
    h. probe
    h. pulse oximeter
    h. retractor
    h. rotary prism
    h. trephine
handholder
    Tupper h.
hand-honed reverse cutting needle
Handi-Cath catheter kit
Handi oxygen sensor
Handisol phototherapy device
handle
    Acufex h.
    autopsy h.
    Bard-Parker h.
    bayonet h.
    Beaver h.
    blade h.
    Bruening esophagoscopy forceps h.
    Chana EZ clean reamer h.
    Cloward crossbar h.
    Cloward double-hinged cervical
      retractor h.
    Corwin knife h.
    Cottle modified knife h.
    Cottle protected knife h.
    DORC h.
    Dynagrip blade h.
    ear knife h.
    Elliot trephine h.
    exchange tip deflecting wire
      guide h.
    exchange-tip deflecting wire
      guide h.
    Gigli saw h.
    Hardy lateral knife h.
    hexagonal h.
    House myringotomy knife h.
    insulated knife h.
    Klein Delrin Luer-Lok h.
    knife h.
    knurled h.
    laryngeal knife h.
    laryngeal mirror h.
    Luikart-Bill traction h.
    Lynch laryngeal knife h.
    Marino rotatable transsphenoidal
      knife h.
    Marlow Primus h.
    Morse instrument h.
    myringotomy knife h.
    Ortho-Grip silicone rubber h.
    Parker-Bard h.
    rotatable transsphenoidal knife h.

safety h.
saw h.
scalpel h.
stone basket screw-mounted h.
Storz ear knife h.
surgical h.
Thera-Band h.
Therap-Loop door h.
traction h.
Transfer Handle support h.
Universal chuck h.
hand-operated suction device
hand-painted lens
handpiece
AMO series 4 phaco h.
Avit h.
B-mode h.
Cavitron I&A h.
Chayes h.
Chill Tip cooling h.
ClearCut 2 electrosurgical h.
CooperVision irrigation/aspiration h.
CUSA system 200 straight
    autoclavable h.
Doriot h.
DynaSurg electric h.
Dynatrak h.
Emesco dental drill and h.
Endo-Gripper endodontic h.
Excalibur h.
fragmentation/aspiration h.
Hexascan computerized
    dermatology h.
infusion h.
INTRA angled surgical h.
KaVo dental h.
Kelman irrigating h.
Kerr M4 safety h.
McIntyre infusion h.
micro bimanual irrigating h.
Micro-Pen h.
micropigmentation h.
Microseal ophthalmic h.
Microstat h.
M4 safety h.
NeoSoniX h.
oral surgery h.
Packer Wick extrusion h.
Permark micropigmentation h.
phacoemulsification h.
PhotoDerm PL h.
Platinum 5000 micropigmentation h.
ProFinesse II ultrasonic h.
reciprocating power h.
Revolution micropigmentation h.
h. round bur
Sabra 45-degree dental h.
Sapphire 2000 micropigmentation h.
soft-tipped extrusion h.

Storz h.
StraightShot Magnum h.
SureScan scanning h.
Surgitek h.
Titan slow-speed h.
W&H h.
Wullstein contraangle h.
Xomed XPS motor and h.
HandPort
H. hand assist device
H. system
hand-powered suction device
hand-pushed tack driver
hand-roller
handset
Force GSU laparoscopic h.
Hands Free knee retractor system
Hands-Off
H.-O. infusion port heparin-coated
    thermodilution catheter with
    TwistLock
H.-O. thermal dilution catheter
hand-switching electrocautery pencil
HandTact instrument set
Handy
H. II articulator
H. nonmydriatic video fundus
    camera
H. video fundus camera
Handy-Buck traction
HandyStep electronic repeating pipette
Haney
H. needle driver
H. retractor
hanger
Adjusta-Rak h.
H. ComfortFlex knee prosthesis
Conveen bag h.
film h.
yoke h.
hanging stirrup
Hang Ups gravity boot
Hanna
H. arcitome
H. trephine
Hann filter
Hanning window
Hansamed strip
Hansatome
Chiron H.
H. microkeratome
H. suction ring
Hansen pin
Hansen-Street
H.-S. nail
H.-S. pin
H.-S. self-broaching nail
H.-S. solid intramedullary nail
Hanson speed bracket

H

Hans Rudolph 3-way valve
Hapad
    H. felt insert
    H. heel pad
    H. heel wedge
    H. longitudinal metatarsal arch pad
    H. metatarsal insole
    H. prefabricated wool felt pad
    H. shoe insert
Hapex bioactive material
haploscope
    mirror h.
Happy podiatric bur
HappySkin acne light
Hapset
    H. bone graft plaster
    H. bone graft plaster material
    H. hydroxyapatite bone graft
      plaster
haptic
    h. area implant
    h. area lens
    modified C-loop h.
    modified J-loop h.
    modified L-loop h.
    modified L loop h.
    h. plate lens
    PMMA h.
    Slant h.
hard
    h. cervical collar
    h. collar
    h. contact lens
    h. mallet
    h. palate retractor
    h. socket
    h. sonolucent plastic cone
    h. tissue replacement malleable
      facial implant
    h. tissue replacement patient-
      matched implant
    h. x-ray imaging spectrometer
Hardesty
    H. tendon hook
    H. tenotomy hook
Hardinge expansion bolt
hardware
    Genesis arthroplasty h.
    TiMesh h.
Hardy
    H. aluminum crutch
    H. bayonet curette
    H. bayonet dressing forceps
    H. bayonet enucleator
    H. bayonet neurosurgical bipolar
      forceps
    H. bivalve speculum
    H. hypophysial curette
    H. lateral knife handle

    H. lensometer
    H. lip retractor
    H. microsurgical bayonet bipolar
      forceps
    H. microsurgical enucleator
    H. pituitary dissector
    H. pituitary spoon
    H. 3-prong fork
    H. punch
    H. ring curette
    H. rongeur
    H. sellar punch
    H. speculum
    H. suction tube
    H. transsphenoidal mirror
Hardy-Cushing retractor
Hardy-Rand-Rittler plate
Hare
    H. compact traction splint
    H. splint device
    H. traction device
harelip
    h. forceps
    h. needle
    h. traction bow
Harken
    H. auricular clamp
    H. ball heart valve
    H. ball valve
    H. forceps
    H. prosthesis
    H. prosthetic valve
    H. rib retractor
    H. rib spreader
    H. valve
    H. valvulotome
Harloff cart
Harman fixation forceps
Harmon chisel
harmonic
    h. attenuation table
    h. scissors
    h. suture
Harmonic Scalpel
Harmonie
    H. Classic Plus brief
    H. underpad
Harmony
    H. PLIF instrument set
    H. surgical suction device
Harm posterior cervical plate
Harms
    H. cage
    H. corneal forceps
    H. microtying forceps
    H. suture-tying forceps
    H. trabeculotome
    H. trabeculotomy probe
    H. tying forceps

Harms-Colibri forceps
Harms-Moss anterior thoracic instrumentation
Harms-Tubingen tying forceps
harness
    figure-of-8 h.
    Heart Hugger sternum support h.
    Kicker Pavlik h.
    Pavlik h.
    Wheaton Pavlik h.
    Zuni h.
Harpenden
    H. calipers
    H. handgrip dynamometer
    H. skinfold calipers
    H. stadiometer
Harpoon suture anchor
Harrington
    H. Deaver retractor
    H. distraction instrumentation
    H. dual square-ended rod
    H. esophageal diverticulectomy
    H. fixation device
    H. forceps
    H. hook clamp
    H. hook driver
    H. lung-grasping forceps
    H. pedicle hook
    H. protractor
    H. retractor
    H. rod
    H. rod clamp
    H. rod and hook system
    H. rod instrumentation
    H. rod instrumentation distraction outrigger device
    H. spinal instrumentation
    H. splanchnic retractor
    H. spreader
    H. thoracic forceps
    H. tonometer
Harrington-Kostuik
    H.-K. distraction device
    H.-K. instrumentation
Harrington-Mayo
    H.-M. scissors
    H.-M. tissue forceps
Harrington-Mixter
    H.-M. thoracic clamp
    H.-M. thoracic forceps
Harris
    H. band
    H. cemented hip prosthesis
    H. center-cutting acetabular reamer
    H. condylocephalic nail
    H. condylocephalic rod
    H. Design-2 implant
    H. dissector
    H. femoral head gauge

    H. footprint mat
    H. Hemi Arm Sling
    H. hemi-arm sling
    H. hip line
    H. hip nail
    H. implant
    H. knotter
    H. medullary nail
    H. Micromini prosthesis
    H. plate
    H. precoat neck osteotomy guide
    H. precoat prosthesis
    H. protrusio shell
    H. segregator
    H. splint sling
    H. suture-carrying forceps
    H. tube
    H. uterine injector (HUI)
    H. wire tier
    H. wire tightener
Harris-Beath footprint mat
Harris-Galante
    H.-G. cup
    H.-G. hip replacement acetabular component
    H.-G. I porous-coated acetabular component
    H.-G. porous acetabular component
    H.-G. porous-coated femoral component
    H.-G. porous hip prosthesis
Harris-Kronner uterine manipulator/injector (HUMI)
Harrison
    H. bone-holding forceps
    H. capsular knife
    H. chalazion retractor
    H. implant
    H. interlocked mesh dressing
    H. interlocked mesh prosthesis
Harrison-Nicolle polypropylene peg
Harrison-Shea curette
Hartman hemostat
Hartmann
    H. adenoidal curette
    H. alligator forceps
    H. biopsy punch
    H. bone rongeur
    H. clamp
    H. ear dressing forceps
    H. ear forceps
    H. ear polyp forceps
    H. ear punch
    H. ear rongeur
    H. ear speculum
    H. eustachian catheter
    H. hemostat
    H. hemostatic mosquito forceps
    H. knife

H

Hartmann (*continued*)
- H. mastoid rongeur
- H. mosquito forceps
- H. mosquito hemostatic forceps
- H. nasal conchotome
- H. nasal-cutting forceps
- H. nasal-dressing forceps
- H. nasal polyp forceps
- H. nasal punch
- H. nasal speculum
- H. tonsillar dissector
- H. tonsillar punch
- H. tonsillar punch forceps
- H. tuning fork
- H. uterine biopsy forceps

Hartmann-Noyes nasal-dressing forceps

Hartmann-Shack
- H.-S. wavefront aberrometer
- H.-S. wavefront sensor system

Hartmann-Weingärtner ear forceps

Hart pediatric 3-mirror lens

Hartshill rectangle

Hartzler
- H. ACS coronary dilation catheter
- H. ACX II catheter
- H. balloon catheter
- H. LPS dilatation catheter
- H. Micro-600 catheter
- H. Micro II angioplasty balloon
- H. Micro II balloon
- H. Micro II catheter
- H. Micro XT catheter
- H. RX-014 balloon catheter
- H. Ultra-Lo-Profile catheter

Harvard
- H. cannula
- H. 2 dual-syringe pump
- H. microbore intravenous extension set
- H. multidetector scanner
- H. needle
- H. pump

harvester
- Brandel cell h.
- multiple automated sample h.
- OsteoHarvester bone h.
- QuickDraw bone h.
- tendon h.
- TomTec cell h.

harvesting pistol

Harvey
- H. Elite stethoscope
- H. vapor sterilizer
- H. wire-cutting scissors

Hashizume endoscopic ligator kit

Hashmat shunt

Hashmat-Waterhouse shunt

Haslinger
- H. bronchoscope
- H. esophagoscope
- H. laryngoscope
- H. palate retractor
- H. retractor
- H. tip forceps

Hasner
- H. lid forceps
- H. valve

Hassan-type port

Hasson
- H. balloon uterine elevator cannula
- H. blunt port
- H. bullet-tip forceps
- H. cannula
- H. grasper
- H. grasping forceps
- H. laparoscope
- H. laparoscopic trocar
- H. needle-nose forceps
- H. open laparoscopy cannula
- H. retractor
- H. ring forceps
- H. spike-tooth forceps
- H. stable access cannula
- H. trocar
- H. uterine manipulator

hat
- measuring h.
- silver thermal h.

Hatch
- H. catheter
- H. chisel
- H. clamp

hatchet
- black h.
- California h.

Hatfield bone curette

Hausmann
- H. vascular clamp
- H. weight rack
- H. Work-Well work hardening system

Haverhill
- H. clamp
- H. dermal abrader
- H. needle

Hawkeye
- H. SPECT application
- H. suture needle
- H. suture needle for arthroscopy

Hawkin hookwire

Hawkins
- H. accordion catheter drainage set
- H. breast localization needle
- H. cervical biopsy forceps

Hawkins-Akins needle

Hawks-Dennen obstetrical forceps

Hawksley random zero mercury sphygmomanometer

Hawley
 H. appliance
 H. bite plate
 H. chart
 H. retainer
 H. table
Hayek oscillator
Hayes
 H. anterior resection clamp
 H. anterior resection forceps
 H. colon clamp
 H. intestinal clamp
 H. vaginal speculum
Haynes-Griffin mandibular splint
Haynes 25 material
Haynes-Stellite implant metal prosthesis
Hays
 H. finger retractor
 H. hand retractor
Hayton-Williams forceps
HBT
 HBT Sleuth
 HBT Sleuth portable hydrogen
  monitor
H buttress support patellofemoral brace
H-1 catheter
HD
 HD II total hip prosthesis
 HD Secura dialyzer
HDI
 HDI ultrasound
 HDI 1000, 3000, 3500, 4000,
  5000 ultrasound imaging system
HDL
 high-density lipoprotein
 AccuMeter HDL
 HDL direct test prefilled cartridge
head
 Aequalis h.
 h. of bed
 Biolox-forte ball h.
 BioPro ceramic TARA h.
 h. box
 h. brace
 4-h. camera
 cobalt-chrome h.
 cobalt-chromium h.
 h. coil
 Continuum bipolar acetabular h.
 Copeland humeral resurfacing h.
 coupling h.
 DePuy Global Advantage CTA
  humeral h.
 DePuy Global Advantage shoulder
  eccentric humeral h.
 h. extractor
 h. fixation device
 forged femoral h.

 h. frame
 Global Advantage CTA humeral h.
 h. halter
 h. halter cervical traction
 h. holder
 J-FX bipolar h.
 h. lamp
 Matroc femoral h.
 h. mirror
 Morse h.
 MRI probe h.
 Omniflex h.
 h. ring
 rotatable coupling h.
 h. sling
 Storz-Bruening diagnostic h.
 Vitox femoral h.
 Ziramic femoral h.
 zirconia orthopaedic prosthetic h.
 Zyranox femoral h.
3-head
 3-h. camera
 3-h. gamma camera-based SPECT
  system
headband
 fiberoptic h.
 imaging h.
 plagiocephaly h.
 Storz face shield h.
headed Bio-Corkscrew
headgear
 horizontal pull h.
 Kloehn h.
 Velstretch/Velcro h.
headholder
 Aesculap h.
 Amsco h.
 Caspar h.
 Derlacki-Juers h.
 Gardner h.
 integrated h.
 Malcolm-Rand carbon composite h.
 Mayfield-Kees h.
 Mayfield radiolucent h.
 Mayfield skull-pin h.
 Methodist Hospital h.
 pin h.
 pinion h.
 radiolucent cranial pin h.
 Sugita h.
headhunter visceral angiography
 catheter
Headisc
headlamp
 Keeler fiberoptic h.
 Keeler Magnalite h.
 Keeler Magnalite fiberoptic h.
 Keeler video h.

H

401

headless
> h. bone screw
> h. bone screw system

headlight
> Clip-Lite clip-on h.
> Cogent LightWear h.
> fiberoptic h.
> Heine UBL 100 h.
> high-beam fiberoptic h.
> Keeler fiberoptic h.
> MultArray h.
> Orascoptic fiberoptic h.
> Quadrilite 6000 fiberoptic h.
> Welch Allyn single-fiber illumination h.
> Welch Allyn Solarc h.

Headliner guidewire

Headmaster collar

head/moisture exchanger

head-mounted
> h.-m. device
> h.-m. instrument
> h.-m. video magnifier LVES

headpiece
> e-Net h.
> Novascan scanning h.

headrest, head rest
> adjustable h.
> doughnut h.
> Freeman surgical h.
> horseshoe h.
> Lempert rongeur h.
> Light h.
> Mayfield-Kees h.
> Mayfield pediatric horseshoe h.
> Mayfield radiolucent h.
> Mayfield swivel horseshoe h.
> McConnell orthopaedic h.
> neurosurgical h.
> pin h.
> pinion h.
> Richards h.
> Timo h.

head-tilt-chin lift

Heaf gun

Healey revision acetabular component

healing
> h. screw
> h. shoe

Healon aspirating cannula

Healos
> H. bone graft substitute
> H. synthetic bone grafting material

HealosMP52 implant

Health
> H. O Meter scale
> H. Scan Assess Plus peak flow meter

HealthCheck One-Step One Minute pregnancy test

Healthdyne
> H. apnea monitor
> H. oximeter
> H. pulse oximeter
> H. ventilator

Healthflex orthotic

Healthier seating cushion

Heal Well night splint

Healy
> H. gastrointestinal forceps
> H. intestinal forceps
> H. suture removing forceps
> H. uterine biopsy forceps

Heaney
> H. clamp
> H. endometrial biopsy curette
> H. hysterectomy forceps
> H. hysterectomy retractor
> H. retractor
> H. suture
> H. tissue forceps
> H. uterine curette
> H. vaginal retractor

Heaney-Simon
> H.-S. hysterectomy forceps
> H.-S. hysterectomy retractor
> H.-S. retractor
> H.-S. vaginal retractor

hearing
> h. aid
> h. aid amplifier
> h. aid battery
> h. aid microphone
> h. protection device
> h. protector

Hearport EndoClamp-ST II aortic catheter

heart
> AbioCor implantable replacement h.
> H. Aid 80 defibrillator
> H. Aide Ezd noninvasive monitoring equipment
> air-driven artificial h.
> Akutsu III total artificial h.
> ALVAD artificial h.
> artificial h.
> h. assist device
> electromechanical artificial h.
> Hershey total artificial h.
> H. Hugger sternum support harness
> implantable artificial h.
> Jarvik 7, 8 artificial h.
> Jarvik 7-70 artificial h.
> Jarvik 2000 artificial h.
> H. laser
> Liotta total artificial h.
> H. nebulizer

h. needle
orthotopic univentricular artificial h.
h. pacemaker
H. pillow
h. pump
H. Rate 1-2-3 monitor
Symbion Jarvik-7 artificial h.
Symbion J-7 70-mL ventricle total
artificial h.
Symbion total artificial h.
H. Technology Rotablator
total artificial h.
Utah total artificial h.
h. valve
heartbeating simulator
HeartCard
H. monitor
H. 3X cardiac event recorder
Heartflo anastomotic device
heart-lung resuscitator
HeartMate
H. implantable pneumatic left
ventricular assist system
H. implantable ventricular assist
device
H. portable pump
H. pump
H. vented electric left ventricular
assist system
Heartport
H. catheter system
H. DirectFlow arterial catheter
H. endoaortic clamp
H. EndoClamp-ST aortic catheter
H. endocoronary sinus catheter
H. Endopledge sinus catheter
H. endopulmonary vent
H. endovascular catheter
H. endovenous drainage cannula
H. Endovent pulmonary catheter
H. Port-Access system
H. Quickdraw venous cannula kit
HeartSaver VAD
Heartscan heart attack prediction test
HeartStart MRx defibrillator
Heartstream
H. FR2 AED with attenuated
defibrillation pad
H. FR2+ defibrillator
Heartstring proximal seal system
HeartView CT cardiac monitor
Heartwave
H. EP
H. EP system
heat
h. exchanger
h. gun
h. and moisture exchanger (HME)

h. pad
H. Plus Massage lower body wrap
**heat-activated recoverable temporary
stent**
heated tracheostomy collar
heater
h. probe
resistance wire h.
SlidePro slide h.
Heath
H. chalazion curette
H. chalazion forceps
H. clip
H. clip-removing forceps
H. clip-removing scissors
H. curette
H. mallet
H. mules
H. nasal forceps
H. punctum dilator
H. suture-cutting scissors
H. suture scissors
H. wire-cutting scissors
**heat-vulcanized silicone elastomer
implant**
Heatwave electrode
heavy
h. cross-slot screwdriver
h. monofilament suture
h. retention suture
h. septal scissors
h. silk retention suture
h. wire suture
heavy-duty standard exchange wire
heavy-gauge suture
heavy-ion medical accelerator
HeavyMed ball
Hebra
H. blade
H. chalazion curette
H. corneal curette
H. curette
H. hook
Hedgehog
Sonic H.
Hedrocel
H. cup
H. proximal tibia augmentation
implant
H. titanium screw
Hedstrom file
heel
CarbonX active h.
h. cup
h. cushion
H. Free splint
H. Hugger therapeutic heel
stabilizer
h. lift

H

403

heel *(continued)*
    H. Minder foot elevator
    h. pillow
    h. posting
    rubber walking h.
    h. sleeve
    solid ankle cushioned h. (SACH)
    H. Spur Special
    H. Spur Special orthosis
    Thomas h.
    walking h.
    wedge adjustable cushioned h.
      (WACH)
Heelbo
    H. decubitus protector
    H. L-Bow arm restraint system
HeelCare cushion
Heeler inflatable heel protector
Heelift
    H. suspension boot
    H. traction boot
HeelWedge healing shoe
Heermann
    H. alligator forceps
    H. ear forceps
Hegar
    H. intrarectal bougie
    H. needle
    H. needle holder
    H. rectal dilator
    H. uterine dilator
Hegar-Baumgartner
    H.-B. needle
    H.-B. needle holder
Hegenbarth
    H. clip
    H. clip-applying forceps
Heidelberg
    H. arm
    H. laser tomographic scanner
    H. retinal flowmeter
    H. retina tomograph
    H. retina tomograph II
Heifitz clip
Heifitz-Weck clip
Heightronic stadiometer
Heilen expressor
Heimlich
    H. catheter
    H. chest drainage valve
    H. heart valve
    H. MicroTrach
    H. tube
Heine
    H. gonioscope
    H. HSL 100 handheld slit-lamp
    H. Lambda 100 retinometer
    H. penlight
    H. UBL 100 headlight

Hein rongeur
Heiss
    H. arterial forceps
    H. flexible endoscopic scissors
    H. hemostatic forceps
    H. retractor
    H. soft tissue retractor
Heister
    II. mouthgag
    H. valve
helical
    h. basket
    h. coil
    h. coil stent
    h. CT scanner
    h. electrode
    h. PTCA dilatation catheter
    h. ridged ureteral stent
    h. suture
    h. tube saw
Helicobacter pylori
    H. p. gII test
helicoid endosteal implant
Helioseal
Helisal Rapid Blood diagnostic kit
Helistat
    H. absorbable collagen hemostatic
      sponge
    H. collagen matrix sponge
Helistent
Helitene absorbable collagen hemostatic agent
helium-filled balloon catheter
helium-neon
    h.-n. aiming laser
    h.-n. beam
    h.-n. laser
helium neon laser
Helix
    H. balloon
    H. camera
    H. endocervical curette
    H. multihead nuclear imaging
      system
    H. PTCA dilation catheter
    H. uterine biopsy curette
Heller
    H. biopsy forceps
    H. probe
helmet
    collimator h.
    cooling h.
    cranial h.
    cranial molding h.
    plagiocephaly h.
    traction h.
Helmholtz
    H. double-surface coil
    H. head coil

H. keratometer
H. ophthalmoscope
H. speculum
Helmstein balloon
Helparm
Swedish H.
Helsper
H. laryngectomy button
H. tracheostomy vent tube
Helveston
H. finder hook
H. Great Big Barbie retractor
H. hook
H. scleral marking ruler
HemaCarotid vascular patch
hemacytometer (*var. of* hemocytometer)
Hemaduct wound drain
hemadynamometer
Hemaflex
H. PTCA sheath with obturator
H. sheath
Hemagard collection tube
HemaPatch vascular graft
Hemaquet
H. introducer
H. PTCA sheath with obturator
Hemaseel APR kit fibrin sealant
Hemashield
H. Finesse cardiovascular patch
H. Gold 1, 4 branch AAA graft
H. Gold Microvel knitted double velour graft
H. Vantage vascular graft
HemAssist blood substitute
Hemastainer
Hemasure r\LS red blood cell filtration system
HemataSTAT Easy Read centrifuge
Hematek 2000 slide stainer
Hematome system
HemCon bandage
hemianopic spectacles
HemiCAP resurfacing system
Hemifield glaucoma test
hemi-implant
cannulated h.-i. (CHI)
hemi-interpositional implant
Hemi-Kock neobladder
hemilaminectomy
h. blade
h. retractor
hemiprosthesis
single-stemmed silicone h.
Hemi sling
hemisphere
H. modular cup
silicone h.

hemispherical
h. pusher
h. reamer
Hemobahn
H. endoprosthesis
H. endovascular prosthesis stent-graft
H. PTFE-covered stent-graft
H. stent
H. stent-graft
Hemoband hemostasis device
Hemoccult
H. II card
H. II test
H. Sensa
H. Sensa developer
H. Sensa slide
Hemochron
H. glass-activated ACT tube
H. monitor
hemoclip
Hx-5LR-1 h.
Samuels h.
hemoclipping application device
hemoconcentrator
Biofilter cardiovascular h.
HemoCue
H. AB hemoglobin measurement device
H. B-Glucose analyzer
H. blood glucose analyzer
H. blood glucose system
H. blood hemoglobin analyzer
H. blood hemoglobin system
H. glucose meter
H. glucose test
H. hemoglobin photometer
H. hemoglobin test
H. hemoglobin test system
H. microcurette
H. photometer
hemocytometer, hemacytometer
Coulter MD 16 h.
Neubauer h.
hemodialysis
h. catheter
personal h. (PHD)
hemodialyzer
Altra-Flux h.
Baxter h.
1550 Baxter h.
2008E h.
Gambro h.
Gambro Lundia Minor h.
hemofilter
HemoGlide long-term hemodialysis catheter
hemoglobin-based therapeutic system

hemoglobin glutamer-250[bovine] oxygen-based therapeutic system
Hemoject
    H. injection catheter
    H. needle
HemoMatic blood collection monitor
Hemophan membrane
Hemopump
    H. cardiac assist system
    Johnson & Johnson H.
    Medtronic H.
    Nimbus H.
Hemopure oxygen-based therapeutic system
hemorrhage occluder pin
hemorrhoidal
    h. clamp
    h. forceps
    h. ligator
    h. needle
HemoSplit
    H. catheter
    H. hemodialysis catheter
    H. long-term dialysis catheter
hemostasis
    h. scalp clip
    h. silver clip
hemostat
    Actifoam h.
    Actifoam active h.
    Allis h.
    Avitene microfibrillar collagen h.
    h. awl
    blunt nose h.
    Carmalt h.
    Collastat OBP microfibrillar collagen h.
    Corboy h.
    Crile h.
    Crile gall h.
    curved h.
    curved Kelly h.
    curved mosquito h.
    Dandy scalp h.
    Dean tonsil h.
    D-Stat flowable h.
    Endo-Assist disposable h.
    Endo-Avitene microfibrillar collagen h.
    fine-tipped mosquito h.
    Halsted h.
    Halsted mosquito h.
    Hartman h.
    Hartmann h.
    Instat collagen absorbable h.
    Instat MCH microfibrillar collagen h.
    Kelly h.
    Kocher h.

    Lahey h.
    Lewis h.
    Lothrop h.
    Lowsley h.
    Mayo h.
    McWhorter h.
    Meigs h.
    microfibrillar collagen h.
    Mixter h.
    mosquito h.
    Nu-Knit absorbable h.
    orthopaedic h.
    Providence Hospital h.
    Rankin h.
    Rochester-Ochsner h.
    Rochester-Péan h.
    Sawtell tonsil h.
    Schnidt h.
    straight mosquito h.
    Surgicel fibrillar absorbable h.
    Surgicel Nu-Knit absorbable h.
    Vitagel surgical h.
hemostatic
    h. bag
    h. catheter
    h. cervical forceps
    h. clamp
    h. clip
    h. clip applier
    h. clip-applying forceps
    h. eraser
    h. forceps
    h. neurosurgical forceps
    h. occlusive leverage device
    h. puncture closure device
    h. suture
    h. tissue forceps
    h. tonsillar forceps
    h. tonsillectome
    h. tracheal forceps
Hemostatix scalpel blade
HemoTec
    H. activated clotting time monitor
    H. ACT machine
Hemovac
    H. drain
    H. Hydrocoat drain
    H. suction device
    H. suction tube
Hendel guided osteotome
Henderson
    H. bone chisel
    H. lag screw
Hendren
    H. clamp
    H. megaureter clamp
    H. self-retaining retractor
    H. ureteral clamp

He-Ne
    H.-N. beam
    H.-N. laser
Henke punch forceps tip
Henke-Stille conchotome
Henley
    H. carotid retractor
    H. dilator
    H. retractor blade
    H. subclavian artery clamp
    H. vascular clamp
Henley-Cohn prosthesis
Henning
    H. cast spreader
    H. instrument set
    H. mallet
    H. meniscal retractor
    H. plaster spreader
Henrotin
    H. vulsellum forceps
    H. weighted vaginal speculum
Henry
    H. cilia forceps
    II. ciliary forceps
    H. instrument tray
    H. Schein excavator
    H. Schein filling instrument
Henschke
    H. afterloader
    H. colpostat
    H. seed applicator
Henson CFS 2000 perimeter
HEPA
    H. filter
    H. filter mask
    H. respirator
Hepacoat stent
heparin arterial filter
heparin-coated Palmaz-Schatz stent
heparin-induced extracorporeal
    lipoprotein precipitation system
HepatAssist
    H. bioartificial liver
    H. bioartificial liver system
    H. liver support system
HEPAtech air purification system
hepatic artery infusion pump
Hepatix device
hepatofugal portosystemic venous shunt
hepatotoxicity
    halothane h.
HER-2/neu serum test
Heraeus LaserSonics laser
Herbert
    H. bone screw
    H. bone screw system
    H. jig
    H. knee prosthesis
    H. scaphoid screw

    H. screw
    H. screw fixator
Herbert-Whipple
    H.-W. bone screw
    H.-W. cannulated screw system
Herbst appliance
HercepTest
    Dako H.
    H. IHC kit
Hercules
    H. mobile x-ray unit
    H. Nd:YAG laser system
    H. plaster shears
    H. power injector
    H. TM drop-adjusting table
Herculite XRV Lab system
Herczel
    H. rib elevator
    H. rib rasp
Heritage hip system
Herman-Taylor gastroscope
Hermes
    H. Evolution tricompartmental knee
    system
    H. total knee system
Hermetic
    H. external ventricular drainage
    system
    H. II drainage management system
hermetically sealed pacemaker
Hernandez-Ros bone staple
hernia
    h. knife
    h. retractor
    h. stapler
Herniamesh
    H. surgical mesh
    H. surgical plug
herniotome
heroin usage
Her Option uterine cryoablation
    therapy system
Heros chiropody sponge
HerpeSelect type specific IgG antibody
    detection kit
Herrick
    H. kidney clamp
    H. kidney forceps
    H. lacrimal plug
    H. pedicle clamp
    H. silicone lacrimal implant
Herring tube
Hersh
    H. LASIK retreatment forceps
    H. LASIK retreatment spatula
Hershey
    H. left ventricular assist device
    H. total artificial heart

H

Hertel
- H. bougie urethrotome
- H. exophthalmometer
- H. kidney stone forceps
- H. ophthalmometer
- H. stone forceps

HES
- HydroCoil embolization system

Hess
- H. capsular forceps
- H. diplopia screen
- H. forceps
- H. iris forceps
- H. lens spoon
- H. screen
- H. spoon

Hessburg
- H. intraocular lens glide
- H. lacrimal needle
- H. vacuum trephine

Hessburg-Barron disposable vacuum trephine

Hessco 300, 500 series hydrotherapy table

Hess-Lee screen

heterograft
- bovine h.
- Hancock porcine h.
- h. implant
- h. prosthesis

heteroscope

Hewlett-Packard (HP)
- H.-P. 177020 A phased-array sector scanner
- H.-P. biplane probe
- H.-P. Codemaster XL defibrillator
- H.-P. color flow imager
- H.-P. defibrillator
- H.-P. ear oximeter
- H.-P. 500, 1000 Echo-Doppler machine
- H.-P. IVUS imaging system
- H.-P. 5 MHz phased-array TEE system
- H.-P. omniplane probe
- H.-P. phased-array sector scanner
- H.-P. phased-array ultrasound imaging system
- H.-P. pressure monitor
- H.-P. scanner
- H.-P. SDN monitor
- H.-P. Sonos 1000, 1500, 2500 ultrasound system
- H.-P. ultrasound
- H.-P. ultrasound unit

Hewson
- H. breakaway pin
- H. ligament drill guide
- H. ligature passer
- H. suture passer
- H. suture retriever

hex
- h. bar
- h. implant
- h. socket wrench

hexagonal
- h. handle
- h. handle osteotome
- h. wrench

Hexalon ACL/PCL screw[7]

Hexascan
- H. computerized dermatology handpiece
- krypton laser with H.
- H. Mark I, II model robotic scanning device
- Nd:YAG laser with H.
- tunable laser with H.

Hexastat

Hexcel
- H. cast dressing
- H. total condylar knee system
- H. total condylar prosthesis

Hexcelite
- H. cast
- H. mesh
- H. sheet splint

Hex-Fix
- H.-F. Add-A-Clamp
- H.-F. monolateral external fixator
- H.-F. system
- H.-F. Universal swivel clamp

hexhead
- h. bolt
- h. pin
- h. screwdriver

Hex-Lock abutment

Hexon illumination system

Heyer-Pudenz valve

Heyer-Schulte
- H.-S. antisiphon device
- H.-S. brain retractor
- H.-S. breast implant
- H.-S. breast prosthesis
- H.-S. catheter
- H.-S. disposal bag
- H.-S. hydrocephalus shunt
- H.-S. rhinoplasty implant
- H.-S. silicone kit
- H.-S. Small-Carrion sizing set
- H.-S. specular microscope
- H.-S. subcutaneous tissue expander
- H.-S. valve
- H.-S. wound drain

Heyman
- H. nasal forceps
- H. nasal scissors

Heyman-Simon
  H.-S. capsule
  H.-S. source
Heyner
  H. dilator
  H. double cannula
  H. double needle
  H. forceps
Heywood-Smith dressing forceps
HF
  HF dialyzer
  HF infrared laser
H-file
  engine H-f.
  Mity engine H-f.
HG
  Cobe Centrysystem dialyzer 400 HG
HGM
  HGM argon green laser
  HGM intravitreal laser
  HGM ophthalmic laser
  HGM Spectrum K1 krypton yellow & green laser
HGP
  HGP II acetabular component
  HGP II acetabular cup
Hi
  All-Purpose Boot Hi
  Darco Body Armor Hi
  Hi Speed Pulse lavage
  Hi Vac tubing
Hibbs
  H. blade
  H. bone chisel
  H. bone curette
  H. bone-cutting forceps
  H. bone gouge
  H. bone-holding forceps
  H. chisel elevator
  H. clamp
  H. costal elevator
  H. curette
  H. fracture appliance
  H. fracture frame
  H. hammer
  H. mallet
  H. osteotome
  H. periosteal elevator
  H. retractor
  H. self-retaining laminectomy retractor
  H. spinal curette
  H. spinal fusion gouge
  H. spinal retractor blade
  H. sponge
Hibiclens antiseptic/antimicrobial skin cleanser
Hibistat germicidal hand rinse

Hi-Care closed suction and pulmonary hygiene system
Hickman
  H. catheter
  H. indwelling right atrial catheter
  H. line
  H. long-term catheter
  H. percutaneous introducer
  H. tunneled indwelling catheter
Hickman-Broviac catheter
Hicor system
Hideaway oxygen conserver
Hieshima microcatheter
Hi-Flex lead
HiFocus electrode
high
  h. air-loss bed
  h. forceps
  h. heat-capacity x-ray tube
  h. muscular resistance bed
  H. Pure PCR product purification kit
  H. Pure PCR template preparation kit
  h. viscosity (HV)
high-beam fiberoptic headlight
high-capacity
  h.-c. fluid warmer
  h.-c. silicone drain
high-compliance latex balloon
high-density
  h.-d. foam
  h.-d. lipoprotein (HDL)
  h.-d. polyethylene
  h.-d. sector basket catheter
  v33W h.-d. endocavity probe
high-diameter dilator
high-efficiency particulate air filter
high-energy
  h.-e. bent-beam linear accelerator
  h.-e. laser
high-fidelity micromanometric catheter
high-field
  h.-f. open MRI scanner
  h.-f. system
high-field-strength scanner
Highflex large stone retrieval basket
high-flow
  h.f. catheter
  h.-f. coaxial cannula
  h.-f. regulator
high-flux dialyzer
high-force Sundt clip system
high-frequency
  h.-f. hemostatic forceps
  h.-f. jet ventilator
  h.-f. miniature probe
  h.-f. miniprobe
  h.-f. oscillation ventilator

high-frequency *(continued)*
    h.-f. oscillatory ventilation
    h.-f. oscillatory ventilator
    h.-f. tweezer-type epilator
    h.-f. ultrasound biomicroscope
high-humidity
    h.-h. face mask
    h.-h. tracheostomy collar
    h.-h. tracheostomy mask
    h.-h. tracheostomy shield
high-impedance low-threshold lead
high-intensity focus ultrasound
highlighter
    Eschenbach h.
highly oxygen-permeable contact lens
high-oscillation ventilator
high-pass filter
high-performance liquid chromatograph
high-pressure
    h.-p. Blue Max balloon
    h.-p. connecting tube
    h.-p. inflatable prosthesis cylinder
    h.-p. liquid chromatograph
    h.-p. mercury arc lamp
high-purity germanium detector
high-resolution
    h.-r. brain SPECT imager
    h.-r. brain SPECT system
    h.-r. collimator
    h.-r. fan-beam collimator
    h.-r. linear-array transducer
    low-energy ultra h.-r. (LEUHR)
    h.-r. multileaf collimator
    h.-r. parallel hole collimator
    h.-r. probe
    h.-r. real-time scanner
high-risk needle
high-sensitivity collimator
high-speed
    h.-s. cutter
    h.-s. dermabrader
    h.-s. diamond 3-tiered depth cutting
      bur
    h.-s. diamond wheel bur
    h.-s. drill
    h.-s. drill system
    h.-s. electrical tissue morcellator
    h.-s. gradient coil
    h.-s. 2-grit bur
    h.-s. microdrill
    h.-s. rotation dynamic angioplasty
      catheter
    h.-s. tungsten carbide bur
HighSpeed CT scanner
HighTide diabetic boot
high-tide walking brace
high-torque
    h.-t. bur
    h.-t. wire

High-Vision surgical telescope
high-voltage
    h.-v. electron microscope
    h.-v. generator
    h.-v. transformer
high-volume evacuator
Hilal
    H. coil
    H. embolization apparatus
    H. embolization microcoil
    H. microcoil
    H. modified headhunter catheter
hilar
    h. clamp
    h. retractor
Hildebrandt uterine hemostatic forceps
Hildreth
    H. cautery
    H. coagulator
    H. electrocautery
Hilger facial nerve stimulator
HiLight Advantage System CT scanner
Hill
    H. Air-Drop HA90C table
    H. Air-Flex table
    H. rectal retractor
Hillis-DeLee fetoscope
Hillis fetal stethoscope
HiLo
    H. BodyTable
    H. MultiPro table
Hi-Lo
    H.-L. Evac endotracheal tube
    H.-L. Jet tracheal tube
Hi-Loo Power lift
hi-lo table
Hilton
    H. self-retaining infusion cannula
    H. sutureless infusion cannula
Hinderer cartilage forceps
hindfoot orthosis
Hind-SITE 20/20 system
hinge
    Adjusta-Wrist h.
    Arizona Health Sciences Center-
      Volz h.
    h. articulator
    Camber axis h.
    Compass h.
    Dee elbow h.
    elbow h.
    Genucentric knee h.
    implant h.
    h. joint
    Kinematic rotating h.
    Kinematic rotation h.
    Lacey h.
    Lacey rotating h.
    Rancho swivel h.

hinged
>h. articulated fixator
>h. articulator
>h. cast
>h. constrained knee prosthesis
>h. great toe replacement prosthesis
>h. implant
>h. implant prosthesis
>h. knee brace
>h. Thomas splint
>h. total knee prosthcsis

hinged-distraction apparatus
Hingson-Edwards needle
Hingson-Ferguson needle
hip
>anthropometric total h.
>h. arthroplasty gouge
>Bio-Groove h.
>Biomet h.
>Corin total h.
>DePuy AML h.
>h. disarticulation prosthesis
>h. distractor
>h. fraction compaction drill
>h. fracture compaction drill bit
>Gemini h.
>h. guidance orthosis
>Gustilo-Kyle total h.
>Howmedica PCA textured h.
>Kinamed anthropometric total h.
>Leinbach head and neck total h.
>Link anatomical h.
>Metasul metal-on-metal h.
>MS-30 h.
>h. orthosis
>PCA total h.
>h. pin
>h. positioner
>Precision Osteolock total h.
>Precision total h.
>h. replacement prosthesis
>h. skid
>h. spica cast
>h. spica dressing

HIPciser abduction splint
Hi-Per
>H.-P. cardiac device
>H.-P. Flex exchange wire

hipGRIP body positioning device
hip-knee-ankle-foot orthosis (HKAFO)
hip-knee-ankle orthosis
hip-knee orthosis
Hipokrat bimodular shoulder system
Hipper twist release coil
hipRAP postsurgical wound wrap
HipSaver protective underwear
Hirsch
>H. hypophysial punch

>H. hypophysis punch forceps
>H. mucosal clamp

Hirschberg magnet
Hirschman
>H. anoscope
>H. anoscope rectal speculum
>H. iris hook
>H. iris spatula
>H. lens forceps
>H. lens manipulator
>H. lens spatula
>H. proctoscope
>H. retractor
>H. spatula
>H. speculum

Hirschowitz
>H. gastroduodenal fiberscope
>H. gastroscope

Hirst
>H. placental forceps
>H. spore trap

His bundle catheter
HiSonic-TRD device
HiSonic ultrasonic bone conduction hearing device
HiSpeed
>H. Advantage helical scanner
>H. Advantage System CT scanner
>H. CT scanner

Hi-Star MRI system
Histoacryl
>H. glue
>H. sealer

Histochoice
Histofine
>H. SAB kit
>H. SAB-PO immunohistochemical staining kit
>H. SAB-PO kit
>H. SAB-PO(M) detector kit

Histofreezer
>H. cryosurgical system
>H. cryosurgical wart treatment kit

histogram
>gray-level h.

Histopaque-1077
histrelin implant
Hitachi
>H. Altaire Open MRI system
>H. 704, 717, 736, 911 analyzer
>H. 737, 747 autoanalyzer
>H. 747-100 cholesterol analyzer
>H. 747 CK/MB analyzer
>H. convex-convex biplane probe
>H. convex ultrasound probe
>H. CT, MR scanner
>H. CT scanner
>H. digital ultrasound
>H. EUB-515C ultrasound console

H

411

Hitachi *(continued)*
  H. EUB-555 diagnostic ultrasound system
  H. EUB 405 imaging system
  H. F-2000 fluorescence spectrophotometer
  H. fingertip ultrasound probe
  H. F-series fluorescence spectrophotometer
  H. 4-head system
  H. H600, H7000 electron microscope
  H. linear ultrasound probe
  H. MR scanner
  H. Open MRI system
  H. Open MRI system scanner
  H. PCT-3600W PET system
  H. rotating detector array system
  H. SPECT 2000H-40 camera
  H. spectrophotometer
  H. transrectal ultrasound probe
  H. transvaginal ultrasound probe
  H. 0.3-T unit scanner
  H. UB 420 digital ultrasound system
  H. ultrasound
  H. U-2000 spectrophotometer
hitch
  ankle h.
  girth h.
Hitchcock stereotactic immobilization frame
Hi-Top
  H.-T. foot/ankle brace
  H.-T. II adjustable walker
  H.-T. shoe
Hi-Torque
  H.-T. balance middleweight universal guide wire
  H.-T. balance middleweight universal guidewire
  H.-T. Floppy exchange guidewire
  H.-T. Floppy guide catheter
  H.-T. Floppy guidewire
  H.-T. Floppy II guidewire
  H.-T. Floppy intermediate guidewire
  H.-T. Floppy with Pro/Pel
  H.-T. Modified J-GW guidewire
  H.-T. Spartacore 14 guidewire
  H.-T. Standard guidewire
  H.-T. Steelcore 18 guidewire
  H.-T. steerable guidewire
  H.-T. Supracore 35 guidewire
Hittenberger prosthesis
HiWire highly elastic nitinol core wire guide
HKAFO
  hip-knee-ankle-foot orthosis

  HKAFO prosthesis
  Rochester HKAFO
HLT-405 instrument adjusting table
HM4 lithotriptor
HME
  heat and moisture exchanger
  Tracheolife HME
HmX
  HmX hematology analyzer
  HmX Hematology flow cytometer
  HmX H20 hematology system
Hobbs
  H. dilatation balloon catheter
  H. needle
  H. polypectomy snare
  H. sheath brush
  H. stent set
  H. stone basket
hockey-stick
  h.-s. catheter
  h.-s. dissector
  h.-s. electrosurgical probe
  h.-s. guiding sheath
Hodge
  H. obstetrical forceps
  H. pessary
Hodgen
  H. apparatus
  H. hip splint
  H. leg splint
hoe
  Hough h.
  Joe's h.
  LASEK epithelial micro h.
  Rhein LASIK epithelial detaching h.
  Sloane micro h.
  stapes h.
Hoefer GS 300 laser densitometer
Hoefflin suture passer
Hoen
  H. dural separator
  H. gouge
  H. intervertebral disc rongeur
  H. laminectomy rongeur
  H. nerve hook
  H. periosteal elevator
  H. pituitary rongeur
Hoffer
  H. corneal marker
  H. forward-cutting knife cannula
  H. optic zone marker
Hoffman
  H. external fixation system
  H. external fixator
Hoffmann
  H. apex fixation pin
  H. clamp
  H. C-series Colles wrist fixator

H. ear punch forceps
H. ear rongeur
H. external fixation device
H. external fixation system
H. external fixator
H. eye implant
H. II compact external fixation component
H. ligament clamp
H. mini-lengthening fixation device
H. traction device
H. transfixion pin
Hoffmann-Steinberg gastric reservoir
Hoffmann-Vidal external fixation device
Hoffman-Pappas total joint prosthesis
Hoff towel clamp
Hofmann-Thornton globe fixation ring
Hofmann T-incision marker
Hogness box
Hohmann
H. bone lever
H. bone retractor
H. clamp
H. osteotome
Hohn central venous catheter
hoist
Hoke
H. lumbar brace/corset
H. osteotome
holder
Abbey needle h.
Adson needle h.
Alvarado knee h.
Anis needle h.
Arruga needle h.
arthroscopic ankle h.
Assistant Free orthopaedic needle h.
Axhausen needle h.
Ayers cardiovascular needle h.
Aztec shoulder h.
Bard leg bag h.
Barraquer baby needle h.
Barraquer eye needle h.
Barraquer needle h.
Barraquer-Troutman needle h.
Baumgartner needle h.
Baum tonsillar needle h.
bayonet needle h.
Bechert-Sinskey needle h.
Belin needle h.
Bethea sheet h.
Bihrle dorsal clamp T-C needle h.
Björk-Shiley heart valve h.
blade h.
Bodkin thread h.
bone h.
bone graft h.
Bookler swivel-ball laparoscope h.

Bookler swivel-ball laparoscopic instrument h.
boomerang needle h.
Bovie h.
Boyce needle h.
Boynton needle h.
Bozeman-Wertheim needle h.
Bra Pocket pump h.
Bunt forceps h.
Cameco syringe h.
Capillary System slide h.
Carb-N-Sert needle h.
cardiovascular needle h.
Castroviejo-Barraquer needle h.
Castroviejo blade h.
Castroviejo-Kalt eye needle h.
Castroviejo-Mayo needle h.
Castroviejo needle h.
Cath-Secure catheter h.
Cath-Secure Dual Tab h.
Charnley trochanter h.
clamp h.
Clerf needle h.
Cohan needle h.
Collier needle h.
Comfit endotracheal tube h.
Converse-Gillies needle h.
Converse needle h.
Corboy needle h.
Craig headrest h.
Crile-Murray needle h.
Crile needle h.
Crile-Wood needle h.
Crile-Wood-Vital needle h.
curved microneedle h.
Dale drainage bulb and G-tube h.
Dale Foley catheter h.
Dale gastrostomy tube h.
Dale nasal dressing h.
Dale secondary wound dressing and h.
Dale tapeless wound dressing h.
Dale tracheostomy tube h.
Dean knife h.
delicate needle h.
DeMartel-Wolfson clamp h.
Derf eye needle h.
diamond grip needle h.
Diamond-Jaw needle h.
Donaghy angled suture needle h.
Drummond hook h.
Ellis needle h.
Endo-Assist disposable needle h.
Endo-Assist endoscopic needle h.
EndoGrip endotracheal tube h.
endoscopic in-line needle h.
Eriksson-Paparella h.
eye h.
eye needle h.

H

holder *(continued)*

E-Z hold adhesive/stretchable strap catheter tube h.
Ferguson bone h.
Ferris-Smith needle h.
Finochietto needle h.
flossAwl floss h.
Floss Rite floss h.
foot h.
Foster needle h.
French needle h.
Gambro dialyzer h.
Gardner needle h.
Gifford needle h.
Gillies needle h.
goniotomy needle h.
GraftAssist vein-graft h.
GraftAssist vein and graft h.
Greenberg instrument h.
green needle h.
Grieshaber needle h.
Hagedorn needle h.
Halsey needle h.
head h.
Hegar-Baumgartner needle h.
Hegar needle h.
hook h.
Huang vein h.
Ilg microneedle h.
instrument h.
intracardiac needle h.
I-tech cannula h.
I-tech needle h.
Jacobson needle h.
Jaffe needle h.
Jako laryngeal needle h.
Jarcho tenaculum h.
Jarit forceps h.
Jarit microsurgical needle h.
Jarit sternal needle h.
Johnson prostatic needle h.
Jones IMA needle h.
Julian needle h.
Kalt-Arruga needle h.
Kalt eye needle h.
Kalt needle h.
Kilner needle h.
Knolle needle h.
Langenbeck needle h.
Lapides h.
laryngoscope chest support h.
laser Heaney needle h.
laser Julian needle h.
leg h.
Leg Thing pump h.
Leonard Arms instrument h.
Lewy chest h.
Lewy laryngoscope h.
Lichtenberg needle h.

LifePort endotracheal tube h.
limb h.
lion jaw bone h.
lion-jaw bone h.
Malis needle h.
Margraf beam-aligning film h.
Marquette 3-channel laser h.
Marsupial Pouch postsurgical drain h.
Mason leg h.
Mason needle h.
mat h.
Mathieu needle h.
Mathieu-Olsen needle h.
Mayo-Hegar needle h.
Mayo needle h.
McAllister needle h.
McIntyre fish-hook needle h.
McPherson microsurgery eye needle h.
McPherson needle h.
Metzenbaum needle h.
MGH needle h.
microneedle h.
microstaple h.
microsurgical needle h.
microvascular needle h.
mirror h.
needle h.
Neivert needle h.
Neo-Fit neonatal endotracheal tube h.
neonatal tracheostomy tube h.
nerve h.
Neuro-smooth needle h.
neurosurgery needle h.
neurosurgical head h.
neurosurgical needle h.
New Orleans needle h.
Nolan needle h.
octopus h.
Olsen-Hegar needle h.
operative leg h.
OSI arthroscopic leg h.
Paton needle h.
pin h.
pinion head h.
Pittman needle h.
3-point head h.
Portmann speculum h.
prostatic needle h.
prosthetic valve h.
Pump-N-Shorts pump h.
Punctur-Guard Revolution safety needle h.
Ramirez EndoFacelift needle h.
razor blade h.
Rhoton needle h.
Rinn XCP film h.

rod h.
Ryder needle h.
Sarot needle h.
Schlein shoulder h.
Shea speculum h.
Sheehan-Gillies needle h.
sheet h.
Sims sponge h.
Sinskey needle h.
smooth jawed needle h.
speculum h.
Spetzler needle h.
S-P needle h.
spring-handled needle h.
spring needle h.
Stangel modified Barraquer
  microsurgical needle h.
Steinmann h.
sterile forceps h.
sternal needle h.
Stevens needle h.
Storz head h.
Stratte needle h.
Sugita head h.
suture h.
tapered-spring needle h.
Taylor catheter h.
T-C needle h.
temporal bone h.
Tennant eye needle h.
Tennant thumb-ring needle h.
Texas Scottish Rite Hospital
  hook h.
The Dale tracheostomy tube h.
Thigh Thing pump h.
Thomas endotracheal tube h.
Thomas long-term endotracheal
  tube h.
Thomas LT endotracheal tube h.
Thomas Quick Block endotracheal
  tube h.
Toennis needle h.
Trake-Fit tracheal tube h.
trochanter h.
Troutman-Barraquer needle h.
Troutman blade h.
Troutman needle h.
Tru-Cut biopsy needle h.
TSRH hook h.
Turner-Warwick needle h.
Universal head h.
Vacutainer h.
valve h.
vascular needle h.
VBH head h.
Vickers needle h.
Vital French eye needle h.
Vital-Heaney needle h.
Vital-Ryder microvascular needle h.

Vogele-Bale-Hohner head h.
Waist It pump h.
Wangensteen needle h.
washer h.
Watson heart valve h.
Webster needle h.
well leg h.
Wertheim needle h.
Wolf-Castroviejo needle h.
Worcester instrument h.
Yasargil bayonet needle h.
Yasargil microneedle h.
Yasargil needle h.
Young boomerang needle h.
Young needle h.

holder/scissors
Assistant Free orthopaedic
  needle h./s.

holding
h. clip
h. forceps
h. mitt

hole
bone hook with cable/wire h.
6-h. mandibular plate
8-h. miniplate
5-h. plate
6-h. plate
7-h. plate

1-hole
1-h. angiographic catheter
1-h. angioplastic catheter

2-hole
2-h. miniplate
2-h. plate
2-h. standard tip

3-hole
3-h. aspiration cannula
3-h. plate
3-h. standard tip

4-hole
4-h. Alta straight plate
4-h. side plate

Holinger
H. anterior commissure
  laryngoscope
H. applicator
H. bronchoscope
H. cannula
H. curved scissors
H. dissector
H. infant bougie
H. infant bronchoscope
H. infant esophageal speculum
H. infant esophagoscope
H. infant laryngoscope
H. slotted laryngoscope
H. ventilating fiberoptic
  bronchoscope

H

Holladay contrast acuity test
Hollander clog
Hollenback carver
Holligard seal closed stoma pouch
Hollister
- H. circumcision device
- H. clamp
- H. collecting device
- H. colostomy bag
- H. colostomy irrigator
- H. disposable convex insert
- H. drainage bag
- H. external catheter
- H. First Choice pouch
- H. Hot/Ice knee blanket
- H. irrigator drain
- H. medial adhesive bandage
- H. replacement filters pouch cover
- H. self-adhesive catheter
- H. urostomy bag
- H. wound exudate absorber

hollow
- h. albumin microsphere
- h. bone
- h. cannula
- h. chisel
- h. cutter
- h. filter dialyzer
- h. mill
- h. needle
- h. needle guide
- h. ribbon
- h. silastic disc heart valve
- h. sphere prosthesis
- h. stainless steel trocar
- h. visceral tonometer

hollow-fiber capillary dialyzer
hollow-object forceps
hollow-sphere implant
Holman
- H. flushing apparatus
- H. lung retractor

Holmes
- H. chisel
- H. fixation forceps
- H. nasopharyngoscope
- H. scissors

holmium
- h. laser
- h. laser lithotriptor

holmium:YAG laser
holmium-yttrium-aluminum-garnet laser
holmium:yttrium-argon-garnet laser
Holofax Oxford retroillumination cataract camera
Hologic
- H. 2000 densitometer
- H. 1000 QDR densitometer

H. 1000 QDR dual-energy absorptiometer
H. QDR 4500 DXA bone densitometer
H. QDR 1000W dual-energy x-ray absorptiometry scanner
H. 2000 scanner

Holtain height stadiometer
Holter
- H. connector
- H. distal peritoneal catheter
- H. elliptical valve
- H. external drainage system
- H. high-pressure valve
- H. hydrocephalus shunt system
- H. in-line shunt filter
- H. introducer
- H. lumboperitoneal catheter
- Marquette 3-channel laser H.
- H. medium-pressure valve
- H. mini-elliptical valve
- H. monitor
- H. Pediatric Pump 903, 907
- H. pump
- H. pump clamp
- H. shunt
- H. straight valve
- H. traction
- H. tube
- H. ventricular catheter
- H. ventriculostomy reservoir

Holter-Hausner
- H.-H. catheter
- H.-H. valve

Holth
- H. corneoscleral punch
- H. cystotome
- H. forceps
- H. punch forceps
- H. scleral punch

Holzheimer skin retractor
home
- h. cardiorespiratory monitor
- H. Care Simplimatt Plus zoned foam mattress
- H. Ranger shoulder pulley
- h. uterine activity monitor

Homepump infusion system
Homerlok needle
Homer needle/wire localizer
HomeStretch lumbar traction
HomeTrac
- Saunders cervical H.

HomMed
- H. monitor
- H. monitoring system

homogenizer
- Potter-Elvehjem h.
- Wheaton tissue h.

homograft
 CryoLife h.
 denatured h.
 h. implant
 h. implant material
 h. prosthesis
homonuclear spin system
Honan
 H. balloon
 H. cuff
 H. manometer
Honeywell recorder
hood
 H. dissector
 extensor h.
 H. Laboratories Eccovision acoustic
  rhinometer
 laminar flow h.
 H. manual dermatome
 oxygen h.
 Oxyhood oxygen h.
 Oxypod oxygen h.
 H. speaking valve
 H. stoma stent
 surgical h.
hooded transilluminator
hook (*See also* buttonhook)
 Adson h.
 Adson blunt dissecting h.
 Adson dissecting h.
 Adson dural h.
 Alio-Kelman IOL h.
 anchor h.
 angled discission h.
 h. approximator
 ASSI fixation h.
 Austin Moore h.
 ball-tip nerve h.
 Barr crypt h.
 Behler LASIK enhancement h.
 Behler LASIK retreatment h.
 Berens scleral h.
 biangled h.
 bifid h.
 h. blocker
 blunt h.
 blunt dissecting h.
 blunt iris h.
 blunt nerve h.
 boat h.
 Bobechko sliding barrel h.
 bone h.
 Bonn iris h.
 Bonn microiris h.
 Boyes-Goodfellow h.
 Braun obstetrical h.
 button h.
 buttressed h.
 calvarial h.

 canted finger h.
 Carroll skin h.
 caudal h.
 C-D h.
 Chavasse strabismus h.
 h. clamp
 clawed pedicle h.
 Clayman iris h.
 closed Cotrel-Dubousset h.
 Cloward dural h.
 cold knife h.
 compression h.
 Converse hinged skin h.
 corneal h.
 Cotrel-Dubousset closed h.
 Cottle double h.
 Cottle-Joseph h.
 Cottle nasal h.
 Cottle skin h.
 Cottle tenaculum h.
 cranial Jacobs h.
 Crawford h.
 Crile nerve h.
 crypt h.
 Culler h.
 Culler muscle h.
 Culler rectus muscle h.
 Cushing dural h.
 Dandy nerve h.
 Day ear h.
 destructive obstetrical h.
 discission h.
 dissecting h.
 distraction h.
 h. distractor
 Dortu phlebectomy h.
 double-hook Tyrell skin h.
 double-pronged Cottle h.
 double-pronged skin h.
 double skin h.
 double tenaculum h.
 down-angle h.
 downsized circular laminar h.
 Drummond h.
 Du Plessis muscle h.
 dura h.
 dura twist skin h.
 ear h.
 Edwards h.
 Edwards-Levine h.
 Effler-Groves h.
 Emmet tenaculum h.
 expressor h.
 h. expressor
 extraction h.
 fenestration h.
 Fenzel angled manipulating h.
 fibroid h.
 finger h.

H

hook *(continued)*

Fisch dural h.
fistula h.
fixation h.
fixation twist h.
flat h.
flat tenotomy h.
Fomon nasal h.
footplate h.
h. forceps
Frazier dura h.
Frazier nerve h.
Frazier-Shepherd skin h.
Frazier skin h.
Freer skin h.
Fukasaku small pupil snapper h.
ganglion h.
gasserian ganglion h.
Gass muscle h.
Gass retinal detachment h.
Gillies bone h.
Gillies-Converse skin h.
Gillies-Dingman tenaculum h.
Gillies dural h.
Gillies nasal h.
Gillies skin h.
Gillies zygoma h.
glide h.
goiter h.
Graefe iris h.
Graefe strabismus h.
Graether button h.
Graether mushroom h.
Graham blunt h.
Graham dural h.
Graham muscle h.
Graham nerve h.
Green muscle h.
Green strabismus h.
Gross ear h.
Guthrie eye fixation h.
Guthrie iris h.
Guthrie skin h.
Hardesty tendon h.
Hardesty tenotomy h.
Harrington pedicle h.
Hebra h.
Helveston h.
Helveston finder h.
H. hemi-harness shoulder
    immobilizer
Hirschman iris h.
Hoen nerve h.
h. holder
Hosmer Dorrance h.
House oval-window h.
House strut h.
House tragus h.
Humby h.

Hunkeler ball-point h.
h. impactor
instant skin h.
intermediate C-D h.
intracapsular lens expressor h.
intraocular h.
iris h.
irrigating iris h.
Isola spinal implant system h.
IUD remover h.
Jackson tracheal h.
Jacobson blunt h.
Jaeger strabismus h.
Jaffe iris h.
Jaffe lens manipulating h.
Jaffe-Maltzman h.
Jameson muscle h.
Jameson strabismus h.
Jannetta h.
Jarit palate h.
jaw h.
jig h.
Johnson skin h.
Jordan h.
Joseph h.
Joseph nasal h.
Joseph sharp skin h.
Joseph single-prong h.
Joseph skin h.
Joseph tenaculum h.
Juers h.
Katena boat h.
Keene compression h.
Kelly uterine tenaculum h.
Kelman irrigation h.
Kelman manipulator h.
Kennerdell-Maroon h.
Kennerdell muscle h.
Kennerdell nerve h.
Kilner h.
Kilner goiter h.
Kilner sharp h.
Kilner skin h.
Kimball nephrostomy h.
Kirby double-fixation muscle h.
Kirby muscle h.
Kleinert-Kutz skin h.
Kleinsasser h.
Knapp iris h.
h. knife
Kratz iris push-pull h.
Krayenbuehl dural h.
Krayenbuehl nerve h.
Krayenbuehl vessel h.
Kuglen manipulating iris h.
Küntscher nail-extracting h.
Lahey Clinic dural h.
Lambotte bone h.
laminar C-D h.

Lange fistular h.
Lange plastic surgery h.
large ball nerve h.
Leader iris h.
Leatherman alar h.
Leatherman compression h.
Leinbach olecranon h.
lens h.
Levy-Kuglen iris h.
Lewicky lens manipulating h.
Lewicky microlens h.
Lillie attic h.
Lillie ear h.
Linton vein h.
Lucae h.
lyre-shaped finger h.
Madden sympathectomy h.
Malgaigne patellar h.
Malis nerve h.
h. manipulator
Marino rotatable transsphenoidal right-angle h.
Martin rectal h.
Maumenee iris h.
Mayo h.
Mayo fibroid h.
McIntyre irrigating iris h.
McReynolds lid-retracting h.
Meyerding skin h.
microball h.
microiris h.
Micro-One h.
microscopic h.
microsurgical ear h.
microvessel h.
Millard thimble h.
Millet phlebectomy h.
Miltex tenaculum h.
mitral h.
Miya h.
modified right-angled h.
Moe alar h.
Moss h.
Muller phlebectomy h.
multispan fracture h.
muscle h.
nail-extracting h.
narrow-blade laminar h.
nasal polyp h.
nerve h.
nerve pull h.
neutral h.
Nugent h.
oblique muscle h.
O'Brien rib h.
Ochsner h.
O'Connor flat h.
O'Connor muscle h.
O'Connor sharp h.

O'Connor tenotomy h.
Oesch h.
Oesch phlebectomy h.
open C-D h.
ophthalmic h.
Osher h.
oval-window h.
palate h.
PCL-oriented placement marking h.
pear-shaped nerve h.
pediatric C-D h.
pediatric TSRH h.
pedicle C-D h.
Pitie-Salpetriere saphenous vein h.
plain ear h.
pocketing h.
Pratt crypt h.
h. probe system
2-pronged dural h.
Pucci-Seed h.
push-and-pull h.
h. pusher
Ramelet phlebectomy h.
recession ophthalmic muscle h.
rectal h.
Rentsch boat h.
retinal detachment h.
h. retractor
retractor h.
retractor handle Cloward dural h.
reversed Sinskey h.
ribbed h.
Richards bone h.
right-angle h.
Rogozinski h.
h. rotary scissors
rotatable transsphenoidal right-angle h.
Sachs dural h.
h. scissors
scleral h.
scleral twist fixation h.
Scobee oblique muscle h.
Scoville blunt h.
Scoville curved nerve h.
Selby I, II h.
sharp h.
Sheets iris h.
Shepard reversed iris h.
side-opening laminar h.
Simon fistula h.
single h.
single-hook Frazier skin h.
Sinskey h.
Sinskey iris h.
Sinskey lens h.
Sinskey lens manipulating h.
skin h.
sliding barrel h.

H

hook *(continued)*
Sluder sphenoidal h.
Smellie obstetrical h.
Smith expressor h.
Smith lid-retracting h.
Smithwick ganglion h.
Smithwick nerve h.
Smithwick sympathectomy h.
spatula h.
h. spatula
split-finger h.
spring h.
square-ended h.
squint h.
Stamler side-port fixation h.
stapes h.
Stevens h.
Stevens tenotomy h.
Stewart crypt h.
Stewart rectal h.
Storz twist h.
strabismus h.
straight nerve h.
strut bar h.
suture pickup h.
sympathectomy h.
tenaculum h.
tendon h.
tenotomy h.
Texas Scottish Rite Hospital
  buttressed laminar h.
Texas Scottish Rite Hospital
  circular laminar h.
Texas Scottish Rite Hospital
  pedicle h.
Texas Scottish Rite Hospital
  trial h.
Tomas iris h.
Tomas suture h.
tonsillar h.
top-entry h.
tracheal h.
tracheostomy h.
tracheotomy h.
traction h.
tragus House h.
transection h.
triple h.
TSRH buttressed laminar h.
TSRH circular laminar h.
TSRH pedicle h.
TSRH trial h.
tubal h.
twist h.
twist fixation h.
Tyrrell iris h.
Tyrrell skin h.
Tyrrell tympanic membrane h.
Universal nerve h.

up-angle h.
Varady phlebectomy h.
vas h.
vessel h.
Vilex Ouchless H.
Visitec angled lens h.
Visitec corneal suture
  manipulating h.
Visitec micro double-iris h.
Visitec microiris h.
Visitec straight lens h.
Volkmann bone h.
von Graefe muscle h.
von Graefe strabismus h.
Welch Allyn h.
Whitaker h.
wide-blade laminar h.
Wiener corneal h.
Wiener scleral h.
Wilder foreign body h.
Y h.
Yasargil spring h.
zygoma h.
Zylik-Joseph h.
hook-and-loop fastener strap
hooked
  h. catheter
  h. intramedullary nail
  h. knife
  h. medullary nail
  h. needle
hook-end intramedullary pin
hook-on
  h.-o. bronchoscope
  h.-o. folding laryngoscope
hook-plate fixation
hook-rod
  Cotrel-Dubousset h.-r.
  Isola h.-r.
  TSRH h.-r.
**hook-to-screw L4-S1 compression
  construct**
hook-type
  h.-t. dermal curette
  h.-t. eye implant
  h.-t. implant
hookwire
  Hawkin h.
  Kopans spring h.
  h. needle
Hooper deep surgery scissors
Hope
  H. continuous & Heliox nebulizer
  H. processor
  H. resuscitation bag
  H. resuscitator
Hopkins
  H. angle-view 30-degree optical
    system

H. aortic forceps
H. aortic occlusion clamp
H. arthroscope
H. dilator
H. direct-vision telescope
H. forceps
H. forward oblique telescope
H. hook-guiding catheter
H. hysterectomy clamp
H. II endoscope
H. II optical system
H. II rod lens
H. lateral telescope
H. nasal endoscopy telescope
H. pediatric telescope
H. plaster knife
H. retrospective telescope
H. rigid telescope
H. rod
H. rod endoscope
H. rod-lens system
H. rod-lens telescope
H. sigmoidoscope
H. straight-view optical system
H. telescope

Horgan
H. center blade
H. retractor

Horizon
H. AutoAdjust CPAP system
H. CPAP device
H. Eclipse spinal system
H. Legacy spinal system
H. LT CPAP system
H. LX scanner
H. LX 1.5-T superconducting magnet
H. nasal CPAP system
H. PFT spirometer
H. prostatic stent
H. Sextant rod insertion set
H. surgical ligating and marking clip
H. temporary stent

horizontal
h. drain attachment device
h. flexible bar retractor
h. gantry cut
h. pull headgear
h. ring curette
h. scissors
h. tube attachment device

horn
bone graft shoe h.
1-h. bridge
H. endootoprobe
H. endootoprobe laser
shoulder h.

horopter
Vieth-Mueller h.

horseshoe
h. headrest
h. heel pad
h. magnet
h. patellofemoral brace
h. therapy table
h. tourniquet

horseshoe-shaped pad

Horsley
H. bone cutter
H. bone-cutting forceps
H. bone rongeur
H. bone wax
H. cranial bone rongeur
H. dural knife
H. dural separator
H. elevator
H. guard
H. spine cutter
H. suture
H. trephine

Horsley-Clarke
H.-C. stereotactic apparatus
H.-C. stereotactic frame

Horsley-Stille
H.-S. bone-cutting forceps
H.-S. rib shears forceps

hose
Juzo h.
TED h.
thromboembolic disease h.
Venosan support h.

Hosford
H. double-ended lacrimal dilator
H. foreign body spud
H. lacrimal dilator
H. spud

hosiery
Spa Ready-To-Wear gradient pressure therapy h.

Hoskins
H. beaked Colibri forceps
H. fine straight forceps
H. fixation forceps
H. lens
H. miniaturized micro straight forceps
H. nylon suture laser lens
H. straight microiris forceps
H. suture forceps

Hoskins-Barkan goniotomy infant lens
Hosmer
H. above-knee rotator
H. Dorrance hook
H. Dorrance voluntary control 4-bar knee mechanism
H. Endurance knee

Hosmer *(continued)*
- H. single-axis friction knee
- H. single-axis locking knee
- H. WALK prosthesis
- H. weight-activated locking knee
- H. weight-activated locking knee prosthesis

Hospal Biospal filter
Hospidex microtiter plate
hospital
- h. bed
- H. Recliner seat
- Texas Scottish Rite H. (TSRH)

host tissue forceps
hot
- h. biopsy forceps
- h. cathode x-ray tube
- h. flexible forceps
- h. knife
- h. laser
- h. moist pack
- h. pack
- h. pad
- h. quartz lamp
- h. quartz vapor lamp
- h. salt sterilizer
- H. Sampler disposable hot biopsy forceps
- H. Tap portable hot shower
- h. water bottle
- h. wet pack

hot/ice
- H./i. cold therapy cooler
- h./i. cold therapy cooler therapy device
- H./i. System III
- H./i. System III knee blanket

Hotline
- H. blood and fluid warmer
- H. fluid warming device

Hotsy high-temperature cautery
Hottentot apron
hot-tip
- h.-t. laser
- h.-t. laser probe

hot-water circulating suit
hot-wire
- h.-w. anemometer
- h.-w. pneumotachometer
- h.-w. respirometer

Hotz-type alveolar molding plate
Hough
- H. anterior crurotomy nipper
- H. curette
- H. drape
- H. drum scraper
- H. gouge
- H. hoe
- H. incision knife
- H. middle ear instrument
- H. scissors
- H. spatula
- H. spatula elevator
- H. Teflon cutter

Hough-Wullstein bur saw
24-hour
- 24-h. ambulatory electrocardiographic recorder
- 24-h. ambulatory gastric pH monitor
- 24-h. esophageal pH probe

hourglass
- h. dressing
- H. vertebral body spacer

House
- H. adapter
- H. alligator crimper forceps
- H. alligator grasping forceps
- H. alligator scissors
- H. alligator strut forceps
- H. cup forceps
- H. detachable blade
- H. dissector
- H. ear curette
- H. ear elevator
- H. ear forceps
- H. ear knife
- H. ear separator
- H. endaural elevator
- H. endolymphatic shunt
- H. endolymphatic shunt tube
- H. endolymphatic shunt tube introducer
- H. Gelfoam pressure forceps
- H. grading system
- H. grasping forceps
- H. handheld double-end retractor
- H. implant
- H. knife blade
- H. lacrimal dilator
- H. lancet knife
- H. malleus nipper
- H. measuring rod
- H. middle ear instrument
- H. middle ear mirror
- H. miniature forceps
- H. myringoplasty knife
- H. myringotomy knife
- H. myringotomy knife handle
- H. obtuse pick
- H. ophthalmic blade
- H. oval-cup forceps
- H. oval-window hook
- H. oval-window pick
- H. pressure forceps
- H. round knife
- H. sickle knife
- H. stapes curette

H. stapes elevator
H. stapes needle
H. stapes speculum
H. strut calipers
H. strut forceps
H. strut guide
H. strut hook
H. strut pick
H. suction tube
H. tragus hook
H. wire
H. wire stapes prosthesis
House-Barbara pick
House-Baron suction tube
House-Bellucci alligator scissors
Housecall transtelephonic monitoring system
House-Crabtree dissector pick
House-Dieter
H.-D. eye forceps
H.-D. malleus nipper
H.-D. nipper
household ambulatory
Houser
H. cul-de-sac irrigator T tube
H. cul-de-sac irrigator tube
House-Rosen
H.-R. knife
H.-R. needle
House-Urban
H.-U. middle fossa retractor
H.-U. tube
housing
x-ray tube h.
Housset-Debray gastroscope
Houston
H. halo cervical traction
H. halo traction cervical collar
Hoveround programmable wheelchair
166Ho in vivo generator
Howard
H. Jones needle
H. stone basket
Howard-Dolman apparatus
Howarth elevator
Howell
H. aspiration needle
H. biliary aspiration needle
H. biopsy aspiration needle
H. needle
H. phoria card
H. Rotatable BII papillotome
H. tibial guide
Howell-Jolly body
Howland lock
Howmedica
H. bone anchor
H. cerclage
H. cerclage cable

H. Duracon implant
H. external bone-lengthening device
H. hip fracture stem
H. HNR system
H. Kinematic II knee prosthesis
H. knee instrumentation
H. Microfixation System drill bit
H. Microfixation System forceps
H. Microfixation System plate cutter
H. Microfixation System pliers
H. monospherical implant
H. monotube
H. monotube external rotator
H. PCA prosthesis
H. PCA textured hip
H. pediatric osteotomy system
H. Simplex P cement
H. slit catheter
H. total ankle system
H. Unitrax hip fracture system
H. Universal compression screw
H. VSF fixation system
Howmedica-Osteonics instrument
Howorth
H. elevator
H. osteotome
H. prosthesis
H. toothed retractor
Howse prosthesis
Howtek Scanmaster DX scanner
Hoya
H. AR-570 autorcfractor
H. HDR objective refractometer
H. MRM objective refractometer
Ho:YAG laser
Hoyer
H. lift
H. snare
HP
Hewlett-Packard
FlexSure HP
HP Sonos imaging catheter
HP Sonos transducer
HP Sonos 5500 ultrasound echocardiography system
HP Sonos 5500 ultrasound imaging system
HP-100
HP-100 prosthetic finger
HP-100 prosthetic finger joint
HP7754 pneumohydraulic capillary infusion system
HPC-2 standard needle knife
HPGe detector
Hp-test
Jatrox Hp-t.
HPU heat probe

H

16HR
Synectics PC Polygraf 16HR
HRR pseudoisochromatic test
Hruby
H. contact implant
H. contact lens
H. implant
H. laser
H. lens
H/S
H/S Elliptosphere catheter
H/S Elliptosphere catheter set
H-series healing shoe
HSG tray
H-shaped
H-s. plate
H-s. tilt tag
HSRA device
HSV Lightning vitrectomy cutter
HTO
HTO fixator
HTO wedge human donor tissue allograft
HTP
Bio-Gel HTP
HTR-MFI
HTR-MFI chin implant
HTR-MFI curved implant
HTR-MFI malar implant
HTR-MFI paranasal implant
HTR-MFI premaxillary implant
HTR-MFI ramus implant
H-TRON insulin pump
H-TRONplus insulin pump
HTR polymer
Huang
H. Universal arm retractor
H. Universal flexible arm
H. vein holder
hub
H. Cap limited wrist fusion plate catheter h.
Hubbard
H. bolt
H. corneoscleral forceps
H. hydrotherapy tank
H. plate
H. retractor
H. side plate
H. tank
Huber
H. point needle
H. probe
Huco diamond knife
Hudson
H. adapter
H. bone bur
H. bone drill
H. bone retractor

H. brace
H. brace bur
H. brace drill
H. brain forceps
H. bur
H. cerebellar attachment
H. cerebellar extension
H. clamp
H. conical bur
H. cranial bur
H. cranial drill
H. cranial forceps
H. dressing forceps
H. forceps
H. Hydrofloat cushion
H. Lifesaver resuscitator
H. Multi-Vent
H. prongs
H. rongeur forceps
H. shank
H. tissue forceps
H. TLSO brace
H. T Up-Draft II disposable nebulizer
Hudson-type oxygen mask
Huene biaxial elbow system
Hueter bandage
Huffman
H. adolescent speculum
H. vaginal speculum
H. vaginoscope
Huffman-Graves vaginal speculum
Hufnagel
H. aortic clamp
H. commissurotomy knife
H. implant
H. low-profile heart prosthesis
H. mitral valve forceps
H. prosthetic valve
Hu-Friedy
H.-F. dental bur
H.-F. elevator
H.-F. PermaSharp suture
H.-F. probe
H.-F. suction-tip aspirator
Hugger
Bair H.
Hughes
H. eye implant
H. fixation
H. implant
HUI
Harris uterine injector
HUI catheter
HUI Mini-Flex
Huibregtse
H. biliary stent
H. biliary stent set

Huibregtse-Katon
- H.-K. ERCP catheter
- H.-K. needle knife
- H.-K. papillotome

Huisman percutaneous drainage set

Hulka
- H. clip
- H. clip applier
- H. clip forceps
- H. tenaculum forceps
- H. uterine cannula
- H. uterine manipulator
- H. uterine tenaculum

Hulka-Clemens clip

human
- h. allograft tissue
- h. demineralized bone matrix
- h. fibroblast-derived dermis
- h. IFN-y quantikine ELISA kit

Human-CFSE Flow kit

Humatrix Microclysmic Gel filler

HumatroPen

Humby
- H. hook
- H. knife

humeral
- h. cutting guide
- h. impactor
- h. reamer
- h. retractor
- h. saw

HUMI
- Harris-Kronner uterine manipulator/injector
- HUMI cannula
- HUMI catheter
- HUMI uterine manipulator/injector

HumidAire heated humidifier

HumidFilter heat and moisture exchanger

humidification
- BiPAP Pro II with heated h.
- REMstar Auto with heated h.
- REMstar Plus with C-Flex and heated h.
- REMstar Pro with C-Flex and heated h.
- h. ventilator

humidified isolette

humidifier
- Bennett Cascade II Servo controlled heated h.
- bubble h.
- cold-mist h.
- electrical air h.
- Fischer & Paykel HC100 heated h.
- Fisher-Paykel heated h.
- HumidAire heated h.
- hygroscopic Condenser h.

- jet h.
- Mistogen passover h.
- Ohio h.
- passover h.
- Respironics Oasis h.
- room h.
- Sullivan HumidAire heated h.
- ThermoFlo h.
- Whisper Mist h.

Hummer
- H. microdebrider
- Stryker H. II
- H. V Sputter coater

Hummingbird wand

hump
- h. forceps
- h. gouge

Humphrey
- H. Atlas 991
- H. Atlas Eclipse corneal topography system
- H. automatic keratometer
- H. automatic refractor
- H. B-scan
- H. field analyzer II
- H. Instruments vision analyzer
- H. lens analyzer
- H. Mastervue corneal topography system
- H. perimeter
- H. retinal imager
- H. videokeratographer
- H. visual field analyzer

Humphriss binocular balance

Hungarian grip plate

Hunkeler
- H. ball-point hook
- H. frown incision marker
- H. intraocular lens
- H. lens

Hunsaker
- H. jet ventilation tube
- H. Mon-Jet tube anesthesia system

Hunstad
- H. hand
- H. infusion needle
- H. system for tumescent anesthesia
- H. tumescent liposuction system

Hunt
- H. angiographic trocar
- H. angled serrated ring forceps
- H. angled tip forceps
- H. bipolar forceps
- H. chalazion forceps
- H. chalazion scissors
- H. clamp
- H. colostomy clamp
- H. forceps
- H. grasping forceps

H

Hunter
  H. open cord tendon implant
  H. 1-piece all-PMMA intraocular
    lens
  H. separator
  H. splinter forceps
  H. tendon rod
Hunter-Sessions balloon
Hunt-Lawrence pouch
Huntleigh bubble pad mattress
Hunt-Limo-Basto gastric reservoir
Hunt-Reich cannula
Hurd
  H. bipolar diathermy electrode
  H. bone-cutting forceps
  H. bone forceps
  H. dissector
  H. pillar retractor
  H. septal bone-cutting forceps
  H. septal elevator
  H. septum-cutting forceps
  H. suture needle
Hurst
  H. bougie
  H. mercury-filled dilator
  H. mercury-filled esophageal bougie
Hurst-type bougie
Hurwitz
  H. catheter
  H. dialysis catheter
  H. intestinal clamp
Husk bone rongeur
Hustead epidural needle
Hutchinson patch
Hutson loop
Huxley respirator
Huygenian eyepiece
Huygens eyepiece
HV
  high viscosity
  HV Nightsplint splint
  HV Softsplint splint
HX-5/6-1 endoscopic clipping device
Hx-5LR-1 hemoclip
hyaline cartilage implant
Hybond
  H. ECL nitrocellulose membrane
  H. N filter
  H. N+ nylon membrane
hybrid
  H. Capture 2 device
  H. Capture 2 HPV DNA test
  H. Capture system
  h. fixation of hip replacement
    component
  H. graft
  h. PET/SPECT camera
  h. prosthesis

HybridFit
  H. total hip system
  H. total knee system
hybridized probe
Hybritech Tandem-R assay kit
Hybriwix probe system
hyCURE
  h. collagen hemostatic wound
    dressing
  h. wound care powder
Hyde
  H. astigmatism ruler
  H. double-curved forceps
  H. irrigator/aspirator unit
Hyde-Osher keratometric ruler
Hydra
  H. Vision Es urological imaging
    system
  H. Vision IV urology system
  H. Vision Plus
  H. Vision Plus DR, ES, HP
    urological imaging system
  H. Vision Plus DR urological
    imaging system
  H. Vision Plus urologic system
HydraClear endoscopic cleansing system
Hydradjust
  H. IV table
  H. urology system
**HydraGlide XL small-caliber silicone
  chest tube catheter**
Hydragran absorption dressing
Hydrasoft contact lens
Hydrasorb foam wound dressing
hydraulic
  h. capillary infusion system
  h. chamber
  h. hand dynamometer
  h. hinge penile prosthesis
  h. knee unit prosthesis
  h. vein stripper
hydraulic-type disc prosthesis
Hydro
  H. Bonnet
  Cutinova H.
  H. Plus
  H. Plus coated guidewire
  H. Plus stent
hydroactive dressing
Hydro-Bell
HydroBlade keratome
**HydroBrader irrigating/aspirating
  dermabrader**
HydroBrush keratome
Hydro-Cast
  H.-C. dental mold
  H.-C. reliner
HydroCath catheter

hydrochopper
Lesieur h.
HydroCoil embolization system (HES)
Hydrocol
H. hydrocolloid dressing
H. sacral wound dressing
H. Thin
H. wound dressing
hydrocollator
h. gel pack
h. heating unit
h. pad
h. steam pack
hydrocolloid
BGC matrix h.
CombiDERM ACD h.
Comfeel h.
Curaderm h.
Cutinova thin h.
DermAssist h.
Dermatell h.
h. dressing
ExuDerm h.
Nu-Derm h.
h. occlusive dressing
RepliCare h.
Restore h.
SignaDress sterile h.
Tegasorb Thin h.
Triad h.
Ultec h.
Hydrocurve lens
HydroDerm transparent dressing
hydrodiascope
hydrodissection
h. cannula
h. tip
hydrodissector
anterior capsule h.
cortical cleaving h.
Nezhat-Dorsey trumpet valve h.
Pearce nucleus h.
hydrodissector/rotator
5195 nucleus h./r.
HydroDot neuromonitoring system
Hydroduct biliary plastic stent
hydrodynamic thrombectomy system
Hydro-Ease
H.-E. II gel flotation mattress
overlay
H.-E. I water flotation mattress
overlay
hydrofiber dressing
Hydroflex
H. penile implant
H. penile implant rod
H. penile prosthesis
H. sphincter
HydroFlex arthroscopy irrigating system

hydrofloat cushion
Hydrofloss electronic oral irrigator
hydrogel
Carrasyn h.
h. dressing
h. intraocular lens
h. plug
h. sheet
Tegagel h.
h. wound dressing
hydrogel-coated slide
HydroGlide guidewire
hydroirrigator
Lindstrom h.
HydroKeratome
h. device
Visijet h.
Hydrokinetic Vichy shower
Hydrolyser
H. hydrodynamic thrombectomy
catheter
H. microcatheter
H. percutaneous thrombectomy
catheter
hydromassage table
HydroMed wound dressing
hydromer-coated
h.-c. central venous catheter
h.-c. micro guidewire
h.-c. polyurethane stent
Hydron
H. burn Bandage
H. lens
hydrophilic
h. acrylic intraocular lens
h. angulated guidewire
h. contact lens
h. dilator
h. guide
h. guidewire
h. hydrogel implant
h. lens
h. polymer-coated steerable
guidewire
h. polyurethane foam dressing
h. tent
h. wire
hydrophilic-coated
h.-c. guidewire
h.-c. guiding catheter
hydrophobic barrier pen
hydrophone
needle h.
hydropolymer pad
HydroSoothe recliner
hydrosphere
hydrostatic
h. bag
h. balloon

H

427

hydrostatic *(continued)*
    h. balloon catheter
    h. bed
    h. dilator
    h. dissector
HydroSteer hydrophilic guidewire
hydrotherapy tub
HydroThermAblator endometrial
  ablation system
Hydro-Tone Bell
HydroTrack
    H. underwater treadmill
    H. underwater treadmill system
Hydroview
    H. foldable IOL
    H. intraocular lens
    H. IOL
    H. lens
hydroxyapatite, hydroxylapatite (HA)
    h. adhesive
    h. bead
    h. block
    h. cement
    h. ceramic implant
    h. implant material
    Interpore h.
    Interpore 200 porous h.
    h. ocular implant
    h. orbital implant
    h. ossicular prosthesis
    PureFix h.
    h. spherical enucleation implant
    h. threaded hexlock implant
hydroxyapatite-coated
    h.-c. implant
    h.-c. porous alumni cement
    h.-c. stem
hydroxyethyl methacrylate implant
hydroxylapatite *(var. of* hydroxyapatite)
HyFil hydrogel dressing
Hyflex X-File instrument
hyfrecator
    Birtcher h.
    H. coagulator
Hy-Gene seminal fluid collection kit
hygroscopic
    h. Condenser humidifier
    h. dilator
    h. heat and moisture exchanger
    h. rod
Hylaform viscoelastic gel
Hylamer
    H. enhanced ultra-high molecular
      weight polyethylene acetabular
      liner
    H. orthopaedic bearing polymer
HylaSine device
Hylin rasp
hyoid cutting forceps

Hypafix retention tape
Hypan test
hyperalimentation
    central h.
hyperbaric
    h. bed
    h. boot
    h. chamber
    h. oxygen chamber
hyperbolic glasses
hyperextension
    h. brace
    cruciform anterior spinal h.
      (CASH)
    h. fracture frame
    h. orthosis
Hyperflex tracheostomy tube
Hypergel hydrogel wound dressing
Hyperion
    H. bordered hydrocolloid dressing
    H. hydrophilic wound gel hydrogel
      dressing
    H. LTK system
    H. thin hydrocolloid dressing
    H. wound cleanser
Hyper-Oxy portable hyperbaric chamber
HyperPACS teleradiology system
Hypobaric
    H. microvalve
    H. transfemoral system
    H. transtibial system
hypodermic
    h. microscope
    h. needle
hypogastric artery forceps
Hypoguard
    H. Advance glucose meter
    H. Advance test strip
Hypo intraosseous needle
hypophysial
    h. curette
    h. forceps
hypothermia
    h. blanket
    h. I-bolt
    h. mattress
    h. oxygen warmer
HyProCure
    H. sinus tarsi implant
    H. sinus tarsi implant block
Hyrax appliance
hysterectomy
    h. clamp
    h. forceps
    h. kit
    h. retractor
hysterofiberscope
    Olympus flexible h.
hysterosalpingography catheter

hysteroscope
    Amsco h.
    Baggish h.
    Baloser h.
    Circon-ACMI h.
    contact h.
    diagnostic h.
    fiberoptic h.
    flexible h.
    French h.
    Fujinon flexible h.
    Galileo rigid h.
    Gynecare Versascope h.
    Hamou h.
    Karl Storz flexible h.
    Karl Storz flexible h.
    Liesegang LM-Flex 7 flexible h.
    MicroSpan h.
    Olympus h.
    Opera Star SL h.
    h. sheath
    Storz h.
    Valle h.
hysteroscopic insufflator
Hy-Tape
    H.-T. adhesive
    H.-T. latex-free surgical tape
    H.-T. surgical tape
    H.-T. waterproof adhesive tape
Hy-Tec automated allergy diagnostic system

H

3i
    3i dental implant
    3i implant
    3i Implant Innovations implant
       system
    3i wide-diameter dental implant
       system

I&A
  irrigation and aspiration
    I&A coaxial cannula
    I&A instrument
    I&A kit
    I&A machine
    McIntyre I&A system
    Simcoe I&A system
    I&A system

I/A
  irrigation and aspiration
    I/A cannula
    steerable I/A

IAB catheter

IABP
  intraaortic balloon pump

IAD
  implantable atrial defibrillator
    Metrix IAD

Iamin
    I. gel wound dressing
    I. hydrating gel wound dressing
    I. hydrogel dressing

IBD First Step test

I-beam
    I-b. cement punch
    I-b. hemiarthroplasty hip prosthesis
    Jergesen I-b.
    I-b. press-fit punch

IBF knee instrument

IBM
    IBM field-cycling research
      relaxometer
    IBM NMR spectrometer

I bolt

I-bolt
    hypothermia I.-b.
    Texas Scottish Rite Hospital I.-b.
    TSRH I.-b.

IBP
  instrumented bone preserving
    IBP elbow system

IBS
  interbody spacer
    IBS allograft

IBT
  inflatable bone tamp

    KyphX Elevate IBT
    KyphX Exact IBT

IC
    Babytherm IC

iCAST covered stent

**i-CAT cone beam 3D dental imaging
  system**

ICD
  implantable cardioverter-defibrillator
  intracervical device
    Angstrom II ICD
    Angstrom MD ICD
    Contour high-voltage can ICD
    Contour II ICD
    Contour LT V-135D ICD
    Contour V-145D ICD
    dual-chamber ICD
    Guardian ICD
    Photon DR dual-chamber ICD
    Res-Q Micron ICD
    Telectronics Guardian ATP II ICD
    transthoracically implanted ICD
    Ventritex Cadence ICD
    Vitatron Diamond ICD

ICD-ATP device

ice
    i. bag
    i. clot evacuator
    Liquid I.
    N'ice Stretch night splint
      suspension system with Sealed I.
    i. pack
    I. Wedge hot/cold therapy wrap

ICE catheter

I.C.E. Down cold pack

**Iceflex Endurance suction suspension
  sleeve**

Iceman
    I. cold therapy pad
    I. continuous cold therapy unit

Iceross
    I. Comfort Plus silicone gel liner
    I. silicone socket
    I. sleeve

Icex socket

Icon
    I. 25 hCG test
    I. pylon

ICP
    ICP Camino bolt
    ICP catheter
    ICP microsensor

ICSI Massachusetts clamp

icterometer

ictometer

ICTP RIA kit
ICV reservoir
Identifit hip prosthesis
IDI-Strep B test
ID-Micro typing system
IDSI scanner
IDXrad radiology information system
iFind handheld device
I-Flow nerve block infusion kit
IgA
    immunoglobulin A
      IgA HIV antibody test
      IgA II-HA assay test kit
Igaki-Tamai stent
Iglesias
    I. continuous flow resectoscope
    I. dilator
    I. electrode
    I. evacuator
    I. fiberoptic resectoscope
    I. microlens resectoscope
Igloo Heatshield system
IgM
    immunoglobulin M
      IgM II-HA assay test kit
iiRAD DR1000C digital radiographic system
Ikeda microcapsulorrhexis forceps
I-knife
    Alcon I-k.
Ikuta
    I. clamp approximator
    I. fixation
    I. fixation device
IL
    IL 1640 blood gas/electrolyte system
    IL Synthesis analyzer
IL-282 co-oximeter
ILA-series stapling device
ileal
    i. artery stent
    i. neobladder urinary pouch
ileoneobladder
    W-shaped i.
ileostomy
    i. appliance
    i. bag
    i. cup
Ilfeld
    I. brace
    I. splint
Ilg
    I. curved micro tying forceps
    I. lens loupe
    I. microneedle holder
iliac
    i. artery stent
    i. clamp

    i. crest dowel
    i. forceps
    i. graft separator
    i. screw
iliofemoral cannula
iliosacral
    i. and iliac fixation construct
    i. implant
    i. screw
Ilizarov
    I. circular external fixator
    I. device
    I. distractor
    I. external fixator
    I. external ring fixator
    I. frame
    I. hybrid fixator
    I. limb-lengthening system
    I. ring
    I. screw
ill-fitting shoe
Illinois needle
illiterate E chart
Illouz
    I. cannula
    I. modified tip
    I. standard tip
    I. suction cannula
Illumena injector
Illumina
    I. Pro Series CO_2 surgical laser system
    I. Pro Series laparoscopic laser
illuminated
    i. probe
    i. St. Mark retractor
    i. suction needle
    i. vaginal speculum
illuminating stylet
illuminator
    BLU-U blue light photodynamic therapy i.
    Cogent XL i.
    fiberoptic i.
    fiberoptic surgical field i.
    intramedullary i.
    Light Commander xenon i.
    LightMat surgical i.
    Luxo surgical i.
    Mammo Mask i.
    Opmi VISU 200 BrightFlex i.
    Pilling fiberoptic i.
    slit i.
    suspended operating i.
    Synergetics endo i.
    XL i.
iLook 15 handheld ultrasound system
ILS stapler
ILUS catheter

IM
- IM Jaws alligator forceps
- IM nail
- IM tendon stripper

IMA
- I. graft
- I. retractor
- I. scissors

image
- i. analysis system
- I. custom external breast prosthesis
- i. intensifier
- i. intensifier tube
- i. Orthicon tube
- I. 1 Pendulum endoscope
- i. reconstruction computer
- I. Titer

Imagecast imaging system
ImageChecker CT CAD software system
ImageMASTER
IMAGEnet 2000 series digital imaging system
image-processing unit
imager
- Acuson 128EP i.
- Agfa LR 3300 laser i.
- DaTSCAN i.
- Digirad 2020tc i.
- Digirad 2020 TC i.
- digital fundus i.
- Digital slit-lamp i.
- Drystar dry i.
- flat-panel megavoltage i.
- GE Advantage i.
- GE EchoSpeed whole-body MR i.
- GE Signa Genesis MR i.
- GE Signa 5.4 Genesis MR i.
- GE Signa Horizon EchoSpeed MR i.
- GE Signa 5.5 Horizon EchoSpeed MR i.
- GE SPECT i.
- Hewlett-Packard color flow i.
- high-resolution brain SPECT i.
- Humphrey retinal i.
- I. II angiographic catheter
- Integris V3000 i.
- iris III i.
- Kodak Digital Science 1200, 3600 distributed medical i.
- Kodak Digital Science 1200, 3600 medical i.
- laser i.
- Lorad digital breast i.
- Magnes 2500 WH i.
- Magnetom SP MRI i.
- NeuroScan 3D i.

- peripheral instantaneous x-ray i. (PIXI)
- Photoshop 6.0 digitized i.
- Signa i.
- Sonata i.
- Sonos 2000, 5500 ultrasound i.
- tesla magnetic resonance i.
- tesla Signa magnetic resonance i.
- tesla Signa MR i.
- I. Torque selective catheter
- Voxar Plug n View 3D i.

imager/spectrometer
- Signa whole-body i./s.
- Signa whole body i./s.

ImageView system
imaging
- i. compatible stereotactic coordinate frame
- i. densitometer
- i. headband
- interventional magnetic resonance i. (iMRI)
- magnetic resonance i. (MRI)

Imagyn
- I. microlaparoscope
- I. surgical stapler

Imatron
- I. C-100 EBT scanner
- I. C-150L EBCT scanner
- I. CT bone mineral phantom
- I. CT scanner
- I. C-100 Ultrafast CT scanner
- I. C-150XL CT scanner
- I. C-100XP CT scanner
- I. Fastrac C-100 cine x-ray CT scanner
- I. system
- I. Ultrafast CT scanner

imbedded microtransducer
IMC
- intramedullary collar

Imed
- I. 430 enteral feeding pump
- I. Gemini PC-2 volumetric controller
- I. Gemini PC-2 volumetric pump
- I. infusion device
- I. infusion pump

Imelab vascular diagnostic system
Imex
- I. antepartum monitor
- I. Pocket-Dop OB Doppler
- I. scleral implant
- I. StethoDop

Imexdop CT Doppler
Immage
- I. Anti-DNaseB
- I. immunochemistry system

ImmEdge pen

immediate
- I. Implant Impression system
- I. Impression implant
- I. Load implant
- i. load prosthesis
- i. postoperative prosthesis
- i. response mobile analysis blood analysis system
- i. response mobile analyzer (IRMA)

immediately detachable coil
immersion bath
immobilization jacket
immobilizer
- Angle-Iron skull i.
- ankle i.
- AP-PA skull i.
- arm and shoulder i.
- cast i.
- Comfort wrist i.
- cross-table leg i.
- DonJoy Ultrasling shoulder i.
- dual leg i.
- external i.
- Ezy Wrap shoulder i.
- Hook hemi-harness shoulder i.
- joint i.
- Kapp Surgical Instrument surgical knee i.
- knee i.
- Kuz-Medics disposable knee i.
- long leg i.
- molded i.
- Olympic Neostraint i.
- Pedi-Wrap i.
- Pigg-O-Stat mechanical i.
- postoperative i.
- QuickCast wrist i.
- sheet i.
- shoulder abduction i.
- single-panel knee i.
- sling i.
- Slingshot shoulder i.
- Sta-Block head i.
- sternal occipital mandibular i. (SOMI)
- sternal-occipital-manubrial i.
- straight-leg i.
- Tab-Strap knee i.
- tomographic skull i.
- Trimline knee i.
- tri-panel knee i.
- Universal sling and swathe shoulder i.
- universal tri-panel knee i.
- Vac-Lok bag i.
- Velcro i.
- Velcro strap i.
- Velpeau shoulder i.

- waist i.
- Watco knee i.
- Y-strap knee i.
- Zimmer knee i.
- Zinco thumb-wrist i.

immobilizing vest
Immulite
- I. 2000 anti-HBc IgM analyzer
- I. 2000 anti-HBs analyzer
- I. 2000 chemiluminescent analyzer
- I. Dynamic Duo analyzer
- I. 2000 HBsAg immunoanalyzer
- I. HBsAg immunoassay analyzer
- I. 1000, 2000, 2500 immunoassay system
- I. 2500 SMS immunoassay system

immunoadsorption column
immunoanalyzer
- Elecsys 1010, 2010 i.
- Elecsys 1010 and 2010 i.
- Immulite 2000 HBsAg i.

immunoassay reagent
Immuno-Brite Fluorospheres
ImmunoCyt cytopathology recurrent bladder cancer test
immunocytometer
ImmunoDip urinary albumin test
ImmunoDOT Mono G, M test kit
immunofluorescent assay kit
immunoglobulin
- i. A (IgA)
- i. M (IgM)

immunomagnetic bead
Immunomedics system
Immuno-mini NJ-2300 microplate reader
Immunomount
immunonephelometer
ImmunoPrep reagent system
immunostain
- Dako hepatocyte i.

immunostainer
- Shandon Cadenza i.
- TechMate 1000 i.
- Ventana automated i.
- Ventana NexES i.
- Ventana TechMate i.

Immunotech
- I. immunoassay component
- I. immunoassay kit

Immuno-trol cell
immunoturbidimetry analyzer
IMP
- IMP bone screw targeter
- IMP knee-positioning triangle
- IMP Steri-Clamp
- IMP surgical leg pedestal
- IMP turnstile casting stand
- IMP Universal lateral positioner

impact
- i. glove
- I. lithotriptor system
- i. mitt
- I. modular porous prosthesis
- I. modular total hip system
- I. on-site drug and alcohol test system
- I. total hip prosthesis
- I. Uni-Vent ventilator

impactor
- Andersen Cascade i.
- Cascade i.
- Cloward bone graft i.
- Cohort spinal i.
- Dawson-Yuhl i.
- electromechanical i.
- femoral i.
- hook i.
- humeral i.
- Judet i. for acetabular cup
- Küntscher i.
- lateral gutter i.
- orthopaedic i.
- i. plate
- i. rod
- rotating air i.
- rotating arm i.
- shell i.
- Smith-Petersen i.
- spondylophyte i.
- vertebral body i.

impactor-extractor
- Fox i.-e.

Impax PACS system
IMP-Capello arm support
impedance
- i. electrode
- i. monitor
- i. phlebograph
- i. threshold valve

impeller basket catheter
impermeable dressing
impervious
- i. sheet
- i. stockinette
- i. U sheet

impingement rod
ImplaMed
- I. gold screw
- I. implant system

implant
- absorbable i.
- accessory cyc i.
- accommodative i.
- accordion i.
- acrylic ball eye i.
- acrylic hydroxyapatite i.
- Acufex-Suretac i.

Acu-Form flexible rod i.
adjustable breast i.
Advent i.
Aequalis humeral head i.
alar-columellar i.
Allen eye i.
Allen orbital i.
AllHear cochlear i.
Alpha I penile i.
alumina i.
aluminum oxide i.
anatomical Tobin malar prosthetic i.
anchor endosteal i.
angle i.
anophthalmic i.
Arenberg-Denver inner-ear valve i.
Arnett LeFort i.
Arroyo i.
Arruga i.
Arruga-Moura-Brazil orbital i.
artificial iris i.
artificial iris diaphragm i.
artificial joint i.
Ascension MCP finger joint i.
Ascension MCP total joint i.
Ashworth-Blatt i.
aspheric i.
Astra Tech dental i.
auditory brainstem i. (ABI)
Avanta i.
Avanta soft skeletal i.
Avanta uHead ulnar head i.
Baerveldt glaucoma i.
Baerveldt glaucoma drainage i.
Baerveldt seton i.
Baha osseointegrated bone conduction i.
BAK/C cervical interbody fusion i.
BAK/Proximity interbody fusion i.
Bankart tack i.
Bannon-Klein i.
Bard i.
Barkan infant i.
Barraquer i.
bent reform i.
Berens conical i.
Berens pyramidal i.
Berens-Rosa scleral i.
Bicon dental i.
bifocal eye i.
bilumen mammary i.
Binder submalar i.
Binkhorst collar stud lens i.
Binkhorst 2-loop intraocular lens i.
Binkhorst 4-loop iris-fixated i.
BioAction great toe i.
bioactive i.
Biocare dental i.

implant *(continued)*
Biocell anatomical reconstructive
mammary i.
Biocell RTV i.
Biocell RTV breast i.
Biocell smooth surface i.
Biocell textured shell surface i.
bioceramic i.
Bioceram 2-stage series II
endosteal dental i.
Biocoral i.
BioCuff bioresorbable screw and
spiked washer i.
BioCuff C bioresorbable cannulated
screw and spike washer i.
BioCuff C bioresorbable spike
washer i.
BioCurve saline-filled breast i.
biodegradable i.
Biodel i.
BioDIMENSIONAL saline-filled i.
Bio-Eye hydroxyapatite ocular i.
Biofix biodegradable i.
Biomatrix ocular i.
Biomet custom i.
Bionic eye microdetector
subretinal i.
bioresorbable i.
BioSorb FX dental i.
BioSphere suture anchor i.
BioStinger absorbable meniscal i.
Bio-Vent i.
bivalve nasal splint i.
blade-form i.
Blair-Brown i.
i. blank
Boberg-Ans lens i.
Bosker transmandibular i.
bovine collagen i.
Boyd orbital i.
BrachySeed Pd-103 i.
Brånemark endosteal i.
Brånemark osseointegration i.
Brawner orbital i.
breast i.
Brink PeriPyriform i.
build-up i.
Bunker i.
Calcitek i.
calcium phosphate ceramic i.
carbon i.
carpal lunate i.
Carrion-Small penile i.
cartilage i.
cartilaginous dorsal i.
Castroviejo acrylic i.
ceramic i.
ceramic endosteal i.
CeraOne abutment i.

Charnley i.
chin i.
Choyce Mark VIII i.
chromium-cobalt alloy i.
ciliary neurotrophic factor capsule
protein eye i.
Clarion hearing i.
Clarion multistrategy cochlear i.
cobalt-chrome alloy and
polyethylene i.
cobalt-chromium i.
cobalt-chromium-molybdenum alloy
metal i.
cobalt-chromium-tungsten-nickel
alloy metal i.
Coburn anterior chamber intraocular
lens i.
cochlear i.
Cogan-Boberg-Ans lens i.
cohesive anatomic silicone gel
breast i.
collagen i.
i. collar
columellar i.
Combi 40 cochlear i.
Complete i.
Concorde lumbar i.
condylar i.
conical i.
Contigen Bard collagen i.
Continuum knee system i.
Contour Profile Natural saline
breast i.
Contour Profile silicone breast i.
contraceptive i.
conventional shell i.
Coonrad-Morrey i.
Cooper i.
Copeland i.
Copeland intraocular lens i.
Corail HA-coated stem hip i.
Core-Vent i.
corneal i.
Corning i.
corrected cosmetic contact shell
eye i.
COR/T i.
cosmetic contact shell i.
CosmoDerm 1, 2 human-based
collagen i.
CosmoPlast human-based collagen i.
Cox-Uphoff i.
CrystaLens model AT-45 i.
C-Stem triple taper stabilized
hip i.
CT-based CAD/CAM revision
femoral i.
CTNF capsule protein eye i.
curvilinear chin i.

Custodis i.
custom-contoured i.
Cutler i.
Cutter i.
cylinder-type i.
3D Accuscan facial i.
Dacron i.
Dacron-backed i.
Dannheim eye i.
DeBakey i.
defibrillator i.
Deflux injectable i.
Deflux system i.
45-degree bent reform i.
dental i.
DePuy C-Stem triple taper
 stabilized hip i.
Dermostat i.
Doherty sphere i.
dorsal columellar i.
dorsal column stimulator i.
double-lumen i.
double-lumen breast i.
double-plate Molteno i.
double-stem silicone lesser MP i.
Dow Corning i.
D-shaped i.
dual-compartment gel-inflatable
 mammary i.
Duracon knee i.
Dura-II concealable penile i.
dural i.
Durallium i.
Durapatite i.
Duros leuprolide i.
Dynaflex penile i.
Edwards Teflon intracardiac i.
i. elastomer shell
electrical i.
endodontic endosteal i.
Endopore i.
endosseous dental i.
endosseous HA i.
endosseous hydroxyapatite i.
Endotine TransBleph i.
Envision TD i.
Envision TD intravitreal i.
epilepsy i.
Epoca RH humeral resurfacing
 head i.
Epstein collar stud acrylic i.
EPTFE i.
esthetic Taylor mandibular angle i.
E-type dental i.
Ewald-Walker knee i.
expandable breast i.
expanded polytetrafluoroethylene i.
expanded polytetrafluoroethylene
 SoftForm facial i.

expansible infrastructure endosteal i.
Extend absorbable synthetic
 punctal i.
extended anatomical high-profile
 malar i.
extraoral bone-anchored i.
eye spherical i.
facial i.
fascia lata i.
feathered extended malar i.
fenestra i.
Ferguson i.
Fibrel gelatin matrix i.
Fine magnetic i.
finger joint i.
Finney penile i.
fixed anatomic patellar i.
fixed bearing knee i.
fixed mandibular i.
flail i.
Flatt i.
Flexblock temporal fossa i.
flexible digital i.
flexible Dualens i.
flexible rod penile i.
flexible silicone i.
Flexi-Flate penile i.
Flexi-Rod II penile i.
Flowers Extended Tear Trough i.
Flowers mandibular i.
Flowers mandibular glove i.
Flowers tear trough i.
FluidVision i.
foldable silicone i.
i. forceps
Fox sphere i.
free i.
freestanding i.
Frey tunneled eye i.
Frialoc transgingival threaded
 dental i.
Friatec i.
front build-up i.
full-dimpled Lucite i.
full-thickness i.
Futura conical subtalar i.
Futura flexible digital i.
Futura metal hemi-toe i.
Future i.
ganciclovir i.
Garcia-Novito eye i.
gel-filled i.
Gelfilm retinal i.
Gemini MKII mobile-bearing
 knee i.
Genesis II mobile-bearing knee i.
gentamicin i.
Geo Rectangles spinal i.
Geristore dental i.

implant *(continued)*

Glasgold Wafer chin i.
glass sphere i.
glass sphere eye i.
Gliadel i.
Global total shoulder i.
gold biocompatible i.
Goldenberg hydroxylapatite i.
gold eyelid i.
gold eyelid load i.
Gold-Mules eye i.
gonioscopic i.
Gore-Tex nasal i.
Gore-Tex SAM facial i.
Gore-Tex vascular i.
Gott i.
great toe i.
grooved silicone i.
HA-coated hip i.
HA-coated Micro-Vent i.
HA-coated root-form dental i.
haptic area i.
hard tissue replacement malleable facial i.
hard tissue replacement patient-matched i.
Harris i.
Harris Design-2 i.
Harrison i.
HealosMP52 i.
heat-vulcanized silicone elastomer i.
Hedrocel proximal tibia augmentation i.
helicoid endosteal i.
hemi-interpositional i.
Herrick silicone lacrimal i.
heterograft i.
hex i.
Heyer-Schulte breast i.
Heyer-Schulte rhinoplasty i.
i. hinge
hinged i.
histrelin i.
Hoffmann eye i.
hollow-sphere i.
homograft i.
hook-type i.
hook-type eye i.
House i.
Howmedica Duracon i.
Howmedica monospherical i.
Hruby i.
Hruby contact i.
HTR-MFI chin i.
HTR-MFI curved i.
HTR-MFI malar i.
HTR-MFI paranasal i.
HTR-MFI premaxillary i.
HTR-MFI ramus i.

Hufnagel i.
Hughes i.
Hughes eye i.
Hunter open cord tendon i.
hyaline cartilage i.
Hydroflex penile i.
hydrophilic hydrogel i.
hydroxyapatite ceramic i.
hydroxyapatite-coated i.
hydroxyapatite ocular i.
hydroxyapatite orbital i.
hydroxyapatite spherical enucleation i.
hydroxyapatite threaded hexlock i.
hydroxyethyl methacrylate i.
HyProCure sinus tarsi i.
3i i.
3i dental i.
iliosacral i.
Imex scleral i.
Immediate Impression i.
Immediate Load i.
Implantech Binder i.
Implantech facial i.
Implantech Flowers i.
Implantech Mittelman i.
Implantech Terino i.
Imtec premounted threaded i.
IMZ i.
I. Innovations titanium screw
Insall-Burstein intracondylar total knee i.
Insall-Burstein total knee i.
Intacs corneal ring i.
Integral Omniloc i.
Interax Integrated Secure Asymmetric mobile-bearing knee i.
Intermedics intraocular lens i.
Interpore i.
Interpore osteointegrated i.
interstitial i.
intracochlear i.
intracorneal i.
intraocular i.
intraorbital i.
intravitreal bioerodible dexamethasone i.
Iowa orbital i.
ITI dental i.
ITI type-F endosseous i.
Ivalon sponge i.
Ivalon sponge eye i.
joint i.
Jonas i.
Jordan eye i.
Joseph valve i.
K i.
Kalix flatfoot i.

keratolens i.
Kimba disc i.
Kinetik great toe i.
Kinetikos joint i.
King orbital i.
Koenig total great toe i.
Koeppe intraocular lens i.
KPS bipolar vitallium-
 polyethylene i.
Kratz i.
Krause-Wolfe i.
Krupin-Denver eye valve-to-disc i.
Lacey total knee i.
LaminOss i.
LaPorta great toe i.
large-pore polyethylene i.
Lash-Loeffler i.
Lawrence first metatarsophalangeal
 joint i.
LCS total knee system i.
Lemoine orbital i.
lens i.
leuprolide acetate i.
Levitt i.
levonorgestrel rod i.
Lifecath peritoneal i.
Lifecore Restore wide-diameter i.
Lincoff scleral sponge i.
Linkow blade i.
Little intraocular lens i.
Liverpool elbow i.
4-loop iris clip i.
4-loop iris fixated i.
Lovac fundal contact lens i.
Lovac 6-mirror gonioscopic lens i.
low bleed i.
low-profile breast i.
LT Mesh i.
Lucite sphere i.
Luhr i.
lumbar anterior root stimulator i.
lunate i.
Macroplastique i.
MacroSorb absorbable plate i.
Maestro i.
i. magnet
magnetic i.
magnetic eye i.
malar i.
malleable i.
malleable facial i.
mammary i.
Mark III TiUnite i.
Marlex mesh i.
i. material
maxillary lateral incisor i.
Maximus dental i.
McCannel i.
McCutchen hip i.

McGhan Biocell anatomical
 breast i.
McGhan eye i.
McGhan facial i.
McGhan smooth saline i.
Medallion intraocular lens i.
MedDev gold eyelid i.
Medical Electronic cochlear i.
Medical Optics eye i.
Medical Optics intraocular lens i.
Medical Optics PC11NB intraocular
 lens i.
Medical Workshop intraocular
 lens i.
Medpor biomaterial i.
Medpor facial i.
Medpor Flexblock i.
Medpor malar i.
Medpor MCOI i.
Medpor reconstructive i.
Medpor surgical i.
Meme i.
Meme mammary i.
Meniscus Arrow i.
Mentor 1600 i.
Mentor H/S Siltex i.
Mentor malleable semirigid
 penile i.
meridional i.
Mersilene i.
meshed ball i.
mesostructure i.
metacarpophalangeal i.
metal-backed acetabular component
 hip i.
metal hemi-toe i.
metal orthopaedic i.
Metasul hip i.
methylmethacrylate i.
methyl methacrylate bead i.
methyl methacrylate eye i.
Microloc knee i.
Micro-Lok dental i.
Micro-Vent i.
Micro-Vent^2 i.
middle ear i.
Mini-Matic i.
Miragel i.
Mittelman i.
3M mammary i.
mobile bearing knee i.
modular i.
Molteno double-plate i.
Molteno drainage eye i.
motility eye i.
MSI i.
Mueller shield eye i.
Mules i.
Mules eye i.

implant *(continued)*
    multichannel cochlear i.
    multifocal i.
    narrow neck i.
    nasal dorsal i.
    Natural-Knee i.
    needle endosteal i.
    Neer II total shoulder system i.
    NeuFlex metacarpophalangeal
      joint i.
    NewIris ocular i.
    NexGen knee i.
    Nexus i.
    Niebauer i.
    Niebauer-Cutter i.
    Nobel Biocare i.
    NobelPerfect dental i.
    Nobelpharma i.
    Novagold mammary i.
    NovaSaline prefilled breast i.
    Nucleus 22 cochlear i.
    Nucleus 24 Contour cochlear i.
    Nucleus 24 multichannel auditory
      brainstem i.
    Nucleus multichannel cochlear i.
    Octa-Hex i.
    Oculo-Plastik ePTFE ocular i.
    O'Malley self-adhering lens i.
    Omniloc dental i.
    onlay i.
    OP-1 i.
    Ophtec occlusion i.
    OP-1 putty spinal fusion i.
    optic i.
    OP-1 TM bone i.
    oral i.
    orbital i.
    orbital floor i.
    Organon percutaneous E2 i.
    orthobiologic i.
    osseointegrated dental i.
    osseointegrated oral i.
    Osseotite 2-stage procedure i.
    osseous i.
    osteochondral i.
    Osteonics HA femoral i.
    Osteoplate i.
    Oxinium hip i.
    Padgett i.
    palatal i.
    paraffin i.
    Paragon Complete i.
    Partnership i.
    patch i.
    patella resurfacing i.
    patient-matched i.
    peanut i.
    pectoralis muscle i.
    pedicle i.

    penile i.
    percutaneous dorsal column
      stimulator i.
    periarticular reduction i. (PE.R.I)
    perichondrial i.
    periosteal i.
    Periotest i.
    PhacoFlex II foldable intraocular
      lens i.
    2-piece dental i.
    piggyback i.
    PIIP hydrogel breast i.
    pin i.
    Pisces i.
    planar I mesh i.
    planoconvex eye i.
    plastic sphere i.
    plastic sphere eye i.
    platform i.
    platinum eyelid i.
    Plexiglas i.
    PMMA i.
    polyethylene i.
    polyethylene sphere i.
    polyglycolide i.
    polylactide i.
    polymer tooth replica i.
    polymethylmethacrylate i.
    Polypin biodegradable pin i.
    Polystan i.
    polytetrafluoroethylene i.
    polyurethane-coated silicone
      breast i.
    polyvinyl sponge i.
    Porex i.
    Porex Medpor i.
    porous i.
    porous-coated i.
    porous orbital i.
    porous polyethylene i.
    porous tantalum i.
    posterior chamber lens i.
    Precision Cosmet intraocular lens i.
    press-fit i.
    processed carbon i.
    Prodisc-C cervical artificial disc i.
    Profix mobile-bearing knee i.
    ProOsteon synthetic bone i.
    Proplast I, II i.
    Proplast preformed facial i.
    Proplast-Teflon disc i.
    protein eye i.
    pseudophake i.
    PTFE i.
    PTFE-containing i.
    pyrocarbon i.
    PyroHemiSphere joint i.
    radiocarpal i.
    ramus blade i.

ramus endosteal i.
Rapid Strand i.
RBM i.
reduced-height i.
reform eye i.
refractive floating i.
refractive phakic i.
Replace system tapered i.
Restore bone i.
Restore cuff tear i.
Restore dental i.
Restore orthobiologic soft-tissue i.
Restore RBM i.
Restore soft tissue i.
Restore threaded i.
ReSTOR vision i.
Retisert intravitreal i.
reverse-shape i.
rHead Recon i.
Ridley anterior chamber lens i.
Ridley Mark II lens i.
Rizzo dorsal i.
Rodin orbital i.
root-form dental i.
Rotaglide knee i.
rotating patellar i.
RZ extended chin i.
RZ jowl i.
saline-filled anatomical breast i.
saline-filled round breast i.
SAM facial i.
Sargon i.
Schocket tube i.
Schuring ossicular i.
Schwaber otologic i.
scleral i.
scleral buckle eye i.
scleral buckler i.
screw-type i.
Screw-Vent i.
Seeburger i.
seed i.
self-aligning mobile-bearing knee i.
self-tapping screw-type i.
semishell i.
Septopal i.
Severin i.
Sgarlato hammertoe i.
Sgarlato toe i.
Shaw-SHIP rod hammertoe i.
Shearing posterior chamber
  intraocular lens i.
shelf-type i.
i. shell
shell i.
shell eye i.
Shepard intraocular lens i.
Ship-Shaw rod hammertoe i.
Shirakabe i.

silastic chin i.
silastic midfacial malar i.
silastic penile i.
silastic scleral buckler i.
silastic silicone rubber i.
silastic subdermal i.
silastic testicular i.
silastic toe i.
Silhouette IC i.
Silhouette Laser-Lok i.
silicone buckling i.
silicone button eye i.
silicone elastomer rubber ball i.
silicone elastomer suspension i.
silicone-filled anatomical breast i.
silicone-filled mammary i.
silicone-filled round breast i.
silicone gel breast i.
silicone MP i.
silicone nasal strut i.
silicone pad eye i.
silicone rod i.
silicone sleeve eye i.
silicone sponge i.
silicone strip eye i.
silicone textured mammary i.
silicone tire eye i.
Silimed i.
Siloxane i.
Siltex breast i.
Siltex mammary i.
Simaplast i.
Simcoe intraocular lens i.
simple button patellar i.
single-channel cochlear i.
single-stage screw i.
single-stage Straumann dental i.
single-tooth subperiosteal i.
Sinskey lens i.
Sinterlock i.
i. site dilator
sizing i.
i. sleeve
sleeve i.
Small-Carrion silastic rod for
  penile i.
Smith orbital floor i.
smooth staple i.
Snellen conventional reform i.
Snellen conventional reform eye i.
SoftForm collagen facial i.
SoftForm facial i.
solid silicone buttock i.
solid silicone with Supramid
  mesh i.
Soundtec Direct system i.
Spectra-System i.
Spectrum Designs facial i.
Spectrum Designs Medical facial i.

implant (*continued*)

sphere i.
spherical i.
spherical eye i.
Sphero Flex i.
spike washer i.
spiral endosteal i.
Spline Twist microtextured
    titanium i.
Spline Twist MTX i.
Spline Twist Ti i.
split-thickness i.
i. sponge
sponge i.
stainless steel i.
standard i.
StarLock multi-purpose submergible
    threaded i.
StarLock press-fit cylinder i.
Star/Vent 1-stage dental screw i.
StayFuse i.
Steri-Oss dental i.
Steri-Oss endosteal dental i.
Steri-Oss Hexlock i.
ST Mesh i.
Straumann Standard Plus i.
subdermal i.
submucosal i.
subperiosteal i.
subtalar MBA i.
I. Support Systems titanium screw
SupraFOIL i.
Supramid i.
Supramid-Allen i.
surface i.
surface eye i.
Surgibone i.
Surgitek mammary i.
Sustain HA-coated screw i.
Sutter i.
Sutter hinged great toe i.
SutureGroove gold eye weight i.
Swanson carpal lunate i.
Swanson carpal scaphoid i.
Swanson finger joint i.
Swanson great toe i.
Swanson metacarpophalangeal i.
Swanson radial head i.
Swanson silastic i.
Swanson small joint i.
Swanson trapezium i.
Swanson wrist joint i.
Swede-Vent TL self-tapping
    external hex i.
SwissPlus 1-stage i.
Syed-Neblett i.
Syed template i.
SynerGraft i.
synthetic i.

synthetic bone i.
tantalum mesh i.
tantalum mesh eye i.
tapered Micro-Vent i.
Taper-Lock external hex i.
tear trough-style i.
Techmedica i.
I. Technology LSF prosthesis
Teflon i.
Teflon mesh i.
Teflon orbital floor i.
Teflon-Proplast TMJ i.
Tegress endoscopic urethral i.
tendon i.
Tennant i.
Tensilon i.
Terino i.
Terino anatomical chin i.
testicular i.
Tevdek i.
TG Osseotite single-stage
    procedure i.
TheraSeed i.
The Wedge bioresorbable
    interference fit i.
The Wedge bioresorbable
    interference-fit i.
thick-walled Dacron-backed i.
ThinProfile eyelid i.
ThreadLoc i.
TiMesh patient configured titanium
    craniomaxillofacial i.
TiOblast dental i.
i. tire
tire i.
TissueTak corkscrew i.
titanium alloy i.
titanium plasma sprayed dental i.
titanium-sprayed IMZ i.
titanium vocal fold medialization i.
TiUnite dental i.
TMI i.
tobramycin-impregnated PMMA i.
total knee i.
total ossicular reconstruction i.
Townley i.
Trac II knee i.
TransBleph i.
transmandibular i.
transosseous i.
transosteal pin i.
trapezium i.
trial i.
Trilucent breast i.
triple-lumen i.
Troutman i.
Troutman eye i.
TruBlock BGS block i.
TruFit BGS plug i.

T-type dental i.
tunneled i.
tunneled eye i.
Twist MTX i.
Twist Ti i.
uHead ulnar head i.
Ultex lens i.
UltraFix RC i.
UltraFix rotator cuff repair i.
ultrasmall incision i.
unicompartmental knee i.
Unilab Surgibone surgical i.
Uniplant contraceptive i.
Unipost i.
Universal i.
unpegged hydroxyapatite i.
ureteral i.
Uribe orbital i.
U-type dental i.
Varilux lens i.
vent-plate i.
Viadur i.
vitallium i.
vitallium eye i.
Vitek interpositional i.
Vitrasert i.
Vitrasert intraocular i.
Vitrasert intravitreal i.
Walter Reed i.
Weber hip i.
Weck-cel i.
Weil i.
Weil modified Swanson i.
Weil-type Swanson-design
  hammertoe i.
Wheeler eye sphere i.
wire mesh i.
wire mesh eye i.
Wolf i.
Wölfe-Krause i.
Wright monoblock titanium i.
Zang metatarsal cap i.
Zeichner i.
Zest i.
Zest subperiosteal i.
Zoladex i.
Zyderm collagen i. (ZCI)
zygomaticus i.
Zymderm collagen i.
Zyplast collagen i.

implantable
i. access catheter
i. artificial heart
i. atrial defibrillator (IAD)
i. automatic cardioverter-defibrillator
i. bone anchor
i. bone anchor device
i. cardioverter-defibrillator (ICD)
i. cardioverter-defibrillator catheter

i. collamer lens
i. contact lens
i. defibrillator
i. gastric stimulator
i. glucose sensor
i. infusion port
i. internal system
i. intraperitoneal pump
i. middle ear hearing device
i. miniature telescope
i. miniaturized telescope
i. neural stimulator
i. neuromodulation system
i. osmotic pump
i. pacemaker
i. pronged unipolar electrode
i. pulse generator
i. silicone microballoon
i. unipolar endocardial electrode
i. vascular access device (IVAD)
i. venous access device

implantation
collared press-fit femoral stem i.
i. forceps
noncollared press-fit femoral
  stem i.

implant-borne prosthesis
Implantech
I. Binder implant
I. facial implant
I. Flowers implant
I. Mittelman implant
I. SE-100 smoke aspiration tip
I. Terino implant

implanted
i. infusion pump
i. NCP
i. pacemaker

implanter
Wallner interstitial prostate i.

implant-retained denture
implant-supported
i.-s. fixed prosthesis
i.-s. overdenture

Implast
I. bone cement
I. bone cement adhesive

Implatome dental tomography system
Import
I. vascular access port
I. vascular access port with Bio-
  Glide

impotence
Esteem advanced vacuum therapy
  for i.

Impra
I. Carboflo ePTFE vascular graft
I. CenterFlex graft

Impra *(continued)*
  I. collagen-impregnated Dacron
    prosthesis
  I. Distaflo bypass graft
  I. Flex vascular graft
  I. graft
  I. microporous PTFE vascular graft
  I. peritoneal catheter
  I. Venaflo vascular graft
impregnated
  i. dressing
  i. electrode
  i. vaginal packing
Impregum impression material
Impress
  I. Softpatch
  I. Softpatch urinary pad
impression
  i. material syringe
  I. mattress
  i. tonometer
ImPressure ultrasound pressure sensor
imprinter
  foot i.
impulse
  I. angiographic catheter
  I. diagnostic catheter
  i. inertial exercise trainer
**ImPulse electronic oxygen-conserving
  device**
IMR
  ischemic mitral ring
iMRI
  interventional magnetic resonance
    imaging
    PoleStar N-10 iMRI
Imtec
  I. BioBarrier membrane
  I. premounted threaded implant
IMx
  IMx analyzer
  IMx PSA system
IMZ
  IMZ implant
  IMZ implant system
in
  In Charge diabetes control system
  in situ tricortical iliac crest block
    bone graft
  in situ valve-cutter kit
  in situ valve scissors
  in vitro fertilization micropipette
4-in-1
  4-i.-1 cutting block
  4-i.-1 positioning block system
inactive electrode
Inamura
  I. race chopper

  I. small incision capsulorrhexis
    forceps
inanimate simulator
In-Bed AFO boot
INC
  inside-the-needle catheter
Inc.
  Kinetic Muscles, I. (KMI)
incandescent
  i. endoscope lamp
  i. lamp
  i. sheath
Incardia valve system
InCare
  I. brace
  I. pelvic floor therapy office
    system
  I. PRES 9300 system
INCA system
Incavo wire passer
incentive spirometer
In-Ceram
  I.-C. Alumina bonding
  I.-C. Alumina dental bonding
    material
  I.-C. Cerestore bonding
  I.-C. Cerestore dental bonding
    material
  I.-C. Dicor dental bonding material
  I.-C. Empress bonding
  I.-C. Empress dental bonding
    material
  I.-C. Fortress bonding
  I.-C. Optec bonding
  I.-C. Optic dental bonding material
  I.-C. Spinell bonding
  I.-C. Spinell dental bonding
    material
incident command system
Incise
  I. drape
  I. pouch
incision
  i. aligner
  i. dilator
  i. knife
  i. retractor
  i. spreader
  i. viewing instrument
Incisor arthroscopic blade
inclinometer
  Baseline Bubble i.
  Dualer Plus i.
InCompass
  I. thoracolumbar fixation system
  I. thoracolumbar spine fixation
    screw
incontinence clamp

incubator
  BOD i.
  double-insulated i.
  double-walled i.
  Forma water-jacketed i.
  Ohmeda Care-Plus i.
  Sagian 180 CO2 i.
incudostapedial joint knife
incus replacement prosthesis
Indeflator
  ACS I.
  I. Plus 20
indentation tonometer
indenter
  diamond pyramid i.
in-department film
independent jaw
in-depth shoe
Indermil tissue adhesive
index
  I. Knobber II massage tool
  I. prosthesis
  volume thickness i. (VTI)
indexed splint
INdGO disposable manual resuscitator
Indiana
  I. Tome carpal tunnel release
    system
  I. Tome carpal tunnel syndrome
    release system
  I. Tome clip
  I. Tome knife
  I. urinary pouch
Indian club needle
India rubber suture
indicator
  AccuAngle i.
  Berens-Tolman ocular
    hypertension i.
  finger i.
  fundamental frequency i.
  gamma ray level i.
  i. paper
  SPI-Lite sleep position i.
  xylol pulse i.
indifferent electrode
Indigo
  I. diffuse fiber
  I. LaserOptic treatment system
  I. Optima laser
  I. Optima laser system
indirect
  i. calorimetry
  i. laser ophthalmoscope
  i. ophthalmoscope
  i. retainer
individual protective equipment
Indomitable scanner

InDuct
  I. breast aspirator
  I. breast microcatheter
inductive coupling device
InductOs collagen sponge
InDuo system
InDura intrathecal catheter and pump
industrial
  i. eye protector
  i. spectacles
Industrial Work brace
indwelling
  i. cannula
  i. catheter
  i. Foley catheter
  i. nonvascular shunt
  i. stent
  i. subclavian catheter
  i. transcutaneous vascular access
    device (ITVAD)
  i. ureteral stent
  i. venous catheter
Inerpan flexible burn dressing
inert allograft biomaterial
inertial suction sampler
In-Exsufflator respiratory device
InfaMyst aerosol spray device
infant
  i. abdominal retractor
  i. abduction splint
  i. airflow and effort sensor
  i. Ambu resuscitator
  i. biopsy forceps
  i. bronchoscope
  i. dilator
  i. esophagoscope
  i. eyelid retractor
  i. female catheter
  I. Flow nCPAP system
  I. Flow noninvasive nasal CPAP
    system
  i. Karickhoff laser lens
  i. male catheter
  i. 3-mirror laser lens
  i. nasal cannula assembly
  i. passive mitt
  i. resuscitation system
  i. rib retractor
  i. rib shears
  I. Star high-frequency ventilator
  i. Star high-frequency ventilator
  I. Star 8000 oscillator
  I. Star ventilator
  i. telescope
  i. urethrotome
  i. urethrotome blade
  i. ventilation monitor
infantometer
  Measure Mat i.

In-Fast bone screw system
infection-prevention device
inferior
 i. mesenteric artery retractor
 i. vena cava catheter
 i. vena cava clip
 i. vena cava umbrella filter
inferoposterior acetabular capsule retractor
infiltration cannula
infiltrator
 Byron i.
 Klein i.
 I. local drug delivery device
 showerhead i.
Infinia Hawkeye nuclear medicine system
Infinitech laser probe
Infiniti
 I. catheter
 I. catheter introducer system
Infinity
 I. hip system
 I. modular hip prosthesis
 I. sensor
Infinix
 I. DP-i vascular x-ray
 I. NB-i vascular x-ray
 I. VC-i vascular x-ray
InFix interbody fusion system
inflatable
 i. ball pessary
 i. bone tamp (IBT)
 i. elbow splint
 i. Foley bag catheter
 i. mammary prosthesis
 i. Mentor penile prosthesis
 i. thoracic lumbosacral orthosis
 i. tourniquet cuff
 i. tracheal tube cuff
inflated
 i. balloon
 i. rubber cylinder
inflator
 LeVeen i.
 rapid cuff i.
InflatoRing
inflow cannula
influenza test
infrapatellar strap
infrared
 i. applicator
 i. camera
 i. coagulator
 i. digitizer
 i. laser Doppler flowmeter
 i. light-reflecting sphere
 i. liver scanner
 i. optometer

 i. ray photocoagulator
 i. thermometer
 i. videoendoscope
infrared-beam diode laser
Infratonic QGM
infratympanic catheter
Infravision imaging system
Infumed pump
infundibular
 i. forceps
 i. punch
Infusaid
 I. catheter
 I. Infuse-a-Port
 I. infusion pump
 I. needle
 I. pump
InfusaSleeve
 I. II catheter
 Kaplan-Simpson I.
 LocalMed I.
InFuse
 I. bone graft
 I. bone graft/LT-Cage lumbar tapered fusion device
Infuse-A-Cath catheter
Infuse-a-Port
 I.-a.-P. catheter
 Infusaid I.-a.-P.
 I.-a.-P. port
 I.-a.-P. pump
 I.-a.-P. vascular access system
infuser, infusor
 Alton Deal pressure i.
 Baxter i.
 BP Cuff pressure i.
 button i.
 IVAC P4000 i.
 MicroFuse I.
 Ohio pressure i.
 Paragon i.
 PCA i.
 pen pump insulin i.
 single-day i.
 Travenol i.
 UROS i.
Infuset T fluid delivery system
Infusible pressure infusion bag
infusion
 i. cannula
 i. catheter
 i. device
 i. handpiece
 i. light pipe
 i. port
 i. pump
 i. suction vitreous cutter
 i. tube
infusion/infiltration cannula

infusor (*var. of* infuser)
Infu-Surg pressure infuser bag
Inge
> I. laminar spreader
> I. laminectomy retractor
> I. spreader

Ingersoll
> I. adenoid curette
> I. tonsillar needle

Ingold M3, M4 glass electrode pH monitor
Ingram
> I. bicycle seat
> I. catheter
> I. trocar

Inhal-Aid bronchodilator
inhalation
> i. breath unit
> i. cannula

inhalator
inhaler
> Aerodose insulin i.
> AERx i.
> AERx electronic i.
> breath-operated i.
> Chiesi powder i.
> Diskhaler i.
> Diskhaler metered-dose i.
> Diskus i.
> dry powder i.
> Easi-Breathe i.
> FOII powder i.
> handheld aerosol i.
> Inhalet i.
> InspirEase i.
> metered-dose i. (MDI)
> metered solution i.
> Nebuhaler i.
> Orion i.
> pressurized metered-dose i.
> Rondo i.
> Spinhaler i.
> Spiral Mark V portable ultrasonic drug i.
> Turbuhaler i.
> ultrasound i.

Inhalet inhaler
inhibited
> ventricular i. (VVI)
> ventricular inhibited, atrial i. (VVI/AAI)

inhibitor
> vaporizing rust i.

Inion
> I. CPS
> I. GTR biodegradable membrane system
> I. S-1 biodegradable anterior cervical system

initial incision retractor
initiator drill
InjecAid system
Injectate probe
injection
> i. cannula
> i. catheter
> i. electrode catheter
> ERxin multicomponent penile i.
> i. gold probe
> i. needle

injector
> Amplatz i.
> Angiomat Illumena i.
> auto i.
> automatic twin syringe i.
> Bioject jet i.
> Biojector 2000 jet i.
> Cordis i.
> Dermo-Jet high-pressure i.
> double-power i.
> Dyonics syringe i.
> Envision CT power i.
> extractor i.
> EZ-Ject i.
> Geuder i.
> Harris uterine i. (HUI)
> Hercules power i.
> Illumena i.
> Injectron CT2 power i.
> Injex i.
> jet i.
> MadaJet XL needle-free i.
> Mark V Plus automatic i.
> Medi-Jector i.
> Medrad automated power i.
> Medrad contrast medium i.
> Medrad Mark IV angiographic i.
> Medrad power angiographic i.
> Mill-Rose esophageal i.
> Mini-Flex flexible Harris uterine i.
> modified Mark IV R-wave-triggered power i.
> Monarch II i.
> MR-compatible power i.
> Olympus i.
> OptiStat handheld power i.
> plunger-type i.
> power i.
> preloaded i.
> pressure i.
> Pulse-Spray i.
> Renovist II i.
> Royale intraocular lens i.
> SciTojet needle-free i.
> SofPort easy-load i.
> Spectris MR-compatible i.
> Spectris power i.
> Stellant D CT i.

injector *(continued)*
    Stellant Sx CT i.
    Syrijet Mark II needleless i.
    Taveras i.
    Teflon i.
    Tubex i.
    uterine i.
    Viamonte-Hobbs dye i.
    Virag i.
injector-aspirator
    double-barreled i.-a.
Injectron CT2 power injector
InjecTx cystoscope
Injex injector
ink
    China i.
inlay
    setting i.
    Sher diabetic shoe i.
InLay Optima ureteral stent
inlet forceps
in-line
    i.-l. blood gas monitor
    i.-l. probe
    i.-l. venous pressure monitor
inline trap
inner
    i. heel wedge
    I. Lok ankle brace
InnerVasc expandable vascular access system
Innerview GI
Innervision MR scanner
InnerVue diagnostic scope system
Innoboot splint
Innoflex variable-stiffness colonoscope
Innomed
    I. arthroplasty measuring system
    I. Assistant Free surgical instrument
    I. bone curette
Innova
    I. feminine incontinence treatment system
    I. 4100 flat-panel detector
    I. 4100 flat-panel x-ray system
    I. home incontinence therapy system
    I. pelvic floor stimulator
Innovasive
    I. bone anchor
    I. device
Innovation
    I. Sports bracing product
    I. Sports bracing support
Innovative
    I. COR/T implant system
    I. Medical Products Steri-Clamp
Innovatome microkeratome

InnoVit
    I. 1800 probe
    I. vitrectomy probe
inorganic dental cement
Inoue
    I. balloon catheter
    I. endovascular stent-graft
    I. self-guiding balloon
    I. triple-branched stent-graft
INOvent delivery system
InPath cervical cancer screening device
InPouch TV subculture kit
input
    i. device
    I. PS introducer
Inquiry
    I. fixed curve diagnostic catheter
    I. His diagnostic catheter
    I. H steerable diagnostic catheter
InQwire guidewire
INR home anticoagulation blood monitoring system
Inro
    I. surgical nail
    I. surgical nail splint
Insall-Burstein
    I.-B. II modular total knee system
    I.-B. intracondylar total knee implant
    I.-B. knee prosthesis
    I.-B. posterior stabilizer
    I.-B. total knee implant
insemination
    i. dish
    intrauterine i. (IUI)
insert
    AirSep Ultimate nasal seal gel i.
    AliMed i.
    articular i.
    Bidet toilet i.
    clamp i.
    Cookie I.
    custom-made i.
    Durasul polyethylene, high wear resistant acetabular i.
    Energy Plus shoe i.
    EverGrip clamp i.
    FemSoft i.
    FemSoft continence i.
    FemSoft urethral i.
    Fogarty i.
    Gel-Sole shoe i.
    Hapad felt i.
    Hapad shoe i.
    Hollister disposable convex i.
    Intacs prescription i.
    Johnson & Johnson PFC cruciate-substituting i.
    Koala vascular i.

New York University orthotic i.
Orthex Relievers shoe i.
Osteonics Scorpio i.
Poly-Dial i.
polyethylene tibial i.
POWERPoint orthotic shoe i.
Profix confirming tibial i.
Reliance urinary control i.
retainer i.
Roho solid seat i.
soft socket i.
Spenco shoe i.
S-ROM Poly-Dial i.
Sur-Fit Natura disposable convex i.
urinary control urethral i.
viscoelastic heel i.
warm-and-form i.

inserter
AC tube i.
AMO PhacoFlex lens and i.
Buck femoral cement restrictor i.
cement restrictor i.
cement spacer i.
DDT lock screw i.
diaphragm i.
Fine III i.
Kirschner wire i.
Lehner II i.
Lens-Eze i.
Moon-Robinson prosthesis i.
Mport lens i.
Prodigy lens i.
Repose screw i.
screw i.
Shaffner orthopaedic i.
spacer i.
subperiosteal glass bead i.
Texas Scottish Rite Hospital
  hook i.
TSRH hook i.
twist-in drain tube i.
ventilation tube i.

insertion forceps
in-shoe transducer
inside-the-needle
i.-t.-n. catheter (INC)
i.-t.-n. infusion catheter

Insight
I. digital camera
I. knee positioning and alignment
  system

InSIGHT manometry system
Insignia Ultra DR, SR pacing system
InSite Her-2/neu kit
insole
Aliplast i.
Anti-Shox gel i.
Apex i.
Bestfoam i.

biomagnetic i.
Comf-Orthotic 3/4-length i.
Comf-Orthotic sports replacement i.
Comf-Orthotic wool felt i.
Darco moldable i.
Diab-A-Foot rocker i.
Diab-A-Pad i.
Diab-A-Sole flat i.
Diab-A-Sole molded i.
Diabetic Diagnostic i.
D-Soles i.
EMED i.
Ever-Flex i.
Flat Foot i.
FlexiTherm diabetic diagnostic i.
Hapad metatarsal i.
Kinetic Wedge molded i.
magnetic i.
molded postpartum i.
Plastazote i.
Plexidure i.
Poron 400 i.
PPT flat i.
PPT MXL soft molded i.
PPT Plastizote i.
PPT RX firm molded i.
ProThotics i.
PumpPals shoe i.
Reflex Comfort i.
Sherform silicone i.
silicone i.
Sof Airr i.
SofSole Airr i.
Sorbothane i.
Spenco i.
S-Soles i.
TechnoGel i.
Viscoped S i.

Insorb subcuticular skin stapler
Inspec-100
**Inspector large-bore inline hemostasis
  valve**
InSpectra tissue spectrometer
Inspiration ventilator system
inspirator
inspiratory limb
Inspire
Medtronic I.
InspirEase
I. device
I. inhaler
inspirometer
Inspiron
I. incentive spirometer
I. nebulizer
I. small inspiratory training device
**InstaCheck Med+ immunoassay for
  drugs of abuse**
InstaGene Matrix resin

Insta-Mold
    I.-M. ear protection device
    I.-M. silicone ear impression
      material
Insta-Nerve device
instant
    i. cold pack
    I. Fever Tester thermometer
    I. Response technology generator
    i. skin hook
InstantPlus
    Accu-Chek I.
Insta-Pulse heart rate monitor
Insta-Putty silicone earplug
InstaScan scanner
Instat
    I. collagen absorbable hemostat
    I. collagen absorbable hemostatic
      agent
    I. collagen matrix sponge
    I. collagen sponge
    I. MCH microfibrillar collagen
      hemostat
Insta-Temp
    Diatek 9000 I.-T.
InstaTrak ENT image-guidance system
Instead feminine protection cup
InStent
    I. EsophaCoil stent
    I. VascuCoil stent
Instron machine
instrument
    Accu-Line distal femoral
      resection i.
    Accu-Line knee i.
    Accu-Line patellar i.
    Accurate Surgical and
      Scientific I.'s (ASSI)
    AccuSharp carpal tunnel release i.
    Achieve computer-assisted i.
    activating adjusting i. (AAI)
    Acufex arthroscopic i.
    Acufex MosaicPlasty i.
    Advia 60, 120 automated cell
      counting i.
    Alcon Surgical i.
    American Hydron i.
    angular screwing i.
    Arthroforce III hand i.
    Arthrotek Ellipticut hand i.
    Ascon i.
    A13 Sequel programmable behind-
      the-ear hearing i.
    ASSI S&T microsurgical i.
    Atlas orthogonal percussion i.
    Auto Ref-keratometer i.
    Autosuture ProTack i.
    AxyaWeld i.
    Ayerst i.

BabyBeat ultrasound i.
backbiter i.
Backlund stereotactic i.
back range of motion i.
Bard BladderScan bladder
  volume i.
Bard Monopty reusable core
  biopsy i.
i. basket
battery-powered i.
bibeveled cutting i.
Biophysic Ophthascan S i.
BIP biopsy i.
bipolar radiofrequency surgical
  ablation i.
body piercing i.
bone abduction i.
Carl Zeiss i.
Cell-Dyn 1200, 3200, 4000
  automated cell-counting i.
Cell-Dyn Sapphire hematology i.
Ceprate SC I. II
cervical range-of-motion i.
Chang Quick Chop combo
  ophthalmic i.
Clarke stereotactic i.
ClearCut 2 i.
Cloward i.
i. coding tape
Collis TDR i.
Command Instrument System
  surgical i.
conization i.
Cooley neonatal i.
Corex i.
Crit-Line i.
cryosurgical i.
Daisy I&A i.
Daniel EndoForehead i.
diamond fraise dermabrasion i.
Diamond-Lite cardiovascular i.
Diamond-Lite titanium i.
digitized i.
Dilamezinsert urologic i.
Disk-Criminator i.
Dolphin i.
DORC backflush i.
double-ended i.
double-plane i.
Dualine digital hearing i.
Duette double-lumen ERCP i.
Dwyer i.
Dyonics arthroscopic i.
EarCheck Pro i.
Ectra carpal tunnel i.
electrosurgical i.
Endoloop chromic ligature suture i.
endosonography i.
Endo Stitch i.

EndoWrist i.
Erbe electrical coagulation i.
Erbe electrical coagulation i.
Erbe electrical cutting i.
Erbe electrical cutting i.
ESI Lite-Pipe fiberoptic i.
ESI Lite-Pipe plastic surgery i.
eXcel-DR disposable/reusable i.
Exprin DQ1 biopsy i.
falloposcope endoscopic i.
Femur Finder i.
FirstStep tibial osteotomy i.
FlashPoint image-guided surgical i.
Forte ES i.
Friatec manual arthroscopy i.
G-C filling i.
Gen-S automated cell-counting i.
Glick i.
GM i.
gnathologic i.
Gobble Plus removal i.
GPX rotary i.
Graefe i.
graft measuring i.
grasping i.
i. grasping forceps
guillotine vitrectomy i.
Halifax fine adjustment i.
Hall large bone i.
Hall Micro E power i.
Hall series 4 large bone i.
Hall-Zimmer power i.
head-mounted i.
Henry Schein filling i.
i. holder
Hough middle ear i.
House middle ear i.
Howmedica-Osteonics i.
Hyflex X-File i.
I&A i.
IBF knee i.
incision viewing i.
Innomed Assistant Free surgical i.
Iolab titanium i.
IOLMaster optical i.
ionization i.
ionizing chamber i.
IOS immunodiagnostic testing i.
IVI i.
Johnson Endobag i.
Jordan middle ear i.
Jordan strut-measuring i.
Karlin cervical microdiscectomy i.
Keeler cryosurgical i.
Keyes biopsy i.
KinetiX i.
Kirkland i.
Kirschner surgical i.
knot-tying i.

Krwawicz cataract cryosurgical i.
Küntscher nail i.
K x-ray fluorescence i.
Ladmore plastic filling i.
LDS i.
Ligaclip ERCA i.
LightCycler polymerase chain
  reaction analysis i.
Lusk i.
Magnum biopsy i.
I. Makar biodegradable interference
  screw
Malis bipolar i.
Marlow Primus i.
Mastel Precision surgical i.
Matsuda titanium surgical i.
matte black i.
MaxCore biopsy i.
McCabe measuring i.
McCall i.
McGee middle ear i.
mechanical radial scanning i.
Medicon i.
3M filling i.
Micro-Aire pneumatic power i.
micro-Doppler i.
Micro-Three microsurgery i.
Midas Rex pneumatic i.
MiniSite laparoscopic i.
Mitek SuperAnchor i.
Mity Roto 360 i.
Mity Roto rotary i.
M4 Kerr Safety Hedstrom i.
MLA-100 coagulation i.
Monogram total knee i.
Monopty biopsy i.
myoma fixation i.
nail fold capillaroscopic i.
NeoKnife electrosurgical i.
Newport medical i.
Nicolet Compass EMG i.
Nova DPM 9003 skin testing i.
oblique forward-viewing i.
Obwegeser orthognathic surgery i.
ophthalmic i.
orthopaedic cutting i.
OrthoVise orthopaedic i.
oscilloscope i.
Ovation cutting i.
Paparella middle ear i.
Partnership i.
passivation metal i.
PCEE automated anastomotic i.
PediGuard freehand vertebral
  pedicle perforation i.
pencil-grip i.
phacofracture ophthalmic i.
pistol-grip i.
PlasmaKinetic i.

instrument *(continued)*

Plastibell compression i.
plastic i.
plugging i.
Pneumoneedle reusable i.
point-search i.
Polaris reusable i.
Polaris reusable laparoscopic i.
polytome i.
PowerTrack II muscle testing i.
Precision tack i.
primer i.
ProFile variable taper rotary i.
ProTack i.
pulsed-range gated Doppler i.
quadriceps-sparing minimally
  invasive total knee i.
Quinton suction biopsy i.
Radionics bipolar i.
Rancho external fixation i.
Rank-Taylor-Hobson-Talysurf i.
reciprocal planing i.
reduction i.
Reichert Ultramatic Rx Master
  Phoroptor refracting i.
Retinomax refractometry i.
i. retrieval container
RingLoc i.
Rizzuti-Bonaccolto i.
Rizzuti-Fleischer i.
Rizzuti-Kayser-Fleischer i.
Rizzuti-Lowe i.
Rizzuti-Maxwell i.
Roboprep G i.
Rosenberg gynecomastia
  dissection i.
rotary cutting i.
Ruggles surgical i.
Rumex titanium i.
Schlesinger i.
ScoliTron i.
screwdriver i.
Semmes-Weinstein monofilament i.
Sensonic plaque removal i.
Sharpoint cutting i.
single-beveled cutting i.
single-headed i.
single-plane i.
single reference point i.
single-use i.
slotted i.
small-diameter endosonographic i.
Snowden-Pencer laparoscopic
  cholecystectomy i.
Sofamor spinal i.
solid-state i.
Sonomed 1500 A-scan i.
spark-gap i.
spring-loaded biopsy i.

i. stabilizer pad
stereotactic i.
stereotaxic i.
STKS automated cell counting i.
Stratus i.
strut measuring i.
Sulzer Orthopaedics i.
Sutcliffe laser shield and
  retracting i.
Sutherland rotatable microsurgery i.
Suture Assistant i.
Suture Tram i.
suturing i.
Sysmex CA-6000 coagulation i.
take-apart i.
Tessier craniofacial i.
test handle i.
topographic scanning/indocyanine
  green angiography combination i.
Ultra-Cut i.
Ultra-Cut Cobb spinal i.
ultrasonic bone-cutting i.
UniPuls electrostimulation i.
Unitech i.
Universal Medical I.'s (UMI)
Universal nasal i. handle
ureteral visualization i.
Uroloop i.
Utas electroretinography i.
Valleylab laparoscopic i.
Vilex plastic surgery i.
WeeFIM i.
Welch Allyn AudioPath Platform
  hearing acuity i.
Wiet graft-measuring i.
XP peritympanic hearing i.
Yasargil-Aesculap i.
Yellow Springs I. (YSI)
Yesavage depression i.

instrumentation

Accu-Line knee i.
advanced breast biopsy i. (ABBI)
AO notched i.
Apofix cervical i.
Baxter V. Mueller laparoscopic i.
biodegradable fixation i.
biofeedback i.
Caspar anterior i.
C-D i.
compression U-rod i.
Cotrel-Dubousset i. (CDI)
Cotrel-Dubousset pedicle screw i.
Cotrel-Dubousset pedicular i.
Cotrel-Dubousset spinal i.
craniofacial i.
distraction i.
double Zielke i.
Dwyer i.
dynamic compression plate i.

Edwards i.
EndoMax endoscopic i.
Gellman i.
halo-Ilizarov distraction i.
Harms-Moss anterior thoracic i.
Harrington distraction i.
Harrington-Kostuik i.
Harrington rod i.
Harrington spinal i.
Howmedica knee i.
interspinous segmental spinal i.
Isola i.
Jacobs locking hook spinal rod i.
Kambin i.
Kaneda anterior spinal i.
Karl Storz i.
Kostuik-Harrington spinal i.
Louis i.
L-rod i.
lumbosacral spine transpedicular i.
Luque II segmental spinal i.
Luque semirigid segmental spinal i.
Miami Moss i.
Microvasive i.
Midas Rex i.
modular i.
Moss i.
Moss-Miami spinal i.
multiple hook assembly C-D i.
Passport i.
PLUS spinal i.
posterior distraction i.
posterior hook-rod spinal i.
powered i.
Putti-Platt i.
rod-sleeve i.
Russell-Taylor interlocking nail i.
sacral spine modular i.
sacral spine Universal i.
segmental spinal i.
skin-contact i.
Smith-Richards i.
Steffee spinal i.
stereotactic i.
Stryker power i.
TAG i.
Tangent spinal i.
TSRH i.
TSRH 3D spinal i.
Zielke pedicular i.
Instrumentation Laboratory system
instrumented bone preserving (IBP)
InstruSponge
I. enzymatic sponge
I. flexible plastic wand
insufflation
i. device
i. needle

i. test set
i. tubing
insufflator
colonic i.
Dyopneumatic i.
Eder i.
gas i.
hysteroscopic i.
Kelly i.
Kidde tubal i.
laparoscopic i.
Op-Pneu i.
Protoco$_2$l automated CO_2 i.
Semm Pelvi-Pneu i.
Sieger i.
Snowden-Pencer i.
variable-flow i.
Weber colonic i.
InsuFilter filter
Insuflon insulin delivery device
insulated
i. bayonet forceps
i. curved scissors
i. electrode needle
i. epidural needle
i. forceps
i. gate field-effect transistor
i. knife handle
i. monopolar forceps
i. straight scissors
i. tissue forceps
insulated-tip electrosurgical knife
insulation-tipped electrosurgical knife
insulin
i. infusion pump
i. pen
insulin-like growth factor
InsulScan
Insul-Sheath vaginal speculum sheath
Insul-Tote
InSync
I. cardiac resynchronization device
I. implantable cardioverter-
defibrillator
I. miniform pad
I. multisite cardiac stimulator
Insyte Autoguard IV shielded catheter
In-Tac bone-anchoring system
Intacs
I. corneal ring
I. corneal ring implant
I. corneal ring segment
I. intrastromal corneal ring
I. prescription insert
I. ring
Intact
I. catheter
I. xenograft valve

Intec
- I. AID cardioverter-defibrillator generator
- I. implantable defibrillator

Integra
- I. artificial skin
- I. catheter
- I. dermal regeneration template
- I. II balloon
- I. Selector ultrasonic aspiration
- I. skin replacement system
- I. tissue expander

integral
- I. distal centralizer
- I. hip system
- I. Interlok femoral prosthesis
- I. Omniloc implant
- i. uniformity scintillation camera

integrated
- I. Ankle orthotic ankle joint
- i. automatic stone-tissue detection system
- i. clinical information system
- I. Core system
- i. headholder
- i. lead system
- i. side port access portal
- I. Wound Manager

integrating spherical power meter

integrator
- Medical Graphics pneumotachograph with volume i.

Integre 532 delivery system

Integris
- I. cardiac imaging system
- I. H5000 digital x-ray imaging system
- I. III-V DSA system
- I. 3000 scanner
- I. V3000 DDSA
- I. V3000 digital subtraction system
- I. V3000 imager

Integrity
- I. acetabular cup
- I. acetabular cup prosthesis
- I. acetabular cup screw
- I. AFx AutoCapture pacing system
- I. AFx DR model 5346 pacemaker
- I. neutral liner
- I. shell

Intelect
- I. Combo stimulator/ultrasound
- I. electric stimulator
- I. laser system device
- I. Legend Combo stimulator and ultrasound unit
- I. Legend stimulator
- I. 600MP microcurrent stimulator

InteliJET fluid management system

Intellicath pulmonary artery catheter

Intelligent Prosthesis Plus prosthesis

Intelliject pump

IntelliTemp insulation material

intensified
- i. radiographic imaging system
- i. radiographic imaging system scanner

intensifier
- C-arm image i.
- image i.
- OEC-Diasonics mobile C-arm image i.

intensifying screen

IntePro large-pore synthetic mesh

Inteq small joint suturing system

Inter
- I. Fix RP threaded spinal fusion cage device
- I. Fix RP threaded spinal fusion device
- I. Fix threaded spinal fusion cage device

Interax
- I. Integrated Secure Asymmetric mobile-bearing knee implant
- I. total knee system

interbody
- i. fusion cage system
- i. fusion rasp
- i. graft tamp
- i. rasp
- i. spacer (IBS)

intercalary allograft

Interceed
- I. absorbable adhesion barrier
- I. barrier material
- I. TC7 absorbable adhesion barrier

Intercept
- I. esophagus microcoil
- I. platelet system
- I. prostate microcoil
- I. urethra microcoil
- I. vascular internal MR coil

Interceptor
- I. M3 triple-channel solid-state monitor
- I. wire distal protection device

interchangeable
- i. plate
- i. vein stripper
- i. vein stripper olive

intercom
- ultrasound i.

intercostal
- i. catheter
- i. drain
- i. trocar

interdental splint

interface
    I. arterial blood filter
    Monarch Mini Mask nasal i.
    ShearBan low-friction i.
    Ultimate Seal gel i.
interference
    i. barrier filter
    i. filter
    i. microscope
    i. screw
interferential stimulator
interferometer
    electron i.
    Zeiss IOL Master laser i.
InterFix
    I. RP threaded spinal fusion cage
    I. titanium threaded spinal fusion cage
interfragmentary
    i. lag screw
    i. minilag screw
    i. plate
InterGard
    I. heparin graft
    I. knitted collagen
    I. Silver vascular graft
    I. vascular graft
Intering vascular graft
interlaminar clamp
Interlink
    I. cannula
    I. injection cap
    I. threaded lock cannula
interlocking
    i. detachable coil
    i. sound
Inter-Lock screw and fixation system
Interlok primary femoral component
Intermate infusion system
intermaxillary wire
intermediate
    i. C-D hook
    i. socket
    i. splint
Intermedics
    I. atrial antitachycardia pacemaker
    I. Cyberlith X multiprogrammable pacemaker
    I. intraocular lens implant
    I. intraocular tonometer
    I. lens
    I. lithium-powered pacemaker
    I. Marathon dual-chamber rate-responsive pacemaker
    I. Marathon VVI single-chamber pacemaker
    I. natural hip system
    I. Natural-Knee knee prosthesis
    I. phaco I/A unit

    Pharmacia I.
    I. Quantum unipolar pacemaker
    I. Res-Q implantable cardioverter-defibrillator
    I. Stride pacemaker
intermittent
    i. extremity pump
    i. flow machine
internal
    i. biliary stent
    i. cardioverter-defibrillator
    i. cervical device
    i. ear prosthesis
    i. fiberoptic cable
    i. fixation device
    i. fixation spring
    i. gel pad
    i. hex-thread connection
    i. mammary artery catheter
    i. monitor
    i. nucleus hydrodelineation needle
    i. reed switch
    i. tibial torsion brace
    i. ureteral stent
internal/external catheter
International
    I. Acoustic Company audiologic assessment room
    I. Biomedical Mode 745-100 microcapillary infusion system
    I. compression system
    I. standard goniometer
    I. 10-20 system
Inter-Op
    I.-O. acetabular prosthesis
    I.-O. acetabular shell
    I.-O. hip prosthesis
interosseous wire
Interpore
    I. bone replacement material
    I. ceramic material
    I. hydroxyapatite
    I. implant
    I. IMZ implant system
    I. osteointegrated implant
    I. 200 porous hydroxyapatite
interprobe system
interproximal stripper
interrogation device
interrupted pledgeted suture
Interseal
    I. acetabular cup
    I. Variant I–IV prosthesis
intersegmental traction chiropractic table
Intersept cardiotomy reservoir
Intersorb
    I. absorptive burn pad
    I. fine mesh gauze

Intersorb *(continued)*
    I. 6-ply absorbent roll stretch gauze
    I. wide mesh gauze
InterSpace
    I. hip spacer
    I. knee spacer
interspace
    i. shaper
    i. width marker
    I. YAG laser lens
interspinous
    i. cable
    i. process decompression (IPD)
    i. segmental spinal instrumentation
    i. spacer device
InterStim device
interstitial implant
Intertach
    I. II pacemaker
    I. II pacer
Intertech
    I. anesthesia breathing circuit
    I. nonrebreathing modified Jackson-Rees circuit
InterTherapy intravascular ultrasound
Intertron therapy microprocessor
intervener
    Love-Gruenwald i.
interventional
    i. catheter
    i. magnetic resonance imaging (iMRI)
intervertebral
    i. curette
    i. disc forceps
    i. disc rongeur
    i. spreader
Interzeag bowl perimeter
intestinal
    i. anastomosis clamp
    i. anastomosis forceps
    i. bag
    i. closing forceps
    i. decompression trocar
    i. holding forceps
    i. occlusion clamp
    i. occlusion retractor
    i. plication needle
    i. resection clamp
    i. ring clamp
    i. tissue forceps
InteXen porcine dermal matrix
in-the-bag lens
in-the-canal hearing aid
in-the-ear
    i.-t.-e. hearing aid
    i.-t.-e. listening device
In-Time retrieval device

INTRA angled surgical handpiece
intraaortic
    i. balloon
    i. balloon assist device
    i. balloon catheter
    i. balloon counterpulsation device
    i. balloon pump (IABP)
    i. counterpulsation balloon
intraarterial
    i. cannula
    i. chemotherapy catheter
Intrabeam intraoperative radiotherapy system
intracanalicular punctum plug
intracapsular
    i. lens expressor
    i. lens expressor hook
    i. lens forceps
    i. lens loupe
intracardiac
    i. accelerometer
    i. cannula
    i. catheter
    i. needle holder
    i. retractor
    i. sucker
    i. sucker guard
    i. suction tube
    i. sump tube
IntraCardiac Echocardiography IVUS catheter
Intracath catheter
intracavitary
    i. afterloading applicator
    i. balloon applicator
    i. transducer
Intracell
    I. mechanical muscle device
    I. myofascial trigger-point device
    I. Sprinter stick
    I. trigger point massager
intracerebral depth electrode
intracervical
    i. bag
    i. device (ICD)
Intrack XT clamp
intracochlear implant
IntraCoil
    I. endoprosthesis
    I. nitinol stent
    I. self-expanding nitinol stent
    I. self-expanding peripheral stent
    I. self-expanding stent
    I. stent
Intracone intramedullary reamer
intracorneal
    i. implant
    i. lens
intracoronal retainer

intracoronary
    i. Doppler flow guidewire
    i. Doppler flow wire
    i. guiding catheter
    i. perfusion catheter
    i. stent
intracranial
    i. pressure catheter
    i. pressure Express digital monitor
    i. pressure microsensor
    i. pressure monitoring device
    i. pressure monitor screw
intracrine negative feedback modulator
IntraDop
    Doppler I.
    I. intraoperative Doppler
    I. probe
Intraducer
    I. peritoneal cannula
    I. peritoneal catheter
intraductal
    i. endoscope
    i. imaging catheter
    i. ultrasound
    i. ultrasound probe
intradural retractor
IntraEAR
    I. microcatheter
    I. Microdose Cath catheter
Intrafix
    I. ACL tibial fastener
    I. screw
Intraflex intramedullary pin
intragastric
    i. balloon
    i. cannula
    i. continuous pH-meter
IntraLase FS30 laser
intraligamentary syringe
intraluminal
    i. probe
    i. reference electrode
    i. stapler
    i. suture
    i. ultrasound
    i. ultrasound catheter
IntraLuminal Safe-Steer system
intrameatal
    i. earphone
    i. electrode
Intramedic polyethylene tubing
intramedullary
    i. alignment rod
    i. ANK nail
    i. bar
    i. broach
    i. brush
    i. canal plug
    i. catheter

    i. collar (IMC)
    i. drill
    i. fixation device
    i. guide
    i. illuminator
    i. nail
    i. nail extractor
    i. pin
    i. reamer
    i. rod
    i. Rush rod
    i. skeletal kinetic distractor
    i. skeletal kinetic distractor system
    i. supracondylar multihole nail
intranasal
    i. bivalve splint
    i. hammer
    i. splint
intraocular
    i. balloon
    i. forceps
    i. hook
    i. implant
    i. irrigating forceps
    i. lens (IOL)
    i. lens cannula
    i. lens dialer
    i. lens folder
    i. lens forceps
    i. lens glide
    i. retinal prosthesis
    i. tension recorder
Intra-Op autotransfusion system
intraoperative
    i. device
    i. film
    i. gamma probe
    i. ultrasonic probe
intraoral
    i. fracture appliance
    i. spacer
    i. stent
    i. titanium mandibular distraction
      device
intraorbital implant
intraosseous
    i. needle
    i. suture anchor
intrapartum monitor
intraperitoneal onlay mesh
intrapleural
    i. catheter
    i. sealed drainage unit
intraportal endovascular ultrasonography
intraprostatic
    i. spiral
    i. stent
IntraSite
    I. dressing

IntraSite *(continued)*
    I. gel
    I. gel wound dressing
    I. hydrogel dressing
IntraSonix TULIP laser device
Intrasound
    Medtronic Pulsor I.
intraspinal drug infusion system
IntraStent
    I. balloon-expanded stent
    I. biliary stent
    I. DoubleStent biliary
       endoprosthesis
    I. DoubleStrut biliary endoprosthesis
    I. DoubleStrut biliary stent
    I. DoubleStrut ParaMount
       premounted stent-biliary system
    I. DoubleStrut ParaMount XS
       premounted stent-biliary system
    I. DS balloon-expanded stent
    I. LD balloon-expanded stent
    I. LP balloon-expanded stent
intrathecal catheter
intrathoracic forceps
intratracheal tube
intraurethral
    i. coil
    i. prostatic bridge catheter
intrauterine
    i. balloon cannula
    i. balloon-type cannula
    i. catheter (IUC)
    i. contraception device
    i. contraceptive progesterone system
    i. device (IUD)
    i. insemination cannula
    i. insemination cannula with
       mandrel
    i. insemination catheter
    i. pessary
    i. pressure catheter
    i. pressure monitor
intravaginal ring
intravascular
    i. accurate control (IVAC)
    i. catheter electrode
    i. Doppler
    i. Doppler-tipped guidewire
    i. oxygenator
    i. stent
    i. ultrasound (IVUS)
    i. ultrasound catheter
intravenous (IV, I.V.)
    i. accurate control device
    i. needle
    i. pacing catheter
    i. ultrasound catheter
    i. urogram

intraventricular pressure monitoring
   catheter
intravitreal
    i. bioerodible dexamethasone
       implant
    i. cryoprobe
    i. laser
Intrepid
    I. balloon catheter
    I. functional knee brace
    I. percutaneous transluminal
       coronary angioplasty catheter
    I. PTCA catheter
intrinsic transverse connector
Introcan Safety IV catheter
introducer
    Agilis steerable i.
    Angestat hemostasis i.
    Angetear tear-away i.
    aortic assist balloon i.
    Atkinson i.
    Avanti i.
    i. cannula
    Cardak i.
    Carter sphere i.
    i. catheter
    catheter i.
    Charnley i.
    Check-Flo i.
    Chiou SP tube i.
    Ciaglia percutaneous
       tracheostomy i.
    Cook micropuncture i.
    Cook Peel-Away i.
    Desilets-Hoffman i.
    Desilets-Hoffman catheter i.
    Edwards IntroFlex i.
    end-hole i.
    endolymphatic shunt tube i.
    entrapment sack i.
    Eschmann endotracheal tube i.
    Excalibur i.
    Fast-Cath Duo i.
    Fastrac i.
    Flexor i.
    Furlow i.
    gum elastic bougie i.
    i. gun
    Hall self-holding i.
    Hemaquet i.
    Hickman percutaneous i.
    Holter i.
    House endolymphatic shunt tube i.
    I. II sheath
    Input PS i.
    IntroFlex i.
    LapSac i.
    LPS Peel-Away i.
    Maximum hemostasis i.

micropuncture Peel-Away i.
Moss T-anchor needle i.
Mullins catheter i.
Nottingham i.
Nottingham KeyMed i.
PD Access with Peel-Away
  needle i.
peel-away i.
percutaneous sheath i.
pull-apart i.
Ramses diaphragm i.
Razi cannula i.
i. sheath
silicone i.
Speck i.
sphere i.
split-sheath i.
stent i.
Storz vent tube i.
SupraFoley suprapubic i.
Taut percutaneous i.
Tuohy-Borst i.
Tuohy-Borst side-arm i.
Ultimum hemostasis i.
UMI transseptal Cath-Seal
  catheter i.
Uni-Shunt with reservoir i.
USCI i.
ventricular catheter i.
Weaver trocar i.
introducer/endoscope
Czaja-McCaffrey rigid stent i./e.
introducing forceps
IntroFlex introducer
Introl bladder neck support prosthesis
Intron Λ multidose pen
intubating
i. laryngeal mask
i. laryngeal mask airway
intubation
i. laryngoscope
i. tube
intussuscepted nipple valve
Invacare
I. APM mattress
I. Comfort-Mate extra cushion
I. manual wheelchair
I. nasal prongs
I. padded shower chair
I. Venture HomeFill complete
  home oxygen system
I. vinyl transfer bench
invaginator
Lempert i.
invalid
i. chair
i. cushion
i. ring
InvertaChair traction device

inverted
i. buttoned device
i. cone bur
i. orthotic
i. U-pouch ileal reservoir
inverter
Mayo-Kelly appendix i.
stereoscopic diagonal i.
Wangensteen tissue i.
Invertertube
Inverter vitrectomy system
Invertrac equipment
Investa suture
INVISx cranial fixation system
Invitrogen TA cloning kit
Invos
I. 3100, 3100A cerebral oximeter
  monitoring system
I. cerebral oximeter
I. 3100 cerebral oximeter
I. transcranial cerebral oximeter
INX stent
Ioban
I. antimicrobial incise drape
I. 2 cesarean sheet
I. drape
I. 2 iodophor cesarean sheet
I. Steri-Drape
I. Vi-Drape
IOBeads magnetic bead
iodine
i. catgut suture
i. cup
Iodoflex
I. absorptive dressing
I. solid gel pad
iodoform
i. gauze
i. gauze packing
iodoform-impregnated plastic sheet
Iodosorb absorptive dressing
IOL
intraocular lens
AC IOL
accommodating IOL
AcrySof single-piece IOL
AMO Array SA40N multifocal
  IOL
AMO Clariflex IOL
apodized diffractive IOL
AquaSense IOL
Artisan IOL
Artisan iris-fixated phakic IOL
blue-filtering IOL
blue filtration hydrophobic IOL
CeeOn Edge foldable IOL
ClariFlex foldable IOL
Crystalens IOL
CV232 square-round-edge IOL

IOL *(continued)*
  IOL dialer
  foldable iris-claw phakic IOL
  foldable 3-piece silicone IOL
  foldable silicone IOL
  Hydroview IOL
  Hydroview foldable IOL
  iris claw phakic IOL
  Kearney side-notch IOL
  KH-3500 IOL
  light-adjustable IOL
  MemoryLens IOL
  MemoryLens prefolded IOL
  modified prolate anterior surface
    IOL
  monofocal IOL
  multifocal phakic IOL
  multifocal silicone IOL
  NewLife IOL
  non-blue filtering IOL
  NuLens accommodating IOL
  parent spherical IOL
  Phakic 6 H2 IOL
  3-piece IOL
  1-piece hydrophilic acrylic IOL
  3-piece hydrophilic acrylic IOL
  piggybacked toric IOL
  plate-haptic IOL
  presbyopia-correcting IOL
  ReZoom multifocal refractive IOL
  SC60B-OUV IOL
  Sensar OptiEdge AR40e IOL
  Sensar OptiEdge foldable acrylic
    IOL
  sharp-edged IOL
  silicone toric IOL
  single-piece acrylic IOL
  single-piece SN60AT IOL
  SoFlex IOL
  soft acrylic IOL
  spherical IOL
  Staar IOL
  Staar low-diopter IOL
  Staar toric IOL
  Synchrony Dual Optic
    Accommodating IOL
  Tecnis acrylic IOL
  Tecnis foldable IOL
  traditional IOL
  UV-absorbing IOL
  Verisyse phakic IOL
  Visian IOL
  wavefront-corrected IOL
  well-centered IOL
Iolab
  I. 108 B lens
  I. irrigating/aspirating
    photocoagulator
  I. irrigating needle

I. taper-cut needle
I. titanium instrument
I. titanium needle
IOLMaster optical instrument
Iomed Phoresor electrode
ion
  i. chromatograph
  i. laser
  i. microscope
  i. pump
Ionalyzer analyzer
Ionescu-Shiley
  I.-S. aortic valve prosthesis
  I.-S. artificial cardiac valve
  I.-S. pericardial patch
  I.-S. pericardial valve
  I.-S. pericardial valve graft
  I.-S. pericardial xenograft
  I.-S. valve prosthesis
  I.-S. vascular graft
Ionescu trileaflet valve
Ionic spine spacer system
iON intraoperative navigation system
ionization
  i. counter
  i. instrument
ionizing chamber instrument
ion-selective electrode
ion-sensitive field-effect transistor
iontophoresis electrode
iontophoretic applicator
IOP monitor
Ioptex TabOptic lens
**IOS immunodiagnostic testing
  instrument**
Iowa
  I. membrane forceps
  I. orbital implant
  I. pudendal needle guide
  I. State fixation forceps
  I. stem
  I. total hip prosthesis
  I. trumpet
  I. trumpet needle guide
  I. University periosteal elevator
Ipas
  I. aspirator
  I. flexible cannula
IPC boot
IPD
  interspinous process decompression
I-plate
  Syracuse anterior I-p.
I-Plus
  I-P. System humeral fracture brace
  I-P. System ulnar fracture brace
IPM wound gel
Ipomax orthosis

ipos
  i. arch support system
  i. forefoot relief orthosis
  i. heel relief orthosis
  i. heel relief shoe
  i. postoperative shoe
IPS total hip system
IQ nasal mask
¹⁹²Ir
  ¹⁹²Ir ribbon
  ¹⁹²Ir wire
Irex
  I. Exemplar ultrasound
  I. Exemplar ultrasound scanner
iridectomy
  i. laser lens
  i. scissors
iridium
  i. needle
  i. prosthesis
iridium-192 stent
iridocapsular intraocular lens
iridocapsulotomy scissors
iridodialysis spatula
iridodilator
iridotomy scissors
iris
  i. bipolar forceps
  i. claw intraocular lens
  i. claw phakic IOL
  i. clip intraocular lens
  I. coronary stent
  i. dilator
  i. expressor
  i. forceps
  i. hook
  i. hook cannula
  i. III imager
  I. II stent
  i. knife
  i. lens manipulator
  I. Medical OcuLight green laser
    system
  I. Medical OcuLight infrared laser
    system
  I. Medical OcuLight SLx
  i. microscissors
  i. needle
  I. OcuLight SLx indirect
    ophthalmoscope delivery system
  I. OcuLight SLx MicroPulse laser
  i. repositor
  i. retractor
  i. scanner
  i. scissors
  i. spatula
  i. suture microforceps
  i. tissue forceps
Iriscorder recorder

iris-fixated lens
IrisMate flexible translimbal iris
  retractor
iris-supported intraocular lens
IRMA
  immediate response mobile analyzer
    IRMA blood gas analysis system
    IRMA SL blood glucose strip
      tester
Irom
  I. bilateral splint
  I. Regal splint
  I. splint with shell
iron
  Böhler i.
  I. Intern retractor
  i. lung
  Pineda LASIK flap i.
Ironman Triathlon Pro-Power massager
IROX endocardial pacing lead
irradiation sterilized graft
irradiator
  MDS-2000 microwave i.
  portable blood i.
Irri-Cath suction system
irrigated coiled catheter
irrigating
  i. axe
  i. catheter
  i. C-hook extractor
  i. chopper
  i. cortex extractor
  i. cystotome
  i. dialer
  i. grasping forceps with curved
    shaft
  i. IOL positioner
  i. iris hook
  i. J-hook cannula
  i. lens loupe
  i. lens manipulator
  i. mushroom retractor
  i. notched spatula
  i. probe
  i. pupil expander
  i. scissors with straight shaft
  i. sheath
  i. tip
  i. uterine curette
  i. vectis loop
  i. vectis loupe
irrigating/aspirating
  i./a. cannula
  i./a. vectis
irrigating-positioning needle
irrigation
  i. and aspiration (I&A, I/A)
  i. catheter
  i. system

irrigation/aspiration cannula
irrigator
> anterior chamber i.
> Arthro-Flo i.
> Brackmann suction i.
> Doss automatic percolator i.
> Dougherty i.
> Endo-Flo i.
> Fox i.
> Gibson i.
> Hollister colostomy i.
> Hydrofloss electronic oral i.
> Irrijet i.
> Kelman i.
> laser-assisted intrastromal
>   keratomileusis flap i.
> LASIK flap i.
> Lukens double-channel i.
> LySonix 250 i.
> LySonix Delta Tip i.
> nasal i.
> olive-tip i.
> Randolph i.
> Seibel LASIK flap i.
> Shambaugh i.
> Shooter Saeed multiband i.
> sinus i.
> Stropko i.
> StrykeFlow PS suction i.
> StrykeFlow 2 suction i.
> Stryker suction i.
> suction i.
> Vidaurri i.
> Waterpik i.

irrigator/aspirator
> LySonix Series 250 i./a.
> Nezhat-Dorsey i./a.

Irrijet
> I. DS irrigation system
> I. DS wound irrigation device
> I. irrigator

Irrivac syringe
Irvine
> I. irrigating/aspirating unit
> I. probe-pointed scissors
> University of California-I. (UCI)

**IS1000 gel documentation imaging
system**
Isch-Dish Plus cushion
ischemic mitral ring (IMR)
ischial
> i. containment socket
> i. lift
> i. strap
> i. weightbearing brace
> i. weightbearing prosthesis

ischial-gluteal weightbearing socket
iScreen photoscreener
iseikonic lens

Iselin forceps
ISG
> ISG viewing wand
> ISG Wand navigation system

Ishihara
> I. IV slit-lamp
> I. plate
> I. pseudoisochromatic plate
> I. test chart book

ISKD system
island wound dressing
Isletest ICA kit
Ismat manual muscle tester
Isobar barostat distension device
Isocam
> I. scintillation imaging system
> I. SPECT imaging system

isochromatic plate
IsoCode Stix device
isocon camera
IsoDyn knee brace
isoelastic
> i. pelvic prosthesis
> i. rip clamp

Isoflex
> I. bed
> I. mattress

Isogard system
isokinetic
> i. resistance apparatus
> i. Unex III exerciser

Isola
> I. fixation system
> I. hook-rod
> I. instrumentation
> I. spinal implant system
> I. spinal implant system accessory
> I. spinal implant system anchor
> I. spinal implant system component
> I. spinal implant system eye rod
> I. spinal implant system hook
> I. spinal implant system iliac
>   screw
> I. spinal instrumentation system
> I. vertebral screw
> I. wire

Isolagen human collagen
Isolar rod
isolation
> i. bag
> i. drape
> i. face mask
> i. forceps

isolator
> Ankle I.
> I. blood culture system
> I. endoscopic ablation device
> I. endoscopic ablation system
> Vickers i.

isolette
 Airshields i.
 double-bubble i.
 humidified i.
 temperature-controlled i.
Isolex 300i magnetic stem cell selection system
IsoMed
 I. constant-flow infusion system
 I. implantable drug pump
Isomet
 I. low-speed saw
 I. Plus precision saw
isometer
 I. bone graft placement site detector
 CA-5000 drill-guide i.
 tension i.
isometric strain gauge
Isoplast adhesive short stretch bandage
Isoprene plastic splint
Iso-Quadron exerciser
Isostation B200
Isostent
 Bx I.
 I. stent
Isotechnologies
 I. B-200 back testing and rehabilitation system
 I. B-200 low back machine
Isotoner glove
isotonic machine
isotope calibrator
IsoTrac brachytherapy needle
isotropic
 i. band
 i. probe
Isovue-370 prefilled syringe
Isovue prefilled syringe
Israel
 I. blunt rake retractor
 I. camera
 I. rasp
 I. retractor
 I. tongue depressor
i-STAT
 i-STAT bedside blood testing device
 i-STAT handheld analyzer
 i-STAT system
iStep FIT digital scanner
Itard eustachian catheter
ITC radiopaque balloon catheter
ITE
 ITE hearing aid
 ITE listening device
I-tech
 I-t. cannula
 I-t. cannula holder
 I-t. cannula tray
 I-t. needle holder
ITI
 ITI dental implant
 ITI dental implant system
 ITI type-F endosseous implant
Ito
 I. laser pen
 I. needle
I-TRAC Plus transfusion system
Itrel
 I. II, III spinal cord stimulation system
 I. II quadripolar pulse generator
 I. I unipolar pulse generator
 I. programmed transmitter-receiver
 I. pulse generator
ITVAD
 indwelling transcutaneous vascular access device
IUC
 intrauterine catheter
IUD
 intrauterine device
 copper T 380A IUD
 ParaGard T380 copper IUD
 Progestasert IUD
 IUD remover hook
 Saf-T-Coil IUD
IUI
 intrauterine insemination
 IUI disposable cannula
 IUI catheter
IV, I.V.
 intravenous
 IV catheter
 IV needle
IVAC
 intravascular accurate control
 IVAC device
 IVAC needleless IV system
 IVAC P4000 infuser
 IVAC Temp Plus II thermometer
 IVAC ventilator
 IVAC volumetric infusion pump
IVAD
 implantable vascular access device
 Thoratec IVAD
Ivalon
 I. compressed patch graft
 I. dressing
 I. embolic sponge
 I. foam
 I. particle
 I. plug
 I. prosthesis
 I. sponge
 I. sponge eye implant
 I. sponge implant

Ivalon *(continued)*
    I. suture
    I. wire coil
Ivan laryngeal applicator
IVA seal
IVC filter
Iverson dermabrader
Ives
    I. anoscope
    I. rectal speculum
IV-Heart nebulizer
IVI instrument

ivory rubber dam clamp
IVU
IVUS
    intravascular ultrasound
        IVUS catheter
Ivy
    I. loop
    I. mastoid rongeur
    I. wire
iWALKfree hands-free crutch
iZon wavefront-guided lens

J

J board
J exchange wire
J guidewire
J & J stent
J needle
J pad
J retention wire
J2 cushion
J-24 cervical orthosis
J-35 hyperextension orthosis
J-45 contraflexion orthosis
J-55
　　J-55 postfusion brace
　　J-55 postfusion orthosis
J-59 Florida brace
J6-HC, J6-MC, J6-MI high capacity centrifuge
Jabaley-Stille Super Cut Scissors
Jaboulay button
Jace
J. continuous passive motion ankle system
J. hand continuous passive motion unit
J. knee brace
J. shoulder exerciser
J. W550 CPM device
jacket
body j.
Boston soft body j.
Calot j.
cervicothoracic j.
Frejka j.
immobilization j.
Kydex body j.
Lexan j.
LS^4 custom spinal j.
Medtronic cardiac cooling j.
Minerva back j.
Minerva plastic j.
Orfizip body j.
Orthoplast j.
plaster of Paris j.
Prenyl j.
Raney j.
Sayre j.
Vitrathene j.
Weathertech EMS 3-in-1 systems j.
Wilmington plastic j.
jacket-type chest dressing
Jack Frost hot/cold pack
Jackman
J. coronary sinus electrode catheter
J. orthogonal catheter

Jacknobber
The J. II
Jackson
J. alligator grasping forceps
J. anterior commissure laryngoscope
J. approximation forceps
J. aspirating tube
J. biopsy forceps
J. bistoury
J. bone clamp
J. broad staple forceps
J. button forceps
J. coil
J. compression test
J. cone-shaped tracheal tube
J. conventional foreign body forceps
J. cross-action forceps
J. cylindrical object forceps
J. dilator
J. double-prong forceps
J. dressing forceps
J. dull rotation forceps
J. endoscopic forceps
J. esophageal dilator
J. esophagoscope
J. fiberoptic slide laryngoscope
J. flexible upper lobe bronchus forceps
J. forward grasping forceps
J. hollow object forceps
J. intervertebral disc rongeur
J. lacrimal intubation set
J. laryngeal applicator
J. laryngeal applicator forceps
J. laryngeal atomizer
J. laryngeal basket forceps
J. laryngeal punch forceps
J. laryngeal ring-rotation forceps
J. laryngectomy tube
J. laryngofissure forceps
J. papilloma forceps
J. ring jaw globular object forceps
J. ring rotation forceps
J. sharp-pointed rotation forceps
J. silver tracheostomy tube
J. sliding laryngoscope
J. spinal surgery and imaging table
J. spine table
J. sponge carrier
J. staging system
J. standard bronchoscope
J. staple bronchoscope
J. steel-stem woven filiform bougie
J. tendon-seizing forceps

Jackson *(continued)*
- J. tracheal bistoury
- J. tracheal hook
- J. tracheal retractor
- J. tracheoscope
- J. triangular brass dilator
- J. tunneler
- J. turbinate scissors
- J. vaginal retractor
- J. vaginal speculum

Jackson-Pratt
- J.-P. bifurcated drain extension
- J.-P. catheter
- J.-P. dissector
- J.-P. drain
- J.-P. flat drain kit
- J.-P. Gold wound drain
- J.-P. Hemaduct drain
- J.-P. hysterectomy kit
- J.-P. large-volume round silicone drain kit
- J.-P. large-volume suction reservoir
- J.-P. PVC kit
- J.-P. round PVC drain
- J.-P. silicone flat drain
- J.-P. silicone round drain
- J.-P. suction drain
- J.-P. suction tube
- J.-P. T-tube drain

Jackson-Rees
- J.-R. apparatus
- J.-R. circuit
- J.-R. endotracheal tube

Jacob capsule fragment forceps
Jacobs
- J. biopsy forceps
- J. cannula
- J. chuck adapter
- J. chuck drill
- J. clamp
- J. distraction rod
- J. locking hook spinal rod
- J. locking hook spinal rod instrumentation
- J. T-handled chuck
- J. uterine tenaculum
- J. vulsellum
- J. vulsellum forceps

Jacobsen template
Jacobson
- J. bladder retractor
- J. blunt hook
- J. bulldog clamp
- J. curette
- J. forceps
- J. hemostatic forceps
- J. microbulldog clamp
- J. mosquito forceps
- J. needle holder

- J. resonator
- J. resonator device
- J. suture pusher
- J. vessel clamp
- J. vessel knife

Jacoby heel splint
Jacques catheter
Jaeger
- J. acuity card
- J. eye chart
- J. keratome
- J. lid plate
- J. lid retractor
- J. metal lid plate
- J. plate
- J. reading chart
- J. retractor
- J. strabismus hook

Jaffe
- J. capsulorrhexis forceps
- J. Cilco lens
- J. intraocular spatula
- J. iris hook
- J. laser blepharoplasty and facial resurfacing set
- J. lens manipulating hook
- J. lens spatula
- J. needle holder
- J. 1-piece all-PMMA intraocular lens
- J. press-fit prosthesis
- J. wire lid retractor

Jaffe-Bechert nucleus rotator
Jaffe-Maltzman
- J.-M. hook
- J.-M. lens manipulator

Jaguar lumbar I/F cage system
Jagwire
- J. guidewire
- J. wire

Jako
- J. clamp
- J. facial nerve monitor
- J. laryngeal forceps
- J. laryngeal knife
- J. laryngeal mirror
- J. laryngeal needle holder
- J. laryngeal probe
- J. laryngeal suction tube
- J. laryngoscope
- J. microlaryngeal cup forceps
- J. microlaryngeal grasping forceps
- J. microlaryngeal scissors
- J. microlaryngoscope
- J. suction-irrigator
- J. transilluminator

Jamar
- J. dynamometer
- J. hand dynamometer

J. hydraulic hand dynamometer
J. hydraulic pinch gauge
Jameson
J. calipers
J. facelift scissors
J. muscle forceps
J. muscle hook
J. muscle recession forceps
J. strabismus forceps
J. strabismus hook
J. strabismus needle
James wound forceps
Jamshidi
J. adult needle
J. liver biopsy needle
J. needle
Janeway
J. gastroscope
J. sphygmomanometer
Jannetta
J. duckbill elevator
J. hook
J. retractor
Jansen
J. bayonet dressing forceps
J. bone curette
J. bone rongeur
J. clamp
J. dissecting forceps
J. dressing forceps
J. ear rongeur
J. mastoid retractor
J. monopolar forceps
J. nasal dressing forceps
J. rasp
J. thumb forceps
Jansen-Middleton
J.-M. nasal cutting forceps
J.-M. punch forceps
J.-M. rongeur
J.-M. scissors
J.-M. septal forceps
J.-M. septal punch
J.-M. septotomy forceps
J.-M. septum cutting forceps
Jansen-Wagner mastoid retractor
Japanese
J. erection ring
J. suction tip
Jaquet apparatus
Jarabak-type archwire
Jarcho
J. pressometer
J. tenaculum forceps
J. tenaculum holder
J. uterine tenaculum
Jarell forceps
Jarit
J. air injection cannula

J. anterior resection clamp
J. bipolar coagulator
J. cartilage clamp
J. disposable cannula
J. disposable trocar
J. dissecting scissors
J. forceps holder
J. intestinal clamp
J. mallet
J. microsurgery scissors
J. microsurgical needle holder
J. microsuture tying forceps
J. mosquito forceps
J. palate hook
J. periosteal elevator
J. peripheral vascular scissors
J. pin cutter
J. 3-prong cast spreader
J. rotator
J. sternal needle holder
J. tendon-pulling forceps
J. tube-occluding forceps
Jarrett side port manipulator
Jarvik
J. 7, 8 artificial heart
J. 7-70 artificial heart
J. 2000 artificial heart
Jarvis
J. pile clamp
J. snare
JAS
joint activated system
JAS elbow motion device
Jasco spectropolarimeter
Jatrox Hp-test
Java arthrodesis system
Javal
J. keratometer
J. ophthalmometer
Javid
J. bypass clamp
J. bypass tube
J. carotid clamp
J. carotid shunt
J. catheter
J. shunt
jaw
end gripping forceps with standard j.
j. exerciser
j. hook
independent j.
j. rongeur
j. spreader
j. spring clip
Jawz disposable biopsy forceps
Jay
J. basic cushion
J. Care wheelchair seating system

Jay *(continued)*
    J. Combi cushion
    J. J2 wheelchair
    J. Rave cushion
    J. Triad cushion
    J. Xtreme cushion
JB1 catheter
Jeanie
    J. Rub
    J. Rub massager
JedMed TRI-GEM microscope
Jeffrey introducer set
jejunal feeding tube
jejunoileal shunt
jejunostomy
    j. catheter
    j. tube
Jelco
    J. catheter
    J. intravenous catheter
    J. intravenous stylet
    J. needle
Jelenko
    J. arch bar
    J. facial fracture appliance
    J. pliers
    J. splint
jelly
    j. dressing
    Wharton j.
    Xylocaine j.
Jelm 2-way catheter
Jelonet dressing
Jeltrate impression material
JEM-100B, 100S electron microscope
JEM-100CX electron microscope
Jennings Loktite mouthgag
Jenning-Streifeneder gastroscope
Jensen
    J. capsule polisher
    J. capsule polisher cannula
    J. capsule scratcher
    J. intraocular lens forceps
    J. polisher/scratcher
Jensen-Thomas I&A cannula
Jeol
    J. 100 CX electron microscope
    J. JSM 35 CF scanning electron
       microscope
    J. 1200 transmission electron
       microscope
Jerald forceps
Jergesen I-beam
Jervey
    J. capsule fragment forceps
    J. iris forceps
Jesberg esophagoscope
jet
    Doppler color j.

    j. humidifier
    j. injector
    j. nebulizer
    J. shield
    j. stylet
    J. Vac cement dispenser
    j. ventilator
Jet-Air splint
Jetco spray cannula
Jeter
    J. lag/position screw
    J. lag screw
Jettmobile Tumble Forms
Jewel
    J. AF implantable arrhythmia
       management device
    J. AF implantable cardioverter-
       defibrillator
    J. AF implantable defibrillator
    J. atrial fibrillation dual-chamber
       device
    J. pacer-cardioverter-defibrillator
    J. PCD
jeweler's
    j. bipolar forceps
    j. forceps
    j. pickup forceps
    j. tweezers
jewelry
    optical j.
Jewett
    J. bar
    J. bone chip packer
    J. bone extractor
    J. contraflexion brace
    J. contraflexion orthosis
    J. double-angled osteotomy plate
    J. driver
    J. electrode
    J. extractor
    J. fracture appliance
    J. frame
    J. gouge
    J. hip nail
    J. hyperextension brace
    J. nail
    J. nail plate
    J. pickup screw
    J. postfusion brace
    J. postfusion orthosis
    J. prosthesis
    J. slotted plate
    J. socket reamer
    J. sound
    J. thoracolumbosacral orthosis
    J. urethral sound
    J. uterine dilator
    J. uterine sound

Jewett-Benjamin
  J.-B. cervical brace
  J.-B. cervical orthosis
JF-200
  JF-200 duodenoscope
JF-1T Olympus adult duodenoscope
JF-20 side-viewing fiberoptic endoscope
JFB III endoscope
JF-IT20 duodenoscope
JF-V10 duodenoscope
J-FX bipolar head
J-hook
  J-h. cannula
  J-h. electrosurgical probe
Jiffy tube
jig
  acrylic j.
  Charnley tibial onlay j.
  customized j.
  cutting j.
  external alignment compression j.
  external-alignment compression j.
  extramedullary tibial alignment j.
  fixation j.
  Herbert j.
  j. hook
  loading j.
  Osteonics j.
  Plexiglas j.
  precompression j.
jigsaw blade
Jimmy
  J. dislodger
  J. dissector
  J. John colonic irrigation system
Jindo tapered peripheral guidewire
Jinotti
  J. closed suctioning system
  J. dual-purpose catheter
JI shunt
J & J
  Johnson & Johnson
JJIS stent
JL
  Judkins left
    JL catheter
JL4
  Judkins left 4
JL5
  Judkins left 5
JL4, JL5 catheter
J-loop
  J-l. electrode
  J-l. PC lens
  J-l. posterior chamber intraocular
    lens
J-Maxx stent

Jobson-Horne
  J.-H. cotton applicator
  J.-H. ear probe
Jobst
  J. air band
  J. appliance
  J. athrombic pump system
  J. athrombotic pump
  J. boot
  J. extremity pump
  J. glove
  J. mammary support dressing
  J. postoperative air-boot
  J. pressure garment
  J. prosthesis
  J. sleeve
  J. Stride support stocking
  J. Stridette support stocking
  J. UlcerCare dressing
  J. Vairox gradient compression
    vascular stocking
  J. VPGS stocking
Joe-Hall-Morris biphasic appliance
Joe's
  J. hoe
  J. hoe retractor
Jography angiographic catheter
Johannson
  J. hip nail
  J. lag screw
Johannson-Stille
  J.-S. cystotomy trocar
  J.-S. lag screw
John
  J. Bunn Mini-Mist nebulizer
  J. Green calipers
  J. Green pendulum scalpel
Johns
  J. Hopkins bulldog clamp
  J. Hopkins coarctation clamp
  J. Hopkins gallbladder forceps
  J. Hopkins gallbladder retractor
  J. Hopkins gall duct forceps
  J. Hopkins hemostatic forceps
  J. Hopkins modified Potts clamp
  J. Hopkins occluding forceps
  J. Hopkins serrefine forceps
  J. Hopkins stone basket
Johnson
  J. brain tumor forceps
  J. canaliculus wire
  J. cervicothoracic orthosis
  J. cheek retractor
  J. coagulation suction tube
  J. dental band
  J. double cannula
  J. Endobag instrument
  J. erysiphake
  J. evisceration knife

Johnson *(continued)*
    J. hockey stick
    J. hook retractor
    J. hydrodelineation cannula
    J. hydrodissection cannula
    J. intestinal tube
    J. & Johnson (J & J)
    J. & Johnson Band-Aid sterile
      drape
    J. & Johnson biliary stent
    J. & Johnson coronary stent
    J. & Johnson dressing
    J. & Johnson gauze sponge
    J. & Johnson Hemopump
    J. & Johnson Interventional
      Systems stent
    J. & Johnson nonstick pads
    J. & Johnson PFC cruciate-
      substituting insert
    J. & Johnson PFC Sigma system
    J. & Johnson saliva ejector
    J. & Johnson tourniquet
    J. & Johnson waterproof tape
    J. Kydex chairback orthosis
    Mead J.
    J. prostatic needle holder
    J. ptosis forceps
    J. ptosis knife
    J. screwdriver
    J. skin hook
    J. spatula
    J. stone dislodger
    J. swab sampler
    J. thoracic forceps
    J. total hip stabilization orthosis
    J. transtracheal oxygen catheter
    J. twin-wire appliance
    J. ureteral stone basket
    J. ventriculogram retractor
Johnson-Elloy accord unconstrained
  prosthesis
Johnston
    J. clamp
    J. fixation ring
    J. gastrostomy plug
    J. infant dilator
    J. LASIK flap applanator
Johnston-Iowa hip prosthesis
joint
    j. activated system (JAS)
    artificial hip j.
    Ascension MCP total j.
    Ascension PIP total j.
    Cam Lock knee j.
    j. cinch
    Clevisphere ankle j.
    j. distraction cuff
    double-action ankle j.

    elastic knee cage with medial and
      lateral contoured knee j.'s
    Fillauer dorsiflexion assist ankle j.
    Fillauer PDC ankle j.
    Gaffney j.
    Gillette j.
    Gillette double-flexure ankle j.
    gliding hinge j.
    hinge j.
    HP-100 prosthetic finger j.
    j. immobilizer
    j. implant
    Integrated Ankle orthotic ankle j.
    Klenzak double-channeled ankle j.
    Klenzak knee j.
    Metasul j.
    Oklahoma ankle j.
    Otto Bock 3R65 children's
      hydraulic knee j.
    Otto Bock 3R45 modular knee j.
    3R80 modular hydraulic knee j.
    Scotty stainless ankle j.
    Select j.
    Sutter silicone
      metacarpophalangeal j.
    Tamarack flexure j.
    temporomandibular j. (TMJ)
    Virtual hip j.
Joint-Jack finger splint
joker
    j. dissector
    j. elevator
Jomed
    J. Flexmaster stent
    J. peripheral stent
    J. peripheral stent-graft
    J. stent
Jonas
    J. implant
    J. penile prosthesis
Jones
    J. abduction frame
    J. adenoid curette
    J. arm splint
    J. brace
    J. cervical knife
    J. compression cast
    J. dissecting scissors
    J. dressing
    J. forceps
    J. forearm splint
    J. hemostatic forceps
    J. IMA diamond knife
    J. IMA epicardial retractor
    J. IMA forceps
    J. IMA kit
    J. IMA needle holder
    J. IMA scissors
    J. keratome

J. lacrimal canaliculus dilator
J. metacarpal splint
J. nasal splint
J. pin
J. punctum dilator
J. Pyrex tube
J. scissors
J. suspension traction
J. tear duct tube
J. thoracic clamp
J. towel clamp
J. towel forceps
J. traction splint
Joplin toe prosthesis
Jordan
J. canal elevator
J. canal incision knife
J. capsular knife
J. eye implant
J. hook
J. middle ear instrument
J. needle
J. perforating bur
J. stapedectomy knife
J. strut forceps
J. strut-measuring instrument
J. wire loop dilator
Jordan-Day
J.-D. cutting bur
J.-D. dermatome
J.-D. drill
J.-D. fenestration bur
J.-D. polishing bur
Jordan-Rosen
J.-R. curette
J.-R. elevator
Jorgenson
J. dissecting scissors
J. gallbladder scissors
J. retractor
J. thoracic scissors
Joseph
J. angular knife
J. antral perforator
J. bayonet saw
J. bistoury knife
J. button-end knife
J. cervical knife
J. chisel
J. double-edged knife
J. guard
J. hook
J. measuring ruler
J. nasal brace
J. nasal elevator
J. nasal hook
J. nasal knife
J. nasal rasp
J. nasal saw

J. nasal scissors
J. nasal splint
J. periosteal elevator
J. periosteal rasp
J. periosteotome
J. punch
J. saw guide
J. saw protector
J. septal bar
J. septal clamp
J. septal fracture appliance
J. septal frame
J. septal splint
J. serrated scissors
J. sharp skin hook
J. single-prong hook
J. skin hook
J. skin hook retractor
J. tenaculum
J. tenaculum hook
J. urodynamics catheter
J. valve implant
J. wound retractor
Joseph-Maltz saw
Josephson
J. quadpolar mapping electrode
J. quadripolar catheter
J. Tip Arrow QuadPolar electrode
catheter
Jostent
J. coronary stent
J. coronary stent-graft
J. covered stent
J. Grafaster
J. graft stent
J. peripheral stent-graft
J. SelfX nitinol stent
Jostra
J. arterial blood filter
J. cardiotomy reservoir
J. catheter
joule counter
Jousto dropfoot splint, skid orthosis
JoyBags therapeutic heat pack
**Joyce-Loebl Magiscan image analysis
system**
J periosteal elevator
JR
Judkins right
JR catheter
JR4
Judkins right 4
JR5
Judkins right 5
Jr.
EpiPen Jr.
JR4, JR5 catheter
J-scope esophagoscope

J-shaped
 J-s. endoscope
 J-s. I&A cannula
 J-s. irrigating/aspirating cannula
 J-s. pacemaker electrode
 J-s. tube
JSM-54 IOLV microscope
JSM-6400 scanning electron microscope
JS Quick-fill system
J-tip guidewire
J-tipped
 J-t. guidewire
 J-t. wire
Jubileum 2.0 single-use gastroesophageal pH probe
Judd
 J. cannula
 J. clamp
 J. cystoscope
 J. forceps
 J. strabismus forceps
 J. suture forceps
 J. trocar
 J. urethroscope
Judd-Allis
 J.-A. clamp
 J.-A. intestinal forceps
 J.-A. intestinal retractor
 J.-A. tissue forceps
Judet
 J. dissector
 J. hip prosthesis
 J. impactor for acetabular component
 J. impactor for acetabular cup
 J. strut
Judkins
 J. catheter
 J. coronary catheter
 J. curve LAD catheter
 J. curve LCX catheter
 J. curve STD catheter
 J. 4 diagnostic catheter
 J. guiding catheter
 J. left (JL)
 J. left 4 (JL4)
 J. left 5 (JL5)
 J. left catheter
 J. left coronary catheter
 J. pigtail left ventriculography catheter
 J. right (JR)
 J. right 4 (JR4)
 J. right 5 (JR5)
 J. right coronary catheter
 J. torque-control catheter
 J. USCI catheter

Judson-Smith manipulator
Juers
 J. crimper forceps
 J. ear curette
 J. hook
 J. lingual forceps
 J. wire crimper
Juers-Lempert
 J.-L. endaural rongeur
 J.-L. rongeur forceps
jugular venous catheter
Julian
 J. cystoresectoscope
 J. needle holder
 J. splenorenal forceps
 J. thoracic artery forceps
 J. thoracic forceps
Julian-Damian clamp
Julstro Self-Treatment system
jumbo
 j. acetabular cup
 j. biopsy forceps
 j. forceps
junctional pacemaker
junction field-effect transistor
Jung
 J. Autostainer XL
 J. CV 5000 Robotic Coverslipper
 J. microtome knife
Junod boot
Jurgan
 J. pin
 J. pin ball
 J. pin ball pin protector
 J. pin ball system
JustVision diagnostic ultrasound system
Jux-A-Cisor exerciser
juxtaglomerular apparatus
Juzo
 J. brace
 J. hose
 J. Patellaligner brace
 J. shrinker
 J. stocking
 J. support
Juzo-Hostess 2-way stretch compression stocking
J-Vac
 J-V. bulb suction reservoir
 J-V. catheter
 J-V. closed wound drainage system
 J-V. drain
J-wire
 J-w. lead
 safety J-w.

K

K blade
K implant
K 54 lead
K needle
K pack
K pad
K reamer
K root canal file
K stylet
K tube
K wire
K x-ray fluorescence instrument

K2

K2 hemi toe implant system
K2 sensation prosthesis

K-2000 surgical saw blade
K3-7991 Thornton 360-degree arcuate marker
K-37 pediatric arterial blood filter
Kaat II Plus intraaortic balloon pump
Kader

K. fishhook needle
K. intestinal spatula

KAFO

knee-ankle-foot orthosis
Generation II KAFO
GII KAFO
KAFO prosthesis

Kager triangle
Kahler

K. bronchial biopsy forceps
K. bronchoscopic forceps
K. bronchus grasping forceps
K. double-action tip
K. forceps
K. laryngeal biopsy forceps
K. polyp forceps

Kahn

K. cannula
K. scissors
K. tenaculum forceps
K. traction tenaculum
K. trigger cannula
K. uterine cannula
K. uterine dilator

Kainox A+ single-lead ICD lead
Kairos pacemaker
Kaleidoscope chair
Kalginate

K. alginate dressing
K. alginate wound cover
K. calcium alginate wound dressing

Kalish

K. Duredge wire cutter
K. Duredge wire extractor

Kalix flatfoot implant
Kallassy

K. ankle support
K. brace
K. orthosis

Kalman

K. filter
K. occluding forceps
K. tube-occluding forceps

Kalostat dressing
Kalt

K. capsular forceps
K. corneal needle
K. eye needle
K. eye needle holder
K. eye spoon
K. forceps
K. needle holder
K. needle holder clamp
K. vein needle

Kalt-Arruga needle holder
Kaltenborn joint mobilization system
Kaltostat

K. alginate dressing
K. dressing
K. Fortex dressing
K. hydrofiber wound packing
K. rope
K. wound packing dressing
K. wound packing material

Kambin instrumentation
Kamdar microscissors
Kamen-Wilkinson endotracheal tube
Kamerling 1-piece all-PMMA intraocular lens
Kamppeter anomaloscope
Kam Vac suction tube
Kanavel

K. apparatus
K. brain exploring cannula
K. cock-up splint
K. conductor

Kandel stereotactic apparatus
Kaneda

K. anterior scoliosis system
K. anterior spinal instrumentation
K. anterior spinal/scoliosis system
K. anterior spinal system
K. anterior spine stabilizing device
K. distraction device
K. distractor
K. plate

Kaneda *(continued)*
K. rod
K. SR spinal system
K. SR threaded rod system
Kane umbilical cord clamp
Kangaroo
K. enteral feeding pump
K. 200, 324, 330 enteral feeding pump
K. feeding pump
K. gastrostomy feeding tube
K. gastrostomy tube
K. infusion pump
K. pump
K. silicone gastrostomy feeding tube
KangarooWeb abdominal retraction device
Kanpolat
K. CT electrode
K. electrode kit
Kansas
K. City band truss
K. fragment lens forceps
K. University corneal forceps
Kantor
K. circumcision clamp
K. forceps
Kantor-Berci videolaryngoscope
Kantrowitz
K. dressing forceps
K. hemostatic clamp
K. pacemaker
K. thoracic clamp
K. thoracic forceps
K. tissue forceps
Kapandji-Sauvé arthrodesis
Kaplan
K. PenduLaser laser
K. PenduLaser 115 laser system
K. resectoscope
K. tracheostomy needle
Kaplan PenduLaser 115
Kaplan-Simpson InfusaSleeve
Kapp
K. clip
K. forceps
K. microclamp
K. Surgical Instrument prosthetic knee
K. Surgical Instrument surgical knee immobilizer
K. Surgical Instrument total hip calipers
K. Surgical Instrument total knee retractor
Kappa
K. CTD finishing system
K. dual-chamber pacemaker

K. 700, 900 pacemaker
K. 700, 900 pacing system
K. 400-series pacemaker
K. SP lens finishing system
Kapp-Beck
K.-B. bronchial clamp
K.-B. coarctation clamp
K.-B. colon clamp
K.-B. forceps
Kaprelian easy-access tweezers
Kara
K. cataract aspirating cannula
K. cataract needle
Karaya
K. adhesive ileostomy appliance
K. dressing
K. electrode
K. seal ileostomy stomal bag
K. self-adhesive conductive material
Karickhoff
K. diagnostic lens
K. double cannula
K. keratoscope
K. laser lens
Karl
K. Storz Calcutript
K. Storz Calcutript endoscope
K. Storz coagulator
K. Storz D-LIGHT AF autofluorescence system
K. Storz D-Light AF autofluorescence system
K. Storz endoscope
K. Storz flexible endoscope
K. Storz flexible hysteroscope
K. Storz flexible ureteropyeloscope
K. Storz instrumentation
K. Storz light source connector
K. Storz lithotriptor
K. Storz-Lutzeyer lithotriptor
K. Storz pediatric bronchoscopy system
K. Storz reusable multifunction valve trocar take-apart scissors forceps
Karlin
K. cervical microdiscectomy instrument
K. microknife
Karman cannula
Karmen catheter
Karmody
K. vascular spring retractor
K. venous scissors
Karp aortic punch
Kartush
K. Hapex implant system
K. incus strut prosthesis
K. insulated retractor

K. stimulus dissection elevator
K. tympanic membrane patcher
Kasai peritoneal venous shunt
Kasdan retractor
Katena
K. boat hook
K. cannula
K. capsulorrhexis forceps
K. depth gauge
K. double-edged sapphire blade
K. iris spatula
K. MicroFinger tip irrigating chopper
K. product
K. quick switch I/A system
K. ring
K. scleral shield
K. soft IOL cutter
K. speculum
K. trephine
Katzen
K. flap unzipper
K. infusion guidewire
K. infusion wire
K. long balloon dilatation catheter
Katzin
K. corneal transplant scissors
K. scissors
K. trephine
Katzin-Barraquer forceps
Kaufman
K. adapter
K. catheter
K. clip applier
K. ENT forceps
K. III anti-incontinence prosthesis
K. incontinence device
K. kidney clamp
K. male urinary incontinence prosthesis
K. type II retractor
K. type II vitrector
K. vitreophage
KaVo
K. dental handpiece
K. oral surgery system
Kawai capsulorrhexis forceps
Kay
K. aortic anastomosis clamp
K. balloon
K. rhinolaryngeal stroboscope
K. scissors
Kayak hydrophilic guidewire
Kaycel towel
Kaye
K. blepharoplasty scissors
K. facelift scissors
K. fine-dissecting scissors
K. nephrostomy tamponade balloon

K. scissors
K. tamponade balloon catheter
Kay-Shiley
K.-S. disc valve prosthesis
K.-S. heart valve
Kay-Suzuki
K.-S. heart valve
K.-S. prosthesis
Kazanjian
K. action-type osteotome
K. bone-cutting forceps
K. cutting forceps
K. guide
K. nasal hump forceps
K. nasal splint
K. scissors
K. T bar
K. tooth button
KC1 Delta coagulation analyzer
K-Centrum anterior spinal fixation system
KDC-Healthdyne nonfluorescent spotlight
KD chin prosthesis
KDF-2.3
KDF-2.3 intrauterine catheter
KDF-2.3 intrauterine insemination cannula
Keane mobility bed
Kearney
K. side-notch intraocular lens
K. side-notch IOL
K. side-notch lens
Kearns
K. bag catheter
K. bladder dilator
K-edge filter
keel
All Poly Deltafit k.
k. bone punch
Deltafit k.
McNaught k.
Montgomery laryngeal k.
k. stent
Keeler
K. binocular indirect ophthalmoscope
K. camera
K. cryoextractor
K. cryosurgical instrument
K. cryosurgical unit
K. extended round tip forceps
K. fiberoptic headlamp
K. fiberoptic headlight
K. intraocular foreign body grasping forceps
K. intravitreal scissors
K. lamp
K. lancet tip
K. Lightsource stand

K

Keeler *(continued)*
- K. loupe
- K. Magnalite fiberoptic headlamp
- K. Magnalite headlamp
- K. micro round tip
- K. microscissors
- K. micro spear tip
- K. panoramic lens
- K. panoramic loupe
- K. panoramic surgical telescope
- K. pantoscope
- K. prism
- K. prosthesis
- K. Pulsair noncontact tonometer
- K. Pulsair tonometer
- K. puncture tip
- K. razor tip
- K. retinoscope
- K. retractable blade
- K. ruby knife
- K. specular microscope
- K. spotlight lens loupe
- K. Tearscope
- K. triple facet tip
- K. ultrasonic cataract removal lancet
- K. video headlamp
- K. wide-angle lens loupe

Keeler-Amoils
- K.-A. curved cataract probe
- K.-A. glaucoma probe
- K.-A. long-shank retinal probe
- K.-A. microcurved cataract probe
- K.-A. ophthalmic cryosystem
- K.-A. ophthalmic long-shank probe
- K.-A. ophthalmic Machemer retinal probe
- K.-A. ophthalmic straight cataract probe
- K.-A. ophthalmic vitreous probe

Keeler-Galilean surgical loupe

Keeler-Konan Specular microscope

Keene
- K. compression hook
- K. obturator

Keen Edge disposable biopsy forceps

keeper
- line k.

Keeper vena cava filter

Kegelcisor

Kegel perineometer

Kehr
- K. gallbladder tube
- K. T tube

Keith
- K. abdominal needle
- K. drain
- K. needle

Keithly DAS-500 series data-acquisition system

Keizer-Lancaster lid retractor

Kelikian foot dressing

Kellan
- K. capsular sparing system
- K. hydrodissection cannula
- K. sutureless incision blade

Kellen capsulorrhexis marker

Kelling gastroscope

Kelly
- K. abdominal retractor
- K. arterial forceps
- K. clamp
- K. curette
- K. cystoscope
- K. direct-vision adenotome
- K. dressing forceps
- K. endoscope
- K. fistular scissors
- K. forceps
- K. hemostat
- K. hemostatic forceps
- K. inflatable T tube
- K. insufflator
- K. intestinal needle
- K. orifice dilator
- K. ovum forceps
- K. placental forceps
- K. polypus forceps
- K. proctoscope
- K. punch
- K. rectal speculum
- K. sigmoidoscope
- K. sphincter dilator
- K. sphincteroscope
- K. stereotactic system
- K. suture
- K. tissue forceps
- K. tube
- K. urethral forceps
- K. uterine dilator
- K. uterine scissors
- K. uterine tenaculum
- K. uterine tenaculum hook
- K. vulsellum
- K. vulsellum forceps

Kelly-Descemet membrane punch

Kelly-Goerss Compass stereotactic system

Kelly-Gray
- K.-G. uterine curette
- K.-G. uterine forceps

Kelly-Murphy forceps

Kelly-Rankin forceps

Kelman
- K. air cystotome
- K. aspirator
- K. cryoextractor

K. cryophake
K. cryosurgical unit
K. cyclodialysis cannula
K. cystotome knife
K. dipstick
K. double-bladed cystotome
K. Duet phakic lens
K. flexible tripod lens
K. II 3-point fixation rigid tripod intraocular lens
K. implantation forceps
K. intraocular forceps
K. iris retractor
K. irrigating/aspirating unit
K. irrigating handpiece
K. irrigation hook
K. irrigator
K. irrigator forceps
K. knife
K. knife-cannula cystotome
K. knife cystotome
K. manipulator hook
K. Multiflex II intraocular lens
K. Multiflex II lens
K. needle
K. Omnifit intraocular lens
K. PC 27LB CapSul lens
K. phacoemulsification unit
K. Phaco-Emulsifier
K. tip
Kelman-Cavitron I&A unit
Kelman-Mackool flare tip
Kelman-McPherson
K.-M. corneal forceps
K.-M. lens-holding forceps
K.-M. microtying forceps
K.-M. suture forceps
K.-M. suturing forceps
K.-M. tissue forceps
K.-M. tying forceps
Kelsey pile clamp
Kempf internal screw fixation
Ken
K. driver
K. screwdriver
K. sliding nail
Kendall
K. A-V impulse system
K. Company Telfa pad
K. compression stocking
K. double-lumen catheter
K. endotracheal tube cuff
K. Foley catheter
K. McGaw Intelligent pump
K. nasal prongs
K. sequential compression device
K. Ventex wound dressing system
Kendrick extrication device
Kenna Knee Scale

Kennedy
K. bar
K. LAD
K. ligament augmentation device
K. sinus pack
K. spillproof cup
K. vulsellum forceps
Kennerdell
K. bayonet forceps
K. medial orbital retractor
K. muscle hook
K. nerve hook
K. spatula
Kennerdell-Maroon
K.-M. elevator
K.-M. hook
Kenny crutch
Kenny-Howard splint
Kensey rotation atherectomy extrusion
Kent deep surgery forceps
Kenwood
K. finger cot
K. laparotomy sponge
Keofeed
K. enteral feeding bag
K. 500 enteral feeding pump
K. II enteral feeding pump
K. II feeding tube
K. tube
Keracor laser
Keramos ceramic/ceramic total hip system
Kerasoft DuraWave lens
keratectomy scissors
keratinocyte fibroblast coculture system
keratoconus contact lens
Keratograph corneal topography system
keratographer
keratoiridoscope scope
keratolens implant
Keratome
K. excimer laser system
K. II Coherent-Schwind excimer laser
keratome, keratotome
Agnew k.
automated disposable k.
Bard-Parker k.
Beaver k.
k. Beaver blade
Berens partial k.
Castroviejo electro k.
Czermak k.
Draeger modified k.
femtosecond laser k.
filamentary k.
Fink-Rowland k.
Fuchs lancet-type k.
Grieshaber k.

K

keratome *(continued)*
  k. guard
  Guyton-Lundsgaard k.
  HydroBlade k.
  HydroBrush k.
  Jaeger k.
  Jones k.
  Kirby k.
  Kirby-Duredge k.
  Lancaster k.
  Landolt k.
  Lichtenberg k.
  Martinez k.
  McReynolds-Castroviejo k.
  McReynolds pterygium k.
  SatinSlit k.
  Storz k.
  Tri-Beeled trapezoidal k.
  UltraShaper k.
  UniShaper single-use k.
  Wiener k.
keratometer
  Autoref k.
  Bausch & Lomb manual k.
  k. calibrator
  Canon automatic k.
  Canon autorefraction k.
  Haag-Streit k.
  Helmholtz k.
  Humphrey automatic k.
  Javal k.
  k. lens
  manual k.
  Marco manual k.
  Osher surgical k.
  OV-1 surgical k.
  10 SL/O Zeiss k.
  surgical k.
  Terry k.
  Topcon k.
keratomileusis
  laser in situ k. (LASIK)
keratophakia lens
Keratoplast tip
keratoplasty scissors
keratoprosthesis
  Dohlman k.
  Eckardt temporary k.
  Lander wide-field temporary k.
  Phema core-and-skirt k.
keratoscope
  Karickhoff k.
  Klein k.
  Klein self-luminous k.
  Placido k.
  Polack k.
  wire-loop k.
keratotome *(var. of* keratome*)*

Keratron
  K. corneal topographer
  K. scout topographer
  K. Scout topography system
  K. videokeratoscope
KeraVision Intacs intracorneal ring
Kerboull acetabular reinforcement device
Kerlix
  K. bandage
  K. bandage roll
  K. cast pad
  K. cast padding
  K. gauze bandage
  K. laparotomy sponge
  K. MD antimicrobial gauze dressing
  K. MD antimicrobial wound dressing
  K. packing sponge
  K. super sponge
  K. wrap
Kern
  K. bone-holding clamp
  K. bone-holding forceps
Kernan-Jackson bronchoscope
Kern-Lane bone forceps
kerotome
Kerpel bone curette
Kerr
  K. abduction splint
  K. clip applier
  K. electrotorque drill
  K. Endopost
  K. hand drill
  K. K-Flex file
  K. M4 safety handpiece
  K. pulp canal sealer
Kerraboot device
Kerrison
  K. bone punch
  K. bone punch kinesthesiometer
  K. cervical rongeur
  K. forceps
  K. laminectomy punch
  K. lumbar rongeur
  K. mastoid rongeur
  K. microrongeur
  K. retractor
  K. rongeur
Kerrison-Costen rongeur
Kershner
  K. butterfly capsulorrhexis forceps
  K. LASIK flap forceps
  K. LRI marker
  K. reversible eyelid speculum
  K. 1-step micro capsulorhexis forceps

Kesling
    K. appliance
    K. tooth-spacing spring
Kessler
    K. external fixator
    K. fixation device
    K. metacarpal distractor
    K. podiatry rasp
    K. prosthesis
    K. suture
    K. traction frame
Kessler-Kleinert suture
Kestrel disinfector
Ketac
    K. Fil cement
    K. liner
    K. Silver cement
Keuch pupil dilator
Kevlar glove
Kevorkian
    K. curette
    K. endocervical curette
    K. endometrial curette
    K. uterine biopsy forceps
Kevorkian-Younge
    K.-Y. cervical biopsy forceps
    K.-Y. endocervical biopsy curette
    K.-Y. uterine applicator
    K.-Y. uterine biopsy forceps
    K.-Y. uterine curette
key
    Allen-type hex k.
    K. elevator
    K. periosteal elevator
    K. rasp
    ResCue K.
    K. wrist brace
keyboard
    ErgoLogic k.
    Kinesis k.
    wave k.
keyed
    k. filling device
    k. supracondylar plate
Keyes
    K. biopsy instrument
    K. bone-splitting chisel
    K. cutaneous biopsy punch
    K. cutaneous trephine
    K. dermatologic punch
    K. lithotrite
    K. punch
    K. skin punch
    K. vulvar punch
keyhole punch
KeyMed
    K. advanced dilator
    K. advanced esophageal dilator set
    K. automatic reprocessor

    K. disposable variceal injection
      needle
    K. esophageal tube
    K. fiberoptic scope
    K. unit
Keystone
    K. PF analyzer
    K. Plus oxygenator concentrator
    K. splint
K-file
    Mity K-f.
    Nitinol K-f.
K-Fix fixator system
K-Flexofile Batt tip
KF ring
KH-3500 IOL
Khan-Jaeger clamp
Khodadad
    K. clamp
    K. clip
    K. microclamp
    K. microclip
    K. microclip forceps
Khouri hydrodissection cannula
kibisitome cystotome
kick bucket
Kicker
    K. Pavlik harness
    K. Pavlik harness hip abduction
      brace
Kidd
    K. cystoscope
    K. trocar
    K. U tube
Kidde
    K. apparatus
    K. nebulizer
    K. tourniquet
    K. tourniquet cuff
    K. tubal insufflator
    K. uterine cannula
Kid glove
Kid-Kart wheelchair
kidney
    Ask-Upmark k.
    k. elevating forceps
    Gambro Lundia Minor artificial k.
    Goldblatt k.
    k. internal splint
    k. internal splint/stent
    k. internal splint/stent catheter
    k. internal stent
    k. internal stent catheter
    k. pedicle clamp
    k. pedicle forceps
    k. punch
    k. retractor
    k. stone forceps
    k. suturing needle

K

KidneyScreen
 K. At·Home mail-in test
 K. At·Home testing kit
Kielland forceps
Kiene bone tamp
Killian
 K. antral cannula
 K. cutting forceps tip
 K. dissector
 K. double articulated forceps tip
 K. frontal sinus chisel
 K. gouge
 K. laryngeal spatula
 K. nasal cannula
 K. nasal speculum
 K. probe
 K. rectal speculum
 K. septal compression forceps
 K. septal elevator
 K. septal speculum
 K. suspension gallows apparatus
 K. tonsillar knife
 K. tube
Killian-Lynch suspension laryngoscope
Kilner
 K. chisel
 K. elevator
 K. goiter hook
 K. hook
 K. malar lever
 K. nasal retractor
 K. needle holder
 K. sharp hook
 K. skin hook
 K. skin hook retractor
 K. suture carrier
Kilner-Dott mouthgag
kiloelectron volt
Kilp lens
KilRoid single-handed ligator
Kimba disc implant
Kimball
 K. catheter
 K. nephrostomy hook
Kim Care contour brief
Kim-Ray Greenfield vena cava filter
Kimura
 K. cartilage graft
 K. platinum spatula
Kimwipes wipe
KinAir
 K. bed
 K. III, TC low-air-loss bed
 K. IV mattress
Kinamed
 K. anthropometric total hip
 K. Exact-Fit ATH system

Kin-Con
 K.-C. device
 K.-C. isokinetic exercise system
Kinder Design pedo forceps
Kindt
 K. arterial clamp
 K. carotid artery clamp
Kinematic
 K. facebow
 K. II condylar and stabilizer total knee system
 K. II rotating-hinge knee system
 K. II rotating-hinge total knee prosthesis
 K. rotating hinge
 K. rotating-hinge total knee
 K. rotation hinge
Kinemax
 K. modular condylar and stabilizer total knee system
 K. Plus knee prosthesis
 K. Plus total knee system
 K. removable fixation peg
 K. spacer
kinescope
kinesiological electromyogram
Kinesis
 K. keyboard
 K. reagent kit
kinestatic charge detector
kinesthesiometer
 Kerrison bone punch k.
Kinetec
 K. clubfoot CPM exerciser
 K. hip CPM machine
kinetic
 k. continuous passive motion device
 k. microplate reader
 K. Muscles, Inc. (KMI)
 k. rehabilitation device
 K. Wedge molded insole
 K. Wedge orthotic
Kinetik
 K. great toe implant
 K. great toe implant system
Kinetikos joint implant
KinetiX
 K. instrument
 K. ventilation monitor
Kinetron muscle strengthening apparatus
King
 K. adenoidal punch
 K. bioptome
 K. cardiac bioptome
 K. cardiac device
 K. cervical brace
 K. clamp

K. connector adapter
K. corneal trephine
K. double umbrella closure system
K. fluff rolls and sponge
K. guiding catheter
K. of Hearts AF recorder
K. of Hearts event recorder
K. of Hearts Express AF recorder
K. of Hearts Express recorder
K. of Hearts Express 3X cardiac event recorder
K. of Hearts Holter monitor
K. of Hearts + recorder
K. interlocking device
K. multipurpose catheter
K. multipurpose coronary graft catheter
K. orbital implant
K. self-retaining goiter retractor
K. suture needle
K. tissue forceps
K. wound forceps
King-Armstrong unit
King-Hurd
K.-H. retractor
K.-H. tonsillar dissector
King-Prince
K.-P. knife
K.-P. muscle forceps
K.-P. recession forceps
Kingsley
K. grasping forceps
K. orthodontic plate
K. splint
K. Steplite foot
kink-resistant peritoneal catheter
Kins
K. all-in-1 cotton brief
K. draw sheet
K. fitted mattress protector
K. liner
K. prefolded flat 100% cotton flannelette diaper
K. pull-on waterproof bloomer
K. pull-on waterproof pant
K. soaker pad
Kirby
K. angulated iris spatula
K. capsular forceps
K. capsule forceps
K. cataract knife
K. corneoscleral forceps
K. curved zonular separator
K. cylindrical zonular separator
K. double-ball separator
K. double-fixation muscle hook
K. eye tissue forceps
K. fixation forceps
K. flat zonular separator

K. hook expressor
K. intracapsular lens expressor
K. intracapsular lens forceps
K. intracapsular lens loupe
K. intracapsular lens spoon
K. intraocular lens loupe
K. iris forceps
K. keratome
K. lens dislocator
K. lid retractor
K. muscle hook
K. refractor
K. scissors
K. tissue forceps
Kirby-Duredge
K.-D. keratome
K.-D. knife
Kirchner retractor
Kirk
K. bone hammer
K. mallet
K. orthopaedic hammer
Kirkland
K. cement
K. cement dressing
K. curette
K. instrument
K. knife
K. periodontal pack
K. retractor
Kirklin
K. atrial retractor
K. fence
K. sternal awl
Kirsch
K. laser
K. stapling device
Kirschenbaum
K. foot positioner
K. retractor
Kirschner
K. abdominal retractor
K. apparatus
K. bone drill
K. boring wire
K. device
K. extension bow
K. femoral canal plug
K. guiding probe
K. hip replacement system
K. II-C shoulder system
K. II-C shoulder system stem
K. integrated shoulder system
K. interlocking intramedullary nail
K. Medical Dimension hip replacement system
K. pin fixation
K. skeletal traction
K. stem

Kirschner *(continued)*
  K. surgical instrument
  K. suture
  K. tightener
  K. total shoulder prosthesis
  K. traction apparatus
  K. traction bow nut
  K. Universal self-centering captive-head bipolar component
  K. wire (K-wire)
  K. wire cutter
  K. wire drill
  K. wire fixation
  K. wire inserter
  K. wire pin
  K. wire splint
  K. wire spreader
  K. wire tightener
  K. wire traction
  K. wire traction bow
  K. wire tractor
Kish
  K. urethral illuminated catheter
  K. urethral illuminated catheter set
Kishi lens
kissing balloon
Kistler force platform
Kistner
  K. speaking valve
  K. tracheal button
kit
  Abbott HCV EIA 2nd generation k.
  Abbott HCV 2.0 test k.
  ABI Prism Dye Terminator Cycle Sequencing Ready Reaction K.
  A1c At·Home testing k.
  Ace bone screw tacking k.
  active total PSA ELISA k.
  AeroGear asthma action k.
  AlaBLOT k.
  Alpha suction attachment block k.
  Amersham Life Science PCR product presequencing k.
  Amersham Life Science Thermo Sequenase sequencing k.
  Amplicor HIV-1 test k.
  Amplicor PCR k.
  Amplicor typing k.
  AnemiaPro Self-Screening K.
  Apdyne phenol applicator k.
  ApopTag Plus k.
  ARROWgard Blue Plus multilumen central venous catheter k.
  Arrow pneumothorax k.
  Ascensia Breeze testing k.
  Ascension RADFx proximal radium fixation k.
  A·S·KMerit safety access k.

Asserachrom D-dimer k.
Assess esophageal testing k.
AsthmaPACK personal asthma care k.
AutoDELFIA PRL molecule k.
AutoDELFIA unconjugated E3 k.
Babystart fertility test k.
Banyan emergency k.
Bard-Stiegmann-Goff variceal ligation k.
Bayer Versant HCV RNA 2.0 assay test k.
BCA-1 protein assay k.
BD-CHEK intestinal inflammation k.
Bergland-Warshawski phaco/cortex k.
BFO K.
Bindazyme ANA screening ELISA k.
Bio-Dermal Hydrogel k.
Bioshaf automated 1-step fertility k.
BioSource Cytoscreen SAA k.
Biotene Dry Mouth K.
BiPort hemostasis introducer sheath k.
Boehringer k.
Boehringer Mannheim DIG-nucleic detection k.
Boehringer Mannheim DIG-oligonucleotide tailing k.
bone fixation k.
Brimms Quik-Fix denture repair k.
brush biopsy k.
cake mix k.
Camino OLM intracranial pressure monitoring k.
Camino postcraniotomy subdural pressure monitoring k.
Carey-Coons biliary endoprosthesis k.
carpal tunnel surgery relief k.
CAS DNA staining k.
Cavilon diabetes foot care k.
Cell Proliferation k.
Centocor CA 125 radioimmunoassay k.
CEP 12 SpectrumOrange DNA probe k.
CEP X, Y SpectrumOrange DNA probe k.
cervical block k.
chemiluminescent substrate k.
Circulon System Step 1, 2 venous ulcer k.
clear PVC tube and connector k.
CloseSure procedure k.
Cloward anterior fusion k.

Cloward PLIF II k.
Cloward posterior lumbar interbody
  fusion k.
Coat-A-Count neonatal 17
  hydroxyprogesterone k.
Codman IMA k.
Coloplast deluxe irrigation k.
Coloplast irrigation k.
combination cone/tube irrigator k.
Concept CTS Relief K.
Confide HIV test k.
ConQuest male continence system
  leg bag k.
contour defect molding k.
Corzyme k.
CPAP k.
CTS Relief k.
Cyfra 21-1 IRMA k.
DakoCytomation EGFR pharmDx
  colorectal cancer diagnostic k.
Dako large volume LSAB2
  alkaline phosphatase k.
Davol sterile female
  catheterization k.
Debut ear piercing k.
Dentifix home denture repair k.
Denver percutaneous access k.
Denver Pleurx pleural catheter/home
  drainage k.
diabetic orthosis k.
Diatest diabetes breath test k.
Digital Care k.
Directigen Flu A + B test k.
DNA labeling k.
DNA polymerase assay k.
DNAzol k.
Dr. Joseph's diabetic foot k.
dye terminator cycle sequencing
  core k.
DynaPak electrode k.
EIA k.
Elastafit tubing k.
Elbow Injury Management K.
Enteryx GERD procedure k.
ERx avulsed tooth k.
Euro-Collins multiorgan
  perfusion k.
Exerball k.
extended wear self-adhering urinary
  external catheter starter k.
Extract-N-Amp Blood PCR k.
EZ Detect colorectal screening
  test k.
E-Z mount disinfectant k.
FastPrep DNA k.
Fergus percutaneous introducer k.
Ferritin IRMA k.
FertilMARQ home diagnostic
  screening test k.

FertilMARQ male fertility screening
  test k.
Fillauer Scottish Rite orthosis k.
First Check Ecstasy test k.
Fix and Perm permeabilizing k.
Flexiflo Inverta-PEG gastrostomy k.
Flexiflo Lap G laparoscopic
  gastrostomy k.
Flexiflo Lap J laparoscopic
  jejunostomy k.
Flexiflo over-the-guidewire
  gastrostomy k.
FlexSure in-office rapid serology
  test k.
Fluorognost HIV-1 IFA assay k.
Fome-Cuf laser k.
Freedom T-tap leg bag k.
Fresenius Euro-Collins k.
Gastrin RIA k. II
GastroPanel assay k.
Gene Clean II k.
GenePhor DNA silver staining k.
Gen-Probe hybridization k.
GenSpin gDNA purification k.
Gentra Systems Puregene DNA
  isolation k.
genuine sheepskin crutches
  accessory k.
GFXTM Genomic blood DNA
  purification k.
Glick hip k.
Glove-n-Gel amniotomy k.
Glucatell beta-glucagon blood
  test k.
Great Smokies Diagnostic
  Laboratories intestinal permeability
  test k.
Hall Osteon drill system k.
Hall Osteon irrigation k.
Handi-Cath catheter k.
Hashizume endoscopic ligator k.
Heartport Quickdraw venous
  cannula k.
Helisal Rapid Blood diagnostic k.
HercepTest IHC k.
HerpeSelect type specific IgG
  antibody detection k.
Heyer-Schulte silicone k.
High Pure PCR product
  purification k.
High Pure PCR template
  preparation k.
Histofine SAB k.
Histofine SAB-PO k.
Histofine SAB-PO
  immunohistochemical staining k.
Histofine SAB-PO(M) detector k.
Histofreezer cryosurgical wart
  treatment k.

K

kit *(continued)*

Human-CFSE Flow k.
human IFN-y quantikine ELISA k.
Hybritech Tandem-R assay k.
Hy-Gene seminal fluid collection k.
hysterectomy k.
I&A k.
ICTP RIA k.
I-Flow nerve block infusion k.
IgA II-HA assay test k.
IgM II-HA assay test k.
ImmunoDOT Mono G, M test k.
immunofluorescent assay k.
Immunotech immunoassay k.
InPouch TV subculture k.
InSite Her-2/neu k.
Invitrogen TA cloning k.
Isletest ICA k.
Jackson-Pratt flat drain k.
Jackson-Pratt hysterectomy k.
Jackson-Pratt large-volume round
    silicone drain k.
Jackson-Pratt PVC k.
Jones IMA k.
Kanpolat electrode k.
KidneyScreen At·Home testing k.
Kinesis reagent k.
Lacrimedics occlusion starter k.
Laitinen high-precision stereotactic-
    assisted radiation therapy k.
Laitinen percutaneous tumor
    biopsy k.
Lang jet adjustor k.
Laserscope discography k.
latex tube and connector k.
Leukotape P combo pack taping k.
Lingeman k.
LUA ELISA test k.
Male FactorPak seminal fluid
    collection k.
Malis brain retractor k.
Mallinckrodt Ultra tag labeling k.
manual CD4 k.
MarBlot test k.
Marlen biliary drainage k.
Massachusetts Vision K.
Master K.
McGhan fill k.
MDI k.
MediCordz rehabilitation k.
MediCordz tubing k.
Melastatin test k.
Merit final flexion k.
MERmaid DNA k.
MERmaid-Spin k.
Metra PS procedure k.
microbicinchoninic acid protein
    assay k.
Micro E irrigation k.

Micro 100 irrigation k.
modular temPPTthotic k.
Moss G-tube PEG k.
neonatal internal jugular
    puncture k.
nerve agent antidote k.
nerve block infusion k.
Nichols IRMA k.
nitrite-thiosulfate k.
No Pour Pak II suction
    catheter k.
No Pour Pak suction catheter k.
OctreoScan k.
Oncor ApopTaq k.
OneTouch Fast Take meter k.
Ortho diaphragm k.
Osteo-Lock endodontic
    stabilization k.
OsteoSet resorbable bead k.
ototome irrigation k.
Otovent autoinflation k.
Ott/Mayo Channel Sampling k.
Oval-8 k.
OvuQuick One-Step ovulation k.
palmar swab k.
parallel pin k.
PathVysion HER-2 DNA probe k.
PAXgene Blood RNA k.
PB-FOxS pediatric femoral
    sensor k.
peel-away sheath cystostomy k.
pelvic reconstruction k.
Percufix catheter cuff k.
percutaneous access k.
percutaneous catheter introducer k.
Per-fit percutaneous tracheostomy k.
PeriVac pericardiocentesis k.
Perkin Elmer rhodamine dye
    terminator k.
PICC k.
PicoGreen dsDNA Quantitation K.
PICP RIA k.
Pierce Micro BCA Assay k.
Pleurx home drainage k.
Pleurx pleural catheter k.
Pleurx pleural catheter/home
    drainage k.
Pneumotest k.
Ponsky pull PEG standard k.
Portex Per-fit tracheostomy k.
Posey bar k.
PowerPlex 1.2 genetic
    identification k.
Predicta TGF-β1 k.
Prep-IM hip bone preparation k.
propHiler urinary pH testing k.
Pros-Check k.
ProteinChip antibody capture k.
Pro-Vent ABG k.

Pro-Vent arterial blood gas k.
Pro-Vent arterial blood sampling k.
PSA IRMA k.
Pulsator dry heparin arterial blood gas k.
Pulse-Pak infusion k.
Puregene DNA isolation k.
PyloriTek *Helicobacter pylori* test k.
QIAamp DNA blood biorobot k.
QIAamp Tissue k.
Qiagen QIAquick gel extraction k.
QIAmp tissue k.
QIAquick PCR 96 purification k.
Quanta Lite ANA ELISA test k.
Quanta Lite CCP ELISA k.
Quanta Lite ELISA autoimmune k.
Quantikine ELISA k.
Quickdraw venous cannula k.
QuickVue *H. pylori* gII test k.
RADFx proximal radium fixation k.
Radifocus introducer B k.
radioimmunoassay k.
Random Primed DNA Labeling k.
Redquant k.
Refrax corneal repair k.
resistive chair exercise k.
Reversecell Ag k.
RIA k.
RLP-Cholesterol Immunoseparation Assay k.
RNA PCR core k.
RNeasy Maxi k.
RNeasy Mini k.
Roche Z gel k.
Russell gastrostomy k.
Sacks-Vine gastrostomy k.
SAFE k.
sensory stimulation k.
Serodia commercial k.
Set-Op myringotomy k.
Shearing cortex suction k.
Shiley distention k.
Shofu porcelain stain k.
shunt k.
Sigma TMB assay k.
Sims Per-fit percutaneous tracheostomy k.
in situ valve-cutter k.
Skin Care k.
Staclot protein S test k.
STA Liatest D-DI coagulation/inflammation test k.
Staller k.
Starlite endodontic implant starter k.
Steigmann-Goff endoscopic ligator k.

stereotactic-assisted radiation therapy k.
Stomate low-profile gastrostomy k.
StoneRisk diagnostic monitoring k.
Sub-4 Platinum Plus wire k.
Tacticon peripheral neuropathy k.
Tago diagnostic k.
Takara Biomedicals One-Step RNA PCR k.
Tandem-R assay k.
Taq DyeDeoxy Terminator Cycle Sequencing k.
Taq Master Mix k.
Taub minute stain k.
TCI OcuLook saliva ovulation tester k.
Tearscope Plus tear film k.
thermodilution catheter introducer k.
Tisseel VH k.
Toomey syringe k.
TriPort hemostasis introducer sheath k.
True test k.
TruKor site preparation k.
tuboplasty surgical k.
UltraTag RBC k.
Universal ISH detection k.
Unna-Flex Plus venous ulcer k.
ureteral brush biopsy k.
Uri-Kit culture k.
Uri-Three urine culture k.
UroVision bladder cancer recurrence k.
UroVysion bladder cancer k.
UroVysion test k.
Vari-Lase endovenous laser procedure k.
vascular access safety k.
Vectastain Elite ABC k.
Ventana alkaline phosphatase blue detection k.
VersaFlex tubing k.
Versa-PEG gastrostomy k.
Vesica percutaneous bladder neck suspension k.
Vesica Sling k.
Vidas Estradiol II assay k.
Vielle menopause home test k.
Vitros HBsAg confirmatory k.
Vitros Immunodiagnostic Products HBsAg Confirmatory K.
Wako NEFA test k.
Wilson-Cook feeding tube k.
Xomed sinus irrigation k.
Xpouch emergency k.
Xtrax DNA commercial extraction k.

K

kit *(continued)*
    You-Bend hemodialysis
      catheterization k.
    ZstatFlu test k.
Kitchen postpartum gauze packer
Kit-Green
Kittner blunt dissector
Kjelland
    K. blade
    K. forceps
    K. obstetrical forceps
Klatskin needle
Klearway oral appliance
Klebanoff
    K. common duct bougie
    K. common duct sound
    K. gallstone scoop
Kleen Needle system
KleenSpec
    K. disposable anoscope
    K. disposable laryngoscope
    K. disposable vaginal speculum
    K. fiberoptic disposable
      sigmoidoscope
    K. forceps
    K. otoscope adapter
Klein
    K. cannula
    K. cannula tip
    K. curved cannula
    K. Delrin Luer-Lok handle
    K. 1-hole infiltrator tip
    K. infiltration needle
    K. infiltrator
    K. keratoscope
    K. multihole infiltrator tip
    K. pump
    K. punch
    K. self-luminous keratoscope
    K. transseptal introducer sheath
    K. ventilation tube
Kleinert-Kutz
    K.-K. bone cutter
    K.-K. bone-cutting forceps
    K.-K. bone file
    K.-K. bone rongeur
    K.-K. clamp
    K.-K. clamp approximator
    K.-K. dissector
    K.-K. elevator
    K.-K. hook retractor
    K.-K. microclip
    K.-K. rasp
    K.-K. rongeur forceps
    K.-K. skin hook
    K.-K. synovectomy rongeur
    K.-K. tendon forceps
    K.-K. tendon-passing forceps

    K.-K. tendon retriever
    K.-K. tendon-retrieving forceps
Kleinert-Ragnell retractor
Kleinert splint
Kleinsasser
    K. anterior commissure
      laryngoscope
    K. hook
    K. knife
    K. lens loupe
    K. microlaryngeal scissors
    K. operating laryngoscope
    K. probe
    K. retractor
Klemm nail
Klenzak
    K. brace
    K. double-channeled ankle joint
    K. double-upright splint
    K. knee joint
Kleppinger bipolar forceps
Kling
    K. adhesive dressing
    K. bandage
    K. fluff roll
    K. gauze
    K. gauze bandage
    K. gauze dressing
    K. sponge
    K. wrap
Klippel retractor set
Kloehn
    K. facebow
    K. headgear
Kloti radiofrequency diathermy needle
**KLS-Martin modular osteosynthesis
  system**
Klutch denture adhesive
KM-1 breast pump
KMI
    Kinetic Muscles, Inc.
    KMI 60 enteral feeding pump
KMP
    KMP femoral stem
    KMP femoral stem prosthesis
Knapp
    K. blade
    K. cataract knife
    K. cataract spoon
    K. cyclodialysis spatula
    K. cystotome
    K. eye speculum
    K. forceps
    K. iris hook
    K. iris knife
    K. iris knife needle
    K. iris probe
    K. iris repositor
    K. iris scissors

K. iris spatula
K. knife needle
K. lacrimal sac retractor
K. lens loop
K. lens loupe
K. lens scoop
K. lens spoon
K. refractor
K. scoop
K. strabismus scissors
K. trachoma forceps

knavel table
Knead-A-Ball exerciser
knee

anatomic modular k.
k. arthrography bolster
Axiom total k.
Biomet Ascent total k.
k. bolster
k. brace splint
Brodie k.
cadaveric k.
k. cage brace
Continuum P/S total k.
DePuy LCS mobile-bearing k.
k. extension orthosis
Genesis unicompartmental k.
GeoFlex k.
Gustilo-Kyle total k.
k. height measuring device
Hosmer Endurance k.
Hosmer single-axis friction k.
Hosmer single-axis locking k.
Hosmer weight-activated locking k.
k. immobilizer
k. immobilizer splint
Kapp Surgical Instrument
  prosthetic k.
Kinematic rotating-hinge total k.
Link Endo-Model rotational k.
k. management orthosis
Mauch Swing and Stance
  hydraulic k.
k. MD brace
Miller-Galante unicompartmental k.
Most Options system rotating hinge
  revision k.
Noiles posterior stabilized k.
Noiles rotating hinge k.
k. orthosis
Otto Bock 3R60 EBS k.
Otto Bock 3R80 modular rotary
  hydraulic k.
Otto Bock Safety constant-
  friction k.
Oxford unicompartmental k.
PCA modular total k.
PCA revision total k.
PCA unicompartmental k.

PC Performer k.
K. Pillo
K. Pillo pillow
pneumatic 4-bar linkage k.
PolymerFriction total k.
k. positioner
press-fit condylar total k.
ProAdvantage k.
K. ProMotion overhead pulley
k. rest
k. retractor
k. saver
Seattle safety k.
self-aligning k.
K. Signature System
single-axis friction k.
single-axis locking k.
K. Sleeve knee support
k. sling
k. splint
Stanmore total k.
Total Knee 2100 prosthetic k.
Ultimate k.
USMC stance locking safety k.
variable-axis k.
voluntary control 4-bar k.
k. wedge
weight-activated locking k.
  (WALK)
knee-ankle-foot orthosis (KAFO)
knee-ankle orthosis
kneecap stabilizer
KneeCrank II
Kneed-It knee guard
knee-positioning triangle
KneeRanger hinged knee brace
kneeRAP wrap
knife, pl. knives

Accutome LRI diamond k.
Accutome side-port diamond k.
ACL graft k.
Agnew canaliculus k.
A-K diamond k.
Alcon A-OK crescent k.
Alcon A-OK ShortCut k.
Alcon A-OK slit k.
amputation k.
angled sapphire k.
angular k.
arachnoid k.
Arthro-Knife sheathed
  arthroscopy k.
arthroscopic k.
arthroscopy k.
Asico multiangled diamond k.
Austin k.
backward-cutting k.
Bailey-Glover-O'Neill
  commissurotomy k.

knife *(continued)*

Ballenger nasal k.
Ballenger swivel k.
Bard-Parker k.
Barkan goniotomy k.
Barraquer corneal k.
Barraquer keratoplasty k.
bayonet k.
BD safety k.
Beaver k.
Beaver cataract k.
Beaver Xstar k.
Beer k.
Beer canaliculus k.
Beer cataract k.
Berens cataract k.
Berens glaucoma k.
Berens keratoplasty k.
Berens ptosis k.
Biomet trigger finger release k.
Bircher meniscus k.
Bishop-Harmon k.
bistoury k.
blade k.
k. blade
Blair k.
Braithwaite skin graft k.
BRVO k.
Buck myringotomy k.
button-end k.
C k.
canal k.
canaliculus k.
cartilage k.
cast k.
Castroviejo discission k.
Castroviejo twin k.
cataract k.
Catlin amputating k.
Catlin amputation k.
Celita elite k.
Celita sapphire k.
central retinal vein occlusion k.
cervical cone k.
chalazion k.
circle k.
clasp k.
clear cornea angled CVD
  diamond k.
ClearCut dual-bevel line k.
ClearCut ophthalmic dual-bevel k.
ClearCut SatinSlit k.
Clearpath corneal diamond k.
cleft palate k.
Cobalt k.
Cobbett skin graft k.
cold k.
Collin k.
Collin amputating k.

Collings electrosurgery k.
Converse nasal k.
corneal k.
Cottle double-edged nasal k.
Cottle nasal k.
crescent CVD diamond k.
Crile gasserian ganglion k.
Cronin palate k.
CRVO k.
CVD diamond k.
k. cystotome
Dean capsulotomy k.
Dean iris k.
Dean tonsillar k.
Desmarres k.
Deutschman cataract k.
Diamatrix trapezoidal diamond k.
diamond blade k.
diamond-dusted k.
diamond laser k.
diamond phaco k.
Diamontek k.
diathermy k.
discission k.
dissection k.
k. dissector
dissector k.
DORC illuminated diamond k.
double-edged sickle k.
Down epiphysial k.
Downing cartilage k.
3D stainless steel k.
Duredge k.
Duredge-Paufique k.
ear furuncle k.
EdgeAhead crescent k.
EdgeAhead microsurgical k.
EdgeAhead phaco slit k.
k. electrode
electronic k.
Elschnig cataract k.
Elschnig corneal k.
Elschnig pterygium k.
epiretinal delamination diamond k.
Esmarch plaster k.
eye k.
facial nerve k.
Farrior-McHugh ear k.
Farrior otoplasty k.
Farrior septal cartilage stripper k.
Feaster radial keratotomy k.
Feather k.
Feather clear cornea k.
Fergusson k.
Fine-Gill corneal k.
Fisher tonsillar k.
flap k.
Foerster capsulotomy k.
Fomon double-edge k.

k. and fork
forward-cutting k.
Fowler-Zollner k.
Freedom k.
Freer nasal k.
Freer nasal submucous k.
Freer septal k.
Freiberg cartilage k.
Friesner ear k.
Fugo plasma k.
Gamma K.
Gandhi k.
Gerzog ear k.
Gerzog-Ralks k.
Gill corneal k.
Gill-Fine corneal k.
Gills pop-up arcuate diamond k.
Gills-Welsh k.
gingivectomy k.
Girard-Swan k.
Glasscock-House k.
Goldman-Fox k.
Goldmann serrated k.
goniopuncture k.
goniotomy k.
Goulian k.
Graefe k.
Graefe cataract k.
Graefe cystitome k.
Graefe iris k.
Green cataract k.
Grieshaber ruby k.
Grieshaber ultrasharp k.
Grover meniscus k.
Guyton-Lundsgaard cataract k.
Haab eye k.
Haab scleral resection k.
Halle dural k.
k. handle
Harrison capsular k.
Hartmann k.
hernia k.
hook k.
hooked k.
Hopkins plaster k.
Horsley dural k.
hot k.
Hough incision k.
House ear k.
House lancet k.
House myringoplasty k.
House myringotomy k.
House-Rosen k.
House round k.
House sickle k.
HPC-2 standard needle k.
Huco diamond k.
Hufnagel commissurotomy k.
Huibregtse-Katon needle k.

Humby k.
incision k.
incudostapedial joint k.
Indiana Tome k.
insulated-tip electrosurgical k.
insulation-tipped electrosurgical k.
iris k.
Jacobson vessel k.
Jako laryngeal k.
Johnson evisceration k.
Johnson ptosis k.
Jones cervical k.
Jones IMA diamond k.
Jordan canal incision k.
Jordan capsular k.
Jordan stapedectomy k.
Joseph angular k.
Joseph bistoury k.
Joseph button-end k.
Joseph cervical k.
Joseph double-edged k.
Joseph nasal k.
Jung microtome k.
Keeler ruby k.
Kelman k.
Kelman cystotome k.
Killian tonsillar k.
King-Prince k.
Kirby cataract k.
Kirby-Duredge k.
Kirkland k.
Kleinsasser k.
Knapp cataract k.
Knapp iris k.
Koi diamond k.
Kyle crypt k.
Ladd k.
Lancaster k.
lancet k.
Landolt eye k.
Lange blade k.
Lange cartilage k.
Langenbeck flap k.
Langenbeck resection k.
Lang eye k.
laryngeal k.
Laseredge microsurgical k.
Lebsche sternal k.
Lee cartilage k.
Lee-Cohen k.
Leksell cobalt-60 Gamma K.
Leksell Gamma K.
Leland-Jones tonsillar k.
Leland tonsillar k.
Lempert k.
Liberator k.
ligamentum teres k.
Lillie tonsillar k.
Lindvall-Stille meniscal k.

K

knife *(continued)*

Lister k.
Liston amputating k.
Liston phalangeal k.
Lothrop tonsillar k.
Lowe-Breck cartilage k.
Lowell glaucoma k.
LRI diamond k.
Lucae ear perforation k.
Lundsgaard k.
Lundsgaard-Burch k.
Lynch obtuse angle laryngeal k.
Lynch right-angle k.
Lynch straight k.
Lynch tonsillar k.
Machemer scleral k.
Maltz cartilage k.
margin-finishing k.
Martinez k.
Martinez corneal dissector k.
Maumenee goniotomy k.
Mayo k.
McCabe canal k.
McGee tympanoplasty k.
McHugh facial nerve k.
McHugh flap k.
McKeever cartilage k.
McPherson-Wheeler eye k.
McPherson-Ziegler k.
McReynolds-Castroviejo
  pterygium k.
McReynolds pterygium k.
Mead lancet k.
meniscal k.
meniscectomy k.
meniscus k.
Merrifield k.
metal k.
Meyer Swiss diamond lancet k.
Meyer Swiss diamond mini-
  angled k.
Meyer Swiss diamond wedge k.
Meyhoefer eye k.
microiris k.
micrometer k.
microsurgical k.
Midas Rex k.
Monahan-Lewis k.
Moncorps k.
Murphy plaster k.
myringoplasty k.
myringotomy k.
nasal k.
k. needle
needle k.
Neff meniscus k.
Optima diamond k.
Orandi k.
orthopaedic k.

Oto-Flex diamond k.
paracentesis k.
Parasmillie k.
Paton corneal k.
Paufique corneal k.
Paufique graft k.
Paufique keratoplasty k.
Phaco-4 diamond step k.
pick k.
plaster k.
platelet-shaped k.
Politzer angular ear k.
preset diamond k.
pterygium k.
ptosis k.
pull k.
pulsed electron avalanche k.
quadruple-bladed k.
Quantum enhancement k.
radial keratotomy k.
razor blade k.
Reese ptosis k.
Reiner plaster k.
retrograde k.
retrograde-cutting hook-shaped k.
Rhein Advantage II diamond
  limbal-relaxing incision k.
Rhein clear corneal diamond k.
Rhein 3D angled trapezoid
  diamond k.
right-angle k.
Rizzuti-Spizziri cannula k.
rocker k.
roentgen k.
roller k.
round ruby k.
ruby diamond k.
Salenius meniscus k.
sapphire k.
SatinCrescent implant k.
SatinShortCut implant k.
SatinSlit implant k.
Sato corneal k.
Scheie goniopuncture k.
Schuknecht roller k.
scleral resection k.
sculp k.
Seibel LRI diamond k.
semilunar cartilage k.
septal k.
serrated fine-cutting k.
Sexton ear k.
sharp k.
Sharpoint microsurgical k.
Sheehy-House k.
Sheehy round k.
Shorti limbal relaxing incision
  diamond k.
Shorti LRI diamond k.

sickle k.
side-port fixation k.
Simon fistula k.
skiving k.
slit blade k.
Smillie cartilage k.
Smith k.
Smith cartilage k.
Smith-Green cataract k.
Spizziri cannula k.
spoon k.
k. spud
stapedectomy k.
Stealth DBO freehand diamond k.
Step-Knife diamond blade k.
sternal k.
stiletto k.
stitch-removing k.
Storz cataract k.
straight sapphire k.
straight tympanoplasty k.
Stryker cartilage k.
swift-cut phaco incision k.
SwissBlade diamond surgical k.
SwissBlade disposable surgical k.
swivel k.
sword k.
tendon k.
teres k.
testing drum k.
thermal k.
Thornton triple micrometer k.
tonsillar k.
Tooke angled corneal k.
trapezoid angled CVD diamond k.
triangle-tipped k.
trifacet diamond k.
trigeminal k.
trigger finger release k.
triple-edge diamond-blade k.
Troutman corneal k.
twin k.
tympanoplasty k.
UltraCision ultrasonic k.
Unicat diamond k.
Universal Pathfinder k.
upward-cutting triangular k.
Vaughan abscess k.
vessel k.
Virchow brain k.
Visitec crescent k.
Visitec EdgeAhead phaco slit k.
Visitec stiletto k.
V-lance eye k.
von Graefe cataract k.
Watson k.
Watson skin graft k.
wave-edge k.

Weber k.
Weck k.
Wheeler discission k.
Wilder cystotome k.
X k.
X-Acto k.
X-Acto utility k.
XKnife k.
Yamanda myelotomy k.
Zaldivar k.
ZAP diamond k.
Ziegler k.
Ziegler iris k.

knife/dissector
Morlet lamellar k./d.

knife-needle

knife-pick

Knight
K. biopsy needle
K. bone-cutting forceps
K. brace
K. nasal-cutting forceps
K. nasal scissors
K. nasal septum-cutting forceps
K. polyp forceps
K. septal forceps
K. septum-cutting forceps
K. turbinate forceps

KnightStar 335 respiratory-support system

Knight-Taylor
K.-T. brace
K.-T. and Williams spinal orthosis

Knit-Rite suspension sleeve

knitted
k. Dacron
k. graft
k. sewing ring
k. Teflon prosthesis
k. vascular prosthesis

knives (*pl. of* knife)

knobber
Original Index K. II

Knobble massager

Knodt distraction rod

Knolle
K. anterior chamber irrigating cannula
K. capsular scraper
K. capsular scratcher
K. capsule polisher
K. dipstick
K. lens cortex spatula
K. lens gauge
K. lens implantation forceps
K. lens nucleus spatula
K. lens speculum
K. needle holder

Knolle-Kelman
  K.-K. cannulated cystotome
  K.-K. sharp cystotome
Knolle-Pearce
  K.-P. cannula
  K.-P. irrigating lens loupe
  K.-P. vectis
Knolle-Shepard
  K.-S. lens forceps
  K.-S. lens-holding forceps
knot
  k. pusher
  k. tier
knot-holding forceps
knotter
  Harris k.
knotting forceps
knot-tying instrument
Knowles
  K. bandage scissors
  K. hip pin
  K. pin nail
Knuckle Bender splint
knurled handle
Knutsson penile clamp
Knuttsen bending film
Koala
  K. intrauterine pressure catheter
  K. vascular clamp
  K. vascular insert
Kobak needle
Kobayashi
  K. retractor
  K. vacuum extractor
Koby Isogard surgical treatment system
Koch
  K. chopper
  K. LRI marker
  K. nucleus hydrolysis needle
  K. nucleus manipulator
  K. phaco manipulator
  K. phaco manipulator/splitter
Kocher
  K. arterial forceps
  K. artery forceps
  K. bladder retractor
  K. bladder spatula
  K. blade retractor
  K. bone retractor
  K. brain spoon
  K. bronchocele sound
  K. clamp
  K. depressor
  K. elevator
  K. forceps
  K. gallbladder retractor
  K. goiter director
  K. goiter dissector
  K. grooved director

  K. hemostat
  K. hemostatic forceps
  K. intestinal clamp
  K. kidney elevating forceps
  K. periosteal dissector
  K. periosteal elevator
  K. probe
  K. rasp
  K. retractor
  K. self-retaining goiter retractor
Kocher-Langenbeck retractor
Koch-Minami chopper
Koch-Salz nucleus splitter
Kock
  K. ileal reservoir
  K. nipple
  K. nipple valve
  K. urinary pouch
Kodak
  K. Digital Science 1200, 3600
    distributed medical imager
  K. Digital Science 1200, 3600
    medical imager
  K. Ektachem autoanalyzer
  K. Ektachem DT-60 cholesterol
    analyzer
  K. Ektachem 700 machine
  K. Ektachem Vitros 250, 750, 950
    cholesterol analyzer
  K. Mammography CAD engine
  K. Min-R film
  K. Min-R screen
  K. RP X-OMAT processor
  K. Surecell Chlamydia test
  K. XAR-5 x-ray film
  K. X-Omatic C-1 cassette
  K. XRP-1 x-ray film
Kodel
  K. polyester elbow protector
  K. sling
Kodex drill
Koeberlé forceps
Koeller illumination system
Koelner Vitaport accelerometer
Koenig
  K. elevator
  K. graft
  K. grooved director
  K. metatarsal broach
  K. MPJ implant and arthroplasty
    system
  K. MPJ prosthesis
  K. nail-splitting scissors
  K. probe
  K. rasp
  K. tonsillar swab
  K. total great toe implant
  K. vascular forceps
  K. vein retractor

Koeppe
- K. diagnostic lens
- K. goniolens
- K. gonioscopic lens
- K. intraocular lens implant
- K. lamp

Koerte
- K. gallstone forceps
- K. retractor

Koffler-Hajek
- K.-H. laminectomy rongeur
- K.-H. sphenoidal punch

Kogan
- K. endocervical speculum
- K. endospeculum
- K. endospeculum forceps
- K. urethra speculum

KOH colpotomizer system
Koi diamond knife
Koken nasal stent
KoKo
- K. Moe pulmonary function filter
- K. Rhythm PC-Based ECG
- K. spirometer

Kold
- K. Kompress cold pack
- K. wrap
- K. Wrap cold compression bandage
- K. Wrap freezable compress
- K. Wrap general use sterile burn dressing & emergency wound cover

Kolibri ENT image-guided system
Kollagen dressing
Kolobow membrane lung
Kolodny
- K. clamp
- K. forceps

Komai stereotactic head frame
Komet
- K. K-2000 surgical saw blade
- K. K-wire/Steinman pin and delivery tray system
- K. medical battery tester
- K. Medical/Brasseler USA XK-95 high-speed drill system

Konan
- K. SP-5500 contact specular microscope
- K. SP8000 image analysis system
- K. SP8000 noncontact specular microscope

Konica KFDR-S laser film scanner
Konigsberg
- K. catheter
- K. 5-channel solid-state catheter assembly
- K. microtransducer

Konno bioptome

Konstram angle
Kontes Pellet Pestle disposable microtissue grinder
Kontron
- K. balloon catheter
- K. electrode
- K. intraaortic balloon
- K. intraaortic balloon pump
- K. TFT 45.6 rotor

Koo
- K. foldable intraocular lens cutter
- K. foldable IOL cutter

Kooijman eye model
Kool Kit cold therapy pack
Koolpak cold pack
Kopan needle
Kopans
- K. needle
- K. spring hookwire

Korex cork sheet
koroscope
Kostuik
- K. internal spine fixation system
- K. rod
- K. screw

Kostuik-Harrington
- K.-H. anterior distraction system
- K.-H. device
- K.-H. distraction system
- K.-H. spinal instrumentation

Kotz modular femur and tibia resection
Kowa
- K. angiographic camera
- K. fluorescein system
- K. FM-500 laser flare meter
- K. hand camera
- K. handheld slit-lamp
- K. laser flare-cell photometer
- K. laser flare photometer
- K. Optimed slit-lamp
- K. PRO II retinal camera
- K. RC-XV fundus camera

Koyle diaper stent
Kozlowski tube
KPS bipolar vitallium-polyethylene implant
Krackow
- K. HTO blade staple
- K. suture

Kraff
- K. capsule polisher
- K. capsule polisher curette
- K. cortex cannula
- K. fixation forceps
- K. hyperopic fixation ring
- K. intraocular utility forceps
- K. lens-holding forceps
- K. lens-inserting forceps

Kraff *(continued)*
   K. LRI marker
   K. nucleus lens loupe
   K. nucleus splitter
   K. suturing forceps
   K. tying forceps
Kraff-Utrata
   K.-U. capsulorrhexis forceps
   K.-U. intraocular utility forceps
   K.-U. tear capsulotomy forceps
Kraft forceps
Krahn exophthalmometry
Kramer
   K. direct-vision telescope
   K. ear speculum
   K. forceps
   K. operating laryngoscope
Kramer-Collins spore trap
Kratz
   K. aspirating speculum
   K. capsular scraper
   K. capsular scratcher
   K. capsule polisher
   K. cystotome
   K. diamond-dusted needle
   K. elliptical-style lens
   K. implant
   K. iris push-pull hook
   K. lens-inserting forceps
   K. modified J-loop intraocular lens
   K. polisher/scratcher
   K. posterior chamber intraocular lens
Kratz-Barraquer wire lid speculum
Kratz-Jensen
   K.-J. capsular scratcher
   K.-J. polisher
Krause
   K. angular oval punch
   K. antral trocar
   K. arm rest
   K. biopsy forceps
   K. ear polyp snare
   K. esophagoscopy forceps
   K. laryngeal snare
   K. nasal polyp snare
   K. nasal snare cannula
   K. oval punch tip
   K. punch forceps
   K. punch forceps tip
   K. square basket tip
   K. universal forceps
Krause-Wolfe
   K.-W. graft
   K.-W. implant
   K.-W. prosthesis
Kraus modified
Krayenbuehl
   K. dural hook

   K. nerve hook
   K. vessel hook
KRD L2000 rehab device
Kreiselman
   K. infant warmer
   K. resuscitation unit
   K. unit
Kremer
   K. corneal fixation forceps
   K. excimer laser
   K. 2-point fixation forceps
   K. triple-optical zone corneal marker
Krentz
   K. gastroscope
   K. photogastroscope
Kretz
   K. Combison 330 ultrasound scanner
   K. 311 ultrasound scanner
   K. ultrasound system
Krieger wide-field fundus lens
Krinkle gauze roll
Kristeller
   K. vaginal retractor
   K. vaginal speculum
Kritzinger-Updegraff
   K.-U. corneal marker
   K.-U. manipulator/elevator
Krogh apparatus spirometer
Kromayer lamp
Kron
   K. bile duct dilator
   K. bile duct probe
Kroner apparatus
Kronfeld
   K. eyelid retractor
   K. micropin forceps
   K. pin
   K. refractor
   K. surface electrode
   K. suturing forceps
Krönlein-Berke retractor
Krönlein hemostatic forceps
Kronner
   K. external fixation device
   K. Manipujector
   K. Manipujector uterine manipulator/injector
   K. ring fixation
KR 7000-P cycloplegic refractor
Krukenberg
   K. pigment spindle forceps
   K. sponge
   K. vein
Krumeich-Barraquer
   K.-B. lasitome
   K.-B. microkeratome

Krupin-Denver
  K.-D. eye valve
  K.-D. eye valve-to-disc implant
  K.-D. valve
Krupin eye disc
Krwawicz
  K. cataract cryosurgical instrument
  K. cataract extractor
krypton
  k. laser
  k. laser with Hexascan
  k. red laser
KS 5 ACL brace
KSO brace
K-Sponge II
KT1000 foot stabilizer
KT1000, 2000 knee ligament arthrometer
K-tome microkeratome
KTP
  KTP laser
  KTP laser probe
KTP/532
  KTP/532 laser
  KTP/532 laser system
  KTP/532 surgical laser
  KTP/532 surgical laser system
KTP/Nd:YAG
  KTP/Nd:YAG laser
  KTP/Nd:YAG XP surgical laser system
KTP/YAG
  KTP/YAG laser
  KTP/YAG surgical laser system
K-Tube hypodermic needle tubing
K-U
  K-U corneal marker
  K-U manipulator/elevator
Kuda
  K. endoscope
  K. laparoscope
  K. retractor
  K. shaver
Kudo elbow component
Kuehne coverglass forceps
Kugel
  K. hernia patch
  K. mesh
Kuglen
  K. angled lens manipulator
  K. irrigating lens manipulator
  K. lens manipulator
  K. lens retractor
  K. manipulating iris hook
  K. nucleus manipulator
  K. refractor
  K. retractor
  K. straight lens manipulator

Kuhlman
  K. cervical brace
  K. cervical traction device
Kuhn
  K. endotracheal tube
  K. mask
  K. tube
Kuhn-Bolger
  K.-B. angled curette
  K.-B. frontal recess curette
  K.-B. seeker
Kuhnt
  K. capsular forceps
  K. corneal scarifier
  K. fixation forceps
  K. gouge
  K. postcentral vein
Kulvin-Kalt
  K.-K. iris forceps
  K.-K. mules
Kulzer inlay system
Kumetrix microneedle technology
Kumpe catheter
Küntscher
  K. cloverleaf nail
  K. drill
  K. extractor
  K. femur guide pin
  K. finisher
  K. hammer
  K. impactor
  K. intramedullary nail
  K. nail driver
  K. nail extender
  K. nail-extracting hook
  K. nail instrument
  K. nail set
  K. rod
  K. shaft reamer
  K. traction apparatus
  K. traction device
Küntscher-Hudson brace
Kurer anchor
Kurosaka interference-fit screw
Kurstin flap-stretching forceps
Kurten vein stripper
Kurze
  K. dissecting scissors
  K. dissector
  K. microscissors
  K. pickup forceps
  K. suction-irrigator
  K. suction tube
Kurzweil reading machine
Kuschkin Ace wheelchair
Kushyfoot sock
Kuske breast template
Küstner
  K. suture

K

Küstner *(continued)*
- K. tenaculum
- K. uterine tenaculum forceps

Kuwabara paper

Kuz-Medics disposable knee immobilizer

Kwik
- K. Board IV and arterial line stabilizer
- K. wax

K-wire
- Kirschner wire
- blunt K.-w.
- K.-w. driver
- K.-w. fixation
- percutaneous K.-w.

Kwitko
- K. conjunctival spreader
- K. lens spatula

Kydex
- K. body jacket
- K. brace
- K. chairback orthosis

Kyle
- K. applicator
- K. crypt knife
- K. nasal speculum

kyphosis brace

KyphX
- K. Elevate IBT
- K. Exact IBT
- K. HV-R bone cement
- K. Xpander inflatable bone tamp

K-Y pliers

L
    L 67 lead
    L stylet
L-25 absorbable surgical suture
Labcath catheter
Labophot-2 microscope
laboratory, pl. **laboratories**
    l. automation system
    computerized speech l.
    surgical simulation virtual reality l.
    University of California
        Biomechanics L. (UCBL)
Laborde
    L. forceps
    L. tracheal dilator
Labotect catheter
Labpette FX pipette
LabraFix system
labstation
Labtician oval sleeve
Labtron stethoscope
lace
    no-tie stretch l.
lace-lock ankle splint
lace-on brace
L.A. cervical orthosis
lace-up RocketSoc ankle brace
Lacey
    L. hinge
    L. prosthesis
    L. rotating hinge
    L. total knee implant
LacriCATH
    L. balloon catheter
    L. lacrimal duct catheter
lacrimal
    l. apparatus
    l. awl
    l. balloon catheter
    l. canaliculus dilator
    l. duct probe
    l. duct T tube
    l. intubation probe
    l. irrigating cannula
    l. needle
    l. osteotome
    l. probe
    l. sac bur
    l. sac chisel
    l. sac gouge
    l. sac retractor
    l. sac rongeur
    l. sound
    l. stent
    l. trephine

Lacrimedics occlusion starter kit
Lacrytest
    L. strip
    L. strips
Lact-Aid nursing trainer system
Lactate Pro LT-1710 portable lactate analyzer
Lactina Select breast pump
Lactomer
    L. copolymer absorbable stapler
    L. skin staple material
LactoSorb
    L. craniofacial plate fixation
        system
    L. craniomaxillofacial fixation
        system
    L. orthopaedic wound material
    L. resorbable craniomaxillofacial
        fixation
    L. resorbable fixation device
    L. resorbable fixation system
    L. trauma plating system
LAD
    ligament augmentation device
    LAD composite graft
    Kennedy LAD
LAD-01 ER:YAG lightweight portable laser unit
LADAR 6000 excimer laser
LADARTracker closed-loop tracking system
LADARVision
    L. excimer laser
    L. excimer laser system
    L. 4000 excimer laser system
LADARWave CustomCornea wavefront system
Ladd
    L. band
    L. calipers
    L. elevator
    L. fiberoptic system
    L. intracranial pressure monitor
    L. intracranial pressure sensor
    L. knife
    L. lid clamp
    L. monitor
    L. rasp
ladder
    finger l.
    shoulder l.
Ladmore plastic filling instrument
Lady Dignity Plus pant
Laerdal
    L. infant resuscitator**

L

Laerdal *(continued)*
    L. mask
    L. resuscitator
LaFaci surgical system
Lafayette skinfold calipers
LaForce
    L. adenotome
    L. adenotome blade
    L. golf club knife spud
    L. hemostatic tonsillectome
LAGB
    Lap-Band adjustable gastric band
    LAGB system
LaGrange
    L. eye scissors
    L. scissors
    L. sclerectomy scissors
lag screw
Lahey
    L. aneurysm needle
    L. arterial forceps
    L. bag
    L. bronchial clamp
    L. Carb-Edge scissors
    L. catheter
    L. clamp
    L. Clinic dural hook
    L. Clinic nerve root retractor
    L. Clinic skull trephine
    L. Clinic spinal fusion gouge
    L. Clinic thin osteotome
    L. delicate scissors
    L. dissecting forceps
    L. dissecting scissors
    L. drain
    L. gall duct forceps
    L. goiter retractor
    L. goiter seizing forceps
    L. goiter tenaculum
    L. goiter vulsellum forceps
    L. hemostat
    L. hemostatic forceps
    L. ligature carrier
    L. ligature passer
    L. lock arterial forceps
    L. operating scissors
    L. scissors
    L. thoracic clamp
    L. thoracic forceps
    L. thyroid retractor
    L. thyroid scissors
    L. thyroid tenaculum forceps
    L. thyroid tissue traction forceps
    L. thyroid traction vulsellum
      forceps
    L. Y tube
Lahey-Babcock forceps
Lahey-Péan forceps
Laidley double-catheterizing cystoscope

Laing H-beam nail
LAIS excimer laser
Laitinen
    L. CT guidance system
    L. high-precision stereotactic-assisted
      radiation therapy kit
    L. percutaneous tumor biopsy kit
    L. stereotactic head frame
    L. stereotactic system
Lakeside
    L. cotton roll
    L. nasal scissors
Lalonde
    L. bone clamp
    L. delicate hook forceps
    L. extra-fine skin hook forceps
    L. hook forceps
    L. oblique fracture large bone
      clamp
    L. oblique fracture medium bone
      clamp
    L. oblique metacarpal fracture bone
      clamp
    L. small bone clamp
    L. tendon approximator
Lambda
    L. Omni Stanicor pacemaker
    L. Physik EMG 103 laser
    L. Plus PDL 1, 2 laser system
    L. Plus PDL1, PDL2 laser
Lambert
    L. aortic clamp
    L. chalazion forceps
    L. hook forceps
Lambert-Kay
    L.-K. anastomosis forceps
    L.-K. aortic clamp
    L.-K. vascular clamp
Lambert-Lowman
    L.-L. bone clamp
    L.-L. chisel
Lambone
    L. cortical bone
    L. demineralized laminar bone
    L. freeze-dried bone
Lambotte
    L. bone chisel
    L. bone-holding clamp
    L. bone-holding forceps
    L. bone hook
    L. elevator
    L. exhaust system
    L. fibular forceps
    L. osteotome
    L. rib rasp
lamellar blade
laminar
    l. air flow unit
    l. C-D hook

l. dissector
l. elevator
l. flow hood
l. flow system
l. spreader
laminaria
l. cervical dilator
l. cervical tent
l. seaweed obstetrical cervical dilator
lamina spreader
laminectomy
l. blade
l. chisel
l. frame
l. rasp
l. rongeur
l. self-retaining retractor
l. wedge sponge
LaminOss
L. implant
L. implant system
LAM IPM wound gel
Lamis
L. infusion system
L. patellar clamp
Lamitrode lead
lamp
Aero-Kromayer l.
Alzheimer l.
Birch-Hirschfeld l.
black light fluorescent l.
black ray l.
carbon arc l.
clamp l.
cold quartz l.
cold quartz lamp germicidal l.
CureLight l.
Derma-Wand germicidal l.
Duke-Elder l.
Edridge-Green l.
examining l.
Finsen l.
fluorescent l.
fluorescent sun l.
gas discharge l.
Hague cataract l.
halogen l.
head l.
high-pressure mercury arc l.
hot quartz l.
hot quartz vapor l.
incandescent l.
incandescent endoscope l.
Keeler l.
Koeppe l.
Kromayer l.
mercury arc l.
mercury vapor l.

miniclip l.
mouth l.
narrowband UVB l.
Nightingale examining l.
Philips 100W TL-01 l.
24, 50 Philips 100W TL-01 l.
portable magnifier lab l.
quartz l.
quartz-iodine l.
sigmoidoscope replacement l.
sun l.
Sunnex Tri-Star l.
tungsten-halogen l.
ultraviolet l.
UVA l.
UVB l.
VisionSaver lab l.
V-slit l.
Wood l.
xenon l.
xenon arc l.
xenon flash l.
Lamprey cannula
Lancaster
L. eye magnet
L. eye speculum
L. keratome
L. knife
L. lid speculum
L. ocular transilluminator
L. red-green screen
L. sclerotome
Lancaster-O'Connor
L.-O. forceps
L.-O. speculum
lance
Rolf l.
lancet
l. blade
Cleanlet l.
Genie l.
Haemolance l.
Keeler ultrasonic cataract removal l.
l. knife
laser l.
Lipectron ultrasonic l.
Meyer Swiss diamond knife l.
Microtainer l.
MPD Pro l.
Pharmacia l.
Phazet l.
Quikheel l.
l. suture
suture l.
Swan l.
TechLite l.
ultrasonic l.
ultrasonic cataract-removal l.

L

lancet-shaped
    l.-s. biopsy forceps
    l.-s. electrode
Landau
    L. dilator
    L. speculum
    L. trocar
    L. vaginal retractor
Landeez all-terrain wheelchair
Landers
    L. biconcave lens
    L. contact lens
    L. irrigating vitrectomy ring
    L. sew-on lens
    L. subretinal aspiration cannula
    L. vitrectomy lens forceps
    L. vitrectomy ring
Landers-Foulks
    L.-F. prosthesis
    L.-F. temporary keratoprosthesis
      lens
Lander wide-field temporary
  keratoprosthesis
Landmark midline catheter
LandmarX system
Landolt
    L. cannula
    L. enucleation scissors
    L. eye knife
    L. keratome
    L. spreader
    L. spreading forceps
Landolt-C
    L.-C acuity chart
    L.-C ring
Landry
    L. vein light
    L. vein light venoscope
Lane
    L. bone-holding clamp
    L. bone-holding forceps
    L. bone lever
    L. bone screw
    L. cleft palate needle
    L. dissector
    L. fracture plate
    L. gastroenterostomy catheter
    L. gastroenterostomy clamp
    L. gastrointestinal forceps
    L. intestinal clamp
    L. intestinal forceps
    L. mouthgag
    L. periosteal elevator
    L. periosteal rasp
    L. plate
    L. quick chopper
    L. rectal catheter
    L. retractor
    L. screwdriver

    L. screw-holding forceps
    L. suturing needle
    L. tissue forceps
    L. towel clamp
    L. ureteral meatotomy electrode
Lanex medium screen
Lang
    L. denture duplicator
    L. dissector
    L. eye knife
    L. eye scoop
    L. eye speculum
    L. iris forceps
    L. jet adjustor kit
    L. suture
Lange
    L. antral punch
    L. approximation forceps
    L. blade
    L. blade knife
    L. bone elevator
    L. bone retractor
    L. cartilage knife
    L. fistular hook
    L. hip reduction
    L. mouthgag
    L. plastic surgery hook
    L. skinfold calipers
Lange-Converse nasal root rongeur
Lange-Hohmann
    L.-H. bone lever
    L.-H. bone retractor
Langenbeck
    L. bone-holding forceps
    L. bone saw
    L. flap knife
    L. metacarpal amputation saw
    L. metacarpal saw
    L. needle holder
    L. periosteal elevator
    L. periosteal rasp
    L. periosteal retractor
    L. rasp
    L. resection knife
    L. retractor
    L. saw
Langendorff apparatus
Langer curette
Langerman
    L. bi-directional phaco chopper
    L. bidirectional phaco chopper
    L. diamond knife system
Langston dual-lumen catheter
language acquisition device
Lanier clinical reporting system
Lantiseptic skin protectant
Lanz
    L. endotracheal tube

L. low-pressure cuff endotracheal tube
L. pressure-regulating valve
L. tracheostomy tube

lap
L. Disc hand access device
l. pad
L. Sac
l. tape
L. Vacu-Irrigator

Laparofan
L. pneumoperitoneum device
L. smoke evacuator

laparoflator
Storz L.
Weck High-Flow l.

Laparolift system
LaparoLith
Laparomed
L. cholangiogram device
L. cholangiogram vacuum system
L. suture applier device

LaparoSAC single-use obturator and cannula
laparoscope
ACMI Transvaginal Hydro l.
AMS autoclavable l.
Cabot Medical Corporation diagnostic l.
Cabot Medical Corporation operating l.
Circon ACMI diagnostic l.
Combilight PDD 5133 l.
3D l.
3-Dscope l.
EL2-LS2 flexible video l.
Elmed diagnostic l.
Elmed operating l.
EL2-TF410 l.
flexible video l.
Fujinon diagnostic l.
Hasson l.
Kuda l.
Lent l.
MiniSite l.
Olympus A5256 l.
Olympus diagnostic l.
Olympus operating l.
Richard Wolf Medical Instruments diagnostic l.
Richard Wolf Medical Instruments operating l.
Storz l.
Storz diagnostic l.
Storz operating l.
Surgiview multi use disposable l.
USA Series Distortion Free Hydro l.
Weerda l.
Wolf l.
Wolf insufflation l.

laparoscopic
l. Allis clamp
l. cannula
l. cholangiography catheter
l. Doppler probe
l. grasper
l. insufflator
l. laser
l. needle driver
l. plasma forceps
l. probe
l. retraction system
l. scissors
l. sleeve
l. stapler
l. tie clip
l. ultrasound probe

Laparoshield laparoscopic smoke filtration system
LaparoSonic coagulating shears
Laparostat
laparotomy
l. pad
l. sponge
l. sponge ring

Lap-Band
L.-B. adjustable gastric band (LAGB)
L.-B. adjustable gastric banding system

Lapides
L. catheter
L. collecting bag
L. holder
L. ileostomy bag
L. needle

Lapidus
L. alternating air-pressure mattress
L. bed

Laplace
L. forceps
L. liver retractor
L. mechanism

LaPorta
L. great toe implant
L. total toe prosthesis

lapping tool
Lapras catheter
Lapra-Ty
L.-T. clip
L.-T. suture

Lapro-Clip
LapSac introducer
LAPSE monitor
LapTie
laptop cushion
Lapwall sponge

L

large
l. angled forceps
l. antral cannula
l. ball nerve hook
l. bowel curette
l. callus Podi-Burr
l. Cobra retractor
l. cup forceps
l. egress cannula
l. field-of-view gamma camera
l. nail Podi-Burr
l. nail spicule bur
l. particle sorting module
l. spot slit lamp adapter
l. trapezoid (LT)
l. uterine curette
L. vena cava clamp
large-base quad cane
large-bore
l.-b. angiocatheter
l.-b. aspiration tube
l.-b. bile duct endoprosthesis
l.-b. biliary endoprosthesis
l.-b. cannula
l.-b. catheter
l.-b. chest tube
l.-b. double-pigtail stent
l.-b. heat probe
l.-b. imaging system scanner
l.-b. intravenous line
l.-b. magnet
l.-b. slotted aspirating needle
l.-b. suction catheter
l.-b. trocar
l.-b. Tuohy-Borst side-arm adapter
large-caliber
l.-c. chest tube
l.-c. nonabsorbable suture
l.-c. tube
large-channel
l.-c. endoscope
l.-c. therapeutic duodenoscope
l.-c. video curvilinear
echocndoscope
large-diameter optics intraocular lens
large-loop electrode
large-lumen catheter
large-pore polyethylene implant
larger-caliber cutting needle
large-tip electrode
large-volume
l.-v. round silicone drain
l.-v. suction reservoir
Lark scooter
LaRoe undermining forceps
Larrey
L. bandage
L. dressing

Larry
L. rectal director
L. rectal probe
Larsen
L. tendon forceps
L. tendon-holding forceps
laryngeal
l. applicator
l. applicator forceps
l. atomizer
l. basket forceps
l. biopsy forceps
l. bronchial grasping forceps
l. cannula
l. curette forceps
l. dilator
l. dissector
l. grasping forceps
l. knife
l. knife handle
l. mask
l. mask airway
l. mirror
l. mirror handle
l. probe
l. punch forceps
l. retractor
l. rotation forceps
l. saw
l. scissors
l. snare
l. sponge carrier
l. sponging forceps
l. stent
l. syringe
l. trocar
laryngeal-bronchial telescope
larynges (*pl. of* larynx)
laryngofissure forceps
Laryngoflex reinforced endotracheal tube
laryngoscope
adult l.
Andrews infant l.
anterior commissure l.
Belscope l.
Benjamin binocular l.
Benjamin binocular slimline l.
Benjamin-Lindholm
microsuspension l.
Benjamin pediatric l.
Benjamin pediatric operating l.
Bizzarri-Giuffrida l.
l. blade
Bullard intubating l.
l. chest support holder
Clerf l.
commissure l.
Dedo laser l.

Dedo-Pilling l.
direct l.
disposable l.
dual distal lighted l.
fiberoptic l.
fiberoptic slide l.
Flagg l.
Flexiblade l.
folding l.
Foregger l.
Garfield-Holinger l.
Guedel l.
Guedel-Negus l.
Haslinger l.
Holinger anterior commissure l.
Holinger infant l.
Holinger slotted l.
hook-on folding l.
intubation l.
Jackson anterior commissure l.
Jackson fiberoptic slide l.
Jackson sliding l.
Jako l.
Killian-Lynch suspension l.
KleenSpec disposable l.
Kleinsasser anterior commissure l.
Kleinsasser operating l.
Kramer operating l.
laser l.
Lewy anterior commissure l.
Lewy suspension l.
Lindholm operating l.
Lynch suspension l.
Machida fiberoptic l.
MacIntosh l.
Magill l.
Miller l.
mirror l.
multipurpose l.
Negus l.
Olympus ENF-P2 l.
Olympus ENF-P series l.
optical l.
Ossoff-Karlan l.
pencil-handled l.
Pentax l.
polio l.
l. profilometer
reverse-bevel l.
Riecker-Kleinsasser l.
rigid l.
rotating l.
self-retaining l.
shadow-free l.
Shapshay-Healy l.
Shapshay/Healy phonatory and
  operating l.
Siker mirror l.
sliding l.

slotted l.
standard Jackson l.
Storz-Hopkins l.
Storz infection ventilation l.
straight-blade l.
suspension l.
Tucker anterior commissure l.
Weerda distending operating l.
Welch Allyn l.
Wisconsin l.
Yankauer l.

LaryngoSeal laryngeal mask
laryngostat
Lewy l.
laryngostroboscope
larynx, pl. **larynges**
artificial l.
Cooper-Rand intraoral artificial l.
electronic artificial l.
Nu-Vois artificial l.
TruTone artificial l.
Western Electric artificial l.
Xomed intraoral artificial l.
Lasag contact lens
Laschal
L. precision suture tome
L. scissors
L. suture scissors
LaseAway
Polytec PI L.
L. ruby laser system
L. ruby and Q-switched Nd:YAG
  laser
L. Smooth Touch laser
LASEK
LASEK alcohol well
LASEK alcohol well and epithelial
  trephine
LASEK bow dissector
LASEK epithelial detaching spatula
LASEK epithelial flap repositioning
  spatula
LASEK epithelial micro hoe
laser
AccuLase excimer l.
acupuncture l.
ADD'Stat l.
Aesculap argon ophthalmic l.
Aesculap excimer l.
Aesculap-Meditec excimer l.
alexandrite l. (ALEXlazr)
ALEXlazr l.
Allegretto wave excimer l.
Allergan Humphrey l.
Altea MicroPor l.
AMO YAG 100 l.
Apex Plus excimer l.
ArF excimer l.
argon l.

laser *(continued)*
  argon blue l.
  argon fluoride excimer l.
  argon green l.
  argon ion l.
  argon/krypton l.
  argon-pumped dye l.
  argon-pumped tunable dye l.
  argon tuneable dye l.
  ArthroProbe arthroscopic l.
  Athos l.
  Atlas-Elite l.
  Atlas ophthalmic l.
  Aura desktop l.
  Aurora diode soft tissue l.
  Autonomous Technologies l.
  l. balloon
  biocavity l.
  Biophysic Medical YAG l.
  Britt argon/krypton l.
  Britt argon pulsed l.
  Britt BL-12 l.
  Britt krypton l.
  Candela l.
  Candela Model MDL 2000 l.
  Candela 405-nm pulsed dye l.
  Candela ScleroLaser l.
  Candela SPTL l.
  carbon dioxide l.
  Carl Zeiss YAG l.
  Cavitron l.
  CB Diode/532 l.
  CB Erbium/2.94 l.
  Ceralas I l.
  char-free carbon dioxide l.
  Chromaser dermatology l.
  L. CHRP rigid fiberscope system
  CHRYS CO_2 l.
  Cilco argon l.
  Cilco Frigitronics l.
  Cilco krypton l.
  Cilco YAG l.
  CLR 2940 erbium l.
  CO_2 l.
  Coherent 7910 l.
  Coherent 920 argon/dye l.
  Coherent CO_2 surgical l.
  Coherent 5000C UltraPulse l.
  Coherent EPIC l.
  Coherent Medical YAG l.
  Coherent model 90-K l.
  Coherent Novus Omni
    multiwavelength l.
  Coherent radiation argon/krypton l.
  Coherent radiation argon model
    800 l.
  Coherent Schwind Keraton 2 l.
  Coherent Selecta 7000 l.
  Coherent UltraPulse 5000C l.

  Coherent UltraPulse CO_2 l.
  cold beam l.
  continuous-wave argon l.
  continuous-wave CO_2 l.
  continuous-wave diode l.
  Contour l.
  cool-tip l.
  Cool Touch l.
  CoolTouch Nd:YAG l.
  CoolTouch Varia l.
  Cooper 2000, 2500 l.
  Cooper Laser Sonics l.
  CooperVision argon l.
  CooperVision YAG l.
  copper bromide l.
  copper vapor l.
  copper vapor pulsed l.
  CO_2 Sharplan l.
  coumarin flashlamp pumped pulsed
    dye l.
  CrTmEr:YAG l.
  CTE:YAG l.
  Cynosure long-pulse infrared l.
  da Vinci femtosecond surgical l.
  l. delivery catheter
  dental diode l.
  Derma 20 l.
  Derma K l.
  Derma K combination l.
  Derma K combination Er:YAG &
    CO_2 l.
  l. digitizer
  diode pumped Nd:YAG l.
  diode-pumped solid-state
    photocoagulation l.
  Diomed l.
  Diomed EVLT l.
  Diomed PDT l.
  Diomed surgical diode l.
  l. disc decompression
  l. Doppler flowmeter
  l. Doppler flowmetry probe
  l. Doppler perfusion monitor
  l. Doppler Periflux PF-3 probe
  l. Doppler velocimeter
  Dornier Medilas H holmium:YAG
    endourology l.
  dye l.
  dye yellow l.
  EC-5000 excimer l.
  Eclipse holmium l.
  Eclipse TMR l.
  EndoLase $C0_2$ l.
  endoscopic l.
  Epic ophthalmic 3-in-1 l.
  EpiLaser hair removal l.
  EpiTouch l.
  erbium l.
  erbium CrystaLase l.

erbium resurfacing l.
erbium:YAG l.
erbium:YAG infrared l.
ErCr:YAG l.
Er:YAG l.
esthetic CO_2 l.
EVLT l.
ExciMed UV200 excimer l.
ExciMed UV200LA l.
excimer l.
excimer cool l.
excimer gas l.
excimer ultraviolet l.
L. Extensometer
FeatherTouch CO_2 l.
femtosecond l.
l. fiber
l. fiber director
FiberLase l.
l. flare meter
flashlamp-pulsed dye l.
flashlamp pulsed Nd:YAG l.
flashlamp-pulsed Nd:YAG l.
flashlamp pumped pulsed dye l.
flash pump dye l.
flashscanner-enhanced CO_2 l.
fluorescence-guided smart l.
frequency doubled double pulse
  ND:YAG l.
frequency doubled nd:YAG l.
frequency doubled
  neodymium:yttrium-aluminum-
  garnet l.
FS30 femtosecond l.
l. fume absorber
gallium-aluminum-arsenide 904-
  nm l.
gallium-arsenide l.
gas l.
Genesis 2000 carbon dioxide l.
GentleLASE l.
25 Gold portable CO_2 l.
green pulsed dye l.
l. Heaney needle holder
Heart l.
helium neon l.
helium-neon l.
helium-neon aiming l.
He-Ne l.
Heraeus LaserSonics l.
HF infrared l.
HGM argon green l.
HGM intravitreal l.
HGM ophthalmic l.
HGM Spectrum K1 krypton yellow
  & green l.
high-energy l.
holmium l.
holmium:YAG l.

holmium-yttrium-aluminum-garnet l.
holmium:yttrium-argon-garnet l.
Horn endootoprobe l.
hot l.
hot-tip l.
Ho:YAG l.
Hruby l.
Illumina Pro Series laparoscopic l.
l. imager
Indigo Optima l.
l. indirect ophthalmoscope (LIO)
infrared-beam diode l.
IntraLase FS30 l.
intravitreal l.
ion l.
Iris OcuLight SLx MicroPulse l.
l. Julian needle holder
Kaplan PenduLaser l.
Keracor l.
Keratome II Coherent-Schwind
  excimer l.
Kirsch l.
Kremer excimer l.
krypton l.
krypton red l.
KTP l.
KTP/532 l.
KTP/Nd:YAG l.
KTP/532 surgical l.
KTP/YAG l.
LADAR 6000 excimer l.
LADARVision excimer l.
LAIS excimer l.
Lambda Physik EMG 103 l.
Lambda Plus PDL1, PDL2 l.
l. lancet
L. Lancet laser device
laparoscopic l.
l. laryngoscope
LaseAway ruby and Q-switched
  Nd:YAG l.
LaseAway Smooth Touch l.
Laserex Era 4106 YAG l.
LaserHarmonic l.
Laserscope KTP/532 l.
Lasertek l.
Lastec System angioplasty l.
Lateralase l.
lateral-firing l.
l. lens
Lightlas 532 green l.
LightMed Lpulsa SYL9000 YAG l.
LightShear diode l.
LightSheer l.
LightSheer SC diode l.
Lightstic 180, 360 fiberoptic l.
liquid organic dye l.
Lithognost flashlamp pulsed dye l.
l. lithotriptor

laser *(continued)*

l. lithotriptor basket
long-pulsed dye l.
long-pulsed potassium-titanyl-phosphate l.
low-dose Excimer 308-nm l.
low-energy l.
low-power l.
LPK-80 II argon l.
Lumonics YAG l.
Luxar NovaPulse l.
Luxar NovaPulse CO_2 l.
LX-20 l.
Lyra l.
Mainster retina l.
Maloney endootoprobe l.
MC-7000 multi-wavelength ophthalmic l.
Medilas fiberTome l.
Medilas Nd:YAG surgical l.
Meditech l.
Meditec MEL-60 excimer l.
MedLite Q-switched neodymium-doped yttrium-aluminum-garnet l.
Medpacific LD 5000 l.
MEL 60, 80 excimer l.
MEL 70 flying spot l.
Melles Griot diode l.
MEL 60 scanning l.
Merrimack 1040 CO_2 l.
l. microlaryngeal cup forceps
l. microlaryngeal grasping forceps
Microlase transpupillary diode l.
Microlight 830 l.
Microprobe l.
l. microprobe mass analyzer
Microprobe ophthalmic l.
l. microscope
microsecond pulsed flashlamp pumped dye l.
MicroSpot l.
l. microtome
midinfrared l.
mid-infrared pulsed l.
miniature excimer l.
l. mirror
mode-locked l.
Moeller l.
molectron l.
Molectron Nd:YAG l.
MultiLase D copper vapor l.
MultiLase Nd:YAG surgical l.
Multipulse cosmetic treatment l.
Nanolas Nd:YAG l.
NaturaLase erbium l.
NaturaLase Er:YAG l.
Nd:YAG l.
neodymium l.
neodymium:YAG l.

neodymium:yttrium-aluminum-garnet l.
neodymium:yttrium garnet l.
neodymium:yttrium lithium fluoride l.
neodymium:yttrium-lithium-fluoride photodisruptive l.
New Star model 130 l.
Nidek EC-1000 excimer l.
Nidek EC-5000 excimer l.
Nidek Laser System l.
NLite l.
NLite nonablative l.
NLite wrinkle reduction l.
308-nm Excimer l.
normal-mode ruby l.
NovaLine excimer l.
NovaPulse CO_2 l.
Novatec LightBlade l.
Novus Spectra l.
Nuvolase 660 l.
OcuLight SL l.
OcuLight SL diode l.
OcuLight SLx l.
OcuLight SLx ophthalmic l.
oculocutaneous l.
Olympus Nd:YAG l.
OmniMed argon-fluoride excimer l.
OmniPulse MAX holmium l.
Opal PDT Photoactivator l.
Ophthalas argon l.
Ophthalas argon/krypton l.
Ophthalas krypton l.
Opmilas CO_2 l.
Opmilas CO_2 multipurpose l.
Opmilas 144 surgical l.
l. optometer
Opus 5, 10, 20 dental l.
Opus 20 dental Er:YAG l.
orange dye l.
orthogonal l.
OtoLAM l.
l. ovary forceps
Palomar E2000 l.
Paragon l.
pattern scan l. (PASCAL)
PBI Medical copper vapor l.
PBI MultiLase D copper vapor l.
Pegasus Nd:YAG surgical l.
Pegasus PIV l.
PerioLase l.
photocoagulation l.
l. photocoagulator
PhotoDerm l.
PhotoDerm PL l.
PhotoDerm T 10 l.
PhotoDerm V l.
PhotoDerm VL l.
photodisrupting l.

PhotoGenica LPIR with TKS l.
PhotoGenica T^{10} l.
PhotoGenica V l.
PhotoGenica VLS pulsed dye l.
PhotoGenica V-Star l.
PhotoPoint l.
photovaporizing l.
pigmented lesion dye l.
Polaris 1.32 Nd:YAG l.
Polytec LaseAway Q-switched
  ruby l.
potassium titanyl phosphate l.
potassium-titanyl-phosphate:YAG l.
Prima l.
Prima KTP/532 l.
Prolase II lateral-firing Nd:YAG l.
Prostalase l.
pulsed carbon dioxide l.
pulsed dye l.
pulsed green l.
pulsed metal vapor l.
pulsed tunable dye l.
pulsed yellow dye l.
PulseMaster l.
Pulsion FS l.
Pulsolith l.
pumped dye l.
Q-LAS 10 Q-switched YAG l.
QRS ruby/YAG l.
QS alexandrite l.
Q-switched l.
Q-switched alexandrite l.
Q-switched Er:YAG l.
Q-switched Nd:YAG l.
Q-switched neodymium:YAG l.
Q-switched neodymium:yttrium
  aluminum-garnet l.
Q-switched ruby l.
Q-switched YAG l.
red l.
red-beam l.
Renaissance erbium l.
rhodamine 6G dye l.
l. rod
ruby l.
l. scalpel
scanning excimer l.
ScleroPlus flashlamp-pumped pulsed
  tunable dye l.
Selecta 7000 l.
S4 excimer l.
Sharplan 710 Acuspot l.
Sharplan argon l.
Sharplan CO$_2$ l.
Sharplan/ESC SilkTouch l.
Sharplan Medilas Nd:YAG
  surgical l.
Sharplan SilkTouch flashscan
  surgical l.

Sharplan SilkTouch Flashscan
  surgical l.
SharpLase Nd:YAG l.
short-pulse l.
side-fire l.
Silhouette endoscopic l.
Silk L.
SilkLaser aesthetic CO$_2$ l.
SilkTouch l.
SilkTouch CO$_2$ l.
l. in situ keratomileusis (LASIK)
Skinlight erbium:YAG l.
Skinlight erbium yttrium-aluminum-
  garnet l.
Skinlight Er:YAG l.
SLS l.
SLT contact MTRL l.
SoftLight l.
solid-state dye l.
Spectranetics l.
Spectra-Physics argon l.
Spectra-Physics microsurgical l.
spectroscopy-directed l.
Spectrum K1 l.
Spectrum ruby l.
SPTL-1a l.
SPTL-1b vascular lesion l.
SPTL vascular lesion l.
Star excimer l.
stereotaxic l.
Storz l.
Summit Apex Plus excimer l.
Summit excimer l.
Summit OmniMed excimer l.
Summit SVS Apex l.
Summit UV 200 ExciMed l.
superpulsed l.
Surgica K6 l.
surgical l.
Surgicenter 40 CO$_2$ l.
Surgilase 150 l.
Surgilase CO$_2$ l.
Surgilase 150 high-powered CO$_2$ l.
Surgilase Nd:YAG l.
Surgilase 55W l.
SurgiPulse XJ l.
Surgipulse XJ 150 CO$_2$ l.
l. system
Takata l.
l. taper
Technolas 217 l.
Technolas 217 excimer l.
Technolas 217z excimer l.
TEC-2100 positioning l.
TEMoo mode beam l.
THC:YAG l.
thulium-holmium-chromium:yttrium-
  aluminum-garnet l.
thulium-holmium:YAG l.

L

laser *(continued)*
    Tissue Technologies TruPulse l.
    titanium:sapphire l.
    TKS l.
    Topaz CO_2 l.
    tracker-assisted PRK l.
    transpupillary l.
    l. trap
    Trimedyne holmium l.
    L. Tripter ureteroscope
    TruPulse l.
    TruPulse carbon dioxide l.
    TruPulse CO_2 skin resurfacing l.
    Tsunami l.
    l. tubal scissors
    l. tube
    tunable dye l.
    tunable pulsed-dye l.
    l. tweezers
    TwiLite l.
    UltraFine erbium l.
    UltraLine l.
    Ultraline l.
    UltraPulse l.
    UltraPulse CO_2 l.
    UltraPulse surgical l.
    ultrasound-guided l.
    ultraviolet l.
    Unilase CO_2 l.
    URAM E2 compact MicroProbe l.
    Urolase l.
    Urolase CO_2 l.
    Urolase fiber l.
    Varia l.
    V-beam pulsed dye l.
    V-beam vascular l.
    VersaLight l.
    VersaPulse l.
    VersaPulse holmium l.
    VersaPulse PowerSuite dual-
      wavelength l.
    VersaPulse PowerSuite holmium l.
    VersaPulse Select l.
    VersaPulse variable pulse-width
      green l.
    Viridis pulsed l.
    visual endoscopically controlled l.
    Visulas 532 l.
    Visulas argon C l.
    Visulas argon/YAG l.
    Visulas Combi 532/YAG l.
    Visulas Nd:YAG l.
    Visulas 690s PDT l.
    Visulas 690s photodynamic
      therapy l.
    Visulas YAG C, E, S l.
    Visulas YAG II plus l.
    VisuMed MEL60 l.
    Visx 20/20 excimer l.

    Visx S2, S3 excimer l.
    Visx Star S2 l.
    Visx Star S3 ActiveTrak l.
    VitaLase Er:YAG l.
    Vitesse Cos l.
    white l.
    Wild l.
    Xanar 20 Ambulase CO_2 l.
    XeCl excimer l.
    xenon chloride excimer l.
    YAG l.
    yellow dye l.
    yttrium-aluminum-garnet l.
    Zeiss MD l.
    Zeiss Opmilas surgical l.
    Zeiss Visulas 532, 532s l.
    Zeiss Visulas YAG II l.
    Zyoptix Infinity l.

laser-adjustable lens
laser-assisted
    l.-a. epithelium keratomileusis pump
    l.-a. intrastromal keratomileusis
      cannula
    l.-a. intrastromal keratomileusis
      cannula eye guard
    l.-a. intrastromal keratomileusis flap
      irrigator
Laserdish
    L. electrode
    L. pacing lead
Laseredge microsurgical knife
Laserex Era 4106 YAG laser
Laserflo
    L. BPM laser Doppler monitor
    L. laser Doppler
Laserflow
    L. blood perfusion monitor
    L. BPM^2 real-time cerebral
      perfusion monitor
    L. Doppler probe
LaserHarmonic laser
Laseridge
    Cilco Hoffer L.
    L. Optics lens
laser-induced thermotherapy
LaserLite system
LaserMed laser pointer
LaserPen
Laserphaco probe
Laserprobe catheter
Laserprobe-PLR Plus
LaserScan LSX excimer laser system
Laserscope
    L. discography kit
    L. disposable Endostat fiber
    L. KTP/532 laser
Laserscope KTP 532
Laserscope YAG 1064

Laser-Shield XII wrapped endotracheal tube
Lasersonic ACMI Ultraline
LaserSonics
    L. EndoBlade
    L. Nd:YAG Laserblade scalpel
Lasertek laser
Lasertripter
    Candela MDA-200 L.
Lasertubus tracheal tube
LaserTweezer
Lasette
    L. laser finger perforator
    L. laser lancing device
    Personal L.
    L. Plus assisted blood sampling device
Lash-Loeffler
    L.-L. implant
    L.-L. penile implant material
    L.-L. penile prosthesis
LASIK
    laser in situ keratomileusis
    LASIK aspiration spoon
    Dishler Excimer Laser System for LASIK
    LASIK eye guard
    LASIK eyelid drape
    LASIK flap irrigator
    LASIK flap manipulator
    LASIK spear
lasitome
    Krumeich-Barraquer l.
lasso
    L. catheter
    guidewire/basket l.
    lens l.
    l. snare
Lastec System angioplasty laser
latent pacemaker
lateral
    l. batten
    l. cervical spine film
    l. guide pin
    l. gutter impactor
    l. lumbar support
    l. mass screw
    l. microlens telescope
    l. osteotome
    l. positioner
    l. rotation mattress
    l. spring-loaded lock
    l. trap suture
    l. wall retractor
Lateralase laser
lateral-firing laser
lateral-viewing endoscope
latex
    l. bag

    l. balloon
    l. catheter
    l. cushion
    l. drain
    l. O band
    l. rubber tourniquet strap
    l. sponge graft
    l. tube and connector kit
    l. wheelchair cushion
Latham
    L. appliance
    L. bowl
LaTIS endovascular laser system
Latitude curette
Laufe
    L. aspirating curette
    L. cervical dilator
    L. divergent outlet forceps
    L. obstetrical forceps
    L. portable uterine evacuator
    L. uterine polyp forceps
Laufe-Novak diagnostic curette
Laufe-Piper
    L.-P. forceps
    L.-P. obstetrical forceps
    L.-P. uterine polyp forceps
Laurer forceps
Laurus ND-260 needle driver
lavage
    bone l.
    bronchoalveolar l.
    bronchopulmonary l.
    diagnostic peritoneal l.
    Easi-Lav gastric l.
    Hi Speed Pulse l.
    pulsatile jet l.
    Pulsavac l.
    pulse l.
    Simpulse pulsing l.
    Simpulse S/I l.
    Waterpik l.
lavaging catheter
LaVeen shunt
Lavoisier retractor
Lawford speculum
Lawrence
    L. Add-a-Cath
    L. deep surgery forceps
    L. device
    L. first metatarsophalangeal joint implant
    L. gastric reservoir
    L. hemostatic forceps
Lawson-Thornton plate
Lawton
    L. corneal scissors
    L. forceps
Layden infant lens
4-layer bandage

L

509

LazerSmile
    L. tooth-whitening device
    L. tooth-whitening system
LB 9501 luminometer
L-buttress plate
LC
    LC Plus reusable nebulizer
    LC Star reusable nebulizer
    LC strip
L-Cath peripherally inserted neonatal catheter
LCP
    locking compression plate
    LCP locking compression plate
LCS
    LCS meniscal bearing semiconstrained prosthesis
    LCS mobile bearing knee system
    LCS rotating platform semiconstrained prosthesis
    LCS substituting semiconstrained prosthesis
    LCS total knee system
    LCS total knee system implant
    LCS universal APG semiconstrained prosthesis
LDD delivery system
LDL direct test prefilled cartridge
LD 400 luminescence detector
LDS
    LDS clip applier
    LDS instrument
Le
    Le Bag
    Le Bag urinary pouch
    Le Blond R diamond dental bur
    Le Fort follower
    Le Fort suture
    Le Grand-Gullstrand eye model
Lea
    monosialosyl L.
    L. shield
    L. Symbol chart
lead
    3.3 l.
    Accufix II DEC pacing l.
    Accufix pacemaker l.
    active fixation pacemaker l.
    Aescula left ventricular l.
    Aescula LV l.
    American Pacemaker Corporation l.
    Angeflex defibrillation l.
    l. apron
    Artisan surgical l.
    Attain bipolar over-the-wire l.
    Axxess spinal cord stimulation l.
    barb-tip l.
    bifurcated J-shaped tined atrial pacing and defibrillation l.

Biocontrol Technology/Coratomic l.
Biopore TM l.
Biotronik l.
l. block
l. bra
capped l.
CapSure cardiac pacing l.
CapSureFix l.
CapSure SP l.
CapSure VDD l.
Cardiac Control Systems l.
CCS endocardial pacing l.
Cordis Ancar pacing l.
CPI endocardial defibrillation rate-sensing pacing l.
CPI/Guidant l.
deep brain l.
dual coil transvenous l.
dual octapolar l.
dual quadrapolar l.
Easytrak coronary venous l.
Elwrite pediatric l.
endocardial cardiac l.
Endotak C tripolar transvenous l.
Endotak DSP l.
Endotak Picotip defibrillation l.
Endotak Reliance l.
epicardial l.
l. extraction system
l. eye shield
Fineline II Sterox l.
finned pacemaker l.
fishhook l.
Flextend pacing l.
Flextend steroid-eluting transvenous pace/sense l.
floating l.
Frank XYZ orthogonal l.
l. hand
Hi-Flex l.
high-impedance low-threshold l.
IROX endocardial pacing l.
J-wire l.
K 54 l.
Kainox A+ single-lead ICD l.
L 67 l.
Lamitrode l.
Laserdish pacing l.
left ventricular transvenous l.
Lewis l.
Lifeline l.
limb l.
l. locking device
Low-Flex l.
Medtronic Transvene endocardial l.
microtip l.
modified chest l.
monitor l.
MR l.

myocardial l.
nonintegrated transvenous
  defibrillation l.
octapolar l.
Oscor pacing l.
Osypka atrial l.
over-the-wire pacing l.
Pacesetter/St. Jude l.
Pacesetter Tendril DX steroid-
  eluting active-fixation pacing l.
pediatric l.
l. pellet marker
permanent cardiac pacing l.
Picotip steroid-eluting endocardial l.
l. pin
Pisces l.
l. plate
Polyflex l.
Polyrox Fractal active fixation l.
PolySafe A-track l.
QuickSite LV l.
reversed arm l.
scalar l.
screw-in l.
screw-on l.
segmented ring tripolar l.
Selute Picotip steroid-eluting
  endocardial l.
silicone l.
single-pass l.
Sorin l.
Sprint Model 6942, 6943
  tachyarrhythmia l.
SRT l.
Stelid II pacing l.
Stelix pacing l.
Stop at Ring l.
Stop at Tip l.
l. suture
SVC l.
Sweet Tip bipolar l.
Sweet Tip Rx pacing l.
Synox fractal pacemaker l.
Telectronics Accufix pacing l.
temporary pervenous l.
Tendril DX implantable pacing l.
Tendril DX steroid-eluting active-
  fixation pacing l.
Tendril SDX model 1688 active-
  fixation pacing l.
Terox RV l.
ThinLine EZ bipolar pacemaker l.
ThinLine EZ pacing l.
TIJ l.
transcutaneous l.
transvenous defibrillator l.
tripolar l.
2-turn epicardial l.
3-turn epicardial l.

3-turn epicardial l.
unipolar J-tined passive fixation l.
unipolar precordial l.
Uni-Silicone l.
Wilson l.
l. wire

LeadCare handheld blood lead analyzer
leader
    tendon l.
Leader iris hook
lead-filled mallet
leading bar
lead-rubber apron
leaf
    l. gauge
    l. splint
leaf-spring
    AFO posterior l.-s.
    l.-s. brace
Leahey chalazion forceps
Leander
    L. chiropractic table
    L. motorized flexion table
LEAP
    Lewis expandable adjustable prosthesis
    LEAP collimator
Learning retinal implant system
Lea's shield female barrier
    contraceptive
leather
    l. lacer gauntlet
    l. orthosis
Leatherman
    L. alar hook
    L. compression hook
    L. trochanteric retractor
Leather retrograde valvulotome
Lebensohn chart
Lebsche
    L. forceps
    L. raspy
    L. rongeur
    L. saw guide
    L. shears
    L. sternal chisel
    L. sternal knife
    L. sternal punch
    L. sternal shears
    L. wire saw
LED
    light-emitting diode
Ledraplastic exercise ball
Lee
    L. bracket
    L. bronchus clamp
    L. cartilage knife
    L. cryoprobe
    L. diamond bur
    L. double-ended retractor

L

Lee *(continued)*
    L. graft
    L. lingual button
    L. microvascular clamp
    L. orthodontic resin
    L. & Westcott needle
leech
    mechanical l.
Lee-Cohen
    L.-C. knife
    L.-C. septal elevator
LEEP Redi-kit
Lees
    L. arterial forceps
    L. nontraumatic forceps
    L. vascular clamp
    L. wedge resection clamp
LeeSpec disposable vaginal speculum
Leff
    L. alloy
    L. forceps
    L. stethoscope
Lefferts
    L. bone-cutting forceps
    L. rib shears
    L. rib spreader
LeFort
    L. dilator
    L. filiform
    L. filiform bougie
    L. filiform guide
    L. male catheter
    L. sound
    L. speculum
    L. urethral catheter
    L. urethral sound
    L. urethral ultrasound
    L. uterine sound
left
    Amplatz l. (AL)
    l. coronary catheter
    l. heart catheter
    Judkins l. (JL)
    Judkins l. 4 (JL4)
    Judkins l. 5 (JL5)
    l. Judkins catheter
    l. long leg brace
    l. ventricular (LV)
    l. ventricular assist device (LVAD)
    l. ventricular assist system
    l. ventricular bypass pump
    l. ventricular sump catheter
    l. ventricular transvenous lead
left-handed cornea scissors
leg
    l. brace
    C-Leg System artificial l.
    l. holder
    l. positioner

    l. sling
    L. Thing pump holder
    l. traction
Legacy
    AdvanTec L.
    L. cannulated implant system
    L. cataract surgical system
    L. Series 2000 Cavitron/Kelman
      phacoemulsifier aspirator
    L. spinal system
Legasus support CPM device
Legend
    L. ACL functional knee brace
    L. high-speed pneumatic system
    L. Hy-Lo adjusting table
    L. PCL functional knee brace
legged
    3-l. cage heart valve
4-legged
    4-l. cage heart valve
    4-l. cage valve
**Leggiero hydrophilic-coated
    microcatheter**
legging
    traction l.
legGRIP body positioning device
legholder
    Alvarado l.
    Arthroplasty Products Consultants
      foot and l.
    arthroscopic l.
    Cherf l.
    lithotomy l.
    Prep-Assist l.
    Surbaugh l.
    SurgAssist surgical l.
leg-holding device
Lehman
    L. aortographic catheter
    L. cardiac device
    L. pancreatic manometry catheter
    L. ventriculography catheter
Lehner
    L. II inserter
    L. II loader
Lehner-Utrata capsulorrhexis forceps
Leibinger
    L. 3D bone plate
    L. E-Z flap
    L. locking system
    L. Micro Dynamic mesh
    L. Micro Plus plate
    L. Micro Plus screw
    L. Micro System drill bit
    L. Micro System plate cutter
    L. Micro System plate-holding
      forceps
    L. miniplate system
    L. Mini Würzburg plate

L. Mini Würzburg screw
L. plating
L. plating system
L. Profyle hand system
L. titanium mini Würzburg implant system
L. titanium Würzburg mandibular reconstruction system
L. Würzburg plate
L. Würzburg screw

Leibinger/Karlis intermaxillary fixation screw system

Leica
L. microscope
L. model 1600 water-cooled diamond saw
L. vibrating knife microtome
L. VT1000 E fully automatic microtome
L. VT1000 M semi-automatic microtome

Leicaflex camera
Leigh capsule forceps
Leinbach
L. device
L. head and neck endoprosthesis
L. head and neck total hip
L. hip prosthesis
L. olecranon hook
L. olecranon screw
L. osteotome

Leisegang colposcope
Leiske lens
Leitz
L. image analysis system
L. microscope
L. periplan photomicroscope
L. 1600 saw microtome

Lejeune
L. cotton applicator
L. thoracic forceps

Leksell
L. apparatus
L. arc
L. bone rongeur
L. cardiovascular rongeur
L. cobalt-60 Gamma Knife
L. D-shaped stereotactic frame
L. Gamma Knife
L. gamma unit
L. grooved director
L. G stereotactic head frame
L. laminectomy rongeur
L. micro-stereotactic system
L. punch
L. rongeur
L. rongeur forceps
L. selector
L. stereotactic device

L. stereotactic gamma unit
L. stereotactic gamma unit lens
L. stereotactic system
L. stereotaxic frame
L. sternal approximator
L. sternal spreader
L. trephine

Leksell-Elekta stereotactic frame
Leksell-Stille thoracic rongeur
Leland
L. refractor
L. tonsillar knife

Leland-Jones
L.-J. forceps
L.-J. tonsillar knife
L.-J. vascular clamp

Lell
L. esophagoscope
L. laryngofissure saw

LeMaitre Glow 'N Tell tape
Lema strap
Lem-Blay circumcision clamp
Lemmon
L. intimal dissector
L. needle
L. rib contractor
L. sternal elevator
L. sternal spreader

Lemoine
L. forceps
L. orbital implant
L. serrefine

Lemoine-Searcy
L.-S. anchor
L.-S. fixation anchor loupe

lemon-squeezer obstetrical elevator
Lempert
L. bone curette
L. bone rongeur
L. diamond-dust polishing bur
L. endaural curette
L. endaural rongeur
L. excavator
L. fenestration bur
L. fine curette
L. heavy elevator
L. invaginator
L. knife
L. malleus cutter
L. malleus nipper
L. malleus punch
L. narrow elevator
L. perforator
L. periosteal elevator
L. retractor
L. rongeur
L. rongeur forceps
L. rongeur headrest

L

Lempert-Colver
   L.-C. endaural speculum
   L.-C. retractor
Lempert-Storz
   L.-S. lens
   L.-S. lens loupe
   L.-S. loupe
Lenard ray tube
Lengemann wire
Lenox bucket
lens
   Abraham contact l.
   Abraham peripheral button
      iridotomy l.
   Abraham YAG laser l.
   AC l.
   Accugel l.
   achromatic l.
   acrylic foldable intraocular l.
   AcrySof foldable intraocular l.
   AcrySof haptic l.
   AcrySof MA60 l.
   AcrySof ReSTOR l.
   AcrySof ReSTOR apodized
      diffractive optic posterior chamber
      intraocular l.
   Acuvue Advance contact l.
   Acuvue bifocal l.
   Acuvue brand toric contact l.
   Acuvue 1-day disposable l.
   Acuvue disposable contact l.
   Acuvue etafilcon A l.
   Acuvue toric contact l.
   Acuvue 2-week UV-blocking
      disposable l.
   adherent l.
   Alan-Thorpe l.
   Alcon AcrySof SA30AL single-
      piece l.
   Alcon intraocular l.
   Alcon MA30BA optic AcrySof l.
   Alien WildEyes l.
   Allen-Thorpe l.
   Allergan AMO Array S155 l.
   all-in-the-bag intraocular l.
   all-PMMA 1-piece C-loop
      intraocular l.
   Amenabar l.
   American Medical Optics Baron l.
   amnifocal l.
   AMO Array foldable intraocular l.
   AMO Array intraocular l.
   AMO Array multifocal ultraviolet-
      absorbing silicone posterior
      chamber intraocular l.
   AMO intraocular l.
   AMO Ioptex Model ACR 360
      foldable acrylic l.

AMO Phacoflex II foldable
   intraocular l.
AMO Sensar intraocular l.
Amsoft l.
angle-fixated l.
Anis staple l.
anterior chamber intraocular l.
   (AC-IOL)
aplanatic l.
apochromatic l.
Aquaflex contact l.
Aquasight l.
Arnott 1-piece all-PMMA
   intraocular l.
Array foldable intraocular l.
Array multifocal intraocular l.
Arruga l.
Artisan myopia l.
aspheric l.
aspherical ophthalmoscopic l.
aspheric cataract l.
aspheric viewing l.
astigmatic l.
auxiliary l.
Azar l.
bag-fixated intraocular l.
Bagolini l.
Baikoff l.
balafilcon A contact l.
bandage contact l.
bandage soft contact l.
Barkan gonioscopic l.
Baron l.
Barraquer l.
Bausch & Lomb Optima l.
Bausch & Lomb Surgical
   L161U l.
8.4 BC disposable l.
Bechert 1-piece all-PMMA
   intraocular l.
Beebe l.
biconcave l.
biconcave contact l.
biconvex intraocular l.
bicylindrical l.
Bietti l.
bifocal l.
bifocal intracorneal l.
Binkhorst-Fyodorov l.
Binkhorst 2-loop l.
Binkhorst modified J-loop
   intraocular l.
BIOM l.
Biomedics contact l.
biomicroscopic indirect l.
Bi-Soft l.
bispherical l.
Bloodshot WildEyes l.
blue filtering l.

blue light-absorbing intraocular l.
Boberg-Ans l.
Boston 7 contact l.
Boston Envision contact l.
Boston EO, ES contact l.
Boston II, IV contact l.
Boston RXD contact l.
Boston XO contact l.
Bowling l.
Boys-Smith laser l.
Burian-Allen contact l.
l. cannula
capsular-style l.
Carl Zeiss l.
cast-molded PMMA intraocular l.
catadioptric l.
CeeOn foldable l.
CeeOn heparin surface-modified l.
CeeOn intraocular l.
CeeOn model 920 foldable
   intraocular l.
central retinal l.
Charles handheld infusion l.
Charles intraocular l.
Chiroflex C11UB l.
Choyce Mark VIII l.
Choyce-Tennant l.
CibaSoft Visitint contact l.
Cibathin l.
CIMA*flex* 411 foldable silicone l.
ClariFlex l.
ClariFlex foldable silicone
   intraocular l.
ClariFlex OptiEdge foldable
   intraocular l.
clariVit central mag l.
clariVit central magnification
   vitrectomy l.
clariVit wide-angle l.
clariVit wide-angle vitrectomy l.
Clayman intraocular l.
ClearView contact l.
l. clip
C-loop posterior chamber l.
Coburn intraocular l.
Collamer intraocular l.
Collamer 1-piece intraocular l.
Collamer 3-piece intraocular l.
colored contact l.
ColorMax color vision
   enhancement l.
L. Comfort ultrasound cleaning and
   disinfecting system
compound l.
compressible acrylic intraocular l.
compression-molded PMMA
   intraocular l.
concave l.
concavoconcave l.

concavoconvex l.
condensing l.
congenital subluxated crystalline l.
contact l.
contact bandage l.
contact low-vacuum l.
contact side field l.
convergent l.
convex l.
convexoconcave l.
convexoconvex l.
Cooper Clear DW contact l.
Cooper Toric contact l.
CooperVision-Cilco-Kelman multiflex
   all-PMMA intraocular l.
CooperVision PMMA-ACL Flex l.
Copeland radial panchamber UV l.
coquille plano l.
corneal l.
Crookes l.
crystalline l.
CSI toric contact l.
cylindric l.
cylindrical l.
Dailies contact l.
daily wear contact l.
Definity contact l.
diagnostic fiberoptic l.
diffractive multifocal l.
diopter l.
direct gonioscopic l.
disc lens intraocular l.
dispersing l.
double concave l.
double convex l.
Doubra l.
Drews l.
dual mechanism l.
Dulaney l.
Durasoft 2 ColorBlends l.
Durasoft 2 contact l.
Durasoft 3 Optifit Toric
   Colorblends contact l.
Durasoft 2 Optifit Toric for light
   eyes contact l.
Dura-T l.
E Clips prescription computer l.
Edge III hydrogel contact l.
El Bayadi-Kajiura l.
Emcee l.
Emery l.
Encore monthly disposable
   contact l.
endocapsular artificial lens
   intraocular l.
EndoView sapphire l.
l. enucleation scoop
Epstein collar stud acrylic l.
Epstein-Copeland l.

lens *(continued)*

Epstein intraocular l.
Epstein posterior chamber l.
ERG-Jet disposable contact l.
Ernest-McDonald soft intraocular l.
Eschenbach Optik l.
etafilcon A disposable contact l.
European in-the-bag l.
l. expressor
extended wear soft contact l.
eye l.
EZ.1 multifocal contact l.
EZVue violet haptic intraocular l.
Falcon l.
Feaster Dualens l.
field l.
Fisher-Price polycarbonate l.
flexible contact l.
flexible fluoropolymer contact l.
flexible-loop anterior chamber
   intraocular l.
flexible-loop posterior chamber
   intraocular l.
Flexlens l.
Flexner-Worst iris claw l.
fluid-ventilated l.
Fluorex 300, 500 contact l.
F/M base curve contact l.
Focus Dailies toric contact l.
Focus Night & Day l.
Focus Night & Day contact l.
foldable acrylic l.
foldable intraocular l.
foldable plate-haptic silicone
   intraocular l.
folding l.
4-footed l.
3-footed intraocular l.
FormFlex l.
foroblique l.
Frenzel l.
Frequency 38 monthly disposable
   contact l.
FreshLook contact l.
Fresnel l.
Friedman handheld Hruby l.
fundus contact l.
fundus focalizing l.
fused bifocal l.
Galand-Knolle modified J-loop
   intraocular l.
Galin intraocular implant l.
gas permeable contact l.
Genesis l.
Gentex PDQ polycarbonate l.
Gill intraocular implant l.
l. glide cutter
glued-on hard contact l.
Goldmann macular contact l.

Goldmann 3-mirror contact
   diagnostic l.
Goldmann 3-mirror gonioscopy l.
Goldmann multi-mirror l.
goniofocalizing l.
gonioscopic l.
Gould intraocular implant l.
Gradal individual customized
   progressive l.
gradient index l.
Gray photochromic l.
Gridley intraocular l.
GRIN l.
Gullstrand l.
handheld Hruby l.
hand-painted l.
haptic area l.
haptic plate l.
hard contact l.
Hart pediatric 3-mirror l.
highly oxygen-permeable contact l.
l. hook
Hopkins II rod l.
Hoskins l.
Hoskins-Barkan goniotomy infant l.
Hoskins nylon suture laser l.
Hruby l.
Hruby contact l.
Hunkeler l.
Hunkeler intraocular l.
Hunter 1-piece all-PMMA
   intraocular l.
Hydrasoft contact l.
Hydrocurve l.
hydrogel intraocular l.
Hydron l.
hydrophilic l.
hydrophilic acrylic intraocular l.
hydrophilic contact l.
Hydroview l.
Hydroview intraocular l.
l. implant
implantable collamer l.
implantable contact l.
l. implantation forceps
infant Karickhoff laser l.
infant 3-mirror laser l.
Intermedics l.
Interspace YAG laser l.
in-the-bag l.
intracorneal l.
intraocular l. (IOL)
Iolab 108 B l.
Ioptex TabOptic l.
iridectomy laser l.
iridocapsular intraocular l.
iris claw intraocular l.
iris clip intraocular l.
iris-fixated l.

iris-supported intraocular l.
iseikonic l.
iZon wavefront-guided l.
Jaffe Cilco l.
Jaffe 1-piece all-PMMA
  intraocular l.
J-loop PC l.
J-loop posterior chamber
  intraocular l.
Kamerling 1-piece all-PMMA
  intraocular l.
Karickhoff diagnostic l.
Karickhoff laser l.
Kearney side-notch l.
Kearney side-notch intraocular l.
Keeler panoramic l.
Kelman Duet phakic l.
Kelman flexible tripod l.
Kelman II 3-point fixation rigid
  tripod intraocular l.
Kelman Multiflex II l.
Kelman Multiflex II intraocular l.
Kelman Omnifit intraocular l.
Kelman PC 27LB CapSul l.
Kerasoft DuraWave l.
keratoconus contact l.
keratometer l.
keratophakia l.
Kilp l.
Kishi l.
Koeppe diagnostic l.
Koeppe gonioscopic l.
Kratz elliptical-style l.
Kratz modified J-loop intraocular l.
Kratz posterior chamber
  intraocular l.
Krieger wide-field fundus l.
Landers biconcave l.
Landers contact l.
Landers-Foulks temporary
  keratoprosthesis l.
Landers sew-on l.
large-diameter optics intraocular l.
Lasag contact l.
laser l.
laser-adjustable l.
Laseridge Optics l.
l. lasso
Layden infant l.
Leiske l.
Leksell stereotactic gamma unit l.
Lempert-Storz l.
Lester notch intraocular l.
Lewicky intraocular l.
Lieb-Guerry cataract implant l.
light adjustable l.
lighthouse l.
Lindstrom Centrex l.
long-wearing contact l.

l. loop
loop-fixated intraocular l.
l. loop forceps
lotrafilcon A contact l.
l. loupe
Lovac 6-mirror gonioscopic l.
low-power optics for myopic
  correction l.
MA30BA intraocular l.
Machemer flat l.
Machemer infusion contact l.
Machemer magnifying vitrectomy l.
macular contact l.
Mainster l.
Mainster-HM retinal laser l.
Mainster retinal laser l.
Mainster-S retinal laser l.
Mainster Ultra Field PRP laser l.
Mainster-WF retinal laser l.
Mainster wide-field l.
Maltese cross l.
Mandelkorn suture laser lysis l.
Mandelkorn suture lysis l.
l. manipulator
March laser l.
Mark IX l.
Maxsight sport-tinted contact l.
Maxsight sport tinted contact l.
McGhan l.
McLean prismatic fundus laser l.
Meditec bandage contact l.
Meditech bandage contact l.
MemoryLens foldable intraocular l.
meniscus l.
meniscus concave l.
meter l.
microincision intraocular l.
MiniQuad XL l.
3M intraocular l.
minus l.
3-mirror contact l.
4-mirror Gonio l.
3-mirror intraocular l.
l. mitral heart valve
modified C-loop intraocular l.
modified J-loop posterior chamber
  intraocular l.
Momose l.
Morgan therapeutic l.
multidrop l.
multifocal l.
Multi-Optics l.
multipiece l.
multiple-piece intraocular l.
narrow l.
Neolens l.
New Orleans l.
NewVues sterile contact l.
Nike Max Rx prescription sun l.

lens *(continued)*
    Nikon aspheric l.
    Nikon SMZ 2T magnifying l.
    noncontact l.
    Nova Aid l.
    Nova Soft II l.
    NuVita l.
    objective l.
    Oculaid l.
    ocular l.
    omnifocal l.
    O2Optix breathable contact l.
    O2Optix contact l.
    L. Opacities Classification System II
    open l.
    open-loop intraocular l.
    Ophtec Co. l.
    Optical Radiation l.
    Optical Radiation intraocular l.
    optic 3-piece intraocular l.
    2-Optifit toric l.
    Optiflex l.
    OptiLOUPE attachable l.
    Optima contact l.
    orthokeratology contact l.
    orthoscopic l.
    O'Shea l.
    Osher gonio/posterior pole l.
    Osher panfundus l.
    Osher surgical gonio/posterior pole l.
    Packard intraocular l.
    panchamber UV l.
    parfocal defraction l.
    PBII blue loop l.
    PC-IOL l.
    Pearce Tripod cataract l.
    Pearce Tripod intraocular l.
    pediatric Karickhoff laser l.
    pediatric 3-mirror laser l.
    periscopic l.
    Permalens l.
    PermaVision intracorneal l.
    Perspex CQ intraocular l.
    Perspex CQ-Shearing-Simcoe-Sinskey l.
    Peyman-Green vitrectomy l.
    Peyman special optics for low vision l.
    Peyman wide-field l.
    PhacoFlex II foldable intraocular l.
    PhacoFlex II SI30NB intraocular l.
    Phakic 6 l.
    Pharmacia Visco J-loop l.
    photochromic l.
    3-piece acrylic intraocular l.
    3-piece hydrophobic acrylic l.

    3-piece hydrophobic acrylic Sensar l.
    4-piece intraocular l.
    3-piece modified J-loop intraocular l.
    3-piece monofocal silicone l.
    3-piece plate-haptic intraocular l.
    1-piece plate-haptic silicone intraocular l.
    1-piece plate haptic silicone intraocular l.
    3-piece silicone intraocular l.
    piggyback contact l.
    plano l.
    planoconcave l.
    planoconvex l.
    planoconvex nonridge l.
    plate-haptic intraocular l.
    Platina clip l.
    plus l.
    plus power l.
    PMMA custom-made calibration contact l.
    PMMA hard contact l.
    PMMA intraocular l.
    Pointer 1-piece all-PMMA intraocular l.
    3-point fixation intraocular l.
    4-point fixation intraocular l.
    polarized l.
    polycarbonate l.
    polypropylene intraocular l.
    Posner diagnostic l.
    posterior chamber intraocular l.
    posterior convex intraocular l.
    Precision Cosmet l.
    presbyopic intraocular l.
    prismatic contact l.
    progressive spectacles l.
    prosthetic l.
    punctal l.
    PureVision extended-wear contact l.
    PureVision toric l.
    l. pusher
    QuadPediatric fundus l.
    Rayner l.
    Red Reflex Lens Systems l.
    refractive l.
    removable keratophakia l.
    retroscopic l.
    Revolution l.
    right-angle l.
    right-angled telescopic l.
    rigid contact l.
    rigid gas permeable l.
    rigid intraocular l.
    Ritch contact l.
    Ritch nylon suture laser l.
    Ritch trabeculoplasty laser l.

Rodenstock panfundus l.
SA60AT intraocular l.
safety l.
sapphire l.
Sarfarazi dual optic intraocular l.
SaturEyes contact l.
Sauflon PW l.
Sauflon PW contact l.
Sauflon PW hydrophilic contact l.
Schachar l.
scleral contact l.
SeeQuence disposable contact l.
self-stabilizing vitrectomy l.
Sensar acrylic intraocular l.
Sensar foldable acrylic posterior
  chamber intraocular l.
Sensar OptiEdge intraocular l.
Severin l.
sewn-in l.
sew-on l.
Sheets l.
Sheets closed loop posterior
  chamber intraocular l.
short C-loop l.
short C-loop intraocular l.
Signet Optical l.
silica contact l.
silicone elastomer l.
silicone hydrogel contact l.
silicone intraocular l.
Silsoft extended wear contact l.
Simcoe C-loop intraocular l.
Simcoe II PC l.
l. simulation sales tool
single-vision l.
Sinskey J-loop intraocular l.
slab-off l.
Slant haptic intraocular l.
Snellen soft contact l.
SofLens contact l.
SofLens66 toric contact l.
SoFlex intraocular l.
SoFlex series l.
SofPort AO aspheric l.
SofPort L161 AO l.
soft contact l.
soft intraocular l.
SoftSITE high add aspheric
  multifocal contact l.
Sola Optical USA Spectralite high-
  index l.
Sovereign bifocal l.
l. spatula
Spectralite Transitions l.
spheric l.
spherocylindric l.
spherocylindrical l.
l. spoon
Staar AA 4207 l.

Staar foldable intraocular l.
Staar implantable contact l.
Staar intraocular l.
Staar toric l.
Staar 4203VF l.
Staar 4207VF l.
Stableflex l.
Stokes l.
Strampelli l.
Style S2 clear-loop l.
subluxated crystalline l.
Super Field NC slit lamp l.
Surefit AC 85J l.
Surevue contact l.
Sutherland l.
T l.
Tano double-mirror peripheral
  vitrectomy l.
Tecnis foldable intraocular l.
Tecnis Z9000 l.
Tek-Clear accommodating
  intraocular l.
Tennant Anchorflex AC l.
Thorpe 4-mirror goniolaser l.
Thorpe 4-mirror vitreous fundus
  laser l.
Thorpe plastic l.
l. threading forceps
Tillyer bifocal l.
tinted l.
T-lens therapeutic contact l.
Tolentino prism l.
Tolentino vitrectomy l.
Topcon aspheric l.
toric l.
toric intraocular l.
Toric-Optima series l.
Touchlite zoom l.
transition l.
trial l.
trial contact l.
trifocal l.
tripod intraocular l.
Trokel l.
Troncoso tubular l.
Trupower aspherical l.
Ultex l.
Ultra mag l.
Ultra View SP slit-lamp l.
ultraviolet-blocking intraocular l.
uniplanar intraocular l.
uniplanar-style PC II l.
Univision low-vision microscopic l.
Urrets-Zavalia retinal surgical l.
uvea-fixated intraocular l.
uvea-supported intraocular l.
Uvex l.
Varigray l.
Varilux Infinity l.

L

lens *(continued)*
 Varilux Pangamic thin plastic l.
 Varilux Plus l.
 Viscolens l.
 Visian implantable collamer l.
 Vision Tech l.
 Visitec Company l.
 Vistakon contact l.
 Volk aspheric l.
 Volk coronoid l.
 Volk G-Series l.
 Volk high-resolution aspherical l.
 Volk 3-mirror ANF+ l.
 Volk panretinal l.
 Volk QuadrAspheric fundal l.
 Volk SuperMacula 2.2 focal
  laser l.
 Volk SuperPupil NC l.
 Volk SuperQuad 160 contact l.
 Volk SuperQuad 160 panretinal l.
 Volk Transequator l.
 Wang l.
 Wesley-Jessen l.
 Wild l.
 Wise iridotomy laser l.
 Wise iridotomy-sphincterotomy
  laser l.
 Wise sphincterotomy laser l.
 Wood l.
 Woods Concept l.
 Worst Claw l.
 Worst Medallion l.
 Yannuzzi fundus laser l.
 Youens l.
 Z-alpha l.
 Zeiss aspheric l.
 Zeiss-Gullstrand l.
LensCheck Advanced Logic lensometer
Lens-Eze inserter
Lensmeter
 L. 701
 L. lensometer
 Zeiss projection L.
lensometer
 Allergan Humphrey l.
 AO Reichert Instruments l.
 Carl Zeiss l.
 Coburn l.
 Hardy l.
 LensCheck Advanced Logic l.
 Lensmeter l.
 Marco l.
 Reichert l.
 Topcon LM P5 digital l.
Lent laparoscope
lentula spiral drill
Leo
 L. Bathlifter
 L. Schwartz sponge-holding forceps

Leon
 L. cobra cannula
 L. cobra tip
Leonard
 L. arm
 L. arm device
 L. Arms instrument holder
 L. catheter
 L. forceps
Lere bone mill
Leriche
 L. hemostatic forceps
 L. spatula
 L. tissue forceps
Lerman
 L. hinge brace
 L. noninvasive halo
LeRoy
 L. clip-applying forceps
 L. infant scalp clip
 L. ventricular catheter
Lesieur hydrochopper
Lesinski Flex-HA PORP ossicular chain prosthesis
Lester
 L. fixation forceps
 L. IOL manipulator
 L. Jones bypass tube
 L. lens manipulator
 L. muscle forceps
 L. notch intraocular lens
Lester-Burch eye speculum
Letournel acetabular fracture bone plate
leucocyte detection strip
LEUHR
 low-energy ultra high-resolution
  LEUHR fan-beam collimator
  LEUHR parallel-hole collimator
leukocyte
 l. depletion filter
 l. removal filter
leukodepletion filter
LeukoNet Filter
LeukoScan
leukoscope
Leukotape
 L. P combo pack taping kit
 L. P Sportstape
 L. P sports tape
 L. P stretch bandage
 L. sports tape
leukotome
 Freeman transorbital l.
 Lewis l.
 Love l.
 McKenzie l.
Leukotrap
 L. RC storage system

L. red cell collector
L. red cell storage system
leuprolide acetate implant
Leur-par collimator
LeVasseur-Merrill retractor
LeVeen
    L. ascites shunt
    L. catheter
    L. dialysis shunt
    L. inflation syringe
    L. inflator
    L. inflator with pressure gauge
    L. peritoneal shunt
    L. peritoneovenous shunt
    L. plaque cracker
    L. plaque-cracker
    L. radiofrequency ablation needle electrode
    L. RF probe
    L. shunt
    L. valve
level
    Albarran deflecting l.
    L. Anchorage appliance
    L. Anchorage system
    L. I normothermic irrigating system
    L. One normothermic IV fluid set
lever
    bone l.
    Buck-Gramcko bone l.
    Hohmann bone l.
    Kilner malar l.
    Lane bone l.
    Lange-Hohmann bone l.
    Murphy-Lane l.
    l. pessary
    Verbrugge-Mueller bone l.
Levin
    L. catheter
    L. drill guide
    L. duodenal tube
    L. thermocouple cordotomy electrode
    L. tube
    L. tube catheter
Levine
    L. curetting spud
    L. foreign body spud
    L. spud
Levitt implant
levonorgestrel rod implant
Levret forceps
Levulin PDT system
Levy
    L. articulating retractor
    L. perineal retractor
    L. & Rappel foot orthosis

Levy-Kuglen
    L.-K. iris hook
    L.-K. lens manipulator
Lewicky
    L. capsular scraper
    L. cortex extractor
    L. formed cystotome
    L. intraocular lens
    L. IOL spatula
    L. lens manipulating hook
    L. microlens hook
    L. needle
    L. self-retaining chamber maintainer
    L. threaded infusion cannula
Lewin
    L. baseball finger splint
    L. bone-holding clamp
    L. bone-holding forceps
    L. bunion dissector
    L. elevator
    L. finger splint
    L. forceps
    L. sesamoidectomy dissector
    L. spinal perforating forceps
Lewin-Stern
    L.-S. finger splint
    L.-S. thumb splint
Lewis
    L. bracket
    L. cystometer
    L. dental mirror
    L. expandable adjustable prosthesis (LEAP)
    L. hemostat
    L. laryngectomy tube
    L. lead
    L. lens loupe
    L. lens scoop
    L. leukotome
    L. nail
    L. nasal rasp
    L. periosteal elevator
    L. periosteal rasp
    L. recording cystometer
    L. retractor
    L. scoop
    L. septal forceps
    L. tongue depressor
    L. tonsillar hemostatic forceps
    L. tonsillar screw
    L. tonsillar snare
    L. ureteral stone isolation forceps
    L. vertical slot bracket
Lewis-Resnik punch
Lewkowitz
    L. lithotomy forceps
    L. ovum forceps
    L. placental forceps

L

Lewy

    L. anterior commissure laryngoscope
    L. chest holder
    L. laryngoscope holder
    L. laryngostat
    L. suspension apparatus
    L. suspension device
    L. suspension laryngoscope
    L. syringe
    L. Teflon glycerine mixture injection needle

Lewy-Rubin needle

Lexan jacket

Lexer

    L. chisel
    L. dissecting scissors
    L. gouge
    L. osteotome
    L. tissue forceps

Leyla

    L. bar
    L. flexible arm
    L. self-retaining brain retractor
    L. self-retaining tractor bar
    L. self-retaining tractor bar lift

L-frame fixator

LGM filter

LHE apparatus

LH 500, 750, 1500 series hematology analyzer

Libbe lower bowel evacuation device

liberator

    l. elevator
    l. knife
    l. locking stylet
    l. universal locking stylet

Liberty

    L. CMC thumb brace
    L. One splint
    L. spinal system
    L. walking stick cane

Lichtenberg

    L. corneal trephine
    L. keratome
    L. needle holder

Lichtwitz

    L. abdominal trocar
    L. antral cannula
    L. antral needle
    L. antral trocar

lid

    l. clamp
    l. crutch spectacles
    l. everter
    l. expressor
    l. forceps
    l. plate
    l. retractor

    l. scalpel
    l. speculum

Liddle aorta clamp

Lido

    L. Active Multijoint system
    L. isokinetic dynamometer
    L. lift
    L. Multi Joint II isokinetic dynamometer
    L. Passive Multijoint system
    L. WorkSET work simulator

Lidoback isokinetic dynamometry system

Lido-Pen Auto-Injector

Liebel-Flarsheim CT 9000 contrast delivery system

Lieberman

    L. abrader
    L. aspirating speculum
    L. fragmentor
    L. K-wire speculum
    L. lens-holding forceps
    L. microfinger
    L. MicroFinger manipulator
    L. micro-ring lens forceps
    L. phaco crusher
    L. proctoscope
    L. sigmoidoscope
    L. suturing forceps
    L. tying forceps
    L. wire aspirating speculum with V-shape blade

Lieberman-type

    L.-t. speculum reversible thin solid blade
    L.-t. speculum thin solid blade
    L.-t. speculum with Kratz open wire blade

Lieb-Guerry

    L.-G. cataract implant lens
    L.-G. forceps

Lieppman

    L. sharp cystotome
    L. spatula

Liesegang LM-Flex 7 flexible hysteroscope

Life

    L. Liner stick and cut-resistant glove
    L. Pulse high-frequency jet ventilator
    L. SoftPac AED companion oxygen unit
    L. Suit

Life-Air 1000 hypothermic therapy system

Lifecare

    L. pump
    L. ventilator

Lifecath
    L. catheter
    L. peritoneal implant
LifeCell AlloDerm acellular dermal graft
Lifecore
    L. Restore wide-diameter implant
    L. Restore wide-diameter implant system
LifeGuide
    L. glucose meter
    L. system
LifeJet catheter
Lifeline
    L. lead
    L. Wall Gym 2000 fitness system
LIFE-Lung system
Lifemed
    L. blood tubing
    L. cannula
    L. catheter
    L. heterologous heart valve
Life-O-Matt
Lifepak
    L. 5 cardiac monitor
    L. defibrillator
    L. 12 defibrillator/monitor
    L. 5, 7 monitor/defibrillator
Lifepath
    L. AAA endovascular graft system
    L. stent-graft
LifePort
    L. endotracheal tube holder
    L. infusion set
Lifesaver disposable resuscitator bag
lifesaving tube
LifeScan
    L. blood glucose meter
    L. blood glucose monitoring system
    L. Profile
    L. Ultra
LifeShirt
    L. ambulatory monitoring system
    L. monitor
LifeSigns
    L. Micro 12 ECG + recorder
    L. Rhythm Check recorder
    L. SP spirometer
LifeSite hemodialysis access system
LifeSpex device
LifeStent
    L. LP SDS biliary stent
    L. NT self-expanding biliary stent
    L. XL SDS biliary stent
Lifestream
    L. centrifugal pump
    L. coronary dilation catheter
Lifestride treadmill

life support
LifeSync wireless ECG system
Life-Tech flowmeter
LifeVest wearable defibrillator
LifeView care station
lift
    BTE dynamic l.
    Calypso l.
    Easy Pivot patient l.
    head-tilt-chin l.
    heel l.
    Hi-Loo Power l.
    Hoyer l.
    ischial l.
    Leyla self-retaining tractor bar l.
    Lido l.
    M/L l.
    plantar l.
    pneumatic chair l.
    Sabina l.
    shoe l.
    VuRyser monitor l.
lifter
    tissue l.
    Totallift-II l.
    Weinstein fixation ring and flap l.
    Yasargil tissue l.
LiF thermoluminescence dosimeter
Ligaclip
    L. applier
    L. ERCA instrument
    Ethicon L.
    L. MCA multiple-clip applier
    L. surgical clip
ligament
    anterior cruciate l. (ACL)
    anterior cruciate ligament/posterior cruciate l. (ACL/PCL)
    l. augmentation device (LAD)
    l. button
    l. clamp
    Dacron synthetic l.
    l. grasping forceps
    Zenotech synthetic l.
ligamentous
    l. anterior dislocation composite graft
    l. control brace
ligamentum
    l. flavum forceps
    l. teres knife
LigaSure vessel sealing system
ligating and dividing stapler
ligation
    l. device
    Linton radical vein l.
ligator
    Bandito endoscopic l.
    Bandito single-band l.

L

ligator *(continued)*
DDV l.
endoscopic band l.
hemorrhoidal l.
KilRoid single-handed l.
McGivney l.
McGivney hemorrhoidal l.
multiple-band l.
O'Regan hemorrhoid l.
RapidFire multiple-band l.
rubber band l.
Rudd l.
Saeed multiband l.
Saeed multiple l.
Saeed six-shooter l.
Saeed six-shooter multi-band l.
Speedband multiple-band l.
Speedband Superview l.
Stiegmann-Goff Clearvue
endoscopic l.
Stiegmann-Goff variceal l.
ligature
l. cannula
l. carrier
l. carrying forceps
l. director
Endoloop l.
l. forceps
l. guide
l. needle
l. passer
l. scissors
Surgiwip suture l.
Tahoe Surgical Instruments l.
l. tie wire
l. tucker
ligatureless bracket
ligature-locking pliers
ligature-tying pliers
light
l. adjustable lens
Amsco l.
Barkan l.
l. beam generator
bili l.
Boyd surgical l.
Brite Lite III l.
l. carrier
Castle examination l.
Castle surgical l.
Clar head l.
cobalt blue l.
Cogent l.
L. Commander xenon illuminator
l. cross-slot screwdriver
CureLight Broadband red l.
curing l.
dermatologic ultraviolet l.
l. electron microscope

l. emitter
floor-standing surgical l.
Floxite mirror l.
Fotofil activator l.
Hanalux Oslo l.
HappySkin acne l.
L. headrest
Landry vein l.
Maglite l.
l. microscope
monochromatic red HeNe laser l.
MultArray l.
overhead l.
l. pen
l. pipe
l. pipe pick
l. pipette
pulsed l.
Right L.
Right Light examination l.
Sabre FreeHand high-intensity
medical pocket l.
scleral fixation l.
Solar Beam medical examination l.
L. Talker device
ultraviolet l.
ultraviolet A l.
l. wand
l. wire appliance
Wood l.
light-adjustable IOL
LightBlade
Novatec L.
light-curing resin
LightCycler
L. polymerase chain reaction
analysis instrument
L. system
lighted
l. flute needle
l. retractor
l. speculum
l. stent
l. stylet
light-emitting diode (LED)
lighthouse
L. ET-DRS acuity chart
l. lens
Lightlas 532 green laser
LightMat surgical illuminator
LightMed Lpulsa SYL9000 YAG laser
light-monitoring probe
LighTouch Neonate thermometer
LightShear diode laser
LightSheer
L. diode laser system
L. diode laser system for
permanent hair removal
L. laser

L. SC diode laser
L. SC laser hair removal system

lightsource
halogen dual l.

LightSpeed
L. CT scanner
L. multidetector CT scanner
L. QX/i scanner
L. Ultra CT system

Lightstic 180, 360 fiberoptic laser

Light-Veley apparatus

LightWare micro retractor

lightweight and portable Sullivan nasal CPAP

Ligmajet syringe

LIH hook pin

Lilienthal
L. probe
L. rib guillotine
L. rib spreader

Lilienthal-Sauerbruch
L.-S. retractor
L.-S. rib spreader

Lillehei-Kaster
L.-K. cardiac valve prosthesis
L.-K. mitral valve prosthesis
L.-K. pivoting disc
L.-K. pivoting-disc prosthetic valve

Lillehei pacemaker

Lillie
L. antral trocar
L. attic cannula
L. attic hook
L. ear hook
L. frontal sinus probe
L. gouge
L. intestinal forceps
L. nasal speculum
L. rectus tendon clamp
L. retractor
L. rongeur
L. tissue-holding forceps
L. tonsillar knife
L. tonsillar scissors

Lillie-Koffler tool

Lilliput neonatal oxygenator

LIMA-Lift tool

LIMA-Loop tool

limb
l. brace
l. and elbow protector
l. gym
l. holder
inspiratory l.
l. lead
l. preservation system (LPS)
Trowbridge TerraRound sports l.

limited compression-dynamic compression plate

limited-contact dynamic compression plate

limiter
Becker 655 motion control l.

LINAC
linear accelerator
LINAC gantry
Varian LINAC

LINAC-based radiosurgical system

Linatrix suture

Lincoff
L. balloon catheter
L. lens sponge
L. scleral sponge implant
L. sponge implant material
L. sponge rod

Lindbergh pump

Linde
L. cryogenic probe
L. cryoprobe
L. Xi-scan

Lindeman
L. self-retaining uterine vacuum cannula
L. transfusion needle

Lindemann
L. bone cutter
L. bur

Lindeman-Silverstein
L.-S. Arrow tube
L.-S. ventilation tube

Lindholm
L. microlaryngoscope
L. operating laryngoscope
L. tracheal tube

Lindner
L. anastomosis clamp
L. corneoscleral suture
L. cyclodialysis spatula
L. cyclodialysis spoon
L. spatula

Lindorf
L. lag screw
L. position screw

Lindstrom
L. arcuate incision marker
L. astigmatic marker
L. Centrex lens
L. hydroirrigator
L. LASIK flap roller
L. LASIK spatula
L. lens-insertion forceps
L. small incision marker
L. Star
L. Star nucleus manipulator
L. Trident ophthalmic splitter

Lindstrom-Chu aspirating speculum

Lindvall-Stille meniscal knife

L

line

Armstrong tube l.
Arrow PICC l.
arterial l.
AxyaWeld product l.
Beacon surgical l.
central l.
central venous l.
Codman ICP monitoring l.
CVD black diamond keratome l.
dial-a-flow IV l.
Freedom Clear long-seal male
  external catheter l.
Freedom Clear LS male external
  catheter l.
Freedom Clear sport-sheath male
  external catheter l.
Freedom Clear SS male external
  catheter l.
Harris hip l.
Hickman l.
l. keeper
large-bore intravenous l.
Nafion dryer l.
oxygen supply l.
peripherally inserted central
  catheter l.
PICC l.
total parenteral nutrition l.
Tycos pressure infusion l.
Wackenheim clivus canal l.

Lineage acetabular cup

linear

l. accelerator (LINAC)
l. accelerator system
l. accelerator unit
l. actuator
l. array echoendoscope
l. array-hydrophone assembly
l. array transrectal ultrasound probe
l. convex array scanner
l. hearing aid
L. hip stem
l. in-line ligature carrier
L. KGT tonometer
l. potentiometer
l. probe
l. scissor punch
l. staple cutter
l. stapler
l. stapling device
L. total hip system
l. transducer
l. variable differential transformer
l. visual analog scale

linear-array

l.-a. B-mode ultrasound transducer
l.-a. convex array scanner
l.-a. echoendoscope

l.-a. probe
l.-a. staple cutter
l.-a. transducer

linear-type echoendoscope

linear-variable-differential transducer

linen suture

liner

acetabular l.
acetabular prosthetic l.
Alpha cushion l.
Alps CustomPro custom l.
cast l.
Cavitec cavity l.
Conveen Security+male external
  catheter & l.
DePuy acetabular l.
DePuy Marathon crosslinked
  polyethylene l.
DePuy Poly-Dial constrained l.
Dignity Plus l.
elevated rim acetabular l.
Enduron acetabular l.
Fillauer prosthesis l.
Fillauer silicone suction l.
Fillauer silicone suspension l.
Gore cast l.
Gore-Tex waterproof cast l.
grommet bone l.
Hylamer enhanced ultra-high
  molecular weight polyethylene
  acetabular l.
Iceross Comfort Plus silicone
  gel l.
Integrity neutral l.
Ketac l.
Kins l.
Marathon crosslinked
  polyethylene l.
Medium-Plus alpha l.
metal acetabular l.
Myerson PermaSoft soft denture l.
OrthoGel l.
Ortho-Wick foam l.
Poly-Dial constrained l.
polyethylene l.
Polysorb l.
polyurethane l.
provisional l.
Pulpdent cavity l.
Reflection l.
RingLoc hip l.
rubber bite l.
SiloLiner gel l.
Silosheath gel l.
SlimLine fitted l.
splint l.
Sticky Thermoliner custom
  locking l.
TEC l.

Teflon l.
Tempo denture l.
Tubulitec cavity l.
USMC luxury l.

Lingeman
L. kit
L. 3-in-1 procedure drape
L. TUR drape

lingoscope

lingual
l. arch
l. bar
l. cortical plate
l. forceps
l. spatula
l. wire

lining
DePuy acetabular l.
Thermold heat moldable shoe l.

Link
L. acetabular cage
L. anatomical hip
L. approximator
L. cementless reconstruction hip
prosthesis
L. custom partial pelvis
replacement system
L. Endo-Model rotational knee
L. Endo-Model rotational knee
prosthesis
L. Endo-Model rotational knee
system
L. Lubinus AP hip system
L. Lubinus SP II hip replacement
system
L. Lubinus SP II total hip
replacement system
L. microporous hip stem
L. MP hip noncemented
reconstruction prosthesis
L. Orthopaedics device
L. Saddle Prosthesis Endo-Model
hip replacement system
L. stack split splint
L. toe splint

Linkow
L. blade implant
L. dental implant material

Link-Plus retention pin

Linnartz
L. forceps
L. intestinal clamp
L. stomach clamp

Linson electronic cell counter

lint-free
l.-f. drape
l.-f. sponge

Linton
L. elastic stocking

L. esophageal tube
L. radical vein ligation
L. splanchnic retractor
L. tourniquet
L. tourniquet clamp
L. tube
L. vein hook
L. vein stripper

Linton-Nachlas tube

lint pledget

Lintro-Scan

Linvatec
L. absorbable screw
L. arthroscopic infusion pump
L. arthroscopy product
L. bioabsorbable interference screw
L. bone anchor
L. cannula
L. débrider blade
L. driver
L. meniscal BioStinger anchor
suture
L. microdebrider
L. wrist arthroscopy traction tower

Linx
L. exchange guidewire
L. extension guidewire
L. extension wire
L. guidewire extension
L. guidewire extension cardiac
device

LIO
laser indirect ophthalmoscope
Coaxial Multicolor LIO

lion
l. forceps
L. hearing aid
l. jaw bone holder
l. jaw tenaculum
L.'s Claw grasper
L.'s Paw grasper

lion-jaw
l.-j. bone holder
l.-j. bone-holding forceps
l.-j. clamp
l.-j. forceps

**Liotta-BioImplant low-profile
bioprosthesis prosthetic valve**

Liotta total artificial heart

lip
l. clamp
l. retractor
l. traction bow

Lipectron ultrasonic lancet

Lipisorb dressing

LipoClear reagent tube

Lipo-Medi girdle

**Lipoprint cholesterol subfraction test
system**

L

527

lipoprotein
   high-density l. (HDL)
liposhaver
Liposorber
   L. cholesterol filter
   L. LA-15 system
   L. LA-15 System lithotriptor
Lipovacutainer canister
Lippes loop intrauterine device
Lippman screw
Lippy modified prosthesis
Lipshultz urology microsurgical set
liquefaction device
LiquiBand tissue adhesive
liquid
   l. crystal display projector
   l. crystal glasses
   L. Embolic system
   L. Ice
   l. nylon
   l. organic dye laser
   l. scintillation counting
   l. scintillation spectrometer
   l. scintillation spectrophotometer
   Sklar Kleen l.
   l. vitreous aspirating cannula
Liquiderm liquid adhesive bandage
Lisco sponge
Lister
   L. bandage
   L. bandage scissors
   L. conjunctival forceps
   L. dressing
   L. forceps
   L. knife
   L. lens manipulator
   L. mules
   L. scissors
Liston
   L. amputating knife
   L. bone-cutting forceps
   L. bone rongeur
   L. phalangeal knife
   L. plaster-of-Paris scissors
   L. shears
   L. splint
Liston-Key bone-cutting forceps
Liston-Key-Horsley
   L.-K.-H. forceps
   L.-K.-H. rib shears
Liston-Littauer
   L.-L. bone-cutting forceps
   L.-L. rongeur
Liston-Stille bone-cutting forceps
Lite
   L. blade
   MedaSonics Fetalgard L.
   Profile L.
   Spinal-Stim L.

   TheraPress DUO L.
   L. Touch lancing device
LiteGait partial weightbearing gait therapy device
Liteguard mini-defibrillator
Lite-Pipe
lithium
   l. iodine battery
   l. pacemaker
lithium-powered pacemaker
lithoclast
   L. ballistic energy generator
   L. endoscopic lithotriptor
   l. miniature pneumatic drill
Lithognost flashlamp pulsed dye laser
lithometer
Lithospec electromagnetic intracorporeal lithotriptor
Lithostar
   L. lithotripsy unit
   L. multiline lithotripsy system
   L. nonimmersion lithotriptor
   L. Plus
   L. Plus electromagnetic lithotriptor bidimensional x-ray focusing system
   Siemens L.
Lithostat
lithotomy
   l. forceps
   l. legholder
lithotripsy table
lithotriptor, lithotripter
   Breakstone l.
   Calcusplit pneumatic l.
   Calcutript electrohydraulic l.
   Circon-ACMI l.
   Diasonics Therasonic l.
   Direx Tripter X-1 l.
   DoLi S extracorporeal shock wave l.
   Dormia gallstone l.
   Dormia waterbath l.
   Dornier compact l.
   Dornier HM3, HM4 electrohydraulic l.
   Dornier HM-series l.
   Dornier MPL 5000 l.
   Dornier MPL 9000 gallstone l.
   DP-1 l.
   dual-pulse l.
   EDAP LT.01 l.
   effective l.
   electrohydraulic l.
   electromagnetic l.
   electropneumatic endoscopic l.
   extracorporeal piezoelectric l.
   extracorporeal shock wave l.
   HM4 l.

holmium laser l.
Karl Storz l.
Karl Storz-Lutzeyer l.
laser l.
Liposorber LA-15 System l.
Lithoclast endoscopic l.
Lithospec electromagnetic
  intracorporeal l.
Lithostar nonimmersion l.
manual l.
Medispec Econolith spark plug l.
Medstone extracorporeal shock
  wave l.
Medstone STS l.
MFL 5000 l.
Modulith SL 20 l.
Northgate SD-3 dual-purpose l.
Olympus BML-3Q, -4Q l.
out-of-scope l.
Pentax l.
percutaneous ultrasonic l.
piezoelectric l.
piezoelectric shock wave l.
Piezolith EPL l.
Piezolith 2300, 2500 model l.
pneumatic endoscopic l.
pneumoballistic l.
l. probe
Pulsolith laser l.
Richard Wolf Piezolith l.
second-generation l.
shock wave l.
Siemens Lithostar Plus System
  C l.
Sonolith 3000 l.
Sonolith Praktis portable l.
Sonotrode l.
Storz Modulith SL20 l.
Swiss Lithoclast l.
Therasonics l.
third-generation l.
tubeless l.
Twinheads shock wave l.
ultrasonic l.
Waltz endoscopic l.
water cushion l.
Wolf Piezolith l.
Wolf Sonolith l.
lithotriptoscope
lithotrite
Keyes l.
Löwenstein l.
Lowsley l.
Marmite l.
Reliquet l.
Rotolith l.
Thompson l.
Wolf l.
Lithovac master suction system

litmus paper
LITT applicator
Littauer
L. bone-cutting forceps
L. cilia forceps
L. dissecting scissors
L. ear dressing forceps
L. ear polyp forceps
L. nasal dressing forceps
L. rongeur
L. scissors
L. stitch scissors
L. suture carrying scissors
Littauer-Liston bone-cutting forceps
Littauer-West
L.-W. cutting forceps
L.-W. rongeur
Littig strut AFO
Little
L. Black Box frequency generator
L. cargo vest
L. intraocular lens implant
L. Ones pediatric urine collector
L. Ones Sur-Fit flexible wafer
L. Ones Sur-Fit pediatric appliance
  belt
L. retractor
Littler
L. dissecting scissors
L. suture-carrying scissors
Littlewood tissue forceps
Littman defibrillation pad
Littmann
L. ECG electrode
L. Galilean magnification changer
L. Master Classic II stethoscope
Litwak cannula
liver
l. biopsy needle
l. coil
l. dialysis unit
HepatAssist bioartificial l.
l. retractor
liver-holding clamp
Livernois
L. lens-holding forceps
L. pickup and folding forceps
Liverpool
L. elbow implant
L. knee prosthesis
live splint
Livewire
L. TC ablation catheter
L. TC steerable electrophysiology
  catheter
living
L. Air unit
l. related conjunctival limbal
  allograft

L

529

Livingskin silicone prosthesis
Livingston
L. forceps
L. intramedullary bar
L. peribulbar wedge
Lixiscope scope
LKB/Wallac
L. automatic gamma counter
L. scintillation counter
LLETZ-LEEP active loop electrode
Llorente dissecting forceps
Lloyd
L. adapter
L. bronchial catheter
L. chiropractic table
L. double catheter
L. esophagoscopic catheter
L. flexion distraction table
L. nail driver
L. nail extractor
Lloyd-Davies
L.-D. clamp
L.-D. occlusion forceps
L.-D. rectal scissors
L.-D. sigmoidoscope
L.-D. stirrup
LMA
LMA Ctrach mask
LMA disposable laryngeal mask
airway
LMA Fastrach laryngeal mask
airway
LMA laryngeal mask
LMA ProSeal laryngeal mask
airway
LMB
LMB finger splint
LMB wire-foam economical resting
splint
L'Nard
L. boot
L. long opponens hand and wrist
orthosis
L. thoracolumbosacral orthosis
LNOP
low noise optical probe
Lo
Lo Bak spinal support
Lo Bak spinal support prosthesis
Darco Body Armor Lo
Lo Rider prosthetic foot
load beam
loader
Lehner II l.
loading jig
Lobana wound cleanser
lobe
l. grasping forceps
l. holding forceps

lobectomy
l. forceps
l. scissors
lobotomy
l. electrode
l. needle
lobster bone-reduction forceps
lobster-type clamp
local gradient coil
LocaLisa cardiac navigation system
localizer
FlashPoint optical l.
Homer needle/wire l.
Risser l.
Roper-Hall l.
Suetens-Gybels-Vandermeulen
angiographic l.
Urrets-Zavalia l.
localizing
l. electrode
l. probe
LocalMed
L. catheter infusion sleeve
L. InfusaSleeve
locator
apex l.
Apit electronic apex l.
ASIS femoral head l.
automatic vehicle l.
Berman foreign body l.
Endex apex l.
foreign body l.
Gill-Thomas l.
Neosono MC apex l.
Odontometer electronic apex l.
Root ZX apex l.
Roper-Hall l.
saddle l.
Staodyn Insight point l.
Sweet l.
locator/stimulator
Neuro-Pulse nerve l./s.
Pointer-Plus l./s.
LOC guidewire extension
lock
Ball knee l.
L. Clamshell device
Codman disposable ICP l.
German l.
Howland l.
lateral spring-loaded l.
Luer cannula l.
l. needle
l. pericardiocentesis set and tray
Ratchet Lock variable flexion
knee l.
sliding l.
suture l.
VariLock socket l.

Lock-A-Card
locked intramedullary osteosynthesis pin
Lockhart-Mummery
    L.-M. probe
    L.-M. retractor
lock-in amplifier
locking
    l. bar
    l. clamp
    l. compression plate (LCP)
    l. device
    l. nut
    l. peg
    l. prosthesis
    l. reconstruction plate
    l. screw
    l. stylet
LockJaw arch bar
lockout suture
Lockwood
    L. clamp
    L. intestinal forceps
    L. tissue forceps
Lockwood-Allis
    L.-A. intestinal forceps
    L.-A. tissue forceps
LoCon-T
    L.-T distal radial plate
    L.-T distal radial plating system
Loctite 15494 ethyl cyanoacrylate glue
Lode BV Excalibur braked cycle
  ergometer
Lo-Fold balloon
Löfqvist tourniquet
Lofstrand crutch
Logan
    L. dissector
    L. lacrimal sac self-retaining
      retractor
    L. lip traction bow
    L. periosteal elevator
Log-a-Rhythm signal acquisition unit
logger
    Digitrapper Gold MK III solid-state
      data l.
Logic
    L. coronary stent
    L. mandibular distraction system
    L. MR transducer
LogiCal pressure transducer system
logMAR chart
LOK
    Swede-O Arch Lok
Lombard-Beyer
    L.-B. forceps
    L.-B. rongeur
Lombard-Boies mastoid rongeur

Lombart
    L. radioscope
    L. tonometer
London
    L. College foil carrier
    L. narrow-bladed retractor
    L. School of Hygiene and Tropical
      Medicine sphygmomanometer
    L. tissue forceps
Lone
    L. Star retractor
    L. Star retractor system
    L. Star self-retractor
long
    l. above-elbow cast
    l. ACE fixed-wire balloon catheter
    l. alignment rod
    l. arm navicular cast
    l. arm splint
    l. atraumatic retractor
    l. axis traction chiropractic table
    l. backboard
    L. Beach pedicle screw
    L. Beach stereotactic robot
    l. below-elbow cast
    l. Brite Tip guiding catheter
    l. coarse bur
    l. double upright brace
    L. Island College Hospital
      placental forceps
    l. leg brace
    l. leg cylinder cast
    l. leg immobilizer
    l. leg plaster
    l. leg plaster cast
    l. leg posterior molded splint
    l. leg walking cast
    l. nail-mounted drill guide
    l. needle
    l. occluder
    l. opponens orthosis
    l. scalpel
    l. skinny over-the-wire balloon
      catheter
    l. stitch scissors
    l. stretch bandage
    l. taper stiff shaft Glidewire
    l. tissue forceps
    l. vascular needle driver
Long45 endocutter
long-bore collimator
Longdwel
    L. catheter needle
    L. Teflon catheter
long-edge medullary nail
Longevity V-Lign hip prosthesis
long-handle
    l.-h. curette
    l.-h. offset gouge

L

long-handled dressing reacher
longitudinal spinal bar
long-jaw
    l.-j. basket forceps
    l.-j. disposable forceps
long-nosed sphincterotome
long-pulsed
    l.-p. dye laser
    l.-p. potassium-titanyl-phosphate
    laser
long/short occluder
long-span rigid plate
long-term
    l.-t. ambulatory physiologic
    surveillance monitor
    l.-t. internal jugular catheter
long-wearing contact lens
Look
    L. capsule polisher
    L. cortex extractor
    L. cystotome
    L. I&A coaxial cannula
    L. irrigating lens loop
    L. irrigating lens loupe
    L. irrigating vectis
    L. micropuncture device
    L. retrobulbar needle
    L. suture
loop (*See also* loupe)
    access l.
    advanced insulin infusion using a
    control l.
    2-angled polypropylene l.
    l. ball electrode
    bipolar cutting l.
    bipolar urological l.
    Blair-Ivy l.
    blind l.
    Bunnell finger l.
    Clayman-Knolle irrigating lens l.
    C-Max cutting l.
    l. curette
    cutting l.
    Duncan l.
    l. electrode
    Electrodes l.
    finger l.
    Flynn lens l.
    foreign body l.
    Gerdy intraauricular l.
    l. and hook strapping
    Hutson l.
    irrigating vectis l.
    Ivy l.
    Knapp lens l.
    lens l.
    Look irrigating lens l.
    maxi-vessel l.
    Meyer-Archambault l.

Meyer temporal l.
l. monitor
nylon l.
Olympus resectoscope l.
perineal l.
physiologic endometrial
    ablation/resection l. (PEARL)
polyglactin monofilament l.
polyglyconate monofilament l.
pressure length l.
Ransford l.
l. retractor
rigid monopolar l.
Roux l.
l. scaler
Schroeder tenaculum l.
l. scissors
l. shunt
soft wire l.
spring wire l.
Sur-Fit l.
Surgitite ligating l.
tenaculum hook l.
toe l.
tonsillar l.
tonsillectomy l.
twisted wire snare l.
unipolar cutting l.
Uresil radiopaque silicone-band
    vessel l.
vaginal speculum l.
Vaper Cut l.
Vapor Cut l.
vascular l.
vectis l.
vessel l.
Wedge l.
wire l.
4-loop
    4-l. iris clip implant
    4-l. iris fixated implant
loop-fixated intraocular lens
loop-over wrap
loop-tipped electrode
loop-type
    l.-t. snare forceps
    l.-t. stone-crushing forceps
Loo punch
loose
    l. body grasper
    l. body suction forceps
Lopez enteral valve
Lo-Por
    L.-P. vascular graft
    L.-P. vascular graft prosthesis
LoPresti fiberoptic esophagoscope
Lo-Profile
    L.-P. balloon
    L.-P. II balloon catheter

L.-P. II catheter
L.-P. steerable dilatation catheter
L.-P. urostomy pouch
Lo-Pro tracheal tube
Lorad
L. digital breast imager
L. full-field digital mammography system
L. StereoGuide
L. StereoGuide prone breast biopsy system
L. StereoGuide stereotactic breast biopsy system
Lord
L. cup
L. total hip arthrodesis
L. total hip prosthesis
Lordan chalazion forceps
Lordex lumbar spine system
lordoticiser
Posture Pump l.
Lore
L. subglottic forceps
L. suction tube
L. suction tube-holding forceps
L. suction tube and tip-holding forceps
Lore-Lawrence trachea tube
Lorenz
L. brace
L. chisel
L. gauze packer
L. Micro-Power dense bone drilling and cutting system
L. night splint
L. osteosynthesis system
L. PC/TC scissors
L. plating system
L. reamer
L. screw
L. temporomandibular prosthetic joint system
L. titanium screws and plate
Lorenz-Rees nasal rasp
lorgnette occluder
Loring ophthalmoscope
Lorna nonperforating towel clamp
Lothrop
L. dissector
L. hemostat
L. ligature forceps
L. tonsillar knife
L. tonsillar retractor
L. uvular retractor
Lotmar Visometer
lotrafilcon A contact lens
Lo-Trau side-cutting needle
Lottes
L. pin

L. reamer
L. triflange intramedullary nail
Lotus unicompartment prosthesis
Louis
L. instrumentation
L. plate
loupe (*See also* loop)
Adler tripronged lens error l.
angled lens l.
angled lens l.
angled nucleus removal l.
Beebe l.
Berens lens l.
Billeau ear l.
binocular l.
Castroviejo lens l.
Denlan magnifying l.
ear l.
Elschnig-Weber l.
fiberoptic l.
Flynn lens l.
Galilean l.
Gill-Welsh-Morrison lens l.
Gullstrand lens l.
Ilg lens l.
intracapsular lens l.
irrigating lens l.
irrigating vectis l.
Keeler l.
Keeler-Galilean surgical l.
Keeler panoramic l.
Keeler spotlight lens l.
Keeler wide-angle lens l.
Kirby intracapsular lens l.
Kirby intraocular lens l.
Kleinsasser lens l.
Knapp lens l.
Knolle-Pearce irrigating lens l.
Kraff nucleus lens l.
Lemoine-Searcy fixation anchor l.
Lempert-Storz l.
Lempert-Storz lens l.
lens l.
Lewis lens l.
Look irrigating lens l.
Magill magnifying l.
l. magnification
magnifying l.
Mark II Magni-Focuser l.
May hook-on lens l.
New Orleans lens l.
nucleus delivery l.
nucleus removal l.
ocular l.
ocular gamboscope l.
operating l.
Opticaid lens l.
panoramic l.
prism l.

loupe *(continued)*
  Simcoe double-end lens l.
  Simcoe II PC nucleus delivery l.
  Simcoe nucleus lens l.
  Snellen lens l.
  surgical l.
  Troutman lens l.
  Visitec nucleus removal l.
  Weber-Elschnig lens l.
  Wilder lens l.
  Wilder lens l.
  Zeiss-Gullstrand l.
  Zeiss lens l.
  Zeiss operating field l.
Lovac
  L. fundal contact lens implant
  L. 6-mirror gonioscopic lens
  L. 6-mirror gonioscopic lens
    implant
Love
  L. leukotome
  L. nasal splint
  L. nasopharyngeal retractor
  L. nerve root retractor
  L. pituitary rongeur
  L. retractor
  L. uvula retractor
Love-Adson periosteal elevator
Love-Gruenwald
  L.-G. alligator forceps
  L.-G. cranial rongeur
  L.-G. intervener
  L.-G. intervertebral disc rongeur
  L.-G. laminectomy rongeur
  L.-G. pituitary forceps
  L.-G. pituitary rongeur
Love-Kerrison
  L.-K. rongeur
  L.-K. rongeur forceps
Lovelace
  L. bladder forceps
  L. gallbladder traction forceps
  L. hemostatic forceps
  L. lung grasping forceps
  L. thyroid traction vulsellum
    forceps
  L. tissue forceps
  L. traction lung forceps
  L. traction tissue forceps
Loving
  L. Comfort maternity support
  L. Comfort postpartum support
Lovitt-Uhler modification of Jewett
  postfusion brace
low
  l. air-loss bed
  l. bleed implant
  l. forceps
  l. noise optical probe (LNOP)

  l. outlet forceps
  l. profile R-K marker
  l. quarter Blucher shoe
Löw-Beer forceps
low-compliance
  l.-c. balloon
  l.-c. perfusion pump
  l.-c. perfusion system
  l.-c. pneumohydraulic pump
low-compliance, fixed diameter balloon
low-contact
  l.-c. dynamic compression plate
  l.-c. stress plate
  l.-c. stress semiconstrained
    prosthesis
low-dose Excimer 308-nm laser
low-dye
  l.-d. strapping
  l.-d. taping
Lowe-Breck cartilage knife
Lowell
  L. glaucoma knife
  L. pleural needle
Löwenberg forceps
low-energy
  l.-e. collimator
  l.-e. laser
  l.-e. ultra high-resolution (LEUHR)
Lowenstein-Jensen plate
Löwenstein lithotrite
lower
  l. gall duct forceps
  l. lateral forceps
  l. limb orthosis
  l. limb prosthesis
low-field
  l.-f. MRI system
  l.-f. MR scanner
Low-Flex lead
low-flow
  l.-f. circuit
  l.-f. regulator
low-grade suction unit
low-heeled shoe
low-impedance thermocouple
low-magnification electron micrograph
Lowman
  L. bone-holding clamp
  L. bone-holding forceps
  L. chisel
  L. hand retractor
  L. rongeur
Lowman-Hoglund
  L.-H. chisel
  L.-H. clamp
low-margin standard abutment
Lown cardioverter
low-pass filter

low-power
    l.-p. laser
    l.-p. optics for myopic correction lens
low-pressure
    l.-p. breast pump
    l.-p. voice prosthesis
low-profile
    l.-p. angioplasty balloon
    l.-p. balloon-positioning catheter
    l.-p. breast implant
    l.-p. dorsal plate
    l.-p. mitral heart valve
    l.-p. plate
    l.-p. port implantable port
    l.-p. prosthesis
    l.-p. R-K marker
    l.-p. walker
low-resistance rolling seal spirometer
Lowsley
    L. grasping forceps
    L. hemostat
    L. lithotrite
    L. prostate retractor
    L. prostatic forceps
    L. prostatic tractor
    L. retractor
    L. retractor with hand-sutured closure
    L. ribbon-gut needle
    L. stone crusher
    L. suprapubic tractor
    L. tractor
    L. urethroscope
Lowsley-Peterson
    L.-P. cystoscope
    L.-P. endoscope
low-speed
    l.-s. Christmas tree diamond bur
    l.-s. rotation angioplasty catheter
    l.-s. tapered carbide bur
low-surface reactive Bioglass
low-tide walking brace
low-viscosity bone cement
low-vision
    l.-v. aid
    l.-v. enhancement system (LVES)
low-weight tonometer
LPI excimer laser system
LPK-80 II argon laser
L-plate
    L-p. plate
    Synthes mini L-p.
LPS
    limb preservation system
    LPS balloon
    DePuy Orthogenesis LPS
    Orthogenesis LPS
    LPS Peel-Away introducer

LP^2 stainless steel delivery system
LP stent
L-resection guide
LRI diamond knife
LR needle
L-rod
    L-r. implant material
    L-r. instrumentation
    Luque L-r.
L&R X-ray film dryer
LS
    LS 6500 liquid scintillation counting system
    LS 100Q/200/230 series laser diffraction particle size analyzer
    LS 13 320 series laser diffraction particle size analyzer
LSC curved-array transducer
LS^4 custom spinal jacket
L-shaped
    L-s. aneurysm clip
    L-s. cautery
    L-s. elevator
    L-s. miniplate
    L-s. plate
LSI silver self-adhesive disposable electrode
LSK
    LSK One disposable microkeratome
    LSK One standard microkeratome
LSM-2100C eye bank specular microscope
LSU
    LSU reciprocation-gait orthosis
    LSU reciprocation-gait orthosis bracc
LT
    large trapezoid
    LT Mesh implant
LTK system
LTX3000 lumbar rehabilitation system
LUA ELISA test kit
lube
    Sklar l.
Lubinus
    L. acetabular component
    L. AP hip system
    L. knee prosthesis
    L. SP II anatomically adapted hip system
Lübke-Berci VersaLight
Lübke uterine vacuum cannula
Lubri-Flex
    L.-F. stent
    L.-F. ureteral stent
    L.-F. urologic stent
Lubriglide-coated guidewire
Luc
    L. ethmoidal forceps

Luc *(continued)*
- L. forceps
- L. nasal cutting forceps
- L. septal forceps
- L. septum cutting forceps

Lucae
- L. bayonet
- L. bayonet dressing forceps
- L. bayonet ear forceps
- L. bayonet tissue forceps
- L. bone hammer
- L. bone mallet
- L. dissecting forceps
- L. dressing forceps
- L. ear perforation knife
- L. ear probe
- L. ear speculum
- L. eustachian catheter
- L. hook
- L. mastoid mallet

Lucas
- L. alveolar curette
- L. chisel
- L. gouge

Lucite
- L. form
- L. sphere implant

Luck
- L. bone drill
- L. bone saw
- L. nail

Lu corneal marker
Ludwig
- L. middle ear applicator
- L. sinus applicator

Luedde exophthalmometer
Luer
- L. bone curette
- L. bone rongeur
- L. cannula lock
- L. connection
- L. connector
- L. curette forceps
- L. double-ended tracheal retractor
- L. eye speculum
- L. hemorrhoidal forceps
- L. mallet
- L. needle
- L. reconstruction plate
- L. retractor
- L. rongeur forceps
- L. speaking tube
- L. S-shaped retractor
- L. suction cannula adapter
- L. syringe
- L. syringe tip
- L. thoracic rongeur
- L. tracheal cannula
- L. tracheal tube
- L. tube

Luer-Lok
- L.-L. adapter
- L.-L. B-D syringe
- L.-L. connector
- L.-L. fitting
- L.-L. jet ventilator connector
- L.-L. male adapter plug
- L.-L. needle
- L.-L. port
- L.-L. stopcock
- L.-L. syringe
- universal L.-L.
- Yale L.-L.

Luer-type syringe
Luer-Whiting
- L.-W. rongeur
- L.-W. rongeur forceps

Luetje stimulating dissector
Luhr
- L. fixation plate
- L. implant
- L. implant screw
- L. mandibular plate
- L. maxillofacial fixation system
- L. microfixation cranial plate
- L. microfixation system
- L. Microfixation System drill bit
- L. microfixation system plate cutter
- L. microfixation system plate-holding forceps
- L. microfixation system pliers
- L. microplate
- L. miniplate
- L. pan fixation system
- L. pan plate
- L. screw
- L. vitallium micromesh plate
- L. vitallium screw

Luikart
- L. dissector
- L. forceps

Luikart-Bill
- L.-B. forceps
- L.-B. traction handle

Luikart-Kjelland obstetrical forceps
Luikart-Simpson obstetrical forceps
Lukens
- L. aspirator
- L. bone wax dressing
- L. cannula
- L. catgut suture
- L. collecting tube
- L. collector
- L. double-channel irrigator
- L. double-ended tracheal retractor
- L. epiglottic retractor
- L. needle

L. orthodontic band
L. thymus retractor
L. trap

Luki
L. aspirating tube
L. specimen trap

Luma-Cath
L.-C. fixed-curve diagnostic catheter
L.-C. steerable curve diagnostic
catheter

Luma cervical imaging system
Lumaguide catheter
Lumax
L. fiberoptic catheter
L. Flex guiding catheter
L. Pro cystometry system

lumbar
l. anterior root stimulator implant
l. aortography needle
l. corset
l. drain
l. drainage catheter
l. I/F Cage
l. intersomatic fusion expandable
cage
l. orthosis
l. pedicle screw
l. peritoneal catheter
l. port
l. puncture needle
l. retractor
l. roll
l. subarachnoid catheter
l. support cushion
l. tapered cage lumbar tapered
fusion device

lumbodorsal support corset
Lumbo 90 home care traction system
lumbosacral
l. brace
l. corset
l. fusion elevator
l. orthosis
l. spine transpedicular
instrumentation
l. support pelvic traction

Lumbotrain lumbosacral support
lumbrical bar
lumen
l. cannula
l. finder

8-lumen
8-l. catheter assembly
8-l. manometric catheter

Lu-Mendez
L.-M. LRI guide
L.-M. LRI guide and fixation ring

Lumenis 950 slit-lamp
4-lumen polyvinyl manometric catheter

Lumex
L. lightweight wheelchair
L. Preferred Care recliner
L. PT fiberoptic cystometry system
L. recliner
L. shower bed
L. shower stretcher
L. Tilt-in-Space reclining
wheelchair
L. Tub-Guard safety rail
L. walker

Lumina
L. guidewire
L. operating telescope
L. rod lens arthroscope

luminal stent
Luminary LASIK light probe
Luminexx
L. biliary stent
L. self-expanding stent

luminometer
LB 9501 l.
Packard l.

luminous retinoscope
Lumiscan LS 85 scanner
Lumisys 20 digital x-ray scanner
Lumonics YAG laser
**Lumos implantable cardioverter-
defibrillator**
Lunar
L. bone density machine
L. DPX densitometer
L. DPX dual-energy absorptiometer
L. DPX total-body scanner
L. Expert densitometer
L. scanner

lunate
l. acrylic cement wrist prosthesis
l. implant
l. prosthesis

Lunax Boot
Lunderquist
L. catheter
L. coat hanger wire
L. exchange guidewire
L. exchange wire
L. extra-stiff wire guide
L. guidewire

Lunderquist-Ring
L.-R. guidewire
L.-R. torque guide

Lundholm
L. plate
L. screw

**Lund prototype unicompartment
prosthesis**
Lundsgaard
L. blade
L. knife

L

Lundsgaard *(continued)*
  L. rasp
  L. sclerotome
Lundsgaard-Burch
  L.-B. corneal rasp
  L.-B. knife
  L.-B. sclerotome
Luneau retinoscopy rack
lung
  artificial l.
  l. dissecting scissors
  l. exclusion clamp
  l. grasping forceps
  l. imaging fluorescence endoscope
  iron l.
  Kolobow membrane l.
  membrane artificial l.
  Penn State intravascular l.
    (PENSIL)
  l. retractor
  Sci-Med Life Systems, Inc.
    membrane artificial l.
  l. tissue forceps
Lungmotor
Luntz-Dodick punch
Luongo
  L. hand retractor
  L. needle
Luque
  L. cerclage wire
  L. fixation device
  L. II fixation system
  L. II plate
  L. II screw
  L. II segmental spinal
    instrumentation
  L. L-rod
  L. rectangle
  L. rod
  L. rod fixation
  L. semirigid segmental spinal
    instrumentation
  L. sublaminar wire
Luque-Galveston rod
Lusk
  L. forceps
  L. instrument
Lusskin bone drill
Luster investment material
lutetium oxyorthosilicate-based PET
  scanner
Luther-Peter retractor
Lutz
  L. automatic reprocessor
  L. septal forceps
Luxar
  L. NovaPulse CO_2 laser
  L. NovaPulse laser

  L. Silhouette noninvasive body
    appearance equipment
Luxator extractor
5 lux color videocamera
Luxo
  L. illuminated magnifier
  L. surgical illuminator
LuXon Journey foot prosthesis
Luxtec
  L. fiberoptic system
  L. illuminated surgical telescope
Luy segregator
LV
  left ventricular
    LV apex cannula
LVAD
  left ventricular assist device
    vented-electric HeartMate LVAD
LVES
  low-vision enhancement system
    head-mounted video magnifier
      LVES
LX
    BiPAP Duet LX
    LX EchoSpeed CV/i, NVi MR
      system
    Millennium LX
    LX needle
LX-20 laser
LX20, LX200, LX2000 PRO clinical
  system
LX4201 clinical system
LXi 725 clinical system
lyer
  side l.
Lyman-Smith
  L.-S. toe drop brace
  L.-S. tractor
lymphangiography
  pedal l.
Lymphapress device
lymphedema
  Meige l.
Lymphoprep tube
LymphoScan
  L. nuclear imaging system
  L. nuclear imaging system scanner
Lynch
  L. blunt dissector
  L. cup-shaped curette forceps
  L. curette
  L. electrode
  L. laryngeal dissector
  L. laryngeal forceps
  L. laryngeal knife handle
  L. mucosa separator plate
  L. obtuse angle laryngeal knife
  L. right-angle knife
  L. scissors

L. septal splint
L. spatula
L. straight knife
L. suspension apparatus
L. suspension laryngoscope
L. tonsillar dissector
L. tonsillar knife

Lynco
L. biomechanical orthotic system
L. foot orthosis

Lynx
L. midurethral sling
L. wrist, hand, finger orthosis arm positioner splint

Lyofoam
L. A, C, T foam dressing
L. Extra foam dressing

Lyo-Ject syringe

Lyon
L. forceps
L. ring
L. tube

Lyra
L. 2020 implantable cardioverter

L. 2020 implantable cardioverter-defibrillator
L. laser
L. laser system

Lyra-i laser system
lyre-shaped finger hook
LySonix
L. 250 aspirator
L. Delta Tip irrigator
L. Diamond Tip scavenger
L. 250 irrigator
L. 2000 Micro ultrasonic surgical system
L. Post-Operative patient system
L. Series 250 irrigator/aspirator
L. Series 250 operative system
L. 2000 standard ultrasonic surgical system
L. TTD cannula system
L. 2000 ultrasonic surgical system
L. 2000 ultrasound device

lysoPC diagnostic ovarian cancer test
Lyte Fit orthotic

L

3M
- 3M Clean Seals waterproof bandage
- 3M Coban LF self-adherent wrap
- 3M CTRS device
- 3M filling instrument
- 3M Healthcare particulate respirator
- 3M Healthcare surgical mask
- 3M intraocular lens
- 3M limb isolation bag
- 3M mammary implant
- 3M matrix tape
- 3M Maxi Driver blade
- 3M Microdon dressing
- 3M Micropore surgical tape
- 3M microvascular anastomotic coupling device
- 3M No Sting barrier film
- 3M Reston self-adhcring foam pad & roll
- 3M scanner
- 3M small aperture Steri-Drape
- 3M small aperture Steri-Drape drape
- 3M SoftCloth adhesive wound dressing
- 3M staple
- 3M Steri-Drape drape
- 3M Tegaderm transparent dressing with absorbent pad
- 3M Tegapore wound contact material
- 3M Tegasorb hydrocolloid dressing
- 3M Vi-drape

M4
- M4 Kerr Safety Hedstrom instrument
- M4 safety handpiece

M-2 anterior plate system
M3-X extremity fixation system
M4-400 freedom blade
M6/C cylinder carrying case
M6 oxygen cylinder
M2A swallowable imaging capsule
MA-1 respirator
MA30BA intraocular lens
Macaluso stent remover
MacAusland
- M. bone mallet
- M. chisel
- M. dissector
- M. finishing ball reamer
- M. finishing cup reamer
- M. hip skid
- M. muscle retractor

Macbeth ColorChecker
MacCarty forceps
MAC cervical collar
Macdonald
- M. dissector
- M. gastric clamp
- M. periosteal elevator

Macewen
- M. drill
- M. saw

MacGregor nasal osteotome
MA 53 2-channel audiometer
Machat
- M. adjustable aspirating wire speculum
- M. double-ended marker
- M. superior flap LASIK marker

Machat-type adjustable aspirating LASIK speculum
Machemer
- M. calipers
- M. diamond dust-coated foreign body forceps
- M. diamond-dusted forceps
- M. flat lens
- M. infusion contact lens
- M. magnifying vitrectomy lens
- M. scleral knife
- M. vitreous cutter

Mach 1 guide catheter
Machida
- M. FCS-ML II magnifying colonoscope
- M. fiber duodenoscope
- M. fiberoptic laryngoscope
- M. flexible endoscope
- M. light source connector

machinable apatite-free glass ceramic
machine
- A2008 ABGII hemodialysis m.
- Accuray Neurotron 1000 m.
- Accuson-128 color flow Doppler m.
- Accu-SPINA cervical decompression m.
- Accu-Tron microcurrent m.
- Acoma portable x-ray m.
- Acuson model 128XP m.
- Aestiva/5 MRI anesthesia m.
- AK-10 dialysis m.
- ankle exercise m.
- Apogee CX100 Interspec ultrasound m.
- BackStrong lumbar extension m.
- Berkeley suction m.

M

machine *(continued)*
Biodex isokinetic testing m.
Bionx servohydraulic testing m.
BiPAP m.
Bird m.
borazone blade cutting m.
Brown-Bovari m.
Brüel & Kjaer 1860 ultrasound m.
Burdick ECG m.
bypass m.
CamStar exercise m.
Catalyst m.
Century heart-lung m.
cobalt megavoltage m.
Cobe-Stöckert heart-lung m.
constant passive-motion m.
 (CPMM)
cooling m.
CooperVision I&A m.
Corometrics-Aloka
 echocardiograph m.
CPAP m.
CPM m.
CPM exerciser m.
Cybex m.
Danniflex CPM m.
2D B-mode ultrasound m.
demand flow m.
Drake-Willock dialysis m.
Echospeed 1.5T MR m.
endoscopic sewing m.
Endotek m.
Euro Precision Technology
 submicron lathe m.
Exerstrider m.
Faxitron x-ray m.
Finapres Dinamap blood
 pressure m.
focused segmented ultrasound m.
Fresenius 2008H hemodialysis m.
Gambro AK10 m.
G5 massage and percussion m.
HemoTec ACT m.
Hewlett-Packard 500, 1000 Echo-
 Doppler m.
I&A m.
Instron m.
intermittent flow m.
Isotechnologies B-200 low back m.
isotonic m.
Kinetec hip CPM m.
Kodak Ektachem 700 m.
Kurzweil reading m.
Lunar bone density m.
Mayo-Gibbon heart-lung m.
MB-900 AC m.
MDA ultrasound-assisted
 lipoplasty m.
Med-Fit Senior Circuit exercise m.

Medicamat ultrasound-assisted
 lipoplasty m.
MedX m.
MedX functional testing m.
MedX knee m.
MedX Mark II lumbar
 extension m.
MedX stretch m.
megavoltage m.
Mentor ultrasound-assisted
 lipoplasty m.
milling m.
Morwel ultrasound-assisted
 lipoplasty m.
Narkomed anesthesia m.
neutron therapy m.
Northland bone density m.
Nova II m.
Orthion traction m.
Orthopantomograph-3, -10
 panoramic x-ray m.
Orthoralix dental x-ray m.
OsseoCare m.
OsteoPower drilling and cutting m.
Panelipse panoramic x-ray m.
Panex-E panoramic x-ray m.
Panorex panoramic x-ray m.
Paramount total body plate-
 loaded m.
PC-1000/Laser 1000 panoramic
 cephalometric x-ray m.
PC-1000 panoramic x-ray m.
Philips ultrasound m.
Phillips ultrasound m.
PhotoDerm m.
PodoFlex m.
Primus prostate m.
remote control afterloading m.
ResMed CPAP Sullivan III m.
Respironics BiPAP m.
Respironics CPAP m.
Respitrace m.
Rife m.
Rosys Plato Gene M.
Sakura Seiki Autosmear automatic
 smear m.
Schwinn elliptical full body
 exercise m.
Sebbin ultrasound-assisted
 lipoplasty m.
Select-a-Fuge microcentrifuge m.
SMEI ultrasound-assisted
 lipoplasty m.
Sono-stat Plus EMG m.
Stat Scrub handwasher m.
Status-X m.
suction m.
Sullivan V Elite Real Time Clock
 CPAP m.

Surgilav m.
Surgitron ultrasound-assisted
  lipoplasty m.
Sysmex SE-9500 m.
Teca Sapphire EMG m.
TECA-TD20 EMG m.
TENS m.
Toshiba echocardiograph m.
Toshiba electrocardiography m.
Ventana ES slide processor m.
Ventana immuno-automated m.
VersaClimber RX exercise m.
Visual-Tech m.
Vivatek ultimate healing m.
Voll m.
Wikco ankle m.

Machlett collimator
MacIntosh
M. blade
M. fiberoptic laryngoscope blade
M. laryngoscope
M. tibial plateau prosthesis
Maciol suture needle set
Mack
M. ear plug
M. lingual tonsillar tonsillectome
M. serrefine
M. tonometer
MacKay-Marg tonometer
MacKenty septal elevator
Mackenzie polygraph
Mackler tube
Mackool
M. capsule retractor
M. system
Mack's earplug
Maclaren mobile buggy
MacNab-English shoulder prosthesis
MacRae flap flipper/retreatment spatula
Macro-5 camera
Macroduct
M. coil
M. collecting system
M. system for sweat stimulation
  and collection
macro-mesh mesh
Macroplastique
M. implant
M. implantable device
MacroPore
M. distraction mesh
M. fixation system
M. mesh fixation
M. OS spinal system
M. screw
MacroSorb absorbable plate implant
Mac stent

macular
m. contact lens
m. photostress
MaculoScope scope
MadaJet
M. XL jet-injection anesthesia
  system
M. XL local anesthesia system
M. XL needle-free injector
Madayag biopsy needle
Maddacare child bath seat
Maddacrawler frame
Maddapult Asissto-Seat
Madden
M. dissector
M. forceps
M. intestinal clamp
M. ligature carrier
M. sympathectomy hook
Madden-Potts
M.-P. intestinal forceps
M.-P. tissue forceps
Maddox
M. caudal needle
M. LASIK spatula
M. prism
M. rod
M. rod occluder
Madduri urethrogram catheter
madreporic hip prosthesis
Madsen OB822 clinical audiometer
Maestro
M. implant
M. implantable cardiac pacemaker
M. surgical drill system
M. system
M. wrist joint replacement system
MAFO
molded ankle-foot orthosis
MAFO cane
MAG-3
TechneScan MAG-3
magazine clip
Magellan
M. electromagnetic navigation
  system
M. monitor
Magerl
M. hook-plate system
M. plate-screw system
M. transarticular screw fixation
Maggi
M. biopsy needle
M. disposable biopsy needle guide
M. disposable biopsy needle guide
  for ultrasound
Magic
M. B1 balloon
M. microcatheter

M

Magic *(continued)*
- M. S/P Wallstent
- M. Torque guidewire
- M. Wallstent
- M. Wallstent stent
- M. Wand vibrator

Magill
- M. catheter forceps
- M. circuit
- M. endotracheal catheter
- M. endotracheal forceps
- M. forceps
- M. laryngoscope
- M. magnifying loupe
- M. orthodontic band
- M. Safety Clear endotracheal tube

Maglinte enteroclysis catheter
Maglite light
MagMag breast pump
Magna-Finder locating device
Magna-Fx
- M.-Fx cannulated screw
- M.-Fx cannulated screw fixation system

MagnaPod pain relief magnet
Magnascanner
- Picker M.
- Picker Vista M.

Magna-Site locating system
Magna-SL scanner
Magnassager
- M. massager
- M. massage tool

Magnatherm
- M. pulsed therapy high-frequency unit
- M. SSP electromagnetic therapy unit

Magnathotic orthotic
Magnatone hearing aid
MagneCore magnetic therapy pad
Magnes
- M. biomagnetometer
- M. biomagnetometer system
- M. 2500 WH imager
- M. 2500 whole-blood scanner

magnesium tuning fork
magnet
- air-core m.
- ankle m.
- m. application over pulse generator
- Atlas-Storz eye m.
- BIOflex medical m.
- bipolar m.
- ceramic m.
- doughnut m.
- ear m.
- Eindhoven m.
- elbow m.

- eye m.
- Fe-Ex orogastric tube m.
- foot m.
- foreign body m.
- GE Signa m.
- Grafco m.
- Gruening eye m.
- Grüning m.
- Gyroscan NT 10 m.
- Gyroscan superconducting m.
- Haab eye m.
- handheld eye m.
- Hirschberg m.
- Horizon LX 1.5-T superconducting m.
- horseshoe m.
- implant m.
- Lancaster eye m.
- large-bore m.
- MagnaPod pain relief m.
- Magnetom SP4000 m.
- Magnex m.
- Mellinger m.
- neodymium m.
- nonenclosed m.
- Norris tip m.
- open m.
- original Sweet eye m.
- Oxford m.
- pancake MRI m.
- passively shimmed superconducting m.
- Philips Gyroscan ACS NT superconducting m.
- Plastiform m.
- Ralks eye m.
- rare earth intraocular m.
- Schumann giant-type eye m.
- shim m.
- shimmed m.
- short-bore m.
- m. splint
- static m.
- Storz m.
- Storz-Atlas hand eye m.
- suction m.
- superconducting m.
- surgical power m.
- Sweet original m.
- taiki m.
- Tectonic m.
- tesla m.
- 1.0T, 1.5T superconducting m.
- tubular m.
- unipolar static m.
- Walker m.
- water m.
- m. wire

magnetic
- m. bead
- m. bed pad
- m. blanket
- m. cup
- m. extractor
- m. eye implant
- m. eye probe
- m. implant
- m. induction device
- m. insole
- m. internal ureteral stent
- m. jaw tracking device
- m. mat pad
- m. mattress pad
- m. microsphere
- m. motion transducer
- m. resonance (MR)
- m. resonance-compatible clip
- m. resonance endoscope
- m. resonance imaging (MRI)
- m. resonance imaging-compatible hollow-fiber bioreactor
- m. resonance imaging–compatible piezoelectric power drill
- m. resonance imaging-guided focused ultrasound sector transducer
- m. resonance marker
- m. retriever
- m. sensor
- m. shielded cabin
- m. stimulator
- m. support belt
- M. Support brace
- M. Surgery system
- m. wrap

magnetically activated cell sorter

magnetocardiogram

Magnetom
- M. Espree open MRI unit
- M. Open scanner
- M. Open system
- M. Sonata 1.5T MR system
- M. SP4000 magnet
- M. SP MRI imager
- M. SP63 scanner
- M. Symphony
- M. Symphony MR scanner
- M. Trio unlimited MRI system
- M. Vision MR imaging system
- M. Vision MR system
- M. Vision MR unit
- M. Vision scanner

magnetometer
- 8-channel whole-head m.
- m. probe

MagnetomSonata MR system

magnet-tipped flexible catheter

Magnex
- M. Alpha MR system
- M. magnet
- M. MR scanner

magnification
- loupe m.

magnifier
- aural m.
- Circline m.
- circline m.
- handheld m.
- Luxo illuminated m.
- Omnivue illuminated m.
- Optelec Passport m.
- optical m.
- projection m.
- right-angle prism m.
- stand m.

magnifying
- m. colonoscope
- m. glasses
- m. loupe

Magnum
- M. bariatric patient system bed
- M. 800 bed
- M. biopsy instrument
- M. chisel
- M. curette
- M. food scale
- M. guidewire
- M. 101 Plus stimulator
- M. 101 Plus table
- M. 100 stimulator
- M. Tiger blade

Magnuson
- M. abduction humeral splint
- M. circular twin saw
- M. double counter-rotating saw
- M. single circular saw
- M. strut
- M. twist drill
- M. valve prosthesis

Magnuson-Cromie prosthesis

Magovern-Cromie
- M.-C. ball-cage prosthetic valve
- M.-C. prosthesis

Magrain

Magrina-Bookwalter
- M.-B. vaginal retractor
- M.-B. vaginal retractor ring

Magstim
- M. Rapid magnetic stimulator
- M. 200 stimulator

Maguire-Harvey vitreous cutter

Mahoney
- M. dilator
- M. intranasal antral speculum

Mahurkar
- M. catheter

M

Mahurkar *(continued)*
    M. curved extension catheter
    M. dual-lumen femoral dialysis
      catheter
    M. fistular needle
Maico Gamma hearing aid
Maico-MA 20 audiometer
Maier
    M. dressing forceps
    M. polyp forceps
    M. sponge forceps
    M. uterine forceps
Maingot
    M. clamp
    M. gallbladder tube
    M. hysterectomy forceps
main pancreatic duct stent
Mainstay urologic soft tissue anchor
Mainster
    M. lens
    M. retina laser
    M. retinal laser lens
    M. Ultra Field PRP laser lens
    M. wide-field lens
Mainster-HM retinal laser lens
Mainster-S retinal laser lens
Mainster-WF retinal laser lens
maintainer
    anterior chamber m.
    Blumenthal anterior chamber m.
    Brierley chamber m.
    filter m.
    Gerber space m.
    Lewicky self-retaining chamber m.
Mainz
    M. pouch
    M. pouch urinary reservoir
    M. urinary pouch
Maisonneuve
    M. bandage
    M. urethrotome
Majestik shielded angiographic needle
major amblyoscope
Makler
    M. cannula
    M. counting chamber
    M. insemination device
    M. reusable semen analysis
      chamber
Malakit *Helicobacter pylori* **Biolab**
malar
    m. implant
    m. periosteum-SMAS flap fixation
      suture
Malcolm-Lynn
    M.-L. C-RXF cervical retractor
      frame
    M.-L. radiolucent spinal retraction
      system

Malcolm-Rand
    M.-R. carbon composite headholder
    M.-R. cranial x-ray frame
    M.-R. radiolucent headrest and
      retraction system
male
    m. catheter
    m. compression girdle
    m. condom
    M. FactorPak seminal fluid
      collection kit
    m. washer
Malecot
    M. catheter
    M. nephrostomy catheter
    M. nephrostomy tube
    M. reentry catheter
    M. self-retaining urethral catheter
    M. silastic catheter
    M. suprapubic catheter
    M. suprapubic cystostomy catheter
    M. tube
    M. 2-wing catheter
    M. 4-wing catheter
    M. 2-wing drain
    M. 4-wing drain
Malgaigne
    M. apparatus
    M. clamp
    M. patellar hook
Malibu cervical orthosis
Malis
    M. angled bayonet forceps
    M. bipolar coagulating/cutting
      system
    M. bipolar coagulation forceps
    M. bipolar cutting forceps
    M. bipolar instrument
    M. bipolar irrigating forceps
    M. bipolar microcoagulator
    M. brain retractor kit
    M. cerebellar retractor
    M. cerebral retractor
    M. clip applier
    M. CMC-II bipolar coagulator
    M. CMC-III electrosurgical system
    M. CMC-II PC bipolar coagulator
    M. cup forceps
    M. curette
    M. dissector
    M. electrocoagulation unit
    M. elevator
    M. hinge clamp
    M. irrigating bipolar CMC-III
    M. irrigating forceps stylet
    M. irrigation tubing set
    M. jeweler's bipolar forceps
    M. ligature passer
    M. needle holder

M. nerve hook
M. neurosurgical scissors
M. scissors
M. solid-state coagulator
M. titanium microsurgical forceps
Malis-Jensen
M.-J. bipolar forceps
M.-J. microbipolar forceps
malleable
m. blade
m. blade retractor
m. copper retractor
m. facial implant
m. implant
m. metal finger splint
m. microsurgical suction device
m. multipore suction tube
m. passing needle
m. probe
m. prosthesis
m. retractor
m. ribbon retractor
m. spatula
m. splint
m. stainless steel retractor
m. stylet
m. sucker
malleolar gel sleeve
MalleoLoc
M. ankle orthosis
M. ankle support
Malleo-Med soft ankle support
Malleotrain ankle support
mallet
Acufex m.
Bergman m.
bone m.
boxwood m.
cervical m.
copper m.
Cottle m.
Crane m.
Doyen bone m.
fiber m.
Gerzog bone m.
Hajek m.
hard m.
Heath m.
Henning m.
Hibbs m.
Jarit m.
Kirk m.
lead-filled m.
Lucae bone m.
Lucae mastoid m.
Luer m.
MacAusland bone m.
Mead m.
Meyerding m.

Miltex m.
nasal m.
Ombrédanne m.
polyethylene-faced m.
Richards m.
Rush m.
slotted m.
solid copper head m.
standard pattern m.
Steinbach m.
surgical m.
Swanson m.
White m.
Williger bone m.
malleus
m. cutter
m. forceps
m. nipper
malleus-footplate assembly
malleus-incus prosthesis
malleus-stapes assembly
Mallinckrodt
M. angiographic catheter
M. endotracheal tube
M. Hi-Care Pulmonary Hygiene
system
M. LaryngoSeal laryngeal mask
M. Laser-Flex tube
M. scanner
M. sensor system
M. Ultra tag labeling kit
M. vertebral catheter
Mallory-Head
M.-H. femoral stem
M.-H. I, II prosthesis
M.-H. Interlok calcar trimmer
M.-H. Interlok primary femoral
component
M.-H. Interlok rasp
M.-H. Interlok reamer
M.-H. modular acetabular template
M.-H. modular calcar system
M.-H. porous primary femoral
prosthesis
M.-H. rasp
M.-H. total hip prosthesis
Mallory prosthesis
Malmö hip splint
Malmstrom
M. cup
M. vacuum extractor
Maloney
M. bougie
M. catheter
M. endootoprobe
M. endootoprobe laser
M. mercury-filled esophageal dilator
M. no-hole lens manipulator
M. nucleus rotator

M

Maloney *(continued)*
    M. tapered mercury-filled esophageal bougie
    M. tapered-tip dilator
Maloney-Hurst dilator
Malström
    M. cup
    M. vacuum extractor
Malström-Westman cannula
Malteno glaucoma artificial valve
Maltese cross lens
maltodextrin
    Calgitrol calcium alginate wound dressing with m.
Maltz
    M. cartilage knife
    M. nasal rasp
    M. needle
    M. rasp
    M. retractor
    M. saw
Maltz-Lipsett nasal rasp
Malvern
    M. analyzer
    M. 2600 Sizer laser diffraction scanner
Mambo polishing towel
mammalian olfactory system
Mammalok localization needle
mammary
    m. implant
    m. prosthesis
    m. support dressing
mammary-coronary tissue forceps
Mammex TR computer-aided mammography diagnosis system
Mammo
    M. Mask dedicated viewer
    M. Mask illuminator
    M. Plus mammography system
mammographic view box
Mammo-Lume
Mammomat C3 mammography system
mammometer
MammoReader
    M. computer-aided detection system
    M. mammogram device
    M. mammography system
MammoScan digital imaging system
mammoscope
    acute-tipped m.
    central blunt-tipped m.
MammoSite
    M. radiation therapy system
    M. radiation therapy system catheter
    M. RTS balloon interstitial device
Mammotest Plus breast biopsy system

mammotome
    Biopsys m.
    M. biopsy system
    M. breast biopsy system
    M. core biopsy device
    M. ultrasound system
Mammotrax
Mammoviewer
Manager
    Cholesterol M.
    Integrated Wound M.
Manan needle
Manche
    M. irrigation cannula
    M. LASIK forceps
    M. LASIK speculum
Manchester
    M. LDR implant system
    M. nasal osteotome
    M. ovoid
Manche-type LASIK irrigating cannula
Mancini plate
Mancke flex-rigid gastroscope
Mandelkorn
    M. gauge/dilator system
    M. suture laser lysis lens
    M. suture lysis lens
mandibular
    m. advancement appliance
    m. advancement device
    m. advancing oral appliance
    m. angle fracture intraoral open reduction microplate
    m. angle fracture intraoral open reduction screw
    m. arch bar
    m. body retractor
    m. bridging plate
    m. mesh
    m. miniplate
    m. notch electrode
    m. orthopaedic repositioning appliance
    m. overdenture
    m. positioning device
    m. repositioner
    m. repositioning oral appliance
    m. sheet
    m. staple bone plate
    m. transosseous staple
mandrel, mandril
    m. graft
    intrauterine insemination cannula with m.
    steam-shaping m.
    threaded m.
mandrin
    m. dilator
    wire m.

Mangat curvilinear chin prosthesis
Mangham piston
Manhattan
    M. Eye & Ear corneal dissector
    M. Eye & Ear probe
    M. Eye & Ear spatula
    M. Eye & Ear suturing forceps
Manhood absorbent pouch
manifold
    3-stopcock m.
    Visiprep solid-phase extraction
      vacuum m.
Manifold II slot-blot apparatus
Manipujector
    Kronner M.
manipulation board
manipulator
    Akahoshi nucleus m.
    angled m.
    Barrett irrigating lens m.
    button lip lens m.
    button-tip m.
    ClearView uterine m.
    4-degree-of-freedom m.
    Drysdale nucleus m.
    Friedman phaco/IOL m.
    Gall-Addison uterine m.
    Grieshaber 2-function m.
    Grieshaber 3-function m.
    Guimaraes implantable contact
      lens m.
    Hasson uterine m.
    Hirschman lens m.
    hook m.
    Hulka uterine m.
    iris lens m.
    irrigating lens m.
    Jaffe-Maltzman lens m.
    Jarrett side port m.
    Judson-Smith m.
    Koch nucleus m.
    Koch phaco m.
    Kuglen angled lens m.
    Kuglen irrigating lens m.
    Kuglen lens m.
    Kuglen nucleus m.
    Kuglen straight lens m.
    LASIK flap m.
    lens m.
    Lester IOL m.
    Lester lens m.
    Levy-Kuglen lens m.
    Lieberman MicroFinger m.
    Lindstrom Star nucleus m.
    Lister lens m.
    Maloney no-hole lens m.
    McIntyre irrigating iris m.
    Microbeam m.
    multi coordinate m.

    Ramirez m.
    Rappazzo intraocular m.
    RUMI uterine m.
    Sinskey IOL m.
    Sinskey lens m.
    uterine m.
    Valtzhev uterine m.
    Visitec m.
    ZUMI uterine m.
manipulator/elevator
    Kritzinger-Updegraff m./e.
    K-U m./e.
manipulator/injector
    Harris-Kronner uterine m./i.
      (HUMI)
    HUMI uterine m./i.
    Kronner Manipujector uterine m./i.
    Rowden uterine m./i. (RUMI)
    Zinnanti uterine m./i. (ZUMI)
manipulator/splitter
    Koch phaco m./s.
Mannerfelt
    M. chisel
    M. gouge
    M. rasp
    M. retractor
Manning
    M. forceps
    M. retractor
Mannis
    M. probe
    M. suture
    M. suture probe
manometer
    aneroid m.
    DeVilbiss CPAP m.
    Dinamap ultrasound blood
      pressure m.
    Honan m.
    mercury m.
    Mercury Medical airway
      pressure m.
    Posey Cufflator tracheal cuff
      inflator and m.
    single-patient use m.
    m. stopcock
    Tycos m.
    ventilator pressure m.
manometer-tipped catheter
manometric
    m. catheter
    m. sensor
manoptoscope
Mansfield
    M. balloon
    M. balloon dilatation catheter
    M. bioptome
    M. forceps
    M. orthogonal electrode catheter

M

Mansfield *(continued)*
    M. Polaris electrode
    M. Scientific dilatation balloon
      catheter
Mansfield-Webster deflectable curved catheter
Manson-Aebli corneal section scissors
Mansson urinary pouch
Mantis retrograde forceps
manual
    m. CD4 kit
    m. defibrillator
    m. dermatome
    m. dermatome brush
    m. dermatome thickness gauge
    m. esthesiometer
    m. gun system
    m. jet ventilator
    m. keratometer
    m. lithotriptor
    m. optic planimeter
    m. osteotome
    m. resuscitation bag
    m. resuscitator
    m. retractor
    m. vacuum aspirator
    m. wheelchair
ManuTrain active wrist support
many-tailed
    m.-t. bandage
    m.-t. dressing
Maple Leaf hip orthosis
Mapleson D breathing system
MapMarkers fluorescent DNA sizing standard
mapping/ablation catheter
mapping catheter
Maquet
    M. operating table
    M. Servo-i ventilator
Maramed
    M. Miami fracture brace system
    M. ThermoFlex
Marathon
    M. crosslinked polyethylene liner
    M. guiding catheter
Marax bronchodilator
MarBlot test kit
March
    M. laser lens
    M. laser sclerostomy needle
Marco
    M. ARK-2000 refractor
    M. chart projector
    M. lensometer
    M. manual keratometer
    M. prism exophthalmometer
    M. radius gauge
    M. refractor

    M. slit-lamp
    M. SurgiScope
Marconi Medical Systems console
Mardis-Dangler ureteral stent set
Mardis soft stent
Marena compression garment
Marex MRI system
marginal
    m. chalazion forceps
    m. clamp
margin-finishing knife
Margraf beam-aligning film holder
Margulies
    M. coil
    M. intrauterine device
marijuana patch
Marino
    M. rotatable transsphenoidal
      enucleator
    M. rotatable transsphenoidal
      horizontal ring curette
    M. rotatable transsphenoidal knife
      handle
    M. rotatable transsphenoidal right-
      angle hook
    M. rotatable transsphenoidal round
      dissector
    M. rotatable transsphenoidal spatula
      dissector
    M. rotatable transsphenoidal vertical
      ring curette
    M. transsphenoidal curette
Marion
    M. drain
    M. oxygen resuscitation system
    M. screw
Mark
    M. II Chandler total knee retractor
    M. II concave total knee retractor
    M. II distal femur distractor
    M. II femoral component extractor
    M. III halo system
    M. III TiUnite implant
    M. II Kodros radiolucent awl
    M. II lateral collateral ligament
      retractor
    M. II Magni-Focuser loupe
    M. II modular weight retractor
    M. II PCL retractor
    M. II Sorrells hip arthroplasty
      retractor system
    M. II S total knee retractor
    M. II Stubbs short-prong collateral
      ligament retractor
    M. II Stulberg hip positioner
    M. II Stulberg leg positioner
    M. II tibial component extractor
    M. II wide PCL knee retractor
    M. II Wixson hip positioner

M. II Z knee retractor
M. IV Moss decompression-feeding catheter
M. IV respiratory pacemaker
M. IX lens
M. VII cooling vest
M. V Plus automatic injector
M. V ProVis injection system

Mark-7 intrauterine sound

Markell

M. brace boot
M. Mobility Health Clog
M. Mobility Shoe
M. open-toe boot
M. open-toe shoe
M. tarso medius straight shoe
M. tarso pronator outflare shoe

marker

Accu-line Products skin m.
Accu-line surgical m.
Akura partial depth astigmatic keratotomy m.
Allskin m.
Amsler scleral m.
Anastomark flexible coronary graft m.
Anis radial m.
Anis suture placement m.
Arrowsmith corneal m.
ASSI triple m.
astigmatic m.
BiomarC tissue m.
bone formation m.
bone resorption m.
Bores optic zone m.
Bores radial m.
Brems astigmatism m.
Castroviejo corneal transplant m.
m. catheter
Chayet corneal m.
Chayet-type corneal LASIK m.
cookie cutter-type areolar m.
corneal transplant m.
D'Assumpeau rhytidoplasty m.
Dell astigmatism m.
Dulaney LASIK m.
Ellis astigmatism m.
facelift D'Assumpcão m.
facelift flap m.
fecal m.
Fechtner trabeculectomy m.
Feldman RK optical center m.
fiducial skin m.
fine-line tissue m.
Freeman cookie cutter areola m.
Friedländer incision m.
Gass scleral m.
Geggel corneal transplant m.
gold ear m.

Gonin m.
Gonin-Amsler scleral m.
Grandon T-incision m.
Green-Kenyon corneal m.
Hoffer corneal m.
Hoffer optic zone m.
Hofmann T-incision m.
Hunkeler frown incision m.
interspace width m.
Kellen capsulorrhexis m.
Kershner LRI m.
Koch LRI m.
Kraff LRI m.
Kremer triple-optical zone corneal m.
Kritzinger-Updegraff corneal m.
K3-7991 Thornton 360-degree arcuate m.
K-U corneal m.
lead pellet m.
Lindstrom arcuate incision m.
Lindstrom astigmatic m.
Lindstrom small incision m.
low-profile R-K m.
low profile R-K m.
Lu corneal m.
Machat double-ended m.
Machat superior flap LASIK m.
magnetic resonance m.
Matos laser axis m.
McDonald optic zone m.
Mendez corneal m.
Mendez hexagon m.
Mendez-type corneal LASIK m.
Mendez type corneal LASIK m.
MicroMark tissue m.
microsatellite m.
Nordan-Ruiz trapezoidal m.
O'Brien m.
O'Connor m.
ocular m.
Ostase bone metabolism m.
oval optical zone m.
Perone LASIK m.
Philips gravity pivot axis m.
Phillips gravity pivot axis m.
Pinnacle R/O II radiopaque m.
polymorphic microsatellite m.
Price radial m.
Probst Smiley LASIK m.
radial keratotomy m.
radiopaque m.
radiopaque end m.
radiopaque gold m.
Rccath bypass graft m.
retroreflective m.
RK m.
roentgenographic opaque m.
round optical zone m.

M

marker *(continued)*
    Ruminson astigmatic gauge and m.
    scleral m.
    Sharpie m.
    Shepard optical center m.
    Simcoe corneal m.
    Sitzmarks radiopaque m.
    skin m.
    Skin Skribe m.
    Soll suture and incision m.
    Spivack axis m.
    Spot endoscopic m.
    Squeeze-Mark surgical m.
    tantalum-ball m.
    tantalum ball m.
    tape m.
    Thornton K3-7991 360-degree arcuate m.
    Thornton low-profile m.
    Thorton optic zone m.
    Thurmond pachymetry m.
    T-incision m.
    TLS surgical m.
    trephine m.
    ulcer m.
    USC m.
    vein graft ring m.
    Visitec RK zone m.
    Vismark surgical skin m.
    window rasp m.
    X-Act cutaneous x-ray m.
    X-Act podiatric m.
    Zaldivar LRI m.

marking
    m. clamp
    m. pen
    m. scissors

Markley
    M. orthodontic wire
    M. retention pin
    M. retractor

Markomanolakis aspirating wire speculum

Markwalder
    M. bone rongeur
    M. rib forceps
    M. rib rongeur

Markwort ankle support

Marlen
    M. biliary drainage kit
    M. colostomy appliance
    M. ileostomy bag
    M. leg bag
    M. SkinShield adhesive skin barrier
    M. UltraLite system
    M. Ultra 1-piece pouch

Marlex
    M. band
    M. bandage
    M. graft
    M. mesh
    M. mesh graft
    M. mesh implant
    M. mesh prosthesis
    M. mesh snare
    M. methyl methacrylate prosthesis
    M. suture

Marlin
    M. cervical collar
    M. cervical orthosis
    M. thoracic catheter

Marlow
    M. disposable cannula
    M. disposable trocar
    M. Primus handle
    M. Primus instrument
    M. Primus shaft
    M. Primus tip

Marmite lithotrite

maroon
    M. lip curette
    m. spoon

Marquardt bone rongeur

Marquest Respirgard II nebulizer

Marquette
    M. Case-12 electrocardiographic system
    M. Case-12 exercise system
    M. 3-channel laser holder
    M. 3-channel laser Holter
    M. electrocardiograph
    M. 8000 Holter monitor
    M. Holter recorder
    M. monitor
    M. Responder 1500 multifunctional defibrillator
    M. Series 8000 Holter analyzer
    M. treadmill

Marritt dilator

MARS
    modular acetabular revision system
    MARS revision acetabular component

marsupial
    M. belt
    m. pouch
    M. Pouch postsurgical drain holder

Martel
    M. clamp
    M. conductor
    M. intestinal clamp

martensitic stainless steel

Martin
    M. abdominal retractor
    M. ballpoint scissors
    M. bandage
    M. bipolar coagulation forceps
    M. blade

M. bur
M. cartilage chisel
M. cartilage clamp
M. cartilage forceps
M. cartilage scissors
M. cheek retractor
M. dermal curette
M. diamond wire cutter
M. endarterectomy stripper
M. hip gouge
M. laryngectomy tube
M. lip retractor
M. meniscal forceps
M. muscle clamp
M. nasopharyngeal biopsy forceps
M. nerve root retractor
M. palate retractor
M. pelvimeter
M. rectal hook
M. rectal hook retractor
M. rectal speculum
M. retractor
M. rubber dressing
M. snare
M. Surefit lens pusher
M. tenaculum
M. throat scissors
M. thumb forceps
M. tracheostomy tube
M. uterine fistula probe
M. uterine needle
M. uterine sound
M. uterine tenaculum forceps
M. vaginal retractor
M. vaginal speculum
M. vigorimeter

Martinez

M. corneal dissector knife
M. corneal transplant centering ring
M. corneal trephine blade
M. disposable corneal trephine
M. dissector
M. double-ended corneal dissector
M. keratome
M. knife
M. scleral centering ring
M. universal perineal interstitial
 template

Martini bone curette

Marx

M. bridging plate system
M. needle

Mary Jane breast pump

Maryland

M. bridge
M. dissector
M. monopolar electrosurgical
 dissector
M. tissue-grasping forceps

Masimo

M. LNOP durable adhesive sensor
M. Set
M. Set home monitor
M. Set pulse oximeter

mask

Accurox m.
Ace detachable m.
AeroChamber face m.
aerosol m.
air entrainment face m.
air entrapment m.
Aquaplast m.
Armstrong CPR m.
bag and m.
bag-valve m.
Bili m.
BiPAP m.
BLB m.
Boothby m.
Cold Compress m.
ComfortClassic nasal m.
ComfortFull nasal m.
ComfortGel nasal m.
ComfortSeal m.
convolution m.
Delaire m.
EasiVent valved holding
 chamber m.
ecchymotic m.
face m.
gel eye m.
GoldSeal nasal m.
HEPA filter m.
high-humidity face m.
high-humidity tracheostomy m.
Hudson-type oxygen m.
intubating laryngeal m.
IQ nasal m.
isolation face m.
Kuhn m.
Laerdal m.
laryngeal m.
LaryngoSeal laryngeal m.
LMA Ctrach m.
LMA laryngeal m.
Mallinckrodt LaryngoSeal
 laryngeal m.
meter m.
3M Healthcare surgical m.
Mirage nasal m.
mouth m.
mouth breathing m.
Nasal-Aire ventilator nasal
 insert m.
nasal and mouth breathing face m.
Nic the Dragon aerosol m.
nonbreather m.
nonrebreather face m.

M

mask *(continued)*
   nonrebreathing m.
   nonrebreathing face m.
   N95 particulate respirator
     surgical m.
   open face m.
   Orfit m.
   oxygen m.
   partial rebreathing m.
   partial rebreathing face m.
   Patil-Syracuse m.
   PEP m.
   Petit facial m.
   Phantom nasal m.
   pocket m.
   Portex soft seal laryngeal m.
   Prohibit antifog face m.
   RBS face m.
   rebreathing m.
   Rendell-Baker face m.
   Rendell-Baker Soucek m.
   Rudolph Full Face m.
   SCRAM face m.
   SealEasy resuscitation m.
   Sullivan Mirage nasal m.
   surgical m.
   Swiss Therapy eye m.
   thermoplastic head m.
   Ultimate nasal m.
   Uvex m.
   ventilated m.
   m. ventilation
   ventilation m.
   Venturi m.
   Vickers Ventimask Mark 2 m.
Masket
   M. capsulorrhexis forceps
   M. phaco spatula
Mason
   M. leg holder
   M. needle holder
   M. splint
   M. suction tube
   M. tonsil suction dissector
   M. vascular clamp
Mason-Allen
   M.-A. hand splint
   M.-A. snare
Mason-Judd
   M.-J. bladder retractor
   M.-J. self-retaining retractor
Mason-Likar 12-lead ECG system
mass
   m. flow controller
   m. spectrometer
   m. spectrophotometer
   m. spectrophotometric detector
Massachusetts Vision Kit

massage
   aqua PT water m.
   m. ball
   Teledyne Water Pik misting m.
   M. Time Pro hydroM. table
massager
   AcuVibe m.
   Body Sticks m.
   Cryocup ice m.
   Equalizer Pro m.
   G5 Fleximatic
     massager/percussor m.
   Intracell trigger point m.
   Ironman Triathlon Pro-Power m.
   Jeanie Rub m.
   Knobble m.
   Magnassager m.
   Medisana M.
   Morfam Quality Jeanie Rub m.
   Omni Roller m.
   Original Backknobber muscle m.
   Original Index Knobber II m.
   Power Pillow cervical m.
   Reach Easy m.
   Saso variable speed m.
   Scrip Muscle Master m.
   T-Bar trigger point m.
   The Original Backknobber
     muscle m.
   Thera Cane m.
massager/percussor
   G5 Vibracare m./p.
Masselon
   M. glasses
   M. spectacles
Massengill douche
Masseran trepan bur
mass-flow anemometer
Massie
   M. II nail
   M. II plate
   M. nail assembly
   M. screwdriver
   M. sliding nail
   M. sliding nail tube
Masson
   M. fascial needle
   M. fascial stripper
   M. fasciotome
MAST
   military antishock trousers
   MAST pants
   MAST suit
   MAST trousers
Mastel
   M. compass-guided arcuate
     keratotomy system
   M. diamond compass

M. Precision surgical instrument
M. trifaceted diamond blade
master
Balance M.
m. cement
Cobra M.
M. Flow Pumpette
M. Flow Pumpette pump
M. Kit
NeuroCom Balance M.
Pro Balance M.
M. screwdriver
Smart Balance M.
M. Step foot prosthesis
MasterFlex fetal perfusion pump
MasterLab Pro pneumotachograph
 spirometer
Masters
M. intestinal clamp
M. series mechanical heart valve
MasterScreen BabyBody plethysmograph
Masterson
M. hysterectomy forceps
M. pelvic clamp
Masters-Schwartz
M.-S. intestinal clamp
M.-S. liver clamp
Master-Stim interferential stimulator
masticatory apparatus
Mastin
M. goiter forceps
M. muscle clamp
M. muscle forceps
Mastisol liquid surgical adhesive
mastoid
m. bur
m. catheter
m. chisel
m. curette
m. dressing
m. gouge
m. probe
m. rongeur
m. searcher
m. self-retaining retractor
m. suction tube
mastopexy form
M2A swallowable imaging capsule
mat
Airex m.
air flow m.
AliMed sensor floor m.
AquaBodyCiser aquatic m.
children's m.
Dermafit massage m.
Easyslide sliding m.
EMED-SF sensor m.
GAITRite m.
Harris-Beath footprint m.

Harris footprint m.
m. holder
Minislide sliding m.
Scoot-Gard m.
silicone-spiked m.
sting m.
m. table
yoga m.
Matarasso facelift scissors
material
Absorb-its m.
acrylic implant m.
Adaptic II dental restorative m.
Advia Centaur HBc IgM
 control m.
Agarloid hydrocolloid
 impression m.
alginate impression m.
Alisoft splinting m.
allogeneic m.
AlloGro bone graft m.
alloplastic graft m.
alpha bone substitute m.
alpha-BSM bone repair m.
alpha-BSM bone substitute m.
Amelogen Plus radiopaque
 restorative m.
Aquaplast alloplastic m.
Aquaplast rapid-setting splint m.
Aquaplast splinting m.
Aquarelle hydrogel nucleus
 viscoelastic m.
Aquasil Smart Wetting
 impression m.
bioactive m.
Biobrane graft m.
bioceramic implant m.
biocompatible spacing m.
Bioglass bone graft substitute m.
BioMend periodontal m.
Bio-Oss corticalis bone graft m.
Bio-Oss spongiosa bone graft m.
Bioplastique augmentation m.
Blu-Mousse polyvinyl
 registration m.
bone grafting m.
bone implant m.
Bone Plast bone replacement m.
bone substitute m. (BSM)
bone-tendon graft m.
Bonfiglio bone replacement m.
Carboplast II sheet orthotic m.
Carbo-Seal graft m.
Carbo-Zinc skin barrier m.
Castorit investment m.
celluloid implant m.
Coe investment m.
collagen hemostatic m.
CollaPlug collagen m.

material *(continued)*
    Coltene impression m.
    Coltex impression m.
    Compafill MH dental restorative m.
    Compalay dental restorative m.
    Compamolar dental restorative m.
    Conduit TCP graft m.
    corundum ceramic implant m.
    Cranioplastic acrylic cranioplasty m.
    Cristobalite investment m.
    Crossfire polyethylene m.
    Curaderm hydrocolloid dressing m.
    Cutinova cavity wound filling m.
    Cymetra nonsurgical soft tissue
      replacement m.
    Dacron synthetic ligament m.
    Dentemp filling m.
    Dermalogen m.
    Dermasil impression m.
    DermAssist hydrocolloid
      dressing m.
    DermAssist wound filling m.
    Dermatell hydrocolloid dressing m.
    dextran-70 barrier m.
    DualMesh m.
    DupliCone silicone dental
      impression m.
    Durafill dental restorative m.
    Durapatite bone replacement m.
    Dur-A-Sil ear impression m.
    Duraval Hook & Loop strap m.
    DYNAfabric m.
    DynaLEAP balloon m.
    Elgiloy clip m.
    Embarc bone repair m.
    Endo-Avitene collagen
      hemostatic m.
    Epicel skin graft m.
    Epoxy Die m.
    Evazote cushioning m.
    expander mammary implant m.
    ExuDerm hydrocolloid dressing m.
    Fermit-N occlusal hole blockage m.
    Fletching femoral hernia
      implant m.
    FlowGel barrier m.
    Fotofil dental restorative m.
    Frosted Flex earmold m.
    G-C Vest investment m.
    glycolide trimethylene carbonate m.
    gold weight and wire spring
      implant m.
    Gore cast liner m.
    Gore S.A.M. patch m.
    Gore subcutaneous augmentation m.
    Gore-Tex alloplastic m.
    Gore-Tex periodontal m.
    Gore-Tex regenerative m.
    Graflex m.

    Grafton bone grafting m.
    Grafton demineralized bone matrix
      putty m.
    Hapex bioactive m.
    Hapset bone graft plaster m.
    Haynes 25 m.
    Healos synthetic bone grafting m.
    homograft implant m.
    hydroxyapatite implant m.
    implant m.
    Impregum impression m.
    In-Ceram Alumina dental
      bonding m.
    In-Ceram Cerestore dental
      bonding m.
    In-Ceram Dicor dental bonding m.
    In-Ceram Empress dental
      bonding m.
    In-Ceram Optic dental bonding m.
    In-Ceram Spinell dental
      bonding m.
    Insta-Mold silicone ear
      impression m.
    IntelliTemp insulation m.
    Interceed barrier m.
    Interpore bone replacement m.
    Interpore ceramic m.
    Jeltrate impression m.
    Kaltostat wound packing m.
    Karaya self-adhesive conductive m.
    Lactomer skin staple m.
    LactoSorb orthopaedic wound m.
    Lash-Loeffler penile implant m.
    Lincoff sponge implant m.
    Linkow dental implant m.
    L-rod implant m.
    Luster investment m.
    MediFlex earmold m.
    Medpor allograft m.
    Medpor alloplastic m.
    Medpor block facial structure
      building m.
    methyl methacrylate implant m.
    MP-35 clip m.
    3M Tegapore wound contact m.
    Mycromesh graft m.
    NeuroCell-HD porcine fetal
      neural m.
    NeuroCell-PD porcine fetal
      neural m.
    Nicoll bone replacement m.
    NovaBone Bioglass bone
      grafting m.
    Omega splinting m.
    Ommaya reservoir implant m.
    Opotow filling m.
    Opteform bone graft m.
    Optisson contrast m.
    OrthoDyn bone substitute m.

Ortho-Glass synthetic m.
OsSatura synthetic bone graft substitution m.
OsteoGen bone grafting m.
Osteogenics BoneSource synthetic bone replacement m.
Osteograf bone grafting m.
Osteograf/D bone grafting m.
Osteograf/LD bone grafting m.
Osteomatrix bone filling m.
Osteomatrix bone restoration m.
Palfique Estelite tooth shade resin m.
Pearman penile implant m.
pericardium membrane m.
PerioGlas m.
PerioGlas bone graft m.
PermaSoft reline m.
Phynox cobalt alloy clip m.
plastic wax m.
Poloxamer 407 barrier m.
polyether implant m.
polyethylene implant m.
polyglactin suture m.
polyurethane implant m.
polyvinyl implant m.
Polyviolene polyester suture m.
PolyWic wound filling m.
Porocoat m.
precollagenous filamentous m.
ProOsteon implant graft m.
Proplast I, II porous implant m.
Protouch m.
Ramitec polyether bite registration m.
Regisil polyvinyl registration m.
reline m.
RepliCare hydrocolloid dressing m.
SAM facial implant m.
SeamGuard staple line reinforcement m.
ShearBan orthotic m.
Shearing posterior chamber implant m.
shell implant m.
ShowerSafe protector m.
Silon silicone thermoplastic splinting m.
Small-Carrion penile implant m.
solid buckling implant m.
solid silicone exoplant implant m.
Spitz-Holter valve implant m.
sponge silicone implant m.
SR-Ivocap denture m.
Stimoceiver implant m.
subcutaneous augmentation m. (SAM)
Surgamid polyamide suture m.

Surgical Nu-Knit absorbable hemostatic m.
Synergy flexible splinting m.
Szulc orbital implant m.
ThermoSKY orthotic m.
tissue mandrel implant m.
titanium implant m.
transcatheter umbrella implant m.
Triangle gelatin-sealed sling m.
Trilon multilayered m.
tubular Gore m.
tunnel-type implant m.
Unigraft bone graft m.
Unilab Surgibone bone replacement m.
Usher Marlex mesh implant m.
vitallium implant m.
Zenotech graft m.
Zorbacel shock-absorbing m.

maternity Si-Loc sacroiliac belt
Mathews
M. drill point
M. hand drill
M. load drill
M. osteotome
M. rectal speculum
Mathieu
M. double-ended retractor
M. foreign body forceps
M. needle
M. needle holder
M. pliers
M. rasp
M. tongue forceps
M. urethral forceps
Mathieu-Horton-Devine flip-flap
Mathieu-Olsen needle holder
Mathys prosthesis
Matic UV-Optimize 555 skin reflectance meter
Matos laser axis marker
M.A.T. postoperative comfort device
matrix
Accell Connexus bone m.
Accell DBM 100 bone m.
Accell TBM bone m.
Accell total bone m.
Accor dental m.
AlloDerm acellular dermal m.
m. band
bilayered cellular m.
Boost demineralized bone m.
m. collagen
Collagraft bone graft m.
demineralized bone m. (DBM, DBX)
DuraGen absorbable dural graft m.
dural graft m.

M

matrix *(continued)*
    Dynafill graft biomedium mineralized bone m.
    Epi-Guide bioresorbable barrier m.
    Graftjacket regenerative tissue m.
    Graftjacket ulcer repair m.
    m. Grafton putty
    human demineralized bone m.
    InteXen porcine dermal m.
    NeoDura m.
    Optefil demineralized bone m.
    Osteovit bone m.
    Pelvicol acellular collagen m.
    PermaMesh hydroxyapatite woven sheet m.
    porous collagen m.
    m. retainer
    m. seating system
    Surgiflo hemostatic m.
    TissueMend soft tissue repair m.
    Walser m.
Matrix2 detachable coil
Matroc femoral head
Matrol femoral head prosthesis
Matson
    M. rasp
    M. rib elevator
    M. rib stripper
Matson-Alexander
    M.-A. rasp
    M.-A. rib elevator
    M.-A. rib stripper
Matson-Mead
    M.-M. apicolysis retractor
    M.-M. periosteum stripper
Matsuda titanium surgical instrument
matte
    m. black forceps
    m. black instrument
Matthew
    M. cross-leg clamp
    M. forceps
matting
    Dycem roll m.
Mattox aorta clamp
mattress
    AccuMax self-adjusting pressure management m.
    Air-O-Ease static air flotation m.
    Airsoft dry replacement m.
    Akros m.
    Akros extended care m.
    Akros pressure m.
    AkroTech m.
    antidecubitus m.
    apnea alarm m.
    Babytherm IC gel m.
    Bedge antireflux m.
    Bio Core therapeutic m.

    chiropractic m.
    Clinisert m.
    convoluted foam m.
    critical care m.
    DeCube m.
    DeCube therapeutic m.
    Dermasoft m.
    Dräger thermal gel m.
    Econo-Float water flotation m.
    eggcrate m.
    EMS Immobile-VAC pediatric universal m.
    FirstStep m.
    foam cube m.
    Geo-Mattress bariatric m.
    Home Care Simplimatt Plus zoned foam m.
    Huntleigh bubble pad m.
    hypothermia m.
    Impression m.
    Invacare APM m.
    Isoflex m.
    KinAir IV m.
    Lapidus alternating air-pressure m.
    lateral rotation m.
    MaxiFloat DFP, EF, LFP m.
    MaxiFloat pressure-reduction m.
    Medline Aeroflow II air m.
    Medline deluxe air m.
    Medline Saf-T-Side m.
    microAIR turn-Q-plus hospital m.
    Neuropedic multidensity m.
    Neuropedic neurolon m.
    NightForm infant sleep m.
    Nirvana m.
    OptiMax Supreme pressure reduction m.
    Orthoderm Convertible m.
    overlay m.
    PressureGuard m.
    Proform maxim pressure reduction m.
    Q-Star IV pressure-relief m.
    Q Star Voyager pressure reduction m.
    Q-Star Voyager pressure-reduction m.
    Rik fluid m.
    Roho m.
    Silhouette therapeutic m.
    Sofcare m.
    Sofflex m.
    Sof Matt pressure relieving m.
    static air m.
    m. suture
    m. system
    Tempur-Med hospital replacement m.
    Tempur-Pedic m.

Tempur-Pedic pressure-relieving
  Swedish m.
T-Foam m.
TheraKair m.
TheraRest m.
Tri-Float pressure reduction m.
UltraForm therapeutic m.
vinyl alternating air m.
Mattrix spinal cord stimulation system
Matt Strap knee strap
Maturna bra system
Mauch
  M. double-sheathed plastic wash
    pipe
  M. GaitMaster system
  M. Swing and Stance hydraulic
    knee
Maumenee
  M. capsular forceps
  M. capsule forceps
  M. corneal forceps
  M. cross-action capsular forceps
  M. erysiphake
  M. forceps
  M. goniotomy knife
  M. iris hook
  M. knife goniotomy cannula
  M. straight-action capsular forceps
  M. tissue forceps
  M. vitreous-aspirating needle
  M. vitreous sweep spatula
Maumenee-Colibri corneal forceps
Maumenee-Park eye speculum
Maunder mouthgag
Maunoir iris scissors
Maverick
  M. balloon catheter
  M. 2 Monorail catheter
  M. OTW catheter
Max
  M. Fine forceps
  M. Fine scissors
  M. Fine tying forceps
  M. Plus MR scanner
  Thera-Band M.
  M. ventilator
Max30 inflation device
MaxCore biopsy instrument
Maxenon xenon light source
MaxForce
  M. balloon dilatation catheter
  M. TTS biliary balloon dilatation
    catheter
  M. TTS high-performance balloon
    dilatation catheter
Maxicamera
MaxiCare
  M. adult disposable contoured brief

  M. adult disposable undergarment
  M. disposable underpad
MaxiFloat
  M. DFP, EF, LFP mattress
  M. pressure-reduction mattress
  M. wheelchair cushion
Maxiflo breathable disposable underpad
Maxi LD PTA dilation catheter
Maxilith
  M. pacemaker
  M. pacemaker pulse generator
maxillary
  m. arch bar
  m. disimpaction forceps
  m. fracture forceps
  m. lateral incisor implant
  m. prosthesis
  m. removable implant-retained
    denture
  m. sinus cannula
maxillofacial
  m. bone screw
  m. osteotome
  m. plating system
maxillomandibular elastic
Maxillume quartz halogen light source
Maxima
  M. II TENS unit
  M. II transcutaneous electrical
    nerve stimulator
  M. Plus plasma resistant fiber
    oxygenator
Maxim modular knee system
Maximum hemostasis introducer
Maximus dental implant
Maxi-Myst
  M.-M. bronchodilator
  M.-M. nebulizer system
  M.-M. vaporizer
Max-I-Probe
  M.-I.-P. endodontic irrigation
    syringe
  M.-I.-P. irrigation probe
Maxisorb test plate
Maxisorp microtiter plate
maxi-vessel loop
MaxLock plate and screw system
Maxm hematology flow cytometer
Maxon absorbable suture
Maxorb
  M. alginate wound cover
  M. alginate wound dressing
Max-Relax pillow
Maxsight
  M. sport tinted contact lens
  M. sport-tinted contact lens
Max-Support abdominal retraction belt
MaxTrax diabetic walker boot

M

Maxum
   M. Carr-Locke angled forceps
   M. reusable endoscopic forceps
   M. reusable forceps
Maxwell
   M. coil
   M. 3D field simulator
maxwellian view optical system
Maxxus orthopaedic latex surgical glove
May
   M. anatomical bone plate
   M. hook-on lens loupe
   M. kidney clamp
   M. ophthalmoscope
Mayer
   M. forceps
   M. nasal splint
   M. orthotic
   M. pessary
   M. speculum
Mayfield
   M. adapter
   M. aneurysm clamp
   M. aneurysm forceps
   M. bayonet osteotome
   M. clip applicator
   M. disposable skull pin
   M. fixation frame
   M. forceps
   M. head clamp
   M. head pin
   M. head rest
   M. malleable brain spatula
   M. miniature clip applier
   M. pediatric horseshoe headrest
   M. pediatric horseshoe pad
   M. 3-pin skull clamp
   M. radiolucent base unit
   M. radiolucent headholder
   M. radiolucent headrest
   M. retractor
   M. skull clamp adapter
   M. skull-pin headholder
   M. spinal curette
   M. surgical headrest system
   M. swivel horseshoe headrest
   M. temporary aneurysm clip
      applier
Mayfield-Kees
   M.-K. clip
   M.-K. headholder
   M.-K. headrest
   M.-K. skull fixation apparatus
   M.-K. table attachment
Mayo
   M. abdominal retractor
   M. bone-cutting forceps
   M. catgut needle
   M. Clinic congruent elbow plate

   M. common duct probe
   M. common duct scoop
   M. conservative hip prosthesis
   M. coronary perfusion cannula
   M. coronary perfusion tip
   M. curved scissors
   M. cystic duct scoop
   M. elbow distraction device
   M. external vein stripper
   M. fibroid hook
   M. gallbladder scoop
   M. gall duct scoop
   M. gallstone scoop
   M. goiter ligature carrier
   M. hemostat
   M. hook
   M. instrument table
   M. instrument tray
   M. intestinal needle
   M. kidney clamp
   M. kidney pedicle forceps
   M. kidney stone probe
   M. knife
   M. linen suture
   M. long dissecting scissors
   M. needle
   M. needle holder
   M. operating scissors
   M. rigid cervical collar
   M. round blade scissors
   M. scissors
   M. semiconstrained elbow
      prosthesis
   M. stand
   M. straight scissors
   M. tissue forceps
   M. total ankle prosthesis
   M. trocar needle
   M. trocar-point needle
   M. ureter isolation forceps
   M. uterine probe
   M. uterine scissors
   M. vessel clamp
Mayo-Adams
   M.-A. appendectomy retractor
   M.-A. self-retaining retractor
Mayo-Collins
   M.-C. appendectomy retractor
   M.-C. double-ended retractor
   M.-C. mastoid retractor
Mayo-Gibbon heart-lung machine
Mayo-Guyon
   M.-G. kidney clamp
   M.-G. vessel clamp
Mayo-Harrington
   M.-H. dissecting scissors
   M.-H. forceps
Mayo-Hegar needle holder
Mayo-Kelly appendix inverter

Mayo-Lexer scissors
Mayo-Lovelace
    M.-L. abdominal retractor
    M.-L. spur crusher
    M.-L. spur crushing clamp
Mayo-Noble dissecting scissors
Mayo-Ochsner
    M.-O. cannula
    M.-O. forceps
    M.-O. trocar
Mayo-Robson
    M.-R. gallstone scoop
    M.-R. gastrointestinal forceps
    M.-R. intestinal clamp
Mayo-Stille operating scissors
Mazzariello-Caprini forceps
MB-900 AC machine
MBA hemostasis valve
MB&J
    MB&J hip drape
    MB&J knee positioner
M-Brace
    M-B. corneal trephine
    M-B. knee brace
    M-B. posterior dynamic stabilization
    device
MBS snap-on orthotic
MC-7000 multi-wavelength opthalmic
  laser
McAllister
    M. needle holder
    M. scissors
MCAS modular clip application
McAtee
    M. apparatus
    M. olecranon compression screw
    device
McBride
    M. cup
    M. femoral prosthesis
    M. pin
    M. plate
    M. tripod pin traction
McBurney
    M. fenestrated retractor
    M. retractor
    M. thyroid retractor
McCabe
    M. antral retractor
    M. canal knife
    M. crurotomy saw
    M. crus guide fork
    M. facial nerve dissector
    M. flap knife dissector
    M. measuring instrument
    M. parotidectomy retractor
    M. perforation rasp
    M. posterior fossa retractor

McCain
    M. TMJ arthroscopic system
    M. TMJ cannula
    M. TMJ curette
    M. TMJ forceps
McCall instrument
McCannel
    M. implant
    M. ocular pressure reducer
    M. suture
McCarthy
    M. bladder evacuator
    M. catheter
    M. coagulation electrode
    M. continuous flow resectoscope
    M. diathermic knife electrode
    M. electrode
    M. endoscope
    M. evacuator
    M. foroblique operating telescope
    M. foroblique panendoscope
    cystoscope
    M. fulgurating electrode
    M. hip distractor
    M. infant electrotome
    M. loop operating electrode
    M. microlens resectoscope
    M. miniature electrotome
    M. miniature loop electrode
    M. miniature resectoscope
    M. miniature telescope
    M. multiple resectoscope
    M. panendoscope
    M. punctate electrotome
    M. visual hemostatic forceps
McCarthy-Campbell miniature
  cystoscope
McCleery-Miller
    M.-M. intestinal anastomosis clamp
    M.-M. locking device
McClintoch brace
McClintock
    M. placental forceps
    M. uterine forceps
McClure iris scissors
McCollough
    M. elevator
    M. internal tibial torsion brace
    M. osteotome
    M. rasp
    M. tying forceps
McConnell
    M. orthopaedic headrest
    M. shoulder positioner
McCoy
    M. septal forceps
    M. septum cutting forceps
McCrea
    M. cystoscope

M

McCrea *(continued)*
  M. dilator
  M. infant sound
McCullough
  M. hysterectomy clamp
  M. retractor
  M. strabismus forceps
  M. suture-tying forceps
  M. suturing forceps
McCutchen
  M. hip implant
  M. SLT hip prosthesis
McDavid
  M. ankle guard
  M. hinged knee guard
  M. knee brace
McDermott
  M. clip
  M. extractor
  M. Surgiclip
McDonald
  M. bone plate
  M. cerclage
  M. dissector
  M. expressor
  M. gastric clamp
  M. lens-folding forceps
  M. optic zone marker
  M. soft IOL folding forceps
  M. stone dissector
McDougal prostatectomy clamp
McDowell needle
McFadden-Kees clip
McGannon
  M. iris retractor
  M. lens forceps
  M. refractor
  M. retractor
McGaw
  M. plastic bottle
  M. skinfold calipers
  M. tape measure
  M. volumetric pump
McGee
  M. canal elevator
  M. ear piston prosthesis
  M. footplate pick
  M. middle ear instrument
  M. oval-window rasp
  M. platinum/stainless steel piston
  M. prosthesis needle
  M. splint
  M. tympanoplasty knife
  M. wire closure forceps
  M. wire crimper
  M. wire-crimping forceps
McGee-Priest wire forceps

McGhan
  M. Biocell anatomical breast implant
  M. breast prosthesis
  M. eye implant
  M. facial implant
  M. fill kit
  M. lens
  M. plastic surgical needle
  M. smooth saline implant
  M. tissue expander
McGill
  M. forceps
  M. neurological percussor
  M. retractor
McGivney
  M. forceps
  M. hemorrhoidal forceps
  M. hemorrhoidal ligator
  M. ligator
McGlamry elevator
McGoon
  M. cannula
  M. coronary perfusion catheter
McGovern nipple
McGregor
  M. conjunctival forceps
  M. needle
McGuire
  M. clamp
  M. conformer
  M. corneal scissors
  M. I&A system
  M. marginal chalazion forceps
  M. pelvic positioner
  M. rib spreader
  M. screw system
  M. suture guide
  M. tendon tucker
McHugh
  M. facial nerve knife
  M. flap knife
  M. oval speculum
McIlwain tissue chopper
McIndoe
  M. bone-cutting forceps
  M. dissecting forceps
  M. dressing forceps
  M. elevator
  M. nasal chisel
  M. rasp
  M. retractor
  M. rongeur forceps
  M. scissors
McIntosh
  M. double-lumen hemodialysis catheter
  M. suture-holding forceps

McIntyre
- M. anterior chamber cannula
- M. coaxial cannula
- M. coaxial I&A system
- M. fish-hook needle holder
- M. guarded cystotome
- M. guarded irrigating cystitome set
- M. I/A needle
- M. I&A system
- M. III nucleus removal system
- M. infusion handpiece
- M. infusion set
- M. irrigating iris hook
- M. irrigating iris manipulator
- M. irrigating spatula
- M. irrigation/aspiration needle
- M. lacrimal cannula
- M. microhook
- M. nylon cannula connector
- M. reverse cystotome
- M. suture tamper
- M. truncated cone

McIntyre-Binkhorst irrigating cannula
McIvor mouthgag
McKee
- M. brace
- M. femoral prosthesis
- M. speculum
- M. table
- M. totally constrained elbow
  prosthesis
- M. tri-fin nail

McKee-Farrar
- M.-F. acetabular cup
- M.-F. hip prosthesis

McKeever
- M. cartilage knife
- M. patellar cap prosthesis
- M. patellar resurfacing device

McKenzie
- M. AirBack inflatable back support
- M. bone drill
- M. cervical roll
- M. clamp
- M. clip applying forceps
- M. cranial drill
- M. enlarging bur
- M. hemostasis clip
- M. leukotome
- M. lumbar roll
- M. night roll
- M. perforating twist drill
- M. Repex table
- M. silver brain clip
- M. V clip

McKernan-Adson forceps
McKernan-Potts forceps
McKesson
- M. mouthgag

- M. mouth probe
- M. pneumothorax apparatus
- M. suction bottle unit

McKie
- M. thumb splint
- M. thumb supinator strap

McKinney
- M. eye speculum
- M. fixation ring

McLane
- M. forceps
- M. obstetrical forceps
- M. pile forceps

McLane-Tucker obstetrical forceps
McLaughlin
- M. carpal scaphoid screw
- M. hip plate
- M. laser mirror
- M. laser vaginal measuring rod
- M. nail
- M. osteosynthesis device
- M. quartz rod
- M. speculum

MCL brace
McLean
- M. capsular forceps
- M. capsulotomy scissors
- M. clamp
- M. muscle-recession forceps
- M. ophthalmic forceps
- M. prismatic fundus laser lens
- M. suture
- M. tonometer

MC-7000 multi-wavelength ophthalmic laser
McNamara
- M. coaxial catheter infusion set
- M. renal exchange wire guide

McNaught keel
McNealey-Glassman-Mixter
- M.-G.-M. clamp
- M.-G.-M. forceps

McNeill-Goldman
- M.-G. blepharostat
- M.-G. blepharostat ring
- M.-G. corneal transplant ring
- M.-G. ring
- M.-G. scleral ring

MCP finger joint prosthesis
McPherson
- M. angled forceps
- M. bent forceps
- M. corneal forceps
- M. corneal section scissors
- M. eye speculum
- M. forceps
- M. iris spatula
- M. irrigating forceps
- M. lens forceps

M

McPherson *(continued)*
    M. microbipolar forceps
    M. microcorneal forceps
    M. microiris forceps
    M. microsurgery eye needle holder
    M. microsuture forceps
    M. needle holder
    M. spatula
    M. speculum
    M. straight bipolar forceps
    M. suture-tying forceps
    M. suturing forceps
    M. trabeculotome
    M. tying iris forceps
McPherson-Castroviejo
    M.-C. corneal section scissors
    M.-C. forceps
    M.-C. microcorneal scissors
McPherson-Pierse
    M.-P. microcorneal forceps
    M.-P. microsuturing forceps
McPherson-Vannas
    M.-V. iris scissors
    M.-V. microiris scissors
McPherson-Westcott
    M.-W. conjunctival scissors
    M.-W. stitch scissors
McPherson-Wheeler
    M.-W. blade
    M.-W. eye knife
McPherson-Ziegler knife
M-C prosthesis
McQuigg
    M. clamp
    M. forceps
McReynolds
    M. driver
    M. extractor
    M. eye spatula
    M. lid-retracting hook
    M. pterygium keratome
    M. pterygium knife
    M. pterygium scissors
    M. spatula
McReynolds-Castroviejo
    M.-C. keratome
    M.-C. pterygium knife
McSpadden compactor
M-cup vacuum extraction device
MC walker brace
McWhorter
    M. hemostat
    M. tonsillar forceps
McXIM file
MD2 Doppler
MDA ultrasound-assisted lipoplasty machine
M/D 4 defibrillator system

MDI
    metered-dose inhaler
    MDI kit
MDILog
    M. compliance monitor
    M. microelectronic monitor
    M. therapy monitoring device
MDS
    microdebrider system
    MDS coil
    MDS MicroDebrider
    MDS microdebrider
    MDS system
MDS-2000 microwave irradiator
Mead
    M. bone rongeur
    M. bridge remover
    M. crown remover
    M. dental rongeur
    M. Johnson
    M. Johnson bottle
    M. Johnson tube
    M. lancet knife
    M. mallet
    M. periosteal elevator
    M. rongeur
Meadox
    M. Dacron mesh
    M. Dardik Biograft
    M. graft
    M. graft sizer
    M. ICP monitor
    M. Microvel arterial graft
    M. Microvel double velour Dacron graft
    M. Surgimed catheter
    M. Surgimed Doppler probe
    M. Teflon felt pledget
    M. vascular graft
    M. woven velour prosthesis
measure
    M. Mat infantometer
    McGaw tape m.
measurer
    Bunnell digital exertion m.
    Pach-Pen corneal thickness m.
measuring
    m. device
    m. gauge
    m. guide
    m. hat
    m. rod
    m. sensor
measuring-mounting catheter
meatal
    m. clamp
    m. dilator
    m. sound
meat hook retractor

meatoscope
meatotome
meatotomy
    m. electrode
    m. scissors
mechanical
    m. articulated arm
    m. assist system
    m. buttress
    m. device
    m. epithelial brush
    m. finger
    m. finger forceps
    m. joint apparatus
    m. leech
    m. longitudinal/sector scanning
      echoendoscope
    m. percussor
    m. prosthesis
    m. radial scanning instrument
    m. respirator
    m. rotating probe
    m. separator
    m. support
    m. support device
    m. ventilator
    m. ventilator actuator
    m. vitrector
mechanically
    m. assisted respirator
    m. detachable platinum coil
mechanical-type disc prosthesis
mechanic's
    m. pin
    m. waste dressing
mechanism
    adjustable leg and ankle
      repositioning m.
    Albarran m.
    4-bar linkage prosthetic knee m.
    Bookwalter Rotilt ratchet m.
    disengagement m.
    fixation m.
    Hosmer Dorrance voluntary control
      4-bar knee m.
    Laplace m.
    MicroStable liner locking m.
    Noiles rotating hinge knee m.
    patient-operated selector m.
    pneumatic splint m.
    rotating m.
    Rotilt ratchet m.
    slider crank m.
    spring m.
    terminal extensor m.
    UHR locking ring m.
mechanized scissors
Meckel rod
meconium aspirator

Mecring acetabluar prosthesis
Mectra
    M. I&A system
    M. irrigation/aspiration system
    M. tissue sample retainer
Medak glove
Medallion
    M. intraocular lens implant
    M. lens expressor
Medarmor puncture-resistant glove
MedaSonics
    M. Fetalgard Lite
    M. first beat ultrasound stethoscope
    M. transcranial Doppler
    M. ultrasound BF4A, BF5A
      stethoscope
    M. Versatone perioperative Doppler
Meda 2500 TENS unit
MedCam Pro Plus videocamera
Meddars cardiac catheterization analysis
    system
MedDev gold eyelid implant
Medela
    M. Apgar timer
    M. Dominant vacuum delivery
      pump
    M. manual breast pump
    M. membrane regulator
Medelec
    M. 5-channel neurophysiological
      device
    M. DMG 50 Teflon-coated
      monopolar electrode
    M. MS91 electromyograph
Medena continent ileostomy catheter
Medevice surgical paws
Medex
    M. coronary C1 stent
    M. Protege 3010 syringe infusion
      pump
    M. Secure system
    M. transducer
Med-Fit Senior Circuit exercise
    machine
MedFlo pain management pump
Medfusion 1001 syringe infusion pump
MedGraphics
    M. body plethysmograph
    M. Cardio O2 system
    M. CPE 2000 electronically braked
      bicycle
    M. CPX/D metabolic cart
Medi
    M. Plus compression stocking
    M. vascular stocking
media
    SonoVue ultrasound contrast m.
medial
    m. bicortical screw

M

medial *(continued)*
> m. heel-and-sole wedge
> m. heel wedge
> m. heel wedge orthosis
> m. malleolar/small bone fragment clamp
> m. nerve protector
> m. sole wedge
> m. sole wedge orthosis
> m. T strap
> m. unicortical screw

mediastinal
> m. cannula
> m. catheter
> m. drain
> m. sump filter
> m. tube

mediastinoscope
> Carlens m.
> Freiburg m.
> Goldberg-MPC m.
> Tucker m.

mediastinoscopy aspirating needle
Medi-Band bandage
medibottle
> Rx m.

MedicAIR
> M. Plus spirometer
> M. Plus spirometry station

medical
> m. adhesive remover
> m. ankle orthosis
> m. cyclotron
> M. Design brace
> M. Dynamics 5990 needle arthroscope
> M. Electronic cochlear implant
> m. equipment set
> m. gas analyzer
> M. genuine sheepskin pad
> M. Graphics Cardiopulmonary Exercise System 2001
> M. Graphics pneumotachograph with volume integrator
> M. Optics eye implant
> M. Optics intraocular lens implant
> M. Optics PC11NB intraocular lens implant
> M. Resources hydrophilic wound dressing
> St. Jude M. (SJM)
> M. Support Systems, Inc.
> M. Workshop intraocular lens implant
> M. Z post-surgery garment

MedicAlert bracelet

Medicamat
> M. ultrasound-assisted lipoplasty machine
> M. ultrasound device

Medicated
> M. Urethral System for Erection

medication monitoring event system
medicinal nebulizer
medicine ball
MediClenze hygiene and water therapy system
Medicon
> M. contractor
> M. instrument
> M. rib retractor
> M. rib spreader
> M. ultrasonic liposuction device
> M. wire twister forceps

Medicopaste bandage
MediCordz
> M. rehabilitation kit
> M. tubing kit

Medicus bed
Medicut
> M. cannula
> M. catheter
> M. intravenous needle

Medi-Duct ocular fluid management system
Medi-Facts system
Medifil collagen
MediFlex earmold material
Mediflex MD-7 endoscopic video system
Mediflow
> M. waterbase pillow
> M. water pillow

Medigraphics 2000 analyzer
Medi-Ject needle-free insulin injection system
Medi-Jector
> M.-J. adapter
> M.-J. Choice
> M.-J. Choice needle-free insulin injection system
> M.-J. injector

Medilas
> M. fiberTome laser
> M. Nd:YAG surgical laser

Medilog
> M. 4000 ambulatory ECG recorder
> M. 9000 polysomnography device

MedImage scanner
Medi-Mist nebulizer
Medina
> M. ileostomy catheter
> M. tube

Medi-Pac rescue seat
Medipad drug delivery system
Medipedic Multicentric knee brace

Medipore
 M. dressing cover
 M. Dress-it dressing
 M. H soft cloth surgical tape
 M. H surgical tape
MediPort
 M. catheter
 M. infusion vascular access device
Medi-Rip dressing
MediRule II measuring device
Medisana Massager
Medisense
 M. Pen 2 blood glucose meter
 M. Pen 2 glucose meter
 M. Pen 2 self blood glucose
  monitor
 M. Precision Xtra
MediSense
 M. 2 Card glucose meter
 M. 2 Pen Sensor glucose meter
 M. Q.I.D. test strip
 M. 2 test strip
Mediskin
 M. hemostatic sponge
 M. porcine biological wound
  dressing
Medison scanner
Medisorb drug delivery system
MediSpacer
 Airlife M.
Medispec Econolith spark plug
 lithotriptor
Medi-Stim stimulator
Medi-Strumpf stocking
Medisystems fistula needle
meditation bench
Meditec
 M. bandage contact lens
 M. MEL-60 excimer laser
Meditech
 M. balloon catheter
 M. bandage contact lens
 M. catheter system
 M. fascial dilator
 M. flexible stiffening cannula
 M. IVC filter
 M. laser
 M. multipurpose basket
 M. sheath
 M. steerable catheter
 M. stone basket
 M. ureteral stent system
 M. wire
Medi-Trace electrode
Meditron EL-100 Endolav
medium
 m. below-elbow cast
 m. callus Podi-Burr
 m. carbide cone bur

 m. fine bur
 m. forceps
 m. nail Podi-Burr
medium-energy collimator
medium-grade drywall sanding screen
Medium-Plus alpha liner
Medi-Vac suction canister system
Medivator automatic reprocessor
Medivent
 M. self-expanding coronary stent
 M. vascular stent
Medix ultrasonic nebulizer
MedJet microkeratome
Medline
 M. Aeroflow II air mattress
 M. Alpha subacute care bed
 M. deluxe air mattress
 M. Derma-Gel dressing
 M. gauze sponge
 M. gel/foam wheelchair cushion
 M. Lap-pal safety cushion
 M. lateral stabilizer
 M. Packing strip
 M. positioner
 M. roll
 M. Saf-T-Side mattress
 M. wedge
MedLite Q-switched neodymium-doped
 yttrium-aluminum-garnet laser
Med-Logics ML microkeratome
Medmetric
 M. knee ligament arthrometer
 M. KT1000 knee laxity arthrometer
Medmont
 M. E300 topographer
 M. M600 perimeter
Med-Neb respirator
MedNext high-speed drill
MedNova
 M. NeuroShield cerebral protection
  system
 M. stent
Medoc-Celestin
 M.-C. endoprosthesis
 M.-C. endoprosthesis prosthesis
 M.-C. tube
Medoff
 M. sliding femoral plate
 M. sliding fracture plate
 M. sliding plate
Medos
 M. Hakim programmable valve
 M. mechanical circulatory support
  system
Medpacific
 M. LD 5000 laser
 M. LD 5000 laser-Doppler
  perfusion monitor

M

Medpor
- M. allograft material
- M. alloplastic material
- M. biomaterial implant
- M. biomaterial wedge
- M. block facial structure building material
- M. facial implant
- M. Flexblock implant
- M. malar implant
- M. MCOI implant
- M. prosthesis
- M. reconstructive implant
- M. surgical implant

Medrad
- M. angiographic catheter
- M. automated power injector
- M. contrast medium injector
- M. infusion pump
- M. Mark IV angiographic injector
- M. MRInnervu endorectal colon probe
- M. MRInnervu endorectal colon probe coil
- M. power angiographic injector

MedSlant
- M. acid reflux wedge pillow
- M. therapeutic pillow

Medspec
- M. MR imaging system
- M. MR imaging system scanner
- M. 30/80 tesla MR scanner

Medstone
- M. extracorporeal shock wave lithotriptor
- M. IRIS system
- M. STS lithotripsy system
- M. STS lithotriptor
- M. STS shock wave generator

MedSystem III multichannel infusion pump

Med Tec Vac Loc immobilization system

Medtronic
- M. Activa tremor control therapy device
- M. Activitrax rate-responsive unipolar ventricular pacemaker
- M. AneuRx stent-graft
- M. automated coagulation timer
- M. AVE S660 coronary stent
- M. balloon catheter
- M. BeStent stent
- M. bipolar pacemaker
- M. cardiac cooling jacket
- M. catheter
- M. Chardack pacemaker
- M. corkscrew electrode pacemaker
- M. 5670 coronary stent
- M. defibrillator implant support device
- M. demand pacemaker
- M. Elite II pacemaker
- M. Evergreen balloon
- M. external cardioverter-defibrillator
- M. external/internal pacemaker
- M. external tachyarrhythmia control device
- M. Gem automatic implantable defibrillator
- M. Hancock II tissue valve
- M. Hemopump
- M. Hemopump cardiac assist device
- M. Hemopump system
- M. infusion pump
- M. Inspire
- M. Inspire implantable device
- M. Intact bioprosthetic valve
- M. Intact porcine bioprosthesis
- M. interactive tachycardia terminating system
- M. InterStim sacral nerve stimulation system
- M. interventional vascular stent
- M. Itrel II neurostimulator
- M. Jewel AF implantable arrhythmia management device
- M. Jewel 7219C, D device
- M. Jewel Plus Active Can defibrillator
- M. Kappa 400 pacemaker
- M. Micro Jewel cardioverter-defibrillator system
- M. Micro Jewel defibrillator
- M. Midas Rex Legend system
- M. MiniMed CGMS system gold
- M. Minix
- M. Minix pacemaker
- M. Mosaic bioprosthetic valve
- M. Octopus tissue stabilizing device
- M. Octopus 2+ tissue stabilizing system
- M. Pacette pacemaker
- M. PCD implantable cardioverter-defibrillator
- M. Pisces Quad Plus
- M. prosthetic valve
- M. pulse generator
- M. 3470 pulse generator
- M. Pulsor Intrasound
- M. radiofrequency receiver
- M. RF 5998 pacemaker
- M. Sequestra 1000 autotransfusion system
- M. Sofamor Danek
- M. spinal cord stimulation system

M. SP 502 pacemaker
M. Symbios pacemaker
M. SynchroMed implantable pump
M. SynchroMed pump
M. Talent prosthesis
M. temporary pacemaker
M. Thera DR pacemaker
M. Thera i-series cardiac
    pacemaker
M. thin flexible antimony electrode
M. tip
M. Transvene 6937 electrode
    catheter
M. Transvene endocardial lead
M. Transvene endocardial lead
    system
M. tremor control therapy device
M. Xtrel neurostimulator
M. Zuma guiding catheter

Medtronic-Hall
M.-H. device
M.-H. heart valve prosthesis
M.-H. monocuspid tilting-disc valve
M.-H. prosthetic heart valve
M.-H. tilting disc valve prosthesis

Medtronic-Hancock device
Medtronics Sequestra 1000
  autotransfusion system
medullary
m. canal reamer
m. nail
m. pin
m. rod

Medweb clinical reporting system
Med-Wick
M.-W. medication delivery system
M.-W. nasal pack

MedX
M. camera
M. functional testing machine
M. knee machine
M. machine
M. Mark II lumbar extension
    machine
M. muscle testing apparatus
M. physical therapy device
M. scanner
M. stretch machine

Meek
M. pelvic traction belt
M. snare

Meeker
M. deep surgery forceps
M. gallbladder forceps
M. gallstone clamp
M. hemostatic forceps
M. intestinal forceps

M. monopolar electrosurgical
    dissector
M. right-angle clamp

Meek-Wall
M.-W. dermatome
M.-W. microdermatome

Mefix adhesive tape
MEG
MEG head-based coordinate system
MEG sensor

Mega-Air bed
MegaDyne
M. arthroscopic hook electrode
M. cautery
M. electrocautery pencil
M. E-Z clean cautery tip

Megalink biliary stent
MEGA-Pouch laparoscopic retrieval
  system
MegaSonics PTCA catheter
Mega Tilt and Turn bed
megaureter clamp
megavoltage
m. computed tomography scanner
m. CT scanner
m. machine

Megazinc Pink adhesive tape
meibomian
m. expressor forceps
m. gland expressor

Meier-Magnum system
Meige lymphedema
Meigs
M. endometrial curette
M. hemostat
M. retractor
M. suture
M. uterine curette

MEI system
MEL
MEL 60, 80 excimer laser
MEL 70 flying spot laser
MEL 60 scanning laser

MelaFind handheld imaging device
Melastatin test kit
Melgisorb alginate dressing
Melker cuffed emergency
  cricothyrotomy catheter
Meller
M. cyclodialysis spatula
M. lacrimal sac retractor

Melles Griot diode laser
Mellinger
M. eye speculum
M. fenestrated blades speculum
M. magnet
M. speculum

Mellinger-Axenfeld eye speculum

M

Meltzer
    M. adenoid punch
    M. nasopharyngoscope
    M. tonsillar punch
Membrane[6]
    Resorbable Collagen M.
membrane
    m. artificial lung
    barrier m.
    BioBarrier m.
    biocompatible m.
    Bio-Gide resorbable barrier m.
    Bio-Gide resorbable bilayer m.
    bioincompatible m.
    BioMend collagen m.
    Biopore m.
    BioSorb collagen resorbable m.
    collagen m.
    cuprophane m.
    m. delamination wedge
    Duralon-UV nylon m.
    elastic silicone m.
    EPTFE augmentation m.
    m. forceps
    Gore Resolut Adapt bioresorbable regenerative m.
    Gore Resolut Adapt LT regenerative m.
    Gore-Tex m.
    Gore-Tex surgical m.
    Guidor m.
    HA m.
    Hemophan m.
    Hybond ECL nitrocellulose m.
    Hybond N+ nylon m.
    Imtec BioBarrier m.
    Mem-Lok collagen resorbable m.
    MSI nylon m.
    Ossix 6-month resorbable collagen m.
    m. oxygenator
    m. peeler
    m. peeler-cutter
    m. peeling forceps
    m. perforator
    polysulfone m.
    Preclude pericardial m.
    Preclude peritoneal m.
    Preclude spinal m.
    m. puncturing forceps
    Regentex GBR-200 m.
    Seprafilm bioresorbable m.
    sodium hyaluronate-based bioresorbable m.
    Sure Blot m.
    m. tack
    TefGen-FD guided tissue regeneration m.
    TefGen-FD plastic m.
    TefGen regenerative m.
    Transwell m.
    ultrafiltration m.
    Viresolve ultrafiltration m.
membrane-covered stent
Meme
    M. breast prosthesis
    M. implant
    M. mammary implant
Mem-Lok collagen resorbable membrane
Memokath catheter
memory
    M. basket
    m. board
    m. catheter
    m. compression staple
    m. exercise card
    M. II cushion
    m. splint
MemoryLens
    M. foldable intraocular lens
    M. IOL
    Mentor ORC M.
    M. prefolded IOL
Memotherm
    M. colorectal stent
    M. endoscopic biliary stent
    M. Flexx biliary stent
    M. nitinol self-expandable stent
    M. nitinol stent
    M. stent
MEMS 6 TrackCap Monitor medication monitoring system
Mendez
    M. astigmatism dial
    M. corneal marker
    M. cystotome
    M. degree calipers
    M. degree gauge
    M. hexagon marker
    M. multipurpose LASIK forceps
    M. type corneal LASIK marker
    M. ultrasonic cystotome
Mendez-type corneal LASIK marker
Menge pessary
Menghini
    M. cannula
    M. liver biopsy needle
    M. needle
Menghini-type coring bevel
meniscal
    m. basket forceps
    m. clamp
    m. curette
    m. cutter
    m. hook scissors
    m. knife
    m. mirror
    m. repair needle

m. retractor
m. spoon
m. staple
m. suture grabber
meniscectomy
m. blade
m. knife
m. probe
m. scissors
meniscotome
Grover m.
Smillie m.
meniscotomy chisel
meniscus
M. Arrow fixation
M. Arrow implant
m. concave lens
m. forceps
m. knife
m. lens
M. Mender II system
m. retractor
m. scissors
menopause home test
MENS
microcurrent electrical neuromuscular stimulator
MENS unit
Mentor
M. absorbent pouch
M. Alpha 1 inflatable penile prosthesis
M. biliary stent
M. Bioflex cylinder
M. bladder pacemaker
M. breast prosthesis
M. B-VAT II BVS contour circles distance stereoacuity test
M. B-VAT II BVS random dot E distance stereoacuity test
M. B-VAT II monitor
M. B-VAT II video acuity tester
M. B-VAT visual acuity chart
M. catheter
M. Contour Genesis ultrasonic assisted lipoplasty system
M. coudé catheter
M. curved eraser
M. Exeter ophthalmoscope
M. female self-catheter
M. fine-focus microscope
M. Foley catheter
M. Foley catheter with comfort sleeve
M. GFS penile prosthesis
M. gun
M. H/S Siltex implant
M. 1600 implant
M. injector gun

M. IPP penile prosthesis
M. malleable penile prosthesis
M. malleable semirigid penile implant
M. Mark II penile prosthesis
M. nonhydrophilic PVC catheter
M. ORC MemoryLens
M. prostate biopsy needle
M. Response VCD
M. Self-Cath soft catheter
M. straight catheter
M. tissue expander
M. ultrasound-assisted lipoplasty machine
M. ultrasound device
M. UroSan external catheter
M. wet-field cautery
M. wet-field cordless coagulator
M. wet-field electrocautery
M. wet-field eraser
Mentor-Piston VCD
Mentor-Touch VCD
Menuet Compact urodynamic testing device
Mephisto Mobils professional shoe
Mepiform self-adherent silicone dressing
Mepilex
M. border dressing
M. foam dressing
M. Lite dressing
M. transfer dressing
Mepitac soft silicone tape
Mepitel
M. contact layer sheet
M. contact layer wound dressing
M. nonadherent silicone dressing
Mepore
M. absorptive dressing
M. Pro dressing
Mercator atrial high-density array catheter
Mercedes
M. cannula
M. tip
M. tip cannula
Mercier
M. catheter
M. sound
Merck respirator
mercury
m. arc lamp
m. bougie
m. manometer
M. Medical airway pressure manometer
m. vapor lamp
mercury-filled
m.-f. dilator
m.-f. esophageal bougie

M

mercury-in-rubber strain gauge plethysmograph
mercury-in-silastic strain gauge
mercury-weighted
  m.-w. dilator
  m.-w. rubber bougie
Meridian
  M. intersegmental table
  M. pacemaker
  M. PA femoral component
  M. ST femoral implant component
  M. TMZF femoral component
meridional
  m. implant
  m. refractometer
Merit-B periodontal probe
Merit final flexion kit
Merlin
  M. arthroscopy blade
  M. bendable blade
MERmaid DNA kit
MERmaid-Spin kit
Mermoud nonpenetrating glaucoma forceps
Merocel
  M. epistaxis packing
  M. lint-free sponge
  M. pack
  M. splint
  M. sponge
  M. surgical spear
  M. tampon
MeroGel
  M. nasal dressing
  M. nasal packing
  M. nasal stent
  M. sinus stent
Merrifield knife
Merrimack 1040 CO$_2$ laser
Merry
  M. Walker
  M. Walker ambulation device
Mershon
  M. band pusher
  M. spring
Mersilene
  M. band
  M. braided nonabsorbable suture
  M. gauze hammock
  M. graft
  M. implant
  M. mesh
  M. mesh dressing
  M. mesh sling
  M. tape
Mersilk black silk suture
Merz-Vienna nasal speculum
Mesalt sodium chloride-impregnated dressing

Mesa spinal system
mesh
  absorbable m.
  Apogee surgical m.
  Avaulta biosynthetic m.
  Bard-Marlex m.
  Bard Sperma-Tex preshaped m.
  Bard Visilex m.
  Brennen biosynthetic surgical m.
  C-QUR bioabsorbable surgical m.
  craniomaxillofacial m.
  Dacron m.
  Dexon m.
  Dexon polyglycolic acid m.
  Dexon surgically knitted m.
  DualMesh hernia m.
  Dumbach mini m.
  Dumbach regular m.
  Dumbach titanium m.
  Ethicon m.
  flared patch m.
  m. glove
  m. graft
  Herniamesh surgical m.
  Hexcelite m.
  IntePro large-pore synthetic m.
  intraperitoneal onlay m.
  Kugel m.
  Leibinger Micro Dynamic m.
  macro-mesh m.
  MacroPore distraction m.
  mandibular m.
  Marlex m.
  Meadox Dacron m.
  Mersilene m.
  mixed m.
  OsteoForm mesh formable craniofacial m.
  OTPS m.
  Parietex composite m.
  PelviSoft m.
  Pelvitex polypropylene m.
  Permacol m.
  Pivit AB surgical m.
  polyamide m.
  polyglactin m.
  polyglycolic m.
  polypropylene m.
  polytetrafluoroethylene m.
  POPmesh polypropylene m.
  Proceed surgical m.
  Prolene m. (PS)
  ProLite surgical m.
  ProLite Ultra surgical m.
  PTFE m.
  sintered titanium m.
  skin graft expander m.
  Sperma-Tex preshaped m.
  stainless steel m.

m. stent
m. stent prosthesis
Supramid polyamide m.
surgical m.
surgical metallic m.
Surgipro m.
Surgipro hernia m.
m. suture
synthetic m.
tantalum m.
Teflon m.
ThermoFX m.
TiMesh cranial m.
TiMesh orbital m.
TiMesh titanium m.
titanium m.
Trelex natural m.
Ultrapro m.
Vicryl m.
Visilex polypropylene m.
meshed ball implant
mesher
Collin m.
skin graft m.
Tanner m.
Zimmer skin graft m.
Mesoft
M. sponge
M. swab
mesonephric drain
mesostructure implant
Messerklinger endoscope
Messing root canal gun
Mestopore continent stoma dressing
Meta
M. DDDR pacemaker
M. II pacemaker
M. MV pacemaker
M. rate-responsive pacemaker
metabolator
metabolic cart
metacarpal
m. broach
m. double-ended retractor
m. saw
metacarpophalangeal
m. implant
m. prosthesis
MetaFluor system
metal
m. acetabular liner
m. adapter
m. ball-tip catheter
m. band
m. band suture
m. bar retractor
m. bucket-handle prosthesis
m. cannula
m. clip

d'Arcet m.
m. femoral head prosthesis
m. foot plate
m. Fox shield
m. frame reinforced plastic bracket
m. hemi-toe implant
m. hybrid orthosis
m. knife
m. needle
m. olive dilator
m. orthopaedic implant
m. oxide semiconductor field-effect transistor
m. pin
m. pusher
m. reconstruction plate
m. ruler
m. scleral shield
m. sewing ring
m. sound
m. splint
m. surface electrode
m. tongue depressor
m. tongue retractor
m. wing clamp
m. Z-stent
metal-backed
m.-b. acetabular component hip implant
m.-b. acetabular shell
m.-b. plastic-on-metal prosthesis
m.-b. socket
metal-coated stent
Metalift crown and bridge removal system
metallic
m. biliary endoprosthesis
m. cage
m. clip
m. endplate
m. frontal needle
m. needle
m. pointer
m. screw
m. staple
m. stent
m. suture
m. tip cannula
metallic-tip catheter
metal-on-metal articulating intervertebral disc prosthesis
metal-tipped stent pusher
Metasul
M. hip implant
M. hip joint component
M. hip prosthesis
M. joint
M. metal-on-metal hip

M

Metasul *(continued)*
    M. metal-on-metal hip prosthesis
        system
metatarsal
    m. cookie
    m. head extractor
    m. stem broach
metatarsophalangeal endoprosthesis
Metcher speculum
meter
    Accu-Chek Active glucose m.
    Accu-Chek Advantage glucose m.
    Accu-Chek Compact glucose m.
    Accu-Chek III blood glucose m.
    Accu-Chek Instant glucose m.
    Accu-Chek Voicemate glucose m.
    Airshields jaundice m.
    Aleo m.
    amperometric m.
    analog rate m.
    AvocetPT rapid prothrombin
        time m.
    BioTrainer exercise m.
    Chemstrip MatchMaker blood
        glucose m.
    clip force m.
    coulometric m.
    Endodontic M. SII
    ExacTech blood glucose m.
    ExacTech RSG glucose m.
    exposure m.
    Fischer compliance m.
    Fisher Accumet pH m.
    FreeStyle Flash blood glucose m.
    FreeStyle Tracker glucose m.
    functional visual acuity m.
    galvanic skin response m.
    Gammex RMI DAP m.
    Geiger-Müller survey m.
    Glucometer Elite R m.
    glucose m.
    GlucoWatch Biographer m.
    Guyton-Minkowski potential
        acuity m.
    Health Scan Assess Plus peak
        flow m.
    HemoCue glucose m.
    Hypoguard Advance glucose m.
    integrating spherical power m.
    Kowa FM-500 laser flare m.
    laser flare m.
    m. lens
    LifeGuide glucose m.
    LifeScan blood glucose m.
    m. mask
    Matic UV-Optimize 555 skin
        reflectance m.
    MediSense 2 Card glucose m.
    Medisense Pen 2 blood glucose m.
    Medisense Pen 2 glucose m.
    MediSense 2 Pen Sensor
        glucose m.
    MicroRint portable airway
        resistance m.
    Miles Encore QA glucose m.
    MultiSPIRO The Peak peak
        flow m.
    neutron m.
    OneTouch blood glucose m.
    OneTouch InDuo glucose m.
    OneTouch SureStep glucose m.
    oxygen saturation m.
    OxySAT oxygen saturation m.
    Parkinson-Cowan dry gas m.
    peak flow m. (PFM)
    pH m.
    photovolt pH m.
    potential acuity m.
    Precision QID glucose m.
    Prestige IQ glucose m.
    Prestige LX glucose m.
    QuickTek glucose m.
    reflectance m.
    ReliOn glucose m.
    retinal acuity m.
    roentgen m.
    sound level m.
    Statham electromagnetic flow m.
    Supreme II blood glucose m.
    SureStep glucose m.
    Synectics 6000 digital pH-meter m.
    TD Glucose m.
    transcutaneous jaundice m.
    urinary drainage bag and urine m.
    US uroflow m.
    van den Berg stray-light m.
    Venturi m.
    Vuero m.
metered-dose inhaler (MDI)
metered solution inhaler
MeterPlus
    Triage M.
method
    Plastibell circumcision m.
Methodist
    M. Hospital headholder
    M. vascular suction tube
methyl
    m. cyanoacrylate glue
    m. methacrylate bead
    m. methacrylate bead implant
    m. methacrylate block
    m. methacrylate cement adhesive
    m. methacrylate cranioplastic plug
    m. methacrylate ear stent
    m. methacrylate eye implant
    m. methacrylate graft

m. methacrylate implant material
m. methacrylate spacer
methylmethacrylate implant
methyltransferase
thiopurine m. (TPMT)
MetraGrasp ligament grasper
MetraPass suture passer
Metra PS procedure kit
Metras catheter
MetraTie knot pusher
Metrecom
M. device
M. digitizer
Metricath
M. 1000 console catheter
M. measurement catheter
metric ophthalmoscope
Metrix
M. atrial defibrillation system
M. Atrioverter
M. IAD
M. implantable atrial defibrillator
M. implantable Atrioverter
metrizamide-filled balloon
metronoscope
METRx
METRx Quadrant retractor
METRx system
METRx X-Tube retraction system
METRx X-Tube retractor
Mettler
M. electrotherapy
M. Trio neuromuscular electrical
stimulator
Metzenbaum
M. chisel
M. dissecting scissors
M. gouge
M. long scissors
M. needle holder
M. operating scissors
M. scissors
M. tonsillar scissors
Metz spatially varying filter
MEVA
M. probe
M. Probe for endovaginal scanning
Mevatron 74 linear accelerator
Mewi-5 side-hole infusion catheter
Mewissen infusion catheter
Meyer
M. cervical orthosis
M. Swiss diamond knife lancet
M. Swiss diamond lancet knife
M. Swiss diamond mini-angled
knife
M. Swiss diamond wedge knife
M. temporal loop
Meyer-Archambault loop

Meyerding
M. bone skid
M. finger retractor
M. mallet
M. osteotome
M. retractor
M. retractor blade
M. self-retaining laminectomy
retractor
M. skin hook
M. skin hook and retractor
Meyer-Schwickerath coagulator
Meyhoefer
M. bone curette
M. chalazion curette
M. eye knife
M-F heel protector
MFL 5000 lithotriptor
MG
MG II knee prosthesis
MG II total knee system
MGH
MGH needle holder
MGH osteotome
M-Glucometer
Miami
M. acute care cervical collar
M. acute collar cervical traction
M. fracture brace
M. J cervical collar
M. J collar cervical traction
M. Modular Orthopaedic Spinal
System
M. Moss instrumentation
M. Star tissue expander
M. TLSO scoliosis brace
MIBB breast biopsy system
Mic
M. bolus gastrostomy tube
M. gastroenteric tube
M. gastrostomy tube
M. jejunal tube
M. jejunostomy tube
M. transgastric jejunal feeding tube
Michel
M. clip
M. clip-applying forceps
M. clip-removing forceps
M. pick
M. scalp clip
M. skin clip
M. suture clip
Michele
M. long-stem prosthesis
M. vertebral trephine
Michelson bronchoscope
Michigan intestinal forceps
Mick
M. afterloading needle

M

Mick *(continued)*
  M. prostate template
  M. seed applicator
  M. TP-200 applicator
Mic-Key
  M.-K. gastrostomy tube
  M.-K. low-profile transgastric-jejunal
    feeding tube
MiCOR machine bone allograft
Micrins microsurgical suture
micro
  m. bimanual irrigating handpiece
  m. Colibri forceps
  M. Delta/Max Delta system
  M. E irrigation kit
  m. guidewire
  m. Halstead arterial forceps
  M. II stent
  M. 100 irrigation kit
  M. Jewel defibrillator
  m. Kerrison rongeur
  M. Link endoscope fiber
  M. Minix pacemaker
  M. Mist nebulizer
  M. One pneumatonometer
  M. Plus plating system
  M. punctum plug
  M. QuickAnchor
  m. round-tip needle
  m. scissors
  M. Series wire driver
  m. Suturelassos
  m. vertical scissors
  m. Westcott scissors
Micro-6 ureteroscope
micro-adaption plate
MicroAir
  M. electronic nebulizer
  M. handheld nebulizer
Micro-Aire
  M.-A. bur
  M.-A. drill
  M.-A. facial plating system
  M.-A. oscillating bone saw
  M.-A. oscillating saw
  M.-A. osteotome
  M.-A. pneumatic power instrument
  M.-A. pulse lavage system
  M.-A. reamer
  M.-A. surgical instrument system
microaire cannula
microAIR turn-Q-plus hospital mattress
micro-Allis forceps
microammeter
**microamperage electrical nerve
  stimulator**
microamps TENS unit

microanalyzer
  electronic m.
  electron probe x-ray m.
microanastomosis
  m. approximator
  m. clip
microarterial
  m. clamp
  m. forceps
microaspirator
microball hook
microballoon
  implantable silicone m.
  m. probe
  Rand m.
microbayonet
  m. forceps
  m. rasp
  m. scoop
microbeam
  P.A.L.M. ultraviolet laser m.
Microbeam manipulator
**microbicinchoninic acid protein assay
  kit**
microbiopsy forceps
microbipolar forceps
MicroBite forceps
microblade
  Sharptome m.
Microblator ArthroWand
microbore Tygon tube
microbronchoscopic tissue forceps
microbulldog
  m. clamp
  m. clip
microcaliper
microcannula
Microcap
  M. handheld capnograph
  M. scalpel
Micro-Cast collimator
microcatheter
  AngiOptic m.
  ball-tip m.
  Cardima Pathfinder mapping m.
  Cordis coaxial m.
  end-hole Tracker m.
  Equinox balloon m.
  Excel-14 m.
  Excel double-tipped m.
  Excelsior 1018 m.
  FasTracker 325 coaxial m.
  FirstCyte m.
  Flow Rider m.
  Hieshima m.
  Hydrolyser m.
  InDuct breast m.
  IntraEAR m.
  Leggiero hydrophilic-coated m.

Magic m.
Microferret m.
20-mm Equinox balloon m.
Pathfinder mini m.
Prowler-14 m.
Prowler double-tipped m.
Rapidtransit m.
Rapid Transit m.
Renegade m.
Renegade Hi-Flo m.
Revelation endocardial m.
Spinnaker Elite flow-directed m.
Terumo SP hydrophilic polymer-coated m.
Tracer m.
Tracker m.
Tracker 10 m.
Tracker Excel m.
UltraLite flow-directed m.
microcautery unit
Microcell
M. alternating pressure pad
M. chamber
microcentrifuge
Compac m.
Microfuge 18 m.
Microfuge 22R refrigerated m.
MicroPrep 2 m.
MicroChamber
MicroChoice electric powered surgical system
microclamp
disposable m.
m. forceps
Kapp m.
Khodadad m.
Microclens wipe
microclip
dural m.
m. forceps
Khodadad m.
Kleinert-Kutz m.
Williams m.
Yasargil m.
microcoagulator
Malis bipolar m.
Polar-Mate bipolar m.
MicroCO carbon monoxide monitor
microcoil
Act M.
complex platinum m.
Dacron-coated m.
endothelin-1 platinum Dacron m.
Hilal m.
Hilal embolization m.
Intercept esophagus m.
Intercept prostate m.
Intercept urethra m.

platinum m.
platinum Dacron m.
microcolpomicrohysteroscope
Hamou m.
microcomputer upper limb exerciser
microconjunctival scissors
microconnector
microcorneal
m. forceps
m. scissors
microCT-20 scanner
microcup pituitary forceps
microcurettage
Accurette m.
microcurette
HemoCue m.
microcurrent
m. electrical neuromuscular stimulator (MENS)
m. electrode
MicroDebrider
MDS M.
Topaz M.
microdebrider
Hummer m.
Linvatec m.
MDS m.
Stryker m.
m. system (MDS)
Topaz m.
Wizard m.
microdensitometer
Vickers m.
microdermabrader
Pelle peel m.
microdermatome
Meek-Wall m.
MicroDigitrapper-HR
MicroDigitrapper-S
MicroDigitrapper-S apnea screening device
MicroDigitrapper-V
microdilution system
microdissecting forceps
microdissector
Eppendorf m.
Rhoton m.
micro-Doppler instrument
Microdose Cath catheter
microdressing forceps
microdrill
high-speed m.
Shea m.
system high-speed m.
microdrilling guide
microelectrode
Eppendorf pO_2 m.
tungsten m.
microelectromechanical system

M

microendoscope
    ophthalmic laser m.
    Toshiba m.
microendoscopic
    m. optical catheter
    m. test card
microexplosive generator
microextractor
    vitreous m.
MicroFerret-18 infusion catheter
Microferret microcatheter
MicroFET2 muscle testing device
microfibrillar
    m. collagen
    m. collagen hemostat
Microfil silicone-rubber injection compound
microfilter
    Minnpure m.
    OmniFilter percutaneous guidewire m.
microfinger
    Lieberman m.
MicroFlo test strip
Micro-Flow compactor
MicroFlow phacoemulsification needle
microfocal direct magnification in vitro x-ray tube
microforceps
    Anis m.
    Eckardt ILM m.
    iris suture m.
    Sparta m.
MicroFrance pediatric backbiter
microfuge
    M. 18 microcentrifuge
    M. 22R refrigerated microcentrifuge
    m. tube
MicroFuse Infuser
MicroGard
MicroGas 7650 transcutaneous monitoring system
Microgel surface-enhanced ventilation tube
Microglass pH electrode
Micro-Glide corneal suture
microgonioscope
micrograft dilator
micrograph
    low-magnification electron m.
micrograsper
Micro-Guide catheter
MicroGuide microelectrode recording system
microguidewire
Microgyn II urinary incontinence device
Micro-Halogen otoscope
microhandpiece
microhemostat

microhook
    McIntyre m.
    Rhoton m.
    Visitec m.
Micro-Hysteroflator
    Hamou M.-H.
microhysteroscope
    Hamou contact m.
microimplant
    Artecoll injectable m.
    Bioplastique injectable m.
    silicone m.
microincinerator
microincision intraocular lens
microinfusion pump
microiris
    m. hook
    m. knife
    m. scissors
microirrigator
    Stryker m.
Microjet-based cutting and débriding device
microkeratome
    ALTK system m.
    Amadeus m.
    automated corneal shaper m.
    Barraquer m.
    Barraquer-Carriazo m.
    BD K-3000 m.
    Carriazo-Barraquer m.
    Carriazo-Pendular m.
    Centurion SES m.
    Chiron ACS m.
    Chiron Hansatome m.
    corneal shaper m.
    Epi-K m.
    FlapMaker disposable m.
    Hansatome m.
    Innovatome m.
    Krumeich-Barraquer m.
    K-tome m.
    LSK One disposable m.
    LSK One standard m.
    MedJet m.
    Med-Logics ML m.
    MK-2000 m.
    Moria automated M2 m.
    Moria M2 m.
    Moria Model One m.
    SCMD m.
    SKBM m.
    Summit Krumeich-Barraquer m.
    Supratome m.
MicroKlenz wound cleanser
microknife
    Karlin m.
    Ultrasharp round blade m.

Microknit
  M. patch graft
  M. vascular graft prosthesis
MicroLap
  M. endoscope
  M. Gold system
microlaparoscope
  Imagyn m.
microlaryngeal scissors
microlaryngoscope
  Jako m.
  Lindholm m.
microlaser
  diode m.
Microlase transpupillary diode laser
microlens
  m. cystourethroscope
  M. foroblique telescope
Microlet Vaculance
Microlight 830 laser
MicroLite suture anchor
Microlith
  M. pacemaker pulse generator
  M. P pacemaker
Microloc
  M. knee implant
  M. knee prosthesis
Micro-Lok dental implant
MicroLoop
  M. curette
  M. II handheld spirometer
microloop curette polisher
microlumbar discectomy retractor
MicroLux videocamera system
MicroLyzer
  M. Gas analyzer
  QuinTron M.
micromanipulator
  microscope-mounted m.
  MicroSpot m.
  self-centering m.
  UniMax laser m.
micromanometer
  m. catheter
  m. catheter system
micromanometer-tipped catheter
MicroMark tissue marker
Micromask
  CPR M.
MicroMax
  M. centrifuge
  M. speed drill
Micromax resorbable suture anchor
**MicroMed DeBakey ventricular assist
  device**
micromesh sheeting
micrometer
  diamond m.
  m. knife

Tolman m.
  ultrasonic m.
micrometric screw
**MicroMewi multiple side-hole infusion
  catheter**
Micro-Mill knee instrument system
micromirror
  Apfelbaum m.
MicroMite anchor suture
micromonitor
  Tracer blood glucose m.
micromosquito
  m. curved scissors
  m. straight scissors
micromultileaf
  m. collimator
  m. collimator system
Micronail intramedullary nail
micronebulizer
MicroNeedle
  Colorado M.
microneedle
  m. holder
  m. holder forceps
micronester platinum embolization coil
microneurosurgical forceps
micron needle
**Micron Res-Q implantable cardioverter-
  defibrillator**
Microny
  M. II SR+ pacemaker
  M. II SR+ pulse generator
  M. K SR pacemaker
  M. SR+ single-chamber rate-
    responsive pulse generator
Micro-One
  M.-O. dissecting forceps
  M.-O. hook
Micro-Pen handpiece
microperimeter
microphone
  2-m. acoustical rhinometer
  Bluetooth remote wireless
    technology m.
  hearing aid m.
  Sennheiser electric condenser m.
    ME 40-3
**MicroPhor iontophoretic drug delivery
  system**
microphthalmoscope
micropick
  vitreoretinal m.
micropigmentation handpiece
micropin
  m. forceps
  Pischel m.
micropipette
  in vitro fertilization m.

M

micropituitary
    m. rongeur
    m. scissors
microplaner
    m. blade
    m. soft tissue shaver
microplate
    AO-Titanium m.
    Luhr m.
    mandibular angle fracture intraoral
        open reduction m.
    m. reader
MicroPlus spirometer
micropoint
    m. needle
    m. suture
MicroPor
    Altea M.
Micropore
    M. dressing
    M. tape
MicroPrep
    M. 2 centrifuge
    M. 2 microcentrifuge
microprobe
    M. integrated laser endoscope
    M. integrated laser and endoscope
        system
    M. laser
    M. ophthalmic laser
    Raman m.
    M. tip
microprocessor
    Intertron therapy m.
micropuncture
    m. guidewire
    m. introducer needle
    m. needle
    m. Peel-Away introducer
microrasp
    Yasargil m.
microretractor
    flexible arm m.
**MicroRint portable airway resistance
    meter**
microrongeur
    Kerrison m.
microruler
microsagittal saw
Microsampler device
microsatellite marker
microsaw
    Zimmer m.
microscalpel
    Oasis feather m.
microscanner
microscissors
    curved conventional m.
    DORC microforceps and m.

iris m.
Kamdar m.
Keeler m.
Kurze m.
round-tip m.
Shutt m.
single-bladed Kurze m.
straight m.
Twisk m.
Yasargil m.
microscope
    Accu-Scope m.
    acoustic m.
    analytical electron m. (AEM)
    beta ray m.
    BHTU m.
    binocular m.
    Bio-Optics specular m.
    Bitumi monobjective m.
    capillary m.
    cellular debris centrifuge
        polarizing m.
    centrifuge m.
    color-contrast m.
    confocal m.
    confocal laser scanning m.
    ConfoScan 3 m.
    ConfoScan slit corneal confocal m.
    ConfoScan 2.0 slit corneal
        confocal m.
    conventional transmission
        electron m.
    CooperVision m.
    corneal m.
    Czapski m.
    dissecting m.
    dual-axis confocal m.
    electron m.
    Elekta robotic surgical m.
    Elmiskop 101 electron m.
    endothelial specular m.
    epi-illuminated m.
    epiluminescent skin surface m.
    Fiberlite m.
    fiberoptic m.
    fluorescence m.
    flying spot m.
    Galilean m.
    Heyer-Schulte specular m.
    high-voltage electron m.
    Hitachi H600, H7000 electron m.
    hypodermic m.
    interference m.
    ion m.
    JedMed TRI-GEM m.
    JEM-100B, 100S electron m.
    JEM-100CX electron m.
    Jeol 100 CX electron m.

Jeol JSM 35 CF scanning
electron m.
Jeol 1200 transmission electron m.
JSM-54 IOLV m.
JSM-6400 scanning electron m.
Keeler-Konan Specular m.
Keeler specular m.
Konan SP-5500 contact specular m.
Konan SP8000 noncontact
specular m.
Labophot-2 m.
laser m.
Leica m.
Leitz m.
light m.
light electron m.
LSM-2100C eye bank specular m.
Mentor fine-focus m.
Moller m.
nailfold capillary m.
Nikon NS-1 slit-lamp m.
Olympus BH2 m.
Olympus BH2-epifluorescence m.
Olympus BH2 epifluorescence m.
Olympus BH2-RFCA reflecting m.
Olympus BHT-2 m.
Olympus CBK fluorescence m.
Olympus Vanox VH-2 m.
Omni 2 m.
OM 2000 operation m.
opaque m.
operating m.
Opmi Pentero surgical m.
Opmi pico diagnostic m.
Opmi pico i m.
Opmi Pro Magis dental m.
Opmi surgical m.
Opmi VISU 200 m.
Opmi VISU 210 m.
Optiphot m.
Optiphot-2UD m.
Optique m.
Pentero surgical m.
phase m.
Philips CM 12 electron m.
Philips 301 electron m.
pneumatic m.
polarizing m.
projection x-ray m.
Pro-Koester wide-field SCM m.
Protégé Plus m.
real-time confocal scanning
laser m.
Reichert Zetopan m.
Rheinberg m.
robotic m.
scanning acoustic m.
scanning electron m.
scanning laser acoustic m.

scanning slit confocal m.
scanning transmission electron m.
scanning tunneling m.
schlieren m.
Seiler MC-M900 surgical m.
slit-lamp m.
SMZ-10A zoom stereo m.
specular m.
stereoscopic m.
Storz m.
stroboscopic m.
surgical m.
SurgiScope robotic m.
tandem scanning m.
tandem scanning confocal m.
Tomey ConfoScan confocal m.
Topcon SP-series noncontact
specular m.
transmission electron m.
ultrasonic m.
Universal electron m.
Urban m.
Vario m.
video-rate laser 2-photon
scanning m.
video specular m.
Weck m.
Welch Allyn LumiView portable
binocular m.
white-light tandem-scanning
confocal m.
Wild m.
Wild operating m.
x-ray m.
x-ray tomographic m.
Zeiss Axiophot m.
Zeiss Axiophot fluorescent m.
Zeiss Axioskop m.
Zeiss Axiovert m.
Zeiss-Barraquer cine m.
Zeiss-Barraquer surgical m.
Zeiss electron m.
Zeiss IDO3 phase-contrast m.
Zeiss/Jena surgical m.
Zeiss LSM-10 laser m.
Zeiss operating m.
Zeiss operating m.
Zeiss Opmi-6 FR m.
Zeiss Opmi Neuro/NC4 surgical m.
Zeiss transmission electron m.
microscope-mounted micromanipulator
microscopic
m. hook
m. scissors
microscrew
Microseal ophthalmic handpiece
microsecond pulsed flashlamp pumped
dye laser

Microsect
    M. curette
    M. shaver
microSelectron rapid delivery system
microsensor
    ICP m.
    intracranial pressure m.
microserrated Tano asymmetrical peeling forceps
MicroShape keratome system
Micro-Sharp blade
microshaver
    Stryker m.
Micros infusion system
MicroSkin ostomy pouch
microsnare
    Amplatz gooseneck m.
Micro-Soft Stream side-hole infusion catheter
MicroSpacer
MicroSpan
    M. capnometer
    M. hysteroscope
    M. microhysterescopy system
    M. sheath
microspatula
microspectroscope
microsphere
    calibrated tris-acryl gelatin m.
    Contour SE m.
    EmboGold m.
    Embosphere m.
    hollow albumin m.
    magnetic m.
    paramagnetic m.
    sodium acrylate and vinyl alcohol copolymer m.
    superabsorbent polymer m.
    Super-Bright m.
    tris-acryl gelatin m.
Microspike
    M. approximator
    M. approximator clamp
Microsponge
    M. delivery system
    M. drug delivery system
    M. Teardrop sponge
microsponge
    Alcon m.
    Weck-cel m.
MicroSpot
    M. laser
    M. micromanipulator
Micross
    M. dilatation catheter
    M. SL balloon
MicroStable liner locking mechanism

microstaple
    Barouk m.
    m. holder
Microstat handpiece
MicroStim 100 TENS device
microstomia prevention appliance
Microstream capnograph
Microsulis microwave endometrial ablation system
microsurgical
    m. biopsy forceps
    m. dissector
    m. ear hook
    m. ear pick
    m. grasping forceps
    m. knife
    m. needle holder
    m. retractor
    m. scissors
    m. tying forceps
microsuture
    Sharpoint m.
microsyringe
MicroTach pneumotach
Microtainer lancet
Microtek
    M. Heine otoscope
    M. ScanMaker 9600XL scanner
micro-thin plastic fiber
Micro-Three microsurgery instrument
microtip
    m. bipolar jeweler's forceps
    m. catheter
    m. lead
    m. phaco tip
    m. pressure transducer
    m. sensor catheter
    m. transducer catheter
microtissue forceps
microtitration plate reader
microtome
    Cryo-Cut m.
    laser m.
    Leica vibrating knife m.
    Leica VT1000 E fully automatic m.
    Leica VT1000 M semi-automatic m.
    Leitz 1600 saw m.
    rocking m.
    Stadie-Riggs m.
microtonometer
Micro-Touch Platex medical glove
MicroTrac direct specimen test
Micro-Tracer portable ECG
MicroTrach
    Heimlich M.

microtransducer
  imbedded m.
  Konigsberg m.
Micro-Transducer catheter
microtrephine
Microtron accelerator
Micro-Two forceps
microtying forceps
MicroTymp2 handheld tympanometer
MicroTymp tympanometric device
MicroVac catheter
microvalve
  Hypobaric m.
microvascular
  m. clamp
  m. clamp-applying forceps
  m. clip
  m. needle holder
  m. scissors
  m. tying forceps
Microvasive
  M. Altertome
  M. angled hydrophilic guidewire
  M. ASAP 18
  M. balloon catheter
  M. biliary device
  M. biliary stent system
  M. CRE esophageal dilator
  M. disposable alligator-shaped
    forceps
  M. Geenen Endotorque guidewire
  M. Glidewire
  M. Glidewire guidewire
  M. Gold probe bipolar
    electrocautery device
  M. instrumentation
  M. minisnare
  M. One-Step button
  M. papillotome
  M. radial-jaw biopsy forceps
  M. retrieval balloon
  M. Rigiflex balloon dilator
  M. Rigiflex through-the-scope
    balloon
  M. Rigiflex TTS balloon
  M. stent
  M. stiff piano wire guidewire
  M. Ultraflex esophageal stent
    system
  M. ultratome
Microvel
  M. double velour graft
  M. prosthesis
Microvena
  M. Amplatz goose neck snare
  M. Das Angel Wings occluder
  M. retrieval device

Micro-Vent
  M.-V. implant
  M.-V. implant system
Micro-Vent^2 implant
MicroVent ventilator
microvessel hook
Microvit
  M. cutter
  M. probe
  M. probe system
  M. scissors
  Storz Premiere M.
  M. vitrector
microvitrector
microvitreoretinal
  m. blade
  m. spatula
microwave
  m. applicator
  m. cardiac ablation system
  m. tissue coagulator
MicroWick system
MicroWrlst
Micro-Z neuromuscular stimulator
Mic-TJ transgastric jejunal tube
micturition bag
Midas
  M. II automated stainer
  M. Rex bur guard
  M. Rex craniotome
  M. Rex drill
  M. Rex instrumentation
  M. Rex instrumentation system
  M. Rex knife
  M. Rex Legend system
  M. Rex pneumatic instrument
  M. Rex Quick-Connect system
MIDCAB system
middle
  m. ear aspirator
  m. ear calipers
  m. ear chisel
  m. ear excavator
  m. ear implant
  m. ear implantable system
  m. ear ring curette
  m. ear strut forceps
  m. ear suction cannula
  m. fossa retractor
middle-caliber needle
midforceps
midgastric electrode
midget MRI scanner
midinfrared laser
mid-infrared pulsed laser
Midland
  M. multifunctional mat platform
  M. tilt table

M

midline
> m. catheter
> M. Hi-Lo Mat platform

Midmark 413 power female procedure chair

midoccipital electrode

midstream aortogram catheter

Miethke dual-switch valve

Mighty Bite Zimmon lateral biopsy cup forceps

Mikaelsson catheter

Mikro-Tip
> M.-T. micromanometer tipped catheter
> M.-T. transducer

Mikulicz
> M. abdominal retractor
> M. bag
> M. drain
> M. pack
> M. packing
> M. pad
> M. peritoneal clamp
> M. peritoneal forceps

Mikulicz-Radecki drain

Milagro interference screw

Milano Shoethotic footwear

Milan uterine curette

Miles
> M. bone chisel
> M. Encore QA glucose meter
> M. punch biopsy forceps
> M. vacuum infiltration processor
> M. vena cava clip
> M. V.I.P. 300 vacuum infiltration processor

Milex
> M. pessary
> M. spatula

military antishock trousers (MAST)

mill
> hollow m.
> Lere bone m.
> Retsch MM200 mixer m.

Millar
> M. catheter-tip transducer
> M. Doppler catheter
> M. micromonometer catheter
> M. Mikro-Tip catheter pressure transducer
> M. MPC-500 catheter
> M. pigtail angiographic catheter
> M. urodynamic catheter

Millard
> M. clamp
> M. mouthgag
> M. thimble hook

Millenia
> M. balloon catheter

> M. portable vital sign monitor
> M. PTCA catheter

Millennium
> M. CX, LX microsurgical system
> M. LX
> M. microsurgical system
> M. oxygen concentrator
> M. transconjunctival standard vitrectomy system
> M. TSV25 light pipe
> M. VG SPECT system
> M. vitreous cutter

Mille Pattes screw

Miller
> M. articulating forceps
> M. blade
> M. blade #0, #1
> M. bone file
> M. cystoscope
> M. dental elevator
> M. double mushroom biliary stent
> M. laryngoscope
> M. ocular disc
> M. 9-prong small rake
> M. rasp
> M. rectal scissors
> M. retractor
> M. septostomy catheter

Miller-Abbott
> M.-A. catheter
> M.-A. double-lumen intestinal tube

Miller-Galante
> M.-G. hip prosthesis
> M.-G. I condylar total knee system
> M.-G. revision knee system
> M.-G. total knee system
> M.-G. unicompartmental knee

Miller-Nadler glare tester

Miller-Senn double-ended retractor

Millesi interfascicular graft

Millet phlebectomy hook

Millex filter

Millex-GS pore-size filter

Millex-GV filter

Millie female urinal

Milliknit
> M. Dacron prosthesis
> M. vascular graft prosthesis

millimeter ruler

Millin
> M. bladder neck spreader
> M. bladder retractor
> M. capsular forceps
> M. forceps
> M. prostatectomy forceps
> M. T clamp

milliner's needle

millinery bag

milling
    m. cutter
    m. machine
Millipore
    M. filter
    M. filtration
    M. ultrafree-CL centrifugal filter
Milli-Q water purification system
Mill-Rose
    M.-R. cytology brush
    M.-R. esophageal injector
    M.-R. flexible endoscopic overtube
    M.-R. RiteBite biopsy forceps
Mills
    M. dressing
    M. valvulotome
Miltex
    M. bone saw
    M. disposable biopsy punch
    M. mallet
    M. nail nipper
    M. retractor
    M. rib spreader
    M. saber-back rhytidectomy scissors
    M. stitch scissors
    M. tenaculum hook
    M. undermining scissors
    M. wire twister
Miltner constraint compliance device
Milwaukee
    M. brace
    M. cervicothoracolumbosacral
      orthosis
    M. orthosis
    M. scoliosis brace
    M. scoliosis orthosis
Mi-Mark
    M.-M. disposable endocervical
      curette
    M.-M. endocervical curette set
MIM card
Mimix bone replacement system
Minardi phaco chopper
Miner osteotome
Minerva
    M. back jacket
    M. cast
    M. cervical brace
    M. collar
    M. orthosis
    M. plastic jacket
    M. robot
    M. system
    M. vest
Mingograf
    M. 62 6-channel electrocardiograph
    M. electroencephalograph
    M. 82 recorder
Mingograph

mini
    m. Acutrak small bone fixation
      system
    m. applier
    M. Bio-Phase suture anchor
    m. cliplamp
    m. condylar plate
    m. Crown stent
    m. GLS anchor
    m. Hoffmann external fixation
      system
    m. Hype-Wipe bleach towelette
    M. II, II+ automatic implantable
      cardioverter-defibrillator
    m. lag screw
    m. lag screw system
    m. Orbita plate
    m. scissors
    m. speech processor
    m. trephine
    m. Vidas automated immunoassay
      system
    m. Würzburg Flexplates
      craniomaxillofacial plating system
    m. Würzburg implant system
    m. Würzburg plate
    m. Würzburg screw
    m. Würzburg standard
      craniomaxillofacial plating system
miniature
    m. blade
    m. bulldog clamp
    m. centrifugal fast analyzer
    m. excimer laser
    m. forceps
    m. glaucoma shunt
    m. Gracey curette
    m. intestinal forceps
    m. loop electrode
    m. probe
    m. sound
    m. ultrasound suction device
    m. ultrasound transmitter
miniaturized ultrasound catheter probe
Mini-Bag Plus container
miniballoon
MiniBard catheter
minibasket
    Shutt m.
miniblade
    Beaver m.
    Beaver ES m.
    SP90 m.
minicamera
    GD-LD-208C m.
mini-C-arm
    XiScan m.-C.-a.
miniclip lamp
minicoil

M

MiniCorr digital oximeter
mini-defibrillator
    Liteguard m.-d.
minidriver
mini-echo sounder
mini-endoscope
mini-excimer
    Compak-200 m.-e.
Mini-Fibralux pocket otoscope
minifixator
    articulated m.
    Pennig m.
Mini-Flex
    M.-F. flexible Harris uterine
      injector
    HUI M.-F.
miniforceps
miniform
minifragment screw
minigraft dilator
Miniguard adhesive patch
MiniHEART low-flow nebulizer
minihelical basket
mini-Hoffmann external fixator
mini-Hohmann retractor
mini-keratoplasty stitch scissors
mini-Kessler external fixator
mini-Lambotte osteotome
minilaparoscope
    Aslan 2-mm m.
    Pixie m.
minilaparotomy Falope ring applicator
mini-Lexer osteotome
Minilith pacemaker pulse generator
miniloop
    Olympus HX-21L detachable m.
Minilux pocket otoscope
minimagnet
minimal incision total hip retractor
minimallet
minimally
    m. invasive access set
    m. invasive breast biopsy
Mini-Matic implant
MiniMed
    M. continuous glucose monitoring
      system
    M. III infusion pump
    M. 508, 511 insulin pump
    M. Paradigm insulin pump
MiniMedBall hand exerciser
Mini-Med tubing
mini-meniscus blade
MiniMite
    M. suture anchor
    M. suture anchor system
Mini-Motionlogger Actigraph
miniophthalmic drape

mini-Orthofix fixator
miniosmotic infusion pump
mini-ovoid applicator
MiniOX
    M. IA oxygen analyzer
    M. I, II, III, 100-IV oxygen
      monitor
    M. 3000 oxygen monitor
    M. V pulse oximeter
Mini-Perc entry set
miniplate
    2-hole m.
    8-hole m.
    L-shaped m.
    Luhr m.
    mandibular m.
    monocortical m.
    resorbable PLLA m.
    Storz m.
    m. strut
    titanium m.
    vitallium m.
minipouch
    Assura closed m.
    closed m.
    Filter Security closed m.
    Premier drainable m.
miniprobe
    high-frequency m.
Mini-Profile catheter
minipump
    Alzer Model 2001 osmotic m.
    osmotic m.
minipuncture sheath
MiniQuad XL lens
MiniQuick
mini-retractor
Mini-Revo
    M.-R. Screws suture anchor
    M.-R. suture anchor
    M.-R. suture anchor system
Mini-ROC anchor
miniscope
    Candela m.
    Circon-ACMI m.
    M. MS-3
    M. MS-3 pocket ECG
    Wolfe m.
MiniSite
    M. laparoscope
    M. laparoscopic instrument
Minislide sliding mat
minisnare
    Microvasive m.
Minispace IUI catheter
MiniSpacer
    Airlife Dual Spray M.

ministaple
    Bio-R-Sorb resorbable poly-L-lactic acid m.
    Richards m.
mini-Stryker power drill
mini-Sugita clip
mini-tip culturette
Mini-Torr Plus NIPB monitor
mini-valve
    Novus m.-v.
mini-Westcott scissors
Mini-Wright peak flowmeter
Minix
    Medtronic M.
Minnesota
    M. retractor
    M. thermal disc temperature testing device
    M. tube
Minnpure microfilter
Minolta LS 110 spot photometer
minus lens
30-minute TUMT
MIP
    MIP anatomic overlay
    MIP reusable cover
Mira
    M. AGL-400
    M. cautery
    M. electrocautery
    M. encircling element
    M. endovitreal cryopencil
    M. female trochanteric reamer
    M. photocoagulator
    M. silicone rod
    M. unit
Miracon
Mirage
    M. hydrophilic guidewire
    M. nasal mask
    M. nasal ventilation mask system
    M. over-the-wire balloon catheter
    M. spinal system
Miragel
    M. episcleral buckle
    M. exoplant
    M. implant
    M. sponge
Miralene suture
Miralva applicator
Mirasorb sponge
Mirena intrauterine device
mirror
    concave m.
    concave dental m.
    contact lens training m.
    convex m.
    curved laryngeal m.
    curved magnifying m.
    DenLite illuminated handheld m.
    fiberoptic lighted m.
    front surface dental m.
    Grafco laryngeal m.
    m. haploscope
    Hardy transsphenoidal m.
    head m.
    m. holder
    House middle ear m.
    Jako laryngeal m.
    laryngeal m.
    m. laryngoscope
    laser m.
    Lewis dental m.
    McLaughlin laser m.
    meniscal m.
    Neovision micro m.
    m. optical system
    plane dental m.
    polygon m.
    rhinoscopic m.
    straight laryngeal m.
    straight magnifying m.
3-mirror
    3-m. contact lens
    3-m. intraocular lens
4-mirror
    4-m. Gonio lens
    4-m. goniolens
Miser tube
Mishler
    M. dual-chamber valve
    M. flushing valve
M.I.S. multi-port illumination system
Mission
    M. vacuum constriction device
    M. vacuum erection device
    M. VCD
    M. VED
Missouri catheter
Misstique female external urinary collector
mist
    M. Eubanks instrument series
    m. tent
Mistifier spray catheter
Misti Gold prosthesis
Mistogen
    M. nebulizer
    M. passover humidifier
Mistral ventilator
Misty-Neb nebulizer
Mitchell
    M. osteotome
    M. viscoclastic removal I/A tip
Mitek
    M. Absolute absorbable interference screw
    M. absorbable bone anchor

M

Mitek (*continued*)
- M. bone anchor
- M. Contack labral anchor
- M. Exojet fluid-jet resection system
- M. Fastin threaded anchor
- M. GII easy anchor
- M. GII Snap-Pak
- M. GII suture anchor
- M. GII suture anchor system
- M. GL anchor
- M. knotless anchor
- M. ligament anchor
- M. micro anchor
- M. Micro QuickAnchor
- M. Mini GII anchor
- M. Mini GLS anchor
- M. Mini QuickAnchor
- M. Panalok RC anchor
- M. QuickAnchor device
- M. rotator cuff anchor
- M. SuperAnchor instrument
- M. Tacit threaded anchor
- M. Vapr tissue removal system

mitochondrial ethanol oxidase system
Mitraflex
- M. Plus foam dressing
- M. Plus wound dressing
- M. SC foam dressing

mitral
- m. hook
- m. valve dilator
- m. valve-holding forceps
- m. valve retractor
- m. valve scissors

Mitrofanoff
- M. tube
- M. valve

Mitroflow
- M. pericardial prosthetic valve
- M. PeriPatch cylinders
- M. Synergy PC stented pericardial valve

Mitsubishi HL7955 CRT screen
mitt
- holding m.
- impact m.
- infant passive m.
- motion control m.
- paraffin m.
- wash m.

Mittelman implant
Mitty-Pollack needle set
Mitutoyo
- M. Digimatic calipers
- M. digital calipers

Mity
- M. engine H-file
- M. Hedström file
- M. K-file
- M. plugger
- M. Roto 360 instrument
- M. Roto rotary instrument
- M. spreader
- M. Turbo file

Mityvac
- M. obstetric vacuum extractor cup
- M. reusable vacuum pump
- M. simple hand pump
- M. Super M cup
- M. vacuum delivery system
- M. vacuum extractor

mixed mesh
mixer
- Genotropin m.

Mixter
- M. baby hemostatic forceps
- M. brain biopsy punch
- M. dilating probe
- M. dissector
- M. forceps
- M. hemostat
- M. irrigating probe
- M. ligature-carrier clamp
- M. mosquito forceps
- M. thoracic forceps
- M. ventricular needle

Miya
- M. hook
- M. hook ligament carrier
- M. hook ligature carrier

Miyoshi chopper
Mizuho
- M. aneurysm sizer-dissector
- M. surgical Doppler

MK-2000
- MK-2000 keratome system
- MK-2000 microkeratome

MKG knee support
MKII automated scanner
MK IV ophthalmoscope
MKS II knee brace
MLA-100 coagulation instrument
Mladick
- M. concave cannula
- M. convex cannula

ML 700 daylight processor
M/L lift
MLR+ camera
ML-Ultra balloon stent
MM-6000 colposcope
M-mode sector transducer
MMS-900
- MMS-900 balancing tool
- MMS-900 microscope balancer

Moberg osteotome
Mobetron
- M. electron beam system

M. intraoperative radiation therapy treatment system
M. mobile, self-shielded electron accelerator

mobile
m. air chair
m. bearing knee implant
m. dilator storage tray
m. electroconvulsive therapy apparatus
m. eye unit
m. response unit
m. spiral computed tomography scanner
600XLE m. surgery table

MobilExcimer laser system
Mobilimb CPM device
mobility film
mobilizer
Derlacki-Hough m.
TheraBite m.

Mobils Professionals Pedorthic footwear
Mobin-Uddin
M.-U. filter
M.-U. sieve
M.-U. umbrella endoluminal device
M.-U. umbrella vena cava filter
M.-U. vena cava filter

MobiTrak
M. automated table
M. moving table

Moblvac suction unit
Modabber thumb orthosis
modality
Fluidotherapy sterile dry heat m.

model
AccuView m.
ClearView m.
dynamic EMG-assisted biomechanical m.
floater eye m.
foot m.
Gullstrand 6-surface eye m.
Kooijman eye m.
Le Grand-Gullstrand eye m.
RapidView m.
tracheostomy anatomical m.
tracheostomy TOM anatomical m.
von Helmholtz eye m.

modeling carver
mode-locked laser
modem
Acculink m.

modified
m. aspirating catheter
m. birdcage coil
m. Blalock-Taussig shunt
m. caulking gun
m. chest lead

m. CIF needle
m. C-loop haptic
m. C-loop intraocular lens
m. Darrach-type elevator
m. electron-beam CT scanner
m. Frost suture
m. Fukuda-type retractor
m. Grace plate
m. Gracey curette
m. Harrington rod
m. human graft umbilical vein graft
m. J-loop haptic
m. J-loop posterior chamber intraocular lens
Kraus m.
m. L loop haptic
m. L-loop haptic
m. Mark IV R-wave-triggered power injector
m. Moore hip locking prosthesis
m. Oppenheimer splint
m. prolate anterior surface IOL
m. Rashkind PDA occluder
m. right-angled hook
m. Robert Jones dressing
m. sclerectomy punch
m. spatula needle
m. submental retractor flared tip
m. suction tube
m. zinc oxide-eugenol cement
m. Z-stent

modifier
multidimensional analysis beam m.

Modulap
modular
m. acetabular revision system (MARS)
m. Austin Moore hip prosthesis
m. calcar replacement stem
m. head remover
m. implant
m. implant system
m. instrumentation
m. internal distraction system
m. Iowa Precoat total hip prosthesis
M. One pneumatonometer
3R80 m. hydraulic knee joint
m. socket
m. S-ROM total hip system
m. stent graft
m. temPPTthotic kit

modulator
intracrine negative feedback m.

module
AIM 7 thermocouple input m.
Allen diagnostic m.
Calyx 2 fluoroscopic tracking m.

M

module *(continued)*
    CUSA electrosurgical m.
    large particle sorting m.
    Nd:YAG m.
    NeuroSight cranial m.
    OmniCell catheter m.
    PDT dye m.
    Peak gait m.
    Research Pneumotach System
      instrumentation m.
    SinuSight ENT m.
    SpinalSight spinal m.
Modulith SL 20 lithotriptor
Modulock posterior spinal fixation
Modulus CD anesthesia system
Moe
    M. alar hook
    M. bone curette
    M. gouge
    M. intertrochanteric plate
    M. modified Harrington rod
    M. osteotome
Moeller laser
Moeltgen flexometer
Moersch
    M. bronchoscope
    M. esophagoscope
Mogen
    M. circumcision
    M. circumcision clamp
    M. clamp
Mohr pinchcock clamp
MoistAir humidifying chamber
moistened fine mesh gauze dressing
moist interactive dressing
moisture
    m. chamber
    m. exchanger
    m. goggles
moisture-retentive dressing
Mojave cataract extraction system
Mojave-Mini dehumidifier
molar bracket
mold
    acrylic m.
    Aquaplast m.
    Biothotic orthotic m.
    Counsellor vaginal m.
    Cryo rubber m.
    filter m.
    flavine wool m.
    Hydro-Cast dental m.
    silastic m.
    silicone m.
    StageOne temporary hip prosthesis
      cement spacer m.
    Swyrls swim m.
    Teflon m.

molded
    m. ankle-foot orthosis (MAFO)
    M. Bulb closed wound drainage
      reservoir
    m. immobilizer
    m. lumbosacral orthosis
    m. postpartum insole
    m. Thomas collar
    m. vacuum pillow
molding
    elastomer skin m.
    m. sock
Mold-In-Place back support
molectron laser
Molectron Nd:YAG laser
molecular
    m. adsorbents recirculating system
    m. sieve
MoleMax
moleskin
    m. bandage
    m. padding
Molestick padding
Molina
    M. mandibular distractor
    M. mandibular distractor set
    M. needle catheter
Moller microscope
Mollison self-retaining retractor
Molnar disc
Molt
    M. curette
    M. mouthgag
    M. No. 4 elevator
    M. periosteal elevator
Molteno
    M. double-plate drainage device
    M. double-plate implant
    M. drainage eye implant
    M. implant drainage device
    M. seton
    M. shunt tube
    M. single-plate drainage device
molybdenum
    m. rotating anode x-ray tube
    m. target tube
molybdenum-99 generator
molybdenum-technetium generator
Momberg tube
Momentum DR pacemaker
Momose lens
MOM tractograph
Monaghan
    M. respirator
    M. ventilator
Monahan-Lewis knife
Monaldi drainage system
Monarch
    M. C cartridge

M. II injector
M. 25 inflation device
M. IOL delivery system
M. knee brace
M. Mini Mask nasal interface
M. spinal system
Monarc transobturator sling
Monark
    M. bicycle
    M. bicycle ergometer
    M. rehab trainer
Mon-a-Therm thermocouple
Moncorps knife
MO needle
monitor
Accucap CO_2/O_2 m.
Accu-Chek Easy glucose m.
Accu-Chek II Freedom blood
  glucose m.
Accucom cardiac output m.
AccuGuide injection m.
Accutorr bedside m.
Accutrackcr II ambulatory blood
  pressure m.
actocardiotocograph m.
Acuson V5M m.
Acuson V5M transesophageal
  echocardiographic m.
Aequitron apnea m.
aerosol inhalation m.
AID-Check m.
AirWatch asthma m.
ambulatory electrogram m. (AEM)
Ami infant apnea m.
antepartum m. (APM)
APM-2000 vital signs m.
apnea m.
Appraise m.
AR+ portable heart m.
Arrhythmia Net arrhythmia m.
Arvee model 2400 infant apnea m.
Ascensia Elite XL diabetes blood
  glucose m.
automatic oscillometric blood
  pressure m.
automatic single-needle m.
AvoSure PT m.
Baby Dopplex 3000 antepartum
  fetal m.
Baby Sense m.
Bear NUM-1 tidal volume m.
Bedfont carbon monoxide m.
Bedfont EC60 Gastrolyzer
  hydrogen m.
bedside m.
Biotrack coagulation m.
BioZ.com cardiac output m.
BioZ heart m.
BladderScan m.

blood perfusion m.
BodyGem metabolism m.
Brevio nerve conduction m.
Brilliance 109 MP PC m.
CA m.
Camino m.
canopy ventilation m.
Capintec nuclear Vest m.
Capnocheck Plus NIPB m.
Capnogard capnograph m.
Capnomac Ultima m.
cardiac m.
cardiac apnea m.
cardiac event m.
CardioBeeper CB-12L cardiac m.
Cardiocap/5 m.
Cardiocap II pressure m.
Cardiocap 5-patient m.
cardiovascular m.
Cardiovit AT-10 m.
CDI 2000 blood gas m.
cerebral function m.
4-channel transcranial Doppler m.
chemical agent m.
Chronicle implantable
  hemodynamic m.
ClearPlan Easy fertility m.
CoaguChek Pro/DM m.
Codman intracranial pressure m.
Colin STBP-780 stress test blood
  pressure m.
Contimed II pelvic floor
  muscle m.
Coremetrics fetal apnea m.
Corometrics m.
Corometrics fctal m.
Corometrics 118 maternal/fetal m.
Corometrics maternal/fetal m.
Cortexplorer cerebral blood
  flow m.
CO Sleuth carbon monoxide m.
CO_2SMO Plus continuous
  noninvasive respiratory profile m.
Criticare comprehensive vital
  sign m.
Criticare $ETCO_2/SpO_2$ m.
Criticare 507N noninvasive blood
  pressure m.
Criticare 507O pulse
  oximeter/NIBP m.
Criticare 507-series noninvasive
  blood pressure m.
Criticare 507S vital sign m.
Crit-Line fluid m.
Cue fertility m.
Datascope Accutor bedside m.
Datex infrared CO_2 m.
Deltatrac II metabolic m.
Diasensor 2000 glucose m.

M

monitor *(continued)*

DigiTrak Plus Holter m.
Digitrapper Mk III sleep m.
Dinamap Accutorr A1, A3 blood pressure m.
Dinamap blood pressure m.
Dinamap Plus m.
Dinamap Plus multiparameter m.
Dinamap Plus vital signs m.
Doppler blood flow m.
Doppler-Cavin m.
Doppler fetal heart m.
Doppler ultrasonic fetal heart m.
Doppler ultrasound m.
Doptone fetal m.
dosimetrist radiation beam m.
Duet glucose control m.
Duo-Care combined blood glucose and wrist blood pressure m.
DynaPulse 5000A ambulatory blood pressure m.
EarCheck m.
EcoCheck oxygen m.
EC50 ToxCO breath carbon monoxide m.
EdenTec 2000W in-home cardiorespiratory m.
electrocardiographic transtelephonic m.
Endotek OM-3 Urodata m.
Endotek UDS-1000 m.
endotracheal cardiac output m.
ETO Sleuth m.
event m.
event recorder m.
external m.
fetal Dopplex m.
fetal heart rate m.
FetalPulse Plus m.
Fetasonde fetal m.
Finapres blood pressure m.
Flo-Stat fluid m.
FreeDop Doppler m.
Gastroreflex ambulatory pH m.
Glucometer DEX blood glucose m.
Glucoscan m.
GlucoWatch bloodless glucose m.
GlucoWatch glucose m.
Gould pressure m.
gray-scale m.
Haemogram blood loss m.
HBT Sleuth portable hydrogen m.
Healthdyne apnea m.
HeartCard m.
Heart Rate 1-2-3 m.
HeartView CT cardiac m.
Hemochron m.
HemoMatic blood collection m.

HemoTec activated clotting time m.
Hewlett-Packard pressure m.
Hewlett-Packard SDN m.
Holter m.
home cardiorespiratory m.
home uterine activity m.
HomMed m.
24-hour ambulatory gastric pH m.
Imex antepartum m.
impedance m.
infant ventilation m.
Ingold M3, M4 glass electrode pH m.
in-line blood gas m.
in-line venous pressure m.
Insta-Pulse heart rate m.
Interceptor M3 triple-channel solid-state m.
internal m.
intracranial pressure Express digital m.
intrapartum m.
intrauterine pressure m.
IOP m.
Jako facial nerve m.
KinetiX ventilation m.
King of Hearts Holter m.
Ladd m.
Ladd intracranial pressure m.
LAPSE m.
laser Doppler perfusion m.
Laserflo BPM laser Doppler m.
Laserflow blood perfusion m.
Laserflow BPM^2 real-time cerebral perfusion m.
m. lead
Lifepak 5 cardiac m.
LifeShirt m.
long-term ambulatory physiologic surveillance m.
loop m.
Magellan m.
Marquette m.
Marquette 8000 Holter m.
Masimo Set home m.
MDILog compliance m.
MDILog microelectronic m.
Meadox ICP m.
Medisense Pen 2 self blood glucose m.
Medpacific LD 5000 laser-Doppler perfusion m.
Mentor B-VAT II m.
MicroCO carbon monoxide m.
Millenia portable vital sign m.
MiniOX I, II, III, 100-IV oxygen m.
MiniOX 3000 oxygen m.

Mini-Torr Plus NIPB m.
Mortara ELI 100 12-lead m.
MRL blood pressure m.
MRM-2 oxygen consumption m.
Multinex ID gas m.
MyoTrac EMG m.
MyoTrac 2 EMG m.
N-Cat N-500 tonometric blood
   pressure m.
Nellcor N-499 fetal oxygen
   saturation m.
Nellcor N-200 home m.
Nellcor N-3000 home m.
Nellcor Puritan Bennett home m.
Nellcor Symphony blood
   pressure m.
Nellcor Symphony N-3100
   noninvasive blood pressure m.
neonatal m.
Neo-trak 515A neonatal m.
Neotrend multiparameter blood
   gas m.
Neotrend premature infant blood
   gas/temperature m.
nerve-integrity m.
NervePace nerve conduction m.
Neurosign 100 nerve m.
Nicolet Elite Doppler m.
Nicolet nerve integrity m.
$NICO_2$ noninvasive cardiac
   output m.
NIM-2 nerve integrity m.
nocturnal penile tumescence m.
noise level m.
noninvasive m.
noninvasive continuous cardiac
   output m.
NOxBOX II m.
Ohmeda 6200, 6300 CO_2 m.
Ohmeda 5250 respiratory gas m.
Omron m.
Omron Hem-601 automatic digital
   wrist blood pressure m.
OneTouch blood glucose m.
OnLine ABG m.
OSD m.
OxiFirst fetal oxygen m.
Oxisensor fetal oxygen
   saturation m.
OxyData Plus oxygen m.
Oxylite oxygen m.
PAM2, PAM3 m.
Paradigm Link blood glucose m.
Paratrend 7 continuous blood
   gas m.
Paratrend 7+ multiparameter blood
   gas m.
Passport bedside m.
patient m.

patient dose m.
peak flow meter m.
perfusion m.
Physios CTM 01 cardiac
   transplant m.
Pick and Go m.
picture-in-picture m.
Pocket-Dop 3 m.
Pocket-Dop fetal heart rate m.
Polar Vantage XL heart rate m.
Polar wrist m.
Porta-Resp m.
Press-Mate model 8800T blood
   pressure m.
Pressurometer blood pressure m.
PrinterNOx nitric oxide/nitrogen
   dioxide m.
ProDynamic m.
Profilomat m.
Propaq Encore vital signs m.
Proview eye pressure m.
Pulse Pro heart rate m.
Puritan-Bennett 7250 metabolic m.
Q-Trak IAQ m.
QuietTrak m.
Quik Connect fetal m.
radiation beam m.
Rascal II anesthetic gas m.
respiratory function m.
RigiScan penile tumescence and
   rigidity m.
RIP portable sleep m.
Scholar II vital sign m.
Sentinel-4 neurological m.
Silverstein facial nerve m.
sleep apnea m.
Sof-Tact diabetes glucose m.
Sof-Tact glucose m.
SpaceLabs Holter m.
SpectRx glucose m.
SpiroFlow peak flow m.
Stat-Temp II liquid crystal
   temperature m.
Steritek ICP mini m.
SureStep glucose m.
Surveyor m.
Tabs Elite mobility m.
TC CO_2 m.
TCM30 transcutaneous oxygen m.
Tensys T-line blood pressure m.
Terumo Doppler fetal heart
   rate m.
Thermograph temperature m.
TINA m.
Toitu MT-810 cardiographic m.
Tokos m.
tonometric blood pressure m.
TrackEASE glucose m.
transcutaneous blood gas m.

M

monitor *(continued)*
    transcutaneous carbon dioxide m.
    transcutaneous oxygen m. (TCOM)
    Transonics laser Doppler
        perfusion m.
    Trans-Scan noninvasive
        physiological m.
    transtelephonic exercise m.
    ultrasound m.
    uterine activity m.
    Vantage Performance m.
    Vasotrax handheld m.
    VentCheck handheld respiratory m.
    VenTrak respiratory mechanics m.
    VersaLab APM2 portable
        antepartum m.
    VEST ambulatory ventricular
        function m.
    Via arterial blood gas and
        chemistry m.
    video m.
    VIP Bird volume m.
    VitaGuard m.
    VitalCare m.
    Vitalograph BreathCO m.
    Vitalograph pulmonary m.
    Xomed Treace nerve integrity m.
monitor/defibrillator
    Lifepak 5, 7 m./d.
monitoring probe
MonitorMate monitor arm
monitor/recorder
    Gastroreflex ambulatory pH m./r.
Monitorr urodynamic measuring system
monoangle chisel
monoblock
    m. femoral component
    m. femoral stem prosthesis
monobloc-type appliance
monocanalicular silicone stent
monochromatic red HeNe laser light
monochromator
    grating m.
monocortical
    m. miniplate
    m. screw
Monocryl suture
monocular
    m. bandage
    m. dressing
    m. indirect ophthalmoscope
    m. patch
monocuspid tilting-disc valve
monodisperse aerosol
Monodos orthosis
monofilament
    m. absorbable suture
    calibrated m.
    m. clear suture

    m. green suture
    m. nonabsorbable suture
    m. nylon suture
    m. polypropylene suture
    m. pressure esthesiometer
    Semmes-Weinstein m.
    Semmes-Weinstein 5.07 m.
    Semmes-Weinstein nylon m.
    m. skin suture
    m. snare wire
    m. steel suture
    m. wire suture
Monofixateur external fixator
monofocal IOL
Monogram total knee instrument
Monoject
    M. hypodermic needle
    M. laceration irrigation tray
Monojector fingerstick device
monolithic
    m. A1203 cup
    m. A1203 cup prosthesis
Monolyth oxygenator
Monoplace hyperbaric chamber
monopolar
    BICAP m.
    m. cathodal stimulator
    m. cautery
    m. coagulating forceps
    m. electrocautery
    m. electrode
    m. insulated forceps
    m. needle electrode
    m. radiofrequency probe
    m. stimulating electrode
    m. temporary electrode
    m. triple-hook active needle
Monopty
    M. biopsy instrument
    M. needle
Monorail
    M. angioplasty catheter
    M. aspiration catheter
    Carotid-Wallstent M.
    M. guidewire
    M. imaging catheter
    M. Piccolino catheter
    M. Speedy balloon
    M. Wallstent self-expanding stent
Monoscopy
    M. locking trocar
    M. locking trocar with Woodford
        spike
monosialosyl Lea
Monospot test
MonoStent monocanalicular stent
Monostrut
    M. Bjödork-Shiley valve

M. cardiac valve prosthesis
M. heart valve
monotube
Howmedica m.
Monotube external fixator system
Mono-Vacc
monoxide
carbon m. (CO)
Monsoon ventilator
Montague
M. proctoscope
M. sigmoidoscope
Monte Carlo photon transport
Montgomery
M. dissector
M. laryngeal keel
M. laryngeal stent
M. Safe-T-Tube
M. salivary bypass tube
M. speaking valve
M. strap
M. strap dressing
M. thyroplasty implant system
M. tracheal cannula
M. tracheal fenestrator
M. tracheal T tube
M. tracheal tube
M. tracheostomy
M. T tube
M. Vent-Trach
Monticelli-Spinelli
M.-S. circular external fixation system
M.-S. distractor
M.-S. frame
Moody fixation forceps
Moon
M. Boot
M. Boot brace
M. rectal retractor
M. Walker
Moon-Robinson prosthesis inserter
Moore
M. bone elevator
M. bone reamer
M. disc
M. gallstone scoop
M. hip endoprosthesis system
M. hip endoprosthesis system stem
M. hip prosthesis
M. measuring rod
M. tracheostomy button
Moorehead cheek retractor
Moore-Wilson hyperopic conformer
MOP-Videoplan morphometric system
Moran
M. enhancement spatula
M. LASIK spatula
Moran-Karaya disc

morcellator
Cook tissue m.
Diva laparoscopic m.
electric tissue m.
electromechanical m.
Gynecare X-Tract tissue m.
high-speed electrical tissue m.
motorized m.
Opera Star m.
rotating m.
Semm m.
Steiner electromechanical m.
tissue m.
X-Tract tissue m.
Morcher
M. Asti disc
M. Cionni capsular tension ring
M. Cionni endocapsular capsular tension ring
M. endocapsular tension ring
M. iris diaphragm ring
M. pupil dilator
Morch respirator
More-Flow long-term high-flow catheter
Moreno gastroenterostomy clamp
Moretsky LASIK hinge protector fixation ring
Moretz clip
Morfam Quality Jeanie Rub massager
Morganstern
M. aspiration/injection system
M. continuous-flow operating cystoscope
Morgan therapeutic lens
Moria
M. automated M2 microkeratome
M. M2 microkeratome
M. Model One microkeratome
M. obturator
M. 1-piece speculum
M. trephine
Morlet lamellar knife/dissector
morphine pump
Morpho Exerciser
morphology system CAS-200
Morrell crown remover
Morris
M. flexible cannula
M. retractor
M. vertical scissors
Morrison-Hurd
M.-H. pillar retractor
M.-H. tonsillar dissector
Morrow Brown needle
Morscher
M. anterior cervical plate
M. cervical plate
M. titanium cervical plate

M

Morse
>M. head
>M. instrument handle
>M. sternal retractor
>M. sternal spreader
>M. stopcock
>M. taper
>M. taper lock of modular hip implant component
>M. taper stem
>M. valve retractor

Mortara ELI 100 12-lead monitor
mortising chisel
Morton toe support
Morwel
>M. ultrasound-assisted lipoplasty machine
>M. ultrasound device

Mosaic
>M. cardiac bioprosthesis
>M. porcine bioprosthetic heart valve

MOS capacitor
Moseley fasciotome
Mosher
>M. bag
>M. dilator
>M. esophagoscope
>M. ethmoid curette
>M. lifesaving tracheal suction tube
>M. nasal speculum

mosquito
>m. clamp
>m. forceps
>m. hemostat
>m. hemostatic clamp
>m. hemostatic forceps
>m. lid clamp

Moss
>M. balloon triple-lumen gastrostomy tube
>M. cage
>M. decompression feeding catheter
>M. feeding tube
>M. fixation system
>M. gastric decompression tube
>M. gastrostomy tube
>M. G-tube PEG kit
>M. hook
>M. instrumentation
>M. Mark IV tube
>M. nasal tube
>M. rod
>M. screw
>M. Suction Buster
>M. Suction Buster catheter
>M. Suction Buster tube
>M. T-anchor introducer gun
>M. T-anchor needle

>M. T-anchor needle introducer
>M. T-anchor needle introducer gun
>M. tube

Mossbauer spectrometer
Moss-Harms basket
Moss-Miami
>M.-M. polyaxial screw
>M.-M. spinal instrumentation
>M.-M. spinal system

Mosso
>M. ergograph
>M. sphygmomanometer

most
>M. Options system
>M. Options system rotating hinge revision knee
>m. versatile patch (MVP)

Motarjeme catheter
mother-baby
>m.-b. endoscope
>m.-b. endoscope system

mother-baby-scope system
mother-daughter endoscope
mother endoscopic retrograde cholangiopancreatoscopy system
Mother Jones dressing
Mother-To-Be
>M.-T.-B. abdominal support
>M.-T.-B. Support maternity support

motility eye implant
motion
>m. artifact rejection system
>continuous passive m. (CPM)
>m. control mitt
>range of m. (ROM)
>total range of m. (TROM)

motion-compensating format converter
Motivator FTR2000 exerciser
motor
>Visuscope m.

motorized
>m. bur
>m. meniscal shaver
>m. morcellator
>m. transducer pullback device

Moto-Tool
>Dremel M.-T.

Mott rasp
mount
>Adamount pocket m.

Mountain View transducer
Mount intervertebral disc forceps
Mount-Mayfield aneurysm forceps
Moure esophagoscope
MouseMitt Keyboarders wrist support
Mouse Nest mouse rest
mouse-tooth
>m.-t. clamp
>m.-t. forceps

moustache dressing
mouth
    m. breathing mask
    m. gag
    m. gag frame
    m. guard
    m. lamp
    m. mask
mouthgag, mouth gag
    Boyle-Davis m.
    Brown-Davis m.
    Crowe-Davis m.
    Davis-Crowe m.
    Davis ring m.
    Denhardt m.
    Denhardt-Dingman m.
    Dingman m.
    Dingman-Millard m.
    Dott m.
    Dott-Kilner m.
    Doyen-Jansen m.
    Ferguson m.
    Ferguson-Brophy m.
    Ferguson-Gwathmey m.
    Fergusson-Ackland m.
    m. frame
    Fulton m.
    Green m.
    Green-Sewall m.
    Heister m.
    Jennings Loktite m.
    Kilner-Dott m.
    Lane m.
    Lange m.
    Maunder m.
    McIvor m.
    McKesson m.
    Millard m.
    Molt m.
    Negus m.
    oral screw m.
    oral speculum m.
    palate-type m.
    Rabbit m.
    Ralks-Davis m.
    Roser-Koenig m.
    Sluder-Jansen m.
    m. tongue depressor blade
    m. tooth plate
    Trousseau m.
    Wesson m.
    Whitehead m.
mouthguard
    oxygenating m.
    Oxyguard oxygenating m.
mouthpiece
    E-Z-Guard m.
    pneumotach disposable m.
    SafeTway pediatric m.

movable core guidewire
Moynihan
    M. artery forceps
    M. clamp
    M. respirator
    M. towel clamp
    M. towel forceps
MP-35 clip material
MPA1 catheter
MPA2 catheter
M-Pact
    M-P. cast cutter
    M-P. cast spreader
    M-P. cast vacuum
    M-P. flexible orthotic
MPC automated intravitreal scissors
MPD
    MPD Pro lancet
    MPD stent
MPM
    MPM antimicrobial wound cleanser
    MPM bandage
    MPM composite dressing
    MPM conductive gel pad
    MPM GelPad impregnated gauze
    MPM hydrogel dressing
Mport
    M. foldable lens placement system
    M. lens inserter
    M. lens insertion system
mPower PET scanner
MP videoendoscopic lens attachment
MR
    magnetic resonance
    MR catheter imaging and
      spectroscopy system scanner
    MR 290 humidification chamber
    MR lead
    nonferromagnetic MR (XGIF-MR30)
    MR simulator
    MR SmartPrep
MR-compatible power injector
MRI
    magnetic resonance imaging
    MRI probe head
MRI-compatible
    MRI-c. electrode
    MRI-c. hollow-fiber bioreactor
    MRI-c. plate and screw system
MRL
    MRL blood pressure monitor
    MRL oximeter
MRM-2 oxygen consumption monitor
MR-trackable intramyocardial injection
  catheter
MS-3
    Miniscope MS-3
MS-30 hip
MS322 muscle stimulator

M

MSC-2001 ECG
MSC cold pack
MS-CIS SV stent
MS Classique balloon dilatation
  catheter
M-scope multibending scope
MSI
    MSI implant
    MSI nylon membrane
MT-100 ECG Holter system
MTA brace
MTC catheter
MTI
    MTI PhotoScreener
    MTI PhotoScreener vision screening
      device
MTL trial frame
MTS electrohydraulic piston
M-type extractor
Mucat cervical sampling device
mucoadhesive
    bioerodible m.
mucosal elevator
mucosector
    oblique aspiration m.
mucotome
mucus
    m. aspirator
    m. clearance device
    m. extractor
Mueller
    M. ATF ankle brace
    M. bur
    M. cautery
    M. curette
    M. electric corneal trephine
    M. electrocautery
    M. electronic tonometer
    M. eye shield
    M. fixation device
    M. hinged knee brace
    M. jumper's knee strap
    M. lacrimal sac retractor
    M. Lite ankle brace
    M. orthopaedic shoulder brace
    M. shield eye implant
    M. speculum
    M. total hip prosthesis
    M. Ultralite brace
    M. vena cava clamp
    M. wrap-around knee brace
Mueller-Charnley hip prosthesis
Mueller-Hinton supplemented agar plate
Muenster cast
Muhlberger orbital prosthesis
Mühlemann periodontometer
Mui Scientific pressurized capillary
  infusion system

Muldoon
    M. lacrimal dilator
    M. lacrimal probe
    M. retractor
mules
    M. eye implant
    M. graft
    Heath m.
    M. implant
    Kulvin-Kalt m.
    Lister m.
    M. scoop
    M. vitreous sphere
Mule upper limb exerciser
Mulholland growth guidance system
Mullan
    M. percutaneous trigeminal ganglion
      microcompression set
    M. wire
Müller
    M. catheter guide
    M. plate
    M. prosthesis
    M. saw
    M. tray
Muller phlebectomy hook
Mullins
    M. cardiac device
    M. catheter introducer
    M. long transseptal sheath
    M. sheath system
    M. transseptal catheter
    M. transseptal catheterization sheath
MultArray
    M. headlight
    M. light
multi
    m. coordinate manipulator
    M. Dopplex II Doppler
    M. Dopplex MDI vascular test
      unit
    M. Podus boot
    M. Podus boot system
    M. Podus foot system
multiaccess catheter
multiaxial screw
multiaxis
    m. accelerometer
    m. foot
    m. prosthesis
multiband ligating device
Multibite multiple sample biopsy
  forceps
MultiBoot orthosis
multicellular stent
multichannel
    m. ABI
    m. cochlear implant

m. discrete analyzer
m. signal averager
multicoil
phased-array m.
Multicor II cardiac pacemaker
multicorneal perfusion chamber
multicoupled loop-gap resonator
multicrystal gamma camera
multidetector
m. CT scanner
m. helical scanner
m. system
Multidex
M. chronic wound treatment
system
M. filler
M. maltodextrin wound dressing
multidimensional analysis beam modifier
multidirectional distractor
multidrop lens
multielectrode
m. basket catheter
m. catheter
m. impedance catheter
m. probe
multi-electrode
ESA Coulochem m.-e.
multifilament steel suture
Multifire
M. clip applicator
M. Endo GIA stapling device
M. Endo hernia clip applier
M. GIA-series stapler
M. TA-series stapler
Multiflex
M. catheter
M. foot prosthesis
Multi-Flex stent
multifocal
m. implant
m. lens
m. phakic IOL
m. silicone IOL
multifrequency
m. probe
m. transducer
Multigon 500M non-contrast-enhanced TCD
multihead detector
multihole collimator
multiincision 10-facet diamond blade
MultiLase
M. D copper vapor laser
M. Nd:YAG surgical laser
multilayer design catheter
multilead electrode
multileaf
m. collimating system

m. collimator
m. collimator device
MultiLight system
Multi-Lig knee brace
Multi-Link
M.-L. Ascent stent
M.-L. coronary stent system
M.-L. Duet stent
M.-L. Frontier coronary stent
system
M.-L. Penta coronary stent system
M.-L. Penta stent
M.-L. Pixel coronary stent system
M.-L. Pixel stent system
M.-L. Solo stent
M.-L. Terra stent
M.-L. Tetra coronary stent system
M.-L. Tristar balloon
M.-L. Zeta coronary stent system
multiload occlusive clip applicator
Multi-Lock
M.-L. hand operating table
M.-L. hip prosthesis
M.-L. knee brace
multilumen
m. manometric catheter
m. probe
Multinex ID gas monitor
Multi-Operatory Dentalaser
Multi-Optics lens
MultiPad absorptive dressing
multiparameter intraarterial sensor
multiparticle cyclotron
multipiece lens
multiplace chamber
multiplanar
m. mandibular distractor
m. transducer
multiplane
m. endovaginal
m. intracavitary probe
m. transducer
multiple
m. automated sample harvester
m. gated acquisition scan
m. hook assembly C-D
instrumentation
m. jointed digitizer scanner
m. parameter telemetry device
m. pinhole occluder
m. point electrode
m. side-hole infusion catheter
m. side-hole infusion system
multiple-band ligator
multiple-dose vial
multiple-electrode probe system
multiple-headed gamma camera
multiple-piece intraocular lens
multiplex catheter

M

MultiPly sponge
multiply tuned coil
multipoint contact plate
multipolar
    m. bipolar cup
    m. electrode catheter
    m. impedance catheter
Multi-Pro 2000 biopsy needle
multiprogrammable
    m. pacemaker
    m. pulse generator
multiprong rake retractor
MultiPro table
Multipulse
    M. 1000 compression pump
    M. cosmetic treatment laser
multipurpose
    m. ball electrode
    m. breathing circuit
    m. catheter
    m. clamp
    m. forceps
    m. laryngoscope
    m. retractor
    m. valve
multiradius unconstrained prosthesis
multirod collimator
multiscope
    roaming optical access m.
multisensor
    m. catheter
    m. structured light-range digitizer
      scanner
multi-sideport
    m.-s. catheter infusion set
    m.-s. infusion catheter
Multisizer 3 Coulter counter
multislice CT scanner
multislit catheter
multispan fracture hook
Multispatula cervical sampling device
Multispect 3 camera
MultiSPIRO
    M. Clear Advantage pulmonary
      function filter
    M. The Peak peak flow meter
Multistar
    M. angiographic unit
    M. Top Plus DSA system
multistrand suture
Multitak
    M. SS system
    M. suture snap system
Multitest cell-mediated immunity system
multitooth forceps
multitrauma dressing
multivane intensity modulation
  compensator

Multi-Vent
    Hudson M.-V.
multiwire
    m. gamma camera
    m. proportional chamber
mummy wrap
Munro brain scissors
Munster cast
Murdock eye speculum
Murdock-Wiener eye speculum
Murless vacuum extractor
Murphy
    M. button
    M. drip
    M. gouge
    M. intestinal needle
    M. kidney punch
    M. nail
    M. osteotome
    M. plaster knife
    M. rake retractor
    M. skid
    M. sling
    M. splint
Murphy-Lane
    M.-L. bone skid
    M.-L. lever
Murphy-Péan hemostatic forceps
Murray fixation
muscle
    m. biopsy clamp
    m. bridge
    m. clamp
    elevator m.
    m. filling
    m. filter
    m. flap
    m. forceps
    m. hook
    Kinetic M.'s, Inc. (KMI)
    m. and neurological stimulation
      electrotherapy device
    m. plate
    m. sheath
    m. slide
    m. sling
    m. spindle
    m. stimulator
    m. tone inhibitor system
muscular
    m. tube
    m. venous pump
Museux
    M. uterine forceps
    M. vulsellum forceps
mushroom
    m. catheter
    m. walker glide
mushroom-tip catheter

music vibration table
muslin
    m. dressing
    m. sling
mustache dressing
Mustang steerable guidewire
Mustarde awl
MVP
    most versatile patch
        Biodex Multi-Joint System 3 MVP
        MVP catheter
MVR blade
MW 2000 microwave delivery system
MX2-300 xenon quality light source
MX-Grafter
MX-Pro R3 ambulance cot
mycobacteria growth indicator tube
Mycromesh
    M. biomaterial
    M. graft material
    M. Plus biomaterial
MycroPhylax implantable cardioverter-
    defibrillator
myelography needle
Myelo-Nate
    M.-N. needle
    M.-N. set
myeloperoxidase-H2O2-halide system
Myerson
    M. laryngeal forceps
    M. PermaSoft soft denture liner
    M. resin
Myles
    M. guillotine
    M. hemorrhoidal clamp
    M. hemorrhoidal forceps
    M. nasal forceps
    M. nasal speculum
Myobock system
myocardial
    m. electrode
    m. lead
    m. protection system

myochronoscope
Myocor Coapsys pacing assist device
Myocure blade
myodynamometer
myoelectric control prosthesis
myograph
    acoustic m.
Myojector
myokinesimeter
Myolift heart retractor
myoma
    m. fixation instrument
    m. screw
myometer
Myoscan sensor
myoscope
MyoSight
    M. dedicated nuclear cardiology
      camera system
    M. imaging system
myosthenometer
Myotest train-of-four nerve stimulator
MYOtherm XP cardioplegia delivery
    system
MyoTrac
    M. EMG
    M. EMG monitor
    M. 2 EMG monitor
Myowire II cardiac electrode
myReader low-vision auto-reading device
myringoplasty knife
myringotome
myringotomy
    m. blade
    m. knife
    m. knife blade
    m. knife handle
    m. scissors
    m. tube
Myrtle leaf probe
Mysono portable ultrasound
Mystique resorbable graft
M-Zole 7 Dual Pack

M

N-180 pulse oximeter
N5 submicron particle size analyzer
N95 particulate respirator surgical mask
Nabatoff vein stripper
Nabers probe
Nachlas gastrointestinal tube
Nachlas-Linton esophagogastric balloon tamponade device
Nada-Chair Back-Up portable back sling
Nadler bipolar coaptation forceps
Naegele obstetrical forceps
Naeser laser home treatment program for the hand
Nafion dryer line
Nagahara
    N. karate chopper
    N. phaco chopper
    N. quick chopper
Nagel anomaloscope
NaI detector
nail
    Alta tibial n.
    antegrade femoral n.
    antegrade/retrograde compression n.
    AP n.
    Augustine boat n.
    Bickel intramedullary n.
    Biomet ankle arthrodesis n.
    blind medullary n.
    Böhler n.
    Böhler hip n.
    Brooker double-locking unreamed tibial n.
    Brooker-Wills n.
    Calandruccio n.
    cannulated n.
    Chandler unreamed interlocking tibial n.
    closed Küntscher n.
    closed unlocked n.
    cloverleaf n.
    crutch and belt femoral closed n.
    Derby n.
    diamond n.
    Dooley n.
    double-ended n.
    double-hollow n.
    n. drill
    elastic stable intramedullary n.
    Ender n.
    Engel-May n.
    extension n.
    femoral neck n.

Fixion intramedullary humeral n.
4-flanged n.
flexible intramedullary n.
fluted Sampson n.
fluted titanium n.
n. fold capillaroscopic instrument
gamma locking n.
Gamma trochanteric locking n.
Green-Seligson-Henry n.
Grosse-Kempf femoral n.
Grosse-Kempf locking n.
Grosse-Kempf tibial n.
GSH n.
Hagie pin n.
Hahn bone n.
half-and-half n.
Hansen-Street n.
Hansen-Street self-broaching n.
Hansen-Street solid intramedullary n.
Harris condylocephalic n.
Harris hip n.
Harris medullary n.
hooked intramedullary n.
hooked medullary n.
IM n.
Inro surgical n.
intramedullary n.
intramedullary ANK n.
intramedullary supracondylar multihole n.
Jewett n.
Jewett hip n.
Johannson hip n.
Ken sliding n.
Kirschner interlocking intramedullary n.
Klemm n.
Knowles pin n.
Küntscher cloverleaf n.
Küntscher intramedullary n.
Laing H-beam n.
Lewis n.
long-edge medullary n.
Lottes triflange intramedullary n.
Luck n.
Massie II n.
Massie sliding n.
McKee tri-fin n.
McLaughlin n.
medullary n.
Micronail intramedullary n.
Murphy n.
Neufeld n.
n. nipper

nail *(continued)*
    Nylok self-locking n.
    open n.
    Orthofix intramedullary n.
    OrthoSorb pin n.
    Palmer bone n.
    PFNA proximal femoral n.
    Pidcock n.
    n. plate
    proximal femoral n. (PFN)
    Recon n.
    retrograde intramedullary n.
    ReVision n.
    R-T n.
    Rush intramedullary n.
    Rush pin n.
    Russell-Taylor delta tibial n.
    Russell-Taylor interlocking
      medullary n.
    Rydell n.
    n. scissors
    Seidel humeral locking n.
    SIGN intramedullary n.
    slotted n.
    Smith-Petersen n.
    Smith-Petersen femoral neck n.
    spring-loaded n.
    Steinmann extension n.
    supracondylar n.
    Sven-Johansson femoral neck n.
    Synthes titanium elastic n.
    Terry n.
    TFN trochanteric fixation n.
    Thompson n.
    Thornton n.
    titanium n.
    titanium elastic n.
    titanium flexible humeral n.
    trochanteric fixation n. (TFN)
    True/Flex intramedullary n.
    Uniflex humeral n.
    Uniflex intramedullary n.
    Vector intertrochanteric n.
    VersaNail tibial n.
    vitallium n.
    V medullary n.
    Watson-Jones n.
    Webb bolt n.
    Williams n.
    Williams interlocking Y n.
    Z fixation n.
    Zickel n.
    Zimmer telescoping n.
nail-bending device
nail-cutting forceps
nail-driving guidewire
nail-extracting
    n.-e. forceps
    n.-e. hook

nailfold capillary microscope
nail-mounted compression device
nail-nipper scissors
nail-pulling forceps
Nakamura brace
Nakao
    N. Ejector biopsy forceps
    N. Snare I, II
Nakayama anastomosis apparatus
Na-K exchange pump
Nalgene
    N. capsule filter
    N. freezer storage rack
    N. PETG media bottle
Namic
    N. angiographic syringe
    N. catheter
**Nanoduct neonatal sweat analysis
  system**
Nanolas Nd:YAG laser
Nanos 01 pacemaker
napkin ring calcar allograft
Naraghi-DeCoster reduction clamp
Narco
    N. Bio-Systems physiograph tracing
    N. Biosystems recorder
    N. Bio-Systems rectilinear recorder
    N. Physiograph-6B recorder
Narcomatic flowmeter
Narins cannula
Narkomed anesthesia machine
narrow
    n. AO dynamic compression plate
    n. Assistant Free retractor blade
    n. band spectrophotometer
    n. Cobra retractor
    n. Deaver retractor
    n. double-prong acetabular retractor
    n. gauze roll
    n. inferior acetabular retractor
    n. lens
    n. neck implant
    n. proximal femoral elevator
    n. washer
narrowband UVB lamp
narrow-base quad cane
narrow-bite bone rongeur
narrow-blade laminar hook
NarrowFlex intraaortic balloon catheter
nasal
    n. alligator forceps
    n. aspirator
    n. bivalve speculum
    n. bone forceps
    n. cannula
    n. cannula pressure transducer
    n. cartilage-holding forceps
    n. catheter
    n. chisel

n. CPAP system
n. curette
n. cutting forceps
n. dilator
n. dissector
n. dorsal implant
n. dressing forceps
n. endoscopic telescope
n. gouge
n. hump-cutting forceps
n. insertion forceps
n. irrigator
n. knife
n. knife blade
n. lower lateral forceps
n. mallet
N. Moist gel
n. and mouth breathing face mask
n. needle holder forceps
n. osteotome
n. pack
n. packing
n. polyp forceps
n. polyp hook
n. probe
n. prongs
n. punch
n. rasp
n. retractor
n. saw
n. saw blade
n. scissors
n. septal forceps
n. septal perforation button
n. snare
n. snare cannula
n. snare wire
n. snare wire carrier
n. speculum
n. splint
n. suction cup
n. suction tube
n. suture needle
n. tampon
n. tamponade
n. tampon sponge
n. telescope
n. tenaculum
n. trumpet
Nasal-Aire
N.-A. I, II continuous positive airway pressure device
N.-A. ventilator nasal insert mask
nasal-tip dressing
nasendoscope, nasoendoscope
Nashold biopsy needle
nasobiliary
n. catheter

n. drain
n. tube
nasocystic
n. catheter
n. drain
n. drainage tube
nasoendoscope (*var. of* nasendoscope)
nasoendotracheal tube
nasoenteric feeding tube
nasofrontal
n. osteotome
n. suture
nasogastric (NG)
n. feeding tube
n. tube
nasojejunal tube
nasolacrimal duct probe
nasomaxillary balloon
nasometer
nasopancreatic catheter
nasopharyngeal
n. airway
n. biopsy forceps
n. electrode
n. fiberscope
n. retractor
n. speculum
nasopharyngolaryngoscope
nasopharyngoscope
flexible n.
Holmes n.
Meltzer n.
Smith & Nephew ENT n.
Ura-1 flexible fiberoptic n.
nasoscope
nasostat
Gottschalk n.
nasotracheal
n. catheter
n. tube
nasovesicular catheter
Natchez Mobil-Trac system
Nathanson liver retractor
National
N. cautery
N. general purpose cystoscope
N. Institutes of Health left ventriculography catheter
N. Institutes of Health marking catheter
N. Institutes of Health mitral valve grasping forceps
N. opal glass transilluminator
natural
n. pacemaker
N. Profile abutment system
N. Selection PLIF wedge and cervical spacer
n. suture

NaturaLase
    N. erbium laser
    N. Er:YAG laser
Natural-Hip
    N.-H. prosthesis
    N.-H. stem
    N.-H. system
    N.-H. titanium hip stem
Natural-Knee
    N.-K. II system
    N.-K. implant
    N.-K. unconstrained prosthesis
Natus
    N. Algo screener
    N. Ear Coupler
Naugle exophthalmometer
Nauth traction device
NavAblator catheter
Navarre universal drainage catheter
Navi Ball guidance system
navicular screw
navigation system
navigator
    N. flexible endoscope
    N. gamma ray detector
    N. power wheelchair
    Zeiss STN surgical tool n.
Navigus
    N. cranial base and cap
    N. cranial electrode system
    N. trajectory guide
Naviport deflectable-tip guiding catheter
Navistar
    N. catheter
    N. Thermocool catheter
Navitrack computer-assisted surgery system
NB200 vascular access device
NBIH catheter
***N*-butyl-2-cyanoacrylate glue**
NC
    NC balloon
    NC Bandit catheter
    NC Raptor over-the-wire coaxial PTCA dilatation balloon catheter
    NC Raptor PTCA dilatation catheter
    NC Stormer Zipper MX noncompliant balloon dilatation catheter
N-Cat N-500 tonometric blood pressure monitor
NCircle nitinol tipless stone extractor
NCompass nitinol stone extractor
NCP
    NeuroCybernetic prosthesis implanted NCP
    NCP system
NC-stat nerve conduction system

N-DEX non-latex glove
Nd:YAG
    Nd:YAG laser catheter
    Nd:YAG laser system
    Nd:YAG laser with Hexascan
    Nd:YAG module
NE-8000 analyzer
Neal
    N. catheter
    N. catheter trocar
near-infrared
    n.-i. electronic endoscope
    n.-i. spectroscope
Nearly Me breast form
Nebuhaler inhaler
nebulization ventilator
nebulizer
    Acorn II n.
    AeroChamber n.
    AeroEclipse breath actuated n.
    AeroSonic personal ultrasonic n.
    AeroTech II n.
    Ailos n.
    air-powered n.
    Babbington-type n.
    baffled jet n.
    Bestneb n.
    Centimist n.
    n. chronolog
    Compu-Neb ultrasonic n.
    DeVilbiss n.
    DeVilbiss Pulmo-Aide n.
    Dura-Neb 2000 portable n.
    Emerson-Segal Medimizer demand n.
    Fisoneb ultrasonic n.
    Fisons n.
    handheld n.
    Heart n.
    Hope continuous & Heliox n.
    Hudson T Up-Draft II disposable n.
    Inspiron n.
    IV-Heart n.
    jet n.
    John Bunn Mini-Mist n.
    Kidde n.
    LC Plus reusable n.
    LC Star reusable n.
    Marquest Respirgard II n.
    medicinal n.
    Medi-Mist n.
    Medix ultrasonic n.
    MicroAir electronic n.
    MicroAir handheld n.
    Micro Mist n.
    MiniHEART low-flow n.
    Mistogen n.
    Misty-Neb n.

Omron compressor n.
Pari LC Plus reusable n.
Pari LC Star reusable n.
Pari Proneb Ultra n.
penicillin n.
PermaNeb reusable n.
Proneb Ultra n.
Pulmo-Aide n.
PulmoMate n.
PulmoSonic ultrasonic n.
Raindrop medication n.
Respirgard II n.
Schuco n.
Shuco-Myst n.
side-arm n.
Sidestream high-efficiency n.
small-volume n.
Sonix 2000 ultrasonic n.
spinning disc n.
Twin Jet n.
Ultra-Neb n.
ultrasonic n.
UniHeart IV universal n.
updraft handheld n.
VixOne small-volume n.
Wright n.

Necelon surgical glove
neck
n. brace
n. component
n. rest
n. roll
n. support
Neckcare pillow
Neck-Hugger cervical support pillow
Neck-Roll aromatherapy hot/cold pack
neck-wrap halter
Nec-Loc cervical collar
needle
Abrams n.
Abrams biopsy n.
abscission n.
Accucore II biopsy n.
Accuhair n.
Accuject sterile disposable
dental n.
ACS n.
AcuMaster acupuncture n.
acupuncture n.
Adair-Veress n.
adjustable-depth gauge n.
Adson aneurysm n.
advancement n.
Agnew tattooing n.
Agrikola tattooing n.
air aspirator n.
Alcon CU-15 n.
Alcon irrigating n.
Alcon reverse cutting n.

Alcon spatula n.
Alcon taper cut n.
Alcon taper point n.
Aldrete n.
Alexander tonsil n.
Allerprick n.
AMC n.
Amersham CDCS A-type n.
Amplatz angiography n.
Amsler aqueous transplant n.
anesthesia n.
anesthetic n.
aneurysm n.
angiography n.
angular n.
antrum exploring n.
aqueous transplant n.
arachnophlebectomy n.
Arrow-Fischell EVAN n.
arterial n.
Articulator injection n.
Asap channel-cut automated
biopsy n.
Asap prostate biopsy n.
aspirating n.
aspiration biopsy n.
Atkinson peribulbar n.
Atkinson retrobulbar n.
Atkinson single-bevel blunt-tip n.
Atkinson tip peribulbar n.
Atraloc n.
Atraucan double-bevel spinal n.
atraumatic n.
atraumatic Sprotte n.
automated biopsy n.
automatic single n. (ASN)
Autovac n.
AV fistula n.
Babcock n.
Backlund biopsy n.
Baldwin perineum n.
Barbara n.
Bard n.
Bard biopsy n.
Bard Biopty cut n.
Barker n.
Barraquer n.
Bassini n.
BD n.
BD bone marrow biopsy n.
BD Safety-Gard n.
BD SafetyGlide shielding
hypodermic n.
Becton-Dickinson n.
Becton-Dickinson Teflon-sheathed n.
bent blunt n.
Bergström n.
beveled n.
beveled thin-walled n.

N

needle *(continued)*
    bicurved n.
    Bier lumbar puncture n.
    Bierman n.
    biopsy n.
    Biopty cut n.
    Biopty-Cut biopsy n.
    Biosearch n.
    BIP high-speed multibiopsy n.
    bipolar n.
    bleeding n.
    blinded acupuncture n.
    blood-containment n.
    blunt n.
    blunt-end sialogram n.
    blunt-tipped epidural n.
    bone marrow biopsy n.
    boomerang bladder n.
    Bovie n.
    Bowman cataract n.
    Bowman stop n.
    brain biopsy n.
    breast localization n.
    BRK series transseptal n.
    Brockenbrough curved n.
    Bunnell tendon n.
    butterfly n.
    BV2 n.
    Calhoun n.
    Calhoun-Hagler lens n.
    cardioplegic n.
    Cardiopoint cardiac surgery n.
    Carpule n.
    Carr-Locke injection n.
    Castroviejo vitreous aspirating n.
    cataract n.
    cataract aspirating n.
    catgut n.
    catheter n.
    caudal n.
    CD-5 n.
    CE-24 n.
    cerebral angiography n.
    cervical suture n.
    cesium n.
    Charles flute n.
    Charles vacuuming n.
    Chiba n.
    Chiba biopsy n.
    Chiba eye n.
    Childs-Phillips intestinal plication n.
    CIF n.
    CIF4 n.
    Cleasby spatulated n.
    cleft palate n.
    coaxial sheath cut biopsy n.
    Cobb-Ragde n.
    Cobe AV fistular n.
    Colapinto n.

Colorado n.
Colorado microdissection n.
concentric n.
cone biopsy n.
Cone ventricular n.
Conrad-Crosby bone marrow
  biopsy n.
conventional cutting n.
Cook percutaneous entry n.
CooperVision irrigating n.
CooperVision spatulated n.
Cope biopsy n.
Cope pleural biopsy n.
copper-clad steel n.
Core bone biopsy n.
corneal n.
Corson n.
couching n.
Cournand n.
Cournand arterial n.
Cournand-Grino angiography n.
Cournand-Potts n.
Craig biopsy n.
Crawford n.
Crown n.
C-type acupuncture n.
CU-8 n.
Culp biopsy n.
Curran knife n.
Curry n.
curved suture n.
curved transjugular n.
CUSALap accessory n.
cut biopsy n.
cut taper n.
cutting n.
cutting LR n.
Daily cataract n.
Davis knife n.
Dean knife n.
DeBakey n.
débridement n.
Deknatel K-n.
Delbet-Reverdin n.
DePuy-Weiss tonsillar n.
DermaGlide n.
Deschamps n.
Deschamps ligature n.
desiccation n.
desiccation-fulguration n.
Desmarres paracentesis n.
diamond point n.
diathermal n.
diathermic precut n.
Dieckmann intraosseous n.
discogram n.
discographic n.
disposable acupuncture n.
disposable aspiration n.

disposable biopsy n.
disposable butterfly n.
disposable injection n.
disposable percutaneous entry
  thinwall n.
disposable suturing n.
n. dissector
DLP cardioplegic n.
docking n.
Dos Santos lumbar aortography n.
double-barreled n.
double-hub emulsifying n.
double-lumen n.
double-tipped center-threading n.
double-webbed n.
dragonhead n.
Drews cataract n.
n. driver
DS-9 n.
D-Tach removable n.
D-Tach removal n.
Duff debridement n.
dumbbell n.
Dupuy-Dutemps n.
Dupuy-Weiss tonsillar n.
dural n.
Durrani dorsal vein complex
  ligation n.
DuVries n.
Echo-Coat ultrasound biopsy n.
echogenic n.
Echotip amniocentesis n.
Echotip Norfolk aspiration n.
Echotip percutaneous entry n.
EchoTip Ultra endoscopic n.
Eclipse blood collection n.
EJ bone marrow biopsy n.
n. electrode
Electrodes n.
electrosurgical n.
Ellis foreign body n.
Elschnig extrusion n.
Emmet n.
Emmet-Murphy n.
Empire n.
enclavation n.
Endopath Pneumoneedle
  insufflation n.
Endopath Ultra Veress n.
n. endosteal implant
Entree disposable CO_2
  insufflation n.
epilation n.
ergonomic vascular access n.
  (EVAN)
Espocan combined spinal/epidural n.
Ethalloy n.
Ethicon BV-75-3 n.
Ethicon ST-4 straight taper-point n.

Ethiguard n.
Euro-Med FNA-21 aspiration n.
EUSN-1 EchoTip n.
eXcel-DR disposable/reusable
  Glasser laparoscopic n.
eXcel-DR Glasser laparoscopic n.
exploring n.
extended round n.
extrusion n.
eyed suture n.
eyeless atraumatic suture n.
EZ-EM cut biopsy n.
fascial n.
FastFill brachytherapy n.
fat-injection n.
Fergie n.
Ferguson n.
Ferguson suture n.
Ferris disposable bone marrow
  aspiration n.
Field-Lee biopsy n.
filiform steel n.
filter n.
fine intestinal n.
Fischer pneumothoracic n.
Fisher eye n.
fishhook n.
fistula n.
flat spatula n.
flexible aspiration n.
flexible biopsy n.
flexible injection n.
Flexitip sclerotherapy n.
flute n.
Flynn extrusion n.
FNA-21 n.
Foltz n.
n. forceps
foreign body n.
Framer tendon-passing n.
Francke n.
Frankfeldt hemorrhoidal n.
Franklin liver puncture n.
Franklin-Silverman prostatic
  biopsy n.
Franseen n.
Franseen liver biopsy n.
Franseen lung biopsy n.
Frazier ventricular n.
Frederick pneumothoracic n.
French-eye n.
French spring-eye n.
Fritz vitreous transplant n.
full-intensity n.
Gallic fascial n.
Gallini bone marrow aspiration n.
GAN-19 n.
Gardner n.
gastrointestinal n.

N

needle *(continued)*
    general closure n.
    Gertie Marx spinal n.
    Gill n.
    Gillmore n.
    GIP/Medi-Globe prototype n.
    Girard anterior chamber n.
    Girard cataract-aspirating n.
    Girard phacofragmatome n.
    Girard-Swan n.
    Gittes n.
    GlideCath entry n.
    gold n.
    Goldenberg Snarecoil bone marrow
        biopsy n.
    Graefe iris n.
    GraNee n.
    Greene n.
    Greenfield n.
    Green-Gould n.
    Greenwald n.
    Grice suture n.
    Grieshaber corneal n.
    Grieshaber iris n.
    Grieshaber ophthalmic n.
    gripper n.
    GS-9 n.
    Guest n.
    Haab knife n.
    Haci n.
    Hagedorn n.
    Hagedorn suture n.
    half-intensity n.
    Halsey n.
    hand-honed reverse cutting n.
    harelip n.
    Harvard n.
    Haverhill n.
    Hawkeye suture n.
    Hawkeye suture n.
    Hawkins-Akins n.
    Hawkins breast localization n.
    heart n.
    Hegar n.
    Hegar-Baumgartner n.
    Hemoject n.
    hemorrhoidal n.
    Hessburg lacrimal n.
    Heyner double n.
    high-risk n.
    Hingson-Edwards n.
    Hingson-Ferguson n.
    Hobbs n.
    n. holder
    n. holder clamp
    n. holder forceps
    hollow n.
    Homerlok n.
    hooked n.

    hookwire n.
    House-Rosen n.
    House stapes n.
    Howard Jones n.
    Howell n.
    Howell aspiration n.
    Howell biliary aspiration n.
    Howell biopsy aspiration n.
    Huber point n.
    Hunstad infusion n.
    Hurd suture n.
    Hustead epidural n.
    n. hydrophone
    hypodermic n.
    Hypo intraosseous n.
    Illinois n.
    illuminated suction n.
    Indian club n.
    Infusaid n.
    Ingersoll tonsillar n.
    injection n.
    insufflation n.
    insulated electrode n.
    insulated epidural n.
    internal nucleus hydrodelineation n.
    intestinal plication n.
    intraosseous n.
    intravenous n.
    Iolab irrigating n.
    Iolab taper-cut n.
    Iolab titanium n.
    iridium n.
    iris n.
    irrigating-positioning n.
    IsoTrac brachytherapy n.
    Ito n.
    IV n.
    J n.
    Jameson strabismus n.
    Jamshidi n.
    Jamshidi adult n.
    Jamshidi liver biopsy n.
    Jelco n.
    Jordan n.
    K n.
    Kader fishhook n.
    Kalt corneal n.
    Kalt eye n.
    Kalt vein n.
    Kaplan tracheostomy n.
    Kara cataract n.
    Keith n.
    Keith abdominal n.
    Kelly intestinal n.
    Kelman n.
    KeyMed disposable variceal
        injection n.
    kidney suturing n.
    King suture n.

Klatskin n.
Klein infiltration n.
Kloti radiofrequency diathermy n.
Knapp iris knife n.
Knapp knife n.
knife n.
n. knife
Knight biopsy n.
Kobak n.
Koch nucleus hydrolysis n.
Kopan n.
Kopans n.
Kratz diamond-dusted n.
lacrimal n.
Lahey aneurysm n.
Lane cleft palate n.
Lane suturing n.
Lapides n.
large-bore slotted aspirating n.
larger-caliber cutting n.
Lee & Westcott n.
Lemmon n.
Lewicky n.
Lewy-Rubin n.
Lewy Teflon glycerine mixture
  injection n.
Lichtwitz antral n.
ligature n.
lighted flute n.
Lindeman transfusion n.
liver biopsy n.
lobotomy n.
lock n.
long n.
Longdwel catheter n.
Look retrobulbar n.
Lo-Trau side-cutting n.
Lowell pleural n.
Lowsley ribbon-gut n.
LR n.
Luer n.
Luer-Lok n.
Lukens n.
lumbar aortography n.
lumbar puncture n.
Luongo n.
LX n.
Madayag biopsy n.
Maddox caudal n.
Maggi biopsy n.
Mahurkar fistular n.
Majestik shielded angiographic n.
malleable passing n.
Maltz n.
Mammalok localization n.
Manan n.
March laser sclerostomy n.
Martin uterine n.
Marx n.

Masson fascial n.
Mathieu n.
Maumenee vitreous-aspirating n.
Mayo n.
Mayo catgut n.
Mayo intestinal n.
Mayo trocar n.
Mayo trocar-point n.
McDowell n.
McGee prosthesis n.
McGhan plastic surgical n.
McGregor n.
McIntyre I/A n.
McIntyre irrigation/aspiration n.
mediastinoscopy aspirating n.
Medicut intravenous n.
Medisystems fistula n.
Menghini n.
Menghini liver biopsy n.
meniscal repair n.
Mentor prostate biopsy n.
metal n.
metallic n.
metallic frontal n.
Mick afterloading n.
MicroFlow phacoemulsification n.
micron n.
micropoint n.
micropuncture n.
micropuncture introducer n.
micro round-tip n.
middle-caliber n.
milliner's n.
Mixter ventricular n.
MO n.
modificd CIF n.
modified spatula n.
Monoject hypodermic n.
monopolar triple-hook active n.
Monopty n.
Morrow Brown n.
Moss T-anchor n.
Multi-Pro 2000 biopsy n.
Murphy intestinal n.
myelography n.
Myelo-Nate n.
nasal suture n.
Nashold biopsy n.
neurography n.
neurosurgical suture n.
Neville ascending aortic air
  vent n.
Nokor n.
noncoring Huber n.
noncutting n.
noncutting suture n.
nonferromagnetic n.
noninsulated n.
Nottingham colposuspension n.

N

needle *(continued)*

nucleus hydrolysis n.
O'Brien airway n.
olive-tipped n.
Olympus NM-K series
  sclerotherapy n.
Olympus NM-L series n.
OmniTip side-firing laser n.
optical n.
oral n.
Osgood bone marrow n.
Osteo-Site bone biopsy n.
Osterballe precision n.
Ostycut bone biopsy n.
palpating n.
paracentesis n.
paracervical nerve block n.
paraPRO n.
Parker-Pearson n.
pediatric biopsy n.
Pencan spinal n.
Pentax prototype n.
PercuCut biopsy n.
PercuCut cut-biopsy n.
percutaneous n.
percutaneous cutting n.
Pereyra n.
peribulbar n.
pericardiocentesis n.
permanent n.
Permark micropigmentation n.
PermaSharp suture and n.
Pharmaseal n.
pilot n.
Pitkin n.
plain eye n.
pleural biopsy n.
plication n.
Plum-Blossom acupuncture n.
Pneumo-Matic insufflation n.
Pneumoneedle insufflation n.
pneumoperitoneum n.
Politzer paracentesis n.
polypropylene n.
polytef-sheathed n.
pop-off n.
positioning n.
postmortem suture n.
Potocky n.
Potts n.
Potts-Cournand n.
PrecisionGlide n.
precision-point n.
Pricker n.
probe n.
n. probe
Probloc regional block
  anesthesia n.
Promex biopsy n.

pronged Franseen-type point n.
prostatic biopsy n.
PS-2 n.
pudendal block anesthesia n.
puncture n.
puncture-tip n.
quartz n.
Quick-Core n.
Quick-Core biopsy n.
Quincke-Babcock n.
Quincke-point spinal n.
Quincke spinal n.
Quintero amniocentesis n.
^{226}Ra n.
radioactive strontium n.
radium ^{226}Ra n.
Ranfac n.
Ranfac soft tissue n.
razor-tip n.
rectal injection n.
renal n.
retrobulbar n.
reusable forceps with n.
Reverdin n.
Reverdin suture n.
reverse cutting n.
rib n.
ribbed n.
ribbon gut n.
Riedel corneal n.
Riley n.
Ring drainage catheter n.
Riza-Ribe grasping n.
R-K n.
Rochester n.
Rosch-Uchida n.
Rosen n.
Rosenthal aspiration n.
Ross n.
Rotex n.
round body n.
Rubin n.
Rutner biopsy n.
Rycroft n.
Sabreloc n.
Sabreloc spatula n.
Safe Step blood collection n.
Safety AV fistula n.
Salah sternal puncture n.
SampleMASTER biopsy n.
Sato cataract n.
SC-1 n.
Scabbard n.
scalp vein n.
Scheie cataract aspirating n.
scleral spatula n.
sclerostomy n.
sclerotherapy n.
screw-tipped intraosseous n.

Securcut aspiration biopsy n.
Sedan-Nashold n.
seeker n.
Seirin acupuncture n.
Seldinger n.
Seldinger arterial n.
Seldinger gastrostomy n.
self-aspirating cut-biopsy n.
septal n.
Septoject dental syringe n.
seton n.
Seven-Star acupuncture n.
Sharpoint Ultra-Guide ophthalmic n.
shattering n.
sheath n.
short n.
short-bevel n.
sialography n.
side-cutting spatulated n.
4-sided cutting n.
side-flattened n.
sidewall holed n.
silicone brush back-flushed n.
silver n.
Silverman biopsy n.
Simcoe anterior chamber
  receiving n.
Simcoe II PC aspirating n.
Simcoe irrigating-positioning n.
Simcoe suture n.
Singer n.
single-wall n.
ski n.
Skinny Chiba n.
Sklar ligature n.
slotted n.
small-bore n.
small-caliber n.
SmallPort n.
SmartNeedle n.
SonoVu US aspiration n.
Sos Pulse-Vu bloodless entry n.
spatula n.
n. spatula
spatula split n.
spatulated n.
spatulated half-circle n.
sphenopalatine ganglion n.
spinal n.
Spinocan Quincke bevel spinal n.
splittable n.
spoon n.
n. spoon
spring-eye n.
spring-hook wire n.
spring-loaded biopsy n.
Sprotte epidural n.
Sprotte spinal n.
spud n.

n. spud
stab n.
Stallerpointe n.
Stamey n.
standard n.
stapes n.
staphylorrhaphy n.
steel-winged butterfly n.
StereoGuide n.
stereotactic n.
stereotactic breast biopsy n.
sternal puncture n.
Stifcore aspiration n.
Stifcore biopsy injection n.
Stifcore transbronchial aspiration n.
Stimuplex block n.
Stocker n.
stop n.
strabismus n.
straight-point n.
straight suturing n.
Straus curved retrobulbar n.
Stylus suture n.
subconjunctival n.
suction biopsy n.
Surecut n.
Sure Shot injection n.
Sur-Fast n.
Surgineedle pneumoperitoneum n.
suturing n.
swaged n.
swaged arthroscopic n.
swaged-on n.
Swan knife n.
Tano diamond-dusted n.
taper n.
Tapercut n.
taper-cut n.
tapered n.
taper-point suture n.
tattoo n.
tattooing n.
tax double n.
Teflon-coated n.
Teflon-coated hollow-bore n.
Teflon-covered n.
Temno biopsy n.
Temno II cutting n.
tendon n.
Terry-Mayo n.
Terumo AV fistula n.
Terumo dental n.
Terumo hypodermic n.
T-fastener delivery n.
TG140 n.
The Painless One acupuncture n.
thermistor n.
n. thermocouple
THI n.

N

needle *(continued)*
thin acupuncture n.
thin-walled n.
thin-walled guiding n.
Thomas n.
thoracentesis n.
Thornton n.
threaded eye n.
through-the-scope injection n.
tie-on n.
tissue desiccation n.
titanium n.
titanium alloy n.
Titus venoclysis n.
TLA n.
TMC n.
Tocantins bone marrow biopsy n.
tonsillar suture n.
transaxillary n.
translocation n.
transpubic n.
transseptal n.
Travenol biopsy n.
n. trephination system
trephine core biopsy n.
triple-lumen n.
trocar n.
Troutman n.
Tru-Cut n.
Tru-Cut biopsy n.
Tru Taper Ethalloy n.
TT-3 n.
tungsten microdissection n.
Tuohy n.
Tuohy aortography n.
Tuohy lumbar puncture n.
Tuohy spinal n.
Turkel n.
Turner biopsy n.
Turner-Warwick n.
ultrasonic cataract-removal lancet n.
Ultra-Vue amniocentesis n.
Uni-Cor biopsy n.
Universal soft-tip cannulated sliding
  extrusion n.
University of Illinois biopsy n.
University of Illinois marrow n.
University of Illinois sternal
  puncture n.
urethroplasty n.
uterine n.
Vacutainer n.
vacuuming n.
VanSonnenberg biopsy n.
Variject n.
Venaflo n.
Venflon n.
venipuncture n.
venous n.

ventricular n.
Veress n.
Veress pneumoperitoneum n.
Veress spring-loaded laparoscopic n.
Vicat n.
Vim-Silverman biopsy n.
Virginia n.
Visitec retrobulbar n.
vitreous aspirating n.
vitreous-aspirating n.
vitreous transplant n.
von Graefe knife n.
Voorhees n.
Wang n.
Wangensteen intestinal n.
Wang transbronchial n.
Waterfield n.
Watson-Williams n.
wedge-line n.
Weeks n.
Weiss n.
Westcott n.
Westcott biopsy n.
Whitacre spinal n.
Wiener eye n.
Williams n.
Williams cystoscopic n.
Wilson-Cook electrode n.
winged steel n.
Wolf-Veress n.
Worst n.
Wright n.
Wright fascia n.
Wright ophthalmic n.
Wright ptosis n.
Wyeth bifurcated n.
Yale Luer-Lok n.
Yang n.
Yueh centesis n.
Zavala lung biopsy n.
NeedleAid
Needle-Ease device
needleholder, needle holder *(See* holder)
needle-knife
  n.-k. fistulotome
  n.-k. papillotome
  n.-k. wire
Needle-Less Suture
needle-nose
  n.-n. rongeur
  n.-n. vise-grip pliers
needlepoint
  n. cautery
  n. electrocautery
**needle-point suture passer/incision
  closure guide**
Needle-Pro needle protection device
needlescope device
Needle's Eye snare

needle-tip catheter
needle-tipped sphincterotome
Neer
  N. I, II shoulder prosthesis
  N. II shoulder system
  N. II total knee system
  N. II total shoulder system implant
Neff
  N. meniscus knife
  N. percutaneous access set
negative
  n. eyepiece
  n. impression cast
  n. pressure device
Negus
  N. bronchoscope
  N. laryngoscope
  N. mouthgag
  N. pusher
Neil-Moore electrode
Neisser syringe
Neitz CT-R cataract camera
Nelvert
  N. knife guide
  N. needle holder
  N. osteotome
Nek-LO
  N.-LO hot & cold pillow
  N.-LO orthopaedic support/comfort
    pillow
Nélaton
  N. bullet probe
  N. catheter
  N. rubber tube drain
  N. urethral catheter
Nellcor
  N. Durasensor adult oxygen
    transducer
  N. FS-10, FS-14 oximeter sensor
  N. FS-10 oximeter sensor
  N. FS-14 oximeter sensor
  N. N-2500 capnograph
  N. N-499 fetal oxygen saturation
    monitor
  N. N-400/FS system
  N. N-200 home monitor
  N. N-3000 home monitor
  N. N20, N200 pulse oximeter
  N. N-20PA pulse oximeter
  N. N-20 pulse oximeter
  N. N200 pulse oximeter
  N. N-series pulse oximeter
  N. Puritan Bennett
  N. Puritan Bennett home monitor
  N. Puritan Bennett ventilator
  N. Symphony blood pressure
    monitor
  N. Symphony blood pressure
    monitoring system
  N. Symphony N-3100 noninvasive
    blood pressure monitor
  N. Symphony N-3000 pulse
    oximeter
  N. Symphony pulse oximeter
Nelson
  N. lobectomy scissors
  N. rib retractor
  N. rib spreader
  N. scissors
  N. tissue forceps
Nelson-Metzenbaum scissors
neobladder
  Hemi-Kock n.
  orthotopic n.
NeoControl pelvic floor therapy system
NeoCure cryoablation system
NeoDerm dressing
NeoDisc cervical replacement device
NeoDura matrix
neodymium
  n. laser
  n. magnet
neodymium:YAG laser
neodymium:yttrium
  n. garnet laser
  n. lithium fluoride laser
neodymium:yttrium-aluminum-garnet
  n.-a.-g. laser
  n.-a.-g. laser system
neodymium:yttrium-lithium-fluoride
  photodisruptive laser
Neo-Fit
  N.-F. neonatal endotracheal tube
    grip
  N.-F. neonatal endotracheal tube
    holder
NeoKnife electrosurgical instrument
Neolens lens
Neolon surgical glove
Neolyte laser indirect ophthalmoscope
Neomed electrocautery
neonatal
  n. cuff
  n. internal jugular puncture kit
  n. monitor
  n. sandbag
  n. scissors
  n. stadiometer
  n. sternal retractor
  n. tracheostomy tube holder
  n. vascular clamp
  n. vascular forceps
Neonatal Y TrachCare
NeoNaze device
neon occipitocervical system
Neoplush foam
neoprene
  n. ankle support

neoprene *(continued)*
    n. back support
    n. dressing
    n. elbow sleeve
    n. fabric
    n. hinged knee brace
    n. Osgood-Schlatter knee brace
    n. shoe
    n. wrist brace
    n. wrist orthosis
    n. wrist strap
Neoprobe
    N. 1000, 1500 portable radioisotope detector
    N. radioactivity detector
    N. 1000 radioisotope detection system
Neoscan
Neo-Sert
    N.-S. umbilical vessel catheter
    N.-S. umbilical vessel catheter insertion set
Neosonic
    N. piezo ultrasonic unit
    N. P-5 SPM super-powered mini retroprep/endo system
NeoSoniX
    N. handpiece
    N. system
Neosono
    N. MC apex locator
    N. Ultima apex locator/pulp tester
neosphincter
    Acticon n.
Ne-Osteo bone morphogenic protein
Neo-Therm neonatal skin temperature probe
Neo-trak 515A neonatal monitor
Neotrend
    N. multiparameter blood gas monitor
    N. premature infant blood gas/temperature monitor
    N. sensor
    N. system
Neotrode II neonatal electrode
NeoV0$_2$R volume-control resuscitator
Neovision micro mirror
nephelometer
nephrolithotomy
    n. forceps
    percutaneous n. (PCNL)
NephroMax
    N. balloon catheter
    N. catheter set
nephroscope
    steerable n.
    Storz n.
    Wolf percutaneous universal n.

nephrostomy
    n. catheter
    n. clamp
    n. tube
nephroureteral stent system
nephroureterostomy stent
Neptune high-pressure PTCA balloon catheter
nerve
    n. agent antidote kit
    n. approximator
    n. block infusion kit
    n. cap
    n. cuff
    n. fiber analyzer
    N. Fiber Analyzer laser ophthalmoscope
    n. holder
    n. hook
    n. pull hook
    n. root retractor
    n. root sheath
    n. separator
    n. separator spatula
    n. stimulator
    n. suture
    n. twig
    n. wrapping
nerve-approximating clamp
nerve-integrity monitor
NervePace nerve conduction monitor
Nervoscope device
Nesbit
    N. cystoscope
    N. resectoscope
nested
    n. step stool
    n. trocar
nester coil
net
    rotatable Roth retrieval n.
    Roth endoscopy retrieval n.
    Roth polyp retrieval n.
    Surgiflex elastic n.
    TubeGauz elastic n.
    ureteric retrieval n.
netting
    Baby Air mesh n.
    Dacron n.
    splint pan n.
Nettleship
    N. canaliculus dilator
    N. iris repositor
Nettleship-Wilder dilator
network
    Surgical Internet Generation N. (SIGN)
Neubauer hemocytometer

Neufeld
> N. apparatus
> N. device
> N. nail
> N. pin
> N. roller traction

NeuFlex metacarpophalangeal joint implant
Neuhann cystotome
Neumann scissors
NeuraGen nerve guide
Neurairtome drill
neural
> n. dissector
> n. prosthesis
> n. tube

Neuroacryl tissue adhesive
Neuro-Aide testing device
neurocalometer thermography device
NeuroCell-HD porcine fetal neural material
NeuroCell-PD porcine fetal neural material
NeuroCom Balance Master
NeuroCybernetic
> N. prosthesis (NCP)
> N. prosthesis system

neurodiagnostic scanner
NeuroDrape surgical drape
neuroendoscope
> NeuroPEN n.
> Neuroview n.

NeuroFOCUS scanner
Neuroform
> N. microdelivery stent system
> N. stent

Neuroform3 microdelivery stent system
neurography needle
Neuroguard
> N. pulsed wave transducer
> N. transcranial Doppler

Neurolac nerve guide
NeuroLink II EEG data acquisition system
neurological
> n. percussion hammer
> n. percussor
> n. sponge
> n. tuning fork

neuromagnetometer
> whole-head n.

NeuroMap system
Neuromeet soft tissue approximator
Neurometer CPT electrodiagnostic device
neuromuscular
> n. electrical stimulator (NMES)
> n. III stimulator

neuropacemaker

Neuropack 4, 8 EMG
Neuropak 8 system
neuropatty
Neuropedic
> N. multidensity mattress
> N. neurolon mattress

NeuroPEN neuroendoscope
NeuroProbe amplifier
neuroprobe pain management system
Neuro-Pulse nerve locator/stimulator
Neuropulse unit
Neuro-Sat frameless isocentric stereotactic system
NeuroScan 3D imager
Neurosector
> N. ultrasound
> N. ultrasound system

NeuroSight cranial module
Neurosign
> N. 100 constant current stimulator
> N. 100 nerve monitor
> N. 100 system

Neuro-smooth needle holder
neurostimulator
> Biotens n.
> Grass n.
> Medtronic Itrel II n.
> Medtronic Xtrel n.
> percutaneous epidural n. (PENS)
> Staodyne EMS+2 n.
> Synergy Versitrel n.
> Versitrel n.

neurosurgery needle holder
neurosurgical
> n. bur
> n. cottonoid
> n. head holder
> n. headrest
> n. needle holder
> n. pledget
> n. scissors
> n. shunt
> n. suture
> n. suture needle

neurosuture
Neurotips neurological examination pin
neurotome
Neurotrac II EEG
neurotransmitter
> excitatory amino acid n.

Neurotrend
> N. continuous multiparameter system
> N. sensor

Neurotube bioabsorbable nerve conduit
NeuroVasx submicroinfusion catheter
Neuroview
> N. integrated visualization system
> N. neuroendoscope

N

neutral
- n. amyloid probe
- n. density filter
- n. electrode
- n. hook
- n. position splint

neutralization screw

neutron
- n. meter
- n. personnel dosimeter
- n. therapy machine

Neviaser portal

Neville
- N. ascending aortic air vent needle
- N. stent
- N. tracheal prosthesis
- N. tracheal reconstruction prosthesis

Neville-Barnes forceps

Nevin ankle brace

Nevyas
- N. double sharp cystotome
- N. drape retractor

New
- N. Beginnings GelShapes silicone gel sheeting
- N. Beginnings topical gel sheeting
- N. England Baptist acetabular cup
- N. England scoliosis brace
- N. Mind Set toe splint
- N. Orleans endarterectomy stripper set
- N. Orleans Eye & Ear fixation forceps
- N. Orleans lens
- N. Orleans lens loupe
- N. Orleans needle holder
- N. Schwinn 900 bicycle
- N. Schwinn elliptical bicycle
- N. speaking tube
- N. Star model 130 laser
- N. suture scissors
- N. tissue forceps
- N. Versaback gym ball
- N. Vision magnification system
- N. York catheter exchange wire guide
- N. York Orthopaedic front-opening orthosis
- N. York University orthotic insert

newborn eyelid retractor

Newell lid retractor

Newington orthosis

NewIris ocular implant

NewLife
- N. Elite concentrator
- N. IOL
- N. oxygen concentrator

Newman
- N. collagen plug inserter forceps
- N. proctoscope

Newport
- N. collar
- N. hip system
- N. MC hip orthosis
- N. MC hip orthosis brace
- N. medical instrument
- N. total hip orthosis
- N. total hip orthosis system
- N. ventilator
- N. Wave ventilator

Newsom side-port nucleus cracker

NewTom CT scanner

Newton
- N. catheter
- N. guidewire

Newvicon camera tube

NewVues sterile contact lens

Nexacryl
- N. cohesive product
- N. tissue adhesive

Nexerciser Plus

NexGen
- N. complete knee replacement system
- N. complete knee system
- N. component
- N. knee component
- N. knee implant
- N. offset stem extension

Nex-Link
- N.-L. implant system
- N.-L. spinal fixation system

NexPill SmartCap medication monitoring system

NexStent carotid stent

Nextep
- N. Contour lower leg walker
- N. knee brace

Nexus
- N. coronary stent
- N. hip prosthesis
- N. implant
- N. 2 linear ablation catheter
- N. wheelchair seating system

Ney articulator

Nezhat-Dorsey
- N.-D. aspirator
- N.-D. irrigator/aspirator
- N.-D. suction-irrigator
- N.-D. trumpet valve
- N.-D. trumpet valve hydrodissector

Nezhat irrigation tubing

NForce nitinol helical stone extractor

NG
- nasogastric
    - NG feeding tube

NG strip nasal tube fastener
NG tube
NHS-activated HiTrap affinity column
Niagara temporary dialysis catheter
Niamtu video imaging system
nibbler
Schultz anterior capsule n.
Nicati foreign body spud
Nic the Dragon aerosol mask
N'ice
N. Stretch night splint
N. Stretch night splint suspension
system with Sealed Ice
Nichamin
N. fixation ring
N. hydrodissection cannula
N. I, II nucleus quick chopper
N. I and II nucleus quick chopper
N. LASIK irrigating cannula
N. quick chopper
N. triple chopper
N. vertical chopper
Nicholas manual muscle tester
Nichols IRMA kit
nickel grid
Nickelplast blank
nickel-titanium file
Nickerson BiGGY vial
Nicola
N. forceps
N. scissors
Nicolet
N. Compass EMG instrument
N. Elite Doppler monitor
N. Elite Doppler ultrasound
N. Elite obstetrical Doppler
N. nerve integrity monitor
N. NMR spectrometer
N. SM-300 stimulator
N. VersaLab APM
N. Viking IIe EMG recorder
N. Viking II electrophysiologic
system
Nicoll
N. bone replacement material
N. rasp
Nicol prism
**NICO$_2$ noninvasive cardiac output
monitor**
Nidek
N. AR-2000 objective automatic
refractor
N. combo laser system
N. 3Dx stereo camera
N. 3Dx stereodisk camera
N. EC-1000 excimer laser
N. EC-5000 excimer laser
N. EC-5000 excimer laser system
N. EchoScan

N. EC-5000 refractive laser system
N. Laser System laser
N. MK-2000 keratome system
Niebauer
N. finger joint replacement
prosthesis
N. implant
Niebauer-Cutter implant
night
n. drainage bag
n. drain bottle
N. Owl pocket polygraph
N. Splint support
NightBird nasal CPAP
NightForm infant sleep mattress
Nightimer carpal tunnel support
Nightingale examining lamp
NIH cardiomarker catheter
Nihon
N. Kohden Neurofax
electroencephalograph
N. Kohden polygraph
N. tocodynamometer
Nike Max Rx prescription sun lens
Nikon
N. aspheric lens
N. D100 digital camera
N. digital camera
N. FS-3 photo slit-lamp
biomicroscope
N. microprocessor-controlled camera
N. NS-1 slit-lamp microscope
N. Retinomax K-Plus autorefractor
N. Retinopan fundus camera
N. SMZ 2T magnifying lens
N. zoom photo slit-lamp
NIM-2 nerve integrity monitor
Nimbus Hemopump
**Ninja FX series over-the-wire coaxial
PTCA dilatation balloon catheter**
Niox
N. nitric oxide breath test system
N. nitric oxide monitoring system
Niplette device
nipper
Amico nail n.
cuticle n.
Dieter-House n.
English anvil nail n.
Hough anterior crurotomy n.
House-Dieter n.
House-Dieter malleus n.
House malleus n.
Lempert malleus n.
malleus n.
Miltex nail n.
nail n.
n. nail drill

N

nipple
>Kock n.
>McGovern n.
>split-cuff n.

NIR
>NIR Elite Monorail system
>NIR Elite OTW stent system
>NIR ON Ranger balloon-expandable stent
>NIR Primo Monorail coronary stent
>NIR Royal Advanced stent
>NIR stent

NIRflex coronary stent
Niro
>N. bone-cutting forceps
>N. wire-twisting forceps

Niroyal Advance balloon-expandable stent
Nirvana mattress
Nishimoto Sangyo scanner
Nishizaki-Wakabayashi suction tube
Nissenkorn stent
Nite
>N. Train'r Alarm
>N. Train'r enuresis conditioning device

Ni-Ti alloy stent
nitinol
>n. basket
>n. guidewire
>N. K-file
>n. mesh-covered frame
>n. mesh stent
>n. petal
>n. self-expandable stent
>n. self-expanding coil stent
>n. shape-memory alloy wire
>n. snare
>n. subglottic stenosis stent
>n. Symphony stent
>n. thermal memory stent
>n. U-clip
>n. U-clips
>n. wire
>n. wire core

Niti-S stent
Nit-Occlud device
Nitrazine paper
Nitrex
>N. ev3 guidewire
>N. nitinol guidewire

nitrile glove
nitrite-thiosulfate kit
nitrocellulose filter paper
nitrogen-phosphorus detector
nitroglycerin transdermal patch
Nitrospray Plus cryosurgical device
nitrovasodilator
Nitro wheelchair

NLite
>N. laser
>N. nonablative laser
>N. wrinkle reduction laser

NM-1000 digital nonmydriatic fundus camera
NMES
>neuromuscular electrical stimulator

NMR
>NMR LipoProfile test
>NMR spectrometer

N-Multistix
No
>No Pour Pak II suction catheter kit
>No Pour Pak suction catheter kit
>No Sting barrier film

Nobel Biocare implant
NobelPerfect dental implant
Nobelpharma
>N. gold prosthetic retaining screw
>N. implant
>N. implant system

Noble forceps
N$_2$O cryosurgical unit
noctograph
nocturnal penile tumescence monitor
Node Seeker surgical radiation detection system
Noga XP cardiac navigation system
Nogenol dental cement
Nogier auriculotherapy device
Noiles
>N. posterior stabilized knee
>N. rotating hinge knee
>N. rotating hinge knee mechanism
>N. rotating hinge total knee prosthesis

noise
>n. level monitor
>n. reduction device

Nokor needle
Nolan
>N. needle holder
>N. system collimator mounted contact shield

Nomad-LE EMG
nonabsorbable surgical suture
nonadherent foam
nonadhering dressing
nonadhesive dressing
nonarcon articulator
nonaspirating ultrasonic phaco chopper tip
non-blue filtering IOL
nonbreather mask
non-child-resistant container
noncollared press-fit femoral stem implantation

noncompliant balloon
nonconductive guidewire
noncontact
    n. corneal esthesiometer
    n. lens
    n. pneumatic esthesiometer
    n. tonometer
noncoring Huber needle
noncrushing
    n. bowel clamp
    n. intestinal clamp
    n. intestinal forceps
    n. vascular clamp
noncutting
    n. blunt threads of resorbable
      screw
    n. needle
    n. suture needle
nondetachable
    n. balloon
    n. balloon catheter
    n. endovascular balloon
    n. occlusive balloon
    n. silicone balloon catheter
nondilated system
nondominant vessel
nonenclosed magnet
nonfenestrated forceps
nonferromagnetic
    n. clip
    n. MR (XGIF-MR30)
    n. MR-compatible frame
    n. MR endoscope
    n. needle
    n. positioning device
nonflow-directed catheter
nonhinged knee prosthesis
Nonin Onyx pulse oximeter
noninsulated needle
nonintegrated transvenous defibrillation
   lead
noninterfering separator
noninvasive
    n. continuous cardiac output
      monitor
    n. extrathoracic ventilator
    n. monitor
    n. temporary pacemaker
nonlatex dental dam
nonmedullated nerve fiber
nonocclusive dressing
nonperforating
    n. towel clamp
    n. towel forceps
nonpneumatic tourniquet
nonporous-coated endoprosthesis
nonrebreather face mask
nonrebreathing
    n. face mask

    n. mask
    n. valve
nonthoracotomy
    n. defibrillation lead system
    n. lead implantable cardioverter-
      defibrillator
    n. system antitachycardia device
nontoothed forceps
nontunneled catheter
nonvalved graft
non-valve plate
nonweightbearing brace
nonwoven sponge
Noon AV fistula clamp
noose
    Dormia n.
Nordan-Ruiz trapezoidal marker
Nordent bone file
NordiCare
    N. Enabler exerciser
    N. Strider exerciser
NordicTrack
    N. motion analyzer
    N. ski exerciser
Nordt knot tightener
Norelco allergen reducer
Norian
    N. skeletal repair system
    N. SRS cement
Norland
    N. bone densitometer
    N. digital oscilloscope
    N. pQCT XCT2000 scanner
    N. XR26 bone densitometer
    N. XR-46 central DXA bone
      densitometry system
normal-mode ruby laser
Normlgel
    N. hydrogel dressing
    N. protective wound dressing
Norm testing and rehabilitation system
Norport pump
Norris tip magnet
Northbent
    N. scissors
    N. suture scissors
Northgate
    N. SD-3 dual-purpose lithotriptor
    N. SD-100 EHL generator
Northland bone density machine
Norton
    N. endotracheal tube
    N. flow-directed Swan-Ganz
      thermodilution catheter
Norwegian system
Norwich press-fit prosthesis
Norwood EyeCare epikeratome

N

no-scalpel
>   n.-s. vasectomy fixator ring clamp forceps
>   n.-s. vasectomy instrument set

nose
>   artificial n.
>   n. clip
>   n. cone
>   n. guard splint

nosecone
>   CEM handswitching n.

no-stretch RocketSoc brace

nostril thermistor

notched ramus retractor

notcher device

notch filter

notchplasty blade

no-tie stretch lace

Noto
>   N. polypus forceps
>   N. sponge forceps

No-Touch delivery and mounting system

Nottingham
>   N. colposuspension needle
>   N. introducer
>   N. KeyMed introducer
>   N. One-Step tapered dilator
>   N. ureteral dilator

Nott vaginal speculum

Nouvisage
>   N. Deep Hydration body patch
>   N. Deep Hydration gloves
>   N. Deep Hydration neck patch

Nova
>   N. Aid lens
>   N. Celltrak 12 hematology analyzer
>   N. DPM 9003 skin testing instrument
>   N. II machine
>   N. II pacemaker
>   N. Microsonics ImageVue system
>   N. Soft II lens
>   N. thermodilution catheter

NovaBone
>   N. Bioglass bone grafting material
>   N. bone graft particulate

NovaBone-C/M bone graft particulate

Novack special extraction/injection set

Novaclip atraumatic spring clip

Novacor
>   N. Diasys cardiac device
>   N. Diasys left ventricular assist device
>   N. Diasys left ventricular assist system
>   N. left ventricular assist device
>   N. left ventricular assist system

>   N. mechanical circulatory support system

Novafil suture

Novagel
>   N. gel sheet
>   N. silicone gel sheeting

Novagold mammary implant

Novak
>   N. biopsy curette
>   N. curette
>   N. uterine curette

NovaLine excimer laser

Novametrix
>   N. combination O_2/CO_2 sensor
>   N. pulse oximeter
>   N. Tidal Wave handheld capnograph

Novapath HIV-1 immunoblot tester

NovaPulse
>   N. CO_2 laser
>   N. laser system

NovaSaline prefilled breast implant

Novascan scanning headpiece

NovaSure impedance controlled endometrial ablation system

Novatec
>   N. LightBlade
>   N. LightBlade laser

Novo-10a CBF measuring device

NovolinPen device

Novoste
>   N. Beta-Cath delivery system
>   N. catheter

Novum system

Novus
>   N. LC threaded interbody fusion cage
>   N. LT titanium threaded interbody fusion cage
>   N. mini-valve
>   N. Omni 2000 photocoagulator
>   N. 2000 ophthalmoscope
>   N. 3000 photocoagulation device
>   N. Spectra laser
>   N. Verdi diode-pumped green photocoagulator

NOxBOX II monitor

Noyes
>   N. ear forceps
>   N. forceps
>   N. iridectomy scissors
>   N. iris scissors
>   N. nasal forceps

Nozovent nasal valve dilator

nozzle
>   suction n.

NP-3S auto chart projector

NPB-295 pulse oximeter

NPB-40 handheld pulse oximeter

NPB-75 handheld capnograph/pulse oximeter
NS2000 bipolar generator system
N-Terface
    N-T. contact layer sheet
    N-T. contact layer wound dressing
    N-T. dressing
    N-T. gauze
    N-T. nonadherent dressing
NTrap
    N. endoscopic entrapment and extraction device
    N. stone retrieval basket
Nu
    Nu Gauze dressing
    Nu Gauze sponge
nuclear
    n. magnetic resonance spectrometer
    n. medicine camera
    n. probe
    n. scanner
    n. stent
nuclear-powered pacemaker
Nucleopore filter
Nucleotome probe
Nucletron
    N. applicator
    N. MicroSelectron/LDR remote afterloader
    N. simulator
nucleus
    N. C124M cochlear implant system
    N. 22 cochlear implant
    N. 24 Contour cochlear implant
    N. 24 Contour cochlear implant system
    N. 24 Contour electrode
    N. Contour electrode array
    n. cracker
    n. delivery cannula
    n. delivery loupe
    n. expressor
    5195 n. hydrodissector/rotator
    n. hydrolysis needle
    N. 24 multichannel auditory brainstem implant
    N. multichannel cochlear implant
    n. removal loupe
    n. rotator
    n. spatula
Nu-Derm
    N.-D. foam island dressing
    N.-D. hydrocolloid
    N.-D. hydrocolloid dressing
Nu-Form truss
Nu-Gel
    N.-G. clear hydrogel wound dressing

    N.-G. hydrogel sheet
    N.-G. hydrogel wound dressing
Nugent
    N. hook
    N. soft cataract aspirator
    N. utility forceps
Nugent-Gradle scissors
Nu-Hope
    N.-H. adhesive
    N.-H. adhesive waterproof skin barrier
    N.-H. drainable 1-piece pouch
    N.-H. hole cutter
    N.-H. Karaya powder
    N.-H. neonatal and preemie pouch
    N.-H. ostomy neonatal pouch
    N.-H. pouch cover
    N.-H. skin barrier strip
    N.-H. tubing
    N.-H. urinary pouch
    N.-H. urine collection bottle
    N.-H. urostomy pouch
Nu-Knit
    N.-K. absorbable hemostat
    Surgicel N.-K.
NuLens accommodating IOL
NuMed intracoronary Doppler catheter
NuMe microdermabrasion and exfoliation system
Nunc cryotube
Nuport PEG tube
NuPulse device
Nurolon suture
Nursette prefilled disposable bottle
NuSmile primary crown
Nussbaum
    N. bracelet
    N. intestinal clamp
    N. intestinal forceps
NuStep
    N. exerciser
    N. total body recumbent stepper
nut
    n. alignment guide
    Kirschner traction bow n.
    locking n.
    nylon n.
    sleeved n.
    traction bow n.
    VDS hex n.
Nu-Tip
    N.-T. disposable scissor tip
    N.-T. laparoscopic scissors
NutraCol hydrocolloid wound dressing
NutraDress zinc-saline dressing
NutraFill hydrophilic dressing
NutraGauze hydrophilic wound dressing
Nu-Trake
    N.-T. cricothyrotomy device

N

Nu-Trake *(continued)*
  N.-T. Weiss emergency airway
    system
NutraPrep food
NutraShield perineal protectant
**NutraStat calcium alginate wound
  dressing**
Nutricath catheter
Nutriflex tube
Nutromat Pad S feeding pump
Nuttall liver retractor
NuvaRing vaginal contraceptive ring
Nuvaseal resin
Nuva-Tach resin
NuVita lens
NUVO barrier film
Nu-Vois artificial larynx
Nuvolase
  N. 660 laser
  N. 660 laser system
**Nuwave transcutaneous electrical nerve
  stimulator**
Nycore
  N. cardiac device
  N. pigtail catheter
Nylatex
  N. strap
  N. wrap

Nylex
  N. diagnostic catheter
  N. flush angiographic catheter
**Nylexogrip cohesive long stretch
  bandage**
Nylok
  N. bolt
  N. self-locking nail
nylon
  n. catheter
  liquid n.
  n. loop
  n. monofilament suture
  n. nut
  n. retention suture
  n. scrub brush
  n. strap
  n. surgical sack
  n. suture
  n. 66 suture
  n. teaspoon
  n. tissue biopsy bag
  Xcelon n.
nystagmograph
nystagmus glasses
Nystar Plus ENG
Nytone enuretic control unit
NYU-Hosmer prehension actuator

O₂
    O₂ Boot
    O₂ disposable boot device
OBrien bone clamp
OAC
    optical aspirating curette
OAdjuster knee brace
OA knee brace
Oasis
    O. collagen plug
    O. dry suction chest drain
    O. feather microscalpel
    O. pusher tube system
    O. stent
    O. thrombectomy catheter
    O. thrombectomy system
    O. triple-lumen catheter
    O. wound dressing
OAsys knee brace
OAT device
OB-10 Comfort bite block
Obagi maintenance program
Oberto mouth prop
obese
    o. bed
    o. support
    o. walker
OBF tonometer
OB Gees maternity orthotic
OB/GYN chair
objective
    o. lens
    o. optometer
oblique
    o. aspiration mucosector
    o. bandage
    o. forward-viewing instrument
    o. mucosectomy device tip
    o. muscle hook
    o. prism
    o. prism device
    o. viewing echoendoscope
    o. viewing endoscope
oblique-viewing echoendoscope
O'Brien
    O. airway needle
    O. fixation forceps
    O. marker
    O. rib hook
    O. scissors
    O. spud
    O. stitch scissors
    O. suture scissors
    O. tissue forceps
Obstbaum lens spatula

obstetrical
    o. forceps
    o. retractor
obstetric forceps
obstructed shunt tube
Obtura II gutta percha system
obturator
    Alcock-Timberlake o.
    o. appliance
    blunt o.
    blunt-tipped o.
    cannulated o.
    Check-Flo sheath o.
    concave o.
    distending o.
    Ellik-Shaw o.
    Endopath Optiview laparoscopic o.
    Endopath Optiview optical
     surgical o.
    Endotrac o.
    esophageal o.
    Fitch o.
    Frazier suction tube o.
    Hemaflex PTCA sheath with o.
    Hemaquet PTCA sheath with o.
    Keene o.
    Moria o.
    Optiview o.
    Optiview optical surgical o.
    palatal o.
    prosthetic o.
    sheath and o.
    suction tube o.
    Thermafil Plus o.
    Timberlake o.
    ureteral catheter o.
    visual o.
Obus back support
Obwegeser
    O. channel retractor
    O. orthognathic surgery instrument
    O. periosteal elevator
    O. retractor
Obwegeser-Dalpont internal screw
    fixation
occipital-cervical-thoracic (OCT)
Occluder
occluder
    air clamp inflatable vessel o.
    Amplatzer duct o.
    Amplatzer septal o.
    aortic o.
    ASDOS umbrella o.
    Bard Clamshell septal o.
    black/white o.

O

occluder *(continued)*
    CardioSEAL o.
    CardioSEAL septal o.
    catheter tip o.
    catheter-tip o.
    Clamshell double umbrella o.
    Clamshell septal o.
    clip-on/tie-on o.
    eye o.
    Flo-Rester vascular o.
    Flo-Rester vessel o.
    Halberg trial clip o.
    long o.
    long/short o.
    lorgnette o.
    Maddox rod o.
    Microvena Das Angel Wings o.
    modified Rashkind PDA o.
    multiple pinhole o.
    Odyssey Parasol punctal o.
    Parasol punctal o.
    Pediatric Cardiology Devices
       Sideris buttoned device o.
    PFO-Star o.
    pinhole o.
    Plus punctal o.
    radiolucent plastic o.
    Rashkind o.
    Rashkind double-disc umbrella o.
    red lens o.
    Rumison side port fixation o.
    short o.
    Sideris buttoned device o.
    single o.
    single/double o.
    square-shaped o.
occluding
    o. clamp
    o. forceps
occlusal rest bar
occlusion
    o. balloon
    o. catheter
    o. coil
occlusive
    o. bandage
    o. clamp
    o. collodion dressing
    o. drain
    o. dressing
    o. semipermeable dressing
occlusor
    Elastoplast eye o.
Ocean water-seal chest drain
Ocelot
    O. stackable cage
    O. stackable cage system
Ochsner
    O. arterial forceps

O. clamp
O. gall duct probe
O. hemostatic forceps
O. hook
O. ring
O. spiral probe
O. tissue/cartilage forceps
O. wire twister
OCL volar splint
Ocoee scalp cleansing unit
O'Connor
    O. abdominal retractor
    O. depressor
    O. drape
    O. flat hook
    O. iris forceps
    O. lid clamp
    O. marker
    O. muscle hook
    O. scleral depressor
    O. sharp hook
    O. sheath
    O. sponge forceps
    O. tenotomy hook
    O. tweezer dexterity test
    O. vaginal retractor
**O'Connor-O'Sullivan abdominal
    retractor**
OCT
    occipital-cervical-thoracic
    osteochondral transplant
       OCT compound
       OCT comprehensive system
       Visante OCT
OctaFix
    O. cervical fixation system
    O. occipital fixation system
octagon roll
Octa-Hex implant
octapolar
    o. catheter
    o. lead
octopus
    O. 101 bowl perimeter
    O. 101, 201 bowl perimeter
    O. 500 EZ
    o. holder
    O. 201 perimeter
    O. retractor
    O. visual field analyzer
OctreoScan
    O. kit
    O. system
Ocu-Guard ophthalmic wrap
Oculab Tono-Pen
Oculaid
    O. capsular tension ring
    O. lens

ocular
    o. blood flow analyzer
    o. cautery
    o. cup
    o. gamboscope loupe
    o. grid
    o. lens
    o. loupe
    o. magnification system
    o. marker
    o. pressure reducer
    o. prosthesis
    o. response analyzer
Oculex drug delivery system
OcuLight
    O. GL photocoagulator
    O. GLx green laser photocoagulator
    Iris Medical O. SLx
    O. SL diode laser
    O. SL laser
    O. SLx laser
    O. SLx ophthalmic laser
oculocutaneous laser
oculogyric stimulator
Oculo-Plastik ePTFE ocular implant
oculoplasty corneal protector
oculoplethysmograph
Oculus
    O. BIOM noncontact lens system
    O. Easyloupes
    O. trial frame
Ocuscan
    Sonometric O.
    O. transducer
Ocutech vision enhancing system
ocutome
    CooperVision o.
    disposable o.
    O'Malley o.
    o. probe
    o. vitrectomy unit
    o. vitrector
Odam defibrillator
Odelca camera unit
ODISsey tissue oximeter
Odman-Ledin catheter
O'Donoghue cystourethroscope
Odontometer electronic apex locator
odor-absorbent dressing
O'Dwyer tube
Odyssey
    O. Parasol punctal occluder
    O. phacoemulsification system
    O. scanner laser ophthalmoscope
OEC
    OEC Mini 6600 imaging system
    OEC series 9600 cardiac system
    OEC splint

OEC-Diasonics
    OEC-D. 9400 fluoroscopy C-arm system
    OEC-D. mobile C-arm image intensifier
Oesch
    O. hook
    O. perforation invagination stripper
    O. phlebectomy hook
OES 4000 resectoscope
office diagnostic rechargeable otoscope
offloading knee brace
offset
    o. cane
    o. suspension feeder
O'Gawa
    O. cataract aspirating cannula
    O. tying forceps
Ogden
    O. Anchor soft tissue device
    O. bone anchor
    O. plate
    O. plate system
    O. tissue reattachment mini system
Ogee acetabular component
Ogura
    O. tissue
    O. tissue/cartilage forceps
O'Hara forceps
Ohio
    O. bed
    O. humidifier
    O. pressure infuser
    O. warmer
Ohl periosteal elevator
Ohmeda
    O. Care-Plus incubator
    O. 6200, 6300 CO_2 monitor
    O. continuous vacuum regulator
    O. handheld oximeter
    O. intermittent suction unit
    O. Minx pulse oximeter
    O. probe
    O. pulse oximeter
    O. 3800 pulse oximeter
    O. 5250 respiratory gas monitor
    O. SoftProbe probe
    O. thoracic suction regulator
ohmmeter
Oh-Spectron prosthesis
oil
    ethiodized o.
oiled silk suture
OIS
    OIS image digitizing system
    OIS WinStation 5000 ophthalmic imaging system
Ojemann cortical stimulator

O

627

Oklahoma
- O. ankle joint
- O. ankle joint orthosis
- O. ankle prosthesis
- O. cable system
- O. iris wire retractor

Olbert
- O. balloon
- O. balloon catheter
- O. balloon dilator

Olcott torque device

Oldberg
- O. intervertebral disc forceps
- O. intervertebral disc rongeur
- O. laminectomy rongeur
- O. pituitary rongeur

Oleeva
- O. fabric scar sheeting
- O. foam
- O. wound care product

Olerud
- O. internal fixator
- O. PSF fixation system
- O. PSF rod
- O. PSF screw

olfactometer

oligometric complex

oligonucleotide
- o. probe
- o. probe TC62

olive
- interchangeable vein stripper o.
- Savary-Gilliard metal o.
- o. wire

Olivecrona
- O. aneurysm clamp
- O. brain spatula
- O. clip applier
- O. clip-applying and removing forceps
- O. conchotome
- O. rasp
- O. silver clip
- O. wire saw

Olivecrona-Toennis clip-applying forceps

Oliver retractor

olive-shaped bur

olive-tip
- o.-t. cannula
- o.-t. irrigator

olive-tipped
- o.-t. bougie
- o.-t. catheter
- o.-t. Magnum wire
- o.-t. needle
- o.-t. plastic dilator

Olivier-Bertrand-Tipal frame

Olk
- O. retinal spatula

- O. vitreoretinal pick
- O. vitreoretinal spatula

Ollier
- O. graft
- O. rake retractor
- O. rasp

Ollier-Thiersch graft

Olsen cholangiogram clamp

Olsen-Hegar needle holder

Olshevsky tube

Olson
- O. calibrated cornea trephine
- O. calibrated cornea trephine system
- O. phaco chopper
- O. quick chopper

Olympia Vacpac support device

Olympic
- O. Neostraint immobilizer
- O. speaking valve
- O. Trach-Talk
- O. Vac positioning system

Olympix II PTCA dilatation catheter

Olympus
- O. A5256 laparoscope
- O. angioscope
- O. AU5200 cholesterol analyzer
- O. automatic reprocessor
- O. BH2 epifluorescence microscope
- O. BH2-epifluorescence microscope
- O. BH2 microscope
- O. BH2-RFCA reflecting microscope
- O. BHT-2 microscope
- O. BML-3Q, -4Q lithotriptor
- O. CBK fluorescence microscope
- O. CD-20Z heater probe
- O. CD-Z-series heat probe thermocoagulator
- O. CF-2301 endoscope
- O. CF-20 fibercolonoscope
- O. CF-HM series magnifying colonoscope
- O. CF-L series flexible sigmoidoscope
- O. CF-MB/LB colonoscope
- O. CF-MB-M colonoscope
- O. CF-MB series colonoscope
- O. CF-OSF series flexible O.
- O. CF24OZI colonoscope
- O. CF-PL series colonoscope
- O. CF-P20S fiberoptic colonoscope
- O. CF100S sigmoidoscope
- O. CF100TL
- O. CF-1T100L colonoscope
- O. CF-T series colonoscope
- O. CF-UM3 colonoscope
- O. CF-UM3 flexible echocolonoscope

O. CF-UM series echoendoscope
O. CF-UM20 ultrasonic endoscope
O. CF-UM20 ultrasound endoscope
O. CF-VL series colonoscope
O. CF-200Z colonoscope
O. CF-200Z endoscope
O. CHF-BP30 transduodenal
choledochofiberscope
O. CHF-P20 choledochoscope
O. CHF-Q10 cholangioscope
O. clip-fixing device
O. CLV-U 20 endoscopic halogen
light source
O. 215-cm enteroscope
O. continuous flow resectoscope
O. CV series
O. CV series endoscope
O. CYF-3 OES cystofiberscope
O. diagnostic laparoscope
O. disposable cannula
O. disposable trocar
O. double-channel therapeutic
videoendoscope
O. echoendoscope
O. endocamera
O. endoscopic ultrasound
O. endoscopic ultrasound scanner
O. endoscopy system
O. Endo-Therapy disposable biopsy
forceps
O. ENF-P2 laryngoscope
O. ENF-P2 scope
O. ENF-P series laryngoscope
O. esophagofiberscope
O. esophagoscope
O. EUM-20 echoendoscope
O. EUM-20 endoscope
O. EU-M30S endoscopic
ultrasonography receiver
O. EU-M30 system
O. Europe ETD automated
endoscope washer
O. EUS series endoscope
O. EVIS color computer chip
system
O. EVIS Q series endoscope
O. EVIS Q-200V
O. EVIS Q-200V endoscope
O. EVIS series endoscope
O. EVIS video colonoscope
O. Evis videocolonoscope
O. Evis videoendoscope
O. EW series fiberoptic
duodenoscope
O. FB-20C endoscopic forceps
O. FB-25K endoscopic forceps
O. FBK-13 forceps
O. FB series biopsy forceps
O. FB-24U biopsy forceps

O. FG-12U wide-mouth forceps
O. fiberoptic bronchoscope
O. fiberoptic cystoscope
O. fiberoptic scope
O. fiberoptic sigmoidoscope
O. FK-13-1 biopsy forceps
O. flexible hysterofiberscope
O. forward-viewing endoscope
O. FS-K series endoscopic suture-
cutting forceps
O. gastrocamera
O. GF-EU1 gastrointestinal
fiberscope
O. GF series echoendoscope
O. GF-UC30P echoendoscope
O. GF-UCT30P linear-array
echoendoscope
O. GF-UM30P echoendoscope
O. GF-UM30P endoscope
O. GF-UM30P linear scanning
probe
O. GF-UM29 radial scanner
echoendoscope
O. GF-UM20 radial scanning
endoscope
O. GF-UM series echoendoscope
O. GF-UM3 ultrasonic endoscope
O. GF-UM20 ultrasound endoscope
O. GF-UM3, -UM20 system
O. GIF-D2 endoscope
O. GIF20 echoendoscope
O. GIF-EUM2 echoendoscope
O. GIF-HM series endoscope
O. GIF-HM-series endoscope
O. GIF-J series endoscope
O. GIF-K series gastroscope
O. GIF-P endoscope
O. GIF-Q200 endoscope
O. GIF-Q30 fiberscope
O. GIF series duodenoscope
O. GIF series echoendoscope
O. GIF 1T10 echoendoscope
O. GIF-2T10 endoscope
O. GIF-2T200 endoscope
O. GIF-2T20 end-viewing
endoscope
O. GIF-T series videoendoscope
O. GIFxP10 gastroscope
O. GIF-XP series endoscope
O. GIF-XP10 video endoscope
O. GIF-XQ240 endoscope
O. GIF-XQ30 flexible gastroscope
O. GIF-XV series endoscope
O. grasping rat-tooth forceps
O. heater probe unit
O. heat probe
O. hot biopsy forceps
O. HX-21L detachable miniloop
O. hysteroscope

O

Olympus *(continued)*

O. injector
O. intracavity transducer
O. JF series video duodenoscope
O. JF1T endoscope
O. JF1T10 fiberoptic duodenoscope
O. JF-T series endoscope
O. JF-TV series endoscope
O. JF-UM20 echoendoscope
O. JF-V series endoscope
O. JF-V series videoduodenoscope
O. light source connector
O. linear-array echoendoscope
O. LUS-1 rigid device
O. LUS-2 ultrasonic energy rigid device
O. MAJ363 FNA needle system
O. MH-908 slim ultrasonic probe
O. Nd:YAG laser
O. NM-K series sclerotherapy needle
O. NM-L series needle
O. N series ultrathin endoscope
O. OES fiberscope
O. OM-1 reflex camera
O. one-step button gastrostomy tube
O. One-Step Button tube
O. operating camera
O. operating laparoscope
O. OSF flexible sigmoidoscope
O. OSF scope
O. OSF sigmoidoscope
O. OSP fluorescence measuring system
O. OTV-S series miniature camera
O. PCF-100, -130 pediatric colonoscope
O. PCF series pediatric colonoscope
O. PJF endoscope
O. PJF series pediatric duodenoscope
O. PJF series pediatric endoscope
O. P series endoscope
O. PW-1L wash catheter
O. PW-5V spray catheter
O. resectoscope loop
O. reusable oval cup forceps
O. SD-5L semicircular snare
O. SD-9L-1 snare
O. side-viewing endoscope
O. SIF-10 enteroscope
O. SIF-M magnifying colonoscope
O. SIF-M series video enteroscope
O. SIF-Q240 enteroscope
O. SIF-SW fiberoptic endoscope
O. SIF-SW series video enteroscope

O. SIF-100 video enteroscope
O. SIF-100 video push endoscope
O. SIF-100 video push enteroscope
O. spray catheter
O. SP series image analyzer
O. S-20-20R probe
O. S20-20R transendoscopic ultrasound probe
O. stone retrieval basket
O. 2T100 endoscope
O. TJF-10, -100, -200 duodenoscope
O. TJF-100 endoscope
O. tripod-type endoscopic forceps
O. 2T-2000 twin-channel therapeutic gastroscope
O. UES series snare cautery device
O. ultrasonic esophagoprobe
O. ultrathin balloon-fitted ultrasound probe
O. UM-F30-20R probe
O. UM-20 radial echoendoscope
O. UM-2R, -3R probe
O. UM-R series miniature ultrasonic probe
O. UM series echoendoscope
O. UM series endoscope
O. UM-S30-25R probe
O. UM-1W endoscopic probe
O. UM-W series endoscopic probe
O. UM-1W transendoscopic ultrasound probe
O. URF-P2 translaparoscopic choledochofiberscope
O. URF-type P2 flexible ureteroscope
O. Vanox VH-2 microscope
O. videocolonoscope
O. video duodenoscope
O. videoduodenoscope
O. videoenteroscope
O. videogastroscope
O. videourology procedure system
O. V series endoscope
O. VU-M2 echoendoscope
O. VU-M2 endoscope
O. VU series echoendoscope
O. XCF series endoscope
O. XCF-XK series endoscope
O. XCHF-37 choledochoscope
O. XGF-UCT30 endoscope
O. XIF series echoendoscope
O. XIF-UM3 echoendoscope
O. XJF-UM20 echoduodenoscope
O. XK-10 endoscope
O. XK series oblique-viewing flexible fiberscope
O. XMP-U2 catheter echoprobe

O. XP series endoscope
O. XQ230 gastroscope
O. XQ series endoscope
O. XQ-200, XQ-230 video endoscope
O. Zoom endoscope
Olympus EVIS 140
OM
OM 2000 operation microscope
OM 4 ophthalmometer
O'Malley
O. jaw fracture splint
O. ocutome
O. self-adhering lens implant
Ombrédanne
O. forceps
O. mallet
Omed vented instrument guard
Omega
O. AcuBase
O. AcuBase system
O. compression hip screw
O. NV angioplasty catheter
O. NV polyethylene balloon catheter
O. splinting material
O. stent
Omega-NV balloon
OmegaPort access port
omental plug
Omiderm transparent adhesive film dressing
Ommaya
O. CSF reservoir
O. reservoir
O. reservoir device
O. reservoir implant material
O. reservoir prosthesis
O. reservoir transensor
O. retromastoid reservoir
O. shunt
O. spinal fluid reservoir
O. suboccipital reservoir
O. ventricular reservoir
O. ventricular tube
Omni
O. analyzer
O. Bloc bite block
O. Flex biliary stent
O. Flush catheter
O. knee brace
O. laser tip
O. 2 microscope
O. press
O. retractor
O. Roller massager
O. Selective 0-3 catheter
Omniace RT3200N electromyographic amplifier

Omnican Piston syringe
Omnicarbon
O. heart valve prosthesis
O. prosthetic heart valve
OmniCath atherectomy catheter
OmniCell
O. catheter module
O. supply system
Omnicor Programmer
Omniderm
O. dressing
O. transparent film
OmniFilter percutaneous guidewire microfilter
Omnifit
O. acetabular cup
O. dual geometry microstructured prosthesis
O. Eon femoral stem
O. HA femoral component
O. HA hip stem
O. HA hip stem prosthesis
O. HA hip system
O. knee prosthesis
O. Plus
O. Plus enhanced offset cemented hip system
O. Plus hip system
O. PSL microstructured prosthesis
Omnifit-C
Osteonics O.-C
Omnifix tape
Omniflex
O. balloon
O. head
OmniFlex knee orthosis
Omni-Flexor
O.-F. device
O.-F. wrist exerciser
Omni-Flow
O.-F. 4000 Plus
O.-F. 4000 Plus medical management system
omnifocal lens
Omni-LapoTract support system
Omnilink biliary stent
Omnilink/Megalink balloon-expanded stent
Omniloc
O. dental implant
O. dental system
OmniMed argon-fluoride excimer laser
OmniMedia XRS scanner
Omni-Park speculum
OmniPhase penile prosthesis
OmniPulse MAX holmium laser
Omniscience
O. single-leaflet cardiac valve prosthesis

O

Omniscience (continued)
- O. tilting disc valve
- O. tilting disc valve prosthesis
- O. valve
- O. valve device

Omnisense
- O. multisite QUS device
- O. 7000S bone sonometer

OmniSight EXcel image-guided surgery system

OmniStent stent

OmniTip side-firing laser needle

Omni-Tract
- O.-T. system
- O.-T. vaginal retractor

Omnivue illuminated magnifier

Omotrain active shoulder support

Omron
- O. compressor nebulizer
- O. Hem-601 automatic digital wrist blood pressure monitor
- O. monitor

Oncometrics Imaging Cyto-Savant image analyzer

On-Command catheter

Oncor
- O. ApopTaq kit
- O. Inform HER2/neu gene amplification detection system

on-demand analgesia computer

One
- O. Action Stent Introduction System
- O. Step Button gastrostomy device
- O. Time sharp debridement tray

one-hole
- o.-h. angiographic catheter
- o.-h. angioplastic catheter

O'Neil vacuum extractor

One-Step
- O.-S. gastric button
- O.-S. hCG combo test

OneTouch
- O. Basic
- O. basic glucometer
- O. blood glucose meter
- O. blood glucose monitor
- O. electrolysis unit
- O. Fast Take meter kit
- O. II hospital blood glucose monitoring system
- O. InDuo glucose meter
- O. Profile
- O. SureStep glucose meter
- O. Ultra test strip

Ong capsulotomy scissors

Ongoing Ambulating AFO boot

Onik-Cohen percutaneous access catheter

onlay implant

OnLine ABG monitor

On-Q
- O.-Q. C-bloc continuous nerve block system
- O.-Q. PainBuster postoperative pain relief system
- O.-Q. pain management infusion system
- O.-Q. pump
- O.-Q. Soaker catheter

OnTrack system

OnTrak TestTcard drug testing device

On-X mechanical bi-leaflet prosthetic heart valve

Onyx
- O. finger pulse oximeter
- O. liquid embolic system

O2Optix
- O. breathable contact lens
- O. contact lens

OP-1
- osteogenic protein-1
- OP-1 bone graft
- OP-1 implant
- OP-1 implant/bone graft
- OP-1 putty
- OP-1 putty spinal fusion implant
- OP-1 TM bone implant

Opal
- O. PDT Photoactivator laser
- O. RF needle ablation device

opaque
- o. canalicular plug
- o. Herrick lacrimal plug
- o. microscope
- o. myringotomy tube
- Sur-Fit Natura closed-end pouch, o.
- o. wire suture

Opdima digital mammography system

OPD-Scan
- OPD-S. diagnostic system
- OPD-S. optical path difference scanning system

open
- o. C-D hook
- o. dressing
- o. electrocautery snare
- o. face mask
- o. lens
- o. magnet
- o. MRI system
- o. nail
- O. Pivot heart valve
- O. Sky MRI scanner
- o. sphincterotome

Open-Cath
- Abbokinase O.-C.

open-celled foam

open-end
 o.-e. aspirating tube
 o.-e. flow-through radiopaque tip
open-ended ureteral catheter
OpenGene automated DNA sequencing system
open-heeled Unna boot
open-loop
 o.-l. insulin delivery system
 o.-l. intraocular lens
OpenPACS system
OpenSail
 O. balloon catheter
 O. coronary dilatation catheter
open-side vaginal speculum
open-tube rigid bronchoscope
Opera
 O. Star morcellator
 O. Star resectoscope
 O. Star SL hysteroscope
 O. system
operating
 o. loupe
 o. microscope
 o. platform
operative
 o. explorer
 o. leg holder
operator
 Boolean o.
Ophtec
 O. Co. lens
 O. occlusion implant
 O. trephine
Ophthalas
 O. argon/krypton laser
 O. argon laser
 O. krypton laser
ophthalmic
 o. blade
 o. calipers
 o. cautery electrode
 o. cup
 o. drill
 o. electrocautery
 o. endoscope
 o. hook
 o. instrument
 o. laser microendoscope
 o. pick
 o. sable brush
 o. sponge
 o. YAG laser system
ophthalmocmicroscope
 binocular indirect o.
ophthalmodynamometer
 Bailliart o.
 dial-type o.

Reichert o.
suction o.
ophthalmometer
 American Optical o.
 Haag-Streit o.
 Hertel o.
 Javal o.
 OM 4 o.
ophthalmomicroscope
 binocular indirect o.
ophthalmoscope
 All Pupil II indirect o.
 AO Reichert Instruments binocular indirect o.
 binocular o.
 binocular indirect o.
 Canon SLO scanning laser o.
 confocal laser scanning o.
 confocal scanning laser o.
 cordless monocular indirect o.
 demonstration o.
 direct o.
 Doran pattern stimulator o.
 Exeter o.
 Fison indirect binocular o.
 Friedenwald o.
 Ful-Vue o.
 Grafco o.
 Gullstrand o.
 halogen o.
 halogen coaxial o.
 Helmholtz o.
 indirect o.
 indirect laser o.
 Keeler binocular indirect o.
 laser indirect o. (LIO)
 Loring o.
 May o.
 Mentor Exeter o.
 metric o.
 MK IV o.
 monocular indirect o.
 Neolyte laser indirect o.
 Nerve Fiber Analyzer laser o.
 Novus 2000 o.
 Odyssey scanner laser o.
 Panoramic200 nonmydriatic o.
 Panoramic200 scanning laser o.
 polarizing o.
 Polle pod attachment for o.
 Propper binocular indirect o.
 Propper-Heine o.
 Propper indirect o.
 Reichert binocular indirect o.
 Reichert Ful-Vue binocular o.
 Rodenstock scanning laser o.
 scanning laser o.
 Schepens-Pomerantzeff o.
 TopSS scanning laser o.

O

ophthalmoscope *(continued)*
    Vantage o.
    Visuscope o.
    Welch Allyn o.
    Zeiss o.
ophthalmotrope
Ophthascan Mini-A scan
Ophthasonic
    O. pachymeter
    O. Ultrasonic Biometer
Ophthimus
    O. High-Pass Resolution perimeter
    O. ring perimeter
Ophtho-Burr foreign body removal system
Opmi
    O. colposcope
    O. microscopic drape
    O. Pentero surgical microscope
    O. pico diagnostic microscope
    O. pico i microscope
    O. Pro Magis dental microscope
    O. surgical microscope
    O. Vario/NC 33 system
    O. VISU 200 BrightFlex illuminator
    O. VISU 200 microscope
    O. VISU 210 microscope
Opmilas
    O. CO_2 laser
    O. CO_2 multipurpose laser
    O. laser system
    O. 144 Plus laser system
    O. 144 surgical laser
Opotow filling material
Oppenheimer
    O. spring wire splint
    O. with reverse knuckle-bender splint
Op-Pneu insufflator
Oppociser
    O. exercise device
    O. hand exerciser
opponens splint
opposed
    o. loop-pair quadrature magnetic resonance coil
    o. loop-pair quadrature NMR coil
Opraflex incise drape
OpSite
    O. drape
    O. dressing
    O. film
    O. Flexifix transparent film dressing
    O. Flexigrid dressing
    O. Flexigrid transparent film
    O. occlusive dressing
    O. Plus composite dressing

    O. postop composite dressing
    O. semipermeable dressing
    O. wound dressing
Opta
    O. 5 angioplasty balloon
    O. balloon stent-graft
    O. 5 catheter
    O. Pro PTA balloon dilatation catheter
    O. Pro PTA dilatation catheter
OptEase permanent vena cava filter
Optec 3000 contrast sensitivity test
Optefil demineralized bone matrix
Opteform
    O. bone graft material
    O. 100HT bone graft
Optelec Passport magnifier
Op-Temp
    O.-T. cautery
    O.-T. disposable electrocautery
Optetrak
    O. comprehensive knee system
    O. total knee replacement system
Opthascan Mini B system
Opti
    O. 1 pH/blood gas analyzer
    O. 1 portable blood analyzer
    O. 1 portable pH/blood gas analyzer
optic
    o. implant
    o. pachymeter
    o. 3-piece intraocular lens
    o. ring
    o. tweezers
Opticaid
    O. lens loupe
    O. spring clip
optical
    o. accessory
    o. aspirating curette (OAC)
    o. biopsy forceps
    o. biopsy system
    O. catheter
    o. digitizer
    o. dispenser
    o. Doppler velocimeter
    o. esophagoscope
    o. jewelry
    o. laryngoscope
    o. magnifier
    o. multichannel analyzer system
    o. needle
    o. pachymeter
    o. parametric oscillator
    o. pedobarograph
    O. Radiation intraocular lens
    O. Radiation lens

O. Sensors stand-alone arterial blood gas monitoring system
o. switch
o. tracking system
o. ureterotome
optically transparent electrode
Opticath oximeter catheter
OptiChamber
O. drug-holding device
O. valved holding chamber
opticociliary shunt vein
OptiCor digital cardiac communication and storage system
optics
American Medical O. (AMO)
confocal o.
o. cup
SinuScope rigid rod lens o.
Wappler cystoscope with microlens o.
Opti-Curve therapeutic pillow
Opti-Fix
O.-F. acetabular cup
O.-F. femoral component
O.-F. II acetabular cup
O.-F. I, II prosthesis
O.-F. total hip system
Optiflex lens
Opti-Flow dialysis catheter
Opti-Gard eye protector
OptiHaler drug delivery system
OptiLOUPE attachable lens
Optima
O. contact lens
O. diamond knife
O. pacemaker
O. preparative ultracentrifuge
O. ureteral stent
OptiMax
O. immunostaining system
O. Supreme pressure reduction mattress
OptiMed glaucoma pressure regulator
Optimizer disposable polypectomy snare
Optimum blade
Option
O. hip system
O. Orthotic Series
Optiphot-2UD microscope
Optiphot microscope
Optiplanimat automated unit
Opti-Plast
O.-P. balloon dilatation catheter
O.-P. XT balloon catheter
Optiplast Centurion balloon
Optipore
O. scrub sponge
O. Sponge wound cleanser

Optipost
Brasseler O.
Optique microscope
Optispike dispensing pin
Optisson contrast material
Optistar MR contrast delivery system
OptiStat handheld power injector
Optiva catheter
Optivac vacuum mixing system
Optiview
O. obturator
O. optical surgical obturator
O. trocar
Optivisor lens plate
Opti-Vue plastic barrel
optoelectric measuring apparatus
Optokinetic stimulator
optometer
infrared o.
laser o.
objective o.
Vernier o.
optomyometer
Optotrak
O. motion-analysis system
O. motion measurement system
O. motion and position measurement system
optotype
Snellen letter o.
Op-Trac retractor
Opus
O. 20 dental Er:YAG laser
O. 5, 10, 20 dental laser
OR1 electronic system
OR-340 imaging system
Oracle
O. delivery system
O. Focus imaging catheter
O. Focus PTCA catheter
O. intravascular ultrasound catheter
O. MegaSonics catheter
O. Micro Plus
O. Micro Plus catheter
O. Micro Plus PTCA catheter
O. PTCA catheter
oral
o. appliance
o. endoscope
o. endotracheal tube
o. esophageal tube
o. implant
o. needle
o. pharyngeal airway
o. rongeur forceps
O. Scan computer imaging system
O. Scan videoimaging system
o. screw
o. screw mouthgag

O

oral *(continued)*
    o. screw tongue depressor
    o. speculum mouthgag
    o. surgery handpiece
    o. temperature device
    o. videoscope
Oral-B soft foam interdental brush
OralScreen
    O. rapid oral fluid screening and test device
    O. 4 substance abuse test
Orandi knife
orange dye laser
OraQuick rapid HIV-1 antibody test
Orascoptic
    O. acuity system
    O. fiberoptic headlight
    O. loupe extension
OraSure
    O. collection device
    O. device
    O. HIV-1 oral specimen collection device
    O. salivary collection device
Orban-type explorer
Orbasone system
orbicular retractor
Orbis-Sigma cerebrospinal fluid shunt valve
orbital
    o. bar
    o. compressor
    o. depressor
    o. floor implant
    o. floor prosthesis
    o. implant
    o. retractor
orbit blade
Orbiter
    O. treadmill
    O. woven atrial mapping diagnostic catheter
orbitonometer
Orbix x-ray unit
Orbscan
    O. II corneal diagnostic system
    O. II corneal topography system
    O. II diagnostic system
    O. II multidimensional diagnostic system
    O. II topography system
    O. pachymeter
    O. system
    O. topography analysis system
Orca
    O. Robot
    O. robot system
OrCel wound dressing

orchidometer
    Prader o.
    punched-out o.
    Test-Size o.
O'Regan hemorrhoid ligator
Oregon prosthesis
Orentreich punch
Oreopoulos-Zellerman catheter
Orfit
    O. mask
    O. splint
Orfizip
    O. body jacket
    O. knee cast
    O. wrist cast
organic
    o. dental cement
    o. liquid scintillator
organization
    World Health O. (WHO)
organizer
    Richard Products fundus camera drug o.
Organon percutaneous E2 implant
Origin
    O. balloon
    O. PDB 1000 balloon
    O. Tacker
    O. trocar
original
    O. Backnobber massage tool
    O. Backnobber muscle massager
    O. Index Knobber II
    O. Index Knobber II massager
    O. Index Knobber II massage tool
    O. Jacknobber II muscle-massage device
    O. Pink Tape waterproof adhesive tape
    o. Sweet eye magnet
O-ring attachment
Orion
    O. anterior cervical plate
    O. balloon
    O. device
    O. electrode
    O. inhaler
    O. laser system
    O. lumbar support
    O. model EA 940 ion analyzer
Orlando hip-knee-ankle-foot orthosis
Orlau
    O. swivel walker
    O. swivel walker orthosis
Ormco appliance
oroendotracheal tube
oroesophageal
    o. overtube
    o. stethoscope

orogastric
  o. Ewald tube
  o. feeding tube
  o. tube
oropharyngeal
  o. airway
  o. pack
orotracheal tube
Orozco plate
Orr automatic reprocessor
Orthair oscillating saw
Orthairtome
  O. II drill
  O. wire driver
Orthawear antiembolism stocking
Orth-evac postoperative transfusion system
Orthex
  O. cannulated bone screw
  O. Relievers shoe insert
Orthicon camera
Orthion traction machine
Ortho
  O. All-Flex diaphragm
  O. diaphragm kit
  O. DX electromedical stimulator
  O. Dx electrotherapy system
  O. HCV ELISA test system second generation
  O. System 20 flow cytometer
  O. Tech performer knee brace
Ortho-Arch II orthotic
orthobiologic implant
Ortho-Biotic recliner
OrthoBlast
  O. osteoinductive bioimplant
  O. paste
Orthoblend
  Grafton DBM O.
OrthoBone pillow
Ortho-Cel pad
Orthoceph x-ray unit
OrthoClast
  O. joint revision system
  Swiss O.
Orthocomp cement
Orthocor II pacemaker
Orthoderm
  O. consummate air therapy bed
  O. Convertible mattress
Orthodoc presurgical planning system
orthodontic
  o. aligner
  o. appliance
  o. band
  o. band driver
  o. band setter
  o. base plate
  o. bracket

  o. cement
  o. impression tray
  o. resin
OrthoDyn bone substitute material
Orthodyne Enhancer unit
Orthofit 9000, 9001 orthotic
Orthofix
  O. Cervical-Stim bone growth stimulator
  O. Cervical-Stim stimulator
  O. external fixation device
  O. intramedullary nail
  O. ISKD device
  O. large-pin fixation
  O. lengthening device
  O. M-100 distractor
  O. monolateral femoral external fixator
  O. Ogden anchor
  O. pin
  O. prosthesis
  O. screw
Orthoflex elastic plaster bandage
Ortho-Foam elbow/heel pad
OrthoFrame external fixation
OrthoGel liner
OrthoGen bone growth stimulator
Orthogenesis
  O. LPS
  O. LPS limb preservation prosthesis system
Ortho-Glass
  O.-G. splint
  O.-G. synthetic material
Orthoglass splint
orthognathic occlusal relator
orthogonal
  o. laser
  o. radiofrequency coil
  o. square Helmholtz coil
Ortho-Grip silicone rubber handle
Ortho-Ice Multipaks system
orthokeratology contact lens
Orthokinetics travel chair
Ortholen sheet
Ortholign spinal orthosis
Ortholoc
  O. Advantim revision knee system
  O. Advantim total knee system
  O. II unconstrained prosthesis
OrthoLogic 1000 bone growth stimulator
Orthomatrix binder
Orthomedics
  O. Stretch and Heel splint
  O. Ultra-Guard hip orthosis
Orthomerica
  O. TC AFO system
  O. UFO

Orthomet
    O. Axiom total knee system
    O. Perfecta total hip system
orthometer
Orthomite resin
Ortho-Mold
    O.-M. lumbar body
    O.-M. splint
OrthOneXT dedicated MRI system
orthopaedic
    o. bone file
    o. broach
    o. bur
    o. cement
    o. chisel
    o. curette
    o. cutting instrument
    o. depth gauge
    o. dynamometer
    o. elevator
    o. fixation device
    o. forceps
    o. goniometer
    o. gouge
    o. hammer
    o. hemostat
    o. impactor
    o. knife
    o. osteotome
    o. pin
    o. plate
    o. positioning seat
    o. propeller
    o. rasp
    o. reamer
    o. rod
    o. rongeur
    o. scissors
    o. screw
    o. staple
    o. stockinette
    o. strap clavicle splint
    o. stretcher
    o. surgical pliers
    o. surgical stripper
    o. trauma plating system (OTPS)
    o. Universal drill
OrthoPak bone growth stimulator system
Ortho-Pal body support
Orthopantomograph-3, -10 panoramic x-ray machine
Orthopantomograph panoramic digital radiography unit
OrthoPAT
    O. blood salvage system
    O. orthopaedic perioperative autotransfusion system
    O. system
Orthopedic Systems Inc. (OSI)
Orthoplast
    O. isoprene splint
    O. jacket
    O. slipper cast
    O. splint
orthoptic eye patch
Orthoralix dental x-ray machine
orthoRaps postsurgical wound wrap
Ortho-Rater
orthoscope
orthoscopic
    o. lens
    o. spectacles
Orthoset
    O. radiopaque bone cement
    O. radiopaque bone cement adhesive
orthosis
    accommodative o.
    adjustable advanced reciprocating gait o.
    AliCork foot o.
    AliMed o.
    Aliplast custom-molded foot o.
    ambulation training o.
    Amfit custom o.
    ankle o. (AO)
    ankle contracture o.
    ankle-foot o. (AFO)
    ankle-foot plastic o.
    anteroposterior control o.
    Anti-Shox o.
    Aspen cervical thoracic o.
    Atlanta-Scottish Rite Hospital o.
    balanced forearm o.
    balance padding o.
    bar-and-shoe o.
    Bauerfeind malleolic ankle o.
    Beaufort seating o.
    Bebax o.
    Bennett o.
    BFO o.
    BioCast wrist/hand o.
    Biothotic foot o.
    Bodi Dynamic o.
    Bodi knee extension o.
    Boston postoperative hip o.
    cable-twister o.
    calcaneal spur cookie o.
    Caligamed ankle o.
    caliper o.
    Canadian knee o.
    carrot finger o.
    cervical o. (CO)
    cervical thoracic o.

cervical-thoracic-lumbar o.
cervical-thoracic-lumbar-sacral o.
cervicothoracic o. (CTO)
cervicothoracolumbosacral o.
chairback lumbosacral o.
clavicle o.
Comfy elbow o.
Comfy knee o.
Controller shoulder o.
copolymer ankle-foot o.
Corrxit foot and ankle o.
Craig-Scott o.
cranial o.
CranioCap custom-made cranial o.
cruciform anterior spinal
  hyperextension o.
Daytona cervical o.
Dermoplast-Plastazote o.
Diabetic D-Sole foot o.
dial-lock o.
dorsiflexion assist ankle joint
  ankle-foot o.
dual-photon electrospinal o.
DuraBoot o.
Dynamic elbow o.
Dynamic knee o.
Dynamic wrist o.
elbow o.
elbow-wrist-hand o. (EWHO)
Engen palmar finger o.
external o.
externally powered tenodesis o.
E-Z arm abduction o.
EZBrace o.
FirmFlex custom o.
Flex Foam o.
flexible o.
foot o.
Foot Levelers o.
Frejka o.
gator plastic o.
Gillette joint o.
Gillette modification of ankle-
  foot o.
GunSlinger shoulder o.
G/W Heel Lift, Inc. o.
hallux valgus o.
halo cervical o.
halo vest o.
hand o.
Heel Spur Special o.
hindfoot o.
hip o.
hip guidance o.
hip-knee o.
hip-knee-ankle o.
hip-knee-ankle-foot o. (HKAFO)
hyperextension o.
inflatable thoracic lumbosacral o.

Ipomax o.
ipos forefoot relief o.
ipos heel relief o.
J-24 cervical o.
J-45 contraflexion o.
Jewett-Benjamin cervical o.
Jewett contraflexion o.
Jewett postfusion o.
Jewett thoracolumbosacral o.
J-35 hyperextension o.
Johnson cervicothoracic o.
Johnson Kydex chairback o.
Johnson total hip stabilization o.
Jousto dropfoot splint, skid o.
J-55 postfusion o.
Kallassy o.
knee o.
knee-ankle o.
knee-ankle-foot o. (KAFO)
knee extension o.
knee management o.
Knight-Taylor and Williams
  spinal o.
Kydex chairback o.
L.A. cervical o.
leather o.
Levy & Rappel foot o.
L'Nard long opponens hand and
  wrist o.
L'Nard thoracolumbosacral o.
long opponens o.
lower limb o.
LSU reciprocation-gait o.
lumbar o.
lumbosacral o.
Lynco foot o.
Malibu cervical o.
MalleoLoc ankle o.
Maple Leaf hip o.
Marlin cervical o.
medial heel wedge o.
medial sole wedge o.
medical ankle o.
metal hybrid o.
Meyer cervical o.
Milwaukee o.
Milwaukee
  cervicothoracolumbosacral o.
Milwaukee scoliosis o.
Minerva o.
Modabber thumb o.
molded ankle-foot o. (MAFO)
molded lumbosacral o.
Monodos o.
MultiBoot o.
neoprene wrist o.
Newington o.
Newport MC hip o.
Newport total hip o.

O

orthosis *(continued)*

New York Orthopaedic front-opening o.
Oklahoma ankle joint o.
OmniFlex knee o.
Orlando hip-knee-ankle-foot o.
Orlau swivel walker o.
Ortholign spinal o.
Orthomedics Ultra-Guard hip o.
passive prehension o.
patellar tendon-bearing o.
patellar tendon weightbearing brace o.
patellar tracking o.
pediatric pressure relief ankle foot o.
pelvic stabilization o.
Phelps o.
pillow o.
plantar arch support o.
plastic o.
polypropylene ankle-foot o.
polypropylene glycol ankle-foot o.
polypropylene glycol thoracolumbosacral orthosis
posterior leaf-spring ankle-foot o.
pressure relief ankle-foot o.
pressure-relieving o.
Profile sitting o.
Pro-glide o.
Progressive ankle o.
Pucci inflatable elbow o.
Pucci inflatable knee o.
Pucci pediatric hand o.
Pucci pediatrics hand o.
Pucci rehab knee o.
reciprocal finger prehension o.
reciprocating gait o.
Respond ROM elbow o.
Respond ROM knee o.
resting o.
rigid o.
Rochester hip-knee-ankle-foot o.
sacroiliac o.
Scott-Craig o.
Scottish Rite hip o.
Seattle o.
Select joint o.
semirigid polypropylene ankle-foot o.
Shaeffer rigid o.
shoulder o.
shoulder-elbow-wrist-hand o.
single-photon electrospinal o.
Slim Option shoe o.
SOLEutions custom o.
SOMI o.
spinal o.
Sport-Stirrup o.

standard shell ankle-foot o.
standing frame o.
static o.
steel sole plate o.
sternooccipital mandibular immobilizer o.
supracondylar knee-ankle o.
supramalleolar o.
Swede-O Universal o.
Tachdjian o.
Taylor thoracolumbosacral o.
tenodesis o.
Thera-Pos elbow o.
Therapy Carrot Finger O.
Thomas collar cervical o.
Thomas heel o.
thoracic o.
thoracolumbosacral o. (TLSO)
thoracolumbosacral spinal o.
Tib-Transformer o.
TIRR foot-ankle o.
ToeOFF o.
tone-reducing ankle-foot o.
Toronto parapodium o.
total contact o.
total contact bivalve ankle-foot o.
total hip stabilization o.
TPE ankle-foot o.
TPE biomechanical foot o.
TRAFO o.
Transpire wrist o.
trunk-hip-knee-ankle-foot o.
turnbuckle wrist o.
UCOlite o.
Ultrabrace knee o.
Universal plantar fasciitis o. (UFO)
upper limb o.
VAPC dorsiflexion assist o.
Vari-Duct hip and knee o.
Viscoheel K, N o.
Viscoheel SofSpot o.
Viscolas o.
weight-relieving o.
Williams o.
Wilmington o.
wrist-driven lateral prehension o.
wrist-driven prehension o.
wrist-driven wrist-hand o.
wrist-hand o.
XPE foot o.
Zinco ankle o.

Orthosleep pillow
OrthoSorb
O. absorbable pin
O. pin fixation
O. pin nail
O. rod
Orthostar surgical table
Orthotech Controller knee brace

Orthotec pressurized fluid irrigation system
orthotic (*See also* orthosis)
    Aerodyn o.
    Alden CDI o.
    Alznner o.
    Amfit o.
    ankle-foot o.
    Arch Rival foot o.
    BIOflex o.
    BIOflex penile o.
    Biofoot o.
    BioSole-GEL o.
    Biothotic o.
    Blake inverted o.
    Blanke inverted tibialis posterior tendon o.
    Blue Line o.
    o. coiled spring twister
    cork, leather, and elastic o.
    custom healing o.
    custom-molded o.
    DesignLine o.
    o. device
    Diab-A-Thotics o.
    Dressflex shoe o.
    DSIS o.
    D-Soles o.
    Dual AFO Boot o.
    Duraleve custom molded foot o.
    Extreme foot o.
    FirmFlex custom o.
    FlexiSport o.
    Foot Levelers custom o.
    Footmaster o.
    functional o.
    Golden Comfort o.
    Golden Fitness o.
    Healthflex o.
    inverted o.
    Kinetic Wedge o.
    Lyte Fit o.
    Magnathotic o.
    Mayer o.
    MBS snap-on o.
    M-Pact flexible o.
    OB Gees maternity o.
    Ortho-Arch II o.
    Orthofit 9000, 9001 o.
    ParFlex Plus o.
    plastizote o.
    o. plate
    Powerstep o.
    PRAFO adjustable o.
    pressure-relief ankle-foot o.
    ProLite Plus runner's o.
    Pro Support Systems o.
    Pucci Air o.
    QuikFormables o.
    Rediform o.
    Sandalthotics postural support o.
    Slimthetics o.
    Sof Sole motion control o.
    Soft Super Sport o.
    Soft Support Preforms o.
    soft-tissue Super Sport o.
    SOLEutions soft plus o.
    SOLEutions sport shell o.
    Sporthotics o.
    Sport Preforms o.
    Sport-Rite o.
    Stratos o.
    Superfeet custom prefabricated o.
    Superform Contours o.
    Super Jock n' Jill store Superfeet o.
    Supralen cradle o.
    Supralen Schaefer o.
    Swiss Balance o.
    ThermoCork o.
    Thermo HK/Rohadur o.
    Thermo HK/Tepefom o.
    Thinline uncovered o.
    total contact shell ankle-foot o.
    UCOheal o.
    UCOlite o.
    UltraStep o.
    Universal plantar fasciitis o.
    Wirefoam o.
    XO soft sole o.
orthotopic
    o. neobladder
    o. univentricular artificial heart
Ortho-Trac adhesive skin traction bandage
Orthotrac pneumatic vest
Orthotripter
    OssaTron O.
Orthotron exerciser
OrthoTurn standing transfer aid
OrthoVise
    O. orthopaedic instrument
    O. with slap hammer
OrthoWedge healing shoe
Ortho-Wick foam liner
Orton enamel cleaver
Ortopad orthoptic patch
OS-5/Plus 2 knee brace
Osada
    O. ENAC-W10 quartz piezoelectric ultrasonic system
    O. portable electric handpiece system
    O. portable handpiece system
    O. saw
    O. XL-S30 electric handpiece system
OSAP appliance

O

Osbon
- O. ErecAid VCD
- O. pressure-point tension ring

Osborne punch

Oscar ultrasonic bone cement removal system

Osciflator balloon inflation syringe

oscillating
- o. blade
- o. Bucky
- o. grid
- o. saw

oscillator
- Babylog 8000 o.
- Hayek o.
- Infant Star 8000 o.
- optical parametric o.
- Stephanie 8000 o.

oscillometric blood pressure cuff

oscilloscope
- cathode ray o.
- o. instrument
- Norland digital o.
- single-channel electromyograph o.
- Tektronix 2214 o.
- Tektronix digital o.
- o. tuning station

Oscor pacing lead

OSD monitor

Osgood bone marrow needle

O'Shea lens

Osher
- O. corneal scissors
- O. foreign body forceps
- O. gonio/posterior pole lens
- O. hook
- O. panfundus lens
- O. superior rectus forceps
- O. surgical gonio/posterior pole lens
- O. surgical keratometer

OSI
- Orthopedic Systems Inc.
- OSI arthroscopic leg holder
- OSI extremity elevator
- OSI modular table system
- OSI well leg support

Osmette osmometer

OsmoCyte
- O. island wound care dressing
- O. PCA pillow wound dressing
- O. pillow
- O. pillow wound dressing

osmometer
- freezing point o.
- Osmette o.
- vapor pressure o.
- Vapro vapor pressure o.

OSMO reverse osmosis unit

osmotic
- o. dilator
- o. minipump

OssaTron
- O. device
- O. noninvasive extracorporeal shock wave therapy device
- O. Orthotripter
- O. shock wave therapy system

OsSatura
- O. BCP
- O. BCP bone graft
- O. BCP bone graft substitute
- O. synthetic bone graft substitution material
- O. TCP bone graft
- O. TCP bone graft substitute

OsseoCare
- O. drilling equipment
- O. machine

osseocartilaginous thoracic cage

Osseofix dental implant system

osseointegrated
- o. dental implant
- o. fixture
- o. oral implant
- o. prosthesis

osseoprosthesis

Osseotite 2-stage procedure implant

osseous
- o. coagulum trap
- o. Coagulum Trap collecting system
- o. implant

ossicle
- Tutoplast auditory o.

ossicle-holding
- o.-h. clamp
- o.-h. forceps

ossicular
- o. chain replacement prosthesis
- o. prosthesis
- o. reconstruction prosthesis

Ossix 6-month resorbable collagen membrane

Ossoff-Karlan laryngoscope

Ostase bone metabolism marker

Ostby dam frame

OsteoAnalyzer
- O. bone densitometry device
- O. densitometer
- O. device

osteoarthritic knee brace

osteoarthritis padded night sleeve brace

osteoarticular allograft

Osteobond copolymer bone cement

Osteocap hip prosthesis

osteochondral
- o. autograft transfer system

o. implant
o. transplant (OCT)
Osteo-Clage cerclage cable system
osteoclast
Collin o.
Rizzoli o.
osteodistractor
Ace/Normed o.
Osteofil allograft paste
OsteoForm mesh formable craniofacial mesh
OsteoGen
O. bone graft
O. bone grafting material
osteogenic
o. protein-1 (OP-1)
o. protein-1 bone graft
Osteogenics BoneSource synthetic bone replacement material
Osteograf
O. binder
O. bone grafting material
Osteograf/D bone grafting material
Osteograf/LD bone grafting material
Osteograf/N
OsteoGraft bone grafting wheel
OsteoGram 2000 densitometer
Osteoguide
OsteoHarvester bone harvester
osteoinductive enhanced graft gel
Osteolock
O. acetabular component
O. HA femoral component
O. hip prosthesis
Precision O.
Osteo-Lock endodontic stabilization kit
Osteomark NTx point-of-care device
Osteomatrix
O. bone filling material
O. bone restoration material
Osteomeasure computer-assisted image analyzer
Osteomed screw
osteomicrotome
Tessier o.
Osteomin
O. freeze-dried bone
O. Thermo-Ashed bone powder
O. Thermo-Ashed bone powder Pulvograft
Osteon
O. bur
O. drill
Osteonics
O. acetabular dome hole plug
O. HA femoral implant
O. jig
O. Omnifit-C
O. Omnifit-C stem

O. Omnifit-HA component
O. Omnifit-HA hip stem
O. prosthesis
O. reamer
O. Scorpio insert
O. Scorpio posterior cruciate retaining total knee system
O. spinal system
Osteopatch
osteophyte elevator
osteoplastic flap clamp
osteoplasty
crossed delivery for o. (CDO)
Osteoplate implant
OsteoPower drilling and cutting machine
Osteo-Rx coaxial curved bone biopsy and infusion set
OsteoSet
O. bone filler
O. bone graft substitute
O. resorbable bead kit
Osteo-Site bone biopsy needle
OsteoStat
O. disposable power tool
O. single-use power surgical equipment
OsteoStim
O. cervical allograft spacer
O. DBM putty
O. implantable bone grown stimulator
O. resorbable bone graft substitute
osteosynthesis
wire o.
OsteoTite bone screw
osteotome
AcuDriver o.
Acufex o.
air compression o.
Alexander costal o.
Anderson-Neivert o.
Andrews o.
API o.
Army o.
Aufranc o.
bayonet o.
Box o.
Burton o.
Cebotome o.
Chermel o.
Cherry o.
Cinelli o.
Clayton o.
Cloward spinal fusion o.
Converse o.
Cook o.
Cottle o.
Cottle crossbar chisel o.

osteotome *(continued)*
    Cottle-Medicon o.
    curved o.
    Dautrey o.
    Dingman o.
    disposable 1-piece o.
    flexible blade o.
    Fomon o.
    French-pattern o.
    guarded o.
    Hendel guided o.
    hexagonal handle o.
    Hibbs o.
    Hohmann o.
    Hoke o.
    Howorth o.
    Kazanjian action-type o.
    lacrimal o.
    Lahey Clinic thin o.
    Lambotte o.
    lateral o.
    Leinbach o.
    Lexer o.
    MacGregor nasal o.
    Manchester nasal o.
    manual o.
    Mathews o.
    maxillofacial o.
    Mayfield bayonet o.
    McCollough o.
    Meyerding o.
    MGH o.
    Micro-Aire o.
    Miner o.
    mini-Lambotte o.
    mini-Lexer o.
    Mitchell o.
    Moberg o.
    Moe o.
    Murphy o.
    nasal o.
    nasofrontal o.
    Neivert o.
    orthopaedic o.
    Padgett o.
    Parkes o.
    Peck o.
    Quisling-Parkes o.
    Rhoton o.
    Rish o.
    Rubin o.
    Rubin nasofrontal o.
    Sheehan o.
    Silver o.
    Silver nasal o.
    sinus lift o.
    Smith-Petersen straight o.
    Stille o.
    straight o.

    Swanson o.
    Tardy o.
    Tessier o.
    Ultra-Cut Hoke o.
    U.S. Army o.
    Ward nasal o.
    West o.
    Zeiss o.
osteotomy pin
Osteotron stimulator for bone union
OsteoView
    O. desktop hand x-ray system
    O. device
    Digital O.
    O. digital bone densitometer
    O. 2000 digital imaging system
    O. 2000 imaging system
    O. 2000 system
    O. x-ray device
Osteovit bone matrix
Osterballe precision needle
Ostia stent
ostium seeker
Ostofresh formula
ostomy
    o. appliance
    o. bag
    o. Shadow Buddy
Ostreg spinal marker system
Ostwald-Folin pipette
Ostycut bone biopsy needle
OSU frame
O'Sullivan-O'Connor
    O.-O. self-retaining abdominal
      retractor
    O.-O. vaginal retractor
    O.-O. vaginal speculum
OSV II Smart Valve system
Osypka atrial lead
Otis
    O. anoscope
    O. bougie à boule
    O. bougie à boule dilator
    O. sound
    O. ureterotome
    O. urethrotome
OTI ultrasound B & A scan
otoabrader
Otocap myringotomy blade
OtoClear disposable tip
otoconial plug
Oto-Flex
    O.-F. carbide bur
    O.-F. crura saw
    O.-F. diamond bur
    O.-F. diamond knife
    O.-F. drill
    O.-F. perforator
    O.-F. trephine

OtoLAM laser
Otomed eye protector
OtoScan ear aeration system
otoscope
    acoustic o.
    Advanced beta 200 o.
    Alpha fiberoptic pocket o.
    Bruening pneumatic o.
    Brunton o.
    Earscope o.
    fiberoptic o.
    Grafco o.
    halogen o.
    Micro-Halogen o.
    Microtek Heine o.
    Mini-Fibralux pocket o.
    Minilux pocket o.
    office diagnostic rechargeable o.
    pneumatic o.
    Politzer air bag o.
    Rica pneumatic o.
    Riester o.
    Sabre All-In-One o.
    Siegel o.
    Siegel pneumatic o.
    Siegle o.
    o. speculum
    StarMed video o.
    surgical o.
    Toynbee o.
    video o.
    Welch Allyn dual-purpose o.
    Welch Allyn operating o.
Ototemp 3000 ear thermometer
ototome irrigation kit
Otovent autoinflation kit
OtoView rod lens endoscope
Oto-Wick
    O.-W. medicated ear sponge
    Pope O.-W.
OTPS
    orthopaedic trauma plating system
    OTPS biodegradable pin
    OTPS mesh
    OTPS mesh system
Otsby dam frame
Ott/Mayo Channel Sampling kit
Otto
    O. Bock 1A30 Greissinger Plus foot
    O. Bock 1D25 Dynamic Plus foot
    O. Bock Mobis mobility system
    O. Bock 3R65 children's hydraulic knee joint
    O. Bock 3R60 EBS knee
    O. Bock 3R45 modular knee joint
    O. Bock 3R80 modular rotary hydraulic knee

    O. Bock Safety constant-friction knee
    O. Bock system electric hand
    O. Bock system electric hands prosthesis
OTW
    over-the-wire
    OTW HighSail coronary dilatation catheter
    OTW perfusion catheter
    OTW thrombolytic brush
Oudin resonator
Oulu neuronavigator system
Outback LTD reentry catheter
outflow
    o. cannula
    o. cardiac patch
outlet
    o. cannula
    o. forceps
out-of-cast ankle brace
out-of-scope lithotriptor
output
    o. device
    o. signal processor
Outrigger
outrigger
    o. splint
    o. wire
outside-the-boot brace
OV-1 surgical keratometer
Oval-8
    O.-8 finger splint
    O.-8 kit
    O.-8 ring splint
    O.-8 sizing set
oval
    o. bur
    o. cup erysiphake
    o. cup forceps
    o. curette
    o. cutting bur
    o. esophagoscope
    o. forceps
    o. open esophagoscope
    o. optical zone marker
    o. piston gauge
    o. snare
    o. speculum
    o. window curette
    o. window pick
oval-window hook
ovary forceps
Ovation
    O. cutting instrument
    O. falloposcopy system
oven
    Coltene o.
    Thermoprep heating o.

O

over-bed table
Overcast cast cover
overcouch tube
overdenture
    bar-supported o.
    implant-supported o.
    mandibular o.
    removable partial o.
overhead
    o. light
    o. projector
    o. zoom (OZM)
Overholt
    O. clip-applying forceps
    O. periosteal elevator
    O. rib rasp
Overholt-Geissendörfer arterial forceps
Overholt-Mixter dissecting forceps
overlapping pincer
overlay
    Airdance alternating o.
    Alamo alternating low air loss
      mattress o.
    Bodyline sleeper mattress o.
    BodyWrap premium o.
    DeRoyal mattress o.'s
    First Step select low-air o.
    Geo-Matt therapeutic foam o.
    Hydro-Ease II gel flotation
      mattress o.
    Hydro-Ease I water flotation
      mattress o.
    o. mattress
    MIP anatomic o.
    PAL pump for air mattress o.
    Stimulite honeycomb mattress o.
    UltraForm mattress o.
    x-ray o.
overprojecting nasal tip
oversensing pacemaker
over-shoulder strap
oversize tennis shoe
over-the-door traction unit
over-the-ear earphones
over-the-endoscope Witzel dilator
over-the-needle infusion catheter
over-the-wire (OTW)
    o.-t.-w. Greenfield filter
    o.-t.-w. pacing lead
    o.-t.-w. PTCA balloon catheter
    o.-t.-w. set
overtube
    flexible endoscopic o.
    Mill-Rose flexible endoscopic o.
    oroesophageal o.
    rotational colonoscope o.
    split o.

    Steigmann-Goff endoscopic
      ligature o.
    Williams varix injection o.
over-tying wire
Oves cervical cap
ovoid
    Delclos o.
    Fleming o.
    Fletcher-Suit tandem and o.
    Manchester o.
    tandem and o.
OvuKIT
ovum
    o. curette
    o. forceps
OvuQuick
    O. One-Step ovulation kit
    O. Self-Test
OvuStick
OV-Watch fertility predictor
Owens
    O. balloon
    O. balloon catheter
    O. gauze dressing
    O. Lo-Profile dilatation catheter
    O. silk
    O. Surgical dressing
Oxford
    O. fixator
    O. large-bore imaging system
      scanner
    O. magnet
    O. meniscal unicompartmental knee
      system
    O. meniscal unicompartment
      prosthesis
    O. uncompartmental device
    O. unicompartmental knee
OxiFirst
    O. fetal monitoring system
    O. fetal oxygen monitor
OxiFlow
OxiLink oximeter probe cover
OxiMax pulse oximetry device
oximeter
    Accusat pulse o.
    Armstrong handheld pulse o.
    AutoCorr portable pulse o.
    AVOXimeter 4000 CO o.
    AVOXimeter 1000E whole
      blood o.
    BCI 3301 handheld pulse o.
    BI-OX III ear o.
    Capnocheck II CO_2/pulse o.
    carbon monoxide o.
    CO_2SMO capnograph/pulse o.
    Cricket recording pulse o.
    Criticare pulse o.
    Criticare 503 pulse o.

Datascope pulse o.
Datascope 300 pulse o.
Datex model CH-S-23 pulse o.
Dinamap monitor/Oxytrak pulse o.
Dinamap pulse o.
ear o.
finger o.
FingerPrint handheld pulse o.
handheld pulse o.
Healthdyne o.
Healthdyne pulse o.
Hewlett-Packard ear o.
Invos cerebral o.
Invos 3100 cerebral o.
Invos transcranial cerebral o.
Masimo Set pulse o.
MiniCorr digital o.
MiniOX V pulse o.
MRL o.
Nellcor N20, N200 pulse o.
Nellcor N-20PA pulse o.
Nellcor N-20 pulse o.
Nellcor N200 pulse o.
Nellcor N-series pulse o.
Nellcor Symphony N-3000 pulse o.
Nellcor Symphony pulse o.
Nonin Onyx pulse o.
Novametrix pulse o.
NPB-75 handheld
  capnograph/pulse o.
NPB-40 handheld pulse o.
NPB-295 pulse o.
N-180 pulse o.
ODISsey tissue o.
Ohmeda handheld o.
Ohmeda Minx pulse o.
Ohmeda pulse o.
Ohmeda 3800 pulse o.
Onyx finger pulse o.
Oxypleth pulse o.
Oxyshuttle pulse o.
OxyTemp handheld pulse o.
Oxytrak pulse o.
Palco Laboratories Model 300, 400
  pulse o.
Palco Laboratories model 300, 400
  pulse o.
PalmSAT digital handheld pulse o.
pulse o.
Pulsox-5 portable pulse o.
Respironics 920P handheld pulse o.
Respironics 930 pulse o.
RPO o.
Satellite Plus pulse o.
SensorMedics SAT-TRAK pulse o.
Somanetics Invos 3100 cerebral o.
SpO$_2$-5001 o.
SpotCheck+ handheld pulse o.

Tidal Wave Sp capnometer/pulse o.
tissue reflectance o.
oximetric catheter
oximetry
  o. catheter
  o. sensor
Oxinium hip implant
Oxiplex/SP
  O. bioresorbable product
  O. gel
Oxiport laryngeal blade
**OxiScan oximetry recording and
  reporting system**
Oxisensor
  O. fetal oxygen saturation monitor
  O. II adult adhesive sensor
  O. II adult sensor
  O. oxygen transducer
  O. transducer
Oxycel
  O. dressing
  O. gauze
OxyData Plus oxygen monitor
Oxydome oxygen therapy system
oxygen
  o. analyzer
  o. disposable boot device
  o. hood
  o. mask
  o. saturation meter
  o. (size D, E, M, G, and H)
    cylinder
  o. supply line
  o. tank
  o. tent
oxygenating mouthguard
oxygenator
  Affinity o.
  Biocor 200 high-performance o.
  bubble o.
  Capiox-E bypass system o.
  Capiox hollow flow o.
  Cobe CML o.
  Cobe Optima hollow-fiber
    membrane o.
  disc o.
  extracorporeal membrane o.
    (ECMO)
  extracorporeal pump o.
  Gambro o.
  intravascular o.
  Lilliput neonatal o.
  Maxima Plus plasma resistant
    fiber o.
  membrane o.
  Monolyth o.
  pump o.
  Sarns membrane o.

O

oxygenator *(continued)*
    Shiley o.
    Spiralgold o.
oxygen-based therapeutic system
Oxyguard
    O. endoscopy bite block
    O. oxygenating mouthguard
Oxy-Holter
Oxyhood
    O. oxygen hood
    O. pressurizer
oxylate dentin bonding system
Oxylator
    O. EM-100 emergency resuscitation device
    O. positive pressure resuscitation and inhalation system
OxyLead interconnect cable
Oxylite
    O. ambulatory oxygen system
    O. oxygen monitor

Oxymatic electronic oxygen conserver
Oxymax aeration system
Oxymizer device
Oxypleth pulse oximeter
Oxypod oxygen hood
oxyquinoline dressing
OxySAT oxygen saturation meter
Oxyshuttle pulse oximeter
OxyTemp handheld pulse oximeter
OxyTip sensor
Oxytrak pulse oximeter
oyster-shell brace
oyster splint
OZM
    overhead zoom
      OZM colposcope

P-700 Color Velocity Imaging system
PA
    PA catheter
    PA portal
PaBA anchor
Pac
    Smart Triage P.
pacchionian
pace
    P. bipolar pacing catheter
    p. card
    P. Plus System scanner
PACE-2C DNA probe test
Paceart complete pacemaker patient testing system
pacemaker
    AAI p.
    AAI/AAIR p.
    AAI single-chamber p.
    AAT p.
    Accufix p.
    Activitrax II p.
    Activitrax single-chamber responsive p.
    Activitrax variable-rate p.
    activity-guided p.
    activity-sensing p.
    Actros p.
    Actros+ p.
    adaptive-rate p.
    Addvent atrioventricular p.
    Aequitron p.
    Affinity p.
    AFP II p.
    AICD p.
    Alcatel p.
    American Optical R-inhibited p.
    antitachycardia p.
    AOO p.
    artificial p.
    Arzco p.
    Astra T4, T6 p.
    ASVIP p.
    atrial-based p.
    atrial demand inhibited p.
    atrial demand triggered p.
    atrial synchronous noncompetitive p.
    atrial synchronous ventricular inhibited p. (ASVIP)
    atrial triggered noncompetitive p.
    Atricor Cordis p.
    atrioventricular junctional p.
    atrioventricular sequential demand p.

Autima II dual-chamber cardiac p.
automated external defibrillator p. (AEDP)
AV junctional p.
AV synchronous p.
Axios p.
Betacel-Biotronik p.
bifocal demand DVI p.
Biorate p.
Biotronik p.
bipolar p.
bladder p.
breathing p.
burst p.
Byrel SX p.
p. can
cardiac p.
Cardiac P., Inc. (CPI)
cardiac resynchronization therapy p. (CRT-P)
Cardio-Control p.
p. catheter
Chardack-Greatbatch p.
Chardack Medtronic p.
Chorus DDD p.
Chorus RM rate-responsive dual-chamber p.
Chronos 04 p.
cilium p.
Circadia dual-chamber rate-adaptive p.
circadian p.
committed mode p.
Contak CD ventricular resynchronization p.
Cook p.
Coratomic R wave inhibited p.
Cordis Atricor p.
Cortomic p.
Cosmos 283 DDD p.
Cosmos II DDD p.
CPI/Guidant p.
CPI Microthin DI, DII lithium-powered programmable p.
crosstalk p.
Cybertach automatic-burst atrial p.
Cybertach 60 bipolar p.
Cylos p.
Daig ESI-II, DSI-III screw-in lead p.
Dash single-chamber rate-adaptic p.
DDD p.
DDI mode p.
demand cardiac p.
Dialog p.

P

pacemaker *(continued)*
   Discovery DDDR p.
   Dromos p.
   dual-chamber AV sequential p.
   dual-chamber Medtronic Kappa
      400 p.
   dual-pass p.
   Durapulse p.
   DVI p.
   Ectocor p.
   electric cardiac p.
   p. electrode
   Electrodyne p.
   electronic p.
   Elema p.
   Elema-Schonander p.
   Elite dual-chamber rate-
      responsive p.
   Encor p.
   endocardial bipolar p.
   Endotak p.
   Enertrax p.
   Enertrax 7l00 p.
   EnRhythm p.
   Enterra gastrointestinal p.
   Entity p.
   epicardial p.
   Ergos O_2 dual-chamber rate-
      responsive p.
   escape p.
   external p.
   external asynchronous p.
   external demand p.
   external-internal p.
   externally controlled noninvasive
      programmed stimulation p.
   external transthoracic p.
   Fast-Pass lead p.
   fixed-rate asynchronous atrial p.
   fixed-rate asynchronous
      ventricular p.
   fully automatic atrioventricular
      Universal dual-channel p.
   GE p.
   General Electric p.
   Genisis dual-chamber p.
   Guardian p.
   Guidant CRM p.
   heart p.
   hermetically sealed p.
   implantable p.
   implanted p.
   Integrity AFx DR model 5346 p.
   Intermedics atrial antitachycardia p.
   Intermedics Cyberlith X
      multiprogrammable p.
   Intermedics lithium-powered p.
   Intermedics Marathon dual-chamber
      rate-responsive p.

   Intermedics Marathon VVI single-
      chamber p.
   Intermedics Quantum unipolar p.
   Intermedics Stride p.
   Intertach II p.
   junctional p.
   Kairos p.
   Kantrowitz p.
   Kappa 700, 900 p.
   Kappa dual-chamber p.
   Kappa 400-series p.
   Lambda Omni Stanicor p.
   latent p.
   Lillehei p.
   lithium p.
   lithium-powered p.
   Maestro implantable cardiac p.
   Mark IV respiratory p.
   Maxilith p.
   Medtronic Activitrax rate-responsive
      unipolar ventricular p.
   Medtronic bipolar p.
   Medtronic Chardack p.
   Medtronic corkscrew electrode p.
   Medtronic demand p.
   Medtronic Elite II p.
   Medtronic external/internal p.
   Medtronic Kappa 400 p.
   Medtronic Minix p.
   Medtronic Pacette p.
   Medtronic RF 5998 p.
   Medtronic SP 502 p.
   Medtronic Symbios p.
   Medtronic temporary p.
   Medtronic Thera DR p.
   Medtronic Thera i-series cardiac p.
   Mentor bladder p.
   Meridian p.
   Meta DDDR p.
   Meta II p.
   Meta MV p.
   Meta rate-responsive p.
   Microlith P p.
   Micro Minix p.
   Microny II SR+ p.
   Microny K SR p.
   Momentum DR p.
   Multicor II cardiac p.
   multiprogrammable p.
   Nanos 01 p.
   natural p.
   noninvasive temporary p.
   Nova II p.
   nuclear-powered p.
   Optima p.
   Orthocor II p.
   oversensing p.
   Pacesetter Synchrony p.
   Pacette p.

Paragon II p.
permanent myocardial p.
permanent rate-responsive p.
permanent transvenous demand p.
  (PTDP)
permanent ventricular p.
Philos DR-T p.
physiologic p.
Pinnacle p.
Programalith A-V p.
Programalith II, III p.
programmable p.
Programmer III p.
Pulsar DDD p.
Pulsar NI implantable p.
P-wave triggered ventricular p.
QT interval sensing p.
Quantum p.
radiofrequency p.
rate-adaptive p.
rate-modulated p.
rate-responsive p.
Reflex 8220 p.
reflex p.
rescuing p.
respiratory-dependent p.
reversion p.
runaway p.
SAVVI p.
screw-in lead p.
sensor p.
sensor-based single-chamber p.
Sequicor II, III p.
shifting p.
Siemens p.
Siemens-Elema
  multiprogrammable p.
single-chamber p.
single-pass p.
sinus node p.
Solar p.
Sorin p.
Spectrax bipolar p.
Spectrax programmable
  Medtronic p.
standby p.
Stanicor p.
Starr-Edwards p.
Symbios 7006 p.
synchronous mode p.
Synergyst DDD p.
Synergyst II p.
tachycardia-terminating p.
Telectronics p.
temperature-sensing p.
temporary p.
temporary transvenous p.
Thera-SR p.
tined lead p.

transcutaneous p.
transmural antitachycardia p.
transpericardial p.
transthoracic p.
transvenous ventricular demand p.
Trilogy DC+ p.
Trilogy SR+ single-chamber p.
Ultra p.
unipolar atrial p.
unipolar atrioventricular p.
unipolar sequential p.
variable-rate p.
VAT p.
VDD p.
Ventak AICD p.
Ventak ECD p.
Ventak PRx p.
ventricular asynchronous p.
ventricular demand p.
ventricular demand-inhibited p.
ventricular demand-triggered p.
ventricular triggered p.
Versatrax cardiac p.
Versatrax II 7000A p.
Vigor DR p.
Vista TRS p.
Vitatron Diamond II p.
VOO p.
VVD mode p.
VVI p.
VVI/AAI p.
VVIR single-chamber rate-
  adaptive p.
VVT p.
wandering atrial p.
Xyrel p.
Zoll M-series defibrillator
  monitor p.
Zoll noninvasive p.
**P/ACE MDQ series capillary
  electrophoresis system**
Paceport catheter
pacer
    Intertach II p.
    PolySafe p.
pacer-cardioverter-defibrillator (PCD)
    Jewel p.-c.-d.
pacer-cardioverter defibrillator
Pacesetter
    P. Affinity SR generator
    P. APS II 3004 programmer
    P. APS pacemaker programmer
    P. knee brace
    P. Synchrony III pulse generator
    P. Synchrony pacemaker
    P. Tendril DX steroid-eluting
      active-fixation pacing lead
    P. Trilogy DR+ pulse generator
Pacesetter/St. Jude lead

P

Pacette pacemaker
PachKnife
Pachmate DGH55 pachymeter
Pach-Pen
    P.-P. corneal thickness measurer
    P.-P. XL pachymeter
    P.-P. XL tonometer
pachymeter, pachometer
    Advent p.
    Alcon ultrasound p.
    Compuscan-P p.
    corneal p.
    DGH 2000 AP ultrasonic p.
    Ophthasonic p.
    optic p.
    optical p.
    Orbscan p.
    Pachmate DGH55 p.
    Pach-Pen XL p.
    Packo pars plana cannula p.
    PalmScan AP2000 portable p.
    Sonogage ultrasound p.
    ultrasonic p.
    ultrasound p.
    Villasensor ultrasonic p.
pachymeter-KMI
    ultrasound p.-KMI
Pachymetric P55 analyzer
Pacific
    P. Coast flexible laminar bone
      strip
    P. Coast hearing aid
pacifier
    sucrose p.
    sugar-dipped p.
    sweetened p.
    water p.
pacing
    p. catheter
    p. counter
    p. esophageal stethoscope
    p. wire
    p. wire electrode
pack
    Adaptic p.
    AeroGear fanny p.
    Arctic Blaze hot/cold p.
    Avitene p.
    Back-Ease aromatherapy hot/cold p.
    barrier p.
    Barrier laparoscopy LAVH p.
    Barrier phaco extracapsular p.
    Baxter personal Von-Loc ice p.
    BodyIce cold p.
    CLO Recirculating Slim P.
    cold p.
    Coldhot p.
    Colpacs p.
    cool p.

Cool Comfort cold p.
CP2 inflatable cold p.
DynaHeat hot p.
E-Z Heat hot p.
First Teeth Infa-dent Combo P.
Flents breast comfort p.
gauze p.
gel p.
Gelfoam p.
Glacier P.
hot p.
hot moist p.
hot wet p.
hydrocollator gel p.
hydrocollator steam p.
ice p.
I.C.E. Down cold p.
instant cold p.
Jack Frost hot/cold p.
JoyBags therapeutic heat p.
K p.
Kennedy sinus p.
Kirkland periodontal p.
Kold Kompress cold p.
Kool Kit cold therapy p.
Koolpak cold p.
Med-Wick nasal p.
Merocel p.
Mikulicz p.
MSC cold p.
M-Zole 7 Dual P.
nasal p.
Neck-Roll aromatherapy hot/cold p.
oropharyngeal p.
PCA periodontal p.
Peri-Cold p.
Peri-Gel p.
Peri-Warm p.
Polar P.
Promise pad and pant trial p.
Rhino Rocket nasal p.
RIK fluid-filled head p.
Slik-Pak nonstick nasal p.
Softouch cold/hot p.
subfascial gauze p.
Swiss p.
TheraBeads microwaveable moist
  heat p.
Thera-Med cold p.
thermal p.
ThermalSoft hot & cold p.'s
Thermophore hot p.
Ultimate Cold N' Hot P.
Unna-Flex Plus venous ulcer
  convenience p.
Vaseline petrolatum p.
Vitros Immunodiagnostic Products
  anti-HBc reagent p.
Whitehall Glacier P.

Packard
P. Auto-Gamma 5650 analyzer
P. intraocular lens
P. luminometer
P. Merlin life-monitoring system
P. radioimmunoassay system
packed bead
packer
Balshi p.
Bernay uterine p.
dental amalgam p.
gauze p.
Jewett bone chip p.
Kitchen postpartum gauze p.
Lorenz gauze p.
P. mosquito forceps
Torpin automatic uterine gauze p.
P. Wick extrusion handpiece
packing
abdominal p.
AlgiDerm wound p.
p. forceps
gelatin sponge p.
Gelfoam p.
impregnated vaginal p.
iodoform gauze p.
Kaltostat hydrofiber wound p.
Merocel epistaxis p.
MeroGel nasal p.
Mikulicz p.
nasal p.
Rhino Rocket nasal p.
SinuSeal nasal p.
p. strip
vaginal p.
Weimert epistaxis p.
wound p.
Packo
P. pars plana cannula
P. pars plana cannula pachymeter
Pacs
Boo-Boo P.
PAD
pressure-applied dressing
pad
Achilles heel p.
Airex balance p.
Airlite support p.
Air-O-Pad p.
Akton p.
Aliplast p.
alternating pressure p.
antidecubitus p.
aperture p.
Aquaflex gel p.
Aquaflex ultrasound gel p.
Aquatech cast p.
Aquatherm bed p.
balance p.

Bauerfeind silicone heel p.
BDP p.
Bichat deep cheek p.
Breathe Easy foam p.
Bumpa Bed crib bumper p.
buttress p.
CairPad incontinence p.
CarraGauze hydrogel wound dressing p.
C.B.T. conductive stretcher p.
C.B.T. nonconductive stretcher p.
C.B.T. Siderail bumper p.
Charnley foam suture p.
Chaston eye p.
Chito-Seal topical hemostasis p.
Cliniguard p.
cloverleaf met foot p.
cold p.
Conform II with Heel-Ease Nature Sleep pressure p.
convoluted mattress p.
crest buttress p.
Curity ABD p.
dancer's p.
decubitus p.
digitizing p.
Dignity Plus Briefmates P.
dinner p.
disposable electrode p.
distal star p.
Elbowlift suspension p.
electrical grounding p.
p. electrode
electrode p.
Envisan dextranomer p.
ESU dispersive p.
Expansion control Waffle mattress p.
eye p.
E-Z hold adhesive catheter tube holder p.
flotation gel p.
fluid control trauma p.
foam p.
gauze p.
gel p.
gelatin sponge p.
Gelfoam p.
grounding p.
Hapad heel p.
Hapad longitudinal metatarsal arch p.
Hapad prefabricated wool felt p.
Heartstream FR2 AED with attenuated defibrillation p.
heat p.
horseshoe heel p.
horseshoe-shaped p.
hot p.

pad *(continued)*
    hydrocollator p.
    hydropolymer p.
    Iceman cold therapy p.
    Impress Softpatch urinary p.
    instrument stabilizer p.
    InSync miniform p.
    internal gel p.
    Intersorb absorptive burn p.
    Iodoflex solid gel p.
    J p.
    Johnson & Johnson nonstick p.'s
    K p.
    Kendall Company Telfa p.
    Kerlix cast p.
    Kins soaker p.
    lap p.
    laparotomy p.
    Littman defibrillation p.
    MagneCore magnetic therapy p.
    magnetic bed p.
    magnetic mat p.
    magnetic mattress p.
    Mayfield pediatric horseshoe p.
    Medical genuine sheepskin p.
    Microcell alternating pressure p.
    Mikulicz p.
    MPM conductive gel p.
    3M Tegaderm transparent dressing with absorbent p.
    Ortho-Cel p.
    Ortho-Foam elbow/heel p.
    Pedifix crest p.
    Pedifix hammertoe p.
    Pen/Alps distal p.
    perineal p.
    polyvinylsiloxane impression p.
    prefabricated wool felt p.
    Presence bladder control p.
    Provide incontinence p.
    Redigrip knee p.
    Relton frame p.
    Roho Dry Flotation wheelchair p.
    Roho heel p.
    scaphoid p.
    Scholl p.
    second skin p.
    sensor p.
    Signa P.
    silicone p.
    Silipos digital p.
    Sleep Guardian foam p.
    SlimLine peach sheet care p.
    Sof-Rol cast p.
    SomaSensor p.
    Sontac gel p.
    Soothies glycerin gel breast p.
    Sorbothane recoil p.
    Spectra p.
    S'port Max stabilization p.
    Staph-Chek p.
    Steri-Pad gauze p.
    Stimulite honeycomb seating p.
    Superstat topical hemostatic wound p.
    Sure Sport p.
    table heating p.
    Tegaderm transparent dressing with absorbent p.
    Telfa adhesive p.
    Tempur-Med x-ray table p.
    Tendersorb ABD p.
    TENS p.
    T-Foam bed p.
    Thermalon heat-cold p.
    Thermapad p.
    Thermophore moist heat p.
    TopiFoam silicone gel adhesive foam p.
    UltraEase ultrasound p.
    ultrasound p.
    Vac-Pac p.
    valgus knee control p.
    varus knee control p.
    ventilated incontinence p.
    wheelchair p.
    wireless handheld Web p.
    Zimfoam p.

padded
    p. aluminum splint
    p. board splint
    p. clamp

padding
    cast p.
    Delta-Rol cast p.
    Dyna-Flex Layer One p.
    Kerlix cast p.
    moleskin p.
    Molestick p.
    pressure relief p.
    Protouch orthopaedic p.
    QuickStick p.
    Reston p.
    Sifoam p.
    splint p.
    SurePress absorbent p.
    Therafoam p.
    Thero-Skin gel p.
    Webril cotton p.

paddle
    compression p.
    defibrillation p.
    defibrillator p.
    Rosen nucleus p.
    spot-compression p.
    spot compression p.

Padgett
    P. dermatome

P. dermatome blade
P. endoscope
P. hydraulic hand dynamometer
P. implant
P. manual dermatome
P. mesh skin graft
P. osteotome
P. prosthesis
Padgett-Hood dermatome
PadKit sample collection system
Padua bladder urinary pouch
pain
p. control infusion pump
p. threshold gauge
PainBuster postoperative pain relief system
Paine carpal tunnel retinaculotome
PainFree pump
pak
Apollo hot/cold p.
pal
Vital-Port Infusion P.
Palacos
P. cement adhesive
P. radiopaque bone cement
P. R bone cement
palatal
p. bar
p. implant
p. lifting device
p. lift prosthesis
p. obturator
p. prosthesis
palate
p. hook
p. retractor
palate-free activator
palate-type mouthgag
palatorrhaphy elevator
Palco
P. enuretic alarm system
P. Laboratories model 300, 400 pulse oximeter
P. Laboratories Model 300, 400 pulse oximeter
Palfique Estelite tooth shade resin material
PAL-Guard postamputation limb guard
Pall
P. ELD-96 Set Saver filter
P. filter PL100KL/50K
P. leukocyte removal filter
P. Leukogard-6 leukocyte reduction arterial blood filter
P. PL100 filter
P. RC100 filter
P. RC50 filter
P. transfusion filter

palmar
p. clip
p. plate
p. swab kit
p. T-plate
p. wrist splint
Palmaz
P. Corinthian biliary stent and delivery system
P. Corinthian stent
P. Genesis balloon-expanded stent
P. Genesis stent
P. large balloon-expanded stent
P. medium balloon-expanded stent
P. P394 stainless steel balloon-expandable stent
P. P564 stent
P. stent
P. 424, 784 stent
P. vascular stent
Palmaz-Schatz
P.-S. balloon-expandable stent
P.-S. biliary stent
P.-S. coronary stent
P.-S. Crown balloon-expandable stent
P.-S. Crown stent
P.-S. long medium balloon-expanded stent
P.-S. PS-204 stent
P.-S. stent
Palmer
P. bone nail
P. ovarian biopsy forceps
palm guard
PalmSAT digital handheld pulse oximeter
PalmScan AP2000 portable pachymeter
P.A.L.M. ultraviolet laser microbeam
PalmVue
P. ECG*stat*
P. system
Palomar
P. E2000 laser
P. EpiLaser
P. E2000 ruby laser hair reduction
P. EsteLux
P. SLP1000 diode laser system
Palpagraph breast mapping device
palpating needle
palpation probe
palpator
blunt p.
PAL pump for air mattress overlay
Paltrinieri-Trentani prosthesis
Palumbo
P. ankle stabilizer
P. knee brace
P. knee support

P

Palumbo (*continued*)
    P. patella tracker
    P. stabilizing brace
    P. stabilizing knee brace
PAM2, PAM3 monitor
Panacryl suture
Panafil
    P. enzymatic débrider
    P. enzymatic débriding agent
Panafil-White
    P.-W. enzymatic débrider
    P.-W. enzymatic débriding agent
Panalok
    P. absorbable suture
    P. absorbable suture anchor
    P. RC QuickAnchor Plus suture
    anchor
Panasol II home phototherapy system
Panasonic
    P. hearing aid
    P. hearing aid battery
pancake MRI magnet
panchamber UV lens
Pancoast suture
pancreatic
    p. duct stent
    p. endoprosthesis
    p. pseudocyst
pancreatoscope
    peroral electronic p.
    ultrathin p.
Pancretec 2000 pump
Panda
    P. gastrostomy feeding tube
    P. nasoenteric feeding tube
Panelipse panoramic x-ray machine
panendoscope
    cap-fitted p.
    flexible forward-viewing p.
    foroblique p.
    McCarthy p.
    Storz p.
    Wolf rigid p.
Panex-E panoramic x-ray machine
panfundoscope
Panje
    P. prosthesis
    P. valve
    P. voice button
    P. voice button prosthesis
panning dish
Pannu-Kratz-Barraquer speculum
PanoGauze
    P. dressing
    P. hydrogel-impregnated gauze
    P. impregnated gauze
Panomat
    P. infusion pump
    P. microinfusion pump

Panoplex hydrogel wound dressing
Panoramic200
    P. nonmydriatic ophthalmoscope
    P. scanning laser ophthalmoscope
    P. ultra-widefield ophthalmic
    imaging device
panoramic loupe
Panorex panoramic x-ray machine
Panosol II home phototherapy device
Panoview
    P. arthroscope
    P. Plus sinuscope
    P. rod-lens ureteroscope
panretinal photocoagulation (PRP)
pant, pl. **pants**
    Conveen net p.
    Dignity easy access p.
    Dignity Plus Briefmates stretch
    mesh p.
    Dignity Plus regular p.
    Endo pants
    Feeln' Sure p.
    First Quality pad insert and p.
    Free & Active incontinence p.
    Kins pull-on waterproof p.
    Lady Dignity Plus p.
    MAST pants
    Promise washable knit p.
    reusable incontinence p.
    Safe & Dry p.
    Soft & Silent diaper p.
pantaloon brace
Panther balloon
pantoscope
    Keeler p.
pantoscopic spectacles
pants (*pl. of* pant)
pantyhose
    Activskin support p.
    Glattelast compression p.
Panzer gallbladder scissors
Papanicolaou smear tray
Paparella
    P. middle ear instrument
    P. myringotomy tube
    P. type II ventilation tube
    P. ventilation tube type II
paper
    blue litmus p.
    p. drape
    filter p.
    indicator p.
    Kuwabara p.
    litmus p.
    Nitrazine p.
    nitrocellulose filter p.
    red litmus p.
    Schirmer filter p.
    test p.

Whatman p.
Whatman filter p.
Whatman No. 1 qualitative-type
filter p.
Papette
P. cervical cell collector
P. cervical collector
P. device
papilla drain
papilloma forceps
papillotome
30-30 p.
Accuratome precurved p.
Bard Companion p.
Cremer-Ikeda p.
double-lumen tapered-tip p.
dual-lumen p.
Erlangen p.
Frimberger-Karpiel 12 o'clock p.
Howell Rotatable BII p.
Huibregtse-Katon p.
Microvasive p.
needle-knife p.
Piggyback needle-knife p.
precut p.
shark fin p.
Swenson p.
Wilson-Cook p.
Wiltek p.
wire-guided p.
Zimmon p.
papillotome/sphincterotome
Swenson wire-guided p./s.
Zimmon p./s.
Papineau bone graft
PapNet
P. automated cervical cystology
system
P. reader
P. testing system
papoose
p. board
p. board restraint
Pap-Perfect
P.-P. plastic spatula
P.-P. supply system
Paquelin cautery
Par
P. 5 acetabular reconstruction
system
P. scissors
PAR CTS corneal topography system
**Parabath paraffin heat treatment
system**
Para-Care paraffin therapy bath
paracentesis
p. knife
p. needle
paracervical nerve block needle

Parachute
Corkscrew P.
parachutist ankle brace
Paradigm
P. insulin pump
P. Link blood glucose monitor
P. ocular blood flow analyzer
paraffin
p. block
p. dressing
p. gauze
p. implant
p. mitt
PARAflow circulatory support system
ParaGard
P. intrauterine device
P. T380 copper IUD
Paragon
P. amalgam
P. ambulatory pump
P. Champion stent
P. Complete implant
P. coronary stent
P. CZE 2000 capillary
electrophoresis system
P. II pacemaker
P. infuser
P. laser
P. laser system
P. nitinol stent
P. PAS stent
P. single-stage dental implant
system
parallel
p. pin kit
p. plate dialyzer
**parallel-hole medium-sensitivity
collimator**
parallel-loop electrode
parallel-plate flow chamber
paramagnetic microsphere
Paramax
P. ACL guide system
P. analyzer
parametrium
p. clamp
p. forceps
Paramount
P. total body plate-loaded machine
P. 3-way press bench
paranasal sinus shaver system
parapodium
Toronto p.
Parapost
P. bur
Whaledent P.
paraPRO needle
Parascan scanning device
Parasmillie knife

P

Parasol punctal occluder
Parastep I system
Paratrend
    P. 7 continuous blood gas monitor
    P. 7 intravenous blood gas
      monitoring system
    P. 7+ multiparameter blood gas
      monitor
    P. 7+ sensor
ParCA catheter
parent spherical IOL
ParFlex Plus orthotic
parfocal defraction lens
Parham-Martin fracture device
Pari
    P. LC Plus reusable nebulizer
    P. LC Star reusable nebulizer
    P. Proneb Turbo compressor
    P. Proneb Ultra nebulizer
parietal
    p. ball
    p. band
Parietex composite mesh
Paris
    P. manual therapy table
    plaster of P. (POP)
    P. ultrasound system
Park
    P. Medical Systems scanner
    P. speculum
Parker-Bard
    P.-B. blade
    P.-B. handle
Parker-Kerr intestinal clamp
Parker-Pearson needle
Parker retractor
Parkes
    P. osteotome
    P. rasp
Park-Guyton-Callahan speculum
Park-Guyton-Maumenee speculum
Park-Guyton speculum
Parkinson-Cowan dry gas meter
Park-Maumenee speculum
Park-O-Tron drill system
Parks
    P. anal retractor
    P. bidirectional Doppler flowmeter
    P. 800 bidirectional Doppler
      flowmeter
Parma band
Parodi catheter
paronychia bur
parotidectomy retractor
parquetry set
parrot-beak basket
partial
    p. denture prosthetics
    p. lower denture

    p. occlusion clamp
    p. occlusion forceps
    p. occlusion inferior vena cava
      clip
    p. ossicular replacement prosthesis
      (PORP)
    p. rebreathing face mask
    p. rebreathing mask
    p. upper denture
    p. zona dissection pipette
partially
    p. implantable catheter
    p. threaded pin
partial-ring bismuth germanate-crystal
    scanner
particle
    Ivalon p.
    PVA foam embolization p.
    Spongel gelatin sponge p.
particulate
    Bioglass synthetic bone graft p.
    NovaBone bone graft p.
    NovaBone-C/M bone graft p.
    p. respirator
Partnership
    P. implant
    P. instrument
    P. system
partograph
Partridge strap
Partsch
    P. bone chisel
    P. chisel
    P. gouge
PAS
    peripheral access system
    PAS Port catheter
    PAS Port proximal anastomosis
      system
    PAS Port system
PASCAL
    pattern scan laser
    PASCAL photocoagulator
Passage
    P. biliary dilatation catheter
    P. hemostasis valve
Passager
    P. device
    P. nitinol self-expandable stent
Passarelli 1-pass capsulorrhexis forceps
Passavant
    P. bar
    P. cushion
passer
    Arthrex Viper suture p.
    Batzdorf cervical wire p.
    Bunnell tendon p.
    Carter-Thomason suture p.
    Charnley wire p.

De Mayo suture p.
dermis-fat p.
Dingman wire p.
ExpresSew suture p.
Framer tendon p.
Furlow cylinder p.
Gore suture p.
Hewson ligature p.
Hewson suture p.
Hoefflin suture p.
Incavo wire p.
Lahey ligature p.
ligature p.
Malis ligature p.
MetraPass suture p.
Protect-a-Pass suture p.
pulley p.
Shuttle Relay suture p.
suture p.
tendon p.
Uni-Shunt catheter p.
Viper suture p.
Wedeen wire p.
wire p.

passing forceps
passivation metal instrument
passive
p. alveolar molding appliance
p. infant oral prosthesis
p. motion device
p. night stretch splint
p. prehension orthosis
p. track detector
p. traction table

passively shimmed superconducting magnet
passover humidifier
Passow chisel
Passport
P. Balloon-on-a-Wire dilatation catheter
P. bedside monitor
P. instrumentation

Passy-Muir
P.-M. O2 adapter
P.-M. tracheostomy speaking valve
P.-M. valve

paste
absorbable collagen p.
bismuth-iodoform-paraffin p. (BIPP)
bone p.
calcium phosphatase bone p.
Coloplast skin barrier p.
Critic-Aid skin p.
DBX bone p.
electrode p.
p. filler
Grafton Plus DBM p.

Grafton Plus DBM demineralized bone graft p.
OrthoBlast p.
Osteofil allograft p.
Regenafil allograft p.
Regenafil injectable bone p.
Regenaform moldable bone p.

Pastegraft
Dembone demineralized cortical powder P.

paster
Pasteur pipette
pastille radiometer
PASV valve
Pasys ST cardiac pacing system
patch
acupuncture point skin p.
Bard Crurasoft p.
Bard Ventralex hernia p.
BioGlue surgical p.
CardioFix pericardium p.
CF indicator system chloride p.
CorRestore implantable p.
Crurasoft p.
Dacron p.
Dacron intracardiac p.
defibrillation p.
Donaldson eye p.
doobie derm p.
p. dressing
Dura-Guard dural repair p.
epicardial defibrillator p.
eye p.
felt p.
Fluoropassiv thin-wall carotid p.
full-time occlusion eye p.
glue p.
Gore HemaCarotid vascular p.
Gore-Tex Acuseal cardiovascular p.
Gore-Tex cardiovascular p.
Gore-Tex soft tissue p.
p. graft
HemaCarotid vascular p.
Hemashield Finesse cardiovascular p.
Hutchinson p.
p. implant
Ionescu-Shiley pericardial p.
Kugel hernia p.
marijuana p.
Miniguard adhesive p.
monocular p.
most versatile p. (MVP)
nitroglycerin transdermal p.
Nouvisage Deep Hydration body p.
Nouvisage Deep Hydration neck p.
orthoptic eye p.
Ortopad orthoptic p.
outflow cardiac p.

P

patch *(continued)*
  polypropylene intracardiac p.
  polytef soft tissue p.
  pot p.
  Prolene hernia system onlay p.
  Prolene hernia system underlay p.
  prophylactic epidural blood p.
  RapiSeal p.
  Rutkow sutureless plug and p.
  salmon p.
  Salonpas pain relief p.
  silastic p.
  SJM pericardial p.
  Snugfit eye p.
  Teflon felt p.
  Teflon intracardiac p.
  Testoderm p.
  Tissue-Guard bovine pericardial p.
  transcatheter p.
  Tutoplast Dura p.
  Ventralex hernia p.
  wicking glue p.
patch-clamp
patcher
  Kartush tympanic membrane p.
  Xomed Kartush tympanic
    membrane p.
patch-graft
  Dacron onlay p.-g.
patella
  p. bone saw
  p. cup
  p. pusher
  p. resurfacing implant
  p. tracker
Patellaligner knee brace
patellar
  p. aligner
  p. band
  p. band knee protector
  p. button
  p. cement clamp
  p. drill guide
  p. planer bushing
  p. plug
  p. reamer guide
  p. resection guide
  p. shaft reamer
  p. stabilizing brace
  p. tendon-bearing below-knee
    prosthesis
  p. tendon-bearing orthosis
  p. tendon socket
  p. tendon weightbearing brace
    orthosis
  p. tracking orthosis
patellofemoral
  p. brace
  p. replacement (PFR)

patent
  p. ductus clamp
  p. ductus forceps
  p. ductus retractor
  p. stent
Pathfinder
  P. exchange guidewire
  P. irrigation device
  P. mini microcatheter
  P. prosthetic foot
  P. wire
PathFinder
  P. pedicle screw
  P. pedicle screw system
  P. percutaneous pedicle fixation
    system
  P. polyaxial screw
pathometer attachment
PathVysion
  P. HER-2 DNA probe
  P. HER-2 DNA probe kit
patient
  p. dose monitor
  p. monitor
  p. self-administration device
  p. state analyzer
patient-controlled anesthesia pump
PatientGuard reusable underpad
patient-matched implant
patient-operated selector mechanism
Patil stereotactic system I, II
Patil-Syracuse mask
Paton
  P. anterior chamber lens implant
    forceps
  P. capsule forceps
  P. corneal knife
  P. corneal transplant forceps
  P. corneal trephine
  P. double spatula
  P. eye shield
  P. needle holder
  P. single spatula
  P. spatula
  P. suturing forceps
  P. transplant spatula
  P. tying/stitch removal forceps
Patrick drill
Patriot
  P. disposable cannula system
  P. moderate support guidewire
pattern scan laser (PASCAL)
PattStrap knee support
patty
  cottonoid p.
Paufique
  P. blade
  P. corneal knife
  P. corneal trephine

P. graft knife
P. keratoplasty knife
P. suturing forceps
Paul lacrimal sac retractor
Paul-Mixter tube
Paulson knee retractor
Paulus
P. chin plate
P. midfacial plate
P. plate
P. trocar system
Pautler infusion cannula
Pavcnik Monodisk device
Pavlik
P. harness
P. harness splint
paws
Medevice surgical p.
PAXgene Blood RNA kit
Payne-Péan arterial forceps
Payne retractor
Payr
P. gastrointestinal clamp
P. grooved director
P. probe
P. pylorus clamp
P. pylorus forceps
P. resection clamp
P. stomach clamp
PB-FOxS pediatric femoral sensor kit
PBI
PBI Medical copper vapor laser
PBI MultiLase D copper vapor
laser
PBII blue loop lens
PbrO₂ monitoring probe
PC
PC Performer knee
PC Performer knee prosthesis
PC Polygraf HR device
PC-1000/Laser 1000 panoramic cephalometric x-ray machine
PC-1000 panoramic x-ray machine
PCA
porous-coated anatomic
PCA acetabular cup
PCA hip component
PCA infuser
PCA modular total knee
PCA modular total knee system
PCA Original prosthesis
PCA periodontal pack
PCA Plus infusion device
PCA pump
PCA revision total knee
PCA Standard prosthesis
PCA system
PCA total hip
PCA total hip stem

PCA unicompartmental knee
WalkMed PCA
PCD
pacer-cardioverter-defibrillator
programmable cardioverter-defibrillator
PCD ICD generator
Jewel PCD
PCD Transvene implantable
cardioverter-defibrillator system
PCEE automated anastomotic instrument
PCF-140L pediatric colonoscope
PC-IOL lens
PCL-oriented placement marking hook
PCNL
percutaneous nephrolithotomy
PCS
platelet concentrate system
PD
PD Access with Peel-Away needle
introducer
PD 2000 defibrillator
PD-10 disposable Sephadex G-25 column
PDA umbrella
PDB preperitoneal distention balloon system
pDEXA x-ray peripheral bone densitometer
PDL intraligamentary syringe
PDN device
PDS
polydioxanone suture
PDS band
PDS II Endoloop suture
PDS II suture
PDS Vicryl suture
PDT
photodynamic therapy
PDT dye module
PDT laser system
PE
PE balloon
PE catheter
PE Plus II peripheral balloon
catheter
PE2100 spectroscope
PE-400 ERG/VEP system
PeaceKeeper
P. cannula
P. extrusion aspiration cannula
eraser
peak
P. anterior compression plate
system
P. fixation system
p. flow meter (PFM)
p. flow meter monitor
p. flow whistle

P

peak *(continued)*
    P. gait module
    P. Motus motion measurement
      system
    P. polyaxial anterior cervical
      fixation system
    P. polyaxial anterior cervical plate
peakometer
Péan
    P. arterial forceps
    P. hemostatic clamp
    P. hemostatic forceps
    P. hysterectomy clamp
    P. hysterectomy forceps
    P. intestinal clamp
    P. intestinal forceps
    P. scissors
    P. sponge forceps
    P. vessel clamp
peanut
    p. dissector
    p. grasping forceps
    p. implant
    p. sponge
    p. sponge-holding forceps
peapod
    p. bead-type forceps
    p. intervertebral disc forceps
    p. intervertebral disc rongeur
    upbiting p.
pear bur
Pearce
    P. coaxial I&A cannula
    P. coaxial irrigating/aspirating
      cannula
    P. nucleus hydrodissector
    P. trabeculectomy
    P. Tripod cataract lens
    P. Tripod intraocular lens
PEARL
    physiologic endometrial
      ablation/resection loop
Pearman
    P. penile implant material
    P. penile prosthesis
    P. transurethral hemostatic bag
pear-shaped
    p.-s. bur
    p.-s. extension tube
    p.-s. nerve hook
Pearson
    P. chisel
    P. flexed-knee apparatus
Pease-Allen Color test
PEC
    PEC modular total knee system
    PEC total hip system
Peck-Joseph scissors
Peck osteotome

pectoral catheter
pectoralis muscle implant
Peczon
    P. I&A cannula
    P. I&A unit
    P. I&A vectis
pedal
    p. exerciser
    p. lymphangiography
pedal-mode ergometer
Pedar
    P. in-shoe measurement system
    P. pressure insole system
    P. pressure measurement system
PED block
Pederson vaginal speculum
pedestal
    IMP surgical leg p.
    p. massage table
    surgical leg p.
pediatric
    p. abdominal retractor
    p. balloon
    p. balloon catheter
    p. biopsy needle
    p. biplane TEE probe
    p. blade-plate
    p. bridge
    p. bulldog clamp
    P. Cardiology Devices Sideris
      buttoned device occluder
    p. C-D hook
    p. circle
    p. circle system
    p. Cotrel-Dubousset rod
    p. drainable pouch
    p. endoscope
    p. esophagoscope
    p. fiberscope
    p. finger clip sensor
    p. Foley catheter
    p. forceps
    p. gastroscope
    p. Hendren retractor blade
    P. Ingesta Scan metal detector
    p. IOL calculator
    p. Karickhoff laser lens
    p. lead
    p. lid speculum
    P. LifeShirt system
    p. mastoid retractor blade
    p. 3-mirror laser lens
    p. perineal retractor ring
    p. pigtail catheter
    p. PRAFO brace
    p. pressure relief ankle foot
      orthosis
    p. Racine adapter
    p. rectal dilator

p. retractor adjustable arm
p. retractor malleable wire hand
p. sandbag
p. self-retaining retractor
p. telescope
p. transfer pouch
p. TSRH hook
p. urostomy pouch
p. vascular clamp
p. vitrectomy lens set
Pedi-cap detector
pedicle
p. awl
p. C-D hook
p. clamp
p. connector
p. finder
p. forceps
p. implant
p. plate
p. screw
p. screw construct
p. screw construct peg
p. sounder
Pedic sponge
Pedifix
P. crest pad
P. forefoot compression sleeve
P. hammertoe pad
pedi-gravity assisted valve
PediGuard freehand vertebral pedicle perforation instrument
Pedilen polyurethane foam
Pedi PEG tube
Pediplast
P. cushion
P. moldable footcare compound
Pedi-Wrap immobilizer
pedobarograph
Biokinetics p.
EMED-SF p.
optical p.
pedometer
Pedors orthopaedic shoe
pedoscope
peel-away
p.-a. banana catheter
p.-a. introducer
p.-a. introducer set
p.-a. introducer sheath
p.-a. sheath
p.-a. sheath cystostomy kit
peeler
membrane p.
peeler-cutter
membrane p.-c.
peel-off catheter

PEEP
PEEP valve
PEEP ventilator
Peep-Keep II adapter
Peers towel clamp
Peeso reamer
Peet
P. forceps
P. nasal rasp
P. splinter forceps
Pee Wee low-profile gastrostomy tube
PEG
percutaneous endoscopic gastrostomy
Bard PEG
PEG bumper
Gauderer-Ponsky PEG
Ponsky-Gauderer type PEG
Sacks-Vine-type PEG
Sandoz Caluso super PEG
PEG self-adhesive elastic dressing
PEG tube
peg
anchoring p.
bone p.
p. electrode
epithelial rete p.
fiber-metal p.
p. flap
glenoid alignment p.
Harrison-Nicolle polypropylene p.
Kinemax removable fixation p.
locking p.
pedicle screw construct p.
polyethylene p.
stringing p.
PEG-400 tube
Pegasus
P. Airwave pressure relief system
P. Nd:YAG surgical laser
P. PIV laser
pegboard
p. lateral positioning device
Purdue p.
peg-coupled prosthesis
pegged tibial prosthesis
pelican biopsy forceps
Pelle peel microdermabrader
pellet
calcium hydroxyapatite p.
radiopaque p.
stainless p.
Pelli-Robson letter chart
Pelorus
P. stereotactic frame
P. stereotactic system
P. surgical system
pelvic
p. band
p. bench

P

pelvic *(continued)*
>   p. block
>   p. brace
>   p. clamp
>   p. floor therapy system
>   p. phased-array coil
>   p. reconstruction kit
>   p. reduction forceps
>   p. snare
>   p. stabilization orthosis
>   p. tissue forceps
>   p. traction belt

Pelvicol acellular collagen matrix
PelviLace
>   P. TO biourethral support system
>   P. transobturator biourethral support
>   system

pelvimeter
>   Baudelocque p.
>   Collin p.
>   Collyer p.
>   DeLee p.
>   DeLee-Breisky p.
>   Martin p.
>   Rica p.

PelviSoft
>   P. acellular collagen biomesh
>   P. mesh

Pelvitex polypropylene mesh
Pemberton
>   P. retractor
>   P. spur-crushing clamp

Pemco retractor
PE-MT balloon dilatation catheter
PE-MV balloon dilatation catheter
pen
>   Accu-Line surgical marking p.
>   ASSI Accu-line surgical marking p.
>   Cardioblate surgical ablation p.
>   Epi E-Z P.
>   Genotropin p.
>   gentian violet marking p.
>   hydrophobic barrier p.
>   ImmEdge p.
>   insulin p.
>   Intron A multidose p.
>   Ito laser p.
>   light p.
>   marking p.
>   Pilot Spotlighter p.
>   p. pump insulin infuser
>   red-beam laser p.
>   Rhein reusable cautery p.
>   skin marking p.
>   Skin Skribe p.
>   STA-Pen writer p.
>   surgical marking p.
>   Surgiscribe surgical marking p.
>   weighted p.

Pen/Alps distal pad
Pencan spinal needle
PenChant coronary stent delivery
system
pencil
>   cataract p.
>   p. cautery
>   Conmed electrosurgical p.
>   p. Doppler probe
>   p. drain
>   p. electron beam
>   electrosurgical p.
>   glaucoma p.
>   hand-switching electrocautery p.
>   MegaDyne electrocautery p.
>   retinal detachment p.
>   solid carbon dioxide p.
>   straight bipolar p.
>   Valleylab p.
>   vitreous p.
>   Wallach cryosurgical p.
>   Weck electrosurgery p.

pencil-grip instrument
pencil-handled laryngoscope
pencil-tip
>   p.-t. cautery
>   p.-t. drill
>   p.-t. electrode

Penco Walker Sleds
pendulum scalpel
penetrating drill
penetrator
>   Arthrex p.

penetrometer
>   Benoist p.

Penfield
>   P. 4 dissector
>   P. retractor

penicillamine
penicillin nebulizer
penile
>   p. biothesiometer
>   p. clamp
>   p. Doppler
>   p. implant

PenInject 2.25 Autoinjector
Pen-Jr
>   Epi E-Z P.-J.

Penlet II Automatic blood sampling
device
penlight
>   Heine p.
>   Welch Allyn halogen p.

Penlon
>   P. infant resuscitator
>   P. vaporizer

Penn
>   P. finger drill
>   P. pouch

P. State intravascular lung
  (PENSIL)
pennate suction catheter
Pennig
P. dynamic wrist fixator
P. minifixator
P. minifixator device
Pennington
P. clamp
P. hemostatic forceps
P. rectal speculum
P. septal elevator
P. tissue forceps
P. tissue grasping forceps
PenRad mammography clinical reporting system
Penrose
P. drain
P. sump drain
P. tube
PENS
percutaneous epidural neurostimulator
PENSIL
Penn State intravascular lung
  PENSIL catheter
Penta balloon
Pentalumen catheter
Pentax
P. bronchofiberscope
P. bronchoscope
P. duodenoscope
P. EC series video endoscope
P. EG-2901, -2940, -3800
  endoscope
P. EG-series videoendoscope
P. ELLB 6000, 6500 ultrasound
  gastroscope
P. EndoNet
P. EndoNet digital endoscope
P. ESI-2000 fiberoptic endoscope
P. EUP-EC series ultrasound
  gastroscope
P. EUP-EC124 ultrasound
  gastroscope
P. FC series colonoscope
P. FG-36-UX linear-array
  echoendoscope
P. FG-36UX linear scanning
  echoendoscope
P. FG-38X endoscope
P. fiberscope
P. flexible endoscope
P. flexible sigmoidoscope
P. laryngoscope
P. light source connector
P. linear-array echoendoscope
P. lithotriptor
P. prototype needle
P. side-viewing endoscope

P. videoendoscope
P. videogastroscope
P. VSB-2000 fiberoptic endoscope
P. VSB-P2900 pediatric
  colonoscope
P. VSB-P series enteroscope
Pentax-Hitachi FG32UA endosonographic system
Pentero surgical microscope
Penthrane analgizer
pentose phosphate shunt
Pentra 60C+ analyzer
PepGen P-15 bone graft
PEP mask
Pepper
P. Medical Antidisconnect Device
  strap
P. Medical tube neck band
Per-C-Cath
Perc-DC SpineWand
Perc-DLG SpineWand
Perc-DLR SpineWand
Perception scanner
Perclose
P. arterial closure device
P. Closer
P. closure device
P. diagnostic device
P. PVS device
P. suture device
P. therapeutic device
P. vascular closure device
P. vascular surgical closure system
Perclose/Prostar device
Perc NCircle rapid atraumatic PCNL stone extractor
Percoll
P. bead
P. filter
Percor Stat-DL intraarotic balloon catheter
PercuCut
P. biopsy needle
P. cut-biopsy needle
Percufix catheter cuff kit
Percuflex
P. Amsterdam stent
P. biliary stent
P. catheter
P. endopyelotomy stent
P. flexible biliary stent
P. nephrostomy catheter
P. Plus stent
P. Plus ureteral stent
P. stent
PercuGuide lesion marking system
percussion hammer
Percuss-O-Matic jackhammer device

P

percussor
  Flimm-Fighter p.
  G5 Flimm-Fighter p.
  G5 Neocussor p.
  McGill neurological p.
  mechanical p.
  neurological p.
  Vibracare p.
Percu-Stay catheter fastener
Percusurg distal protection device
PercuSurge
  P. GuardWire
  P. recovery system device
percutaneous
  p. access kit
  p. arterial closure device
  p. atherectomy
  p. atherectomy device
  p. brachial sheath
  p. cardiopulmonary bypass support
  p. catheter introducer kit
  p. central venous catheter
  p. cholecystotomy catheter
  p. cutting needle
  p. discoscope
  p. dorsal column stimulator implant
  p. drainage catheter
  p. endoscopic gastrostomy (PEG)
  p. endoscopic gastrostomy tube
  p. epidural electrode
  p. epidural nerve stimulator
  p. epidural neurostimulator (PENS)
  p. femoral venous catheter
  p. intraaortic balloon
    counterpulsation
  p. intraaortic balloon
    counterpulsation catheter
  p. K-wire
  p. mechanical thrombectomy system
  p. needle
  p. nephrolithotomy (PCNL)
  p. nephrostomy Malecot catheter
  p. nephrostomy tube
  p. pencil Doppler probe
  p. pin
  p. radiofrequency catheter
  p. rotational thrombectomy catheter
  p. sheath introducer
  p. spinal endoscope
  p. stent
  p. stick
  p. suture-mediated arteriotomy
    closure device
  p. suture-mediated closure device
  p. thrombolytic device
  p. transhepatic biliary drainage
    catheter
  p. transhepatic pigtail catheter
  p. transluminal angioplasty (PTA)

  p. transluminal angioplasty balloon
  p. transluminal coronary angioplasty
    catheter
  p. ultrasonic lithotriptor
  p. ventricular assist device (pVAD)
Percy
  P. amputating saw
  P. amputation retractor
  P. bone retractor
  P. clamp
  P. intestinal forceps
  P. plate
  P. tissue forceps
**PerDUCER percutaneous pericardial
  access device**
Pereyra
  P. ligature cannula
  P. needle
  P. needle driver
Pereyra-Raz ligature carrier
Perez-Castro forceps
Perfect
  P. Pupil dilator
  P. Pupil expansion device
Perfecta
  P. femoral stem
  P. HA coated stem
  P. hip prosthesis
  P. I, II prosthesis
  P. IMC stem
  P. PDA calcar replacement stem
  P. RS stem
  P. total hip system
PerfectCapsule
  P. irrigation device
  P. system
**Perfectprep Plasmid 96 VAC direct
  bind purification system**
Per-fit percutaneous tracheostomy kit
PerFix
  P. hernia plug
  P. Marlex mesh plug
PerFixation
  P. screw
  P. system
Perflex
  P. delivery system
  P. stainless steel balloon-expandable
    stent
  P. stainless steel stent
  P. stainless steel stent and delivery
    system
perfluorocarbon coaxial I/A cannula
perforating
  p. bur
  p. forceps
  p. twist drill
perforation rasp

perforator
    Aesculap skull p.
    AmniHook amniotic membrane p.
    Anspach cranial p.
    Baylor amniotic p.
    Boyd p.
    cranial p.
    Dodd p.
    p. drill
    Joseph antral p.
    Lasette laser finger p.
    Lempert p.
    membrane p.
    Oto-Flex p.
    Politzer ear p.
    powered automatic skull p.
    Smellie obstetrical p.
    spondylophyte anular dissector p.
    tympanum p.
    Williams p.

Performa
    P. acoustic imaging system
    P. diagnostic catheter
    P. diagnostic ultrasound imaging system
    P. mammography system
    P. ultrasound
    P. ultrasound system

Performance
    P. knee prosthesis
    P. modular total knee system
    P. unicompartmental knee system
    P. Wrap knee support

Performer Ultralight knee brace
perfused needle applicator
perfusion
    p. balloon catheter
    p. cannula
    p. catheter
    p. monitor
    p. O ring

perfusor
PE.R.I
    periarticular reduction implant
Pe.R.I.
    P. plate system
    P. tongs

periapical curette
periaqueductal gray electrode
periareolar retractor
periarticular reduction implant (PE.R.I)
peribulbar needle
pericarbon
    p. bioprosthesis
    p. pericardial prosthesis

pericardial snare
pericardiocentesis needle
pericardiotomy scissors
pericardium membrane material

perichondrial implant
Peri-Cold pack
Periflow peripheral balloon angioplasty infusion catheter
Periflux PF 1 D blood flowmeter
Perigee
    P. prolapse repair system
    P. vaginal vault system

Peri-Gel pack
Peri-Guard
    P.-G. vascular graft
    P.-G. vascular graft guard

Peri-Loc prosthesis
Perimed PeriFlux Doppler probe system
perimeter
    AccuMap multifocal objective p.
    automated hemisphere p.
    Brombach p.
    Canon p.
    CooperVision imaging p.
    Ferree-Rand p.
    Goldmann p.
    Henson CFS 2000 p.
    Humphrey p.
    Interzeag bowl p.
    Medmont M600 p.
    Octopus 1-2-3 p.
    Octopus 201 p.
    Octopus 101 bowl p.
    Octopus 101, 201 bowl p.
    Ophthimus High-Pass Resolution p.
    Ophthimus ring p.
    Peritest p.
    projection p.
    Schweigger hand p.

Perimount
    P. RSR pericardial bioprosthesis
    P. Theon mitral replacement system

perineal
    p. bandage
    p. loop
    p. pad
    p. pouch
    p. prostatectomy retractor
    p. self-retaining retractor
    p. surgical apron

perineometer
    Kegel p.
    Peritron p.

periodontal
    p. attachment system
    p. probe
    p. prosthesis

periodontometer
    Mühlemann p.

PerioGlas
    P. bone graft material

P

PerioGlas *(continued)*
 P. material
 P. synthetic bone graft
PerioLase laser
perioperative autotransfusion system
periosteal
 p. button
 p. elevator
 p. implant
 p. rasp
periosteotome
 Alexander costal p.
 Alexander-Farabeuf p.
 Alexander-Farabeuf costal p.
 Brown p.
 costal p.
 elevator p.
 Ferris-Smith-Lyman p.
 Fomon p.
 Freer p.
 Joseph p.
Periotemp electronic probe
Periotest
 P. implant
 P. Implant Innovations gold screw
 P. system
PerioWise probe
peripheral
 p. access system (PAS)
 p. AngioJet system
 p. atherectomy catheter
 p. atherectomy system
 p. blood vessel forceps
 p. indwelling intermediate infusion device
 p. instantaneous x-ray imager (PIXI)
 p. interface adapter
 p. iridectomy forceps
 p. long-line catheter
 p. nerve glove
 p. vascular clamp
 p. vascular forceps
 p. vascular retractor
 p. vein catheter
peripherally
 p. inserted catheter
 p. inserted central catheter (PICC)
 p. inserted central catheter line
 p. inserted central venous catheter (PICVC)
periscopic
 p. lens
 p. spectacles
peristaltic pump
Peri-Strips
Peritest perimeter
peritoneal
 p. button

 p. clamp
 p. dialysis catheter
 p. forceps
 p. reflux control catheter
peritoneoscope
Peritron perineometer
periumbilical port
PeriVac pericardiocentesis kit
Peri-Warm pack
Perkin-Elmer
 P.-E. Cetus 480, 9600 DNA thermocycler
 P.-E. model 5000 atomic absorption spectrophotometer
Perkin-Elmer DNA Thermal Cycler 480
Perkin Elmer rhodamine dye terminator kit
Perkins
 P. applanation tonometer
 P. traction
Per-Lee ventilation tube
Perlon suture
PermaClip clip applier
Permacol mesh
Perma-Flow coronary bypass graft
Perma-Hand braided silk suture
Permalens lens
Permalock
 Weber P.
Permalume covering
PermaMesh hydroxyapatite woven sheet matrix
Perman cartilage forceps
PermaNeb reusable nebulizer
permanent
 p. cardiac pacing lead
 p. myocardial pacemaker
 p. needle
 p. rate-responsive pacemaker
 p. silicone catheter
 p. transvenous demand pacemaker (PTDP)
 p. ventricular pacemaker
PermaRidge
 P. alveolar ridge augmentation
 P. delivery syringe
Permark
 P. Enhancer III pigmenting unit
 P. micropigmentation handpiece
 P. micropigmentation needle
 P. micropigmentation system
Perma-Seal dialysis access graft
PermaSharp
 P. PGA suture
 P. suture and needle
PermaSoft reline material
PermaVision intracorneal lens
PermCath
 P. catheter

P. dual-lumen catheter
Quinton P.
permucosal implant system
Perneczky aneurysm clip
Perneczky-designed microscope-assisting
endoscope
Perone
P. LASIK flap forceps
P. LASIK marker
peroral
p. electronic pancreatoscope
p. endoprosthesis
p. gastroscope
p. pancreatoscope system
PerQ
P. SANS
P. SANS system
Per-Q-Cath percutaneously inserted
central venous catheter
Perroncito apparatus
Perry
P. exchange dilator
P. sensor
Persist skin prep swab
person
1-p. stretcher
2-p. stretcher
personal
p. air sampler
P. Best peak flowmeter
P. Catheter 100% silicone
intermittent catheter
P. EMG trainer
p. heart device
p. hemodialysis (PHD)
P. Lasettc
p. protective equipment
P. Scanner TM 18 bedside real-
time ultrasonography system
Personna
P. Plus disposable Teflon scalpel
P. prep blade
P. steel blade
P. surgical blade
Perspective dental imaging system
Perspex
P. block
P. CQ intraocular lens
P. CQ-Shearing-Simcoe-Sinskey lens
P. rod
P. tube
Perthes
P. reamer
P. sling
pervenous catheter
pessary
Albert-Smith p.
Biswas Silastic vaginal p.

bladder neck support p.
blue ring p.
cube p.
cup p.
diaphragm p.
doughnut p.
Dumas p.
Dumontpallier p.
Dutch p.
Emmett-Gellhorn p.
Findley folding p.
Gariel p.
Gehrung p.
Gellhorn p.
globe prolapsus p.
Hodge p.
inflatable ball p.
intrauterine p.
lever p.
Mayer p.
Menge p.
Milex p.
Prentif p.
Prochownik p.
retroversion p.
ring p.
Smith p.
Smith-Hodge p.
stem p.
vaginal p.
Zwanck p.
PET
positron emission tomography
PET balloon
PET balloon atherectomy device
PET full-ring scanner
petal
nitinol p.
PET/CT scanner
PET/Eurotech Generation 2000 table
Petit
P. facial mask
P. tourniquet
petri
P. cast
p. dish
Petroff-Hauser counting chamber
petrolatum
p. gauze
p. gauze dressing
Pettigrove
P. irrigation cannula
P. laser-assisted intrastromal
keratomileusis set
P. LASIK irrigating cannula
P. LASIK set
PETT VI PET scanner

P

Peyman
>P. special optics for low vision lens
>P. wide-field lens

Peyman-Green
>P.-G. vitrectomy lens
>P.-G. vitreous forceps

Pezzer
>P. catheter
>P. drain
>P. mushroom-tipped catheter
>P. self-retaining urethral catheter
>P. suprapubic cystostomy catheter
>P. tube

PF
>PF Night Splint II splint
>PF Universal solder

PF-8P peroral pancreatoscope system

PFA
>platelet function analyzer

PFA-100 system

PFC
>PFC component
>PFC curved unconstrained prosthesis
>PFC femoral prosthesis
>PFC modular total knee system
>PFC offset tibial tray
>PFC Sigma knee system
>PFC Sigma total knee system
>PFC TC3 modular knee system
>PFC total hip replacement system

Pfizer 200 FS 400 scanner

PFM
>peak flow meter
>TruZone PFM

PFN
>proximal femoral nail

PFNA
>proximal femoral nail antirotation
>PFNA proximal femoral nail

PFO-Star occluder

PFR
>patellofemoral replacement

PFT traction brace

PGA synthetic absorbable suture

PGK stereotactic device

PGS-3000 pulsed galvanic stimulator

pH
>p. manometry probe
>p. meter
>p. probe

phaco
>p. emulsifier Cavitron unit
>p. sleeve
>p. tip

Phaco-4 diamond step knife

phacoblade

phacoemulsification
>p. handpiece
>p. system

Phaco-Emulsifier
>Cavitron P.-E.
>Kelman P.-E.

PhacoFlex
>P. II foldable intraocular lens
>P. II foldable intraocular lens implant
>P. II SI30NB intraocular lens

phacofracture ophthalmic instrument

Phacojack phaco system

phacolase
>Er:YAG p.

phacoscope

Phakic
>P. 6 H2 IOL
>P. 6 lens

phakofragmatome
>Girard p.

phalangeal
>p. broach
>p. clamp
>p. forceps

Phaneuf
>P. clamp
>P. hysterectomy forceps
>P. peritoneal forceps
>P. uterine artery forceps

phantom
>3-dimensional SPECT p.
>p. frame
>Imatron CT bone mineral p.
>P. interference screw
>P. nasal mask
>P. nasal mask CPAP

Pharmacia
>P. corneal trephine
>P. Intermedics
>P. lancet
>P. Visco J-loop lens

Pharmaseal
>P. catheter
>P. closed drain
>P. disposable cervical dilator
>P. disposable uterine sound
>P. needle

PharmChek sweat patch drug detection system

pharyngeal
>p. airway
>p. retractor
>p. tracheal lumen airway

pharyngometer
>Eccovision acoustic p.

pharyngoscope

pharyngotympanic tube

phase
    p. difference haloscope
    3-p. generator
    p. microscope
phased-array
    p.-a. color-flow ultrasound system
    p.-a. multicoil
    p.-a. probe
    p.-a. receiver coil
    p.-a. sector transducer
    p.-a. torso coil
    p.-a. ultrasonographic device
phase-sensitive detector
Phazet lancet
PHD
    personal hemodialysis
    PHD personal hemodialysis system
Phelps
    P. brace
    P. orthosis
    P. splint
Phema core-and-skirt keratoprosthesis
Phemister
    P. elevator
    P. rasp
Phenergan
Phenol EZ swab
pheresis catheter
Philadelphia
    P. cervical collar
    P. collar
    P. collar cervical traction
    P. rigid collar
Philips
    P. Angiodiagnostics 96 apparatus
    P. CM 12 electron microscope
    P. DVI 1 system
    P. EasyGuide navigation system
    P. 301 electron microscope
    P. follower dilator and catheter
    P. gravity pivot axis marker
    P. Gyroscan
    P. Gyroscan ACS, NT, NT5, NT15, S5, T5 scanner
    P. Gyroscan ACS NT superconducting magnet
    P. Gyroscan NT-series scanner
    P. Integris 3000 biplane digital subtraction angiography device
    P. Integris 5000 digital subtraction angiography system
    P. linear accelerator
    P. Medical Systems Tomoscan AVE1 CT spiral scanner
    P. Medical Systems Tomoscan SR 7000 CT spiral scanner
    P. 1.5 NT-Intera scanner
    P. SensorTouch temple thermometer
    P. spiral CT scanner

    P. 1.5-T NT MR scanner
    P. toe force gauge
    P. Tomoscan
    P. Tomoscan 310 CT scanner
    P. Tomoscan 350, SR 6000 CT scanner
    P. Tomoscan SR 6000 CT scanner
    P. 4.7-T small-bore system scanner
    P. ultrasound machine
    P. 100W TL-01 lamp
Phillips
    P. fixation forceps
    P. gravity pivot axis marker
    P. recessed-head screw
    P. rectal clamp
    P. screwdriver
    P. ultrasound machine
Philly
    P. Bloc-Head cervical collar
    P. bolt
    P. 1-piece cervical collar
PHILOS
    proximal humerus internal locking system
    PHILOS fixation system
Philos DR-T pacemaker
phimosis forceps
pH-Informer Deltron probe
phlebodissector
phlebograph
    impedance p.
pH-meter
    intragastric continuous pH-m.
Phoenix
    P. ancillary valve
    P. Anti-Blok ventricular catheter
    P. cruciform valve
    P. fifth ventricle system
    P. Outrigger splint
Phonagel collagen
Phonate speaking valve
phone
    Picasso telemedicine p.
phonologic acquisition device
phonometer
    Tektronix digital p.
Phoresor
    P. II iontophoretic drug delivery system
    P. PM900 iontophoresis system
PhorMax CR desktop workstation system
phorometer
phoro-optometer
phoroptor
    P. retractor
    Ultramatic Rx Master p.
phosphate
    biphasic calcium p. (BCP)

P

phosphonated dimethacrylate/phosphated
  bis-GMA system
PhosphorImager system
phosphor plate
photocatalytic air filtration system
photocathode
photochromic
    p. lens
    p. spectacles
photocoagulation
    p. laser
    panretinal p. (PRP)
photocoagulator
    argon laser p.
    Coherent p.
    Coherent argon laser p.
    continuous-wave p.
    EyeLite p.
    green laser light p.
    infrared ray p.
    Iolab irrigating/aspirating p.
    laser p.
    Mira p.
    532nm Green laser p.
    Novus Omni 2000 p.
    Novus Verdi diode-pumped
      green p.
    OcuLight GL p.
    OcuLight GLx green laser p.
    PASCAL p.
    sapphire crystal infrared p.
    semiconductor GaAIAs infrared
      diode laser p.
    Ultima p.
    Viridis p.
    Viridis Lite p.
    xenon arc p.
    Zeiss p.
    Zeiss xenon arc p.
PhotoDerm
    P. bright light delivery system
    P. filtered flashlamp-pumped light
      source
    P. laser
    P. machine
    P. MultiLight system
    P. PL handpiece
    P. PL laser
    P. PL pulsed light device
    P. PL, VL pulsed light device
    P. T 10 laser
    P. V laser
    P. VL device
    P. VL laser
    P. VL light source
    P. VL/PL hair removal system
photodiode
photodisplay unit

photodisrupting laser
photodisruptor
    Aura Nd:YAG p.
photodynamic
    p. therapy (PDT)
    p. therapy laser system
photoelectric multiplier tube
photogastroscope
    Krentz p.
PhotoGenica
    P. laser system
    P. LPIR with TKS laser
    P. T^{10} laser
    P. T laser system
    P. T^{10} tattoo removal system
    P. V laser
    P. VLS pulsed dye laser
    P. V-Star laser
photogrammeter
photographer
    Tearscope Plus p.
photographic radiometer
photohemotachometer
photoionization detector
photokeratoscope
    Allergan Humphrey p.
    Allergan Medical Optics p.
    CooperVision refractive surgery p.
    CorneaScope 9-ring p.
    Tomey TMS-1 p.
photolaparoscope
photometer
    Anthos ht II automatic p.
    flame p.
    flicker p.
    Förster p.
    HemoCue p.
    HemoCue hemoglobin p.
    Kowa laser flare p.
    Kowa laser flare-cell p.
    Minolta LS 110 spot p.
    reflectance p.
    Spectra-Pritchard p.
    TUR-Cue p.
photomicroscope
    Leitz periplan p.
    Zeiss IIIRS p.
photomultiplier
    EMI 9813B p.
    p. tube
photon
    P. DR dual-chamber ICD
    p. laser phacolysis probe
    P. Micro DR/VR implantable
      cardioverter defibrillator
    P. ocular surgery system
    p. radiosurgery system
photon-activated drug delivery system

photonic
  p. radiosurgical system
  p. stimulator
Photopic Imaging ultrasound system
PhotoPoint laser
photoptometer
  Förster p.
photoreceptor
  rod p.
photoscanner
PhotoScreener
  MTI P.
  P. pediatric camera
photoscreener
  iScreen p.
photoselective vaporization (PV)
photosensor
Photoshop 6.0 digitized imager
photostress
  macular p.
phototherapy
  p. bulb
  UVB p.
phototimer
Phototome System 2700
Phototome system
phototube output circuit
photovaporizing laser
photovolt pH meter
phrenicectomy forceps
phrenic retractor
pH-sensitive radiotelemetry capsule
pHydrion strip
Phylax
  P. AV dual-chamber implantable
    cardioverter-defibrillator
  P. 06 implantable cardioverter-
    defibrillator
Phynox cobalt alloy clip material
physial bar
physical therapy table
Physio-Control Lifestat
  sphygmomanometer
PhysioGymnic exercise ball
physiologic
  p. endometrial ablation/resection
    loop (PEARL)
  p. pacemaker
Physio-Roll-R-Cise
Physio-Roll VisuaLiser exercise ball
Physios
  P. CTM 01 cardiac transplant
    monitor
  P. CTM 01 noninvasive cardiac
    transplant monitoring system
  P. CTM 01 noninvasive
    telemonitor
Physio-Stim Lite bone growth
  stimulator

physiotherapy
  aqua PT dry p.
Phytis stent
pi
  pi plate
  pi plate dorsal distal radius plate
PI-30 stapler
piano-wire dorsiflexion brace
Picasso telemedicine phone
PICC
  peripherally inserted central catheter
    Arrow PICC
    Groshong NXT PICC
    PICC kit
    PICC line
    Vaxcel PICC
Piccolino
  P. balloon
  P. Monorail balloon device
  P. Monorail catheter
Piccolo blood chemistry analyzer
pick
  Burch p.
  Burch fixation p.
  P. chisel
  Crane dental p.
  dental p.
  Desmarres fixation p.
  double-ended root tip dental p.
  fiberoptic p.
  fixation p.
  footplate p.
  P. and Go monitor
  Guilford-Wright footplate p.
  House-Barbara p.
  House-Crabtree dissector p.
  House obtuse p.
  House oval-window p.
  House strut p.
  p. knife
  light pipe p.
  McGee footplate p.
  Michel p.
  microsurgical ear p.
  Olk vitreoretinal p.
  ophthalmic p.
  oval window p.
  posterior footplate p.
  Rhein p.
  Rice p.
  right-angle p.
  scleral p.
  Sinskey p.
  slightly curved ear p.
  stapedectomy footplate p.
  stapes p.
  strut p.
  Synergetics Awh serrated p.

P

Picker
- P. camera
- P. CS, CT, MR scanner
- P. Dyna Mo collimator
- P. Eclipse MR unit
- P. Edge 1.5-T scanner
- P. Magnascanner
- P. MR scanner
- P. PQ 2000 CT scanner
- P. PQ 5000 helical CT scanner
- P. PQ helical CT scanner
- P. PQ 2000 spiral CT scanner
- P. Prism 3000 PET scanner
- P. scanner
- P. Synerview 600 scanner
- P. system
- P. Vista HPQ MRI scanner
- P. Vista Magnascanner
- P. Vista MagnaScanner scanner
- P. Vistar image analysis system
- P. Voxel image analysis system

Pickford-Nicholson anomaloscope
pickle fork cannula
pickup
- Adson p.
- DeBakey p.
- p. forceps
- p. noncrushing forceps
- rat-tooth p.
- Shoch foreign body p.
- p. spatula suture
- toothed p.
- p. tube

PicoGreen dsDNA Quantitation Kit
Picotip
- Endotak P.
- P. steroid-eluting endocardial lead

PICP RIA kit
pictograph
picture
- p. archival communication system
- p. archiving and communication system

picture-in-picture monitor
PICVC
- peripherally inserted central venous catheter

Pidcock nail
Pie
- P. Medical CAAS II analysis system
- P. Medical ultrasound
- P. Medical ultrasound system

piece
- 2-p. dental implant
- 4-p. intraocular lens
- pole p.
- Y p.

1-piece
- 1-p. hydrophilic acrylic IOL
- 1-p. plate-haptic silicone intraocular lens
- 1-p. plate haptic silicone intraocular lens
- 1-p. shunt

3-piece
- 3-p. acrylic intraocular lens
- 3-p. hydrophilic acrylic IOL
- 3-p. hydrophobic acrylic lens
- 3-p. hydrophobic acrylic Sensar lens
- 3-p. IOL
- 3-p. modified J-loop intraocular lens
- 3-p. monofocal silicone lens
- 3-p. plate-haptic intraocular lens
- 3-p. silicone intraocular lens

Pierce
- P. antral trocar
- P. coaxial I&A cannula
- P. elevator
- P. I&A unit
- P. I&A vectis
- P. Micro BCA Assay kit

Pierce-Donachy Thoratec ventricular assist device
Pierse
- P. corneal Colibri-type forceps
- P. eye speculum
- P. fixation forceps
- P. tip forceps

Pierse-Colibri corneal utility forceps
piesimeter, piezometer
- Hales p.

piezoelectric
- p. accelerometer
- p. crystal
- p. generator
- p. lithotriptor
- p. shock wave lithotriptor
- p. snore sensor
- p. transducer
- p. ultrasound transducer

piezoelectrical stimulator
Piezolith
- P. EPL
- P. EPL lithotriptor
- P. 2300, 2500 model lithotriptor

piezometer (*var. of* piesimeter)
piezo PLM sensor
piezo-resistive transducer
Piezosurgery device
Piffard dermal curette
Pigg-O-Stat
- P.-O.-S. immobilization device
- P.-O.-S. mechanical immobilizer

P.-O.-S. pediatric immobilizer and positioner

piggyback

    p. contact lens
    p. implant
    P. needle-knife papillotome
    p. probe

piggybacked toric IOL
pigmented lesion dye laser
pigskin graft
pigtail

    p. biliary stent
    p. catheter
    p. endoprosthesis
    p. explorer
    p. nephrostomy catheter
    p. nephrostomy drain
    p. nephrostomy tube
    p. probe
    p. rotation catheter
    p. stent
    p. tendon stripper

PIIP hydrogel breast implant
Pik

    Grossan nasal irrigator tip with Water P.
    P. Stik Reacher

pile clamp
pillar

    p. grasping forceps
    P. palatal implant system
    p. retractor

pillar-and-post microsurgical retractor
Pillcam ESO video capsule
pill counter
Pillet hand prosthesis
Pilliar prosthesis
Pilling

    P. bronchoscope
    P. fiberoptic illuminator
    P. retractor
    P. Weck Y-stent forceps

Pilling-Wolvek sternal approximator
Pillo

    Knee P.
    P. Pro dressing

Pillo-Boot lower leg positioning device
Pillo-Pedic cervical traction pillow
Pillo-Pump alternating pressure system
pillow

    abduction p.
    air p.
    antibacterial p.
    Bedge p.
    Bodynapper comfort p.
    Capello slim-line abduction p.
    Carter p.
    Carter foam p.
    cervical p.

cervical skull p.
cervical sleep p.
p. collar
Comfort Club tub p.
Comfort-U total body p.
Crescent p.
Crescent Complete Sleeper p.
Crescent memory p.
Crescent-Pillo p.
D-Core support p.
dream p.
Flip-Flop p.
foam vacuum p.
foot p.
Fossfill health p.
Frejka p.
Frejka hip p.
Heart p.
heel p.
Knee Pillo p.
Max-Relax p.
Mediflow water p.
Mediflow waterbase p.
MedSlant acid reflux wedge p.
MedSlant therapeutic p.
molded vacuum p.
Neckcare p.
Neck-Hugger cervical support p.
Nek-LO hot & cold p.
Nek-LO orthopaedic support/comfort p.
Opti-Curve therapeutic p.
OrthoBone p.
p. orthosis
Orthosleep p.
OsmoCyte p.
Pillo-Pedic cervical traction p.
Pillo-Wedge p.
positioning p.
Pron p.
Richard p.
Sand-Eze EGD p.
shoulder abduction p.
Silicore foot p.
snooze p.
Softeze water p.
Tempur-Pedic pressure-relieving Swedish p.
T-Foam p.
Theracloud p.
Therapeutica sleeping p.
TherArc p.
Therasleep cervical p.
Tri-Core cervical support p.
vacuum p.
Wal-Pil-O neck p.

Pillo-Wedge pillow
pillow-shaped balloon

Pil-O-Splint

    P.-O-S. elbow splint
    P.-O-S. wrist splint

pilot

    P. audiometer
    p. bur
    p. drill
    p. needle
    p. point screw
    P. Spotlighter pen
    P. suturing guide

pin

    absorbable polyparadioxanone p.
    Ace p.
    Acufex distractor p.
    Allofix freeze-dried cortical
      bone p.
    AO guide p.
    apex p.
    Arthrex zebra p.
    arum fixation p.
    Asnis p.
    p. ball system
    Beath p.
    bevel-point Rush p.
    Biofix system p.
    biphasic p.
    Böhler p.
    Böhler-Knowles hip p.
    Böhler-Steinmann p.
    breakaway p.
    buttress p.
    cancellous p.
    p. chuck
    p. clamp
    cloverleaf p.
    Co-Cr-Mo p.
    cortical p.
    cranial p.
    p. crimper
    Crowe pilot point on Steinmann p.
    DCS p.
    Delitala T p.
    Denham p.
    DePuy FRS SOC p.
    DePuy Rockwood clavicle p.
    derotational p.
    distraction p.
    Fahey p.
    Fahey-Compere p.
    femoral guide p.
    Fisher half p.
    fixation p.
    freeze-dried bone p.
    friction lock p.
    Gouffon hip p.
    p. guard
    guide p.
    p. guide

Hagie p.
Hahnenkratt root canal p.
half p.
Hansen p.
Hansen-Street p.
p. headholder
p. headrest
hemorrhage occluder p.
Hewson breakaway p.
hexhead p.
hip p.
Hoffmann apex fixation p.
Hoffmann transfixion p.
p. holder
hook-end intramedullary p.
p. implant
Intraflex intramedullary p.
intramedullary p.
Jones p.
Jurgan p.
Kirschner wire p.
Knowles hip p.
Kronfeld p.
Küntscher femur guide p.
lateral guide p.
lead p.
LIH hook p.
Link-Plus retention p.
locked intramedullary
  osteosynthesis p.
Lottes p.
Markley retention p.
Mayfield disposable skull p.
Mayfield head p.
McBride p.
mechanic's p.
medullary p.
metal p.
Neufeld p.
Neurotips neurological
  examination p.
Optispike dispensing p.
Orthofix p.
orthopaedic p.
OrthoSorb absorbable p.
osteotomy p.
OTPS biodegradable p.
partially threaded p.
percutaneous p.
rasp p.
resorbable polydioxanon p.
resorbable polymer p.
restorative p.
ReUnite orthopaedic p.
revolving Ge-68 p.
Rockwood clavicle p.
Rush intramedullary fixation p.
safety p.
Schanz p.

self-broaching p.
self-tapering p.
skeletal p.
p. sleeve
SmartPin/PLLA p.
Smillie p.
Smith-Petersen p.
smooth p.
Snap fixation p.
SOC p.
spring p.
sprue p.
stabilizing guide p.
5-p. staple
7-p. staple
7-p. staple
Steinmann p.
Steinmann calibrated p.
Steinmann fixation p.
strut-type p.
Surgin hemorrhage occluder p.
p. suture
Synthes guide p.
tapered p.
threaded guide p.
tibial guide p.
titanium half p.
trochanteric p.
Turner p.
Tutofix cortical p.
union broach retention p.
p. vise
Walker micro p.
Watanabe p.
Webb p.
p. wheel
Z p.
ZAAG guide and p.
Zimmer p.

Pinard
P. fetal stethoscope
P. fetoscope
pin-bending forceps
pincer
overlapping p.
pinch
p. forceps
p. gauge
P. Gauge and Jackson Strength
Evaluation System
p. tree
pinchcock clamp
pinch-handle scissors
pinchometer
Prestop p.
pin-deburring die
pineapple contouring bur
Pineda LASIK flap iron

pinhole
p. camera
p. collimator
p. occluder
pin-index safety system
pinion
p. head holder
p. headholder
p. headrest
pink
p. dressing
p. twisted cotton suture
Pinkerton balloon catheter
Pinky ball
Pinnacle
P. acetabular cup system
P. contact Nd:YAG fiber
P. Destination guiding sheath
P. Destination renal guiding sheath
P. introducer sheath
P. pacemaker
P. reusable underpad
P. R/O II radiopaque marker
Pinn-ACL guide system
**Pinn anterior cruciate ligament guide
system**
PinPoint stereotactic arm
pin-seating forceps
Pinto
P. cannula
P. dissector tip
P. distractor
P. superficial dissection cannula
pin-to-bar clamp
pinwheel
Cleanwheel disposable
neurological p.
Safe-T-Wheel p.
p. sensation gauge
Wartenberg p.
Pinwheel System
PIP/DIP strap
pipe
effusion light p.
endoscopic washing p.
fiberoptic light p.
flute p.
infusion light p.
light p.
Mauch double-sheathed plastic
wash p.
Millennium TSV25 light p.
Storz disposable fiberoptic light p.
p. tree
Pipeline access system
Pipelle
P. biopsy
P. de Cornier endometrial suction
curette

Pipelle *(continued)*
    P. endometrial curette
    P. endometrial suction catheter
    Unimar P.
Piper obstetrical forceps
pipette
    air-displacement p.
    Eppendorf Repeater Pro p.
    Flexipet micro-manipulation p.
    HandyStep electronic repeating p.
    Labpette FX p.
    light p.
    Ostwald-Folin p.
    partial zona dissection p.
    Pasteur p.
    positive-placement p.
    SoftGrip p.
    Unopette p.
    zona drilling p.
pirbuterol acetate inhalation aerosol
Pisces
    P. electrode
    P. implant
    P. lead
    P. spinal cord stimulation device
    P. spinal cord stimulation system
Pisces-Quad electrode
Pischel micropin
Pistofidis cervical biopsy forceps
pistol
    Cameco syringe p.
    harvesting p.
pistol-grip instrument
piston
    Causse p.
    De La Cruz p.
    Mangham p.
    McGee platinum/stainless steel p.
    MTS electrohydraulic p.
    p. stapes prosthesis
    Teflon p.
    Velegrakis p.
    p. wire
Pitanguy
    P. flap demarcator
    P. marking clamp
Pitie-Salpetriere saphenous vein hook
Pitkin
    P. needle
    P. syringe
Pitot tube
Pittman
    P. IMA retractor system
    P. needle holder
Pittsburgh triangular frame
Pitt talking tracheostomy tube
pituitary
    p. curette
    p. forceps

    p. rongeur
    p. spoon
Pivit AB surgical mesh
pivot
    Accu-Line dual p.
    p. aneurysm clip
    P. balloon
    p. clip applier
    p. link universal system (PLUS)
    P. MIS system posterior
      stabilization system
    P. Plate rehabilitation plate
    P. Pole walking device
pivoting
    p. surgical arm board
    p. table
PixCell II laser capture microdissection
  system
Pixel coronary stent
PIXI
    peripheral instantaneous x-ray imager
    PIXI bone densitometer
    PIXI peripheral densitometer
Pixie minilaparoscope
Pixsys
    P. FlashPoint camera
    P. FlashPoint digitizer
PK
    PlasmaKinetic
    PK Plasma-CISE
    PK Plasma-V
    PK Super-Sect
PK110 centrifuge
PKS-25 apparatus stapler
PLA anchor
PLAC coronary heart disease test
placement
    p. forceps
    ultrasound-assisted PEG p.
    variable screw p. (VSP)
placental
    p. clamp
    p. curette
placenta previa forceps
Placer guidewire
Placido
    P. da Costa disc
    P. disc
    P. keratoscope
    P. ring
    P. 25-ring cone
Placido-disc videokeratoscopy system
plagiocephaly
    p. headband
    p. helmet
plain
    p. catgut suture
    p. collagen suture
    p. ear hook

p. ear spoon
p. eye needle
p. forceps
p. gauze
p. gut suture
p. pattern plate
p. rib shears
p. rotary scissors
p. screwdriver
p. vesical trocar
p. wire speculum
plain-end grooved director
plain-line articulator
Plak-Vac oral suction brush
planar
p. circular coil
p. I mesh implant
Planarm Haag Streit attachment
plane dental mirror
planer
calcar p.
Rubin bone p.
Rubin cartilage p.
USC scleral p.
Plange spud
planimeter
manual optic p.
planner
Visx refractive p.
plano
p. lens
p. T bandage
planoconcave lens
planoconvex
p. eye implant
p. lens
p. nonridge lens
planoconvex-shaped disc
Planoscan treatment system
Planostretch stocking
plantar
p. arch support orthosis
p. fasciitis night splint
p. lift
p. plate
plaque
cobalt-60 eye p.
p. retriever
ruthenium-106 ophthalmic p.
plaque-cracker
LeVeen p.-c.
plasma
p. blade
p. clot diffusion chamber
p. dissector
P. ICP-AES unit
p. prothrombin conversion
accelerator
p. scalpel

Plasma-CISE
PK P.-CISE
Plasma-CUT^T
Plasmaflo plasma separator
PlasmaKinetic (PK)
P. instrument
Plasma-Plex bottle
Plasma-V
PK P.-V.
Plastazote
P. arch support
P. blank
P. cervical collar
P. foam
P. foot bed
P. insole
plaster
p. bandage
below-knee walking p.
Hapset bone graft p.
Hapset hydroxyapatite bone graft p.
p. knife
long leg p.
p. pants dressing
p. of Paris (POP)
p. of Paris bandage
p. of Paris cast
p. of Paris dressing
p. of Paris jacket
p. of Paris splint
p. saw
p. shears
p. slab splint
p. sole
p. spatula
p. spreader
Zoroc p.
Plastibell
P. circumcision clamp
P. circumcision device
P. circumcision method
P. compression instrument
plastic
p. bracket
p. cannula
p. collar
p. connector
p. corneal protector
p. curette
p. disposable irrigating vectis
p. drape
p. dressing
p. end cap
p. endoprosthesis
p. endosurgical system
Erkoflex p.
p. eye shield
p. femoral plug
p. forceps

P

plastic *(continued)*
    p. instrument
    p. mouth guard
    p. orthosis
    p. premilled bar
    p. prism
    p. scalp clip
    p. sewing ring
    p. sphere eye implant
    p. sphere implant
    p. stent
    p. strip
    p. surgery scissors
    p. suture
    p. Tiemann catheter
    p. utility scissors
    p. Vortex Port system
    p. wax material
PlastiCast adjustable joint cast system
plastic-covered hydrogel disc
plastic-cuffed tracheostomy tube
Plastiform magnet
plastipore partial ossicular replacement
    prosthesis
Plastiport
    P. TORP
    P. TORP prosthesis
plastizote
    p. cervical collar
    p. orthotic
    p. orthotic device
    p. shoe
Plast-O-Fit
    P.-O-F. thermoplastic bandage
    P.-O-F. thermoplastic bandage
      system
plate
    absorbable p.
    acetabular reconstruction p.
    AcroMed VSP p.
    Acumed congruent clavicle p.
    alar p.
    alloplastic p.
    Alta condylar buttress p.
    Alta distal fracture p.
    Alta femoral p.
    Anchor p.
    Ant-Cer dynamic cervical p.
    anterior cervical p.
    AO/ASIF compression p.
    AO dynamic compression p.
    AO reconstruction p.
    AO semitubular p.
    AO spoon p.
    Armstrong p.
    ASIF T p.
    axial p.
    Balser hook p.
    base p.

Becton Colles fracture p.
p. bender
Bimler elastic p.
biodegradable p.
BioPress p.
Blackstone anterior cervical p.
blood agar p.
BodyForm thoracolumbar p.
bone p.
bone flap fixation p.
Boyd side p.
breast p.
bridging p.
broad AO dynamic compression p.
buccal cortical p.
buttress p.
buttress-type p.
Calcanea calcaneal fracture p.
Caspar cervical p.
cervical p.
cobra-head p.
compression p.
Concise side p.
condylar lag screw p.
connecting p.
Continuum total knee base p.
contoured anterior spinal p.
cortical oral p.
craniocervical p.
Crosslink p.
C-shaped p.
p. cutter
3D p.
Danek cervical fusion p.
deck p.
depth p.
2D flat p.
3D flat Lactosorb p.
Doc cervical p.
dorsal p.
double-angled blade p.
double-H p.
Doughty tongue p.
2D railed p.
3D railed p.
Driessen hinged p.
p. driver
DuPont distal humeral p.
Dwyer-Hall p.
DyNA block 1000 microtiter p.
dynamic bridging p.
dynamic compression p.
Dynex Immulon 1B microtiter p.
eccentric dynamic compression p.
Eggers bone p.
Envision[2] anterior cervical p.
fenestrated compression p.
fiberoptic absorbable p.
finger p.

flat p.
Foley p.
Fresnel zone p.
frontal p.
fusion p.
gait p.
Gallannaugh bone p.
Galveston p.
Gelfilm p.
genial advancement p.
Haid cervical p.
Haid Universal bone p.
half-circle p.
Hardy-Rand-Rittler p.
Harm posterior cervical p.
Harris p.
Hawley bite p.
2-hole p.
3-hole p.
5-hole p.
6-hole p.
7-hole p.
4-hole Alta straight p.
6-hole mandibular p.
4-hole side p.
Hospidex microtiter p.
Hotz-type alveolar molding p.
H-shaped p.
Hubbard p.
Hubbard side p.
Hub Cap limited wrist fusion p.
Hungarian grip p.
impactor p.
interchangeable p.
interfragmentary p.
Ishihara p.
Ishihara pseudoisochromatic p.
isochromatic p.
Jaeger p.
Jaeger lid p.
Jaeger metal lid p.
Jewett double-angled osteotomy p.
Jewett nail p.
Jewett slotted p.
Kaneda p.
keyed supracondylar p.
Kingsley orthodontic p.
Lane p.
Lane fracture p.
Lawson-Thornton p.
L-buttress p.
LCP locking compression p.
lead p.
Leibinger 3D bone p.
Leibinger Micro Plus p.
Leibinger Mini Würzburg p.
Leibinger Würzburg p.
Letournel acetabular fracture
  bone p.

lid p.
limited compression-dynamic
  compression p.
limited-contact dynamic
  compression p.
lingual cortical p.
locking compression p. (LCP)
locking reconstruction p.
LoCon-T distal radial p.
long-span rigid p.
Lorenz titanium screws and p.
Louis p.
low-contact dynamic compression p.
low-contact stress p.
Lowenstein-Jensen p.
low-profile p.
low-profile dorsal p.
L-plate p.
L-shaped p.
Luer reconstruction p.
Luhr fixation p.
Luhr mandibular p.
Luhr microfixation cranial p.
Luhr pan p.
Luhr vitallium micromesh p.
Lundholm p.
Luque II p.
Lynch mucosa separator p.
Mancini p.
mandibular bridging p.
mandibular staple bone p.
Massie II p.
Maxisorb test p.
Maxisorp microtiter p.
May anatomical bone p.
Mayo Clinic congruent elbow p.
McBride p.
McDonald bone p.
McLaughlin hip p.
Medoff sliding p.
Medoff sliding femoral p.
Medoff sliding fracture p.
metal foot p.
metal reconstruction p.
micro-adaption p.
mini condylar p.
mini Orbita p.
mini Würzburg p.
modified Grace p.
Moe intertrochanteric p.
Morscher anterior cervical p.
Morscher cervical p.
Morscher titanium cervical p.
mouthgag tooth p.
Mueller-Hinton supplemented
  agar p.
Müller p.
multipoint contact p.
muscle p.

plate *(continued)*
  nail p.
  narrow AO dynamic
    compression p.
  non-valve p.
  Ogden p.
  Optivisor lens p.
  Orion anterior cervical p.
  Orozco p.
  orthodontic base p.
  orthopaedic p.
  orthotic p.
  palmar p.
  Paulus p.
  Paulus chin p.
  Paulus midfacial p.
  Peak polyaxial anterior cervical p.
  pedicle p.
  Percy p.
  phosphor p.
  pi p.
  pi plate dorsal distal radius p.
  Pivot Plate rehabilitation p.
  plain pattern p.
  plantar p.
  Plexiglas p.
  Polar p.
  polydioxanone p.
  PolyMedics p.
  Polytechnic foot-pressure
    measuring p.
  Pro-Bind U-Bottom microfilter p.
  Profile anterior spinal p.
  Profil-O-Plastic preshaped chin p.
  Profil-O-Plastic preshaped
    midfacial p.
  pseudoisochromatic p.
  p. reader
  reconstruction p.
  resorbable p.
  resorbable poly-L-lactide p.
  Richards-Hirschhorn p.
  Rohadur gait p.
  roof p.
  round hole p.
  Roy-Camille p.
  safety p.
  SC-AcuFix ThinLine p.
  Schwartz p.
  Sensititre *Streptococcus pneumoniae*
    HPB susceptibility p.
  serpentine bone p.
  Sherman bone p.
  side p.
  silastic p.
  Simmons p.
  Skirrow agar p.
  skull p.
  slotted bone p.

  small stature cervical p. (SSP)
  Smith genioplasty p.
  Smith-Petersen intertrochanteric p.
  snap-on inserter p.
  spring p.
  stabilization p.
  stainless steel AO p.
  staple bone p.
  stay p.
  Steffee pedicle p.
  Steffee screw p.
  Steinhauser p.
  Stilling p.
  Storz p.
  straight compression p.
  Strasburger cell p.
  superior border p.
  supracondylar p.
  Sur-Fit Natura irrigation adapter
    face p.
  Swift dynamic anterior cervical p.
  symmetrical sacral p.
  symmetrical thoracic vertebral p.
  Synthes AO reconstruction p.
  Synthes dorsal distal radius p.
  Synthes maxillofacial locking
    reconstruction p.
  Synthes maxillofacial titanium p.
  Synthes stainless steel
    minifragment p.
  Synthes titanium minifragment p.
  Tacoma sacral p.
  tantalum p.
  T-buttress p.
  tectal p.
  Teflon p.
  tendon p.
  ThermoFX mesh bioabsorbable
    fixation p.
  thoracolumbosacral p.
  Thornton p.
  THORP-type mandibular
    reconstruction p.
  tibial p.
  TiMesh orthognathic strap p.
  titanium p.
  titanium AO p.
  titanium hollow osseointegrated
    reconstruction p.
  titanium hollow osseointegrating
    reconstruction p.
  titanium hollow-screw
    osseointegrated reconstruction p.
  titanium mandibular p.
  toe p.
  tongue p.
  trach p.
  tracheostomy p.
  trimandibular p.

trochanteric p.
T-shaped AO p.
tubular p.
twisted p.
Universal bone p. (UBP)
V blade p.
vestibular oral p.
vitallium p.
vitallium Luhr p.
V nail p.
volar p.
volar buttress p.
VSP p.
Weber antiglide p.
Whitman p.
Wilson spinal fusion p.
Wright knee p.
Würzburg p.
x-shaped p.
Yaeger p.
Y bone p.
Y-shaped p.
Z p.
Z-shaped p.
Zuelzer hook p.

plate-guided
p.-g. distraction device
p.-g. distractor

plate-haptic
p.-h. intraocular lens
p.-h. IOL

plate-holding forceps

platelet
p. concentrate system (PCS)
p. function analyzer (PFA)
p. plug

platelet-derived growth factor
platelet-shaped knife
plate-spacer washer
PlateTrak automated microplate processing system

platform
Alfonso cutting p.
Aspen ultrasound p.
Complete stent delivery p.
p. forceps
p. implant
Kistler force p.
Midland multifunctional mat p.
Midline Hi-Lo Mat p.
operating p.
positioning p.
Profile p.
PSI TEC aspiration/irrigation p.
Selecta 1064 laser p.
StealthStation treatment guidance p.
TomTec echo p.
transcatheter intravascular ring p.
wedge-shaped p.

Platina clip lens
plating
Caspar p.
eccentric dynamic compression p.
Gotfried percutaneous compression p.
Leibinger p.
variable spinal p. (VSP)

platinum
p. coil
p. Dacron microcoil
p. embolization coil
p. eyelid implant
p. microcoil
P. 5000 micropigmentation handpiece
p. microwire electrode
p. oxygen electrode
P. Plus guidewire
p. probe spatula
p. ring
P. stationary table
p. tip guidewire
p. wire

platinum-iridium electrode
platinum-marked stent
Playmaker
P. functional knee brace
P. knee brace
P. support

PlayTuf knee brace
PLC-50 linear stapler
Pleatman
P. pouch
P. sac
P. sack

pledget
cotton p.
cottonoid p.
gelatin sponge p.
Gelfoam p.
lint p.
Meadox Teflon felt p.
neurosurgical p.
p. sponge
p. suture
Teflon p.
tetracaine p.
wool p.

pledgeted
p. Ethibond suture
p. mattress suture

PlegiaGuard pressure relief valve
Plester retractor
plethysmograph
air p.
BPXG body p.
face-out whole-body p.
MasterScreen BabyBody p.

P

plethysmograph *(continued)*
>MedGraphics body p.
>mercury-in-rubber strain gauge p.
>pressure p.
>venous p.

pleural
>p. biopsy needle
>p. biopsy needle shears
>p. biopsy punch
>p. dissector
>p. tube

Pleura-Stay
pleurectomy forceps
Pleur-evac
>P.-e. autotransfusion system
>P.-e. chest catheter
>P.-e. device
>P.-e. suction tube

Pleurx
>P. catheter
>P. home drainage kit
>P. indwelling pleural catheter
>P. pleural catheter
>P. pleural catheter/home drainage kit
>P. pleural catheter kit

Plexidure insole
Plexiglas
>P. base
>P. implant
>P. jig
>P. plate
>P. spacer
>P. tissue equivalency block
>P. tube

PlexiPulse intermittent pneumatic compression device
Plexis bone void filling system
Pley
>P. capsular forceps
>P. extracapsular forceps

PLI-100 pico-injector pipette system
pliable earplug
plication needle
pliers
>Becker-Parkin p.
>bending p.
>College p.
>Compaction p.
>crown-crimping p.
>debonding p.
>dental p.
>extraction p.
>fisherman's p.
>Howmedica Microfixation System p.
>Jelenko p.
>K-Y p.
>ligature-locking p.

>ligature-tying p.
>Luhr microfixation system p.
>Mathieu p.
>needle-nose vise-grip p.
>orthopaedic surgical p.
>Power-Grip p.
>Schwarz arrow-forming p.
>slip-joint p.
>Sontec p.
>square-end p.
>Storz Microsystems p.
>Synthes Microsystems p.
>vise-grip p.

PLIF
>posterior lumbar interbody fusion

PL100KL/50K
>Pall filter P.

PLLA anchor
PLM device
plotter
>X-Y p.

PLR
>proximal loading revision
>PLR spine revision hip stem

plug
>arrow-shaft silicone punctal p.
>Avina female urethral p.
>biodegradable collagen p.
>Biomet p.
>blue opaque Herrick lacrimal p.
>bone femoral p.
>bone graft p.
>brass scleral p.
>Buck p.
>capsular p.
>Catamaran swim p.
>catheter p.
>collagen p.
>Coloplast 1-piece Conseal p.
>Coloplast 2-piece Conseal p.
>Corner p.
>p. cutter
>Dittrich p.
>dome hole p.
>DuraPlug synthetic extended temporary punctal/canalicular p.
>Eagle FlexPlug punctum p.
>EaglePlug tapered-shaft punctum p.
>EagleVision Freeman punctum p.
>Exeter intramedullary bone p.
>Extend punctal p.
>FCI Ready-Set punctal p.
>femoral p.
>Form Fit intracanalicular p.
>Freeman punctum p.
>gamma-irradiated p.
>gastrostomy p.
>glass vaginal p.

Grafton DBM matrix demineralized bone graft p.
Herniamesh surgical p.
Herrick lacrimal p.
hydrogel p.
intracanalicular punctum p.
intramedullary canal p.
Ivalon p.
Johnston gastrostomy p.
Kirschner femoral canal p.
Luer-Lok male adapter p.
Mack ear p.
methyl methacrylate cranioplastic p.
Micro punctum p.
Oasis collagen p.
omental p.
opaque canalicular p.
opaque Herrick lacrimal p.
Osteonics acetabular dome hole p.
otoconial p.
patellar p.
PerFix hernia p.
PerFix Marlex mesh p.
plastic femoral p.
platelet p.
polypropylene p.
ProLong absorbable long-term p.
ProLoop mesh p.
punctum p.
Ready-Set punctum p.
R-Med p.
scleral p.
sealing window p.
self-seating p.
Sharpoint UltraPlug punctum p.
Shiley decannulation p.
silicone p.
Smart Plug lacrimal p.
Soft Plug punctal p.
Super Eagle punctum p.
Super Flex punctum p.
Super punctum p.
tapered-shaft punctum p.
TearSaver punctum p.
Teflon p.
Teflon Bardic p.
TruFit BGS p.
umbrella punctum p.
Woodson p.
Xsorb punctal p.
plug-finishing bur
plugged telescoping catheter
plugger
amalgam p.
Bredall amalgam p.
endodontic p.
Mity p.
Schilder p.
serrated amalgam p.

plugging instrument
PlugStation earplug station
Plum-Blossom acupuncture needle
PlumeSafe Whisper 602 smoke evacuation system
Plummer bougie
Plummer-Vinson apparatus
plunger
dome p.
plunger-type
p.-t. femoral pressurizer
p.-t. injector
PLUS
pivot link universal system
PLUS spinal instrumentation
plus
Betadine PrepStick P.
Bio Gard P.
BIS Sensor P.
Cutifilm P.
Cytobrush P.
Decal P.
ENTrak P.
GentleLASE P.
GrowTrak P.
GuardWire P.
Hydra Vision P.
Hydro P.
Laserprobe-PLR P.
p. lens
Lithostar P.
Medtronic Pisces Quad P.
Nexerciser P.
Omnifit P.
Omni-Flow 4000 P.
Oracle Micro P.
Pneu Care P.
p. power lens
P. punctal occluder
REMstar P.
Richards Solcotrans P.
RX Herculink p.
Siemens Lithostar P.
Siemens Somatom P.
Sonicare P.
Steri-Cuff P.
Suture Strip P.
Synergy P.
The Pigment Peel P.
Therevac P.
Track P.
Plyoback Rebounder
Plyo-Sled exerciser
PMMA
polymethylmethacrylate
PMMA centering sleeve
PMMA centralizer
PMMA custom-made calibration contact lens

P

PMMA *(continued)*
    PMMA haptic
    PMMA hard contact lens
    PMMA implant
    PMMA intraocular lens
PMT
    PMT AccuSpan tissue expander
    PMT halo system
    PMT halo system brace
    PMT robotic fulcrumless
      tomographic system
PMV
    PMV speaking valve
    PMV valve
Pneu
    P. Care Plus
    P. Knee brace
PneuGel
    P. ankle brace
    P. ankle wrap
    P. posterior leg splint
    P. shoulder wrap
pneumatic
    p. ankle tourniquet
    p. antiembolic stocking
    p. antishock garment
    p. bag
    p. balloon catheter
    p. balloon dilator
    p. 4-bar linkage knee
    p. chair lift
    p. compression boot
    p. compression sleeve
    p. compression stocking
    p. cuff
    p. cylinder
    p. endoscopic lithotriptor
    p. garment
    p. microscope
    p. otoscope
    p. peripheral circulation
     improvement device
    p. splint
    p. splint mechanism
    p. tonometer
    p. tourniquet
    p. walker
pneumatic-otoscope
pneumatonograph
pneumatonometer, pneumotonometer
    Digibind p.
    Micro One p.
    Modular One p.
PneuMicro small bone power system
Pneumo
    P. disposable pneumotachometer
    P. Sleeve
pneumoballistic lithotriptor
pneumocapillary infusion pump

pneumodissector
**pneumohydraulic capillary infusion
  system**
Pneumo-Matic insufflation needle
Pneumoneedle
    P. insufflation needle
    P. reusable instrument
pneumootoscope
pneumoperitoneum needle
pneumoscope
Pneumo-Sleeve
pneumostatic dilator
pneumotach
    p. disposable mouthpiece
    MicroTach p.
pneumotachograph
    Fleisch p.
    flow-sensing p.
pneumotachometer
    hot-wire p.
    Pneumo disposable p.
Pneumotest kit
pneumothoracic apparatus
pneumotonometer *(var. of*
  pneumatonometer)
Pneumo-Wrap
Pneupac
    P. resuscitator
    P. ventilator
pneuPAC
    p. resuscitator
    p. ventilator
PneuSplint
    P. splint
    STI Medical Products P.
Pneu-trac
    P.-t. cervical collar
    P.-t. neck brace
**PneuView ventilator testing and
  training system**
PNS Unna boot
POC
    POC balloon
    POC Bandit catheter
pocket
    p. mask
    p. probe
    p. red filter
PocketChem UA analyzer
Pocket-Dop
    P.-D. fetal heart rate monitor
    P.-D. fetal stethoscope
    P.-D. II
    P.-D. 3 monitor
Pockethaler
    Vancenase P.
pocketing hook
PocketPeak peak flowmeter
POCT device

podiatric bur
Podiatry Institute rasp
PodiAxis orthopaedic sole
Podi-Burr
    large callus P.-B.
    large nail P.-B.
    medium callus P.-B.
    medium nail P.-B.
    P.-B. nail bur
PodoFlex
    P. machine
    P. reflexology device
Pogon chair
point
    Crowe pilot p.
    2-p. discriminator
    drill p.
    p. electrode
    p. forceps
    gutta-percha p.
    6-p. knee brace
    Mathews drill p.
    powered automatic stopping drill p.
    Rancy-Crutchfield drill p.
    self-stopping drill p.
    Staller p.
    Starlite p.
    Universal drill p.
3-point
    3-p. fixation frame
    3-p. fixation intraocular lens
    3-p. head holder
    3-p. spreader bag
4-point
    4-p. cervical brace
    4-p. fixation intraocular lens
    4-p. IROM brace
    4-p. IROM splint
    4-p. restraint
    4-p. spreader bag
    4-p. SuperSport functional knee
      brace
    4-p. walker
pointed
    p. awl
    p. cone bur
    p. cystotome tip
    p. tip electrode
pointer
    LaserMed laser p.
    metallic p.
    P. 1-piece all-PMMA intraocular
      lens
    Z-Touch ENT laser p.
    Z-Touch laser p.
Pointer-Plus locator/stimulator
point-of-reduction clamp
point-search instrument
Polack keratoscope

polar
    P. Bair forced-air active cooling
      device
    P. Care 500 cryotherapy device
    p. coordinate system
    P. Electro sport tester
    P. enteral feeding bag
    P. Pack
    P. plate
    P. Vantage XL heart rate monitor
    P. wrist monitor
PolarCath
    P. balloon catheter
    P. peripheral dilatation system
polarimeter
    confocal scanning laser p.
    GDx Access scanning laser p.
    GDx scanning laser p.
    GDx VCC scanning laser p.
    scanning laser p.
Polaris
    P. camera system
    P. CPAP system
    P. grasper
    P. knee rehab brace
    P. LE catheter
    P. 1.32 Nd:YAG laser
    P. position tracker
    P. reusable cutter
    P. reusable dissector
    P. reusable forceps
    P. reusable grasper
    P. reusable instrument
    P. reusable laparoscopic instrument
    P. X steerable diagnostic catheter
polariscope
Polaris-Dx steerable diagnostic catheter
polarized lens
polarizing
    p. microscope
    p. ophthalmoscope
Polar-Mate
    P.-M. bipolar coagulator
    P.-M. bipolar microcoagulator
    P.-M. coagulator
polarographic needle electrode
Polaroid
    P. HealthCam system
    P. instant endocamera
    P. vectograph slide
Polaron sputter coater
Polarus
    P. humeral rod
    P. Plus humeral fixation system
    P. positional humeral fixation
      system
pole
    Exerstrider walking p.
    p. piece

P

pole *(continued)*
    p. tip
    walking p.
PoleStar N-10 iMRI
Polhemus
    P. 3D digitizer
    P. 3D digitizer scanner
    P. 3Space digitizer
policeman
    p. glass stirring rod
    p. tip
    p. transfer tool
poliglecaprone 25 suture
polio laryngoscope
polish
    Sklar instrument p.
polisher
    Anis capsule p.
    Buedding squeegee cortex extractor
     and p.
    capsule p.
    Drews capsule p.
    Freeman capsule p.
    Jensen capsule p.
    Knolle capsule p.
    Knolle capsule p.
    Kraff capsule p.
    Kratz capsule p.
    Kratz-Jensen p.
    Look capsule p.
    microloop curette p.
    squeegee capsule p.
    Terry silicone capsule p.
    Yaghouti LASIK p.
polisher/scratcher
    Jensen p./s.
    Kratz p./s.
polishing
    p. brush
    p. bur
    p. strip
Politzer
    P. air bag
    P. air bag otoscope
    P. air syringe
    P. angular ear knife
    P. ear perforator
    P. ear speculum
    P. paracentesis needle
Polk finger goniometer
**Pollack bead chain cystourethrography
  set**
**Polle pod attachment for
  ophthalmoscope**
Pollock
    P. forceps
    P. punch
Pollock-Dingman elevator
Polly power grip

Poloxamer 407 barrier material
poloxamer-based gel
Poly
    P. CS device
    P. GIA stapler
polyacrylamide bead
polyamide
    p. mesh
    p. suture
**polyanhydride biodegradable polymer
  wafer**
polyaxial
    p. cervical screw
    p. screw
    p. system
polybutester suture
polycarbonate
    p. ballistic protective eyewear
    p. lens
polycarboxylate cement
Poly-Cath catheter
polycationic histochemical probe
polycentric
    p. hinged ulnar deviation splint
    p. knee prosthesis
    p. unconstrained prosthesis
**Poly-Chem automated chemistry-
  immunoassay system**
Polydek suture
Polyderm
    P. border with Covaderm tape
    P. foam dressing
    P. foam wound dressing
    P. hydrophilic polyurethane foam
     dressing
Poly-Dial
    P.-D. constrained liner
    P.-D. insert
polydioxanone
    p. plate
    p. sheet
    p. suture (PDS)
polyene thread
polyester fiber suture
polyether implant material
polyethylene
    ArCom compression-molded p.
    ArCom processed p.
    p. button
    p. cannula
    carbon fiber-reinforced p.
    p. catheter
    p. collar button
    p. drain
    Durasul p.
    p. endoprosthesis
    extruded bar p.
    p. feeding tube
    p. foam

p. graft
high-density p.
p. implant
p. implant material
p. intravenous catheter
p. liner
p. liner implant component
p. peg
p. socket
p. sphere implant
p. stent
p. strut
p. suture
p. talar prosthesis
p. terephthalate balloon
p. tibial insert
p. T tube
p. tube
p. tubing
ultrahigh molecular weight p. (UHMWPE)

polyethylene-faced
p.-f. driver
p. f. mallet

polyfilament suture
Polyflex
P. lead
P. stent

Polyflux S dialyzer
Polyform splint
polygalactic acid suture
polyglactin
p. mesh
p. monofilament loop
p. suture
p. 910 suture
p. suture material

polyglecaprone 25 suture
polyglycolate suture
polyglycolic
p. acid conduit
p. acid suture
p. mesh

polyglycolide implant
polyglyconate
p. monofilament loop
p. staple
p. suture

polygon mirror
polygraph
Gould p.
Mackenzie p.
Night Owl pocket p.
Nihon Kohden p.

polylactic acid arrow
polylactide
p. absorbable screw
p. implant

Poly-Lock bonding

PolyMax resorbable fixation system
PolyMedics plate
PolyMem
P. adhesive surgical wound dressing
P. alginate dressing
P. alginate wound cover
P. foam dressing
P. foam wound dressing
P. wound care dressing

polymer
biodegradable synthetic p.
Bioplastique p.
HTR p.
Hylamer orthopaedic bearing p.
superabsorbent p.
p. tooth replica implant

PolymerFriction total knee
polymeric
p. biomaterial
p. endoluminal paving stent

polymethylmethacrylate (PMMA)
p. biomaterial
p. bone cement
p. ear splint
p. ear splint
p. implant

polymorphic microsatellite marker
polyolefin copolymer balloon
polyorganophosphazene-coated stent
polyp
p. forceps
p. grasper
p. retriever

polypectomy snare
polyphase generator
Polypin biodegradable pin implant
polypropylene
p. ankle-foot orthosis
p. button
p. button suture
p. catheter
p. glycol ankle-foot orthosis
p. glycol thoracolumbosacral orthosis
p. hand brush
p. intracardiac patch
p. intraocular lens
p. mesh
p. needle
p. plug
p. stent
p. suture

polypus forceps
Polyrox Fractal active fixation lead
PolySafe
P. A-track lead
P. pacer

polysiloxane cast

Polyskin
- P. II dressing
- P. II transparent film
- P. M.R. transparent film

polysomnograph 20-channel EEG recorder

Polysorb
- P. absorbable staple
- P. heel cup
- P. liner
- P. meniscal stapler XLS
- P. 55 stapler
- P. suture

Polystan
- P. cardiotomy reservoir
- P. implant
- P. perfusion cannula
- P. venous return catheter

Polystim electrode

polysulfone
- p. dialyzer
- p. membrane

Polytec
- P. LaseAway Q-switched ruby laser
- P. PI LaseAway

Polytechnic foot-pressure measuring plate

PolyTech nonlatex urinary external catheter

polytef-sheathed needle

polytef soft tissue patch

polytetrafluoroethylene (PTFE)
- p. covered stent
- expanded p. (EPTFE)
- p. implant
- p. mesh
- p. prosthesis
- p. sock
- p. stent graft
- p. suture

polytome instrument

Polytron DSA equipment

polyurethane
- p. bandage
- p. catheter
- p. dilator
- p. dressing
- p. foam embolus
- p. graft
- p. implant material
- p. liner
- p. nasoenteric catheter
- p. stent

polyurethane-coated silicone breast implant

polyurethane-covered metallic stent

polyvinyl
- p. alcohol foam
- p. alcohol splint
- p. alcohol sponge
- p. bougie
- p. chloride balloon
- p. chloride catheter
- p. chloride endotracheal tube
- p. curette
- p. dilator
- p. drain
- p. graft
- p. implant material
- p. prosthesis
- p. sponge
- p. sponge implant
- p. tubing

polyvinylsiloxane
- p. impression pad
- p. putty

Polyviolene polyester suture material

PolyWic
- P. dressing
- P. filler
- P. wound filling material

Pomeroy ear syringe

pommel cushion

poncho restraint

Pond adjustable splint

Ponsky
- P. PEG tube
- P. pull
- P. pull PEG standard kit

Ponsky-Gauderer
- P.-G. gastrostomy tube
- P.-G. type PEG

pontoon spica cast

pool
- AquaMotion p.
- aquatic therapy p.
- Endless Pool physical therapy p.
- Ferno custom therapy p.
- SwimEx p.

Poole
- P. abdominal suction tube
- P. suction tube
- P. trocar

POP
- plaster of Paris
- POP bandage
- POP cast

Pope
- P. night splint
- P. Oto-Wick
- P. Oto-Wick medicated ear sponge
- P. wick

popliteal retractor

POPmesh polypropylene mesh

pop-off
- p.-o. needle

p.-o. suture
p.-o. valve
Pop-On self-adhering male external catheter
Poppen
    P. forceps
    P. Gigli saw guide
    P. intervertebral disc forceps
    P. intervertebral disc rongeur
    P. suction tube
poppet
    prosthetic p.
    silastic p.
porcelain
    Vitadur Alpha p.
porcine
    p. bioprosthesis
    p. graft
    p. heart valve
    p. prosthesis
    p. valve
Porex
    P. drainage system
    P. implant
    P. Medpor implant
Porges Neoflex dilator
Porocoat material
Poro-in-between sole
Poron
    P. cellular urethane
    P. 400 insole
porous
    p. calcium phosphate cube
    p. collagen matrix
    p. hydroxyapatite sphere
    p. implant
    p. metallic stent
    p. orbital implant
    p. polyethylene implant
    p. sheet
    p. surfaced prosthesis
    p. tantalum implant
porous-coated
    p.-c. acetabular cup
    p.-c. anatomic (PCA)
    p.-c. anatomic knee prosthesis
    p.-c. implant
PORP
    partial ossicular replacement prosthesis
    Richards hydroxyapatite PORP
port
    A-Port implantable p.
    BardPort implanted p.
    BardPort low-profile p.
    BardPort MRI full-size p.
    butterfly needle infusion p.
    CathLink 20 implanted p.
    Celsite implanted p.
    Cordis multipurpose access p.

    endoscopic access p.
    endoscopic threaded imaging p.
    EndoTIP imaging p.
    Gills-Welsh guillotine p.
    Hassan-type p.
    Hasson blunt p.
    implantable infusion p.
    Import vascular access p.
    Infuse-a-Port p.
    infusion p.
    low-profile port implantable p.
    Luer-Lok p.
    lumbar p.
    OmegaPort access p.
    periumbilical p.
    p. protector
    Quinton Q-Port vascular access p.
    2-p. radial tip
    3-p. radial tip
    SEA p.
    self-sealing injection p.
    side-arm pressure p.
    single p.
    tangential p.
    Thora-Port p.
    titanium VasPort p.
    totally implantable access p.
    treatment p.
    Universal catheter access p.
    venous access p.
    Vortex Clear-Flow p.
    X-Port Duo dual-lumen implantable p.
    X-Port Inline implantable p.
portable
    p. aerosol delivery device
    AutoSet P. II
    p. blood irradiator
    p. insulin dosage-regulating apparatus
    p. insulin infusion pump
    p. magnifier lab lamp
    p. monitoring device
    p. perfused manometric system
    p. PT100 noncontact tonometer
    p. radio adaptor
    p. respirator
    p. stretcher
    p. suction aspirator
    p. suction device
    p. topical hyperbaric oxygen extremity chamber
    p. volume ventilator
Port-A-Cath
    P.-A-C. catheter
    P.-A-C. device
    P.-A-C. implantable catheter
    P.-A-C. implantable catheter system

P

691

portacaval
> p. H graft
> p. H-graft shunt
> p. shunt

Port-Access
> St. Jude Medical P.-A.

PortaFlo urine collection system

Port-A-Germ anaerobic transport vial

portal
> AP p.
> AP/PA p.
> p. cannula
> p. catheter
> fixed-beam p.
> integrated side port access p.
> Neviaser p.
> PA p.
> P. Pro 2 treatment chair
> p. vein
> Wilmington arthroscopic p.

portal-phased spiral CT scan

Porta-Lung noninvasive extrathoracic ventilator

PortalVision radiation oncology system

Porta Pulse 3 portable defibrillator

Porta-Resp monitor

Porta-Stat cephalostat

portasystemic shunt

port-catheter system

Portex
> P. Blue Line tracheostomy tube
> P. chorionic villus sampling catheter
> P. nasopharyngeal airway
> P. Per-fit tracheostomy kit
> P. Per-fit tracheostomy tube
> P. preformed blue line tracheal tube
> P. soft seal laryngeal mask
> P. Thermovent heat and moisture device
> P. Thermovent heat and moisture exchanger
> P. XL endotracheal tube cuff

Portmann speculum holder

Portnoy DPV device

portogram
> SMA p.

portosystemic shunt

Porto-Vac suction tube

PortSaver PercLoop device

Porzett splint

Posey
> P. bar kit
> P. bed cradle
> P. belt
> P. Cufflator tracheal cuff inflator and manometer
> P. drop seat

> P. grip
> P. palm cone
> P. restraint
> P. SkinSleeves
> P. sling
> P. snare

Posicam HZ PET scanner

Positex knee wedge

position
> P. Plus cushion
> 5-p. turret

positional feedback stimulation trainer

positioner
> Allen arthroscopic elbow p.
> Allen arthroscopic knee p.
> Allen arthroscopic wrist p.
> arm p.
> Assistant Free Stulberg leg p.
> Bareskin knee p.
> basilar block skull p.
> beach chair p.
> Biomet Second Assistant knee p.
> body p.
> BodyCushion p.
> CAS-8000V general angiography p.
> Cook stent p.
> cup p.
> De Mayo hip p.
> dual lateral hand p.
> dual oblique hand p.
> Foot Waffle p.
> Grasshopper p.
> hip p.
> IMP Universal lateral p.
> irrigating IOL p.
> Kirschenbaum foot p.
> knee p.
> lateral p.
> leg p.
> Mark II Stulberg hip p.
> Mark II Stulberg leg p.
> Mark II Wixson hip p.
> MB&J knee p.
> McConnell shoulder p.
> McGuire pelvic p.
> Medline p.
> Pigg-O-Stat pediatric immobilizer and p.
> Prep-Assist p.
> Profex arthroscopic leg p.
> Schlein shoulder p.
> shoulder abduction p.
> Stulberg hip p.
> Stulberg Mark II leg p.
> SurgAssist leg p.
> Ther-A-Shapes p.
> Thornton anterior p.
> TMJ head p.
> Universal knee p.

Universal lateral p.
Vac-Pac p.
vacuum beanbag p.
Waters p.
Wixson hip p.
Zimfoam pad and patient p.
positioning
p. needle
p. pillow
p. platform
position-sensing catheter
positive
p. eyepiece
p. support ventilator
positive-placement pipette
Positrap
P. miniretrieval basket
P. 3-prong nonretracting grasping forceps
P. retriever
Positrol
P. cardiac device
P. II catheter
P. USCI catheter
positron
p. camera
p. emission tomography (PET)
p. emission tomography balloon
p. emitter
p. scintillation camera
Posner
P. diagnostic gonioprism
P. diagnostic lens
P. slit-lamp
P. surgical gonioprism
Possis AngioJet Xpeedior catheter
post
Caspar retraction p.
FibreKor p.
P. forceps
Hahnenkratt root canal p.
surgical instrument p.
transosseous p.
P. washing cannula
postauricular
p. ear dressing
p. hearing aid
p. retractor
poster
2-p. brace
4-p. frame
posterior
p. capsule scrubber
p. chamber intraocular lens
p. chamber lens implant
p. convex intraocular lens
p. distraction instrumentation
p. footplate pick
p. forceps

p. fossa retractor
p. glenoid elevator
p. hook-rod spinal instrumentation
p. leaf-spring ankle-foot orthosis
p. lumbar interbody fusion (PLIF)
p. neck surface coil
p. reduction device
p. rod system
p. thigh bar
p. urethral retractor
posterior-anterior screw
postgadolinium scan
posting
heel p.
strip p.
wedge p.
postmortem suture needle
postnasal
p. balloon
p. balloon tamponade
p. dressing
p. sponge forceps
postoperative
p. flexor tendon traction brace
p. immobilizer
p. mammary support
p. shoe
postprostatectomy hemostatic catheter
postpyloric feeding tube
Postura wheelchair cushion
Posture
P. Curve lumbar cushion
P. Pump lordoticiser
P. Pump spine trainer
P. S'port
P. Wedge seat cushion
Posture-Rite lap desk
Pos-T-Vac
P.-T.-V. vacuum erection device
P.-T.-V. VCD
Potain
P. apparatus
P. aspirator
potassium titanyl phosphate laser
potassium-titanyl-phosphate:YAG laser
potential acuity meter
potentiometer
linear p.
Potocky needle
pot patch
Potter-Bucky diaphragm
Potter-Elvehjem
P.-E. handheld tissue grinder
P.-E. homogenizer
Potts
P. aortic clamp
P. bronchial forceps
P. bulldog forceps
P. dental elevator

P

Potts *(continued)*
    P. elevator
    P. forceps
    P. needle
    P. scissors
    P. shunt
    P. tenotomy scissors
    P. thumb forceps
    P. vascular scissors
Potts-Cournand needle
Potts-Smith
    P.-S. bipolar forceps
    P.-S. dissecting scissors
    P.-S. dressing forceps
    P.-S. monopolar forceps
    P.-S. reverse scissors
    P.-S. tissue forceps
pouch
    Active Life 1-piece drainable p.
    Active Life 1-piece precut closed-
      end p.
    Assura convex drainable p.
    Assura convex urostomy p.
    Assura pediatric p.
    Assura standard drainable p.
    Bard closed-end adhesive p.
    Bard drainage adhesive p.
    Bard security p.
    bladder replacement urinary p.
    Bongort 1-piece drainable p.
    Bongort 1-piece ostomy p.
    Camey urinary p.
    Cardio-Cool myocardial
      protection p.
    Coloplast closed p.
    Coloplast drainable p.
    Coloplast 1-piece small
      drainable p.
    Coloplast 2-piece small
      drainable p.
    Coloplast 2-piece small
      urostomy p.
    Coloplast 1-piece standard
      drainable p.
    ConvaTec ostomy p.
    ConvaTec urostomy p.
    Dansac Contour 1 mini 1-piece p.
    Dansac Contour 1 oval 1-piece p.
    Dansac standard F 1-piece p.
    Denis Browne p.
    female urinary p.
    FirstChoice closed p.
    FirstChoice drainable p.
    FirstChoice postoperative
      drainable p.
    FirstChoice urostomy p.
    Florida p.
    Florida urinary p.
    Fobi p.

    Holligard seal closed stoma p.
    Hollister First Choice p.
    Hunt-Lawrence p.
    ileal neobladder urinary p.
    Incise p.
    Indiana urinary p.
    Kock urinary p.
    Le Bag urinary p.
    Lo-Profile urostomy p.
    Mainz p.
    Mainz urinary p.
    Manhood absorbent p.
    Mansson urinary p.
    Marlen Ultra 1-piece p.
    marsupial p.
    Mentor absorbent p.
    MicroSkin ostomy p.
    Nu-Hope drainable 1-piece p.
    Nu-Hope neonatal and preemie p.
    Nu-Hope ostomy neonatal p.
    Nu-Hope urinary p.
    Nu-Hope urostomy p.
    Padua bladder urinary p.
    pediatric drainable p.
    pediatric transfer p.
    pediatric urostomy p.
    Penn p.
    perineal p.
    Pleatman p.
    preemie p.
    Premier drainable p.
    Premier urostomy p.
    Premium closed p.
    Premium drainable p.
    RapiSeal p.
    Reality vaginal p.
    Rowland p.
    sigma rectum p.
    Squibb urostomy p.
    Studer p.
    Sur-Fit Natura flexible wafer and
      drainable p.
    Sur-Fit Natura mini p.
    Sur-Fit Natura urostomy p.
    Tena p.
    vaginal p.
Pouchkins
    P. pediatric ostomy belt
    P. pediatric ostomy system
pouch-type sling
Pourchez XpressO hemodialysis catheter
powder
    absorption p.
    Arglaes p.
    p. blower
    p. board
    Chronicure protein hydrolysate p.
    Comfeel p.
    Cranioplastic p.

Dembone cortical bone p.
Dembone demineralized cortical p.
demineralized cortical bone p.
hyCURE wound care p.
Nu-Hope Karaya p.
Osteomin Thermo-Ashed bone p.
Royl-Derm protectant p.
Sklar Kleen p.
Stomahesive p.
Surgifoam absorbable p.
Tru-Stain acrylic p.
Ultimatics demineralized cortical
  bone p.
Vitadur-N porcelain p.
Powell wand
power
  p. adapter
  p. amplifier
  P. Anthro shoe
  p. cannula
  p. Doppler
  p. Doppler ultrasonography
  p. Doppler ultrasound
  p. drill
  P. Grip stent
  p. injector
  p. peak filter
  P. Pillow cervical massager
  P. Pogo stationary exerciser
  p. rasp
  p. router
  P. Trainer cycle
  P. Trak 6000 gradient
  P. Web hand exerciser
  P. Web Jr. exerciser
  p. wheelchair
Powerbelt exercise system
PowerCut drill blade
power-driven reamer
powered
  p. automatic skull perforator
  p. automatic-stopping drill
  p. automatic stopping drill point
  p. instrumentation
Powerflex
  P. CMP exerciser
  P. Extreme PTA balloon catheter
  P. P3 high-pressure balloon
    catheter
  P. tape
Power-Grip pliers
PowerGrip stent delivery system
Powerheart
  P. AECD
  P. automatic external cardioverter-
    defibrillator
  P. external defibrillator
Powerlink endoluminal graft system
Powermatic table

**PowerPICC power injector peripherally
  inserted central catheter**
PowerPlex 1.2 genetic identification kit
POWERPoint orthotic shoe insert
**PowerProxi Sonic interdental toothbrush
  system**
PowerStar bipolar scissors
Powerstep
  P. foot support
  P. orthotic
**PowerTrack II muscle testing
  instrument**
PowerVision ultrasound
Pozzi
  P. tenaculum
  P. tenaculum forceps
P55 pachymetric analyzer
PPCID
  PPCID sequential foot compression
    device
  PPCID slipper
PPG probe
PPH stapler
PPT
  PPT flat insole
  PPT insole system
  PPT MXL soft molded insole
  PPT Plastizote insole
  PPT RX firm molded insole
  PPT sheet
PQ
  PQ 5000 CT scanner
  PQ premium heel cup
pQCT scanner
Prader
  P. calipers
  P. orchidometer
^{32}P radioactive stent
PRAFO
  PRAFO adjustable orthotic
  PRAFO PKA KAFO attachment
Pratt
  P. anoscope
  P. crypt hook
  P. dilator
  P. ethmoid curette
  P. rectal probe
  P. rectal speculum
  P. urethral sound
  P. uterine dilator
preamplifier
  Arzco p.
  epoxy-mounted p.
preassembled metal-backed socket
precalibrated pointing device
prechopper
  Akahoshi combo p.
  Akahoshi hybrid combo p.

P

prechopper *(continued)*
    Akahoshi phaco p.
    Akahoshi Universal p.
pre-chopping forceps
Precise
    P. anastomotic coupler
    P. disposable skin stapler
    P. nitinol transhepatic biliary stent
    P. RX transhepatic biliary stent
    P. self-expanding stent
    P. stapler
Precision
    P. Cosmet intraocular lens implant
    P. Cosmet lens
    P. digital x-ray
    P. Extra
    P. hip system
    P. office TUNA system
    P. Osteolock
    P. Osteolock femoral component
    P. Osteolock femoral component
        system
    P. Osteolock femoral prosthesis
    P. Osteolock hip prosthesis
    P. Osteolock stem
    P. Osteolock total hip
    P. QID glucose meter
    P. QID glucose monitoring system
    P. refractor
    P. SpeedTac transvaginal anchor
        system
    P. spinal cord stimulator
    P. Strata hip system
    P. tack instrument
    P. Tack transvaginal anchor system
    P. total hip
    P. Twist transvaginal anchor
        system
    P. Xtra advanced diabetes
        management system
    P. Xtra test strip
PrecisionGlide needle
Precisionist Thirty Thousand cataract
    removal system
Pre-Cision miniature and
    microminiature scalpel
precision-point needle
Precisor
    P. Broncho pulmonary disposable
        biopsy forceps
    P. Direct Bite biopsy forceps
    P. disposable biopsy forceps
PreClean soak system
Preclude
    P. dura substitute prosthesis
    P. IMA sleeve
    P. MVP dura substitute
    P. PDX dura substitute
    P. pericardial membrane

    P. peritoneal membrane
    P. spinal membrane
Precoat
    P. hip prosthesis
    P. Plus femoral prosthesis
precollagenous filamentous material
precompression jig
precontoured unit rod
precordial stethoscope
precurving endosonic file
precut papillotome
Predator PTCA catheter
Predicta TGF-β1 kit
predictor
    Corazonix P.
    OV-Watch fertility p.
preemie pouch
prefabricated
    p. composite flap
    p. wool felt pad
preformed clasp
Pre-Gen 26 colorectal cancer test
preloaded injector
PremiCron nonabsorbable suture
Premier
    P. anterior cervical plate system
    P. drainable minipouch
    P. drainable pouch
    P. I&A unit
    P. press fit prosthesis
    P. press-fit prosthesis
    P. urostomy pouch
Premium
    P. CEEA circular stapler
    P. CEEA circular stapling device
    P. closed pouch
    P. drainable pouch
    P. Plus CEEA disposable stapler
    P. stapler
premounted stent
Prentif
    P. cavity-rim cervical sap
    P. pessary
Prenyl jacket
Prep-Assist
    P.-A. legholder
    P.-A. positioner
preperitoneal distension balloon
preperitoneal dilator balloon
Prep-IM hip bone preparation kit
prepuce forceps
presbyopia-correcting IOL
presbyopia glasses
presbyopic intraocular lens
Presbyterian
    P. Hospital occluding clamp
    P. Hospital tubing clamp
Prescott wireless foot switch
Presence bladder control pad

Preservation unicompartmental knee system
preserving
    instrumented bone p. (IBP)
preset diamond knife
preshaped catheter
press
    Call-Press graft p.
    CamStar power leg p.
    Omni p.
    Shuttle MVP leg p.
    tissue graft p.
press-button chuck
press-fit
    p.-f. condylar component
    p.-f. condylar total knee
    p.-f. femoral component
    p.-f. implant
    p.-f. prosthesis
    p.-f. stem
    p.-f. total condylar knee system
press-in
    p.-i. bone anchor
    p.-i. bone anchor system
Press-Mate model 8800T blood pressure monitor
pressometer
    Jarcho p.
press-on prism
PresSsion pneumatic garment
pressure
    p. algometer
    Alladin InfantFlow nasal continuous positive air p.
    p. bandage
    bilevel positive airway p. (BiPAP)
    central venous p.
    continuous positive airway p. (CPAP)
    p. controller
    p. cuff
    p. earring
    p. equalization tube
    p. forceps
    p. gauge
    p. glove
    p. guide pressure wire
    p. injector
    p. length loop
    p. patch dressing
    p. phosphene tonometer
    p. plethysmograph
    p. relief ankle-foot orthosis
    p. relief padding
    p. relief shoe
    p. relief valve
    p. ring
    p. sensor

P. Sentinel intramedullary reaming system
P. Sentinel reamer
p. shield
p. sling
p. sore status tool
p. splint
p. support ventilator (PSV)
p. transducer
p. transducer
p. transducer airflow sensor
p. transducer-monitor system
variable positive airway p. (VPAP)
p. ventilator
pressure-activated safety valve
pressure-applied dressing (PAD)
pressure-cycled ventilator
pressure-detachable silicone balloon
Pressurefuse automatic constant pressure device
pressure-gradient wire system
PressureGuard mattress
pressure-point tension ring
pressure-preset ventilator
pressure-producing earring
pressure-relief
    p.-r. ankle-foot orthotic
    p.-r. cushion
pressure-relieving orthosis
pressure-specified sensory device
PressureWire
    P. guidewire
    P. sensor
PressureWire-3 sensor
pressurized
    p. cement
    p. metered-dose inhaler
pressurizer
    Oxyhood p.
    plunger-type femoral p.
pressurizing system (PS)
Pressurometer blood pressure monitor
Prestige
    P. advanced cataract extraction system
    P. IQ glucose meter
    P. Lite Touch lancing device
    P. LX glucose meter
    P. Smart System test strip
Presto-Flash spirometry system
Preston
    P. ligamentum flavum forceps
    P. overhead pulley
    P. pinch gauge
    P. screw
    P. Traveler CPM exerciser
Prestop pinchometer
Presto spirometry system
pretapped Synthes lag screw

P

697

pretarget filtration system
pretibial buttress
Prevacare Total Solution skin care spray
Prevail
  P. protective underwear
  P. steerable catheter
PreVue III digitizing system
Price
  P. corneal punch
  P. corneal transplant system
  P. donor cornea punch set
  P. radial marker
Pricker needle
Priessnitz
  P. bandage
  P. dressing
Priestley-Smith retinoscope
Prima
  P. KTP/532 laser
  P. laser
  P. Laser catheter
  P. laser guidewire
  P. Series LEEP speculum
  P. total occlusion device
  P. total occlusion system
Primaloc cementless hip system
Primapore tape and gauze wound dressing
Primaria tissue culture flask
primary
  p. clip
  p. hydroxyapatite-coated sleeve
Primbs suturing forceps
Prime ECG mapping system
primer
  p. compression wrap
  p. flexible Unna boot
  p. instrument
  p. leg compression dressing
  p. modified Unna boot
PrimeTime
  P. disposable underpad
  P. Plus adult disposable brief
primordial catheter tube
Primus
  P. flexible great toe
  P. prostate machine
Prince
  P. advancement forceps
  P. cautery
  P. electrocautery
  P. muscle clamp
  P. muscle forceps
  P. trachoma forceps
PrinceStar electrophysiologic imaging study system

PrinterNOx
  P. nitric oxide/nitrogen dioxide monitor
  P. nitric oxide with MKII analyzer
Prio video display terminal vision tester
prism
  Allen-Thorpe gonioscopic p.
  AO rotary p.
  bar p.
  base-down p.
  BD p.
  Becker gonioscopic p.
  Berens p.
  diopter p.
  Fresnel p.
  Goldmann contact lens p.
  gonioscopic p.
  handheld rotary p.
  P. 3-head system
  Keeler p.
  p. loupe
  Maddox p.
  P. mixing bowl
  Nicol p.
  oblique p.
  plastic p.
  press-on p.
  Risley rotary p.
  scanning p.
  square p.
  P. 2000XP gamma camera
Prisma digital hearing aid
prismatic
  p. contact lens
  p. spectacles
Pristine-100 allergy control product
Pritchard
  P. elevator
  P. II elbow prosthesis
  P. total elbow prosthesis
Private Practice vibration reminder disc
Prizm
  P. Electro-Mesh Sock electrode
  P. Electro-Mesh Z-Stim II stimulator
  P. keratome blade
PRO
  PRO infusion catheter
  PRO traction table
Pro
  P. Balance Master
  P. Osteon 500 bone graft substitute
  P. Support Systems orthotic
Pro-8 ankle brace
ProAdvantage knee
ProAire portable rotation system

**Pro-Bal protected balloon-tipped
 catheter**
proband
probe

ABCFlex argon beam GI p.
Accurus 2500 p.
acoustic impedance p.
acridinium ester-labeled nucleic
 acid p.
Acufex p.
AcuNav steerable phased vector-
 array ultrasound catheter p.
ADD side-directed p.
afterloading p.
Alcon vitrectomy p.
Aloka MP-PN ultrasound p.
Aloka SSD ultrasound system
 and p.
alpha p.
ambulatory ventricular function p.
Amussat p.
Anel lacrimal p.
AngeLase combined mapping-
 laser p.
angled p.
antisense RNA p.
Arbuckle sinus p.
Arthro-BST arthroscopic p.
back-stop laser p.
Bakes p.
Balectrode pacing p.
p. balloon catheter
Barr fistular p.
p. beam
4-beam laser Doppler p.
beta-actin cDNA p.
BICAP p.
BICAP bipolar hemostasis p.
BiLAP bipolar cutting p.
BiLAP bipolar laparoscopic p.
biliary balloon p.
Bilitec 2000 intraluminal
 fiberoptic p.
biometry p.
biopsy p.
biplane intracavitary p.
biplane sector p.
bipolar circumactive p. (BICAP)
Bipolar EndoStasis p.
bipolar hemostasis p.
blind endosonography p.
blood flow p.
blunt p.
blunt lacrimal p.
blunt-tip p.
Bodian lacrimal pigtail p.
Bowman p.
Bowman lacrimal p.
Brackett dental p.

brain p.
Brüel & Kjaer transvaginal
 ultrasound p.
Brymill cryosurgical p.
Buck ear p.
Buie fistula p.
bullet p.
Bunnell dissecting p.
Bunnell forwarding p.
calibrated p.
cardiac p.
Cardiac View p.
Castroviejo lacrimal sac p.
cataract p.
catheter p.
catheter-based ultrasound p.
catheter ultrasound p.
cDNA p.
Chandler V-pacing p.
chemiluminescent p.
Circon-ACMI electrohydraulic
 lithotriptor p.
Clark p.
coagulation p.
CO_2 laser p.
common duct p.
conical p.
contact p.
Contact Laser convex p.
Contact Laser round p.
continuously perfused p.
convex p.
coronary artery p.
Corson needle electrosurgical p.
cryoablation p.
cryogenic p.
cryopexy p.
cryotherapy p.
C-Trak p.
C-Trak handheld gamma p.
curved laser p.
curved retinal p.
cytochemical p.
dedicated Doppler p.
Desjardins gall duct p.
digoxigenin-labeled
 oligonucleotide p.
dilating p.
p. dilator
dilator p.
disposable p.
dissecting p.
Dobbhoff bipolar coagulation p.
Dodick photolysis p.
Doppler p.
Doppler 4-beam laser p.
Doppler flow p.
Doppler flow echocardiographic p.
Doppler ultrasonic p.

P

probe *(continued)*

dot-plotted p.
double-ended silver p.
drum p.
dual color p.
ear p.
echocardiographic p.
EHL p.
electric p.
electrohydraulic p.
electrohydraulic lithotripsy p.
electrohydraulic lithotriptor p.
electromagnetic flow p.
electromagnetic focusing field p.
electrosurgical monopolar spatula p.
Ellis foreign body spud needle p.
end-fire transrectal p.
endocavitary p.
endocervical p.
EndoENT p.
endolaser p.
Endopath needle-tip
  electrosurgery p.
endoscopic heat p.
endoscopic ultrasound p.
Endosound ultrasound p.
EndoStasis p.
Endotrac p.
Envision endocavity p.
Esmarch p. with Myrtle leaf end
extended sector ultrasonic p.
eye p.
Fenger gall duct p.
fiberoptic p.
filiform bougie p.
Fish sinus p.
fistula p.
flexible endosonography p.
flow p.
Fluhrer bullet p.
Fluhrer rectal p.
fluorescent p.
fluoroptic thermometry p.
Fogarty biliary balloon p.
foreign body p.
fragmentation p.
Fränkel sinus p.
freehand p.
free-spinning p.
French lacrimal p.
Frigitronics freeze-thaw cryopexy p.
frontal sinus p.
gall duct p.
gallstone p.
galvanic p.
gamma p.
gamma-detecting p.
gamma detection p.
gear shift pedicle p.

general p.
genomic p.
GE proton head coil p.
Gilmore p.
Girdner p.
Glider articular cartilage p.
Gold P.
Goldman-Fox p.
G3PDH CDNA p.
p. and groove director
handheld p.
handheld exploring electrode p.
handheld mapping p.
Harms trabeculotomy p.
heater p.
Heller p.
Hewlett-Packard biplane p.
Hewlett-Packard omniplane p.
high-frequency miniature p.
high-resolution p.
Hitachi convex-convex biplane p.
Hitachi convex ultrasound p.
Hitachi fingertip ultrasound p.
Hitachi linear ultrasound p.
Hitachi transrectal ultrasound p.
Hitachi transvaginal ultrasound p.
hockey-stick electrosurgical p.
hot-tip laser p.
24-hour esophageal pH p.
HPU heat p.
Huber p.
Hu-Friedy p.
hybridized p.
illuminated p.
Infinitech laser p.
Injectate p.
injection gold p.
in-line p.
InnoVit 1800 p.
InnoVit vitrectomy p.
IntraDop p.
intraductal ultrasound p.
intraluminal p.
intraoperative gamma p.
intraoperative ultrasonic p.
irrigating p.
isotropic p.
Jako laryngeal p.
J-hook electrosurgical p.
Jobson-Horne ear p.
Jubileum 2.0 single-use
  gastroesophageal pH p.
Keeler-Amoils curved cataract p.
Keeler-Amoils glaucoma p.
Keeler-Amoils long-shank retinal p.
Keeler-Amoils microcurved
  cataract p.
Keeler-Amoils ophthalmic long-
  shank p.

Keeler-Amoils ophthalmic
Machemer retinal p.
Keeler-Amoils ophthalmic straight
cataract p.
Keeler-Amoils ophthalmic
vitreous p.
Killian p.
Kirschner guiding p.
Kleinsasser p.
Knapp iris p.
Kocher p.
Koenig p.
Kron bile duct p.
KTP laser p.
lacrimal p.
lacrimal duct p.
lacrimal intubation p.
laparoscopic p.
laparoscopic Doppler p.
laparoscopic ultrasound p.
large-bore heat p.
Larry rectal p.
laryngeal p.
laser Doppler flowmetry p.
laser Doppler Periflux PF-3 p.
Laserflow Doppler p.
Laserphaco p.
LeVeen RF p.
light-monitoring p.
Lilienthal p.
Lillie frontal sinus p.
Linde cryogenic p.
linear p.
linear-array p.
linear array transrectal
ultrasound p.
lithotriptor p.
localizing p.
Lockhart-Mummery p.
low noise optical p. (LNOP)
Lucae ear p.
Luminary LASIK light p.
magnetic eye p.
magnetometer p.
malleable p.
Manhattan Eye & Ear p.
Mannis p.
Mannis suture p.
Martin uterine fistula p.
mastoid p.
Max-I-Probe irrigation p.
Mayo common duct p.
Mayo kidney stone p.
Mayo uterine p.
McKesson mouth p.
Meadox Surgimed Doppler p.
mechanical rotating p.
Medrad MRInnervu endorectal
colon p.

meniscectomy p.
Merit-B periodontal p.
MEVA p.
microballoon p.
Microvit p.
miniature p.
miniaturized ultrasound catheter p.
Mixter dilating p.
Mixter irrigating p.
monitoring p.
monopolar radiofrequency p.
Muldoon lacrimal p.
multielectrode p.
multifrequency p.
multilumen p.
multiplane intracavitary p.
Myrtle leaf p.
Nabers p.
nasal p.
nasolacrimal duct p.
p. needle
needle p.
Nélaton bullet p.
Neo-Therm neonatal skin
temperature p.
neutral amyloid p.
nuclear p.
Nucleotome p.
Ochsner gall duct p.
Ochsner spiral p.
ocutome p.
Ohmeda p.
Ohmeda SoftProbe p.
oligonucleotide p.
Olympus CD-20Z heater p.
Olympus GF-UM30P linear
scanning p.
Olympus heat p.
Olympus MH-908 slim
ultrasonic p.
Olympus S-20-20R p.
Olympus S20-20R transendoscopic
ultrasound p.
Olympus ultrathin balloon-fitted
ultrasound p.
Olympus UM-F30-20R p.
Olympus UM-2R, -3R p.
Olympus UM-R series miniature
ultrasonic p.
Olympus UM-S30-25R p.
Olympus UM-1W endoscopic p.
Olympus UM-W series
endoscopic p.
Olympus UM-1W transendoscopic
ultrasound p.
palpation p.
PathVysion HER-2 DNA p.
Payr p.
$PbrO_2$ monitoring p.

P

probe *(continued)*
pediatric biplane TEE p.
pencil Doppler p.
percutaneous pencil Doppler p.
periodontal p.
Periotemp electronic p.
PerioWise p.
pH p.
phased-array p.
pH-Informer Deltron p.
pH manometry p.
photon laser phacolysis p.
piggyback p.
pigtail p.
pocket p.
polycationic histochemical p.
PPG p.
Pratt rectal p.
Probex p.
pulpal microdialysis p.
quartz fiberoptic p.
Quickert-Dryden p.
Radiometer p.
rectal p.
Reddick/Saye Lav-1 irrigating and
  aspirating p.
reflectance spectrophotometric p.
right-angle blunt p.
rigid endosonography p.
Ritleng p.
RNA p.
Robicsek vascular p.
Rolf lacrimal p.
Rollet lacrimal p.
rotating Bruel and Kjaer p.
Sandhill p.
Sarns temperature p.
scintillation p.
scissors p.
p. sheath
p. shield
side-firing p.
side-hole cannulated p.
Siemens-Elema AB pulse
  transducer p.
Siemens linear p.
silver p.
Silverstein stimulator p.
Simpson lacrimal p.
Sims uterine p.
sinus p.
Skillern sphenoidal p.
Softflo fiberoptic p.
Somnus p.
Sonablate transrectal p.
Sonocath ultrasound p.
p. spatula
spatula p.
spatula electrosurgical p.

spear-ended chrome p.
Spectraprobe-Max p.
Spencer p.
Spencer labyrinth exploration p.
sphenoidal p.
SpineStat side-directed
  discectomy p.
spinning p.
spiral p.
standard hook electrosurgical p.
stimulation p.
straight retinal p.
StrykeProbe suction irrigator p.
suction p.
Surgiflex Wave XP
  suction/irrigation p.
Swiss Lithoclast pneumatic
  lithotripsy p.
Synergetics directional laser p.
tactile p.
Teflon p.
telephone p.
temperature p.
TempTouch home infrared
  temperature p.
Theobald sinus p.
thermistor p.
through-the-scope catheter p.
thyroid uptake p.
tin-bullet p.
trabeculotomy p.
transcranial Doppler p.
transesophageal echo p.
transesophageal echocardiography p.
Transonic flow p.
Transonics Flow p.
Transonics Systems flow p.
transrectal p.
triple-frequency p.
truncated NMR p.
tulip p.
tumor p.
Ultra-Precision ultrasonic p.
ultrasonic p.
ultrasonic lithotriptor p.
ultrasound p.
ultrasound catheter p.
Universal vaginal p.
USCI p.
uterine p.
Vasoscope 3 Doppler p.
Versadopp ultrasonic Doppler p.
vertebrated p.
ViraType p.
virtual colonoscopy side fire
  APC p.
vitrector p.
Vivacare TPS p.
v33W high-density endocavity p.

Vygantas-Wilder retinal drainage p.
Vysis p.
water p.
Welch Allyn rectal p.
Werb right-angle p.
WHO p.
Williams p.
Williams lacrimal p.
wire p.
Woodson p.
Worst double-ended pigtail p.
Worst pigtail p.
Xomed rectal p.
Yellow Springs p.
YSI Foley p.
YSI neonatal temperature p.
Ziegler p.

probe-ended grooved director
Probex probe
Pro-Bind U-Bottom microfilter plate
probing sheath exchange catheter
Probloc regional block anesthesia needle
ProBond dentin bonding agent
Probst Smiley LASIK marker
Procase Ankle-Lock brace
Procath electrophysiology catheter
procedure

p. drape
selective tubal occlusion p. (STOP)

Proceed surgical mesh
Procera system
process

AuTolo cure p.
BioCleanse tissue sterilization p.
SoftLight laser/skin resurfacing p.
Zimmer PMMA precoat p.

processed carbon implant
processor

array p.
Clarion CII behind-the-ear sound p.
Clarion CII BTE sound p.
Clarion Platinum BTE sound p.
Cobe 2991 cell p.
conventional p.
daylight p.
ESPrit ear level speech p.
Hope p.
Kodak RP X-OMAT p.
Miles vacuum infiltration p.
Miles V.I.P. 300 vacuum infiltration p.
mini speech p.
ML 700 daylight p.
output signal p.
Procomat small-tank semiautomatic p.
RP X-OMAT p.
Sakura Finetek Tissue-Tek VIP 300E automatic tissue p.

sound p.
SPrint speech p.
Tempo+ modular ear-level speech p.
ThinPrep 2000 p.
video image p.
wearable speech p.

Prochownik pessary
Pro-Clude

P.-C. transparent film
P.-C. transparent wound dressing

Procomat small-tank semiautomatic processor
ProComp Infiniti system
ProCon incontinence device
PRO/Covers ultrasound probe sheath
ProCross

P. Rely balloon
P. Rely over-the-wire balloon catheter

Proctor-Livingston endoprosthesis
Proctor retractor
proctoscope

Boehm p.
Gabriel p.
Hirschman p.
Kelly p.
Lieberman p.
Montague p.
Newman p.
Salvati p.
Tuttle p.
Vernon-David p.
Welch Allyn p.

proctosigmoidoscope

ACMI fiberoptic p.
fiberoptic p.

Procyon digital infrared pupillometer
ProCyte

P. transparent adhesive film dressing
P. transparent dressing
P. transparent film

Pro-Designed wrist guard
Prodigy

P. bone densitometer
P. lens inserter
P. total hip system

Prodisc-C cervical artificial disc implant
Prodisc spinal disc prosthesis
product

AllerCare allergy control p.
Aloe Vesta moisturizing skin care p.
BioBypass gene-based drug delivery p.
Body Glove orthopaedic p.
CFC-free p.

P

product *(continued)*
 Fortitude Ti titanium spinal
  fixation p.
 Fortitude Vue titanium spinal
  fixation p.
 Innovation Sports bracing p.
 Katena p.
 Linvatec arthroscopy p.
 Nexacryl cohesive p.
 Oleeva wound care p.
 Oxiplex/SP bioresorbable p.
 Pristine-100 allergy control p.
 Pro-PredictRx diagnostic p.
 Repliform alternative p.
 Sensi-Care skin care p.
 SPP color deficiency testing p.
 standard pseudoisochromatic plates
  color deficiency testing p.
 viscoelastic p.
ProDynamic monitor
Profemur R revision prosthesis
Profex
 P. arthroscopic leg positioner
 P. arthroscopic tourniquet
ProFile
 P. file
 P. orifice shaper
 P. variable taper rotary instrument
profile
 P. anterior plate system
 P. anterior spinal plate
 P. hip prosthesis
 LifeScan P.
 P. Lite
 P. mammography system
 P. MD implantable cardioverter-
  defibrillator
 OneTouch P.
 P. pediatric polypectomy snare
 P. platform
 P. Plus balloon dilatation catheter
  reduced p. (RP)
 P. sitting orthosis
 P. total hip system
 ultralow p. (ULP)
Profile-II ER drug screening device
Profilomat monitor
profilometer
 laryngoscope p.
Profil-O-Plastic
 P.-O.-P. preshaped chin plate
 P.-O.-P. preshaped midfacial plate
ProFinesse II ultrasonic handpiece
Profix
 P. confirming tibial insert
 P. metaphysial tibial stem
 P. mobile-bearing knee implant
 P. nonporous tibial base

 P. porous femoral component
 P. total knee replacement system
Proflex 5 catheter
ProFlex wrist support
Profore
 P. bandage system
 P. Four-Layer bandage system
 P. 4-layer bandage
 P. 4-layer wound dressing
 P. leg compression dressing
 P. wound dressing
ProForma prosthesis
**Proform maxim pressure reduction
 mattress**
PRO/Gel ultrasound transmission gel
Progestasert
 P. intrauterine device
 P. IUD
Pro-glide
 P.-g. orthosis
 P.-g. splint
Prograft bifurcated endograft
program
 Obagi maintenance p.
Programalith
 P. A-V pacemaker
 P. II, III pacemaker
 P. III pulse generator
programmable
 p. cardioverter-defibrillator (PCD)
 p. implantable medication system
 p. pacemaker
 p. pulse generator
 p. pump
 p. valve
 p. VariGrip II prosthetic control
  system
 p. ventricular shunt valve
programmer
 P. III pacemaker
 Omnicor P.
 Pacesetter APS II 3004 p.
 Pacesetter APS pacemaker p.
 p. wand
programming wand
progressive
 P. ankle orthosis
 P. palm guard
 p. spectacles lens
progressively larger reamer
Progress splint
Prohibit antifog face mask
projection
 p. magnifier
 p. perimeter
 p. x-ray microscope
Project-O-Chart
 AO Reichert Instruments P.-O.-C.
 Ultramatic P.-O.-C.

projector
- acuity visual p.
- Eletrohome Marquee 8500 Ultra graphics p.
- fiberoptic light p.
- liquid crystal display p.
- Marco chart p.
- NP-3S auto chart p.
- overhead p.
- Tagarno 3SD cineangiography p.
- Topcon chart p.

ProKera amniotic membrane graft
Pro-Koester wide-field SCM microscope
prolapse coil
Prolase
- Cytocare P. II
- P. fiber
- P. II lateral-firing Nd:YAG laser

Prolene
- P. hernia system
- P. hernia system connector
- P. hernia system onlay patch
- P. hernia system underlay patch
- P. mesh (PS)
- P. mesh sheet
- P. mesh silo
- P. polypropylene suture
- P. suture

Prolieve
- P. microwave therapy system
- P. thermodilation system

Proline Stomatex shoulder brace
ProLite
- P. Plus runner's orthotic
- P. surgical mesh
- P. Ultra surgical mesh

ProLong absorbable long-term plug
ProLumen thrombectomy device
Promex biopsy needle
Promise
- P. brief
- P. pad and pant system
- P. pad and pant trial pack
- P. washable knit pant

Promogran matrix wound dressing
Promos modular shoulder system
pronation/spring control (PSC)
pronation spring-control device
pronator drill
prone
- p. board
- p. cranial support device
- p. stander

Proneb Ultra nebulizer
Pronex
- P. home traction
- P. patient-controlled pneumatic traction device
- P. pneumatic cervical traction

prong
3-prong
- 3-p. fork
- 3-p. grasping forceps
- 3-p. rake blade retractor

4-prong
- 4-p. finger speculum
- 4-p. finger splint
- 4-p. retractor

5-prong
- 5-p. rake blade
- 5-p. rake blade retractor

pronged
- p. Franseen-type point needle
- p. retractor

2-pronged
- 2-p. dural hook
- 2-p. stem finger prosthesis

3-pronged
- 3-p. grasper
- 3-p. polyp retriever
- 3-p. rake blade

6-prong rake retractor
prongs
- Allegiance nasal p.
- binasal p.
- Hudson p.
- Invacare nasal p.
- Kendall nasal p.
- nasal p.
- Pro-Tech nasal p.
- Sims nasal p.
- Uno nasal p.

Pronova suture
Pron-Pillo head positioning device
Pron pillow
Pronto
- P. cement
- P. V3 extraction catheter

Pronto-Short extraction catheter
ProOsteon
- P. implant 500 coralline hydroxyapatite bone void filler
- P. implant graft material
- P. Implant 500 granule
- P. synthetic bone implant

Pro-Osteon 500 bone implant graft
prop
- Oberto mouth p.
- rubber mouth p.

Propac
- Champ Insulated P. II

Propaq Encore vital signs monitor
Pro/Pel
- P./P. coating cardiac device
- Hi-Torque Floppy with P./P.

Propel cannulated interference screw
propeller
- orthopaedic p.

P

propHiler urinary pH testing kit
prophy cup
prophylactic
>p. epidural blood patch
>p. IVC filter
>p. taping

Proplast
>P. graft
>P. HA
>P. I, II implant
>P. I, II porous implant material
>P. preformed facial implant
>P. prosthesis

Proplast-Teflon disc implant
Propper
>P. binocular indirect
>   ophthalmoscope
>P. indirect ophthalmoscope
>P. retinoscope

Propper-Heine ophthalmoscope
Pro-PredictRx
>P.-P. diagnostic product
>P.-P. diagnostic test
>P.-P. Enzact
>P.-P. TPMT

Prop'R Toes hammertoe cushion
proptometer
propylene
>p. dressing
>fluorinated ethylene p.

Pro-Q skin protectant
ProROM walker
Proscan
>P. ultrasound imaging system
>P. ultrasound unit

Pros-Check kit
Pro-Scrub
>Zila P.-S.

ProSeal laryngeal mask airway
ProSeries laparoscopic laser system
Proshield
>P. collagen corneal shield
>P. Plus skin protectant

Prosorba column
ProSound ultrasound
ProSpeed CT scanner
Prostacoil stent
ProstaJect ethanol injection system
Prostakath urethral stent
Prostalac
>P. temporary hip prosthesis
>P. total hip prosthesis

Prostalase
>P. laser
>P. laser system

ProstaLund CoreTherm system
Prostaprobe catheter

Prostar
>P. percutaneous vascular surgery
>   system
>P. Plus percutaneous closure device
>P. Plus percutaneous vascular
>   surgical device
>P. XL hemostatic puncture closure
>   device
>P. XL percutaneous closure device
>P. XL 8, 10 suture-mediated
>   closure device

**Prostar-Techstar suture-mediated closure
device**
ProstaScint
>P. scan
>P. system

prostate
>transurethral resection of p.
>   (TURP)

prostatectomy
>p. bag
>p. forceps

Prostathermer
>P. device
>P. prostatic hyperthermia system

prostatic
>p. biopsy needle
>p. bridge catheter
>p. dissector
>p. driver
>p. lobe forceps
>p. needle holder
>p. retractor
>p. stent
>p. tractor

Prostatron
>P. microwave system
>P. transurethral thermotherapy
>   device

prosthesis
>Accolade hip p.
>acetabular p.
>ACS Gemini p.
>ACS Profile p.
>ACS Star p.
>AcuMatch M series modular
>   femoral hip p.
>Advance PS total knee p.
>Advantim total knee p.
>Advantim unconstrained p.
>Aequalis humeral p.
>Aequalis reversed shoulder p.
>Aesculap-PM noncemented
>   femoral p.
>AGC femoral p.
>AGC knee p.
>AGC tibial p.
>AHP digital p.
>AHSC elbow p.

Airlite p.
Airprene hinged knee p.
Allurion foot p.
alumina cemented total hip p.
alumina-on-alumina total hip p.
Alvarez p.
Ambicor inflatable p.
Ambicor penile p.
AMC total wrist p.
American Heyer-Schulte-Radovan
  tissue expander p.
American Medical Systems
  penile p.
AMK unconstrained p.
AML Plus p.
AML total hip p.
AMS Ambicore penile p.
AMS 700CX-series penile p.
AMS Hydroflex penile p.
AMS inflatable penile p.
AMS inflatable 700 penile p.
AMS malleable penile p.
AMS 3-piece inflatable penile p.
AMS Sphincter 800 urinary p.
Amsterdam-type p.
AMS Ultrex penile p.
Anatomic Precoat hip p.
anchor peg glenoid all-
  polyethylene p.
Anderson acetabular p.
Angelchik antireflux p.
antibiotic-loaded acrylic cement
  total joint p.
antireflux p.
Apollo hip p.
Apollo knee p.
Applebaum incus replacement p.
APR acetabular p.
APR femoral p.
APR II p.
Aptis distal radial ulna joint p.
Armstrong p.
arterial graft p.
Arthropor II acetabular p.
articulated chin p.
Ashley breast p.
Atkinson p.
Atlas modular humeral p.
Attenborough total knee p.
auditory p.
Aufranc cobra hip p.
Aufranc-Turner hip p.
auricular p.
Austin Moore hip p.
Autophor femoral p.
Avanta MCP joint implant
  finger p.
Avanta metacarpophalangeal
  implant p.

Avanta uHead ulnar head p.
Averill press-fit p.
Axtion foot p.
Balance hip p.
ball-and-cage p.
ball-and-socket ankle p.
ball-type disc p.
ball valve p.
Bankart shoulder p.
Bantam CDH p.
Barnard mitral valve p.
4-bar polycentric knee p.
Bateman UPF II shoulder p.
BDH p.
Beachcomber waterproof p.
bead-blasted p.
Beall mitral valve p.
Bechtol shoulder p.
Becker breast p.
Becker hand p.
Becker tissue expander p.
Becker tissue expander/breast p.
Beck-Steffee total ankle p.
below-knee prosthesis
Bi-Angular shoulder p.
Biaxial Weave composite p.
bicondylar ankle p.
bifurcated aortofemoral p.
bifurcated seamless p.
bifurcation p.
bileaflet p.
Bi-Metric hip p.
Bio-Chromatic hand p.
Bioclad with pegs reinforced
  acetabular p.
Bio-Groove acetabular p.
Bio-Groove Macrobond HA
  femoral p.
Biomet AGC knee p.
Biomet hip p.
Biometric p.
Biomet total toe p.
Bio-Modular shoulder p.
Bionic ear p.
bisque-baked p.
Bivona-Colorado voice p.
Björk p.
Björk-Shiley aortic valve p.
Björk-Shiley convexoconcave 60-
  degree valve p.
Björk-Shiley floating disc p.
Björk-Shiley mitral p.
BK p.
bladder neck support p.
Blauth knee p.
Blom-Singer tracheoesophageal p.
Blom-Singer voice p.
Bock knee p.
Bojrab Hapex universal p.

P

707

prosthesis *(continued)*
  bone p.
  Bordeaux p.
  bovine collagen material p.
  Braunwald-Cutter ball valve p.
  breast p.
  Bristol disc p.
  Bryan cervical disc p.
  Buechel-Pappas total ankle p.
  Caffinière p.
  caged ball valve p.
  calcar replacement femoral p.
  Calnan-Nicolle
    metatarsophalangeal p.
  Calnan-Nicolle synthetic joint p.
  camouflage p.
  Canadian hip disarticulation p.
  Capello press-fit p.
  CarboMedics cardiac valve p.
  Carbon Copy high-performance
    foot p.
  Carbon Copy II foot p.
  Carbon Copy II Light p.
  Carbon Copy II light p.
  Carbon Copy II lightweight p.
  Carbo-Seal ascending aortic p.
  Carpentier-Edwards aortic valve p.
  Carpentier-Edwards glutaraldehyde-
    preserved porcine xenograft p.
  Cartwright heart p.
  Cathcart orthocentric hip p.
  Causse partial ossicular
    replacement p.
  Celestin p.
  cementless p.
  Centralign precoat hip p.
  ceramic femoral head p.
  ceramic ossicular p.
  Ceramion p.
  Ceravital incus replacement p.
  CFS hip p.
  Charnley cemented hip p.
  Charnley-Hastings p.
  Charnley hip p.
  Charnley-Mueller hip p.
  Charnley total hip p.
  CHD p.
  Cinch instant suction p.
  Cinch instant suction B.K. p.
  Cintor knee p.
  Cirrus foot p.
  clamshell p.
  Clayton p.
  cleft palate p.
  C-Leg lower limb p.
  Cloutier unconstrained knee p.
  coated p.
  cobalt-chromium alloy p.
  Co-Cr-Mo p.

  collar p.
  College Park TruStep foot p.
  combination gel and inflatable
    mammary p.
  complete denture p.
  composite p.
  conoidal ankle p.
  conservative anatomic p. (CAP)
  constrained hinged knee p.
  constrained nonhinged knee p.
  Continuum unconstrained p.
  p. contourer
  conventional single-axis knee p.
  Cooley-Bloodwell mitral valve p.
  Coonrad-II p.
  Coonrad-Morrey total elbow p.
  Corail press-fit p.
  C-2 OsteoCap hip p.
  covered self-expanding p.
  CPT p.
  crimped Dacron p.
  crimped wire p.
  Cronin silastic mammary p.
  Cross-Jones disc valve p.
  cruciate condylar unconstrained p.
  cruciate-retaining p.
  cruciate-sacrificing p.
  CUI artificial breast p.
  CUI gel mammary p.
  Cummins disc p.
  p. cup
  custom-threaded p.
  custom total alloplastic TMJ
    reconstruction p.
  Cutter aortic valve p.
  Cutter-Smeloff aortic valve p.
  Cutter-Smeloff cardiac valve p.
  CXM p.
  CX Plus p.
  Dacron p.
  Dacron arterial p.
  Dacron bifurcation p.
  Dacron vessel p.
  DANA shoulder p.
  Deane unconstrained knee p.
  DeBakey ball valve p.
  DeBakey Vasculour-II vascular p.
  debonded femoral stem p.
  de la Caffinière
    trapeziometacarpal p.
  DeLaura knee p.
  DeLaura-Verner knee p.
  Delrin frame of valve p.
  DePuy hip p. with Scuderi head
  De Vega p.
  Dilamezinsert penile p.
  Dimension-C femoral stem p.
  Dimension hip p.
  direct-impact p.

distal radioulnar joint p.
double-pigtail p.
DRUJ p.
drum-to-footplate total ossicular
  reconstruction p.
dual-lock total hip p.
duckbill voice p.
Duocentric p.
Duocondylar knee p.
Duo-Lock hip p.
Duracon p.
Dura-II positionable penile p.
Duraloc p.
Duraphase inflatable penile p.
Duromedics valve p.
Dycor Geriatric ADL single-axis
  foot p.
Dynaflex p.
Dynaflex penile p.
dynamic penile p.
ear pinna p.
ear piston p.
Edwards seamless p.
E-2 foot p.
Eftekhar long-stem p.
Endo-Model hinged knee p.
Endo-Model rotating knee joint p.
Endo-Model sled p.
Endo sled p.
energy-storing foot p.
Engh porous metal hip p.
Englehardt femoral p.
English-McNab shoulder p.
Entegra p.
Epoch hip p.
EPTFE graft p.
ERCP conventional p.
Eriksson knee p.
EsophaCoil p.
esophageal p.
Evolution hip p.
Exeter-Femora press-fit p.
expandable p.
extraoral p.
facial p.
fascia lata p.
femorofemoral crossover p.
Fett carpal p.
p. fin
Finney Flexirod penile p.
Finn hinged knee p.
Finn knee revision p.
fixed detachable mandibular p.
fixed expansion p.
fixed femoral head p.
flanged revision p.
Flatt finger p.
Flex-Foot Modular III p.
Flex H/A total ossicular p.

Flexi-Flate I, II penile p.
Flexirod penile p.
Flex-Sprint p.
Flex-Walk p.
Flex-Walk II p.
fluid p.
forged cobalt-chromium alloy p.
fossa eminence p.
Fox p.
Fox-Blazina p.
Fredricks mammary p.
Free-Flow system p.
Freeman high-neck press-fit p.
Freeman modular total hip p.
Freeman-Samuelson knee p.
Freeman-Swanson knee p.
fully constrained tricompartmental
  knee p.
Gaffney ankle p.
Galante hip p.
gel-filled p.
gel-saline Surgitek mammary p.
Gemini hip system p.
Genesis knee p.
GeoFlex knee p.
Geometric total knee p.
Georgiade breast p.
GFS Mark II inflatable penile p.
Gianturco p.
Gianturco expandable self-expanding
  metallic biliary p.
Gilfillan humeral p.
Giliberty acetabular p.
Gillette joint p.
Girard keratoprosthesis p.
glass penile p.
Global conservative anatomic p.
glottic p.
Golaski-UMI vascular p.
Gold Medal foot p.
golf tee-shaped polyvinyl p.
Gore-Tex knee p.
Gott-Daggett heart valve p.
Gott low-profile p.
Greifer p.
Greissinger foot p.
grit-blasted p.
Groningen voice p.
GSB elbow p.
GSB knee p.
Guepar II hinged knee p.
Gustilo knee p.
Gustilo unconstrained p.
Hall-Kaster tilting disc valve p.
Hammersmith mitral p.
Hammersmith mitral valve p.
Hancock aortic valve p.
Hancock mitral valve p.
hand-glove p.

P

prosthesis *(continued)*

Hanger ComfortFlex knee p.
Harken p.
Harris cemented hip p.
Harris-Galante porous hip p.
Harris Micromini p.
Harrison interlocked mesh p.
Harris precoat p.
Haynes-Stellite implant metal p.
HD II total hip p.
Henley-Cohn p.
Herbert knee p.
heterograft p.
Hexcel total condylar p.
Heyer-Schulte breast p.
hinged constrained knee p.
hinged great toe replacement p.
hinged implant p.
hinged total knee p.
hip disarticulation p.
hip replacement p.
Hittenberger p.
HKAFO p.
Hoffman-Pappas total joint p.
hollow sphere p.
homograft p.
Hosmer WALK p.
Hosmer weight-activated locking
  knee p.
House wire stapes p.
Howmedica Kinematic II knee p.
Howmedica PCA p.
Howorth p.
Howse p.
Hufnagel low-profile heart p.
hybrid p.
hydraulic hinge penile p.
hydraulic knee unit p.
hydraulic-type disc p.
Hydroflex penile p.
hydroxyapatite ossicular p.
I-beam hemiarthroplasty hip p.
Identifit hip p.
Image custom external breast p.
immediate load p.
immediate postoperative p.
Impact modular porous p.
Impact total hip p.
implant-borne p.
implant-supported fixed p.
Implant Technology LSF p.
Impra collagen-impregnated
  Dacron p.
incus replacement p.
Index p.
Infinity modular hip p.
inflatable mammary p.
inflatable Mentor penile p.
Insall-Burstein knee p.

Integral Interlok femoral p.
Integrity acetabular cup p.
Intelligent Prosthesis Plus p.
Intermedics Natural-Knee knee p.
internal ear p.
Inter-Op acetabular p.
Inter-Op hip p.
Interseal Variant I–IV p.
intraocular retinal p.
Introl bladder neck support p.
Ionescu-Shiley aortic valve p.
Ionescu-Shiley valve p.
Iowa total hip p.
iridium p.
ischial weightbearing p.
isoelastic pelvic p.
Ivalon p.
Jaffe press-fit p.
Jewett p.
Jobst p.
Johnson-Elloy accord
  unconstrained p.
Johnston-Iowa hip p.
Jonas penile p.
Joplin toe p.
Judet hip p.
KAFO p.
Kartush incus strut p.
Kaufman III anti-incontinence p.
Kaufman male urinary
  incontinence p.
Kay-Shiley disc valve p.
Kay-Suzuki p.
KD chin p.
Keeler p.
Kessler p.
Kinematic II rotating-hinge total
  knee p.
Kinemax Plus knee p.
Kirschner total shoulder p.
KMP femoral stem p.
knitted Teflon p.
knitted vascular p.
Koenig MPJ p.
Krause-Wolfe p.
K2 sensation p.
Lacey p.
Landers-Foulks p.
LaPorta total toe p.
Lash-Loeffler penile p.
LCS meniscal bearing
  semiconstrained p.
LCS rotating platform
  semiconstrained p.
LCS substituting semiconstrained p.
LCS universal APG
  semiconstrained p.
Leinbach hip p.

Lesinski Flex-HA PORP ossicular chain p.

Lewis expandable adjustable p. (LEAP)

Lillehei-Kaster cardiac valve p.

Lillehei-Kaster mitral valve p.

Link cementless reconstruction hip p.

Link Endo-Model rotational knee p.

Link MP hip noncemented reconstruction p.

Lippy modified p.

Liverpool knee p.

Livingskin silicone p.

Lo Bak spinal support p.

locking p.

Longevity V-Lign hip p.

Lo-Por vascular graft p.

Lord total hip p.

Lotus unicompartment p.

low-contact stress semiconstrained p.

lower limb p.

low-pressure voice p.

low-profile p.

Lubinus knee p.

lunate p.

lunate acrylic cement wrist p.

Lund prototype unicompartment p.

LuXon Journey foot p.

MacIntosh tibial plateau p.

MacNab-English shoulder p.

madreporic hip p.

Magnuson-Cromie p.

Magnuson valve p.

Magovern-Cromie p.

malleable p.

malleus-incus p.

Mallory p.

Mallory-Head I, II p.

Mallory-Head porous primary femoral p.

Mallory-Head total hip p.

mammary p.

Mangat curvilinear chin p.

Marlex mesh p.

Marlex methyl methacrylate p.

Master Step foot p.

Mathys p.

Matrol femoral head p.

maxillary p.

Mayo conservative hip p.

Mayo semiconstrained elbow p.

Mayo total ankle p.

M-C p.

McBride femoral p.

McCutchen SLT hip p.

McGee ear piston p.

McGhan breast p.

McKee-Farrar hip p.

McKee femoral p.

McKee totally constrained elbow p.

McKeever patellar cap p.

MCP finger joint p.

Meadox woven velour p.

mechanical p.

mechanical-type disc p.

Mecring acetabluar p.

Medoc-Celestin endoprosthesis p.

Medpor p.

Medtronic-Hall heart valve p.

Medtronic-Hall tilting disc valve p.

Medtronic Talent p.

Meme breast p.

Mentor Alpha 1 inflatable penile p.

Mentor breast p.

Mentor GFS penile p.

Mentor IPP penile p.

Mentor malleable penile p.

Mentor Mark II penile p.

mesh stent p.

metacarpophalangeal p.

metal-backed plastic-on-metal p.

metal bucket-handle p.

metal femoral head p.

metal-on-metal articulating intervertebral disc p.

Metasul hip p.

MG II knee p.

Michele long stem p.

Microknit vascular graft p.

Microloc knee p.

Microvel p.

Miller-Galante hip p.

Milliknit Dacron p.

Milliknit vascular graft p.

Misti Gold p.

modified Moore hip locking p.

modular Austin Moore hip p.

modular Iowa Precoat total hip p.

monoblock femoral stem p.

monolithic A1203 cup p.

Monostrut cardiac valve p.

Moore hip p.

Mueller-Charnley hip p.

Mueller total hip p.

Muhlberger orbital p.

Müller p.

multiaxis p.

Multiflex foot p.

Multi-Lock hip p.

multiradius unconstrained p.

myoelectric control p.

Natural-Hip p.

Natural-Knee unconstrained p.

Neer I, II shoulder p.

P

711

prosthesis *(continued)*
neural p.
NeuroCybernetic p. (NCP)
Neville tracheal p.
Neville tracheal reconstruction p.
Nexus hip p.
Niebauer finger joint
  replacement p.
Noiles rotating hinge total knee p.
nonhinged knee p.
Norwich press-fit p.
ocular p.
Oh-Spectron p.
Oklahoma ankle p.
Ommaya reservoir p.
Omnicarbon heart valve p.
Omnifit dual geometry
  microstructured p.
Omnifit HA hip stem p.
Omnifit knee p.
Omnifit PSL microstructured p.
OmniPhase penile p.
Omniscience single-leaflet cardiac
  valve p.
Omniscience tilting disc valve p.
Opti-Fix I, II p.
orbital floor p.
Oregon p.
Orthofix p.
Ortholoc II unconstrained p.
osseointegrated p.
ossicular p.
ossicular chain replacement p.
ossicular reconstruction p.
Osteocap hip p.
Osteolock hip p.
Osteonics p.
Otto Bock system electric hands p.
Oxford meniscal unicompartment p.
Padgett p.
palatal p.
palatal lift p.
Paltrinieri-Trentani p.
Panje p.
Panje voice button p.
partial ossicular replacement p.
  (PORP)
passive infant oral p.
patellar tendon-bearing below-
  knee p.
PCA Original p.
PCA Standard p.
PC Performer knee p.
Pearman penile p.
peg-coupled p.
pegged tibial p.
Perfecta hip p.
Perfecta I, II p.
Performance knee p.

pericarbon pericardial p.
Peri-Loc p.
periodontal p.
PFC curved unconstrained p.
PFC femoral p.
Pillet hand p.
Pilliar p.
piston stapes p.
plastipore partial ossicular
  replacement p.
Plastiport TORP p.
polycentric knee p.
polycentric unconstrained p.
polyethylene talar p.
polytetrafluoroethylene p.
polyvinyl p.
porcine p.
porous-coated anatomic knee p.
porous surfaced p.
Precision Osteolock femoral p.
Precision Osteolock hip p.
Preclude dura substitute p.
Precoat hip p.
Precoat Plus femoral p.
Premier press fit p.
Premier press-fit p.
press-fit p.
Pritchard II elbow p.
Pritchard total elbow p.
Prodisc spinal disc p.
Profemur R revision p.
Profile hip p.
ProForma p.
2-pronged stem finger p.
Proplast p.
Prostalac temporary hip p.
Prostalac total hip p.
prosthetic antibiotic-loaded acrylic
  cement total joint p.
Protek p.
provisional fixed p.
Provox voice p.
PTFE p.
pyrocarbon p.
Quantum Foot p.
Quattro mitral valve p.
Ranawat-Burstein hip p.
Rancho external fixation p.
Randelli shoulder p.
Rashkind double-disc occluder p.
Reflection I p.
Reflection Interfit p.
reflection V p.
Re-Flex VSP p.
removable expansion p.
Repiphysis p.
retinal p.
reversed shoulder p.
Richards hip p.

Richards hydroxyapatite PORP p.
Richards hydroxyapatite TORP p.
Richards maximum-contact cruciate-
  sparing p.
Richards maximum contact cruciate-
  sparing p.
Richards zirconia femoral head p.
Ring UPM press-fit p.
Robert Brigham semiconstrained p.
Robinson stapes p.
Roper-Day p.
Rosen inflatable urinary
  incontinence p.
rotating femoral head p.
rotating-hinge knee p.
Rothman Institute femoral p.
Roy-Camille p.
SACH p.
sacral segmental nerve stimulation
  implantable neural p.
saddle p.
SAF p.
Sarmiento STH-2 hip p.
Sbarbaro tibial p.
Schuknecht Teflon wire piston p.
Scott AMS inflatable penile p.
Scuderi p.
Seattle foot p.
Secur-Fit HA PSL X'tra p.
Select ankle p.
Select modular shoulder p.
self-articulating femoral p.
self-centering p.
self-centering Universal hip p.
Sense-of-Feel p.
SensorHand p.
shaft p.
Shaw-Sgarlato hammertoe
  implant p.
Shea Teflon piston p.
Sheehan knee p.
Sheehy incus replacement p.
shoulder p.
shoulder disarticulation p.
silastic ball spacer p.
silastic chin p.
silastic mammary p.
silastic penile p.
silastic testicular p.
Silflex intramedullary p.
silicone elastomer p.
silicone gel p.
silicone self-expanding p.
silicone trapezium p.
Siloxane p.
Siltex Becker 50 breast p.
Singer-Blom p.
single-axis ankle p.
single-cylinder penile p.

single-disc p.
Sinterlock implant metal p.
SKI knee p.
Small-Carrion penile p.
Smeloff-Cutter ball-valve p.
Smith total ankle p.
p. smooth wire
solid ankle cushioned heel foot p.
solid silicone orbital p.
Solution p.
Sorin Bicarbon bileaflet aortic
  valve p.
Sorin mitral valve p.
Souter-Strathclyde elbow p.
Spectron p.
Speed radius cap p.
spherocentric knee p.
spinal disc p.
Springlite II foot p.
Springlite lower limb p.
S-ROM Arthropor I–III p.
S-ROM Arthropor oblong p.
S-ROM femoral stem p.
S-ROM hip p.
S-ROM super cup p.
S-ROM ZZT I, II p.
Stanmore shoulder p.
stapedectomy p.
Star ankle joint p.
Starr-Edwards aortic valve p.
Starr-Edwards ball valve p.
Starr-Edwards cardiac valve p.
Starr-Edwards disc valve p.
Starr-Edwards heart valve p.
Starr-Edwards mitral p.
stemmed tibial p.
stentless porcine aortic valve p.
St. Georg fully constrained p.
St. Georg sledge
  unicompartment p.
St. Jude heart valve p.
St. Jude Medical valve p.
St. Jude mitral valve p.
Subrini penile p.
suction suspension p.
Sulzer p.
SuperCup acetabular cup p.
Sure-Flex p.
Surgitek mammary p.
Sutter double-stem silicone
  implant p.
Sutter MCP finger joint p.
Swanson finger joint p.
Swanson great toe p.
Swanson metacarpal p.
Swanson metatarsal p.
Swanson wrist p.
Syme amputation p.
Syme foot p.

P

prosthesis *(continued)*
TARA total hip p.
Target p.
TCCK unconstrained knee p.
Techmedica p.
Teflon trileaflet p.
Teflon woven p.
temporary p.
temporomandibular joint fossa
 eminence p.
tendon p.
Tevdek p.
Thackray hip p.
Tharies hip replacement p.
Thompson femoral head p.
Thompson femoral neck p.
threaded titanium acetabular p.
thrust plate p. (TPP)
Ti-Bac II hip p.
tibial plateau p.
Tilastin hip p.
tilting disc aortic valve p.
titanium p.
TMJ fossa eminence p.
TMJ fossa-eminence p.
toe p.
TORP p.
TORP ossicular p.
torque-type p.
total alloplastic TMJ
 reconstruction p.
Total Concept ankle/foot p.
total condylar III fully
 constrained p.
total ossicular p.
total ossicular replacement p.
 (TORP)
Total Shock p.
Townley horizontal platform p.
TPR ankle p.
Trac II knee p.
transfemoral modular p.
trapeziometacarpal joint
 replacement p.
trapezoidal-28 p.
trial p.
triaxial p.
triaxial semiconstrained elbow p.
Tricon-M cruciate-sparing p.
Tricon-M patellar p.
trileaflet p.
Tri-Lock press-fit p.
Trilogy p.
Tronzo p.
Trowbridge TerraRound all-
 terrain p.
trunnion-bearing hip p.
TruStep foot p.
TTAP-ST acetabular p.

TT Pylon p.
Turner p.
Tygon esophageal p.
UCBL p.
UCI unconstrained p.
uHead ulnar head p.
UHMWPE p.
Ultimate knee p.
Ultraflex esophageal p.
ultra low-resistance voice p.
Ultrex Plus penile p.
umbrella-type p.
unconstrained p.
unicondylar p.
Uni-Flate penile p.
Universal I, II p.
upper extremity myoelectric p.
upper limb p.
urinary incontinence p.
UroLume endourethral Wallstent p.
UroLume urethral p.
Utah arm electronic p.
vaginal prolapse p.
Valls hip p.
valved voice p.
vascular graft p.
Vascutek vascular p.
VerSys p.
VerSys Beaded FullCoat Plus
 hip p.
Viladot p.
Viscoheel K, N p.
Viscoheel SofSpot p.
vitallium Moore self-locking p.
voice p.
VoiceMaster indwelling voice p.
Wagner resurface p.
Wallstent esophageal p.
Warsaw hip p.
Wayfarer modifiable foot p.
1-way valved silicone voice p.
Weavenit p.
Wehrs incus p.
Weller total hip joint p.
Whitesides total knee p.
Wiles p.
Wilson-Cook esophageal balloon p.
Wilson-Cook plastic p.
wire-fat ear p.
Wire-Gelfoam p.
wire stapes p.
wire-vein p.
Wolf p.
woven Teflon p.
woven-tube vascular graft p.
Wright knee p.
Wright titanium p.
Xenophor femoral p.
Young hinged knee p.

Zimaloy femoral head p.
Zimmer Centralign Precoat hip p.
Zimmer hip p.
Zimmer M/L taper hip p.
Zimmer shoulder p.
Zimmer tibial p.
Ziramic femoral head p.
zirconia femoral head p.
zirconia orthopaedic p.
zirconium oxide ceramic p.
Z-stent p.
ZTT I, II acetabular cup p.
Zweymuller cementless hip p.
Zweymuller hip p.

prosthetic
p. antibiotic-loaded acrylic cement
p. antibiotic-loaded acrylic cement
  total joint prosthesis
p. appliance
p. ball valve
p. buttock contour
Cirrus foot p.
p. cone
p. cup
p. device
p. foam
full denture p.'s
p. graft
p. heart valve
p. lens
p. obturator
partial denture p.'s
p. poppet
p. socket
p. speech aid
St. Jude composite p.
p. support
p. valve holder
p. valve sewing ring
ProStretch exerciser
ProSys leg bag comfort strap
Protg
P. GPS self-expanding Nitinol
  stent-biliary system
P. GPS stent
P. self-expanding stent
ProTack
P. instrument
P. stapler
P. tacking device
ProTech instrument protection tray
Pro-Tech nasal prongs
Pro-Tec patellar tendon strap
ProTect abutment
ProtectaCap cap
Protectaid contraceptive sponge
protectant
Lantiseptic skin p.
NutraShield perineal p.

Pro-Q skin p.
Proshield Plus skin p.
Protect-a-Pass suture passer
protected specimen brush
protection
Caldwell p.
EarPlanes flight ear p.
P. Plus belted undergarment
P. Plus brief
P. Plus disposable underpad
venous/arterial management p.
protective
p. bandage
p. dressing
p. eye shield
p. glasses
p. mattress cover
p. spectacles
p. sports eye wear
protector
Air-Limb amputation p.
Alvarado collateral ligament p.
Arroyo p.
autogenous corneal p.
Bandage Gard cast p.
bite p.
breast implant p.
Buratto flap p.
Cast Gard cast p.
Cottle alar p.
Crouch corneal p.
dural p.
Elbowlift elbow p.
EpiFlex heel and elbow p.
eye p.
genuine sheepskin elbow p.
genuine sheepskin heel p.
p. guide
hearing p.
Heelbo decubitus p.
Heeler inflatable heel p.
industrial eye p.
Joseph saw p.
Jurgan pin ball pin p.
Kins fitted mattress p.
Kodel polyester elbow p.
limb and elbow p.
medial nerve p.
P. meniscus suturing system
M-F heel p.
oculoplasty corneal p.
Opti-Gard eye p.
Otomed eye p.
patellar band knee p.
plastic corneal p.
p. plus wire
port p.
pulse oximetry p.

P

protector *(continued)*
    Ramirez EndoForehead right and left p.'s
    Ramirez EndoForehead right and left p.
    Roho heel p.
    Seal-Tight cast p.
    ShowerSafe waterproof cast and bandage p.
    Terumo transducer p.
    The Heeler inflatable heel p.
    tissue p.
    toe p.
    X-tend back p.
Protégé
    P. Plus microscope
    P. self-expanding stent
    P. 3010 syringe infusion pump
Protege manual flexion distraction table
protein
    bone morphogenic p.
    p. characterization system
    extracellular matrix p.
    p. eye implant
    Ne-Osteo bone morphogenic p.
protein-1
    osteogenic p.-1 (OP-1)
protein-based bone graft substitute
ProteinChip
    P. antibody capture kit
    P. Biomarker DU, PA system
    P. System Series 4000 biomarker/assay system
    P. test
Protek prosthesis
ProteomeLab
    P. DU, PA 800 protein characterization system
    P. PF 2D protein fractionation system
    P. XL-A, XL-I protein characterization system
Pro-Tex face shield
Protex swivel adapter
prothelen set
ProThotics insole
ProTime
    P. INR test device
    P. microcoagulation system
    P. prothrombin time test system
protocol
Protoco$_2$l automated CO$_2$ insufflator
Protocult stool sampling device
proton-density axial MR scan
ProTon portable tonometer
prototype cholangioscope
Protouch
    P. material
    P. orthopaedic padding

ProTrac
    P. ACL tibial guide
    P. cruciate reconstruction measurement device
    P. cruciate reconstruction system
    P. measurement device
protractor
    arthrodial p.
    cephalometric p.
    Demariniff p.
    dexterity p.
    Harrington p.
    triplanar p.
    Zimmer p.
protrusio
    p. cage
    p. shell
Pro-Vent
    P.-V. ABG kit
    P.-V. arterial blood gas kit
    P.-V. arterial blood sampling kit
Provide
    P. incontinence pad
    P. underpad
Providence
    P. clamp
    P. Hospital arterial forceps
    P. Hospital clamp
    P. Hospital hemostat
    P. scoliosis system
Provider 6000 ambulatory dual-channel infusion pump
Proview eye pressure monitor
ProVis injection system
provisional
    P. Fixation TC-100 plating system
    p. fixed prosthesis
    p. liner
Provocative sensitivity balloon
Provox
    P. speaking valve
    P. tracheoesophageal speaking valve
    P. voice prosthesis
Prowater guidewire
Prowler
    P. double-tipped microcatheter
    P. Plus catheter
Prowler-14 microcatheter
Proxiderm wound closure system
Proxi-Floss
    P.-F. cleaning appliance
    P.-F. interproximal cleaner
proximal
    p. cement spacer
    p. femoral nail (PFN)
    p. femoral nail antirotation (PFNA)
    p. humerus internal locking system (PHILOS)
    p. loading revision (PLR)

p. over-shoulder strap
p. thigh band
Proximate
    P. disposable skin stapler
    P. flexible linear stapler
    P. II, III stapler
    P. ILS curved intraluminal stapler
    P. ILS SDH circular stapler
    P. linear cutter
    P. RH stapler
Proxi-Strip suture
PRP
    panretinal photocoagulation
Prudoxin cream
Pruitt
    P. anoscope
    P. irrigation catheter
    P. occlusion catheter
Pruitt-Inahara
    P.-I. carotid shunt
    P.-I. vascular shunt
PRx implantable cardioverter-defibrillator
Pryor-Péan vaginal retractor
PS
    pressurizing system
    Prolene mesh
        Gynemesh PS
        PS Medical Flow Control valve
        PS 153 stent
PS-2 needle
PSA
    PSA IRMA kit
    PSA stationary oxygen system
PSC
    pronation/spring control
P-Series sleep monitoring system
pseudocyst
    pancreatic p.
pseudoisochromatic plate
pseudophake implant
PSG LOC guidewire extension
PSI chromosome analysis system
PSI-TEC aspiration/irrigation platform
psoas retractor
PSV
    pressure support ventilator
        Quantum PSV
PTA
    percutaneous transluminal angioplasty
PTB brace
PTBD catheter
PTCA catheter
PTDP
    permanent transvenous demand pacemaker
pterygium
    p. knife
    p. scissors

pterygoid chisel
PTFE
    polytetrafluoroethylene
        PTFE Gore-Tex graft
        PTFE implant
        PTFE mesh
        PTFE prosthesis
        PTFE shunt
        PTFE stent
        PTFE stent graft
PTFE-containing implant
PTFE-covered Palmaz stent
PTHC catheter
PtL airway
ptosis
    p. clamp
    p. forceps
    p. knife
    p. scissors
    p. snare
PT tilt table
public access defibrillator
PU catheter
Pucci
    P. Air orthotic
    P. inflatable elbow orthosis
    P. inflatable knee orthosis
    P. pediatric hand orthosis
    P. pediatrics hand orthosis
    P. rehab knee orthosis
    P. splint
Pucci-Seed
    P.-S. hook
    P.-S. spatula
Puck film changer
Puddu
    P. drill guide
    P. osteotomy system
pudendal
    p. block anesthesia needle
    p. needle guide
Pudenz
    P. connector
    P. flushing chamber
    P. peritoneal catheter
    P. reservoir
    P. shunt
    P. tube
    P. valve-flushing shunt
    P. ventricular catheter
Pudenz-Heyer
    P.-H. clamp
    P.-H. vascular catheter
Pudenz-Schulte shunt
Puestow guidewire
Pugh tractor
Puig
    P. Massana annuloplasty ring
    P. Massana-Shiley annuloplasty ring

P

Puig-Massana-Shiley anuloplasty valve
Puka chisel
Pul-Ez
>P.-E. exerciser
>P.-E. shoulder pulley

pull
>p. knife
>Ponsky p.
>p. rasp
>p. screw

pull-apart introducer
pullback atherectomy device
puller
>Ultra-Drive plug p.

pulley
>Flex Ranger stretch cable with p.
>Home Ranger shoulder p.
>Knee ProMotion overhead p.
>p. paser
>Preston overhead p.
>Pul-Ez shoulder p.
>Range-Master p.
>Saba p.
>shoulder p.

pull-out button
pull-type gastrostomy tube
Pulmanex
>P. PAC pulmonary assist circuit
>P. resuscitator

Pulmicort Turbuhaler
Pulmo-Aide
>P.-A. aerosol compressor/nebulizer
>P.-A. nebulizer
>P.-A. Traveler
>P.-A. ventilator

Pulmo-Aid ventilator
Pulmo-Graph
PulmoMate
>P. aerosol compressor/nebulizer
>P. nebulizer

Pulmo-Mist compressor
pulmonary
>p. arterial catheter
>p. arterial clamp
>p. arterial forceps
>p. arterial snare
>p. artery balloon pump
>p. artery catheter
>p. artery sling
>p. autograft valve
>p. balloon
>p. embolism clamp
>p. flotation catheter
>p. nodulectomy clamp
>p. retractor
>p. thermodilution catheter
>p. triple-lumen catheter
>p. vessel clamp
>p. vessel forceps

Pulmonet spirometer
Pulmonex dynamic air therapy unit
pulmonic stenosis clamp
PulmoSonic ultrasonic nebulizer
Pulmowrap
pulp
>p. canal file
>P. Canal Sealer EBT sealer
>p. cavity

pulpal microdialysis probe
Pulpdent cavity liner
pulped muscle dressing
pulpit spectacles
Pulsair tonometer
Pulsar
>P. DDD pacemaker
>P. infusion pump
>P. Max II DR pacing system
>P. Max II SR pacing system
>P. Max sensor
>P. NI implantable pacemaker
>P. obstetrical 2-channel TENS unit

pulsatile
>p. assist device
>p. jet lavage

pulsating low-air-loss bed
Pulsatome cataract emulsifier
Pulsator
>P. anaerobic syringe
>P. dry heparin arterial blood gas kit
>P. syringe

Pulsatron
>P. II handheld nerve stimulator
>P. unit

Pulsavac
>P. III wound débridement system
>P. lavage
>P. Plus wound debridement system

pulse
>p. amplifier
>p. generator
>2010 P. Holter system
>p. lavage
>p. oximeter
>p. oximetry device
>p. oximetry protector
>12-p. 3-phase p.
>6-p. 3-phase generator
>P. Pro heart rate monitor
>P. Pro heart rate monitor watch
>p. spray catheter
>p. volume recording
>p. wave Doppler

PULSEcdc compact gamma camera
pulsed
>p. carbon dioxide laser
>p. Doppler
>p. Doppler flowmeter

p. Doppler ultrasonic flowmeter
p. Doppler ultrasound
p. dye laser
p. electron avalanche knife
p. galvanic stimulator
p. green laser
p. light
p. metal vapor laser
p. pump
p. tunable dye laser
p. ultrasonic velocity detector
p. wave Doppler
p. yellow dye laser

PulseDose
    P. EX2000D oxygen conserver
    P. portable compressed oxygen
      system

pulsed-range gated Doppler instrument
pulsed-wave Doppler transducer
pulse-height analyzer
PulseMaster laser
Pulse-Pak infusion kit
Pulse-Spray
    P.-S. injector
    P.-S. pulsed infusion system
PulseSpray infusion system
Pulse-Spray/PRO infusion catheter
Pulsion FS laser
Pulsolith
    P. laser
    P. laser lithotriptor
Pulsox-5 portable pulse oximeter
PulStarFRAS device
pulverizer
    Thermovac tissue p.
Pulvertaft weave suture
Pulvograft
    Dembone demineralized cortical
      powder P.
    Osteomin Thermo-Ashed bone
      powder P.
pumice stone
pump
    Aalzet continuous infusion
      osmotic p.
    Abbott infusion p.
    Abbott LifeCare p.
    Acat 1 intraaortic balloon p.
    Advanced Collection breast p.
    Affinity blood p.
    air p.
    Alpha 1 p.
    Alzet continuous infusion
      osmotic p.
    AMO HPF 500 p.
    angle port p.
    Animas R-1000 insulin p.
    ankle rehabilitation p.
    aortic balloon p.

arthroscopic p.
ASID Bonz PP infusion p.
AutoCAT intraaortic balloon p.
Avco balloon p.
A-V Impulse foot p.
Axiom double sump p.
balloon p.
Bard PCA p.
Barron p.
Basis breast p.
battery-operated breast p.
Baxter PCA p.
Baxter volumetric infusion p.
bilateral breast p.
Bio-Medicus p.
Bio-Medicus centrifugal p.
Bio-Pump p.
Biosearch 7000 enteral feeding p.
blood p.
Bluemle p.
Breg pain care infusion p.
BVS p.
CADD-Plus external volumetric
    programmable p.
CADD-Plus intravenous infusion p.
CADD-TPN p.
cardiac balloon p.
cardiopulmonary bypass p.
Carones LASEK p.
Carrel-Lindbergh p.
centrifugal p.
Chicco breast p.
Clarus model 5169 peristaltic p.
Clarus peristaltic p.
Cobe double blood p.
Companion feeding p.
Compat 199205 enteral feeding p.
compression p.
computer-controlled infusion p.
continuous subcutaneous insulin
    infusion p.
continuous-wave arthroscopy p.
Cordis Secor implantable p.
Cormed ambulatory infusion p.
CRS-series alternating overlay
    with p.
Cub R-200 enteral feeding p.
Dana Diabecare insulin p.
Datascope System 90 intraaortic
    balloon p.
DeBakey VAD continuous-axial-
    flow p.
Deltec-Pharmacia CADD p.
DeVilbiss suction p.
Disetronic Diaport p.
Disetronic Dihedi 25 insulin p.
Disetronic D-Tron insulin p.
drug infusion p.
D-Tron insulin p.

pump *(continued)*
dual aspiration p.
Dura-Neb portable nebulizer p.
Dyonics 25 p.
ECMO p.
efflux p.
Egnell breast p.
elastomeric p.
Elmed peristaltic irrigation p.
Emerson p.
Endo Irrigator p.
Enteroport feeding p.
extracorporeal bypass p.
extremity p.
EZ hand p.
Felig insulin p.
flexible p.
Flexiflo Companion enteral
  feeding p.
Flexiflo II enteral feeding p.
Flocare 500 feeding p.
Flo-Gard p.
flow-based p.
Flowtron DVT p.
frame-mounted p.
Frenta Mat feeding p.
Frenta System II feeding p.
Gomco p.
Gomco thoracic drainage p.
Grafco breast p.
Graseby anesthesia p.
Gynkotek p.
Harvard p.
Harvard 2 dual-syringe p.
heart p.
HeartMate p.
HeartMate portable p.
hepatic artery infusion p.
Holter p.
Holter Pediatric P. 903, 907
H-TRON insulin p.
H-TRONplus insulin p.
Imed 430 enteral feeding p.
Imed Gemini PC-2 volumetric p.
Imed infusion p.
implantable intraperitoneal p.
implantable osmotic p.
implanted infusion p.
InDura intrathecal catheter and p.
Infumed p.
Infusaid p.
Infusaid infusion p.
Infuse-a-Port p.
infusion p.
insulin infusion p.
Intelliject p.
intermittent extremity p.
intraaortic balloon p. (IABP)
ion p.

IsoMed implantable drug p.
P. It Up pneumatic socket volume
  management system
IVAC volumetric infusion p.
Jobst athrombotic p.
Jobst extremity p.
Kaat II Plus intraaortic balloon p.
Kangaroo p.
Kangaroo enteral feeding p.
Kangaroo 200, 324, 330 enteral
  feeding p.
Kangaroo feeding p.
Kangaroo infusion p.
Kendall McGaw Intelligent p.
Keofeed 500 enteral feeding p.
Keofeed II enteral feeding p.
Klein p.
KM-1 breast p.
KMI 60 enteral feeding p.
Kontron intraaortic balloon p.
Lactina Select breast p.
laser-assisted epithelium
  keratomileusis p.
left ventricular bypass p.
Lifecare p.
Lifestream centrifugal p.
Lindbergh p.
Linvatec arthroscopic infusion p.
low-compliance perfusion p.
low-compliance pneumohydraulic p.
low-pressure breast p.
MagMag breast p.
Mary Jane breast p.
MasterFlex fetal perfusion p.
Master Flow Pumpette p.
McGaw volumetric p.
Medela Dominant vacuum
  delivery p.
Medela manual breast p.
Medex Protege 3010 syringe
  infusion p.
MedFlo pain management p.
Medfusion 1001 syringe infusion p.
Medrad infusion p.
MedSystem III multichannel
  infusion p.
Medtronic infusion p.
Medtronic SynchroMed p.
Medtronic SynchroMed
  implantable p.
microinfusion p.
MiniMed III infusion p.
MiniMed 508, 511 insulin p.
MiniMed Paradigm insulin p.
miniosmotic infusion p.
Mityvac reusable vacuum p.
Mityvac simple hand p.
morphine p.
Multipulse 1000 compression p.

muscular venous p.
Na-K exchange p.
Norport p.
Nutromat Pad S feeding p.
On-Q p.
p. oxygenator
pain control infusion p.
PainFree p.
Pancretec 2000 p.
Panomat infusion p.
Panomat microinfusion p.
Paradigm insulin p.
Paragon ambulatory p.
patient-controlled anesthesia p.
PCA p.
peristaltic p.
pneumocapillary infusion p.
portable insulin infusion p.
programmable p.
Protégé 3010 syringe infusion p.
Provider 6000 ambulatory dual-
  channel infusion p.
pulmonary artery balloon p.
Pulsar infusion p.
pulsed p.
Quantum enteral p.
rapid infusion p.
Reitan catheter p.
reverse osmosis p.
roller p.
Salem p.
Sarns 7000 MDX roller p.
Sarns Siok II blood p.
Sartorius breast p.
scroll p.
sequential extremity p.
Shiley Infusaid p.
Sigma 6000+ infusion p.
Space Saver volumetric p.
Stat 2 Pumpette disposable IV p.
stomach p.
subcutaneous morphine p.
suction p.
sump p.
surgical suction p.
SynchroMed implantable p.
SynchroMed programmable p.
syringe p.
syringe-type infusion p.
Thoratec p.
Tonkaflo p.
TransAct intraaortic balloon p.
Travenol infusion p.
Travenol Infusor p.
unicare breast p.
Vacumix vacuum p.
vacuum-based p.
VentrAssist heart p.
Venturi p.

Verifuse ambulatory infusion p.
Versaflow peristatic p.
volumetric infusion p.
VTR-300 enteral feeding p.
Wells Johnson p.
pumped dye laser
Pumpette
  Master Flow P.
  Stat 2 P.
Pump-It-Up pneumatic socket
Pump-N-Shorts pump holder
PumpPals shoe insole
Pump-Vac III system
punch
  Abrams pleural biopsy p.
  Accuderm p.
  adenoid p.
  Anderson biopsy p.
  aortic p.
  Australian p.
  baby Tischler biopsy p.
  backbiting bone p.
  backward-biting ostrum p.
  Baker p.
  Baker-Cummings p.
  Barron donor p.
  Barron donor corneal p.
  Barron marking corneal p.
  Berens corneoscleral p.
  biopsy p.
  p. block
  bone graft p.
  bone hole p.
  Carpel trabeculectomy p.
  Caspari suture p.
  Casselberry suture p.
  Castroviejo corneoscleral p.
  cervical p.
  Charnley femoral prosthesis
    neck p.
  Cloward bone p.
  Cone skull p.
  Conquest meniscal crescent p.
  corneal p.
  corneoscleral p.
  Cottingham p.
  cruciate p.
  cutaneous p.
  Descemet membrane p.
  Deyerle p.
  Disposa-Derm skin p.
  Dyonics suction p.
  Dyovac suction p.
  endoscopic suture p.
  Eppendorfer biopsy p.
  ethmoidal p.
  Euro-Med biopsy p.
  Fehling TOP ejector p.
  Ferris-Smith p.

P

punch *(continued)*
    Ferris-Smith-Kerrison p.
    finned stem p.
    fluted stem p.
    p. forceps
    Gass corneoscleral p.
    Gass scleral p.
    Gass sclerotomy p.
    Gelfoam p.
    Gibbs eye p.
    Goosen vascular p.
    Graham-Kerrison p.
    p. guide
    hair transplant p.
    Hardy p.
    Hardy sellar p.
    Hartmann biopsy p.
    Hartmann ear p.
    Hartmann nasal p.
    Hartmann tonsillar p.
    Hirsch hypophysial p.
    Holth corneoscleral p.
    Holth scleral p.
    I-beam cement p.
    I-beam press-fit p.
    infundibular p.
    Jansen-Middleton septal p.
    Joseph p.
    Karp aortic p.
    keel bone p.
    Kelly p.
    Kelly-Descemet membrane p.
    Kerrison bone p.
    Kerrison laminectomy p.
    Keyes p.
    Keyes cutaneous biopsy p.
    Keyes dermatologic p.
    Keyes skin p.
    Keyes vulvar p.
    keyhole p.
    kidney p.
    King adenoidal p.
    Klein p.
    Koffler-Hajek sphenoidal p.
    Krause angular oval p.
    Lange antral p.
    Lebsche sternal p.
    Leksell p.
    Lempert malleus p.
    Lewis-Resnik p.
    linear scissor p.
    Loo p.
    Luntz-Dodick p.
    Meltzer adenoid p.
    Meltzer tonsillar p.
    Miltex disposable biopsy p.
    Mixter brain biopsy p.
    modified sclerectomy p.
    Murphy kidney p.

    p. myringotomy system
    nasal p.
    Orentreich p.
    Osborne p.
    pleural biopsy p.
    Pollock p.
    Price corneal p.
    Ramirez EndoForehead p.
    Rathke p.
    p. rongeur
    Rothman Gilbard corneal p.
    Schlesinger cervical p.
    Schubert uterine biopsy p.
    scleral p.
    sclerectomy p.
    sclerotomy p.
    sellar p.
    side-biting ostrum p.
    skin p.
    skull p.
    Spencer triangular adenoid p.
    sphenoidal bone p.
    Spurling-Kerrison laminectomy p.
    Stammberger antral p.
    Storz corneoscleral p.
    Stough p.
    suction p.
    Tanne corneal p.
    Thoms-Gaylor biopsy p.
    Thomson adenoidal p.
    Tischler cervical biopsy p.
    Tischler-Morgan biopsy p.
    Tomey trabeculectomy p.
    tonsillar p.
    Townsend biopsy p.
    p. trephine
    Troutman p.
    Turkel p.
    uterine biopsy p.
    vessel p.
    Walser corneoscleral p.
    Walton p.
    Walton corneoscleral p.
    Watson-Williams ethmoidal p.
    Wilde nasal p.
    Wittner biopsy p.
    Wittner cervical biopsy p.
    Woolley tibia p.
    Yankauer p.
    Yeoman biopsy p.
punched-out orchidometer
punctal
    p. dilator
    p. lens
punctate electrode
punctum
    p. dilator
    p. plug

puncture
    p. needle
    p. transducer
puncture-proof glove
puncture-tip needle
Punctur-Guard Revolution safety needle holder
Puno-Winter-Byrd system
Puntenney forceps
pupil
    artificial p.
    p. dilator
    p. dilator ring
    p. spreader/retractor forceps
pupillary membrane scissors
pupillograph
pupillometer
    Colvard handheld infrared p.
    ForSite p.
    Procyon digital infrared p.
    Pupilscan II p.
pupilloscope
pupillostatometer
Pupilscan II pupillometer
PuraPly wound dressing
Pura-Vario-AL stent
Pura-Vario-AS stent
Pura-Vario-A stent
Pura-Vario stent
Purdue pegboard
PureFix hydroxyapatite
Puregene
    P. DNA extraction system
    P. DNA isolation kit
PureVision
    P. extended-wear contact lens
    P. toric lens
Puri-Clens wound cleanser
purification
    Wizard plasmid p.
purifier
    Air Supply air p.
    Air Supply wearable air p.
    Bemis air p.
Puritan
    P. all-purpose compressor
    P. Bennett Aeris 590 oxygen concentrator
    P. Bennett KnightStar ventilator
    P. Bennett ventilator
    P. Bubble-Jet
    P. swab
Puritan-Bennett 7250 metabolic monitor
Purkinje image tracker
Puros
    P. Accugraft
    P. Accugraft ALIF allograft system
    P. Accugraft allograft

purpose-built silicone rubber multilumen manometric assembly
Pursuer
    P. CBD helical stone basket
    P. minihelical stone basket
Pursuit
    P. balloon angioplasty catheter
    P. system
push
    p. cuff
    p. enteroscope
    P. medical brace
    p. rasp
pushable coil
push-and-pull hook
Push-Ease
    P.-E. Quad Cuff
    P.-E. wheelchair glove
pusher
    Aker lens p.
    p. catheter
    Clarke-Reich knot p.
    De La Vega lens p.
    Endo-Assist endoscopic knot p.
    Endo-Assist reusable knot p.
    endoscopic knot p.
    Fresnel lens p.
    Gazayerli knot p.
    hemispherical p.
    hook p.
    Jacobson suture p.
    knot p.
    lens p.
    Martin Surefit lens p.
    Mershon band p.
    metal p.
    metal-tipped stent p.
    MetraTie knot p.
    Negus p.
    patella p.
    Ranfac knot p.
    Reddick-Saye macro knot p.
    Revo loop handle knot p.
    p. tube
    Visitec lens p.
    p. wire
push-pull catheter
push-type enteroscopy
push-up block
pus tube
Puth abduction splint
Putterman
    P. levator resection clamp
    P. ptosis clamp
Putti
    P. bone file
    P. bone rasp

P

Putti-Platt
    P.-P. arthroplasty
    P.-P. instrumentation
putty
    AliMed p.
    AlloFuse DBM p.
    AlloMatrix bone graft p.
    AlloMatrix injectable p.
    Bishop p.
    Blue Brand Therapy P.
    color-coded therapy p.
    DBX bone p.
    DynaGraft p.
    Flexi-Grip exercise p.
    Grafton DBM p.
    Grafton moldable p.
    matrix Grafton p.
    OP-1 p.
    OsteoStim DBM p.
    polyvinylsiloxane p.
    Thera-Plast p.
    Thera-Putty exercise p.
    Therapy P.
PV
  photoselective vaporization
    PV foam
pVAD
  percutaneous ventricular assist device
    TandemHeart pVAD
PVA foam embolization particle
PVC
    PVC catheter
    PVC drain
    PVC tubing
PVD dressing
P-wave triggered ventricular pacemaker

PWB transpedicular spine fixation system
pyeloureteral catheter
pyknometer
pylon
    AirStance p.
    dynamic p. (DP)
    Icon p.
    P. intramedullary nail system
    Stratus impact-reducing p.
    vertical shock p.
pyloric stenosis dilator
PyloriTek
    P. *Helicobacter pylori* test kit
    P. reagent strip
pylorus clamp
Pynchon suction tube
Pyramesh cage
pyramid
    p. attachment
    p. cannula
    suction p.
    p. Toomey tip
pyramidal
    p. tip
    p. tip trocar
Pyrex
    P. eye sphere
    P. glass tube
    P. T tube
pyrocarbon
    p. implant
    p. prosthesis
PyroHemiSphere joint implant
pyrolytic carbon device
pyxigraphic device

Q
Q band
Q Star Voyager pressure reduction
mattress
Q200 gastroscope
QAD-1
Doppler QAD-1
QAD-1 sonography unit
Q-cath catheterization recording system
QCT bone densitometry system
QDR-1500, -2000 bone densitometer
QDR 1000 densitometer absorptiometer
QGM
Infratonic QGM
QIAamp
Q. DNA blood biorobot kit
Q. Tissue kit
Qiagen QIAquick gel extraction kit
QIAmp tissue kit
QIAquick PCR 96 purification kit
Q-LAS 10 Q-switched YAG laser
**Qlicksmart scalpel blade removal
system**
Q-Maxx side-firing laser device
Q-Prep system
Q-Ray bracelet
QRS
QRS pulsating magnetic field
system
QRS ruby/YAG laser
QSAC
quadrant-sparing acetabular component
QSAC acetabular component
QS alexandrite laser
Q-Star
Q-S. IV pressure-relief mattress
Q-S. Voyager pressure-reduction
mattress
Q-Stress
Q-S. treadmill
Q-S. treadmill stress test
Q-switched
Q-s. alexandrite laser
Q-s. Er:YAG laser
Q-s. laser
Q-s. Nd:YAG laser
Q-s. neodymium:YAG laser
Q-s. neodymium:yttrium aluminum-
garnet laser
Q-s. ruby laser
Q-s. YAG laser
QT interval sensing pacemaker
Q-Trak IAQ monitor
QT-Watch messaging wristwatch

quad
q. board
Q. electrode
Q. 7000, 12000 high-field open
MRI scanner
q. resonance NMR probe circuit
Quadcat wire
QuaDDS-QP2 stent
QuaDDS stent
QuadPediatric fundus lens
QuadPolar electrode
quad-ported LASIK irrigating cannula
Quadra-Coil ureteral stent
Quadracut ACL shaver system
Quadrant
Q. advanced shoulder brace
Q. retractor
**quadrant-sparing acetabular component
(QSAC)**
quadrature
q. birdcage coil
q. body coil
q. cervical spine coil
q. head coil
q. phase detector
q. radiofrequency receiver coil
q. surface coil
q. surface coil MRI system
q. surface coil system stem
q. terminal latency surface coil
q. transmit/receive head coil
quadriceps De Lorme boot
**quadriceps-sparing minimally invasive
total knee instrument**
**quadricusp stentless mitral bioprosthetic
valve**
**quadrilateral ischial weightbearing
socket**
Quadrilite 6000 fiberoptic headlight
quadriplegic standing frame
quadripolar
q. cutting forceps
q. diagnostic catheter
q. diagnostic electrophysiology
catheter
q. electrode catheter
q. Itrel 2 pulse generator
q. pacing catheter
q. Quad electrode
q. steerable electrode catheter
q. steerable mapping/ablation
catheter
q. thermocouple-equipped ablation
catheter

quadrisected
    q. graft dilator
    q. minigraft dilator
quadruple-bladed knife
QuaDS drug-eluting stent
Quadtro
    Q. cushion
    Q. cushion with Isoflap valve
QualCare knee brace
QualCraft
    Q. ankle support
    Q. short elastic wrist support
    Q. splint
    Q. strap
Quanta
    Q. Lite ANA ELISA test kit
    Q. Lite CCP ELISA kit
    Q. Lite ELISA autoimmune kit
QuantiFERON-TB test
Quantikine ELISA kit
Quantimet 500 analyzing system
quantitative sweat measurement system
Quantrex Sweep 650 ultrasonic cleansing system
Quantronic resonance system
Quantum
    Q. biliary inflation device
    Q. enhancement knife
    Q. enteral pump
    Q. Foot prosthesis
    Q. hearing aid
    Q. inflation device
    Q. Maverick balloon catheter
    Q. pacemaker
    Q. PSV
    Q. PSV ventilator
    Q. traction
    Q. TTC balloon dilator
    Q. TTC biliary balloon
    Q. TTC biliary balloon dilator
Quant-X color quantification imaging tool
quarantine drain
Quartet system
quartz
    q. fiber dosimeter
    q. fiberoptic probe
    q. lamp
    q. needle
    q. rod
    q. transducer
quartz-glass container
quartz-iodine lamp
Quartzo device
Quattro mitral valve prosthesis
Quengel device
Quervain abdominal retractor

Quest
    Q. MPS myocardial protection system
    Tranquility Q.
Questek laser tube
QueST stent
Quevedo fixation forceps
quick
    q. catheter
    q. connector
    Q. Connect twist drill
    Q. CT9800 scanner
    Q. Slide automated stainer
QuickAnchor
    Micro Q.
    Mitek Micro Q.
    Mitek Mini Q.
    Resolve Q.
Quickanchor Plus small bone anchor
Quickbox container
QuickCast
    Q. splint
    Q. wrist immobilizer
Quickclip
Quick-Core
    Q.-C. biopsy needle
    Q.-C. biopsy system
    Q.-C. needle
Quick-Cross catheter
Quickdraw
    Q. venous cannula
    Q. venous cannula kit
QuickDraw bone harvester
Quickert
    Q. grooved director
    Q. suture
Quickert-Dryden probe
Quick-Fix maxillomandibular fixation system
QuickFlash arterial catheter
QuickFlow
    Q. DPS
    Q. DPS distal perfusion system
    Q. DPS foot
QuickFurl
    Q. DL
    Q. SL balloon
Quickie
    Q. Carbon wheelchair
    Q. EX wheelchair
    Q. GPS wheelchair
    Q. GP Swing-Away wheelchair
    Q. GPV wheelchair
    Q. Kidz wheelchair
    Q. Recliner wheelchair
    Q. Ti wheelchair
QuicKlamp hemostasis device
QuickLance lancing device

QuickRinse automated instrument rinse system
QuickSeal femoral arterial closure system
Quick-Sil silicone system
QuickSilver hydrophilic-coated guidewire
QuickSite LV lead
QuickStart
    Beckman Coulter Q.
QuickStick padding
Quickswitch irrigation/aspiration ophthalmic system
QuickTack periosteal fixation system
Quick-Tap paracentesis system
QuickTek
    Q. glucose meter
    Q. test strip
QuickVue
    Q. Advance *Gardnerella vaginalis* test
    Q. *Chlamydia* test
    Q. *H. pylori* gII test
    Q. *H. pylori* gII test kit
    Q. In-Line One-Step Strep A test
    Q. one-step hCG-Combo pregnancy test
    Q. UrinChek urine test strip
    Q. UrinChek 10+ urine test strip
Quiet interference screw
QuietTrak monitor
Quik
    Q. Connect fetal monitor
    Q. splint
Quik-Chek external pacer tester
Quik-Coff electrical cough stimulator
QuikFormables orthotic
Quikheel lancet
Quik-Stitch endoscopic suturing system
Quik-Temp thermometer
quill sheath
Quimby
    Q. implant system
    Q. scissors

Quincke-Babcock needle
Quincke-point spinal needle
Quincke spinal needle
Quinones-Neubüser uterine-grasping forceps
Quinones uterine-grasping forceps
Quintero amniocentesis needle
Quinton
    Q. catheter
    Q. central venous catheter
    Q. dual-lumen catheter
    Q. peritoneal catheter
    Q. PermCath
    Q. PermCath catheter
    Q. Q-Port vascular access port
    Q. single-port scissor valve
    Q. suction biopsy instrument
    Q. Synergy cardiac information management system
    Q. tube
Quinton-Mahurkar dual-lumen peritoneal catheter
Quinton-Scribner shunt
QuinTron
    Q. AlveoSampler
    Q. MicroLyzer
    Q. Microlyzer 12 chromatograph
Quips genetic imaging system
Quire
    Q. foreign body forceps
    Q. mechanical finger forceps
    Q. mechanical finger snare
Quisling intranasal hammer
Quisling-Parkes osteotome
QuPID pregnancy test
QUS-2 calcaneal ultrasonometer
Q-200V
    Olympus EVIS Q-200V
QWIKLoad
    CardioSEAL septal occlusion system with Q.
QwikStrip adhesive bandage

R1 rapid exchange balloon dilatation catheter
R2L rapid exchange balloon dilatation catheter with extended pressure range
Raaf dual-lumen catheter
Raaf-Oldberg intervertebral disc forceps
Rabbit mouthgag
Rabiner neurological hammer
Rabinov cannula
Racer
    R. over-the-wire biliary stent
    R. over-the-wire biliary stent system
Racestyptine cord
rack
    Hausmann weight r.
    Luneau retinoscopy r.
    Nalgene freezer storage r.
RackBeta liquid scintillation counter
Racz Tun-L-Kath catheter
Rad airway laryngeal blade
RADenoid adenoidectomy blade
RADFx proximal radium fixation kit
radial
    r. arterial catheter
    r. artery catheter
    r. hinged ulnar deviation splint
    r. iridotomy scissors
    R. Jaw biopsy forceps
    R. Jaw bladder biopsy forceps
    R. Jaw hot biopsy forceps
    R. Jaw III Max Capacity 1589 biopsy forceps
    R. Jaw III Max Capacity with needle biopsy forceps
    R. Jaw III single-use biopsy forceps
    r. keratotomy knife
    r. keratotomy marker
    r. nerve glove
    r. sector scanning echoendoscope
    r. sponge
radial-sector scan transducer
radiant
    r. heat device
    r. heat warmer
    r. warmer
radiation
    r. beam monitor
    r. detector
    r. seed
    r. simulator
    r. therapy planning system
    r. therapy system (RTS)

    r. treatment system
    ultraviolet r. (UVR)
    ultraviolet autoblood r. (UVAR)
radiative hyperthermia device
Radifocus
    R. catheter guidewire
    R. Glidewire
    R. guidewire
    R. hydrophilic coated guidewire
    R. introducer B kit
    R. wire
Radii-T catheter
radioactive
    r. stent
    r. strontium needle
radiocarpal implant
radiofrequency (RF)
    r. ablation (RFA)
    r. ablator
    r. balloon
    r. coil
    r. diathermy device
    r. generator
    r. head coil
    r. hot balloon
    r. interstitial tissue ablation system
    r. needle electrode system
    r. pacemaker
radiofrequency-generated thermal balloon catheter
radiograph
    Velpeau axillary r.
    West Point axillary lateral r.
radiographic
    r. grid
    r. image processing system
    r. imaging system
radioimmunoassay kit
radioisotope
    r. calibrator
    r. camera
    r. capsule
    r. stent
radiologic portacaval shunt
radiolucent
    r. cranial pin headholder
    r. operating room table extension
    r. plastic occluder
    r. sound
    r. spine frame
    r. splint
    r. wrist fixation system
radiometer
    R. ABL 500 blood gas analyzer
    pastille r.

R

radiometer *(continued)*
>photographic r.
>R. probe

Radionics
>R. articulated arm system
>R. bipolar coagulation unit
>R. bipolar instrument
>R. CRW stereotactic head frame
>R. radiofrequency generator
>R. radiofrequency lesion generator

radionuclide
>r. camera
>r. carrier system
>r. generator

radiopaque
>r. bone cement
>r. end marker
>r. ERCP catheter
>r. gold marker
>r. marker
>r. nitinol stent
>r. pellet
>r. silastic catheter
>r. tantalum stent

radioscope
>Lombart r.

radiotranslucent rod
Radi pressure wire
RadiStop radial compression system
radium ^{226}**Ra needle**
Radius
>R. enteral feeding tube
>R. self-expanding stent

Radix anchor
RadNet radiology information system
Radovan
>R. subcutaneous tissue expander
>R. tissue expander tip

RadPICC catheter
RadStat hemostasis device
RAE endotracheal tube
Ragnell
>R. double-ended retractor
>R. retractor
>R. scissors
>R. undermining scissors

Ragnell-Davis double-ended retractor
Ragnell-Kilner scissors
rail
>Bed-Bar support r.
>Lumex Tub-Guard safety r.
>Railguard bed r.

Railguard bed rail
railway catheter
Raimondi
>R. catheter
>R. hemostatic forceps
>R. peritoneal catheter
>R. scalp hemostatic forceps
>R. ventricular catheter

Rainbow
>R. drill
>R. vacuum

Raindrop medication nebulizer
Rainey Ultra-Flex compression wear
Rainin
>R. air injection cannula
>R. lens spatula

Rains stent
rake
>Miller 9-prong small r.
>r. retractor
>Senn r.

Ralks
>R. adapter
>R. eye magnet

Ralks-Davis mouthgag
Raman microprobe
Ramelet phlebectomy hook
Ramirez
>R. EndoFacelift dissector
>R. EndoFacelift elevator
>R. EndoFacelift needle holder
>R. EndoForehead A/M dissector
>R. EndoForehead A/M scissors
>R. EndoForehead curved dissector
>R. EndoForehead flap dissector
>R. EndoForehead forceps
>R. EndoForehead grasper
>R. EndoForehead parietal elevator
>R. EndoForehead punch
>R. EndoForehead right and left
> protector
>R. EndoForehead right and left
> protectors
>R. EndoForehead spreader
>R. EndoForehead straight dissector
>R. EndoForehead suction coagulator
>R. EndoForehead T dissector
>R. EndoPlastic tape
>R. manipulator
>R. periosteal elevator
>R. shunt
>R. Silastic cannula
>R. telescoping cannula

Ramitec polyether bite registration material
RAMP
>RAMP biological test system
>RAMP myoglobin test

ramp
>Graftech anterior r.
>Graftech posterior r.
>Graftech structural allograft
> anterior r.
>Graftech structural allograft
> posterior r.

Rampart EMS clinical support tool
Rampley
    R. sponge forceps
    R. sponge-holding forceps
Rampton facebow
Ramsden eyepiece
Ramses
    R. diaphragm
    R. diaphragm introducer
Ramstedt pyloric stenosis dilator
ramus
    r. blade
    r. blade implant
    r. endosteal implant
    r. stripper
Ranawat-Burstein
    R.-B. hip prosthesis
    R.-B. porous stem
    R.-B. total hip system
Rancho
    R. ankle-foot control device
    R. cube
    R. Cube system
    R. external fixation instrument
    R. external fixation prosthesis
    R. external fixation system
    R. swivel hinge
Randall stone forceps
Randelli shoulder prosthesis
Rand microballoon
Randolph
    R. cyclodialysis cannula
    R. irrigator
random
    R. Primed DNA Labeling kit
    r. zero sphygmomanometer
Randot
    R. circle
    R. Stereo Smile test
^{226}Ra needle
Raney
    R. clip
    R. flexion jacket brace
    R. jacket
    R. saw guide
    R. scalp clip
    R. scalp clip applier
    R. scalp clip-applying forceps
Raney-Crutchfield
    R.-C. drill point
    R.-C. skull tongs
Ranfac
    R. cannula
    R. cholangiographic catheter
    R. disposable cholangiography catheter
    R. knot pusher
    R. needle
    R. soft tissue needle

range
    D2L OTW balloon dilatation catheter with extended pressure r.
    r. of motion (ROM)
    R2L rapid exchange balloon dilatation catheter with extended pressure r.
range-gated transducer
Range-Master pulley
range of motion (ROM)
range-of-motion brace
Ranger
    R. balloon
    R. over-the-wire balloon catheter
Rankin
    R. anastomosis clamp
    R. hemostat
Rankin-Crile forceps
Rank-Taylor-Hobson-Talysurf instrument
Ransford loop
RAP cannula
Rapicide
rapid
    r. cuff inflator
    r. exchange (RX)
    r. exchange balloon catheter
    r. exchange Flowtrack catheter
    r. infusion pump
    R. One single dipstick system
    R. One single drug screen dipstick
    R. Rhino device
    R. Rhino gel knit nasal dressing
    r. screen
    R. Strand implant
    R. Transit catheter
    R. Transit microcatheter
    r. urease test
Rapide wound suture
RapidFire multiple-band ligator
Rapidlab 800 Critical Care system
RapidMist metered-dose spray applicator
Rapido-mat
Rapidpoint
    R. access
    R. 400 critical care analyzer
RapidScreen
    R. digital CAD
    R. RS-2000 CAD
    R. RS-2000 x-ray equipment
Rapidtransit microcatheter
RapidView model
RapidVUE particle shape and size analyzer
RapiSeal
    R. patch
    R. pouch
RAP-n-roll
Rappaport-Sprague stethoscope

R

Rappazzo
- R. intraocular foreign body forceps
- R. intraocular manipulator

Raptor
- R. PTCA balloon
- R. PTCA dilatation catheter

Raptorrail PTCA dilatation catheter
rare earth intraocular magnet
Rascal
- R. II anesthetic gas monitor
- R. scooter

Rashkind
- R. balloon
- R. cardiac device
- R. double-disc occluder prosthesis
- R. double-disc umbrella occluder
- R. double umbrella device
- R. hooked device
- R. occluder
- R. septostomy balloon catheter
- R. umbrella

Rasor blood pumping system
rasp, raspatory (*See also* raspatory, raspatory)
- Aagesen disposable r.
- Alexander-Farabeuf r.
- Aufricht glabellar r.
- Aufricht nasal r.
- Bankart r.
- bell r.
- Black r.
- bone r.
- Bristow r.
- Brown r.
- cleft palate r.
- compound curved r.
- Converse r.
- convex r.
- Cottle r.
- Cottle-MacKenty elevator r.
- Cottle nasal r.
- Davidson-Mathieu rib r.
- Davidson-Sauerbruch rib r.
- diamond r.
- down-curved r.
- Doyen costal r.
- Doyen rib r.
- ear r.
- Edwards-Verner r.
- Endotrac r.
- Epstein bone r.
- facet r.
- Farabeuf bone r.
- Farabeuf-Collin r.
- Farabeuf-Lambotte r.
- FeatherTouch automated r.
- femoral r.
- Fischer nasal r.
- Fomon r.

Fomon nasal r.
Forman diamond r.
frontal sinus r.
Gallagher r.
Georgiade r.
glabellar r.
Good r.
hand surgery r.
Herczel rib r.
Hylin r.
interbody r.
interbody fusion r.
Israel r.
Jansen r.
Joseph nasal r.
Joseph periosteal r.
Kessler podiatry r.
Key r.
Kleinert-Kutz r.
Kocher r.
Koenig r.
Ladd r.
Lambotte rib r.
laminectomy r.
Lane periosteal r.
Langenbeck r.
Langenbeck periosteal r.
Lebsche r.
Lewis nasal r.
Lewis periosteal r.
Lorenz-Rees nasal r.
Lundsgaard r.
Lundsgaard-Burch corneal r.
Mallory-Head r.
Mallory-Head Interlok r.
Maltz r.
Maltz-Lipsett nasal r.
Maltz nasal r.
Mannerfelt r.
Mathieu r.
Matson r.
Matson-Alexander r.
McCabe perforation r.
McCollough r.
McGee oval-window r.
McIndoe r.
microbayonet r.
Miller r.
Mott r.
nasal r.
Nicoll r.
Olivecrona r.
Ollier r.
orthopaedic r.
Overholt rib r.
Parkes r.
Peet nasal r.
perforation r.
periosteal r.

Phemister r.
r. pin
Podiatry Institute r.
power r.
pull r.
push r.
Putti bone r.
rib r.
Rubin r.
Rubin oblique r.
Sayre periosteal r.
Sédillot r.
Semb rib r.
side-cutting r.
snow plow r.
Stenstrom r.
straight r.
Sullivan sinus r.
surgical general r.
Thompson r.
Thompson stem r.
triangular r.
ulnar r.
Watson-Williams sinus r.
Wiener antral r.
Wiener nasal r.
Williger r.
window r.
Woodward antral r.
Zollner r.

raspatory
Doyen r.
rib r.

Rastelli
R. conduit
R. graft

ratchet
r. clamp
r. flexor tenodesis splint
R. Lock variable flexion knee lock
r. tourniquet

ratcheting T-handle
ratchet-type brace
rate-adaptive
r.-a. device
r.-a. pacemaker

rate-modulated pacemaker
rate-responsive
r.-r. pacemaker
r.-r. pulse generator
ventricle-paced, ventrical-sensed
inhibited, r.-r. (VVIR)

Rathke punch
Rath treatment table
RatioVision
AttoFluor R.
R. digital fluorescent imaging
system

rat-tail catheter
rat-tooth
r.-t. forceps
r.-t. Olympus FG 8L grasping
forceps
r.-t. pickup

rature
r. detector
r. surface coil system

Rauchfuss sling
Raulerson introducer syringe
Ray
R. pituitary curette
R. RRE-TM thermistor electrode
R. TFC threaded fusion cage
R. threaded fusion cage

Rayner lens
Rayport muscle clamp
**Ray-Tec x-ray detectable surgical
sponge**
Raz
R. anterior vaginal wall sling
R. double-prong ligature carrier

Razi cannula introducer
razor
Bard-Parker r.
r. blade
r. bladebreaker
r. blade holder
r. blade knife
r. blade trephine
Castroviejo r.
Credo r.
Detroit Receiving Hospital r.
r. scalpel

razor-tip needle
RazorVac ArthroWand
RBM implant
R&B portable pneumothorax apparatus
RBS face mask
RC1, RC2 catheter
RC-2 fundus camera
**RDX coronary radiation catheter
delivery system**
reabsorbable suture
Reach
R. Easy massager
R. revision stem
R. revision system
R. & Roll cart

reach-and-pin forceps
Reacher
E-Z R.

reacher
Double Duty cane r.
E-Z R.
long-handled dressing r.
Pik Stik R.

733

reactor
> breeder r.
> fast-breeder r.

Read
> R. facial curette
> R. gouge

reader
> AC 3 plate r.
> Affinity multimode plate r.
> AutoPap r.
> Bio-kinetics r.
> Bio-Tek EIx800 plate r.
> Fisher microcapillary tube r.
> Immuno-mini NJ-2300 microplate r.
> kinetic microplate r.
> microplate r.
> microtitration plate r.
> PapNet r.
> plate r.
> screen r.

Readit SNP genotyping system
Ready-Set punctum plug
reagent
> immunoassay r.
> Vector Elite R.

Real-EaSE neck and shoulder relaxer
Reality vaginal pouch
real-time
> r.-t. B scanner
> r.-t. confocal scanning laser microscope
> r.-t. 2-dimensional Doppler flow-imaging system
> r.-t. 4D ultrasound imaging system
> r.-t. format converter
> r.-t. low-intensity x-ray
> r.-t. position management tracking system
> r.-t. sonographic unit
> r.-t. ultrasound
> r.-t. videoprocessor

reamer
> acorn r.
> Aequalis r.
> Arthrex coring r.
> bone r.
> canal r.
> cannulated 4-flute r.
> chamfer r.
> Charnley deepening r.
> Charnley expanding r.
> Charnley taper r.
> Charnley trochanter r.
> congruous cup-shaped r.
> Con-Nex r.
> core r.
> debris-retaining acetabular r.
> deepening r.

> end-cutting r.
> endodontic r.
> expanding r.
> femoral head bone removal r.
> femoral shaft r.
> final-cut acetabular r.
> flexible r.
> flexible-wire bundle r.
> fluted r.
> grater-type r.
> Gray r.
> Gray flexible intramedullary r.
> grooving r.
> Hall Versipower r.
> Harris center-cutting acetabular r.
> hemispherical r.
> humeral r.
> Intracone intramedullary r.
> intramedullary r.
> Jewett socket r.
> K r.
> Küntscher shaft r.
> Lorenz r.
> Lottes r.
> MacAusland finishing ball r.
> MacAusland finishing cup r.
> Mallory-Head Interlok r.
> medullary canal r.
> Micro-Aire r.
> Mira female trochanteric r.
> Moore bone r.
> orthopaedic r.
> Osteonics r.
> patellar shaft r.
> Peeso r.
> Perthes r.
> power-driven r.
> Pressure Sentinel r.
> progressively larger r.
> Richards r.
> Rispi Micromega r.
> Rush awl r.
> shaft r.
> shelf r.
> spherical r.
> spiral trochanteric r.
> spot face r.
> straight r.
> Swanson r.
> tapered r.
> T-handle r.
> triangular bone r.

reaming awl
rear-entry ACL drill guide
rear-tip extender
Rebar-18 micro catheter
Rebounder
> Plyoback R.

rebreathing
  r. bag
  r. mask
Récamier uterine curette
Recath bypass graft marker
receive-only circular surface coil
receiver
  Medtronic radiofrequency r.
  Olympus EU-M30S endoscopic
    ultrasonography r.
receptacle
  C-TUB instrument r.
recessed balloon septostomy catheter
recession
  r. clamp
  r. forceps
  r. ophthalmic muscle hook
reciprocal
  r. finger prehension orthosis
  r. planing instrument
reciprocating
  r. cannula
  r. gait orthosis
  r. power handpiece
  r. saw
Recklinghausen tonometer
recliner
  r. air chair
  HydroSoothe r.
  Lumex r.
  Lumex Preferred Care r.
  Ortho-Biotic r.
reclining chair
reclining-frame wheelchair
Recon nail
reconstruction plate
reconstructive cell/polymer construct
recorder
  blood pressure r.
  cardiac output r.
  circadian event r.
  Cordigital MicroER r.
  Cordigital MicroLR r.
  Del Mar Avionics 3-channel r.
  Digitrapper Mk III portable
    digital r.
  Digitrapper portable pH r.
  DM-400 Holter ECG cassette r.
  Dopcord r.
  event r.
  Gould-Brush 481 8-channel r.
  Gould ES 1000 r.
  graphic level r.
  HeartCard 3X cardiac event r.
  Honeywell r.
  24-hour ambulatory
    electrocardiographic r.
  intraocular tension r.
  Iriscorder r.

King of Hearts + r.
King of Hearts AF r.
King of Hearts event r.
King of Hearts Express r.
King of Hearts Express AF r.
King of Hearts Express 3X cardiac
  event r.
LifeSigns Micro 12 ECG + r.
LifeSigns Rhythm Check r.
Marquette Holter r.
Medilog 4000 ambulatory ECG r.
Mingograf 82 r.
Narco Biosystems r.
Narco Bio-Systems rectilinear r.
Narco Physiograph-6B r.
Nicolet Viking Iie EMG r.
polysomnograph 20-channel EEG r.
Rectigraph-8K r.
rectilinear r.
Respitrace r.
Reveal Plus insertable loop r.
Sandhill-800 TDS chart r.
Sekomic SS-100F r.
sensory nerve action potential
  sleep r.
SnoreSat sleep r.
Sony video r.
Toshiba ERVF 1A video floppy r.
video r.
Visipitch digital tape r.
VitaGuard event r.
recording
  r. electrode
  pulse volume r.
  2120 R. Spirometer
Recovery
  R. filter
  R. nitinol filter
  R. protrusio cage
  R. vena cava filter
rectal
  r. balloon
  r. barostat
  r. catheter
  r. cautery snare
  r. cautery wire
  r. clamp
  r. curette
  r. dilator
  r. expander
  r. finger cot
  r. forceps
  r. hook
  r. hook retractor
  r. injection cannula
  r. injection needle
  r. multiplane transducer
  r. probe
  r. snare insulated stem

R

rectal *(continued)*
    r. snare stem brush
    r. speculum
    r. tip
    r. trocar
    r. tube
rectangle
    Hartshill r.
    Luque r.
rectangular
    r. awl
    r. blade
    r. brain spatula
    r. wire
rectifier
    full-wave r.
    r. tube
Rectigraph-8K recorder
rectilinear
    r. biphasic waveform
    r. recorder
    r. scanner
rectoscope
    Storz continuous-flow r.
rectosigmoidoscope
recumbent
    r. bicycle
    r. cycle
    r. infant board
recurrent bandage
red
    R. Cross adhesive dressing
    R. Cross freeze-dried allograft
    r. laser
    r. lens occluder
    r. litmus paper
    R. Reflex Lens Systems lens
    r. Robinson catheter
    r. rubber catheter
    r. rubber endotracheal tube
    r. rubber Robinson catheter
    R. system
red-beam
    r.-b. laser
    r.-b. laser pen
Reddick cystic duct cholangiogram catheter
Reddick-Saye
    R.-S. macro knot pusher
    R.-S. screw
Reddick/Saye Lav-1 irrigating and aspirating probe
Redfield IRC 2100 infrared coagulator
red-free filter
Redha-cut catheter
Redi-Around finger splint
Rediform orthotic

Redigrip
    R. knee pad
    R. pressure bandage
Rediguard IAB catheter
RED II system
Redi-kit
    LEEP R.-k.
Redi-Trac traction device
Redi-Vac cast cutter
Redi-Vacette wound drainage system
Redivac suction drain
Redi-Vu teleradiology system
Redi+Wash cleansing system
Redon drain
Redquant kit
red-tip aspirator
reduced
    r. profile (RP)
    r. Snellen card
reduced-height implant
reducer
    Cloward cervical dislocation r.
    McCannel ocular pressure r.
    Norelco allergen r.
    ocular pressure r.
reducing
    r. fracture frame
    r. stent
reduction
    Aston cartilage r.
    r. instrument
    Lange hip r.
    Palomar E2000 ruby laser hair r.
    r. ring
Redy
    R. hemodialysis system
    R. 2000 hemodialysis system
    R. sorbent dialysis system
Reebok
    R. Slide system
    R. Step system
Reece
    R. orthopaedic shoe
    R. osteotomy guide
Reed cast belt
reedswitch
Reeh scissors
reel
    r. aspiration cannula
    suture tension adjustment r.
reelin immunoreactive band
reentrant well chamber
Rees
    R. facelift serrated scissors
    R. lighted retractor
Reese
    R. dermatome
    R. muscle forceps

R. ptosis knife
R. stimulator
Reeves stretcher
reference
r. catheter
r. coordinate system
r. electrode
Refinity Coblation system
Ref-Keratometer
Canon R-5+ Auto R.-K.
reflectance
r. meter
r. photometer
r. spectrophotometer
r. spectrophotometric probe
r. TS-200 spectrum analyzer
reflecting retinoscope
Reflection
R. ceramic acetabular system
R. Interfit prosthesis
R. I prosthesis
R. I, V, FSO acetabular cup
R. liner
R. V prosthesis
reflectometer tuning unit
Reflec UV instant camera
reflex
R. Comfort insole
R. exercise and rehabilitation equipment
r. exercise and rehabilitation equipment
r. gun
r. hammer
r. pacemaker
R. 8220 pacemaker
R. skin stapler
R. steerable guidewire
Re/Flex filter
ReFlexion first MPJ implant system
Reflexion steerable catheter
reflexology sock
ReFlex Ultra 45, 55 channeling wand
Re-Flex VSP prosthesis
reform eye implant
Refractec ViewPoint CK System
refractionometer
refractive
r. floating implant
r. lens
r. phakic implant
refractometer, refractionometer
Abbe r.
Hoya HDR objective r.
Hoya MRM objective r.
meridional r.
Speedy-1 Auto r.
8000 Supra Series auto r.

Topcon RM-A2300 auto r.
Zeiss vertex r.
refractor
Agrikola r.
AR 1000 r.
ARK-Juno r.
automated r.
Berens r.
Canon r.
Castroviejo r.
Coburn r.
CooperVision diagnostic imaging r.
Desmarres r.
Elschnig r.
Goldstein r.
Graether r.
Green r.
Humphrey automatic r.
Kirby r.
Knapp r.
Kronfeld r.
KR 7000-P cycloplegic r.
Kuglen r.
Leland r.
Marco r.
Marco ARK-2000 r.
McGannon r.
Nidek AR-2000 objective automatic r.
Precision r.
Reichert r.
Remote Vision electronic r.
SR-IV programmed subjective r.
Stevenson r.
Topcon r.
Refrax corneal repair kit
Ref-Star EP catheter
Regain home EMG trainer
Regal Acrylic/Stretch prosthetic sock
Regan-Lancaster dial
Regan low-contrast acuity chart
Regenafil
R. allograft paste
R. injectable bone paste
Regenaform moldable bone paste
Regency SR, SR+ pulse generator
regeneration
guided tissue r. (GTR)
Regentex GBR-200 membrane
Regent mechanical heart valve
Regisil polyvinyl registration material
regulator
aluminum oxygen r.
Boehringer suction r.
Easy Dial Reg oxygen r.
high-flow r.
low-flow r.
Medela membrane r.
Ohmeda continuous vacuum r.

regulator *(continued)*
    Ohmeda thoracic suction r.
    OptiMed glaucoma pressure r.
    suction Regugauge r.
    Vacutron suction r.
Regulus frameless stereotactic system
rehabilitator
    Ankle Isolator ankle r.
Rehab TROM brace
Rehfuss
    R. duodenal tube
    R. stomach tube
Reichert
    R. binocular indirect
      ophthalmoscope
    R. camera
    R. fiberoptic sigmoidoscope
    R. flexible sigmoidoscope
    R. Ful-Vue binocular
      ophthalmoscope
    R. Ful-Vue spot retinoscope
    R. lensometer
    R. noncontact tonometer
    R. ophthalmodynamometer
    R. radius gauge
    R. refractor
    R. slit-lamp
    R. stereotaxy system
    R. Ultramatic Rx Master Phoroptor
      refracting instrument
    R. Zetopan microscope
Reichert-Jung Ultracut ultramicrotome
Reichert-Mundinger
    R.-M. apparatus
    R.-M. stereotactic device
    R.-M. stereotactic head frame
Reichert-Mundinger-Fischer stereotactic
  frame
Reichling corneal scissors
Reich-Nechtow
    R.-N. clamp
    R.-N. hysterectomy forceps
Reid sleeve
reimplanted electrode
Reiner
    R. bone rongeur
    R. plaster knife
Reiner-Beck snare
Reiner-Knight forceps
reinforced tracheostomy tube
reinforcement
    Gore-Tex sling r.
    r. ring
    Wilson-Cook metal r.
Reisinger lens-extracting forceps
Reitan catheter pump
ReJuveness
    R. pure silicone sheeting
    R. scar silicone sheet

Rekow system
[188]Re-labeled self-expanding nitinol stent
relative shunt
relator
    orthognathic occlusal r.
Relax-a-Cizor
relaxer
    Real-EaSE neck and shoulder r.
RelaxMate
    Shealy R.
Re-Lax-O chiropractic table
relaxometer
    Bruker r.
    Bruker PC-10 r.
    Bruker TC-10 r.
    IBM field-cycling research r.
Relay suture delivery system
releasable compression suture
Release
    R. catheter
    R. non-adhering dressing
reliable wave front sensor
Relia-Flow device
Reliance
    R. CM femoral implant component
    R. urinary control insert
    R. urinary control insert catheter
ReliefBand electrostimulating device
reline material
reliner
    Coe-Rect denture r.
    Coe-Soft denture r.
    Hydro-Cast r.
ReliOn
    R. glucose meter
    R. test strip
Reliquet lithotrite
Relton frame pad
ReLume system
Remac system
Remak band
Remedy sleep therapy system
remote
    r. access perfusion cannula
    r. afterloading system
    r. control afterloading machine
Remote Vision electronic refractor
removable
    r. expansion prosthesis
    r. keratophakia lens
    r. partial denture
    r. partial overdenture
removal
    LightSheer diode laser system for
      permanent hair r.
    r. mesh silo
Removatron epilator
remover
    adhesive tape r.

Atwood bridge r.
Atwood crown r.
Bard adhesive and barrier film r.
Biomet Ultra-Drive cement r.
clip r.
Crown-A-Matic crown and
bridge r.
Detachol adhesive r.
foreign body r.
Macaluso stent r.
Mead bridge r.
Mead crown r.
medical adhesive r.
modular head r.
Morrell crown r.
Richwil bridge r.
Richwil crown r.
Tott ring r.
Universal clip r.
Wölfe-Böhler cast r.
**REM PolyHesive II patient return
electrode**
REMstar
R. Auto
R. Auto with heated humidification
R. CPAP system
R. Plus
R. Plus with C-Flex
R. Plus with C-Flex and heated
humidification
R. Pro with C-Flex
R. Pro with C-Flex and heated
humidification
Remy separator
Renaflo hollow-fiber dialyzer
Renaissance
R. crown system
R. erbium laser
R. spirometry system
renal
r. artery clamp
r. artery forceps
r. kallikrein-kinin system
r. needle
r. pedicle clamp
r. sinus retractor
r. sympathetic nerve activity
recording electrode
R. System HF250 filter
Renalin dialyzer
Renalyzer
Renata battery
Renatron
R. dialyzer
R. II dialyzer reprocessing system
Rendell-Baker
R.-B. face mask
R.-B. Soucek mask

Renegade
R. Hi-Flo microcatheter
R. microcatheter
**Renessa stress urinary incontinence
system**
Renew spinal cord stimulation system
renin-angiotensin system
Renolux convertible car seat
renovascular stent
Renovist II injector
Rentrop catheter
Rentsch boat hook
Rep Band exercise band
repeater
Repel bioresorbable barrier film
**Repel-CV bioresorbable adhesion-barrier
film**
reperfusion catheter
Repiphysis prosthesis
Replace
R. implant system
R. system tapered implant
replaceable blade
replacement
r. collection bag
patellofemoral r. (PFR)
Vanguard Uni unicompartmental
knee r.
replant splint
RepliCare
R. hydrocolloid
R. hydrocolloid dressing
R. hydrocolloid dressing material
R. Thin hydrocolloid dressing
R. wound dressing
replicator
Steers r.
Replica total hip replacement system
Repliderm
Repliform alternative product
Replogle
R. suction catheter
R. sump tube
Re-Ply TENS electrode
reporter
Rosetta-Lt 12-lead r.
Repose
R. screw inserter
R. system
repositioner
mandibular r.
Wilson-Cook prosthesis r.
repositor
iris r.
Knapp iris r.
Nettleship iris r.
Sloane flap r.
reprocessor
AER+ automatic endoscope r.

R

reprocessor *(continued)*
American Endoscopy automatic r.
automated endoscope r.
automatic endoscopic r.
Bard automatic r.
Custom Ultrasonic automatic r.
ECI automatic r.
KeyMed automatic r.
Lutz automatic r.
Medivator automatic r.
Olympus automatic r.
Orr automatic r.
Steris automatic r.
Repro head halter
ResCue Key
rescue screw
rescuing pacemaker
**Research Pneumotach System
  instrumentation module**
resection
r. clamp
r. intestinal forceps
Kotz modular femur and tibia r.
resector
Accu-Line distal femoral r.
Accu-Line femoral r.
Accu-Line tibial r.
Dyonics full-radius r.
femoral r.
full-radius r.
Gator r.
Stryker r.
tibial r.
resectoscope
ACMI r.
r. adapter
continuous-flow Wolfe r.
Elite System rotating r.
foroblique r.
foroblique microlens r.
Iglesias continuous flow r.
Iglesias fiberoptic r.
Iglesias microlens r.
Kaplan r.
McCarthy continuous flow r.
McCarthy microlens r.
McCarthy miniature r.
McCarthy multiple r.
Nesbit r.
OES 4000 r.
Olympus continuous flow r.
Opera Star r.
r. sheath
specialized tissue aspirating r.
Stern-McCarthy electrotome r.
Storz r.
Storz laser r.
Timberlake obturator r.

USA Elite System GYN rotating
  continuous flow r.
Wappler r.
reservoir
Biocor softshell venous r.
Braden flushing r.
Camey r.
cardiotomy r.
contiguous spinal fluid r.
CSF r.
double-bubble flushing r.
double-dome r.
flat bottom r.
flushing r.
Foltz flushing r.
Hoffmann-Steinberg gastric r.
Holter ventriculostomy r.
Hunt-Limo-Basto gastric r.
ICV r.
Intersept cardiotomy r.
inverted U-pouch ileal r.
Jackson-Pratt large-volume
  suction r.
Jostra cardiotomy r.
J-Vac bulb suction r.
Kock ileal r.
large-volume suction r.
Lawrence gastric r.
Mainz pouch urinary r.
Molded Bulb closed wound
  drainage r.
Ommaya r.
Ommaya CSF r.
Ommaya retromastoid r.
Ommaya spinal fluid r.
Ommaya suboccipital r.
Ommaya ventricular r.
Polystan cardiotomy r.
Pudenz r.
Resipump pump r.
retromastoid Ommaya r.
Rickham r.
Sci-Med extracorporeal silicone
  rubber r.
side-port flat-bottomed Ommaya r.
suboccipital Ommaya r.
Uni-Shunt with elliptical r.
William Harvey cardiotomy r.
wound drainage r.
W-stapled urinary r.
resin
Aneuroplastic r.
Bondeze r.
Bowen r.
Celay Tech light-curing r.
r. cement
Chelex r.
Concise r.
diacrylate r.

Directon r.
Dynabond r.
Effapoxy r.
Endur r.
Genie r.
InstaGene Matrix r.
Lee orthodontic r.
light-curing r.
Myerson r.
Nuvaseal r.
Nuva-Tach r.
orthodontic r.
Orthomite r.
Solo-Tach r.
r. sphere
Spurr r.
Technovit acrylic r.
ultraviolet light-polymerized r.
unfilled r.
Visioform light-curing r.
Zapit r.
Resipump pump reservoir
Resist-A-Band exercise band
resistance wire heater
Resist-A-Tube exercise band
resistive
r. chair exercise kit
r. exerciser
r. exercise table
ResMed CPAP Sullivan III machine
resolution element
Resolution ultrasonic catheter
Resolve QuickAnchor
resonance
r. generator
magnetic r. (MR)
resonator
birdcage r.
bridged loop-gap r.
crossed loop r.
detunable elliptic transmission
   line r.
Faraday shielded r.
flexible surface coil-type r.
Jacobson r.
multicoupled loop-gap r.
Oudin r.
resorbable
R. Collagen Membrane[6]
r. copolymer PGA/PLLA-Lactosorb
   miniplate fixation system
r. graft containment system
r. plate
r. plate and screw
r. PLLA miniplate
r. polydioxanon pin
r. poly-L-lactide plate
r. polymer pin
r. polymer screw

r. scaffold
r. thread clip applicator
ReSound
R. CC4 hearing aid
R. Digital 2000 hearing aid
R. Digital 5000 hearing device
RESPeRATE interactive breathing
   device
Resp-EZ piezoelectric sensor
Respiradyne pulmonary function device
respiration bronchoscope
respiratometer
Collins r.
respirator (*See also* ventilator)
Ambu r.
BABYbird r.
BABYbird II r.
Babylog 8000 r.
Bath r.
Bear r.
Bennett r.
Bird Mark 8 r.
Bourns electronic adult r.
Bourns infant r.
Bragg-Paul r.
Breeze r.
Clevedon positive pressure r.
cuirass r.
Drinker tank r.
Emerson r.
Emerson cuirass r.
Engstrom r.
Gill r.
HEPA r.
Huxley r.
MA-1 r.
mechanical r.
mechanically assisted r.
Med-Neb r.
Merck r.
3M Healthcare particulate r.
Monaghan r.
Morch r.
Moynihan r.
particulate r.
portable r.
Sanders jet r.
Stephan HF 300 r.
volumetric diffusive r.
respirator/ventilator
respiratory
r. chamber
r. function monitor
respiratory-dependent pacemaker
Respirex incentive spirometer
Respirgard
R. II
R. II nebulizer
Respirgard II

R

respirometer
    Dräger r.
    Fraser Harlake r.
    Haloscale r.
    hot-wire r.
    Wright r.

Respironics
    R. BIPAP bilevel ventilator
    R. BiPAP machine
    R. CPAP machine
    R. Oasis humidifier
    R. 920P handheld pulse oximeter
    R. 930 pulse oximeter

Respitrace
    R. machine
    R. recorder

Respond
    R. ROM elbow orthosis
    R. ROM knee orthosis
    R. wire

Responder emergency vehicle car seat
Response
    R. electrophysiology catheter
    R. rehabilitation and fitness
      equipment

Res-Q
    R.-Q ACD implantable cardioverter-
      defibrillator
    R.-Q arrhythmia control device
    R.-Q Micron ICD
    R.-Q Micron implantable
      cardioverter-defibrillator

ResQPOD circulatory enhancer
Res-Q-Vac
    R.-Q-V. emergency suction system
    R.-Q-V. handheld emergency
      suction

rest
    Adson head r.
    cervical r.
    Chan wrist r.
    Chiroflow back r.
    Core Hibak R.
    Core Lobak R.
    Core Sitback R.
    face r.
    foot r.
    knee r.
    Krause arm r.
    Mayfield head r.
    Mouse Nest mouse r.
    neck r.

Restcue
    R. bed
    R. CC dynamic air therapy unit

resting
    r. foot sling
    r. orthosis

    r. pan splint
    r. splint

Reston
    R. dressing
    R. foam dressing
    R. foam wound dressing
    R. padding
    R. polyurethane foam
    R. sponge

Restoration
    R. acetabular system
    R. GAP acetabular cup
    R. Secur-Fit X'tra acetabular shell

Restoration-HA hip system
restorative pin
Restore
    R. ACL guide system
    R. alginate dressing
    R. alginate wound cover
    R. alginate wound dressing
    R. bone implant
    R. CalciCare dressing
    R. close tolerance dental implant
      system
    R. cuff tear implant
    R. Cx wound care dressing
    R. dental implant
    R. extra-thin dressing
    R. hydrocolloid
    R. hydrocolloid dressing
    R. hydrogel dressing
    R. impregnated gauze
    R. neurostimulation system
    R. orthobiologic soft-tissue implant
    R. Plus wound care dressing
    R. RBM implant
    R. soft tissue implant
    R. threaded implant
    R. wound cleanser

ReSTOR vision implant
restrainer
    Gulani globe stabilizer and flap r.
restraint
    r. calipers
    Circumstraint r.
    foam-padded Velcro r.
    papoose board r.
    4-point r.
    poncho r.
    Posey r.
    universal canvas body r.
    vacuum-operated viscous r.

restrictor
    Biostop G cement r.
    cement r.
    femoral canal r.

Resume electrode

resurfacing
Skinlight erbium:YAG laser system for skin r.
Resuscitaire birthing room warmer
resuscitation cart
resuscitator
active compression-decompression r.
Ambu infant r.
Ambu Spur disposable r.
BagEasy disposable manual r.
bag-valve r.
BVM r.
CAREvent ALS handheld r.
CAREvent BLS handheld r.
First Response manual r.
Fisher and Paykel RD1000 r.
Fisher-Paykel RD1000 r.
heart-lung r.
Hope r.
Hudson Lifesaver r.
INdGO disposable manual r.
infant Ambu r.
Laerdal r.
Laerdal infant r.
manual r.
NeoVO$_2$R volume-control r.
Penlon infant r.
Pneupac r.
pneuPAC r.
Pulmanex r.
retainer
continuous bar r.
direct r.
extracoronal r.
eyeglass r.
Hawley r.
indirect r.
r. insert
intracoronal r.
matrix r.
Mectra tissue sample r.
space r.
Thermoskin heat r.
Tofflemire r.
tongue r.
viscera r.
retaining
r. device
r. retractor
RetCam 120 fiberoptic fundus camera
retention
r. bar
r. catheter
r. suture bolster
r. suture bridge
reticle
handheld magnifying r.
reticONE system
reticule

retina
artificial silicone r.
retinaculotome
Paine carpal tunnel r.
retinal
r. acuity meter
r. camera
r. detachment hook
r. detachment pencil
r. detachment syringe
r. ellipsometer
r. fundus camera
r. probe sleeve
r. prosthesis
RetinaLyze system
Retinomax
R. autorefractor
R. 2 autorefractor
R. cordless handheld autorefractor
R. K-Plus autorefractor/keratometer
R. refractometry instrument
retinometer
Heine Lambda 100 r.
Retinopan 45 camera
retinoscope
Copeland streak r.
electric r.
Ful-Vue spot r.
Ful-Vue streak r.
Keeler r.
luminous r.
Priestley-Smith r.
Propper r.
reflecting r.
Reichert Ful-Vue spot r.
spot r.
streak r.
Welch Allyn standard r.
Welch Allyn streak r.
Retisert intravitreal implant
retractable
r. blade
r. stylet
retracting rod
retraction
r. ring
Schink metatarsal r.
retractor
Abadie self-retaining r.
abdominal ring r.
abdominal vascular r.
Ablaza-Blanco aortic wall r.
acetabular r.
Adson r.
Adson-Beckman self-retaining r.
Adson cerebellar r.
Adson hemilaminectomy r.
Agrikola lacrimal sac r.
Airlift balloon r.

retractor *(continued)*
    alar r.
    Alexander-Ballen r.
    Allen r.
    Allison lung r.
    Allport r.
    Alm wound r.
    amputation r.
    anal r.
    Anderson-Adson self-retaining r.
    Andrews r.
    angled decompression r.
    angled iris r.
    angled vein r.
    aortic valve r.
    APC hip r.
    appendectomy r.
    appendiceal r.
    arm r.
    Army-Navy r.
    Arruga elevator r.
    Arruga orbital r.
    Assistant Free long prong collateral
      ligament r.
    Assistant Free Shubbs short prong
      collateral ligament r.
    Assistant Free wide PCL r.
    Aston nasal r.
    Aston submental r.
    atrial septal r.
    Aufranc cobra r.
    Aufricht fiberoptic light r.
    Aufricht nasal r.
    automatic skin r.
    baby Balfour r.
    baby Weitlaner self-retaining r.
    Badgley laminectomy r.
    Balfour pediatric abdominal r.
    Balfour self-retaining r.
    Ballen-Alexander orbital r.
    ball-type r.
    Bankart r.
    Bankart rectal r.
    Barbie r.
    Bauer r.
    Beaver r.
    beavertail r.
    Bechert-Kratz cannulated nucleus r.
    Beckman-Adson laminectomy r.
    Beckman-Eaton laminectomy r.
    Beckman-Weitlaner laminectomy r.
    Bennett bone r.
    Bennett tibial r.
    bent Hohman r.
    bent malleable r.
    Berens lid r.
    Berens mastectomy skin flap r.
    Bergen r.
    Berkeley-Bonney r.

    Bernstein nasal r.
    Bertin hip r.
    bifurcated r.
    biliary r.
    Bishop r.
    bivalved r.
    bladder r.
    r. blade
    Blair r.
    Blair 4-prong r.
    Blount knee r.
    blunt rake r.
    Bodnar r.
    bone r.
    Bookwalter r.
    Bookwalter-Goulet r.
    Bookwalter-Hill-Ferguson rectal r.
    Bookwalter ring r.
    Bookwalter-St. Mark deep pelvic r.
    bowel r.
    brain r.
    Breisky-Navratil straight r.
    Breisky vaginal r.
    Brewster phrenic r.
    Brinker tissue r.
    Brompton Hospital r.
    Brophy tenaculum r.
    Brown uvula r.
    buccal r.
    Buchwalter r.
    Budde halo neurosurgical r.
    Budde halo ring r.
    Burford-Finochietto rib r.
    Busenkell posterior hip r.
    Byrd EndoPlastic r.
    Cairns scalp r.
    Campbell nerve root r.
    capsule r.
    cardiovascular r.
    Carroll-Bennett finger r.
    Carroll hand r.
    Caspar r.
    Caspar cervical r.
    Castroviejo lid r.
    Cat's Paw r.
    cerebellar r.
    cerebral r.
    cervical disc r.
    Cer-View lateral vaginal r.
    Chandler knee r.
    channel r.
    Charnley horizontal r.
    Charnley initial incision r.
    Charnley knee r.
    Charnley self-retaining r.
    cheek r.
    claw r.
    Clayman lid r.
    r. clip

Cloward blade r.
Cloward brain r.
Cloward cervical r.
Cloward dural r.
Cloward nerve root r.
Cloward self-retaining r.
Cloward tissue r.
cobra-head r.
Cohen r.
Cole duodenal r.
Coleman r.
collapsible tissue r.
collar-button iris r.
Collin abdominal r.
Collin-Hartmann r.
Collis-Taylor r.
condylar neck r.
contour scalp r.
Converse blade r.
Converse double-ended r.
Converse double-ended alar r.
Converse nasal r.
Conway lid r.
Cook rectal r.
Cooley atrial r.
Cooley atrial valve r.
Cooley-Merz sternum r.
Cooley rib r.
corner r.
corrugated forehead r.
Coryllos r.
Cosgrove r.
Cosgrove mitral valve r.
Cottle alar r.
Cottle-Joseph r.
Cottle knife guide and r.
Cottle nasal r.
Cottle-Neivert r.
Cottle 4-prong r.
Cottle sharp-prong r.
Cottle soft palate r.
Cottle thumb hook r.
Cottle upper lateral r.
cranial r.
crank frame r.
Crawford aortic r.
Crego r.
Crile angle r.
Crile malleable r.
Crile right-angle r.
Crockard hard palate r.
Crowe-Davis mouth r.
Cushing angled decompression r.
Cushing bivalve r.
Cushing-Kocher r.
Cushing nerve r.
Cushing straight r.
Cushing subtemporal r.
Cushing vein r.

Danek self-retaining r.
Darrach r.
David-Baker eyelid r.
Davidson scapular r.
Davis double-ended r.
Davis pillar r.
Davis self-retaining scalp r.
Deaver r.
Deaver pediatric r.
DeBakey-Balfour r.
DeBakey chest r.
DeBakey-Cooley r.
decompressive r.
deep r.
deep blunt rake r.
Delaney phrenic r.
de la Plaza transconjunctival r.
DeLee corner r.
DeLee Universal r.
Denis Browne pediatric r.
dental r.
D'Errico r.
D'Errico-Adson r.
Desmarres r.
Desmarres eyelid r.
Desmarres lid r.
Devine-Millard-Aufricht r.
digital self-retaining r.
Di-Main r.
Dingman-Senn r.
Dingman zygoma hook r.
disposable iris r.
Doane knee r.
dog chain r.
Dohn-Carton brain r.
double bent Hohmann acetabular r.
double cobra r.
double crank r.
double-ended breast r.
double fishhook r.
Doyen child abdominal r.
Doyen vaginal r.
Dozier radiolucent Bennett r.
Drews-Rosenbaum iris r.
dual nerve root suction r.
dull r.
dull-pronged r.
dural suction r.
Eastman vaginal r.
East-West soft tissue r.
Eccentric Y adjustable finger r.
Elias lid r.
Eliasoph lid r.
Elite Farley r.
Elschnig r.
Emory EndoPlastic r.
endaural r.
EndoPlastic r.
Endo Retract r.

R

retractor *(continued)*
- endoscopic r.
- Endotrac r.
- epicardial r.
- epiglottis r.
- erector spinae r.
- ESI light-weight narrow mammaplasty r.
- ESI long narrow mammaplasty r.
- ESI mammary r.
- esophageal r.
- examination r.
- external r.
- extra-depth posterior acetabular r.
- extra-large hip r.
- extraoral sigmoid notch r.
- eyelid r.
- facelift r.
- fan elevator r.
- fan-type laparoscopic r.
- Farabeuf double-ended r.
- Farley Elite spinal r.
- Farr self-retaining r.
- Farr spring r.
- Farr wire r.
- Fasanella double-ended iris r.
- fat pad r.
- femoral neck r.
- Ferguson anal r.
- Ferguson-Moon rectal r.
- Ferris-Smith r.
- Ferris-Smith orbital r.
- Ferris-Smith-Sewall orbital r.
- fiberoptic smoke evaluating r.
- finger rake r.
- Finochietto r.
- Finochietto-Geissendorfer rib r.
- Finochietto hand r.
- Finochietto infant rib r.
- Finsen r.
- Fisch dural r.
- Fisher double-ended r.
- Fisher fenestrated lid r.
- Fisher lid r.
- Fisher-Nugent r.
- Fisher tonsillar r.
- fixed ring r.
- flexible translimbal iris r.
- FlexPosure endoscopic r.
- Fomon hook r.
- Fomon nasal r.
- Fomon nostril r.
- force fulcrum r.
- Ford-Deaver r.
- Forder r.
- Forker r.
- Franklin malleable r.
- Franz abdominal r.
- Frazier-Fay r.
- Frazier laminectomy r.
- Freer skin r.
- Freer submucous r.
- French-Stern-McCarthy r.
- Friedman vaginal r.
- Fritsch r.
- Fritsch abdominal r.
- Fukuda humeral head r.
- Fukushima r.
- Fulton r.
- gallbladder r.
- gallows-type r.
- Garrett peripheral vascular r.
- gastric resection r.
- Gauthier r.
- Gazayerli endoscopic r.
- Gazayerli-Mediflex r.
- Gelpi r.
- Gelpi abdominal r.
- Gelpi perineal r.
- Gelpi self-retaining r.
- Gelpi vaginal r.
- general r.
- Gerow-Harrington heart-shaped distal end r.
- Gibson-Balfour abdominal r.
- Gifford r.
- Gifford-Jansen mastoid r.
- Gifford mastoid r.
- Gillies single-hook skin r.
- Gil-Vernet renal sinus r.
- Glaser laminectomy r.
- Goelet double-ended r.
- goiter r.
- Goldstein r.
- Goldstein lacrimal sac r.
- Goligher r.
- Goligher modification of Berkeley-Bonney r.
- Goligher sternal-lifting r.
- Gomez gastric r.
- Gooch r.
- Good r.
- Gosset abdominal r.
- Gosset appendectomy r.
- Gosset self-retaining r.
- Gott malleable r.
- Gradle eyelid r.
- Graether r.
- Gray surgical r.
- great big Barbie r.
- Greenberg-Sugita r.
- Greenberg Universal r.
- Green thyroid r.
- Greenwald r.
- Greishaber self-retaining r.
- Grieshaber-Balfour r.
- Grieshaber flexible iris r.
- Grieshaber self-retaining r.

Gross-Pomeranz-Watkins r.
Guardian vaginal r.
Guthrie r.
Guttmann obstetrical r.
Guttmann vaginal r.
Haight baby r.
Hajek antral r.
Hajek lip r.
halo r.
hand r.
handheld r.
r. handle Cloward dural hook
Haney r.
hard palate r.
Hardy-Cushing r.
Hardy lip r.
Harken rib r.
Harrington r.
Harrington Deaver r.
Harrington splanchnic r.
Harrison chalazion r.
Haslinger r.
Haslinger palate r.
Hasson r.
Hays finger r.
Hays hand r.
Heaney r.
Heaney hysterectomy r.
Heaney-Simon r.
Heaney-Simon hysterectomy r.
Heaney-Simon vaginal r.
Heaney vaginal r.
Heiss r.
Heiss soft tissue r.
Helveston Great Big Barbie r.
hemilaminectomy r.
Hendren self-retaining r.
Henley carotid r.
Henning meniscal r.
hernia r.
Heyer-Schulte brain r.
Hibbs r.
Hibbs self-retaining laminectomy r.
hilar r.
Hill rectal r.
Hirschman r.
Hohmann bone r.
Holman lung r.
Holzheimer skin r.
r. hook
hook r.
Horgan r.
horizontal flexible bar r.
House handheld double-end r.
House-Urban middle fossa r.
Howorth toothed r.
Huang Universal arm r.
Hubbard r.
Hudson bone r.

humeral r.
Hurd pillar r.
hysterectomy r.
illuminated St. Mark r.
IMA r.
incision r.
infant abdominal r.
infant eyelid r.
infant rib r.
inferior mesenteric artery r.
inferoposterior acetabular capsule r.
Inge laminectomy r.
initial incision r.
intestinal occlusion r.
intracardiac r.
intradural r.
iris r.
IrisMate flexible translimbal iris r.
Iron Intern r.
irrigating mushroom r.
Israel r.
Israel blunt rake r.
Jackson tracheal r.
Jackson vaginal r.
Jacobson bladder r.
Jaeger r.
Jaeger lid r.
Jaffe wire lid r.
Jannetta r.
Jansen mastoid r.
Jansen-Wagner mastoid r.
Joe's hoe r.
Johns Hopkins gallbladder r.
Johnson cheek r.
Johnson hook r.
Johnson ventriculogram r.
Jones IMA epicardial r.
Jorgenson r.
Joseph skin hook r.
Joseph wound r.
Judd-Allis intestinal r.
Kapp Surgical Instrument total
    knee r.
Karmody vascular spring r.
Kartush insulated r.
Kasdan r.
Kaufman type II r.
Keizer-Lancaster lid r.
Kelly abdominal r.
Kelman iris r.
Kennerdell medial orbital r.
Kerrison r.
kidney r.
Kilner nasal r.
Kilner skin hook r.
King-Hurd r.
King self-retaining goiter r.
Kirby lid r.
Kirchner r.

R

retractor *(continued)*
Kirkland r.
Kirklin atrial r.
Kirschenbaum r.
Kirschner abdominal r.
Kleinert-Kutz hook r.
Kleinert-Ragnell r.
Kleinsasser r.
Knapp lacrimal sac r.
knee r.
Kobayashi r.
Kocher r.
Kocher bladder r.
Kocher blade r.
Kocher bone r.
Kocher gallbladder r.
Kocher-Langenbeck r.
Kocher self-retaining goiter r.
Koenig vein r.
Koerte r.
Kristeller vaginal r.
Kronfeld eyelid r.
Krönlein-Berke r.
Kuda r.
Kuglen r.
Kuglen lens r.
lacrimal sac r.
Lahey Clinic nerve root r.
Lahey goiter r.
Lahey thyroid r.
laminectomy self-retaining r.
Landau vaginal r.
Lane r.
Lange bone r.
Lange-Hohmann bone r.
Langenbeck r.
Langenbeck periosteal r.
Laplace liver r.
large Cobra r.
laryngeal r.
lateral wall r.
Lavoisier r.
Leatherman trochanteric r.
Lee double-ended r.
Lempert r.
Lempert-Colver r.
LeVasseur-Merrill r.
Levy articulating r.
Levy perineal r.
Lewis r.
Leyla self-retaining brain r.
lid r.
lighted r.
LightWare micro r.
Lilienthal-Sauerbruch r.
Lillie r.
Linton splanchnic r.
lip r.
Little r.

liver r.
Lockhart-Mummery r.
Logan lacrimal sac self-retaining r.
London narrow-bladed r.
Lone Star r.
long atraumatic r.
loop r.
Lothrop tonsillar r.
Lothrop uvular r.
Love r.
Love nasopharyngeal r.
Love nerve root r.
Love uvula r.
Lowman hand r.
Lowsley r.
Lowsley prostate r.
Luer r.
Luer double-ended tracheal r.
Luer S-shaped r.
Lukens double-ended tracheal r.
Lukens epiglottic r.
Lukens thymus r.
lumbar r.
lung r.
Luongo hand r.
Luther-Peter r.
MacAusland muscle r.
Mackool capsule r.
Magrina-Bookwalter vaginal r.
Malis cerebellar r.
Malis cerebral r.
malleable r.
malleable blade r.
malleable copper r.
malleable ribbon r.
malleable stainless steel r.
Maltz r.
mandibular body r.
Mannerfelt r.
Manning r.
manual r.
Mark II Chandler total knee r.
Mark II concave total knee r.
Mark II lateral collateral
  ligament r.
Mark II modular weight r.
Mark II PCL r.
Mark II S total knee r.
Mark II Stubbs short-prong
  collateral ligament r.
Mark II wide PCL knee r.
Mark II Z knee r.
Markley r.
Martin r.
Martin abdominal r.
Martin cheek r.
Martin lip r.
Martin nerve root r.
Martin palate r.

Martin rectal hook r.
Martin vaginal r.
Mason-Judd bladder r.
Mason-Judd self-retaining r.
mastoid self-retaining r.
Mathieu double-ended r.
Matson-Mead apicolysis r.
Mayfield r.
Mayo abdominal r.
Mayo-Adams appendectomy r.
Mayo-Adams self-retaining r.
Mayo-Collins appendectomy r.
Mayo-Collins double-ended r.
Mayo-Collins mastoid r.
Mayo-Lovelace abdominal r.
McBurney r.
McBurney fenestrated r.
McBurney thyroid r.
McCabe antral r.
McCabe parotidectomy r.
McCabe posterior fossa r.
McCullough r.
McGannon r.
McGannon iris r.
McGill r.
McIndoe r.
meat hook r.
Medicon rib r.
Meigs r.
Meller lacrimal sac r.
meniscal r.
meniscus r.
metacarpal double-ended r.
metal bar r.
metal tongue r.
METRx Quadrant r.
METRx X-Tube r.
Meyerding r.
Meyerding finger r.
Meyerding self-retaining
  laminectomy r.
Meyerding skin hook and r.
microlumbar discectomy r.
microsurgical r.
middle fossa r.
Mikulicz abdominal r.
Miller r.
Miller-Senn double-ended r.
Millin bladder r.
Miltex r.
mini-Hohmann r.
minimal incision total hip r.
Minnesota r.
mitral valve r.
modified Fukuda-type r.
Mollison self-retaining r.
Moon rectal r.
Moorehead cheek r.
Morris r.

Morrison-Hurd pillar r.
Morse sternal r.
Morse valve r.
Mueller lacrimal sac r.
Muldoon r.
multiprong rake r.
multipurpose r.
Murphy rake r.
Myolift heart r.
narrow Cobra r.
narrow Deaver r.
narrow double-prong acetabular r.
narrow inferior acetabular r.
nasal r.
nasopharyngeal r.
Nathanson liver r.
Nelson rib r.
neonatal sternal r.
nerve root r.
Nevyas drape r.
newborn eyelid r.
Newell lid r.
notched ramus r.
Nuttall liver r.
obstetrical r.
Obwegeser r.
Obwegeser channel r.
O'Connor abdominal r.
O'Connor-O'Sullivan abdominal r.
O'Connor vaginal r.
Octopus r.
Oklahoma iris wire r.
Oliver r.
Ollier rake r.
Omni r.
Omni-Tract vaginal r.
Op-Trac r.
orbicular r.
orbital r.
O'Sullivan-O'Connor self-retaining
  abdominal r.
O'Sullivan-O'Connor vaginal r.
r. oval sprocket frame
palate r.
Parker r.
Parks anal r.
parotidectomy r.
patent ductus r.
Paul lacrimal sac r.
Paulson knee r.
Payne r.
pediatric abdominal r.
pediatric self-retaining r.
Pemberton r.
Pemco r.
Penfield r.
Percy amputation r.
Percy bone r.
periareolar r.

R

retractor *(continued)*

perineal prostatectomy r.
perineal self-retaining r.
peripheral vascular r.
pharyngeal r.
Phoroptor r.
phrenic r.
pillar r.
pillar-and-post microsurgical r.
Pilling r.
Plester r.
popliteal r.
postauricular r.
posterior fossa r.
posterior urethral r.
Proctor r.
4-prong r.
pronged r.
6-prong rake r.
3-prong rake blade r.
5-prong rake blade r.
prostatic r.
Pryor-Péan vaginal r.
psoas r.
pulmonary r.
Quadrant r.
Quervain abdominal r.
Ragnell r.
Ragnell-Davis double-ended r.
Ragnell double-ended r.
rake r.
rectal hook r.
Rees lighted r.
renal sinus r.
retaining r.
retropubic prostatectomy r.
rib r.
ribbon r.
Richardson abdominal r.
Richardson appendectomy r.
Richter vaginal r.
Rigby abdominal r.
Rigby bivalve r.
Rigby rectal r.
Rigby vaginal r.
right-angle r.
Rizzuti iris r.
R-Med mini r.
Robin-Masse abdominal r.
Rochard r.
Rollet r.
Rollet lacrimal sac r.
Rollet skin r.
Rosenbaum-Drews iris r.
Rosenbaum-Drews plastic r.
Roux r.
Rowe humeral head r.
Rowe orbital floor r.
Sanchez-Bulnes lacrimal sac r.

Sato lid r.
Sawyer rectal r.
scalp self-retaining r.
scapular r.
Schepens orbital r.
Schink metatarsal r.
Scholten sternal r.
Schuknecht r.
sciatic nerve r.
Scott r.
Scoville cervical disc self-
  retaining r.
Scoville nerve root r.
Seeburger r.
Seldin dental r.
self-adhering lid r.
self-retaining r.
self-retaining abdominal r.
self-retaining brain r.
self-retaining ring r.
self-retaining skin r.
self-retaining spring r.
Senn r.
Senn-Dingman r.
Senn double-ended r.
Senn-Green r.
Senn-Miller r.
serrated r.
serrefine r.
Sewall r.
Shambaugh r.
sharp-pronged r.
Sherwin knee r.
short Heaney r.
sigmoid notch r.
Silverstein lateral venous sinus r.
Simon vaginal r.
Sims rectal r.
Sims vaginal r.
single-blade r.
single-hook r.
single-prong broad acetabular r.
Sistrunk r.
skin flap r.
skin hook r.
skin self-retaining r.
Sluder r.
small rake r.
small tissue r.
Smillie knee r.
Smillie knee joint r.
Smith anal r.
Smithwick r.
soft palate r.
soft tissue blade r.
Soft-Wand balloon r.
Spacekeeper r.
Space-OR flexible internal r.
spike r.

spinal cord r.
splanchnic r.
spoon r.
spring r.
spring-loaded self-retaining r.
spring-wire r.
S-shaped brain r.
Stamey dorsal vein apical r.
standard 2-inch blade r.
standard 4-inch blade r.
stereotactic r.
sternal r.
sternotomy r.
Stevens muscle hook r.
Stevenson r.
Stevenson lacrimal sac r.
Stookey r.
Storz r.
straight r.
Strandell-Stille r.
submucous r.
Sugita r.
surgical r.
sweetheart r.
table-fixed r.
Tang r.
Taylor Britetrac r.
Taylor spinal r.
T-bar r.
Tebbetts ribbon r.
Teflon iris r.
Temple-Fay laminectomy r.
Terino facial implant r.
Tew cranial r.
Theis rib r.
Theis self-retaining r.
thin glenoid r.
Thomas r.
Thompson r.
thumb r.
Thurmond iris r.
thymus r.
thyroid r.
tibial r.
tissue r.
titanium wound r.
T-model endaural r.
Toennis r.
tongue r.
tonsillar pillar r.
toothed r.
tracheal r.
transconjunctival r.
transoral r.
Tuffier abdominal r.
Tuffier rib r.
Tupper handholder and r.
Ullrich self-retaining laminectomy r.
Ultramatic Rx Master phoroptor r.

umbrella r.
Universal r.
Upper Hands r.
Upper Hands self-retaining r.
upper lateral exposing r.
U.S. Army double-ended r.
U-shaped r.
uvular r.
vacuum r.
vaginal r.
vagotomy r.
Vaiser-Cibis muscle r.
Vasco-Posada orbital r.
vein r.
vein hook r.
ventriculogram r.
Verbrugge-Hohmann bone r.
vertical self-retaining bone r.
vesical r.
vessel r.
Villalta r.
Visitec iris r.
Volkmann finger r.
Volkmann rake r.
Walden-Aufrecht nasal r.
Walker r.
Walter nasal r.
Webb r.
weighted posterior r.
Weinberg vagotomy r.
Weitlaner r.
Weitlaner brain r.
Weitlaner hinged r.
Weitlaner microsurgery r.
Weitlaner self-retaining r.
Welsh iris r.
Wexler r.
Wexler abdominal r.
Wexler-Bantam r.
Wexler deep spreader blade
  abdominal r.
Wexler large-frame abdominal r.
Wexler lateral side-blade
  abdominal r.
Wexler malleable-blade
  abdominal r.
Wexler self-retaining r.
Wexler vaginal r.
Wichman r.
Wickham r.
Wieder r.
Wieder dental r.
Wieder pillar r.
Wiet r.
Wilder scleral self-retaining r.
Wilkes self-retaining r.
Wilkinson-Deaver blade
  abdominal r.
Wilkinson ring-frame abdominal r.

retractor *(continued)*
- Wilkinson self-retaining abdominal r.
- Williams microlumbar r.
- Wills eye lacrimal r.
- Wilmer cryosurgical iris r.
- wiring r.
- Wishbone r.
- Wishbone Omni-Track r.
- Wishbone table-mounted r.
- Woodward r.
- Wullstein r.
- Wullstein self-retaining ear r.
- Wylie renal vein r.
- Yasargil r.
- Young anterior prostatic r.
- Young bifid r.
- Young bladder r.
- Young bulb r.
- Young lateral prostatic r.
- Young prostatic r.
- Yu-Holtgrewe prostatic r.
- Z r.
- Zalkind-Balfour center-blade r.
- Zalkind lung r.
- Zenker r.

retractor-endoscope complex
Retract-O-Tape
retrievable IVC filter
retrieval
- r. balloon
- r. basket
- r. device
- r. forceps

retriever
- Blitz suture r.
- Carroll tendon r.
- Conquest suture r.
- Endopouch r.
- Golden R.
- Hewson suture r.
- Kleinert-Kutz tendon r.
- magnetic r.
- plaque r.
- polyp r.
- Positrap r.
- 3-pronged polyp r.
- snail-headed catheter r.
- Soehendra stent r.
- stone r.
- Stryker Conquest suture r.
- ureteral stone r.
- Utrata r.

retrobulbar needle
retroflexed cystoscopy sheath
retrograde
- r. Beaver blade
- r. intramedullary nail
- r. knife
- r. occlusion balloon catheter
- r. urography
- r. valvulotome

retrograde-cutting hook-shaped knife
retromastoid Ommaya reservoir
Retromax endopyelotomy stent
retroperfusion catheter
Retroplast filling
retroprep tip
retropubic prostatectomy retractor
retroreflective marker
Retroscan
retroscopic lens
RetroScrew system
retrospective bronchoscopic telescope
retrotip
- ultrasonic r.

retroversion pessary
Retsch MM200 mixer mill
Retzius system
Reu curette
ReUnite
- R. hand fixation
- R. orthopaedic pin
- R. orthopaedic screw
- R. resorbable orthopaedic fixation system

reusable
- r. forceps with needle
- r. incontinence pant
- r. laparoscopic electrode
- r. Sorensen canister
- r. vein stripper
- r. and washable adult pin-style diaper
- r. and washable adult snap diaper
- r. and washable underpad

Reuter
- R. suprapubic trocar and cannula system
- R. tip deflecting wire guide
- R. tube

Reuter-Bobbin tube
revascularization
- Biosense-guided laser myocardial r.
- r. system

Reveal
- R. MLR+ camera
- R. Plus insertable loop recorder
- R. single lens reflex camera
- R. XVI PET/CT imaging system

Revelation
- R. endocardial microcatheter
- R. hip system

Reverdin
- R. graft
- R. needle
- R. suture needle

reverse
  r. cutting needle
  r. cutting scissors
  r. cystotome
  r. knuckle-bender splint
  r. last shoe
  r. osmosis pump
  r. scissors
reverse-action hypophysectomy forceps
reverse-angle skid curette
reverse-bevel laryngoscope
Reversecell Ag kit
reverse-curve adenoid curette
reversed
  r. arm lead
  r. shoulder prosthesis
  r. Sinskey hook
reverse-shape implant
reverse-threaded screw
reversible lid speculum
reversion pacemaker
revised
  r. Salzburg lag screw system
  r. Würzburg mandibular
    reconstruction system
ReVision
  R. nail
  R. nail system
revision
  r. hip stem
  proximal loading r. (PLR)
  Zimmer modular r. (ZMR)
Revitalizer Soft-Start nasal CPAP
Revo
  R. loop handle knot pusher
  R. retrievable cancellous screw
  R. rotator cuff repair system
  R. suture anchor
Revolution
  R. lens
  R. micropigmentation handpiece
  R. XR/d digital detector
revolving Ge-68 pin
Rexton hearing aid
Reynolds dissecting scissors
Rezaian
  R. external fixation device
  R. interbody device
  R. spinal fixator
ReZoom multifocal refractive IOL
RF
  radiofrequency
  RF ablation system
  RF coil
  RF Marinr catheter
  RF needle electrode system
  RF vacuum ablation system
RF2000 Radiofrequency Generator

RFA
  radiofrequency ablation
R&F camera
RF-generated thermal balloon catheter
RF-shielded cupboard
R-Hab lighter weight ankle
rHead
  r. implant system
  r. Recon implant
Rhein
  R. Advantage II diamond limbal-
    relaxing incision knife
  R. Artisan lens-holding forceps
  R. aspiration cannula
  R. blade cleaning system
  R. capsulorrhexis cystotome forceps
  R. clear corneal diamond knife
  R. 3D angled trapezoid diamond
    knife
  R. 3D trapezoid diamond blade
  R. fine foldable lens-insertion
    forceps
  R. irrigation cannula
  R. LASIK epithelial detaching hoe
  R. LASIK epithelial detaching
    spatula
  R. LASIK flap elevator and
    stromal spatula
  R. LASIK flap forceps
  R. LASIK flap repositioning
    spatula
  R. pick
  R. reusable cautcry pen
Rheinberg microscope
Rheolog device
rheolytic
  r. catheter
  r. mechanical thrombectomy device
  r. thrombectomy catheter
rheometer
  Haake r.
Rheuma wrist and thumb support
Rhino
  R. Rocket dressing
  R. Rocket nasal pack
  R. Rocket nasal packing
  R. Triangle brace
  R. Triangle polypropylene hip
    abduction brace
rhinolaryngoscope
**Rhinoline endoscopic sinus surgery
  system**
rhinomanometer
  Storz r.
rhinometer
  Eccovision acoustic r.
  Hood Laboratories Eccovision
    acoustic r.
  2-microphone acoustical r.

rhinoplasty
    r. diamond bur
    r. scissors
rhinoprobe
rhinoscope
rhinoscopic mirror
Rhinotec shaver
Rhinotherm
rhodamine 6G dye laser
rhodium filter
Rhoton
    R. blunt-ring curette
    R. elevator
    R. microdissector
    R. microhook
    R. needle holder
    R. osteotome
Rhoton-Merz suction tube
Rhythm catheter
RhythmScan
rhytidectomy scissors
RIA kit
rib
    r. approximator
    r. contractor
    r. cutter
    r. drill
    r. elevator
    r. forceps
    r. guillotine
    r. needle
    r. rasp
    r. raspatory
    r. retractor
    r. rongeur forceps
    r. shears
    r. spreader
    vertical expandable prosthetic
      titanium r. (VEPTR)
ribbed
    r. hook
    r. needle
    r. sterile tubing
ribbed-sole shoe
ribbon
    r. arch appliance
    r. blade
    r. gauze dressing
    r. gut needle
    hollow r.
    ^{192}Ir r.
    r. retractor
    seed r.
RiboPrinter microbial characterization
  system
riboprobe
    EBER1 r.
    U6 r.

Rica
    R. clip-applying forceps
    R. ear curette
    R. mastoid suction tube
    R. pelvimeter
    R. pneumatic otoscope
    R. rongeur
    R. surgical catgut
    R. vaginal speculum
    R. vessel clamp
Rice pick
Richard
    R. pillow
    R. Products fundus camera drug
      organizer
    R. Wolf arthroscope
    R. Wolf Medical Instruments
      diagnostic laparoscope
    R. Wolf Medical Instruments
      operating laparoscope
    R. Wolf model 2271.004 ultrasonic
      energy rigid device
    R. Wolf nasal epistaxis system
    R. Wolf Piezolith lithotriptor
    R. Wolf videoresectoscope
Richards
    R. angle guide
    R. bone hook
    R. classic compression hip screw
    R. fixation staple
    R. fixator system
    R. headrest
    R. hip endoprosthesis system
    R. hip prosthesis
    R. hydroxyapatite PORP
    R. hydroxyapatite PORP prosthesis
    R. hydroxyapatite TORP prosthesis
    R. lag screw compression device
    R. lag screw device
    R. locking rod
    R. mallet
    R. maximum contact cruciate-
      sparing prosthesis
    R. maximum-contact cruciate-sparing
      prosthesis
    R. ministaple
    R. modular hip system
    R. reamer
    R. Solcotrans orthopaedic drainage-
      reinfusion system
    R. Solcotrans Plus
    R. Solcotrans Plus drainage system
    R. tamp
    R. zirconia femoral head prosthesis
Richards-Hirschhorn plate
Richardson
    R. abdominal retractor
    R. appendectomy retractor

Riches
  R. artery forceps
  R. diathermy forceps
Richie brace
Rich-Mar external ultrasound
Richmond
  R. bolt
  R. subarachnoid screw
  R. subarachnoid screw sensor
Richter
  R. scissors
  R. vaginal retractor
Richter-Heath clip-removing forceps
Richwil
  R. bridge remover
  R. crown remover
Rickett golden ruler
Rickham reservoir
rickshaw
  r. rehab exerciser
  r. rehabilitation exerciser
Rider-Moeller cardiac dilator
ridge forceps
Ridley
  R. anterior chamber lens implant
  R. Mark II lens implant
Riechert-Mundinger
  R.-M. stereotactic device
  R.-M. stereotactic system
Riecken PQ premium heel cup
Riecker-Kleinsasser laryngoscope
Riedel corneal needle
Rienhoff-Finochietto rib spreader
Ries suction elevator
Riester otoscope
Rife machine
Rigby
  R. abdominal retractor
  R. bivalve retractor
  R. rectal retractor
  R. vaginal retractor
right
  r. ankle bur
  r. coronary catheter
  r. heart catheter
  Judkins r. (JR)
  Judkins r. 4 (JR4)
  Judkins r. 5 (JR5)
  r. Judkins catheter
  R. Light
  R. Light examination light
  r. ventricular assist device (RVAD)
  r. ventricular coil
  r. ventricular copulsation balloon
  r. ventricular ejection fraction
    catheter
  r. ventricular wall device
right-angle
  r.-a. bipolar cautery

  r.-a. blunt probe
  r.-a. booster clip
  r.-a. bronchoscopic telescope
  r.-a. chest catheter
  r.-a. chest tube
  r.-a. clamp
  r.-a. colon clamp
  r.-a. curette
  r.-a. drill
  r.-a. electrode
  r.-a. elevator
  r.-a. erysiphake
  r.-a. examining telescope
  r.-a. forceps
  r.-a. hook
  r.-a. knife
  r.-a. lens
  r.-a. pick
  r.-a. prism magnifier
  r.-a. retractor
  r.-a. scissors
  r.-a. screwdriver
right-angled
  r.-a. isosceles triangle board
  r.-a. telescopic lens
right-handed corneal scissors
right/left corneoscleral scissors
right-to-left intracardiac shunt
rigid
  r. biopsy forceps
  r. cantilever beam construct
  r. collar
  r. contact lens
  r. curette
  r. endosonography probe
  r. external distraction system
  r. gas permeable lens
  r. holding rod
  r. internal fixation device
  r. intranasal endoscope
  r. intraocular lens
  r. kidney stone forceps
  r. laryngoscope
  r. monopolar loop
  r. open-tube endoscope
  r. orthosis
  r. pedicle screw
  r. postoperative brace
  r. rod-lens endoscope
  r. scope
  r. sigmoidoscope
  r. sound
  r. splint
  r. suction catheter
  r. ventriculoscope
**Rigidfix anterior cruciate ligament
  cross-pin system**
rigid-frame wheelchair

rigidometer
 Digital Inflection R.
Rigiflator handheld inflation/deflation device
Rigiflex
 R. ABD balloon dilatation catheter
 R. achalasia balloon
 R. achalasia balloon dilator
 R. achalasia dilator
 R. balloon
 R. biliary balloon dilatation catheter
 R. esophageal TTS
 R. esophageal TTS balloon catheter
 R. OTW balloon dilatation catheter
 R. TTS balloon
 R. TTS balloon catheter
 R. TTS balloon dilatation catheter
 R. TTS balloon dilator
RigiScan
 R. device
 R. penile tumescence and rigidity monitor
 R. Plus rigidity assessment system
RIGS
 R. system
 R. system stem
RIGScan CR49
Rik
 R. fluid mattress
 R. FootHugger fluid heel boot
RIK fluid-filled head pack
Riley needle
ring
 Ace-Colles half r.
 acetabular reinforcement r.
 aniridia r.
 AnnuloFlex flexible annuloplasty r.
 AnnuloFlo annuloplasty r.
 r. applicator
 atrioventricular valve r.
 r. bayonet Rand curette
 R. biliary drainage catheter
 r. biliary stent
 biofragmentable anastomotic r. (BAR)
 Bloomberg SuperNumb anesthetic r.
 Bores twist fixation r.
 Brown-Roberts-Wells base r.
 Budde halo r.
 Buzard-Thornton fixation r.
 capsular tension r.
 Carpentier r.
 Carpentier-Edwards Physio annuloplasty r.
 Carpentier-McCarthy-Adams IMR ETlogix annuloplasty r.
 cataract mask r.
 r. cataract mask eye shield

 centering r.
 Charnley centering r.
 Cionni capsular tension r.
 circumaortic venous r.
 Coloplast skin barrier r.
 confidence r.
 constriction r.
 Cook continence r.
 corneal transplant centering r.
 Cosman-Roberts-Wells stereotactic r.
 r. curette
 r. cushion
 r. cutter
 deep abdominal r.
 Dell fixation r.
 double-flanged valve sewing r.
 R. drainage catheter needle
 Duran annuloplasty r.
 Edwards MC^3 r.
 elastic O r.
 r. electrode
 endocapsular equator r.
 Estrace VR intravaginal r.
 Estring estradiol vaginal r.
 Estring silicone vaginal r.
 external abdominal r.
 Falope r.
 Fine crescent fixation r.
 Fine-Thornton scleral fixation r.
 fixation r.
 Fleischer r.
 Flieringa-Kayser fixation r.
 Flieringa-LeGrand fixation r.
 Flieringa scleral fixation r.
 foam r.
 r. forceps
 Gimbel stabilization r.
 Gimbel stabilizing r.
 Girard scleral expander r.
 gold r.
 R. guidewire
 half r.
 halo r.
 Hansatome suction r.
 head r.
 Hofmann-Thornton globe fixation r.
 Ilizarov r.
 Intacs r.
 Intacs corneal r.
 Intacs intrastromal corneal r.
 intravaginal r.
 invalid r.
 ischemic mitral r. (IMR)
 Japanese erection r.
 Johnston fixation r.
 Katena r.
 KeraVision Intacs intracorneal r.
 KF r.
 knitted sewing r.

Kraff hyperopic fixation r.
Landers irrigating vitrectomy r.
Landers vitrectomy r.
Landolt-C r.
laparotomy sponge r.
r. lens expressor
Lu-Mendez LRI guide and
fixation r.
Lyon r.
Magrina-Bookwalter vaginal
retractor r.
Martinez corneal transplant
centering r.
Martinez scleral centering r.
McKinney fixation r.
McNeill-Goldman r.
McNeill-Goldman blepharostat r.
McNeill-Goldman corneal
transplant r.
McNeill-Goldman scleral r.
metal sewing r.
Morcher Cionni capsular tension r.
Morcher Cionni endocapsular
capsular tension r.
Morcher endocapsular tension r.
Morcher iris diaphragm r.
Moretsky LASIK hinge protector
fixation r.
Nichamin fixation r.
NuvaRing vaginal contraceptive r.
Ochsner r.
Oculaid capsular tension r.
optic r.
Osbon pressure-point tension r.
pediatric perineal retractor r.
perfusion O r.
r. pessary
Placido r.
plastic sewing r.
platinum r.
pressure r.
pressure-point tension r.
prosthetic valve sewing r.
Puig Massana annuloplasty r.
Puig Massana-Shiley annuloplasty r.
pupil dilator r.
reduction r.
reinforcement r.
retraction r.
r. rotation forceps
r. scanner
Schatzki r.
scleral expander r.
Sculptor flexible annuloplasty r.
Seguin annuloplasty r.
sewing r.
silastic r.
silicone elastomer r.

sizing r.
SJM Seguin annuloplasty r.
SJM Tailor annuloplasty r.
sponge r.
Stableyes capsular tension r.
Suarez continence r.
suction r.
supraannular suture r.
suture r.
sutureless biofragmentable r.
symblepharon r.
Tano r.
tantalum r.
tantalum O r.
Thornton-Fine r.
Thornton globe fixation r.
Thornton limbal fixation r.
Thorton globe fixation r.
r. tip forceps
Tolentino r.
r. tongue blade
Tourni-Cot elastic r.
R. transjugular intrahepatic access
set
T-shaped constriction r.
Turner-Warwick adult retractor r.
R. UPM press-fit prosthesis
vacuum fixation r.
vaginal r.
Valtrac absorbable biofragmentable
anastomosis r.
Valtrac anastomosis r.
vascular r.
Villasenor-Navarro fixation r.
Walsh pressure r.
Weinstein fixation r.
Whitten fixation r.
Yoon r.
zipper r.
ring-cutting saw
ring-handled bulldog clamp
ring-jawed holding clamp
RingLoc
R. acetabular series
R. hip liner
R. instrument
Ring-MacLean sump
Ring-McLean
R.-M. catheter
R.-M. sump drainage set
R.-M. sump tube
ring-type
r.-t. imaging system
r.-t. rigidity measuring device
Rinn
R. XCP film holder
R. XCP radiographic paralleling
device

RinoFlow
- R. ENT wash unit
- R. nasal wash and sinus system

rinse
- Hibistat germicidal hand r.

rip-cord suture
RIP portable sleep monitor
Rish osteotome
Risley rotary prism
Rispi Micromega reamer
Risser
- R. brace
- R. frame
- R. localizer
- R. localizer cast
- R. localizer scoliosis cast

Risser-Cotrel body cast
RITA system
Ritch
- R. contact lens
- R. nylon suture laser lens
- R. trabeculoplasty laser lens

Ritchie
- R. brace
- R. catheter
- R. cleft palate tenaculum
- R. nail starter

RiteBite biopsy forceps
Ritleng probe
Ritter
- R. Bovie
- R. coagulator electrosurgical unit

Ritter-Bantam Bovie electrosurgical unit
Riva-Rocci sphygmomanometer
Riverbank Laboratories tuning fork
rivet gun
Rivetti-Levinson intraluminal shunt
Riza-Ribe grasping needle
Rizzo dorsal implant
Rizzoli osteoclast
Rizzuti
- R. graft carrier spoon
- R. iris retractor
- R. rectus forceps

Rizzuti-Bonaccolto instrument
Rizzuti-Fleischer instrument
Rizzuti-Kayser-Fleischer instrument
Rizzuti-Lowe instrument
Rizzuti-Maxwell instrument
Rizzuti-Spizziri cannula knife
RJL model 10 bioelectrical impedance analyzer
RK-5000
RK marker
R-K needle
RLP-Cholesterol Immunoseparation Assay kit
RMC knee replacement device

R-Med
- R-M. mini retractor
- R-M. plug

RMI antegrade cardioplegia catheter
RNA
- R. PCR core kit
- R. probe

RNAzol
- R. Reagent Extractor

RNeasy
- R. Maxi kit
- R. Mini kit

Roach ball precision attachment
Roadmapper
- FluoroPlus R.

Roadrunner
- R. extra-support wire guide
- R. NaviGuide guidewire
- R. wire

roaming optical access multiscope
ROAM right-angled endoscope
Roane bullet tip
Robbins
- R. Acrotorque hand engine
- R. automatic tourniquet

Robert
- R. Brigham semiconstrained prosthesis
- R. Jones bandage
- R. Jones bulky soft compressive dressing
- R. Jones splint

Robertazzi nasopharyngeal airway
Roberts
- R. arterial forceps
- R. folding esophagoscope
- R. oval esophagoscope

Robertshaw tube
Robicsek vascular probe
Robin chalazion clamp
Robin-Masse abdominal retractor
Robinson
- R. arthrometer
- R. catheter
- R. stapes prosthesis
- R. urethral catheter

Robles cutting point cannula
Rob-Nel catheter
Robodoc
- R. robot
- R. system

Roboprep G instrument
robot
- Aesop 2000, 3000 endoscopic stabilizer r.
- automated endoscopic system for optimal positioning surgical r.
- Evolution 1 precision r.
- Long Beach stereotactic r.

Minerva r.
Orca R.
Robodoc r.
Zeus r.
robotic-automated assist device
robotic microscope
robotics-controlled stereotactic frame
Robson intestinal forceps
ROC
ROC anchor
ROC XS suture fastener
Rocabado posture gauge
Rochard retractor
Roche
R. Septi-Chek blood culture system
R. Sysmex hematology system
R. Z gel kit
Rochester
R. bone trephine
R. bone trephine device
R. harvest bone cutter
R. hip-knee-ankle-foot orthosis
R. HKAFO
R. Kocher clamp
R. lamina elevator
R. Medical self-adhering male
external catheter
R. Medical 100% silicone Foley
catheter
R. needle
R. oral tissue forceps
R. Péan clamp
R. recipient bone cutter
R. Russian tissue forceps
R. spinal elevator
Rochester-Carmalt forceps
Rochester-Ochsner
R.-O. forceps
R.-O. hemostat
Rochester-Péan
R.-P. forceps
R.-P. hemostat
R.-P. hysterectomy forceps
Rochette bridge
Rock
R. ankle exercise board
R. & Roller exercise board
rocker
r. balance square
r. board
r. knife
Uniplane r.
rocker-bottom cast boot shoe
rocket dilator
RocketSoc ankle brace
rocking microtome
Rockwood
R. AC screw

R. clavicle pin
R. shoulder screw
rocky boat exerciser
rod
alignment guide r.
Alta advance tibial/humeral r.
Alta CFX reconstruction r.
Alta humeral r.
Alta intramedullary r.
Alta reconstruction r.
Alta tibial r.
Alta tibial/humeral r.
Amset R-F r.
analyzing r.
Auer r.
auto-reinforced polyglycolide r.
r. bender
Bickel intramedullary r.
Biofix absorbable r.
Biofix fixation r.
cloverleaf r.
colostomy r.
compression r.
compression U r.
condyle r.
Cotrel-Dubousset pediatric r.
r. cutter
degradable polyglycolide r.
delta r.
distraction r.
Doc cervical dynamic r.
double-L spinal r.
dual square-ended Harrington r.
Edwards D-L modular screw r.
Edwards-Levine r.
Edwards Universal r.
r. electrode
enamel r.
Enneking r.
ferromagnetic r.
Fixateur Interne r.
flared spinal r.
Harrington r.
Harrington dual square-ended r.
Harris condylocephalic r.
r. holder
Hopkins r.
House measuring r.
Hunter tendon r.
Hydroflex penile implant r.
hygroscopic r.
impactor r.
impingement r.
intramedullary r.
intramedullary alignment r.
intramedullary Rush r.
Isolar r.
Isola spinal implant system eye r.
Jacobs distraction r.

R

759

rod *(continued)*
    Jacobs locking hook spinal r.
    Kaneda r.
    Knodt distraction r.
    Kostuik r.
    Küntscher r.
    laser r.
    Lincoff sponge r.
    long alignment r.
    Luque r.
    Luque-Galveston r.
    Maddox r.
    McLaughlin laser vaginal
      measuring r.
    McLaughlin quartz r.
    measuring r.
    Meckel r.
    medullary r.
    Mira silicone r.
    modified Harrington r.
    Moe modified Harrington r.
    Moore measuring r.
    Moss r.
    Olerud PSF r.
    orthopaedic r.
    OrthoSorb r.
    pediatric Cotrel-Dubousset r.
    Perspex r.
    r. photoreceptor
    Polarus humeral r.
    policeman glass stirring r.
    precontoured unit r.
    quartz r.
    radiotranslucent r.
    retracting r.
    Richards locking r.
    rigid holding r.
    round-ended distraction r.
    round extension r.
    Rush r.
    Russell-Taylor delta r.
    scleral sponge r.
    screw alignment r.
    Selby I, II r.
    semirigid silicone plastic r.
    Shaw-SHIP r.
    Sheffield r.
    silastic r.
    silicone r.
    silicone flexor r.
    SinuScope rigid r.
    slotted intramedullary r.
    spinal r.
    square-ended distraction r.
    sterile transverse r.
    Sur-Fit Natura loop ostomy r.
    surgical r.
    R. TAG suture anchor system
    telescoping r.

    r. template
    thermoluminescent dosimeter r.
    threaded r.
    U Luque vertebral r.
    unit spinal r.
    VDS compression r.
    VSF r.
    Williams r.
    Wiltse system spinal r.
    Wissinger r.
    Zickel supracondylar r.
    Zielke r.
Rodenstock
    R. panfundus lens
    R. scanning laser ophthalmoscope
    R. slit-lamp
    R. system
rod-hook construct
Rodin orbital implant
rod-lens system
rod-sleeve instrumentation
Roeder
    R. forceps
    R. manipulative aptitude test device
    R. towel clamp
roentgen
    r. knife
    r. knife stereotactic radiosurgical
      device
    r. meter
    r. tube
roentgenograph
roentgenographic opaque marker
Rogan teleradiology system
Roger
    R. Anderson external fixation
      apparatus
    R. Anderson external fixation
      device
    R. Anderson fixation
    R. Anderson fixation bar
    R. Anderson pin fixation appliance
    R. Anderson stabilization device
    R. forceps
    R. septal elevator
    R. system
    R. wire-cutting scissors
Rogozinski
    R. hook
    R. screw system
    R. spinal rod system
Rohadur gait plate
Roho
    R. bed
    R. Dry Flotation wheelchair pad
    R. heel pad
    R. heel protector
    R. high-profile cushion
    R. mattress

R. Pack-It cushion
R. pediatric seating system
R. solid seat insert

Rolf

R. forceps
R. lacrimal probe
R. lance

roll

absorbable gelatin film r.
Celluron dental r.
cervical r.
r. control bolster
Dutchman's r.
Fluftex gauze r.
gauze r.
Kerlix bandage r.
Kling fluff r.
Krinkle gauze r.
Lakeside cotton r.
lumbar r.
McKenzie cervical r.
McKenzie lumbar r.
McKenzie night r.
Medline r.
3M Reston self-adhering foam pad & r.
narrow gauze r.
neck r.
octagon r.
silver mylar r.
Skillbuilder half r.
Stretch gauze r.
Tensor elastic bandage r.
therapy r.
Tumble Forms r.

Roll-A-Bout

R.-A-B. mobility device
R.-A-B. 4-wheel walker

Rollator Nova walker

roller

r. bandage
r. electrode
r. forceps
r. knife
Lindstrom LASIK flap r.
r. pump
Sorbothane rice sheller r.
Toledo r.
tubing hand r.

RollerBack self-massage device

rollerball

rollerbar electrode

roller-barrel electrode

RollerLoop vaporizing loop electrode

Rollet

R. chisel
R. irrigating/aspirating unit
R. lacrimal probe
R. lacrimal sac retractor

R. retractor
R. skin retractor

rolling membrane Wallstent cobalt-based alloy balloon-expandable stent

roll-in stretcher

Rollocane

Rolloscope II

Rolyan

R. AquaForm wrist and thumb spica splint
R. arm elevator
R. D-ring wrist brace
R. foot support
R. Gel Shell spica splint
R. Reach-N-Range pulley system
R. TakeOff Sprint brace
R. TakeOff thumb support

Rolz

R. device
R. massage tool

ROM

range of motion
ROM knee brace
ROM walker brace

Romano

R. curved drilling system
R. curved surgical drill
R. surgical curved drilling system

romanoscope

Romhilt-Estes point scoring system

Rommel electrocautery

Rondo inhaler

rongeur

Adson bone r.
Adson cranial r.
aortic valve r.
Bacon bone r.
Bacon cranial bone r.
Baer bone r.
Bailey aortic valve r.
Bane bone r.
Bane-Hartmann bone r.
Bane mastoid r.
Belz lacrimal sac r.
Beyer bone r.
Beyer laminectomy r.
Blumenthal bone r.
Böhler r.
Boies-Lombard mastoid r.
bone-biting r.
bone-cutting r.
bone punch r.
Caspar r.
cervical r.
Cicherelli bone r.
Cintor bone r.
Citelli r.
Citelli sphenoid r.
Cleveland bone r.

rongeur *(continued)*

Cloward intervertebral disc r.
Cloward pituitary r.
Codman-Kerrison laminectomy r.
Codman-Leksell laminectomy r.
Cohen r.
Colclough laminectomy r.
Converse-Lange r.
Converse nasal root r.
Corbett bone r.
Cottle-Jansen r.
Cottle-Kazanjian r.
Cottle nasal-biting r.
Cushing bone r.
Cushing disc r.
Cushing intervertebral disc r.
Cushing pituitary r.
Dale first rib r.
Dean r.
Dean bone r.
Defourmentel bone r.
delicate intervertebral disc r.
dental r.
DeVilbiss cranial r.
disc r.
double-action r.
down-cutting r.
duckbill r.
Echlin bone r.
Echlin duckbill r.
Echlin-Luer r.
end-biting blunt-nosed r.
Falconer r.
Ferris-Smith-Gruenwald r.
Ferris-Smith intervertebral disc r.
Ferris-Smith-Kerrison disc r.
Ferris-Smith-Kerrison
  laminectomy r.
Ferris-Smith-Kerrison
  laminectomy r.
Ferris-Smith pituitary r.
Ferris-Smith-Spurling disc r.
Ferris-Smith-Takahashi r.
Fisch bone r.
flat-bottomed Kerrison r.
FlexTip intervertebral r.
r. forceps
Friedman bone r.
Frykholm bone r.
Fukushima r.
Fulton laminectomy r.
Goldman-Kazanjian r.
gooseneck r.
Guleke bone r.
Hajek antral r.
Hardy r.
Hartmann bone r.
Hartmann ear r.
Hartmann mastoid r.

Hein r.
Hoen intervertebral disc r.
Hoen laminectomy r.
Hoen pituitary r.
Hoffmann ear r.
Horsley bone r.
Horsley cranial bone r.
Husk bone r.
intervertebral disc r.
Ivy mastoid r.
Jackson intervertebral disc r.
Jansen bone r.
Jansen ear r.
Jansen-Middleton r.
jaw r.
Juers-Lempert endaural r.
Kerrison r.
Kerrison cervical r.
Kerrison-Costen r.
Kerrison lumbar r.
Kerrison mastoid r.
Kleinert-Kutz bone r.
Kleinert-Kutz synovectomy r.
Koffler-Hajek laminectomy r.
lacrimal sac r.
laminectomy r.
Lange-Converse nasal root r.
Lebsche r.
Leksell r.
Leksell bone r.
Leksell cardiovascular r.
Leksell laminectomy r.
Leksell-Stille thoracic r.
Lempert r.
Lempert bone r.
Lempert endaural r.
Lillie r.
Liston bone r.
Liston-Littauer r.
Littauer r.
Littauer-West r.
Lombard-Beyer r.
Lombard-Boies mastoid r.
Love-Gruenwald cranial r.
Love-Gruenwald intervertebral
  disc r.
Love-Gruenwald laminectomy r.
Love-Gruenwald pituitary r.
Love-Kerrison r.
Love pituitary r.
Lowman r.
Luer bone r.
Luer thoracic r.
Luer-Whiting r.
Markwalder bone r.
Markwalder rib r.
Marquardt bone r.
mastoid r.
Mead r.

R

Mead bone r.
Mead dental r.
micro Kerrison r.
micropituitary r.
narrow-bite bone r.
needle-nose r.
Oldberg intervertebral disc r.
Oldberg laminectomy r.
Oldberg pituitary r.
orthopaedic r.
peapod intervertebral disc r.
pituitary r.
Poppen intervertebral disc r.
punch r.
Reiner bone r.
Rica r.
Röttgen-Ruskin bone r.
round-nosed r.
Ruskin r.
Ruskin bone r.
Ruskin-Liston bone r.
Ruskin mastoid r.
Ruskin-Rowland bone r.
Schell bone r.
Schlesinger cervical r.
Schlesinger intervertebral disc r.
Selverstone intervertebral disc r.
Semb bone r.
Semb-Stille bone r.
Shearer r.
side-cutting r.
single-action r.
SMIC r.
Spence intervertebral disc r.
Spurling intervertebral disc r.
Spurling-Kerrison upbiting and
  downbiting r.
Spurling laminectomy r.
Spurling pituitary r.
Stille bone r.
Stille-Horsley bone r.
Stille-Liston r.
Stille-Luer angular duckbill r.
Stille-Luer bone r.
Stille-Luer duckbill r.
Stille-Luer-Echlin r.
Stille-Ruskin bone r.
Stookey cranial r.
Super Cut laminectomy r.
synovectomy r.
taper-jaw r.
Tobey ear r.
Universal Kerrison r.
Wagner r.
Watson-Williams intervertebral
  disc r.
Weil-Blakesley intervertebral disc r.
Weil pituitary r.

Whiting mastoid r.
Wilde intervertebral disc r.
Zaufel-Jansen bone r.

roof
r. plate
r. wedge

roof-reinforcement ring hip arthroplasty component

Rooke perioperative boot

room
Allender vertical laminar flow r.
decontaminating r.
r. humidifier
International Acoustic Company
  audiologic assessment r.

root
r. canal broach
r. canal file
r. canal spreader
r. high-pull facebow
r. rubber dam clamp
R. ZX apex locator
R. ZX ultrasonic unit

root-form
r.-f. dental implant
r.-f. device

rope
Bard AlgiDERM r.
Kaltostat r.
r. stretching device

Roper alpha-chymotrypsin cannula

Roper-Day prosthesis

Roper-Hall
R.-H. localizer
R.-H. locator

rosary bougie

Rosch hepatic catheter

Rosch-Thurmond fallopian tube catheterization set

Rosch-Uchida
R.-U. liver access set
R.-U. needle
R.-U. transjugular liver access set

Rosebud dissector

rosehead bur

Rosen
R. bur
R. curved guidewire
R. elevator
R. guidewire
R. inflatable urinary incontinence
  prosthesis
R. needle
R. nucleus paddle
R. phaco splitter
R. splint
R. suction tube
R. wire

Rosenbaum-Drews
 R.-D. iris retractor
 R.-D. plastic retractor
Rosenbaum pocket vision screener
Rosenberg
 R. dissecting cannula
 R. dissector tip
 R. gynecomastia dissection
 instrument
Rosenmüller
 R. curette
 fossa of R.
Rosenthal aspiration needle
Rosenthal-French nebulization dosimeter
Rosenwasser
 R. irrigating endothelial stripper
 R. lamellar donor shovel
 R. medium-curve scissors
 R. strong-curve scissors
Roser-Koenig mouthgag
Rosetta-Lt 12-lead reporter
rosette
 r. Beaver blade
 r. blade
Rosette strain gauge
Rosner tonometer
Ross
 R. needle
 R. pulmonary porcine valve
Rosser signature series
Rosys Plato Gene Machine
Rotablator
 R. atherectomy device
 R. burr catheter
 Heart Technology R.
 R. rotating bur
 R. system
 R. wire
Rotacamera
Rotacaps
 Ventolin R.
Rotacs system
Rotadisk
Rotafix lumbar cage
Rotaflex exerciser
Rotaglide
 R. knee implant
 R. total knee system
Rotahaler
**RotaLink Plus rotational atherectomy
 device**
rotary
 r. cutting instrument
 r. hub saw
rotatable
 r. coupling head
 r. pigtail catheter
 r. polypectomy snare
 r. Roth retrieval net

 r. transsphenoidal enucleator
 r. transsphenoidal horizontal ring
 curette
 r. transsphenoidal knife handle
 r. transsphenoidal right-angle hook
 r. transsphenoidal round dissector
 r. transsphenoidal spatula dissector
 r. transsphenoidal vertical ring
 curette
rotating
 r. adapter
 r. air impactor
 r. anode tube
 r. arm impactor
 r. basket shaver
 r. Bruel and Kjaer probe
 r. brush
 r. endoprobe
 r. endoscissors
 r. femoral head prosthesis
 r. forceps
 r. gamma camera
 r. hemostatic valve
 r. laryngoscope
 r. mechanism
 r. morcellator
 r. patellar implant
 r. speculum anoscope
 r. transilluminator
 r. turner
 r. wire brush
rotating-hinge knee prosthesis
rotating-type cutter
rotational
 r. atherectomy device
 r. colonoscope overtube
 r. dynamic angioplasty catheter
rotation-stop washer
rotator
 Bechert nucleus r.
 r. cuff advancer
 r. cuff buttress
 Espaillat-Deblasio nucleus r.
 Hosmer above-knee r.
 Howmedica monotube external r.
 Jaffe-Bechert nucleus r.
 Jarit r.
 Maloney nucleus r.
 nucleus r.
 R. polypectomy snare
 Tennant nuclear ball r.
rotatory variable-differential transducer
RotaWire Floppy Gold guidewire
Rotex needle
Roth
 R. endoscopy retrieval net
 R. Grip-Tip suture guide
 R. polyp retrieval net

Rothbarth
- R. Uni-Flo infusion catheter
- R. Uni-Flo infusion set

Rothman
- R. Gilbard corneal punch
- R. Institute femoral prosthesis
- R. Institute porous femoral component

roticulating endograsper

roticulator
- r. 55 stapler
- r. stapling device

Rotilt ratchet mechanism

Roto
- R. Kinetic bed
- R. Rest delta kinetic therapy treatment table

RotoClix

rotoextractor
- Douvas r.

Rotograph
- R. Plus imaging system
- R. Plus panoramic dental tomography imaging system

Rotolith lithotrite

roto-osteotome

rotor
- Beckman JE-10X elutriation r.
- Kontron TFT 45.6 r.
- Ti r.

Roto-Rest bed

RotorloC absorbable rotator cuff suture anchor

Rotorod sampler

rotoslide

Röttgen-Ruskin bone rongeur

Roubin infusion catheter

Roughton-Scholander
- R.-S. apparatus
- R.-S. syringe

round
- r. body needle
- r. bur
- r. cutting bur
- r. diamond bur
- r. dissector
- r. end cutter
- r. extension rod
- r. forceps
- r. Gigli saw
- r. hole plate
- r. optical zone marker
- r. punch forceps
- r. ruby knife
- r. speculum
- r. tapper

round-ended distraction rod

round-handled forceps

round-loop electrode

round-nosed rongeur

round-tip
- r.-t. catheter
- r.-t. microscissors

round-tipped periosteal elevator

round-wire electrode

Rousek
- R. extender
- R. extractor

Rousseau chin-lift stabilizer

router
- power r.
- Vortex r.

Roux
- R. loop
- R. retractor
- R. spatula

Roveda lid everter

Rowden uterine manipulator/injector (RUMI)

Rowe
- R. blanket
- R. disimpaction forceps
- R. glenoid reaming forceps
- R. humeral head retractor
- R. maxillary forceps
- R. modified Harrison forceps
- R. orbital floor retractor

Rowe-Harrison bone-holding forceps

Rowe-Killey forceps

Rowen
- R. spatula
- R. white-to-white corneal gauge

Rowland
- R. double-action forceps
- R. pouch

Royal
- R. disposable skin stapler
- R. Flush angiographic flush catheter
- R. Flush pigtail catheter
- R. Flush Plus high-flow angiographic flush catheter
- R. Marsden Hospital staging system

Royale intraocular lens injector

Roy-Camille
- R.-C. plate
- R.-C. prosthesis

Roylan ergonomic hand exerciser

Royl-Derm
- R.-D. hydrogel wound dressing
- R.-D. hydrogel wound nonadherent dressing
- R.-D. protectant powder

RP
- reduced profile
- RP X-OMAT processor

R

RPM
>RPM tracking system
>RPM tracking system/catheter

RPO oximeter

R-Port implantable vascular access system

R. Quétin Bone-Mill

R-Stent stent

RT
>RT Advantage ultrasound
>RT 3200 Advantage ultrasound scanner
>RT ultrasound
>RT 6800 ultrasound scanner

R-Test Evolution

R-T nail

RTS
>radiation therapy system

Rub
>Jeanie R.

rubber
>r. acorn tip
>r. airway
>r. band ligator
>r. bite liner
>r. catheter
>r. dam clamp
>r. dam drain
>r. drain
>r. finger cot
>r. mouth prop
>r. shod clamp
>silicone r.
>r. sole cast walker
>r. spa bowl
>r. spacer
>r. sponge
>r. suture
>r. walking heel

Rubbermaid adjustable bath/shower seat

rubber-reinforced bandage

rubber-sheathed clamp

rubber-shod
>r.-s. catheter
>r.-s. forceps

Rubenstein LASIK cannula

Rubenstein-type LASIK irrigating cannula

Rubin
>R. blade
>R. bone planer
>R. cartilage planer
>R. gouge
>R. nasal chisel
>R. nasofrontal osteotome
>R. needle
>R. oblique rasp
>R. osteotome

>R. rasp
>R. tube

Rubinstein cryoprobe

ruby
>r. diamond knife
>r. laser

Rudd
>R. Clinic hemorrhoidal forceps
>R. ligator

Rudolph
>R. Full Face mask
>R. 1-way respiratory valve

Ruedemann lacrimal dilator

Ruel
>R. aorta clamp
>R. forceps

Ruggles surgical instrument

rule
>Van Praagh loop r.

ruler
>Bio-Pen biometric r.
>calibration r.
>r. calipers
>r. catheter
>centimeter subtraction r.
>Helveston scleral marking r.
>Hyde astigmatism r.
>Hyde-Osher keratometric r.
>Joseph measuring r.
>metal r.
>millimeter r.
>Rickett golden r.
>Scott curved r.
>stainless steel flexible r.
>steel r.
>Thornton double corneal r.
>Thornton limbal incision r.
>ulnar r.

Rumel
>R. cardiovascular tourniquet
>R. rubber clamp

Rumel-Belmont tourniquet

Rumex titanium instrument

RUMI
>Rowden uterine manipulator/injector
>RUMI uterine manipulation system
>RUMI uterine manipulator

Ruminson astigmatic gauge and marker

Rumison side port fixation occluder

runaway pacemaker

Runner
>Sprint R.

runoff film

RUPS-100 liver access set

ruptured disc curette

Rusch
>R. bag
>R. bougie
>R. catheter

R. coudé catheter
R. endotracheal tube cuff
R. external catheter
R. laryngectomy tube
R. leg bag
R. red rubber rectal tube
R. stent
**Ruschelit polyvinyl chloride
endotracheal tube**
Rusch-Foley catheter
Rush
R. awl reamer
R. driver-bender-extractor
R. intramedullary fixation pin
R. intramedullary nail
R. mallet
R. pin nail
R. pin reamer awl
R. rod
Ruskin
R. bone-cutting forceps
R. bone rongeur
R. mastoid rongeur
R. rongeur
R. rongeur forceps
Ruskin-Liston
R.-L. bone-cutting forceps
R.-L. bone rongeur
Ruskin-Rowland
R.-R. bone-cutting forceps
R.-R. bone rongeur
Russell
R. gastrostomy kit
R. gastrostomy tray
R. peel-away sheath dilator
Russell-Taylor
R.-T. delta rod
R.-T. delta tibial nail
R.-T. femoral interlocking nail
system
R.-T. interlocking medullary nail
R.-T. interlocking nail
instrumentation
R.-T. screw
Russian Péan forceps
Rust amputation saw
ruthenium-106 ophthalmic plaque

Rutkow sutureless plug and patch
Rutner
R. biopsy needle
R. Foley-Tractor
R. stone extractor
R. wedge catheter
Rutzen ileostomy bag
RVAD
right ventricular assist device
RVAD centrifugal right ventricular
assist device
R-Value exercise ball
RX
rapid exchange
RX Acculink carotid stent system
RX CrossSail coronary dilatation
catheter
RX Herculink 14 biliary stent
system
RX Herculink plus
RX Herculink Plus biliary stent
system
RX Multilink coronary stent
system
RX perfusion catheter
RX stent delivery system
RX Streak balloon catheter
Rx
Rx Comfort sock
Rx medibottle
Rx5000 cardiac pacing system
Rx90 smooth femoral system
**RxFISH DNA probe and analysis
system**
RX Herculink 14
Rycroft
R. cannula
R. needle
R. tying forceps
Rydell nail
Ryder needle holder
Ryle tube
RZ
RZ extended chin implant
RZ jowl implant
RZ mandibular angle
RZ mandibular matrix system

S7

S. AVE stent
S. coronary stent

S660

S660 coronary stent
S660 coronary stent system
S660 small vessel coronary stent
S660 with Discrete Technology
coronary stent system

S670

S670 coronary stent
S670 over-the-wire coronary stent
S670 stent
S670 with Discrete Technology
coronary stent system

**S-1 biodegradable anterior cervical
system**
S4 excimer laser
SA60AT intraocular lens
Saalfield expressor
Saba pulley
Sabel cast walker
Saber

S. Bisector ArthroWand
S. BT blunt-tip surgical trocar
S. lumbar I/F cage system

saber-back scissors
saber-toothed cannula
Sabina lift
sable

s. brush
S. PTCA balloon catheter

Sabolich

S. above-knee socket system
S. socket

Sabra

S. 45-degree dental handpiece
S. OMS 45

Sabre

S. All-In-One otoscope
S. FreeHand high-intensity medical
pocket light
S. sling

Sabreloc

S. needle
S. spatula needle

**SabreSource realtime imaging guidance
system**
sac

entrapment s.
Lap S.
Pleatman s.

SACH

solid ankle cushioned heel
SACH foot

SACH foot adapter
SACH orthopaedic appliance
SACH prosthesis

Sachs

S. dural hook
S. dural separator
S. nerve separator
S. spatula
S. tissue forceps

sack

entrapment s.
nylon surgical s.
Pleatman s.

Sacks

S. QuickStick catheter
S. Single-Step catheter

Sacks-Vine

S.-V. gastrostomy kit
S.-V. PEG system
S.-V. PEG tube

Sacks-Vine-type PEG
sacral

s. alar screw
S. DISH pressure relief back
cushion
s. docking sheath
s. pedicle screw
s. segmental nerve stimulation
implantable neural prosthesis
s. spine modular instrumentation
s. spine Universal instrumentation
s. support

sacroiliac

s. cinch belt
s. orthosis

saddle

basal block cervical s.
cervical s.
s. clamp
Cloward surgical s.
s. coil
s. locator
s. prosthesis

saddlebag

Seidel s.

Saeed

S. multiband ligator
S. multiple ligator
S. six-shooter
S. six-shooter ligator
S. six-shooter multi-band ligator
S. ten-shooter

Saenger ovum forceps
Safar bronchoscope
Saf-Clens wound cleanser

S

Safe
    S. & Dry diaper
    S. & Dry pant
    S. & Dry undergarment
    S. & Dry underpad
    S. Ear curette
    S. Step blood collection needle
SafeCrit microhematocrit tube
Safe-Cuff blood pressure cuff
SafeFlo IVC filter
Safeguard post-hemostasis device
SAFE kit
Safescraper bone scraper
Safeset blood sampling system
Safe-Steer
    S.-S. guidewire
    S.-S. support catheter
    S.-S. system
Safestretch incontinence system
Safetex tube
Safe-T-Flex enteral feeding container
Safe-T Mate anti-rollback device
Safe-T-Tube
    Montgomery S.-T-T.
SafeTway pediatric mouthpiece
Safe-T-Wheel pinwheel
safety
    S. AV fistula needle
    s. belt
    S. Clear Plus endotracheal tube
    s. glasses
    s. guidewire
    s. handle
    s. J-wire
    s. lens
    s. pin
    s. pin closer
    s. pin splint
    s. plate
    s. spectacles
SafetySure transfer gurney
Safe-Wrap gauze
Saf-Gel hydrogel dressing
SAFHS
    sonic accelerated fracture healing system
    SAFHS 2000 sonic accelerated
      fracture healing system
    SAFHS ultrasound device
Safil synthetic absorbable surgical suture
SAF prosthesis
Safsite
    S. IV therapy system
    S. valve
Saf-T-Coil
    S.-T.-C. intrauterine device
    S.-T.-C. IUD
Saf-T E-Z set

Saf-T-Intima intravenous catheter safety system
SAF-T shield
Sage driver-extractor
Sager
    S. Combo-Pac adult/child and
      infant splint
    S. S304 bilateral splint
    S. S300 infant bilateral splint
    S. 2301 single splint
    S. traction splint
Sagian 180 CO2 incubator
sagittal oscillating saw
Sahara
    S. clinical bone sonometer
    S. portable bone densitometer
    S. super-absorbent reusable
      underpad
Sakura
    S. Finetek Tissue-Tek VIP 300E
      automatic tissue processor
    S. Seiki Autosmear automatic
      smear machine
Salah sternal puncture needle
SAL catheter
Salem
    S. pump
    S. sump double-lumen polyvinyl
      tube
    S. sump drain
    S. sump tube
Salenius meniscus knife
SalEst preterm labor test system
SaliCept freeze-dried dressing
saline
    s. dressing
    Dulbecco phosphate buffered s.
    Grossan nasal irrigator tip with
      Water Pik and s.
saline-filled
    s.-f. anatomical breast implant
    s.-f. expander
    s.-f. round breast implant
saline-saturated wool dressing
salivary bypass tube
Salman FES stent
salmon patch
Salonpas pain relief patch
salpingograph
    Schultze s.
Salter sling
Salubria nerve cuff
Salute fixation system
Salvati proctoscope
Salzburg
    S. biconcave washer
    S. screw
Salz nucleus splitter

SAM
subcutaneous augmentation material
SAM facial implant
SAM facial implant material
SAM OnScene patient assessment guide
SAM splint
SAM system

Sam
S. Jr. posture analyzer
S. Roberts esophagoscope
S. Sling pelvic belt
S. splint

Samadhi cushion
SAMBA imaging system
Sammons biplane goniometer
SampleMASTER biopsy needle
sampler
Accellon s.
air s.
Cervex-Brush cervical cell s.
Cordguard umbilical cord s.
Cytobrush Plus endocervical cell s.
Digene cervical s.
Endocell endometrial cell s.
Endopap endometrial s.
inertial suction s.
Johnson swab s.
personal air s.
Rotorod s.
Sartorious air s.
Sartorius air s.
SelectCells Mini endometrial s.
Wallach Endocell endometrial cell s.

Samsung Medical Center-type collimator cone
Samuels
S. forceps
S. hemoclip
S. hemoclip-applying forceps

Sanchez-Bulnes lacrimal sac retractor
Sanchez-Perez cassette changer
sandal
Benefoot & Birkenstock orthotic s.
Dr. Scholl's exercise s.
exercise s.

Sandalthotics
Foot Levelers S.
S. postural support orthotic

sandbag
neonatal s.
pediatric s.

Sanders
S. bed
S. jet respirator
S. Venturi injector system

Sanders-Castroviejo suturing forceps
Sand-Eze EGD pillow

Sandhill
S. esophageal motility system
S. probe

Sandhill-800 TDS chart recorder
Sandman system
Sandow apparatus
Sandoz
S. balloon replacement tube
S. balloon replacement tube
S. Caluso PEG gastrostomy tube
S. Caluso super PEG
S. feeding/suction tube
S. nasogastric feeding tube
S. suction/feeding tube

sandpaper dermabrader
Sandt forceps
sandwich-type splint
Sani-Cloth
S.-C. HB disposable wipe
S.-C. Plus germicidal disposable wipe

Sani-Grinder
Sani-Spec vaginal speculum
Sani Vac
Sano clip applier
SANS
Stoller afferent nerve stimulation system
PerQ SANS

Santa Barbara thumb splint
Santyl
S. enzymatic débrider
S. enzymatic débriding agent

sap
Prentif cavity-rim cervical s.

saphenous vein cannula
SAPHfinder surgical balloon dissector
SaphLITE saphenous vein system
SAPHtrak
S. balloon dissection system
S. balloon dissector

sapphire
s. crystal infrared photocoagulator
s. knife
s. lens
S. 2000 micropigmentation handpiece
S. table
S. View arthroscope

Saratoga
S. cycle
S. sump catheter

Sarfarazi dual optic intraocular lens
Sargon implant
Sarmiento
S. brace
S. cast
S. STH-2 hip prosthesis

Sarns
S. aortic arch cannula

Sarns (*continued*)
S. electric saw
S. intracardiac suction tube
S. 7000 MDX roller pump
S. membrane oxygenator
S. Siok II blood pump
S. soft-flow aortic cannula
S. 2-stage cannula
S. temperature probe
S. venous drainage cannula
S. ventricular assist device
S. wire-reinforced catheter

Sarot
S. arterial clamp
S. arterial forceps
S. bronchus clamp
S. needle holder

Sartorious air sampler
Sartorius
S. air sampler
S. breast pump

Sartorius SM 111
SAS
Ethicon SAS
SAS II brace
SAS Rota test
SAS shoe

Saso variable speed massager
**SA 3100 surface area and pore size
analyzer**
**Sat-A-Lite contoured wedge seat
cushion**
Satalite cushion by Bodyline
Satellite
S. Plus pulse oximeter
S. spirometer

Saticon vacuum chamber pickup tube
SatinCrescent
S. implant knife
S. tunneler

SatinShortCut implant knife
Satinsky
S. anastomosis clamp
S. aortic clamp
S. clamp
S. forceps
S. pediatric clamp
S. vascular clamp
S. vena cava clamp
S. vena caval scissors

SatinSlit
S. implant knife
S. keratome

Sato
S. cataract needle
S. corneal knife
S. lid retractor

Satterlee
S. amputating saw

S. aseptic saw
S. bone saw
S. bone saw blade

Sattler advancement forceps
saturated calomel electrode
SaturEyes contact lens
Saturn carpal tunnel splint
Satvioni cryptoscope
Saucony shoe
Sauer
S. corneal débrider
S. infant eye speculum
S. suture forceps
S. suturing forceps

Sauerbruch
S. rib elevator
S. rib forceps

Sauflon
S. PW contact lens
S. PW hydrophilic contact lens
S. PW lens

Sauna
Aromist Personal Steam S.

Saunders
S. cervical HomeTrac
S. cervical HomeTrac traction
S. mobilization wedge
S. sacroiliac belt
S. traction

Saupe cilia forceps
Sauvage filamentous velour graft
SAV
supraanular valve

Savage intestinal decompressor
Savant
S. imaging system
S. Speed-Vac drier

Savary
S. bronchoscope
S. dilator
S. esophageal dilator
S. tapered thermoplastic dilator

Savary-Gilliard
S.-G. dilator
S.-G. esophageal dilator
S.-G. metal olive
S.-G. over-the-wire dilator
S.-G. Silastic flexible bougie
S.-G. tip
S.-G. wire guide
S.-G. wire-guided bougie

Save-A-Tooth tooth preserving system
saver
Cell S.
Haemonetics Cell S.
knee s.

Saverburger irrigation/aspiration tip
SAVVI pacemaker
Savvy PTA dilatation catheter

saw

Accutome low-speed diamond s.
Adams s.
Adson wire s.
Aesculap s.
air s.
air-driven oscillating s.
amputation s.
aseptic s.
Bailey wire s.
band s.
Bergman plaster s.
Bier amputation s.
bone s.
Buehler Isomet low-speed s.
cast s.
chain s.
Charriere amputation s.
Charriere aseptic metacarpal s.
Charriere bone s.
Clerf laryngeal s.
Converse nasal s.
Cottle s.
Cottle-Joseph s.
Cottle Universal nasal s.
crown s.
Delrin-handle bone s.
DeMartel wire s.
diamond wafering s.
electric laryngofissure s.
Engel plaster s.
Farabeuf s.
Farrior-Joseph bayonet s.
Farrior-Joseph nasal s.
fine-tooth electric s.
finger ring s.
Gigli s.
Gigli solid-handle s.
Gigli-Strully s.
Gigli wire s.
gold s.
Goldman s.
Gottschalk transverse s.
Guilford-Wright bur s.
Guilford-Wullstein bur s.
Hall sagittal s.
Hall Versipower oscillating s.
Hall Versipower reciprocating s.
s. handle
helical tube s.
Hough-Wullstein bur s.
humeral s.
Isomet low-speed s.
Isomet Plus precision s.
Joseph bayonet s.
Joseph-Maltz s.
Joseph nasal s.
Langenbeck s.
Langenbeck bone s.

Langenbeck metacarpal s.
Langenbeck metacarpal
  amputation s.
laryngeal s.
Lebsche wire s.
Leica model 1600 water-cooled
  diamond s.
Lell laryngofissure s.
Luck bone s.
Macewen s.
Magnuson circular twin s.
Magnuson double counter-rotating s.
Magnuson single circular s.
Maltz s.
McCabe crurotomy s.
metacarpal s.
Micro-Aire oscillating s.
Micro-Aire oscillating bone s.
microsagittal s.
Miltex bone s.
Müller s.
nasal s.
Olivecrona wire s.
Orthair oscillating s.
Osada s.
oscillating s.
Oto-Flex crura s.
patella bone s.
Percy amputating s.
plaster s.
reciprocating s.
ring-cutting s.
rotary hub s.
round Gigli s.
Rust amputation s.
sagittal oscillating s.
Sarns electric s.
Satterlee amputating s.
Satterlee aseptic s.
Satterlee bone s.
Seltzer s.
Shrady s.
single-sided bone s.
Skil s.
Sklar bone s.
Slaughter s.
spinal s.
sternal s.
sternum s.
Stiwer finger-ring s.
Stryker s.
Stryker autopsy s.
surgical s.
threadwire s.
triton reciprocating s.
Tuke s.
Weiss amputation s.
Wigmore plaster s.
wire s.

S

saw *(continued)*
    Xomed micro-oscillating s.
    Zimmer Micro 100 reciprocating s.
Sawa shoulder brace
sawblade
    Stablecut s.
sawdust bed
Sawtell
    S. artery forceps
    S. tonsil hemostat
Sawtell-Tobold laryngeal applicator
saw-toothed curette
Sawyer
    S. extractor
    S. rectal retractor
    S. rectal speculum
Sayre
    S. double-end periosteal elevator
    S. elevator
    S. jacket
    S. periosteal rasp
    S. suspension apparatus
    S. suspension traction
Sbarbaro tibial prosthesis
SBI Universal Hand System
SC-1 needle
SC-210 sidestream capnograph
SC-300 portable capnograph
SC60B-OUV IOL
Scabbard needle
SC-AcuFix
    SC-A. anterior cervical plate system
    SC-A. ThinLine plate
scaffold, scaffolding
    bioabsorbable mesh s.
    biodegradable s.
    biodegradable polymer s.
    collagen s.
    3-dimensional biocompatible s.
    Graftjacket acellular periosteum replacement s.
    Graftjacket rotator cuff tendon reinforcement s.
    resorbable s.
scalar lead
scale
    Attache food s.
    balance beam s.
    bedside s.
    dBA s.
    electronic s.
    Health O Meter s.
    Kenna Knee S.
    linear visual analog s.
    Magnum food s.
    Scotty the Scale stand-on s.
scaler
    Amdent ultrasonic s.

    Cavitron SPS ultrasonic s.
    Columbia s.
    dental s.
    loop s.
    sickle s.
    Steele s.
    straight sickle s.
    Titan s.
    ultrasonic s.
    ultrasonic piezoelectric s.
    Younger-Good s.
scaling device
scalp
    s. clip-applying forceps
    s. electrode
    s. hemostasis clip
    s. self-retaining retractor
    s. vein needle
scalpel
    ASR s.
    Bard-Parker s.
    blade s.
    bone s.
    Bowen double-bladed s.
    carbon dioxide laser s.
    Cobalt s.
    Contact Laser s.
    disposable s.
    s. electrode
    Electrodes s.
    electrosurgical s.
    Endo-Assist retractable s.
    Endotron-Lipectron ultrasonic s.
    Epitome s.
    Feather s.
    s. guard
    s. handle
    Harmonic S.
    John Green pendulum s.
    laser s.
    LaserSonics Nd:YAG Laserblade s.
    lid s.
    long s.
    Microcap s.
    pendulum s.
    Personna Plus disposable Teflon s.
    plasma s.
    Pre-Cision miniature and microminiature s.
    razor s.
    sculpturing s.
    Shaw hemostatic s.
    UltraCision harmonic s.
    ultrasonic s.
    ultrasonically activated s.
    ultrasonic harmonic s.
    ultrasonic suction s.
    water s.

scan
    cine s.
    color Doppler s.
    dipyridamole thallium-201 s.
    fluorescence-activated cell sorter s.
    gadolinium s.
    multiple gated acquisition s.
    Ophthascan Mini-A s.
    OTI ultrasound B & A s.
    S. Pattern generator
    portal-phased spiral CT s.
    postgadolinium s.
    ProstaScint s.
    proton-density axial MR s.
    septal hyperperfusion on thallium s.
    S. spray dressing
    T2-weighted s.
    S. ultrasound gel
    US-2000 echo s.
    ZeroRad MRI s.
Scanditronix
    S. 1024-7B camera
    S. MLC system
    S. PET scanner
Scanlan aneurysm clip
Scanlan-Crafoord contractor
ScanLite scanner
ScanMaker 4 flatbed scanner
Scanmaster
    S. D, DX x-ray film digitizer
    S. DX system
    S. DX x-ray film digitizer scanner
scanned-slot detector system
scanner
    AccuScan CO_2 laser s.
    Acoma s.
    Acuson 128EP s.
    Acuson Sequoia 512 s.
    Acuson ultrasound s.
    Advanced NMR Systems s.
    Agfa Medical s.
    All-Tronics s.
    Aloka 650 s.
    Aloka SSD-720 real-time s.
    Aloka 650 ultrasound s.
    Aloka ultrasound linear s.
    Aloka ultrasound sector s.
    American Shared-CuraCare s.
    ANMR Insta-scan MR s.
    Aquilion combined CT-
      fluoroscopy s.
    Aquilion plus V-detector CT s.
    Artoscan MRI s.
    ATL-HDL color-flow Doppler s.
    ATL Mark 600 real-time sector s.
    ATL Neurosector real-time s.
    Aura Laser helical s.
    Aurora MR breast imaging
      system s.

    Bergmann Optical laser s.
    BioSpec MR imaging system s.
    BladderManager portable
      ultrasound s.
    BladderScan BVI2500 ultrasound s.
    Brüel & Kjaer ultrasound s.
    Bruker s.
    Canon s.
    CardiArc SPECT s.
    Cardio Data MK3 Holter s.
    cardiovascular computed
      tomographic s.
    Cemax/Icon s.
    Cencit facial s.
    Cencit surface s.
    charge-coupled device s.
    cine CT s.
    C-150 LXP EBT s.
    combined CT-fluoroscopy s.
    conventional static s.
    Corometrics Doppler s.
    C-PET s.
    CT9000, 9800 s.
    CT body s.
    CTI 933/04 ECAT s.
    CTI 931 PET s.
    CTI positron emission
      tomography s.
    CT Max 640 s.
    CT Twin s.
    dedicated head s.
    dedicated PET s.
    Delarnette s.
    Del Mar Avionics s.
    DermaTemp DT-1000 infrared
      temperature s.
    Diasonics ultrasound s.
    digital slide s.
    Dine digital s.
    Discovery LS, ST^4 PET/CT s.
    Dornier s.
    3D surface digitizer s.
    dual-probe rectilinear s.
    DuPont s.
    dynamic spatial reconstructor s.
    Eastman Kodak s.
    EBT s.
    ECAT 951/33 PET s.
    Echospeed Signa LX s.
    electron beam CT s.
    8000-element linear array CCD s.
    Elscint Excel 905 s.
    Elscint MR s.
    Elscint Twin CT s.
    EMED s.
    EMI 7070 s.
    EMI brain s.
    EMI CT 500 s.
    Epson 3200 Perfect S.

S

scanner *(continued)*

Esaote extremity s.
EUB-405 ultrasound s.
Evolution s.
Evolution CT s.
Evolution XP s.
Flexart MRI s.
Fonar-360 MRI s.
Fonar Quad MRI s.
Fonar Stand-Up MRI s.
full ring s.
Galen Scan s.
gamma ray s.
Gammex RMI s.
gated CT s.
GE Advance PET s.
GE 9800 CT s.
GE CT Advantage s.
GE CTI 9800 s.
GE CTI single detector s.
GE CT Max s.
GE CT Pace s.
GE 8800 CT/T s.
GE CT/T7 s.
GE CT/T 8800 s.
GE Genesis CT s.
GE GN 500-MHz s.
GE 9800 high-resolution CT s.
GE HiSpeed Advantage helical
  CT s.
GE HiSpeed single detector s.
GE Lightspeed CT s.
GE MR Max s.
GE MR Signa s.
GE MR Vectra s.
General Electric Signa s.
GE Omega 500-MHz s.
GE Pace CT s.
GE QE 300-MHz s.
GE Quest 300-H s.
GE Signa s.
GE Signa Horizon SR 120 whole-
  body s.
GE Signa 4.7 MRI s.
GE Signa 5.2 with SR-230 3-axis
  EPI gradient upgrade s.
GE Spiral CT s.
GE Vectra MR s.
GF-UM3 s.
Gyroscan ACS-NT MR s.
Gyroscan ACS-NT MRI s.
Gyroscan Interna s.
Gyroscan S15 s.
Harvard multidetector s.
Heidelberg laser tomographic s.
helical CT s.
Hewlett-Packard s.
Hewlett-Packard 177020 A phased-
  array sector s.

Hewlett-Packard phased-array
  sector s.
high-field open MRI s.
high-field-strength s.
high-resolution real-time s.
HighSpeed CT s.
HiLight Advantage System CT s.
HiSpeed Advantage helical s.
HiSpeed Advantage System CT s.
HiSpeed CT s.
Hitachi CT s.
Hitachi CT, MR s.
Hitachi MR s.
Hitachi Open MRI system s.
Hitachi 0.3-T unit s.
Hologic 2000 s.
Hologic QDR 1000W dual-energy
  x-ray absorptiometry s.
Horizon LX s.
Howtek Scanmaster DX s.
IDSI s.
Imatron C-100 EBT s.
Imatron C-150L EBCT s.
Imatron CT s.
Imatron C-100 Ultrafast CT s.
Imatron C-150XL CT s.
Imatron C-100XP CT s.
Imatron Fastrac C-100 cine x-ray
  CT s.
Imatron Ultrafast CT s.
Indomitable s.
infrared liver s.
Innervision MR s.
InstaScan s.
Integris 3000 s.
intensified radiographic imaging
  system s.
Irex Exemplar ultrasound s.
iris s.
iStep FIT digital s.
Konica KFDR-S laser film s.
Kretz Combison 330 ultrasound s.
Kretz 311 ultrasound s.
large-bore imaging system s.
LightSpeed CT s.
LightSpeed multidetector CT s.
LightSpeed QX/i s.
linear-array convex array s.
linear convex array s.
low-field MR s.
Lumiscan LS 85 s.
Lumisys 20 digital x-ray s.
Lunar s.
Lunar DPX total-body s.
lutetium oxyorthosilicate-based
  PET s.
LymphoScan nuclear imaging
  system s.
3M s.

Magna-SL s.
Magnes 2500 whole-blood s.
Magnetom Open s.
Magnetom SP63 s.
Magnetom Symphony MR s.
Magnetom Vision s.
Magnex MR s.
Mallinckrodt s.
Malvern 2600 Sizer laser
  diffraction s.
Max Plus MR s.
MedImage s.
Medison s.
Medspec MR imaging system s.
Medspec 30/80 tesla MR s.
MedX s.
megavoltage computed
  tomography s.
megavoltage CT s.
7.5 MHz sector s.
microCT-20 s.
Microtek ScanMaker 9600XL s.
midget MRI s.
MKII automated s.
mobile spiral computed
  tomography s.
modified electron-beam CT s.
mPower PET s.
MR catheter imaging and
  spectroscopy system s.
multidetector CT s.
multidetector helical s.
multiple jointed digitizer s.
multisensor structured light-range
  digitizer s.
multislice CT s.
neurodiagnostic s.
NeuroFOCUS s.
NewTom CT s.
Nishimoto Sangyo s.
Norland pQCT XCT2000 s.
nuclear s.
Olympus endoscopic ultrasound s.
OmniMedia XRS s.
Open Sky MRI s.
Oxford large-bore imaging
  system s.
Pace Plus System s.
Park Medical Systems s.
partial-ring bismuth germanate-
  crystal s.
Perception s.
PET/CT s.
PET full-ring s.
PETT VI PET s.
Pfizer 200 FS 400 s.
Philips Gyroscan ACS, NT, NT5,
  NT15, S5, T5 s.
Philips Gyroscan NT-series s.

Philips Medical Systems Tomoscan
  AVE1 CT spiral s.
Philips Medical Systems Tomoscan
  SR 7000 CT spiral s.
Philips 1.5 NT-Intera s.
Philips spiral CT s.
Philips 1.5-T NT MR s.
Philips Tomoscan 310 CT s.
Philips Tomoscan 350, SR 6000
  CT s.
Philips Tomoscan SR 6000 CT s.
Philips 4.7-T small-bore system s.
Picker s.
Picker CS, CT, MR s.
Picker Edge 1.5-T s.
Picker MR s.
Picker PQ 2000 CT s.
Picker PQ helical CT s.
Picker PQ 5000 helical CT s.
Picker PQ 2000 spiral CT s.
Picker Prism 3000 PET s.
Picker Synerview 600 s.
Picker Vista HPQ MRI s.
Picker Vista MagnaScanner s.
Polhemus 3D digitizer s.
Posicam HZ PET s.
PQ 5000 CT s.
pQCT s.
ProSpeed CT s.
Quad 7000, 12000 high-field open
  MRI s.
Quick CT9800 s.
real-time B s.
rectilinear s.
ring s.
RT 3200 Advantage ultrasound s.
RT 6800 ultrasound s.
Scanditronix PET s.
ScanLite s.
ScanMaker 4 flatbed s.
Scanmaster DX x-ray film
  digitizer s.
scintillation s.
scintiscanner s.
SCU-1200, SCU-2200 digital color
  ultrasound s.
SDCT s.
sector s.
SFP s.
Shimadzu CT s.
Shimadzu MR s.
Siemens DRH CT s.
Siemens Ecat EXACT HR+ CTI
  PET s.
Siemens ECAT 951/31R PET s.
Siemens Impact Expert MRI s.
Siemens Impact Expert Tesla s.
Siemens Magnetom s.
Siemens Magnetom GBS II s.

scanner *(continued)*
Siemens Magnetom Harmony s.
Siemens Magnetom SP 4000 s.
Siemens Magnetom Vision s.
Siemens One Tesla s.
Siemens Plus 4 Volume Zoom
multidetector s.
Siemens Somaform 512 CT s.
Siemens Somatom DR CT s.
Siemens Somatom DR2, DR3
whole-body s.
Siemens Somatom Plus 4A s.
Siemens Somatom Plus CT s.
Siemens Sonoline Elegra
ultrasound s.
Siemens Symphony s.
Siemens Vision s.
SieScape ultrasound s.
Signa s.
Signa Horizon LX SR 77
gradients MR s.
Signa LX s.
Signa MRI s.
Signa superconducting magnetic
resonance imaging s.
Signa VH/i3.0-T MR s.
SilkTouch CO_2 laser s.
single-detector helical s.
single-detector row s.
small-bore s.
Somatom DR CT s.
Somatom Plus S whole body s.
SonoHeart s.
Sonoline Siemens ultrasound s.
Sonos 1500, 2500 s.
spiral CT s.
spiral CT, XCT s.
spiral XCT s.
supercam scintillation s.
Swissray s.
Symbia TruePoint SPECT-CT s.
TCT900S helical CT s.
Technicare Delta 2020 s.
Tecmag Libra-S16 system s.
tesla GE Signa whole-body s.
thermographic s.
tomographic multiplane s.
Tomoscan AVEU spiral CT s.
Tomoscan SR 7000 s.
Toshiba s.
Toshiba brain s.
Toshiba helical CT s.
Toshiba MR s.
Toshiba 900S helical CT s.
Toshiba 900S/XII s.
Toshiba TCT-80 CT s.
Toshiba Xpress SX helical CT s.
Toshiba X-Vigor s.
Toshiba Xvision s.

Trionix s.
4T whole-body GI Signa MRI s.
twin Flash s.
ultrafast computed tomographic s.
ultrafast computed tomography s.
ultrafast CT s.
Ultramark s.
ultrasound bone imaging s. (UBIS)
UltraSure DTU-1 ultrasound s.
UM 4 real-time sector s.
Varian CT s.
Vidar s.
Vision Siemens MRI s.
Vision Ten V-scan s.
whole-body digital s.
whole-body MRI system s.
whole-body Siemens Vision s.
whole-body Tesla s.
Xpress/SW helical CT s.
Xpress/SX helical CT s.
X-Vigor CT s.
Zeiss-Humphrey UBM s.

scanning
s. acoustic microscope
s. arm
s. beam digital system
s. electron microscope
s. excimer laser
s. fluorometer
s. laser acoustic microscope
s. laser ophthalmoscope
s. laser polarimeter
MEVA Probe for endovaginal s.
s. prism
s. slit confocal microscope
s. transmission electron microscope
s. tunneling microscope

scanning-beam digital x-ray

Scanpor
S. acrylate adhesive
S. surgical tape
S. tape

Scanzoni forceps

scapel

scaphoid
s. pad
s. screw guide

Scappa frame

scapular retractor

scarf bandage

Scar Fx lightweight silicone sheeting

scarifier
Berkeley s.
Graefe s.
Kuhnt corneal s.

scarifying curette

scarlet red gauze dressing

scattergram

scatter grid

scattering
s. foil
s. foil compensator
s. system
scavenger
LySonix Diamond Tip s.
scavenging
s. device
s. tube
SCD
sequential compression device
SCD stocking
Scepter system
Schaaf foreign body forceps
Schachar lens
Schachne-Desmarres lid everter
Schachowa spiral tube
Schaedel
S. clip
S. cross-action towel clamp
Schaltenbrand-Wahren stereotactic atlas
Schamberg
S. comedo extractor
S. expressor
Schanz
S. pin
S. Scheie blade
S. screw
Schatzker fracture classification system
Schatzki ring
Schatz-Palmaz intravascular stent
Schede bone curette
Scheie
S. anterior chamber cannula
S. blade
S. cataract aspirating needle
S. electrocautery
S. goniopuncture knife
Scheie-Westcott corneal section scissors
Scheimpflug camera
Schell bone rongeur
Schenck arcuate splint
Schepens
S. forceps
S. orbital retractor
S. retinal detachment unit
S. scleral depressor
S. spoon
Schepens-Pomerantzeff ophthalmoscope
Schick back support
Schiek Belt
Schilder plugger
Schindler esophagoscope
Schink
S. dermatome
S. metatarsal retraction
S. metatarsal retractor

Schiötz
S. tonofilm
S. tonometer
Schirmer
S. filter paper
S. tear test strip
Schlein
S. clamp
S. shoulder holder
S. shoulder positioner
Schlesinger
S. cervical punch
S. cervical punch forceps
S. cervical rongeur
S. clamp
S. instrument
S. intervertebral disc forceps
S. intervertebral disc rongeur
S. rongeur forceps
schlieren microscope
Schmidt optics system
Schmitt fan
Schmitz-Rode catheter
Schneider
S. driver-extractor
S. enteral stent
S. esophageal Wallstent
S. extractor-driver
S. Guider catheter
S. Speedy stent
S. stent
S. Wallstent
S. Wallstent biliary endoprosthesis
Schneider-Meier-Magnum system
Schnidt
S. clamp
S. hemostat
S. thoracic forceps
Schoborg nephrostomy catheter/stent
Schocket
S. scleral depressor
S. tube implant
Schoemaker
S. intestinal clamp
S. scissors
Schoemaker-Loth scissors
Scholander apparatus
Scholar II vital sign monitor
Scholl pad
Scholten
S. biopsy forceps
S. endomyocardial biopsy forceps
S. endomyocardial bioptome
S. sternal retractor
Schonander film changer
SchonCath chronic dialysis catheter
Schoonmaker multipurpose catheter
Schott lid speculum

S

Schroeder
    S. tenaculum loop
    S. uterine curette
    S. uterine tenaculum
    S. uterine vulsellum forceps
    S. vulsellum
Schroeder-Braun uterine forceps
Schrötter catheter
Schrudde rotational flap
Schubert
    S. cervical biopsy forceps
    S. uterine biopsy forceps
    S. uterine biopsy punch
Schuco nebulizer
Schueler Model 200 Aspirator
Schuknecht
    S. retractor
    S. roller knife
    S. suction tube
    S. Teflon wire piston prosthesis
    S. wire-cutting scissors
Schultz anterior capsule nibbler
Schultze
    S. salpingograph
    S. scissors
Schumacher
    S. biopsy forceps
    S. sternal shears
    S. umbilical cord scissors
Schumann giant-type eye magnet
Schuring ossicular implant
Schwaber otologic implant
Schwarten
    S. LP guidewire
    S. Microglide LP balloon
Schwartz
    S. clamp
    S. clip-applying forceps
    S. plate
    S. temporary clamp-applying
        forceps
Schwartze chisel
Schwarz
    S. arrow-forming pliers
    S. bow-type activator
    S. finger extension bow
Schweigger
    S. capsule forceps
    S. hand perimeter
Schwinn
    S. Airdyne bicycle
    S. bi-directional Windjammer upper
        body cycle
    S. elliptical full body exercise
        machine
    S. Fitness Advisor
    S. Spinner bicycle
    S. 900 stationary bicycle
sciatic nerve retractor

Sci-Med
    S.-M. Express Monorail balloon
    S.-M. extracorporeal silicone rubber
        reservoir
    S.-M. Life Systems, Inc. membrane
        artificial lung
Scimed
    S. angioplasty catheter
    S. guiding catheter
    S. stent
scimitar blade
**Scinticore multicrystal scintillation
    camera**
scintigraphic balloon
scintillation
    s. camera
    s. counter
    s. probe
    s. scanner
    s. spectrometer
scintillator
    benzene s.
    cyclohexane s.
    organic liquid s.
**scintimammography prone breast
    cushion**
scintiscanner scanner
Scintiview nuclear computer system
Scintron IV nuclear computer system
scissors (*See also* shears)
    abdominal s.
    Adson ganglion s.
    Aebli corneal s.
    alligator s.
    angled cartilage s.
    angular s.
    Anis corneal s.
    anterior chamber synechia s.
    AROSupercut s.
    arteriotomy s.
    Arthroforce hook s.
    Aslan endoscopic s.
    Assistant Free orthopaedic s.
    Atkinson corneal s.
    Aufricht s.
    Babcock wire-cutting s.
    baby Metzenbaum s.
    ball tipped s.
    bandage s.
    Bantam wire-cutting s.
    Barraquer corneoscleral s.
    Barraquer iris s.
    Barraquer vitreous strand s.
    bayonet s.
    beaded-tip s.
    Beall circumflex artery s.
    Becker corneal section spatulated s.
    Becker septal s.
    Beckman nasal s.

Beebe wire-cutting s.
Bellucci s.
Bellucci alligator s.
Berens corneal transplant s.
Berens iridocapsulotomy s.
bipolar cautery s.
bipolar electrosurgical s.
blepharoplasty s.
blunt Metzenbaum s.
blunt-tipped Vannas s.
Boettcher tonsil s.
Bonn iris s.
brain s.
Braun episiotomy s.
Braun-Stadler episiotomy s.
Brophy s.
bulldog s.
Busch umbilical cord s.
calcified tissue s.
canalicular s.
cannular s.
Caplan nasal bone s.
capsulotomy s.
cardiovascular s.
cartilage s.
Castanares facelift s.
Castroviejo anterior synechia s.
Castroviejo corneal section s.
Castroviejo corneal transplant s.
Castroviejo iridocapsulotomy s.
Castroviejo keratoplasty s.
Castroviejo synechia s.
Castroviejo-Troutman s.
Castroviejo-Vannas capsulotomy s.
cataract s.
Chadwick s.
Church deep surgery s.
circumflex artery s.
Classon pediatric s.
Codman s.
Cohan-Vannas iris s.
Cohan-Westcott s.
Cohney s.
cold s.
collar s.
collar and crown s.
conjunctival s.
Converse nasal tip s.
Converse plastic surgery s.
Converse-Wilmer conjunctival s.
Cooley arteriotomy s.
Cooley cardiovascular s.
corneal section spatulated s.
corneal transplant s.
corneoscleral s.
coronary artery s.
Cottle angular s.
Cottle bulldog s.
Cottle dorsal s.

Cottle dressing s.
Cottle heavy septal s.
Cottle nasal s.
Crafoord lobectomy s.
Crafoord thoracic s.
craniotomy s.
crown s.
curved iris s.
curved-on-flat s.
curved operating s.
curved tenotomy s.
curved turbinate s.
curved turbinectomy s.
cuticle s.
Dandy neurosurgical s.
Dandy trigeminal s.
Davis rhytidectomy s.
Dean s.
Dean dissecting s.
Dean tonsillar s.
Deaver operating s.
DeBakey endarterectomy s.
DeBakey-Metzenbaum s.
DeBakey-Potts s.
delicate operating s.
Dennis dissecting s.
de Wecker s.
de Wecker iris s.
diamond-edge Supercut s.
diathermy s.
Diethrich-Hegemann s.
dissecting s.
dissection s.
dorsal angled s.
Doyen abdominal s.
Doyen dissecting s.
Doyen-Ferguson s.
dressing s.
Dubois decapitation s.
Duffield cardiovascular s.
dural s.
ear s.
Edelstein s.
Electroscope disposable s.
electrosurgical curved s.
endarterectomy s.
endoscopic s.
enterotomy s.
enucleation s.
episiotomy s.
Esmarch bandage s.
esophageal s.
Evershears bipolar curved s.
Evershears bipolar laparoscopic s.
eye stitch s.
eye suture s.
facelift s.
facial plastic surgery s.
Ferguson abdominal s.

S

781

scissors *(continued)*
    Ferguson-Metzenbaum s.
    Fine suture s.
    Finochietto thoracic s.
    Fiskars s.
    fistula s.
    F. L. Fischer microsurgical
      neurectomy bayonet s.
    Fomon angular s.
    Fomon facelift s.
    Fomon lower lateral s.
    Fomon saber-back s.
    Fomon upper lateral s.
    s. forceps
    Frazier dural s.
    Freeman rhytidectomy s.
    Freeman-Schepens s.
    Frost s.
    gallbladder s.
    ganglion s.
    gauze s.
    Gene s.
    general utility s.
    Gibbs-Gradle s.
    Giertz-Stille s.
    Gill s.
    Gillies s.
    Gillies suture s.
    Gills-Welsh s.
    Girard corneoscleral s.
    goiter s.
    Goldman-Fox gum s.
    Goldman-Fox wound debridement s.
    Good-Reiner s.
    Gorney facelift s.
    Gorney-Freeman straight facelift s.
    Gorney rhytidectomy s.
    Gorney septal s.
    Gorney straight facelift s.
    Gorney turbinate s.
    Gradle s.
    Gradle stitch s.
    Graham deep surgery s.
    Graham pediatric s.
    Grieshaber vertical cutting s.
    Grieshaber vitreous s.
    Guggenheim-Schuknecht s.
    Guilford s.
    Guilford-Schuknecht wire-cutting s.
    guillotine s.
    Halsey nail s.
    Halsted strabismus s.
    harmonic s.
    Harrington-Mayo s.
    Harvey wire-cutting s.
    Heath clip-removing s.
    Heath suture s.
    Heath suture-cutting s.
    Heath wire-cutting s.

    heavy septal s.
    Heiss flexible endoscopic s.
    Heyman nasal s.
    Holinger curved s.
    Holmes s.
    hook s.
    hook rotary s.
    Hooper deep surgery s.
    horizontal s.
    Hough s.
    House alligator s.
    House-Bellucci alligator s.
    Hunt chalazion s.
    IMA s.
    insulated curved s.
    insulated straight s.
    iridectomy s.
    iridocapsulotomy s.
    iridotomy s.
    iris s.
    Irvine probe-pointed s.
    Jabaley-Stille Super Cut S.
    Jackson turbinate s.
    Jako microlaryngeal s.
    Jameson facelift s.
    Jansen-Middleton s.
    Jarit dissecting s.
    Jarit microsurgery s.
    Jarit peripheral vascular s.
    Jones s.
    Jones dissecting s.
    Jones IMA s.
    Jorgenson dissecting s.
    Jorgenson gallbladder s.
    Jorgenson thoracic s.
    Joseph nasal s.
    Joseph serrated s.
    Kahn s.
    Karmody venous s.
    Katzin s.
    Katzin corneal transplant s.
    Kay s.
    Kaye s.
    Kaye blepharoplasty s.
    Kaye facelift s.
    Kaye fine-dissecting s.
    Kazanjian s.
    Keeler intravitreal s.
    Kelly fistular s.
    Kelly uterine s.
    keratectomy s.
    keratoplasty s.
    Kirby s.
    Kleinsasser microlaryngeal s.
    Knapp iris s.
    Knapp strabismus s.
    Knight nasal s.
    Knowles bandage s.
    Koenig nail-splitting s.

Kurze dissecting s.
LaGrange s.
LaGrange eye s.
LaGrange sclerectomy s.
Lahey s.
Lahey Carb-Edge s.
Lahey delicate s.
Lahey dissecting s.
Lahey operating s.
Lahey thyroid s.
Lakeside nasal s.
Landolt enucleation s.
laparoscopic s.
laryngeal s.
Laschal s.
Laschal suture s.
laser tubal s.
Lawton corneal s.
left-handed cornea s.
Lexer dissecting s.
ligature s.
Lillie tonsillar s.
Lister s.
Lister bandage s.
Liston plaster-of-Paris s.
Littauer s.
Littauer dissecting s.
Littauer stitch s.
Littauer suture carrying s.
Littler dissecting s.
Littler suture-carrying s.
Lloyd-Davies rectal s.
lobectomy s.
long stitch s.
loop s.
Lorenz PC/TC s.
lung dissecting s.
Lynch s.
Malis s.
Malis neurosurgical s.
Manson-Aebli corneal section s.
marking s.
Martin ballpoint s.
Martin cartilage s.
Martin throat s.
Matarasso facelift s.
Maunoir iris s.
Max Fine s.
Mayo s.
Mayo curved s.
Mayo-Harrington dissecting s.
Mayo-Lexer s.
Mayo long dissecting s.
Mayo-Noble dissecting s.
Mayo operating s.
Mayo round blade s.
Mayo-Stille operating s.
Mayo straight s.
Mayo uterine s.

McAllister s.
McClure iris s.
McGuire corneal s.
McIndoe s.
McLean capsulotomy s.
McPherson-Castroviejo corneal
    section s.
McPherson-Castroviejo
    microcorneal s.
McPherson corneal section s.
McPherson-Vannas iris s.
McPherson-Vannas microiris s.
McPherson-Westcott conjunctival s.
McPherson-Westcott stitch s.
McReynolds pterygium s.
meatotomy s.
mechanized s.
meniscal hook s.
meniscectomy s.
meniscus s.
Metzenbaum s.
Metzenbaum dissecting s.
Metzenbaum long s.
Metzenbaum operating s.
Metzenbaum tonsillar s.
micro s.
microconjunctival s.
microcorneal s.
microiris s.
microlaryngeal s.
micromosquito curved s.
micromosquito straight s.
micropituitary s.
microscopic s.
microsurgical s.
microvascular s.
micro vertical s.
Microvit s.
micro Westcott s.
Miller rectal s.
Miltex saber-back rhytidectomy s.
Miltex stitch s.
Miltex undermining s.
mini s.
mini-keratoplasty stitch s.
mini-Westcott s.
mitral valve s.
Morris vertical s.
MPC automated intravitreal s.
Munro brain s.
myringotomy s.
nail s.
s. nail drill
nail-nipper s.
nasal s.
Nelson s.
Nelson lobectomy s.
Nelson-Metzenbaum s.
neonatal s.

S

scissors *(continued)*
    Neumann s.
    neurosurgical s.
    New suture s.
    Nicola s.
    Northbent s.
    Northbent suture s.
    Noyes iridectomy s.
    Noyes iris s.
    Nugent-Gradle s.
    Nu-Tip laparoscopic s.
    O'Brien s.
    O'Brien stitch s.
    O'Brien suture s.
    Ong capsulotomy s.
    orthopaedic s.
    Osher corneal s.
    Panzer gallbladder s.
    Par s.
    Péan s.
    Peck-Joseph s.
    pericardiotomy s.
    pinch-handle s.
    plain rotary s.
    plastic surgery s.
    plastic utility s.
    Potts s.
    Potts-Smith dissecting s.
    Potts-Smith reverse s.
    Potts tenotomy s.
    Potts vascular s.
    PowerStar bipolar s.
    s. probe
    pterygium s.
    ptosis s.
    pupillary membrane s.
    Quimby s.
    radial iridotomy s.
    Ragnell s.
    Ragnell-Kilner s.
    Ragnell undermining s.
    Ramirez EndoForehead A/M s.
    Reeh s.
    Rees facelift serrated s.
    Reichling corneal s.
    reverse s.
    reverse cutting s.
    Reynolds dissecting s.
    rhinoplasty s.
    rhytidectomy s.
    Richter s.
    right-angle s.
    right-handed corneal s.
    right/left corneoscleral s.
    Roger wire-cutting s.
    Rosenwasser medium-curve s.
    Rosenwasser strong-curve s.
    saber-back s.
    Satinsky vena caval s.

Scheie-Westcott corneal section s.
Schoemaker s.
Schoemaker-Loth s.
Schuknecht wire-cutting s.
Schultze s.
Schumacher umbilical cord s.
Seiler turbinate s.
septal s.
serrated s.
serrated iris s.
Seutin s.
Shea vein graft s.
Shield iridotomy s.
Shortbent s.
Shortbent stitch s.
Shortbent suture s.
Shutt s.
sickle s.
Sims uterine s.
Sistron s.
Sistrunk s.
Sistrunk dissecting s.
in situ valve s.
Slip-N-Snip s.
Smart enucleation s.
Smellie obstetrical s.
Smith bandage s.
Snowden-Pencer Supercut s.
Spencer s.
Spencer stitch s.
spring-handled s.
Spring iris s.
StaySharp Supercut s.
Stevens eye s.
Stevens tenotomy s.
Stille dissecting s.
Stille Super Cut s.
stitch s.
Storz stitch s.
Storz wire-cutting s.
strabismus s.
straight iris s.
straight tenotomy s.
Strulle s.
Strully dissecting s.
Supercut s.
superior radial tenotomy s.
surgical s.
Sutherland s.
Sutherland eye s.
suture s.
suture wire-cutting s.
Sweet esophageal s.
take-apart s.
Taylor brain s.
Taylor dural s.
tenotomy s.
thin-shaft nasal s.
Thomas s.

thoracic s.
Thorek thoracic s.
Thorpe s.
Thorpe-Westcott s.
tissue s.
Toennis-Adson dural s.
Toennis dissecting s.
tonsillar s.
trigeminal s.
Troutman-Castroviejo corneal
  section s.
Troutman conjunctival s.
Troutman-Katzin corneal
  transplant s.
Troutman microsurgical s.
Troutman suture s.
tubal s.
turbinate s.
turbinectomy s.
Turner-Warwick diathermy s.
umbilical s.
Universal wire s.
upper lateral s.
U.S. Army gauze s.
U.S. Army umbilical s.
uterine s.
utility s.
utility bandage s.
Vannas capsulotomy s.
Vannas corneal s.
Vannas iridocapsulotomy s.
vascular s.
Verhoeff s.
vertical spreading s.
vibrating s.
Vital-Metzenbaum s.
vitreous strand s.
Waldman episiotomy s.
Walker s.
Walker-Apple s.
Walker-Atkinson s.
Walker corneal s.
Walton s.
Webster meniscectomy s.
Wecker iris s.
Weck iris s.
Weck microsuture cutting s.
Weller cartilage s.
Werb s.
Wertheim deep surgery s.
Westcott conjunctival s.
Westcott double-end s.
Westcott micro s.
Westcott stitch s.
Westcott tenotomy s.
Westcott utility s.
White s.
Wiet otologic s.
Willauer thoracic s.

Williamson-Noble s.
Wilmer conjunctival s.
Wilmer conjunctival and utility s.
Wilmer iris s.
Wilson intraocular s.
Wincor enucleation s.
wire s.
wire-cutting s.
wire-cutting suture s.
Witherspoon vertical s.
Wong-Stall s.
Wullstein ear s.
Yankauer s.
Yasargil bayonet s.
Yasargil microvascular bayonet s.
Zaldivar iridectomy s.
Z-Scissors hysterectomy s.
SciTojet needle-free injector
scleral
  s. blade
  s. buckle
  s. buckle eye implant
  s. buckler implant
  s. buckling catheter
  s. contact lens
  s. depressor
  s. expander ring
  s. expansion band
  s. fixation light
  s. hook
  s. implant
  s. marker
  s. pick
  s. plug
  s. punch
  s. resection knife
  s. shell
  s. shield
  s. shortening clip
  s. spatula needle
  s. sponge rod
  s. twist fixation hook
  s. twist-grip forceps
sclerectomy punch
ScleroLaser
  Candela S.
  S. laser system
ScleroPlus
  S. flashlamp-pumped pulsed tunable
    dye laser
  S. HP laser system
  S. LongPulse dye laser system
sclerostomy needle
sclerotherapy needle
sclerotome
  Alvis-Lancaster s.
  Atkinson s.
  s. blade
  Curdy s.

S

sclerotome *(continued)*
> Lancaster s.
> Lundsgaard s.
> Lundsgaard-Burch s.
> s. pain chart
> Walker-Lee s.

sclerotomy punch
SCMD microkeratome
Scobee oblique muscle hook
SCOI shoulder brace
scoliometer
scoliosis overlap brace
ScoliTron instrument
scoop
> abdominal s.
> abortion s.
> Arlt s.
> Beck abdominal s.
> S. 1, 2 catheter
> Councill stone s.
> cystic duct s.
> Daviel s.
> Daviel lens s.
> Desjardins gallstone s.
> s. dish
> duct s.
> enucleation s.
> Ferguson gallstone s.
> Ferris common duct s.
> French s.
> gall duct s.
> gallstone s.
> Klebanoff gallstone s.
> Knapp s.
> Knapp lens s.
> Lang eye s.
> lens enucleation s.
> Lewis s.
> Lewis lens s.
> Mayo common duct s.
> Mayo cystic duct s.
> Mayo gallbladder s.
> Mayo gall duct s.
> Mayo gallstone s.
> Mayo-Robson gallstone s.
> microbayonet s.
> S. model polyurethane intratracheal catheter
> Moore gallstone s.
> Mules s.
> Snellen lens s.
> s. stretcher
> S. transtracheal catheter
> uterine s.
> Volkmann s.
> Weber lens s.
> Wells enucleation s.
> Wilder s.

> Wilder lens s.
> Yasargil s.

scooter
> s. board
> Lark s.
> Rascal s.

Scoot-Gard mat
scope
> Augustine guide and s.
> baby s.
> Doppler s.
> Electro-Acuscope s.
> ENT s.
> fixed-focus s.
> flexible s.
> keratoiridoscope s.
> KeyMed fiberoptic s.
> Lixiscope s.
> MaculoScope s.
> M-scope multibending s.
> Olympus ENF-P2 s.
> Olympus fiberoptic s.
> Olympus OSF s.
> rigid s.
> SinuScope s.
> Smart S.
> variable-focus s.
> Welch Allyn pocket s.

ScopeGuide
> S. magnetic resonance imaging device
> S. MRI device

Scopette device
Scopix Laser film
Scorpio total knee system
Scotchcast
> S. 2 cast tape
> S. length splinting system

scotograph
scotomagraph
scotometer
> Bjerrum s.

scotoscope
Scott
> S. AMS inflatable penile prosthesis
> S. ankle splint
> S. cannula
> S. chronic wound care system
> S. curved ruler
> S. double-strap ankle support
> S. elastic ankle strap
> S. hinged knee support
> S. lens-insertion forceps
> S. retractor
> S. Uniform tennis elbow splint
> S. wrist wrap

Scott-Craig orthosis

Scottish
    S. Rite brace
    S. Rite hip orthosis
Scott-RCE osteotomy guide
Scotty
    S. the Scale stand-on scale
    S. stainless ankle joint
Scoville
    S. blunt hook
    S. cervical disc self-retaining
     retractor
    S. clip
    S. clip-applying forceps
    S. curved nerve hook
    S. nerve root retractor
    S. ruptured disc curette
Scoville-Greenwood bayonet
  neurosurgical bipolar forceps
Scoville-Lewis clamp
SCRAM face mask
scraper
    amalgam s.
    Bradley femoral canal
     preparation s.
    Charnley acetabular s.
    diamond-dusted s.
    diamond-dusted membrane s.
     (DDMS)
    drum s.
    epithelial s.
    Hough drum s.
    Knolle capsular s.
    Kratz capsular s.
    Lewicky capsular s.
    Safescraper bone s.
    Simcoe capsular s.
    Tano s.
    Tano membrane s.
scraping brush
scratcher
    Jensen capsule s.
    Knolle capsular s.
    Kratz capsular s.
    Kratz-Jensen capsular s.
screen
    AlaTOP inhalant allergy s.
    Biosafe PSA4 s.
    Bjerrum s.
    drywall sanding s.
    ether s.
    Fast Lanex rare earth s.
    Grey-Hess s.
    Hess s.
    Hess diplopia s.
    Hess-Lee s.
    intensifying s.
    Kodak Min-R s.
    Lancaster red-green s.
    Lanex medium s.

    medium-grade drywall sanding s.
    Mitsubishi HL7955 CRT s.
    rapid s.
    s. reader
    split s.
    Synthes titanium mesh s.
    tangent s.
    titanium mesh s.
    Ultra vision rapid s.
screener
    Algo newborn hearing s.
    AutoPap 300 QC automatic Pap s.
    Natus Algo s.
    Rosenbaum pocket vision s.
    Smart Screener infant hearing s.
    SureSight vision s.
screenless mammography film
Screenoscope
    Topcon S.
screw[7]
    Hexalon ACL/PCL s.
screw
    Absolute absorbable s.
    Absolute absorbable interference s.
    Ace s.
    Ace cortical bone s.
    Ace TiMAX titanium captured
     hip s.
    AcroMed s.
    Acutrak s.
    alar s.
    s. alignment bar
    s. alignment rod
    Alta supracondylar s.
    Ambi hip s.
    amputation s.
    Amset R-F s.
    anchor s.
    AO/ASIF s.
    AO spongiosa s.
    Arthrex sheathed interference s.
    Arthrex TransFix biointerference s.
    ASIF malleolar s.
    Asnis guided s.
    Asnis 2 guided s.
    Asnis III cannulated s.
    Aten olecranon s.
    Auto-Drive self-drilling s.
    Autogenesis automator for
     Ilizarov s.
    axial anchor s.
    Barouk cannulated bone s.
    bicortical superior border s.
    Bilok interference s.
    bioabsorbable interference s.
    Biocryl TCP/PLA s.
    BioCuff C bioresorbable
     cannulated s.
    biodegradable polylactide s.

screw *(continued)*
    Biofix absorbable s.
    Bio-Interference tibial s.
    Biologically Quiet interference s.
    Bionx absorbable cannulated s.
    Bionx self-reinforced PLLA
      smart s.
    BioRCI bioabsorbable s.
    BioScrew absorbable interference s.
    BioSorb endoscopic browlift s.
    BioSorbFX SR self-reinforced plate
      and s.
    Biosteon wedge interference s.
    Bold compression s.
    bone s.
    bone mulch s.
    Bosworth coracoclavicular s.
    brow lift suspension s.
    Buttress thread s.
    Calcitek retaining s.
    Camino subdural s.
    cancellous s.
    cancellous bone s.
    cannulated s.
    cannulated cancellous lag s.
    Caspar cervical s.
    CD Horizon M8 multiaxial s.
    cervical pedicle s.
    chrome-cobalt s.
    Clearfix s.
    Clearfix meniscal s.
    Cohort bone s.
    compression hip s. (CHS)
    s. compressor
    Concise compression hip s.
    cortex s.
    cortical s.
    cortical ASIF s.
    cortical bone s.
    Cotrel pedicle s.
    Coventry s.
    cover s.
    dental implant cover s.
    Dentatus s.
    s. depth gauge
    DePuy FRS s.
    DePuy FRS twist-off s.
    DePuy interference s.
    DePuy Mitek Biocryl TCP/PLA s.
    DePuy Rockwood AC s.
    Deyerle interlocking s.
    DHS s.
    distal locking s.
    distraction s.
    Doyen myoma s.
    Doyen tumor s.
    Duo-Drive cortical s.
    dynamic condylar s.
    dynamic hip s.
    ECT bone s.
    Edwards sacral s.
    encased s.
    endocardial s.
    Endofix absorbable interference s.
    Endofix bioabsorbable
      interference s.
    Endo-FixL s.
    expansion s.
    Fabian s.
    Fixateur Interne s.
    fixation s.
    fixed-head s.
    foreign body s.
    FRS twist-off s.
    Garden s.
    Gentle Threads interference s.
    Glasser fixation s.
    glenoid fixation s.
    s. grip
    Guardsman femoral interference s.
    Hahn s.
    headless bone s.
    healing s.
    Hedrocel titanium s.
    Henderson lag s.
    Herbert s.
    Herbert bone s.
    Herbert scaphoid s.
    Herbert-Whipple bone s.
    Howmedica Universal
      compression s.
    iliac s.
    iliosacral s.
    Ilizarov s.
    ImplaMed gold s.
    Implant Innovations titanium s.
    Implant Support Systems
      titanium s.
    InCompass thoracolumbar spine
      fixation s.
    s. inserter
    Instrument Makar biodegradable
      interference s.
    Integrity acetabular cup s.
    interference s.
    interfragmentary lag s.
    interfragmentary minilag s.
    intracranial pressure monitor s.
    Intrafix s.
    Isola spinal implant system iliac s.
    Isola vertebral s.
    Jeter lag s.
    Jeter lag/position s.
    Jewett pickup s.
    Johannson lag s.
    Johannson-Stille lag s.
    Kostuik s.
    Kurosaka interference-fit s.

lag s.
Lane bone s.
lateral mass s.
Leibinger Micro Plus s.
Leibinger Mini Würzburg s.
Leibinger Würzburg s.
Leinbach olecranon s.
Lewis tonsillar s.
Lindorf lag s.
Lindorf position s.
Linvatec absorbable s.
Linvatec bioabsorbable
  interference s.
Lippman s.
locking s.
Long Beach pedicle s.
Lorenz s.
Luhr s.
Luhr implant s.
Luhr vitallium s.
lumbar pedicle s.
Lundholm s.
Luque II s.
MacroPore s.
Magna-Fx cannulated s.
mandibular angle fracture intraoral
  open reduction s.
Marion s.
maxillofacial bone s.
McLaughlin carpal scaphoid s.
medial bicortical s.
medial unicortical s.
metallic s.
micrometric s.
Milagro interference s.
Mille Pattes s.
minifragment s.
mini lag s.
mini Würzburg s.
Mitek Absolute absorbable
  interference s.
monocortical s.
Moss s.
Moss-Miami polyaxial s.
multiaxial s.
myoma s.
navicular s.
neutralization s.
Nobelpharma gold prosthetic
  retaining s.
noncutting blunt threads of
  resorbable s.
Olerud PSF s.
Omega compression hip s.
oral s.
Orthex cannulated bone s.
Orthofix s.
orthopaedic s.
Osteomed s.

OsteoTite bone s.
PathFinder pedicle s.
PathFinder polyaxial s.
pedicle s.
PerFixation s.
Periotest Implant Innovations
  gold s.
Phantom interference s.
Phillips recessed-head s.
pilot point s.
s. placement C-guide
polyaxial s.
polyaxial cervical s.
polylactide absorbable s.
posterior-anterior s.
Preston s.
pretapped Synthes lag s.
Propel cannulated interference s.
pull s.
Quiet interference s.
Reddick-Saye s.
rescue s.
resorbable plate and s.
resorbable polymer s.
ReUnite orthopaedic s.
reverse-threaded s.
Revo retrievable cancellous s.
Richards classic compression hip s.
Richmond subarachnoid s.
rigid pedicle s.
Rockwood AC s.
Rockwood shoulder s.
Russell-Taylor s.
sacral alar s.
sacral pedicle s.
Salzburg s.
Schanz s.
Selby I, II s.
self-tapping s.
self-tapping bone s.
self-tapping Leibinger lag s.
self-tapping mini s.
self-tapping V-shaped threads of
  metal s.
SemiFix s.
set s.
Sharpey s.
Sherman bone s.
silk s.
small fragment s.
small-headed s.
Smith & Nephew s.
Spiessel position s.
stainless steel s.
Steffee plate and s.
Steinhauser s.
step s.
Storz s.
Stryker lag s.

S

screw *(continued)*
    Stryker universal wedge s.
    subarachnoid s.
    subarticular s.
    Summit bone s.
    superior thoracic pedicle s.
    syndesmotic s.
    Synthes compression hip s.
    Talon compression hip s.
    s. tap
    4-tap s.
    Texas Scottish Rite Hospital pedicle s.
    thoracolumbar pedicle s.
    ThreadLoc driver mount s.
    ThreadLoc retaining s.
    Ti alloy s.
    tibial head s.
    TiMAX titanium captured hip s.
    TiMesh s.
    TiMesh emergency s.
    titanium s.
    titanium cancellous bone s.
    s. toggle
    tonsillar s.
    Townley bone graft s.
    TPS-coated s.
    traction tongs s.
    transarticular s.
    TransFix bio-interference s.
    transfixing s.
    transfixion s.
    translaminar facet s.
    transmaxillary s.
    transpedicular s.
    transpedicular cannulated s.
    triangulated pedicle s.
    Trinion meniscus s.
    TSRH pedicle s.
    tulip pedicle s.
    Tunneloc bone mulch s.
    twist-off s.
    unicortical s.
    Universal fixation s.
    universal wedge s.
    Uppsala s.
    Vari-Angle s.
    VDS s.
    Vilex cannulated s.
    Vilex F-Series dual-thread s.
    vitallium s.
    VSF s.
    Wiltse pedicle s.
    Wood s.
    Woodruff s.
    Würzburg s.
    Zielke s.
    Zimmer s.
screw-and-keel fixation

screw-cup container
screwdriver
    Allen head s.
    AutoDriver s.
    automatic s.
    Bio-Interference s.
    Bosworth s.
    cannulated s.
    cross-slot s.
    cruciform s.
    Hall s.
    heavy cross-slot s.
    hexhead s.
    s. instrument
    Johnson s.
    Ken s.
    Lane s.
    light cross-slot s.
    Massie s.
    Master s.
    Phillips s.
    plain s.
    right-angle s.
    Sherman s.
    single cross-slot s.
    skull plate s.
    Stab-and-Grab s.
    straight hex s.
    Stryker s.
    Trinkle s.
    Universal hex s.
    VDS s.
    White s.
    Williams s.
    Woodruff s.
    Zimmer s.
screw-holding forceps
screw-in
    s.-i. ceramic acetabular cup
    s.-i. epicardial electrode
    s.-i. lead
    s.-i. lead pacemaker
    s.-i. sutureless myocardial electrode
screw-on lead
screw-rod
    Wiltse s.-r.
screw-thread stent
screw-tipped intraosseous needle
screw-to-screw compression construct
screw-type implant
Screw-Vent
    S.-V. implant
    S.-V. implant system
Scribner shunt
Scrip Muscle Master massager
scroll pump
scrotal
    s. dressing
    s. truss

scrub
> s. brush
> Sklar s.

scrubber
> Amoils epithelial s.
> posterior capsule s.
> Simcoe anterior chamber capsule s.
> Simcoe posterior capsule s.

SCU-1200, SCU-2200 digital color ultrasound scanner
Scudder intestinal forceps
Scuderi prosthesis
Scully
> S. Hip S'port
> S. Hip S'port device
> S. Hip S'port hip device

sculp
> Concise cementing s.
> s. knife

Sculptor flexible annuloplasty ring
Sculptured Endostat
sculpturing scalpel
scultetus
> s. bandage
> S. binder
> s. binder dressing

SDCT scanner
SDI-BIOM wide angle viewing system
SDS
> stent delivery system

SD sorb staple
Sea-Band acupressure wristband
Seabands
Sea-Clens wound cleanser
seal
> Asherman chest s.
> IVA s.
> Ultimate Seal CPAP mask s.
> watertight s.

sealant
> Beriplast fibrin s.
> 2-component s.
> CoSeal resorbable synthetic s.
> Crosseal fibrin s.
> dental s.
> DuraSeal s.
> fibrin s.
> fibrin adhesive s.
> fissure s.
> FloSeal matrix hemostatic s.
> FocalSeal-L surgical s.
> FocalSeal-S surgical s.
> Hemaseel APR kit fibrin s.
> Tisseel fibrin s.
> Tissucol fibrin s.

SealEasy resuscitation mask
sealed capsule irrigation device
sealer
> AH-26 silver-free s.

> Calasept s.
> calciobiotic root canal s.
> epoxy resin s.
> Histoacryl s.
> Kerr pulp canal s.
> Pulp Canal Sealer EBT s.
> tear-strength eugenol-based s.

sealing window plug
Seal-Tight cast protector
SeamGuard staple line reinforcement material
seamless graft
seam-sealer gun
SEA port
Seaquence stent
searcher
> Allport-Babcock s.
> Allport mastoid s.
> mastoid s.
> Shea s.
> stone s.

Searcy
> S. anchor/fixation
> S. chalazion trephine
> S. fixation

SeaSorb
> S. alginate wound cover
> S. alginate wound dressing

seat
> antithrust s.
> Backjoy s.
> belt-position booster s.
> Carrie car s.
> Comfy toilet lift s.
> Dream Ride car s.
> Hospital Recliner s.
> Ingram bicycle s.
> Maddacare child bath s.
> Medi-Pac rescue s.
> orthopaedic positioning s.
> Posey drop s.
> Renolux convertible car s.
> Responder emergency vehicle car s.
> Rubbermaid adjustable bath/shower s.
> Snug s.
> Spelcast car s.
> Tall-ette toilet s.
> Tubsider kneeling s.
> Tumble Forms feeder s.

Scated Cable Row exerciser
Seattle
> S. foot prosthesis
> S. orthosis
> S. safety knee
> S. splint

S

Sebbin
    S. ultrasound-assisted lipoplasty machine
    S. ultrasound device
Sebileau periosteal elevator
Secca radiofrequency system
Sechrist
    S. hyperbaric ventilator
    S. infant ventilator
    S. monoplace hyperbaric chamber
    S. neonatal ventilator
second
    s. Look breast imaging device
    s. Look CAD system
    s. skin pad
second-generation lithotriptor
second-stage garment
Secor system
sector scanner
Securcut aspiration biopsy needle
Secure
    S. Balance
    S. Yet Gentle surgical dressing system
SecureStrand
    S. cable
    S. cervical fusion system
Secur-Fit HA PSL X'tra prosthesis
Security
    S. carpal tunnel release system clip
    S. clip enclosed carpal tunnel release system
Security+ self-sealing Urisheath external catheter
Securline blood band
Sedan
    S. cannula
    S. goniometer
Sedan-Nashold needle
Sédillot
    S. periosteal elevator
    S. rasp
sedimentation tube
sediment tube
Seeburger
    S. implant
    S. retractor
seed
    BrachySeed brachytherapy s.
    BrachySeed palladium-103 s.
    s. implant
    radiation s.
    s. ribbon
    Vaccaria press s.
SeedNet
    S. cryotherapy system
    S. gold ultrathin CryoNeedle
    S. system

seeker
    ball-tipped s.
    S. guidewire
    Kuhn-Bolger s.
    s. needle
    ostium s.
SeeQuence disposable contact lens
segment
    capsular tension s.
    Intacs corneal ring s.
segmental
    s. buckle
    s. compression construct
    s. spinal correction system
    s. spinal instrumentation
segmented
    s. orthopaedic system total hip and knee system
    s. ring tripolar lead
Segond hysterectomy forceps
Segond-Landau hysterectomy forceps
segregator
    Cathelin s.
    Harris s.
    Luy s.
Seguin annuloplasty ring
Séguin formboard
Segura CBD basket
Segura-Dretler laser basket
Sehrt
    S. clamp
    S. compressor
Seibel
    S. double-ended LASIK flap lifter and spatula
    S. 3D speculum
    S. LASIK flap irrigator
    S. LASIK flap irrigator and squeegee cannula
    S. LASIK flap squeegee cannula
    S. LRI diamond knife
    S. nucleus chopper
    S. paracentesis valve adjuster
    S. vertical safety quick chopper
Seidel
    S. humeral locking nail
    S. intramedullary fixation
    S. saddlebag
Seiff frontalis suspension set
Seiler
    S. MC-M900 surgical microscope
    S. turbinate scissors
Seirin acupuncture needle
Seitzinger tripolar cutting forceps
seizing forceps
Sekomic SS-100F recorder
Selby
    S. I, II fixation system
    S. I, II hook

S. I, II rod
S. I, II screw
Seldin
S. dental retractor
S. elevator
Seldinger
S. arterial needle
S. gastrostomy needle
S. needle
Selec-3 IV set
Select
S. ankle prosthesis
S. GT blood glucose system
S. joint
S. joint orthosis
S. modular shoulder prosthesis
Selecta
S. Duet combination laser system
S. Duet glaucoma laser system
S. Duo ophthalmic laser system
S. 7000 glaucoma laser system
S. II glaucoma laser system
S. 7000 laser
S. 1064 laser platform
S. Trio glaucoma laser system
Select-a-Fuge microcentrifuge machine
SelectCells Mini endometrial sampler
selective
s. tubal occlusion procedure (STOP)
s. tubal occlusion procedure system
Selectively Lockable knee brace
Select-Lite lancing device
selector
Leksell s.
sleeve s.
Selector ultrasonic aspirator
Selectron system
Selenia imaging system
selenium-based digital chest system
selenium-drum-detector system
self-adherent bandage
self-adhering
s.-a. lid retractor
s.-a. varus/valgus wedge
self-adjusted glasses
self-adjusting suture
self-aligning
s.-a. knee
s.-a. mobile-bearing knee implant
self-articulating femoral prosthesis
self-aspirating cut-biopsy needle
self-broaching pin
Self-Cath
S.-C. closed cathetcrization system
S.-C. closed system catheter
S.-C. coudé tipped catheter
S.-C. HydroGel catheter
S.-C. soft catheter

S.-C. straight-tipped female catheter
S.-C. straight-tipped pediatric catheter
S.-C. straight-tipped soft catheter
self-catheter
Mentor female s.-c.
self-centering
s.-c. bone-holding forceps
s.-c. micromanipulator
s.-c. prosthesis
s.-c. Universal hip prosthesis
self-contained
s.-c. breathing apparatus
s.-c. underwater breathing apparatus
self-drainage catheter
self-expandable
s.-e. metallic stent
s.-e. metal stent
s.-e. stainless steel braided endoprosthesis
s.-e. stent
self-expanding
s.-e. coil stent
s.-e. covered stent
s.-e. Easy Wallstent
s.-e. metallic endoprosthesis
s.-e. metallic stent
s.-e. open mesh stent
s.-e. stainless steel stent
s.-e. stent
s.-e. stent-graft
s.-e. tulip sheath
s.-e. Wallstcnt endoprosthesis
self-gelling glue
self-guiding catheter
self-inflating
s.-i. bulb
s.-i. tissue expander
self-opening
s.-o. forceps
s.-o. rigid snare
self-propelling wheelchair
self-quenched counter tube
self-retaining
s.-r. abdominal retractor
s.-r. bone forceps
s.-r. brain retractor
s.-r. catheter
s.-r. clamp
s.-r. coil stent
s.-r. Cope loop pigtail catheter
s.-r. infusion cannula
s.-r. irrigating cannula
s.-r. laryngoscope
s.-r. retractor
s.-r. retractor blade
s.-r. ring retractor
s.-r. skin retractor
s.-r. spring retractor

S

self-retractor
  Lone Star s.-r.
self-sealing
  s.-s. cannula
  s.-s. injection port
  s.-s. latex balloon
self-seating plug
self-stabilizing vitrectomy lens
self-stopping drill point
self-tapering pin
self-tapping
  s.-t. bone screw
  s.-t. Leibinger lag screw
  s.-t. mini screw
  s.-t. screw
  s.-t. screw-type implant
  s.-t. V-shaped threads of metal
    screw
self-test
  Gluco-Protein OTC s.-t.
  OvuQuick S.-t.
sellar punch
Sellheim
  S. elevating spoon
  S. uterine catheter
Sellors rib contractor
Selman tissue forceps
Seltzer saw
**Selute Picotip steroid-eluting endocardial
  lead**
Selverstone
  S. carotid artery clamp
  S. intervertebral disc forceps
  S. intervertebral disc rongeur
  S. rongeur forceps
  S. Semmes curette sensor
Semb
  S. bone-cutting forceps
  S. bone forceps
  S. bone-holding forceps
  S. bone rongeur
  S. bronchus clamp
  S. ligature forceps
  S. rib forceps
  S. rib rasp
  S. shears
Semb-Stille bone rongeur
semiadjustable articulator
semiautomated external defibrillator
semicircular gouge
semicompressive dressing
semiconductor
  complementary metal oxide s.
  s. detector
  s. GaAIAs infrared diode laser
    photocoagulator
semierect film
SemiFix screw
semiflat tip electrode

semiflexible endoscope
semiinvasive electrode
semilunar cartilage knife
semilunar-tip blade
semiocclusive moisture-retentive dressing
semipermeable
  s. dressing
  s. hollow-fiber catheter
  s. membrane dressing
Semi-Q hCG combo test
semirigid
  s. catheter
  s. endoscope
  s. fiberglass cast
  s. polypropylene ankle-foot orthosis
  s. silicone plastic rod
semishell implant
semitubular blade-plate
Semken
  S. dressing forceps
  S. forceps
  S. thumb forceps
  S. tissue forceps
Semm
  S. morcellator
  S. Pelvi-Pneu insufflator
  S. uterine vacuum cannula
Semmes-Weinstein
  S.-W. monofilament
  S.-W. 5.07 monofilament
  S.-W. monofilament instrument
  S.-W. nylon monofilament
  S.-W. pressure aesthesiometer
    filament
  S.-W. pressure anesthesiometer
SEM stent
send-receive phased-array extremity coil
**SenDx 100 blood gas and electrolyte
  analysis system**
Sengstaken
  S. balloon
  S. nasogastric tube
Sengstaken-Blakemore
  S.-B. esophageal balloon
  S.-B. esophagogastric tamponade
    tube
  S.-B. tube
Senn
  S. double-ended retractor
  S. rake
  S. retractor
Senn-Dingman retractor
Senn-Green retractor
**Sennheiser electric condenser
  microphone ME 40-3**
Senn-Miller retractor
Senographe
  S. 2000D digital mammography
    system

S. 2000D mammography system
S. DMRt mammography system
S. DS mammography system
SenoScan
S. full-field digital imaging system
S. full-field digital mammography system
S. mammography system
Sensa
Hemoccult S.
Sensability breast self-examination aid
Sensaire spirometer
Sensar
S. acrylic intraocular lens
S. foldable acrylic posterior chamber intraocular lens
S. OptiEdge AR40e IOL
S. OptiEdge foldable acrylic IOL
S. OptiEdge intraocular lens
Sens-A-Ray
S.-A.-R. dental imaging system
S.-A.-R. 2000 dental imaging system
S.-A.-R. digital dental imaging system
Sensatec endoscope
Sensation
S. intraaortic balloon catheter
S. Short Throw snare
Sense-of-Feel prosthesis
Sensi-Care skin care product
SensiCare synthetic powder-free surgical glove
SensiCath
S. blood gas measurement system
S. optical sensor
S. system
sensing
s. catheter
s. circuit
s. coil
Sensitire _Streptococcus pneumoniae_ HPB susceptibility plate
sensitizer
Gd-Tex radiation s.
sensitometer
electroluminescent s.
Sensiv endotracheal tube
Senso listening device
Sensonic plaque removal instrument
sensor
acoustic respiratory motion s.
anal EMG PerryMeter s.
Animas R-1000 s.
anterior aspect esophageal s.
BioZtect s.
BIS S.
Bispectral Index S. (BIS)

BreastAlert differential temperature s.
capacitive s.
Capnostat CO_2 s.
CardioSearch s.
catheter-based s.
ClipTip reusable s.
Cross Top replacement oxygen s.
DC SQUID s.
Dentsleeve sleeve s.
DermaTemp infrared thermographic s.
Diasensor 1000 s.
differential temperature s.
3-dimensional magnetic s.
disposable Doppler-constant thermocouple s.
Dymedix sleep s.
electromyogram s.
Endex apex s.
fiberoptic s.
fiberoptic PCO_2 s.
FilterWatch s.
finger clip s.
flat tube pressure s.
Flexisensor s.
GlucoNIR glucose s.
GlucoWatch Biographer transdermal s.
Handi oxygen s.
implantable glucose s.
ImPressure ultrasound pressure s.
infant airflow and effort s.
Infinity s.
Ladd intracranial pressure s.
magnetic s.
manometric s.
Masimo LNOP durable adhesive s.
measuring s.
MEG s.
multiparameter intraarterial s.
Myoscan s.
Nellcor FS-10, FS-14 oximeter s.
Nellcor FS-10 oximeter s.
Nellcor FS-14 oximeter s.
Neotrend s.
Neurotrend s.
Novametrix combination $0_2/C0_2$ s.
oximetry s.
Oxisensor II adult s.
Oxisensor II adult adhesive s.
OxyTip s.
s. pacemaker
s. pad
Paratrend 7+ s.
pediatric finger clip s.
Perry s.
piezoelectric snore s.
piezo PLM s.

sensor *(continued)*
    pressure s.
    pressure transducer airflow s.
    PressureWire s.
    PressureWire-3 s.
    S. PTFE-nitinol guidewire with
      hydrophilic tip
    Pulsar Max s.
    reliable wave front s.
    Resp-EZ piezoelectric s.
    Richmond subarachnoid screw s.
    Selverstone Semmes curette s.
    SensiCath optical s.
    Servo Pro force s.
    sleeve s.
    SpiroSense flow s.
    Stat-Shell disposable pulse
      oximeter s.
    telemetric intracranial pressure s.
    Therasense subcutaneous glucose s.
    TouchTrak glucose s.
    ultrasonic tactile s.
    VTI oxygen monitor with
      disposable polarographic oxygen s.
    Watson angular rate s.
sensor-based single-chamber pacemaker
SensorHand prosthesis
SensorMedics
    S. generator
    S. mass flow sensor heated wire
      flowmeter
    S. 2900 metabolic cart
    S. pressure transducer
    S. SAT-TRAK pulse oximeter
    S. ventilator
sensory
    s. nerve action potential sleep
      recorder
    s. stimulation kit
SensoScan mammography system
Sentalloy wire
Sentinel
    S. ICD device
    S. 2010 implantable cardioverter-
      defibrillator
    S. Seal pleural drainage unit
Sentinel-4 neurological monitor
**Sentron pigtail microtip-manometer
  catheter**
Sentry
    S. balloon catheter
    Sleep S.
Sepacell RZ-2000 device
separating strip
separator
    abduction knee s.
    acrylic s.
    Akahoshi nucleus s.
    Allen stereo s.

    Amicus blood collection s.
    Benson baby pylorus s.
    blood cell s.
    Cobe blood cell s.
    diamond wound s.
    Dorsey dural s.
    dural s.
    Fenwal CS 3000 Plus cell s.
    Ferrier s.
    finger s.
    Hoen dural s.
    Horsley dural s.
    House ear s.
    Hunter s.
    iliac graft s.
    Kirby curved zonular s.
    Kirby cylindrical zonular s.
    Kirby double-ball s.
    Kirby flat zonular s.
    mechanical s.
    nerve s.
    noninterfering s.
    Plasmaflo plasma s.
    Remy s.
    Sachs dural s.
    Sachs nerve s.
    Smith s.
    stem spoon s.
    synovial s.
    True s.
    s. tube
    Woodson dural s.
Sephadex
    S. bead
    S. G-25 column
Seprafilm bioresorbable membrane
Sepramesh biosurgical composite
septal
    s. bone forceps
    s. chisel
    s. clamp
    s. compression forceps
    s. dissector
    s. elevator
    s. forceps
    s. hyperperfusion on thallium scan
    s. knife
    s. needle
    s. perforator branch
    s. ridge forceps
    s. scissors
    s. straightener
SeptiCare wound cleanser
Septi-Chek blood culture system
Septi-Soft skin care cleanser
Septisol soap dressing
Septobal bead
Septoject dental syringe needle
Septopal implant

septostomy balloon catheter
septum cutting forceps
septum-straightening forceps
Sep-T-Vac suction canister
Sequel compression system
sequencer
    automated laser-fluorescence s.
    automatic gas s.
sequencing bead patterns set
sequential
    s. circulator
    s. compression device (SCD)
    s. compression stocking
    s. extremity pump
    s. multiple analyzer
    S. Multiple Analyzer Computer
      (SMAC)
    s. multiple analyzer plus computer
Sequenza immunostaining system
Sequestra
    S. 1000 blood processing system
    S. 1000 system
sequestrum forceps
Sequicor II, III pacemaker
Sequoia
    S. Acuson system
    S. echocardiography system
    S. ultrasound system
Serdarevic
    S. speculum
    S. suture adjuster
Serena
    S. Mx apnea recorder/analyzer
    S. Mx handheld apnea detection
      device
SERFAS
    Stryker Endoscopy radiofrequency
    ablation system
    SERFAS endoscopic system
series
    Accurun 515 drug-resistant mutant
      control s.
    Bioceram 2-stage s. II
    s. 5 forceps
    Mist Eubanks instrument s.
    Olympus CV s.
    Option Orthotic S.
    RingLoc acetabular s.
    Rosser signature s.
    St. Jude medical heart valve
      hemodynamic plus s.
    Unitech cannula s.
    Universal cannula s.
Serodia commercial kit
SeroJet needle-free injection system
Serola sacroiliac belt
Seroma-Cath
    S.-C. catheter
    S.-C. drainage tube

S.-C. feeding tube
S.-C. system
S.-C. wound drainage catheter
S.-C. wound drainage system
Serono SR1 FSH analyzer
Sero-Strip HIV test
serpentine bone plate
Serralnyl suture
Serralsilk suture
serrated
    s. amalgam plugger
    s. blade
    s. catheter
    s. conjunctival forceps
    s. curette
    s. fine-cutting knife
    s. forceps
    s. iris scissors
    s. retractor
    s. scissors
    s. suture
    s. T spatula
serrefine
    ASSI s.
    s. clamp
    Dieffenbach s.
    s. forceps
    Lemoine s.
    Mack s.
    s. retractor
serum pregnancy assay cartridge
Servo
    S. power amplifier
    S. Pro force sensor
    S. Screen 390 ventilator monitoring
      device
    S. ventilator
    S. ventilator
servohydraulic test frame
Servo-i ventilator
servomechanism sphincter
Servox
    S. amplifier
    S. device
    S. electronic speech aid
    S. Inton speech aid
sesamoid clamp
sesamoidectomy dissector
set
    access s.
    Acland-Banis arteriotomy s.
    ACL guide s.
    ACS percutaneous introducer s.
    Amplatz dilator s.
    Arrow high-flow infusion s.
    Assura deluxe irrigation s.
    Assura economy irrigation s.
    Atala-Shepard coaxial balloon
      follower s.

S

set (continued)

Bankart shoulder repair s.
Bio-Medicus percutaneous cannula s.
Bloomberg trabeculotome s.
Boehm rectal diagnostic and treatment s.
Borst side-arm introducer s.
Bremer halo crown traction s.
Brown-Mueller T-fastener s.
Bruening otoscope s.
Brunner ligature s.
Bush DL ureteral illuminating catheter s.
Bush SL ureteral illuminating catheter s.
Carriazo-Barraquer instrument s.
Catalano intubation s.
Catalyst anterior instrument s.
CD Horizon Sextant rod insertion s.
Ciaglia Blue Rhino percutaneous tracheostomy introducer s.
Ciaglia percutaneous tracheostomy introducer s.
Cliniset infusion s.
Cloward cervical retractor s.
coaxial micropuncture introducer s.
coaxial micropuncture needle s.
Codman Cranioplastic Type 1 Slow S.
Codman external drainage ventricular s.
Colapinto transjugular biopsy s.
Coloplast economy irrigation s.
Coloplast hospital irrigation s.
Coloplast 2-piece sterile post-op s.
Contiplex catheter s.
Cook drainage pouch s.
Cope gastrointestinal suture anchor s.
Corpak enteral Y extension s.
Cotton-Huibregtse biliary stent s.
Cotton-Leung biliary stent s.
Crampton-Tsang percutaneous endoscopic biliary stent s.
Crawford lacrimal intubation s.
Curry intravascular retriever s.
Dansac colostomy irrigation s.
Desilets-Hoffman introducer s.
Diethrich coronary artery s.
DORC subretinal instrument s.
Dotter intravascular retrieval s.
Dujovny microsuction dissection s.
Echosight Jansen-Anderson intrauterine catheter s.
Echosight Patton coaxial catheter s.
Echotip Baker amniocentesis s.
Echotip coaxial needle biopsy s.

Echotip Kato-Asch needle s.
Echotip Mennuti sampling needle s.
Eliminator nasobiliary catheter s.
Embryon GIFT transfer catheter s.
Entrex small joint arthroscopy instrument s.
Fine bimanual handpiece s.
Flexor Check-Flo introducer s.
Fuhrman pleural drainage s.
Grandon cortex extractor s.
Greenberg retractor s.
grid maze s.
Guardian 1-piece ostomy system sterile drainage OR s.
Guibor canaliculus intubation s.
hand evaluation s.
HandTact instrument s.
Harmony PLIF instrument s.
Harvard microbore intravenous extension s.
Hawkins accordion catheter drainage s.
Henning instrument s.
Heyer-Schulte Small-Carrion sizing s.
Hobbs stent s.
Horizon Sextant rod insertion s.
H/S Elliptosphere catheter s.
Huibregtse biliary stent s.
Huisman percutaneous drainage s.
insufflation test s.
Jackson lacrimal intubation s.
Jaffe laser blepharoplasty and facial resurfacing s.
Jeffrey introducer s.
KeyMed advanced esophageal dilator s.
Kish urethral illuminated catheter s.
Klippel retractor s.
Küntscher nail s.
Level One normothermic IV fluid s.
LifePort infusion s.
Lipshultz urology microsurgical s.
Maciol suture needle s.
Malis irrigation tubing s.
Mardis-Dangler ureteral stent s.
Masimo S.
McIntyre guarded irrigating cystitome s.
McIntyre infusion s.
McNamara coaxial catheter infusion s.
medical equipment s.
Mi-Mark endocervical curette s.
minimally invasive access s.
Mini-Perc entry s.
Mitty-Pollack needle s.

Molina mandibular distractor s.
Mullan percutaneous trigeminal ganglion microcompression s.
multi-sideport catheter infusion s.
Myelo-Nate s.
Neff percutaneous access s.
Neo-Sert umbilical vessel catheter insertion s.
NephroMax catheter s.
New Orleans endarterectomy stripper s.
no-scalpel vasectomy instrument s.
Novack special extraction/injection s.
Osteo-Rx coaxial curved bone biopsy and infusion s.
Oval-8 sizing s.
over-the-wire s.
parquetry s.
pediatric vitrectomy lens s.
peel-away introducer s.
Pettigrove laser-assisted intrastromal keratomileusis s.
Pettigrove LASIK s.
Pollack bead chain cystourethrography s.
Price donor cornea punch s.
prothelen s.
Ring-McLean sump drainage s.
Ring transjugular intrahepatic access s.
Rosch-Thurmond fallopian tube catheterization s.
Rosch-Uchida liver access s.
Rosch-Uchida transjugular liver access s.
Rothbarth Uni-Flo infusion s.
RUPS-100 liver access s.
Saf-T E-Z s.
s. screw
Seiff frontalis suspension s.
Selec 3 IV s.
sequencing bead patterns s.
Sextant rod insertion s.
Shamrock Safety Winged S.
Shuttle-SL Flexor Tuohy Borst side-arm introducer s.
Simcoe lens-positioning s.
SinoJect puncture s.
Sippy esophageal dilating s.
SmartPin instrument s.
Steinert laser-assisted intrastromal keratomileusis s.
Steinert LASIK s.
STENTube lacrimal intubation s.
Stille bone drill s.
Stille-pattern trephine and bone drill s.
Storz ear knife s.

Sur-Fit Natura night drainage container s.
Sur-Fit Natura Visi-Flow irrigation starter s.
Sur-Fit night drainage container s.
Surflo winged infusion s.
Surgimedics/TMP multiperfusion s.
Sykes Endobrowlift instrument s.
Tangent posterior impacted instrument s.
Tebbetts rhinoplasty s.
telescopic bougie s.
Tender subcutaneous infusion s.
The Foot screw s.
Thomas subretinal instrument s. II
Tissomat application device and spray s.
Toomey surgical steel instrument s.
Topel endoscopic cyst aspirator s.
Turkel bone biopsy trephine s.
U-Mid-O$_2$ Jet S.
Universal laminectomy s.
Van Sonnenberg chest drain s.
variable-power cross-cylinder lens s.
vari-balance board s.
Visi-Flow irrigation starter s.
volumeter s.
Weber human genome screening s.
Wilson-Cook Carey capsule s.
Wilson-Cook low-profile esophageal prosthesis s.
Wissinger s.
Wylie endarterectomy s.
Yudkoff-Okun periodontal instrument s.
Zimmon endoscopic biliary stent s.
Zimmon endoscopic pancreatic stent s.
Zimmon esophagogastric balloon tamponade s.

Setguard antireflux valve
seton
 s. drain
 s. drainage device
 Molteno s.
 s. needle
 s. suture
Set-Op myringotomy kit
Setopress
 S. dressing
 S. high-compression bandage
setter
 orthodontic band s.
S.E.T. thrombectomy system catheter
setting inlay
Set-Up
 AMO S.-U.
Seutin
 S. bandage

Seutin *(continued)*
    S. plaster shears
    S. scissors
Seven-Star acupuncture needle
severance transurethral bag
Severin
    S. implant
    S. lens
Severinghaus electrode
Sevrain cranial clamp
Sewall retractor
sewing ring
sewn-in
    s.-i. lens
    s.-i. waterproof drape
sew-on
    s.-o. electrode
    s.-o. lens
Sew-Right suturing device
Sextant
    S. II surgical instrumentation
        system
    S. rod insertion set
Sexton ear knife
S-file
    engine S-f.
S-finder
S-F Precise stent
SFP scanner
Sgarlato
    S. device
    S. hammertoe implant
    S. toe implant
S-G catheter
SGIA knifeless clamp
Shaaf cilia foreign body forceps
Shack-Hartmann aberrometer
Shadow
    S. balloon
    S. over-the-wire balloon catheter
shadow-free laryngoscope
Shadow-Line ACF spine retractor
  system
Shaeffer rigid orthosis
Shaffner orthopaedic inserter
shaft
    Adante Monorail catheter s.
    s. catheter
    Cloward drill s.
    irrigating grasping forceps with
        curved s.
    irrigating scissors with straight s.
    Marlow Primus s.
    s. prosthesis
    s. reamer
    UniTrack s.
Shah
    S. aural dressing

    S. grommet
    S. permanent tube
Shahinian lacrimal cannula
Shallcross cystic duct forceps
Shambaugh
    S. adenoidal curette
    S. irrigator
    S. retractor
    S. reverse adenotome
Shamrock Safety Winged Set
Shandon
    S. Cadenza immunostainer
    S. Cytospin chamber
shank
    Hudson s.
Shannon bur
shape
    S. Maker system
    s. memory alloy stent
shaper
    automated corneal s. (ACS)
    Chiron automated corneal s.
    interspace s.
    ProFile orifice s.
Shapleigh
    S. curette
    S. wax curette
Shapshay-Healy laryngoscope
Shapshay/Healy phonatory and
  operating laryngoscope
shark
    S. disposable biopsy forceps
    s. fin papillotome
    S. pediatric wheelchair
shark-mouth cannula
shark-tip cannula
sharp
    s. dermal curette
    s. elevator
    s. hook
    s. knife
    s. loop curette
    S. point-tip cystotome
    s. trocar
sharp-edged
    s.-e. IOL
    s.-e. tip
sharpening test stick
Sharpey screw
Sharpie marker
Sharplan
    S. 710 Acuspot laser
    S. argon laser
    S. CO_2 laser
    S. Erbium SilkLaser
    S. FeatherTouch SilkLaser
    S. Medilas Nd:YAG surgical laser
    S. sight system

S. SilkTouch Flashscan surgical laser
S. SilkTouch flashscan surgical laser
S. Ultra ultrasonic aspirator
S. USA ultrasonic surgical aspirator
Sharplan/ESC SilkTouch laser
SharpLase Nd:YAG laser
Sharpoint
S. cutting instrument
S. microsurgical knife
S. microsuture
S. ophthalmic microsurgical suture
S. spoon blade
S. Ultra-Glide corneal transplant suture
S. Ultra-Glide ophthalmic transplant suture
S. Ultra-Guide ophthalmic needle
S. UltraPlug punctum plug
S. V-lance blade
sharp-pointed forceps
sharp-pronged retractor
SharpShooter tissue repair system
Sharptome
S. crescent blade
S. microblade
Sharpx needle destruction unit
Shar-Tek foot positioning grid
Sharvelle side port splitter
shattering needle
shaver
arthroscopic s.
Concept s.
Cuda s.
DORC vitreous s.
dragon s.
Gator s.
Grierson meniscal s.
Kuda s.
microplaner soft tissue s.
Microsect s.
motorized meniscal s.
Rhinotec s.
rotating basket s.
Stryker s.
sucker s.
USC scleral s.
videoarthroscopic s.
Xomed skimmer s.
Shaw hemostatic scalpel
Shaw-Sgarlato hammertoe implant prosthesis
Shaw-SHIP
S.-SHIP rod
S.-SHIP rod hammertoe implant
Shea
S. curette

S. forceps
S. microdrill
S. searcher
S. speculum
S. speculum holder
S. Teflon piston prosthesis
S. vein graft scissors
Shea-Anthony
S.-A. bag
S.-A. balloon
Shealy RelaxMate
ShearBan
S. low-friction interface
S. orthotic material
Shearer
S. chicken-bill forceps
S. forceps
S. rongeur
Shearing
S. cortex suction kit
S. posterior chamber implant material
S. posterior chamber intraocular lens implant
shear-off device
shears (*See also* scissors)
ADC Medicut s.
airplane s.
Baer rib s.
bandage plaster s.
Bethune-Coryllos rib s.
Bethune rib s.
biarticular bone s.
Brunner rib s.
Collin rib s.
Cooley rib s.
Coryllos-Bethune rib s.
Coryllos-Shoemaker rib s.
Duval-Coryllos rib s.
Endo S.
Esmarch plaster s.
Felt s.
first rib s.
Frey-Sauerbruch rib s.
Giertz rib s.
Giertz-Shoemaker rib s.
Giertz-Stille rib s.
Gluck rib s.
Hercules plaster s.
infant rib s.
LaparoSonic coagulating s.
Lebsche s.
Lebsche sternal s.
Lefferts rib s.
Liston s.
Liston-Key-Horsley rib s.
plain rib s.
plaster s.
pleural biopsy needle s.

S

shears *(continued)*
    rib s.
    Schumacher sternal s.
    Semb s.
    Seutin plaster s.
    Shoemaker rib s.
    sternal s.
    Stille-Aesculap plaster s.
    Stille-Horsley s.
    Tudor-Edwards rib s.
    UltraCision harmonic laparoscopic
     cutting s.
    utility s.
    Weck s.
sheath
    Acucise access s.
    Amplatz Teflon s.
    angioplasty s.
    AquaGuide ureteral access s.
    Arrow s.
    ArrowFlex s.
    Avanti s.
    Avanti transradial s.
    Bakelite cystoscopy s.
    blue Cook s.
    cardiogenic s.
    carotid s.
    catheter s.
    check-valve s.
    Colapinto s.
    compensated s.
    concave s.
    Cook peel-away s.
    Cordis s.
    Cordis Bioptome s.
    Daig s.
    Desilets-Hoffman s.
    s. and dilator system
    double-channel operating s.
    Endius bipolar s.
    ERA resectoscope s.
    excimer s.
    femoral introducer s.
    fiberoptic s.
    Futura resectoscope s.
    GlideCath s.
    Glidesheath introducer s.
    Hemaflex s.
    hockey-stick guiding s.
    hysteroscope s.
    incandescent s.
    Insul-Sheath vaginal speculum s.
    introducer s.
    Introducer II s.
    irrigating s.
    Klein transseptal introducer s.
    Meditech s.
    MicroSpan s.
    minipuncture s.

    Mullins long transseptal s.
    Mullins transseptal catheterization s.
    muscle s.
    s. needle
    nerve root s.
    s. and obturator
    O'Connor s.
    peel-away s.
    peel-away introducer s.
    percutaneous brachial s.
    Pinnacle Destination guiding s.
    Pinnacle Destination renal
     guiding s.
    Pinnacle introducer s.
    probe s.
    PRO/Covers ultrasound probe s.
    quill s.
    resectoscope s.
    retroflexed cystoscopy s.
    sacral docking s.
    self-expanding tulip s.
    short monorail polyethylene
     imaging s.
    SL1 s.
    Spectranetics laser s.
    Storz s.
    straight guiding s.
    subclavian peel-away s.
    Super ArrowFlex catheterization s.
    tear-away introducer s.
    Teflon s.
    tendon s.
    Terumo Pinnacle s.
    Terumo Pinnacle R/OII radiopaque
     marker introducer s.
    Terumo Radiofocus s.
    threaded s.
    transseptal s.
    tulip s.
    Universal s.
    ureterorenoscope procedure s.
    vascular s.
    water-filled balloon s.
    s. with side-arm adapter
sheathed flexible sigmoidoscope
Sheathes ultrasound probe cover
sheath/liner
    Silipos Distal Dip prosthetic s./l.
Sheedy disparometer
Sheehan
    S. chisel
    S. gouge
    S. knee prosthesis
    S. osteotome
Sheehan-Gillies needle holder
Sheehy
    S. collar button
    S. collar button ventilating tube
    S. incus replacement prosthesis

S. Pate Collector
S. round knife
Sheehy-House
S.-H. curette
S.-H. knife
Sheehy-Urban sliding lens adapter
Sheen
S. graft
S. tip graft
sheepskin
s. boot
s. dressing
sheet
AcryDerm hydrogel s.
Alpha flat s.
Antishear gel s.
Aquasorb hydrogel s.
autologous oral mucosal
    epithelium s.
barrier s.
barrier lower extremity s.
Biobrane s.
casting wax s.
ClearSite hydrogel s.
Conformant contact layer s.
s. cork
Curagel hydrogel s.
Dacron-impregnated silastic s.
Derma-Gel hydrogel s.
Dermanet contact layer s.
Elasto-Gel hydrogel s.
Flexderm hydrogel s.
foil s.
Grafton flexible s.
s. holder
hydrogel s.
s. immobilizer
impervious s.
impervious U s.
Ioban 2 cesarean s.
Ioban 2 iodophor cesarean s.
iodoform-impregnated plastic s.
Kins draw s.
Korex cork s.
mandibular s.
Mepitel contact layer s.
2nd Skin hydrogel s.
Novagel gel s.
N-Terface contact layer s.
Nu-Gel hydrogel s.
Ortholen s.
polydioxanone s.
porous s.
PPT s.
Prolene mesh s.
ReJuveness scar silicone s.
silastic s.
silicone s.
Silk Skin s.

sterile s.
Supramid s.
Teflon s.
Tegagel hydrogel s.
Tegapore contact layer s.
Telfa Clear contact layer s.
Temper foam s.
THINSite hydrogel s.
Transorbent hydrogel s.
U s.
Vigilon hydrogel s.
wet s.
sheeting
Avogel hydrogel s.
Carboplast II s.
Cica-Care topical gel s.
DermaSof gel s.
Epi-Derm silicone gel s.
gel s.
micromesh s.
New Beginnings GelShapes silicone
    gel s.
New Beginnings topical gel s.
Novagel silicone gel s.
Oleeva fabric scar s.
ReJuveness pure silicone s.
Scar Fx lightweight silicone s.
silicone gel s.
Silon silicone elastomer s.
Sheets
S. closed loop posterior chamber
    intraocular lens
S. iris hook
S. irrigating vectis
S. irrigating vectis cannula
S. lens
S. lens glide
S. lens spatula
Sheets-McPherson
S.-M. angled forceps
S.-M. tying forceps
Sheffield
S. gamma unit
S. rod
S. splint
Sheldon
S. catheter
S. clamp
shelf reamer
shelf-type implant
shell
AFO standard s.
chest s.
elastomer s.
s. eye implant
fibrous s.
Harris protrusio s.
s. impactor
s. implant

S

shell *(continued)*
    implant s.
    implant elastomer s.
    s. implant material
    Integrity s.
    Inter-Op acetabular s.
    Irom splint with s.
    metal-backed acetabular s.
    protrusio s.
    Restoration Secur-Fit X'tra
      acetabular s.
    scleral s.
    S-ROM contained s.
    Terino malar s.
shellac-covered catheter
shelter
    Unifold s.
Shenstone tourniquet
Shepard
    S. grommet
    S. grommet ventilation tube
    S. incision depth gauge
    S. incision irrigating cannula
    S. intraocular lens forceps
    S. intraocular lens-holding forceps
    S. intraocular lens implant
    S. optical center marker
    S. radial keratotomy irrigating
      cannula
    S. reversed iris hook
    S. tying forceps
Shepard-Reinstein forceps
Shepherd
    S. internal screw fixation
    S. Tomahawk chopper
shepherd's
    s. hook catheter
    s. hook explorer
    s. hook-shaped angiographic
      catheter
Shepp-Logan filter function
Sher diabetic shoe inlay
Sherform silicone insole
Sherlock
    S. bone screw suture/anchor system
    S. threaded suture anchor
Sherman
    S. bone plate
    S. bone screw
    S. remote podiatric vacuum system
    S. screwdriver
Sherpa guiding catheter
Sherwin knee retractor
Sheth adnexa hysterectomy clamp
ShiatsuBACK back support
shield
    aluminum eye s.
    AME PinSite s.
    AME pin site s.

Barraquer eye s.
bili mask eye s.
BioElectric S.
bronchoscopic face s.
Buller eye s.
bunion s.
CapSure continence s.
Carapace disposable face s.
Cartella eye s.
Cath-Gard catheter contamination s.
circumcisional s.
Clear View hydrophilic s.
collagen s.
contact s.
corneal light s.
Cox II ocular laser s.
Dalkon s.
dental s.
dual eye s.
Durette dental s.
Durette external laser s.
eye s.
face s.
Face-It protective s.
Faraday s.
Fox aluminum s.
Fox aluminum eye s.
Fox eye s.
Fuller s.
gastric s.
gonad s.
Grafco eye s.
Green eye s.
Guibor s.
high-humidity tracheostomy s.
S. iridotomy scissors
Jet s.
Katena scleral s.
Lea s.
lead eye s.
metal Fox s.
metal scleral s.
Mueller eye s.
Nolan system collimator mounted
    contact s.
Paton eye s.
plastic eye s.
pressure s.
probe s.
Proshield collagen corneal s.
protective eye s.
Pro-Tex face s.
ring cataract mask eye s.
SAF-T s.
scleral s.
Sof-Gel palm s.
Soft Shield collagen corneal s.
Sportelli system collimator mounted
    contact s.

Stevanovsky metal eye s.
Surety S.
Surgical Patient Arm s.
surgical patient arm s.
thyroid s.
Trelles metal scleral s.
tungsten eye s.
tungsten syringe s.
Universal eye s.
Visitec corneal s.
Weck eye s.
wrap-a-round eye s.

shielded

s. gradient coil
s. open-end cone

shielding block
Shields forceps
shifter

AliMed Conductive Patient S.
frequency s.

shifting pacemaker
Shikani-French speaking valve
Shikani middle meatal antrostomy stent
Shiley

S. catheter
S. catheter distention system
S. convexoconcave heart valve
S. cuffless fenestrated tube
S. cuffless tracheostomy tube
S. decannulation plug
S. disposable cannula low-pressure
cuffed tracheostomy tube
S. distention kit
S. extra-length single-cannula
tracheostomy tube
S. fenestrated low-pressure cuffed
tracheostomy tube
S. guiding catheter
S. Infusaid pump
S. irrigation catheter
S. laryngectomy tube
S. low-pressure cuffed tracheostomy
tube with pressure relief valve
S. monostrut heart valve
S. neonatal tracheostomy tube
S. oxygenator
S. pediatric tracheostomy tube
S. Phonate speaking valve
S. pressure-relief adapter
S. saphenous vein irrigation and
pressurization device
S. single-cannula cuffed
tracheostomy tube
S. TracheoSoft XLT tracheostomy
tube
S. tracheostomy tube

shim

s. coil

3/8-inch s.
s. magnet

Shimadzu

S. cardiac ultrasound
S. CT scanner
S. DAR-2400 coronary
arteriographic analyzer
S. HeadTome Set-031 camera
S. HeadTome system
S. IIQ ultrasound
S. MR scanner
S. RF-5301 PC spectrometer
S. ultrasound system

shimmed magnet
Shimstock occlusion foil
Shiner radiopaque tube
Shin-Nippon autorefractor
Shin Nippon SRW-5000 autorefractor
Shinobi radiolucent steerable guidewire
Ship-Shaw rod hammertoe implant
Shirakabe implant
Shirley

S. drain
S. sump wound drain
S. wound drain

Shirodkar suture
shirt

EZ "T" orthopaedic s.

Shoch

S. foreign body pickup
S. suture

shock

s. block
s. wave lithotriptor

shock-absorbent sole
shock-absorbing shoe
shock-advisory defibrillator
Shockmaster heel cushion
shoe

accommodative s.
AccuTread s.
Acor Quikform I, II s.
Ambulator H1200 healing s.
Ambulatory s.
Anywear s.
Apex Ambulator s.
Ariat s.
arthritic s.
Asics Gel-MC s.
Balmoral s.
Birkenstock s.
Blucher low-quarter s.
broad-toed s.
Brooks s.
Canfield s.
cast s.
Comed postoperative s.
corrective s.
custom-made s.

S

805

shoe *(continued)*
    custom-molded s.
    Dansko s.
    Darby surgical s.
    Darco Medical-Surgical s.
    Darco OrthoWedge healing s.
    Darco Softie s.
    Darco surgical s.
    Darco wedge s.
    decubitus boot s.
    depth inlay s.
    Depth orthopaedic s.
    diabetic pressure relief s.
    Dynaslipper night s.
    extended steel-shank s.
    extra-depth s.
    GaitKeeper cast s.
    Gard-all boot s.
    GentleStep s.
    Goldenberg footplate s.
    healing s.
    HeelWedge healing s.
    Hi-Top s.
    H-series healing s.
    ill-fitting s.
    in-depth s.
    ipos heel relief s.
    ipos postoperative s.
    s. lift
    low-heeled s.
    low quarter Blucher s.
    Markell Mobility S.
    Markell open-toe s.
    Markell tarso medius straight s.
    Markell tarso pronator outflare s.
    Mephisto Mobils professional s.
    neoprene s.
    OrthoWedge healing s.
    oversize tennis s.
    Pedors orthopaedic s.
    plastizote s.
    postoperative s.
    Power Anthro s.
    pressure relief s.
    Reece orthopaedic s.
    reverse last s.
    ribbed-sole s.
    rocker-bottom cast boot s.
    SAS s.
    Saucony s.
    shock-absorbing s.
    Shoethotic s.
    Softie s.
    stiff-soled s.
    straight last s.
    s. stretcher
    Terrmocork diabetic s.
    Thera-Medic s.
    therapeutic s.
    Tru-Fit custom-molded s.
    Tru-Mold s.
    Urban Walkers s.
    Viking postoperative s.
    WACH s.
    wedge adjustable cushioned heel s.
    Xsensibles s.
    Xtra Depth s.
    Zimmer postoperative s.
    Zohar s.
shoehorn speculum
Shoemaker
    S. intraocular lens forceps
    S. rib shears
Shoethotic shoe
Shofu
    S. dental cement
    S. porcelain stain kit
Shooter Saeed multiband irrigator
short
    s. above-elbow cast
    s. arm cylinder cast
    s. arm navicular cast
    s. arm plaster splint
    s. arm posterior molded splint
    s. arm splint
    s. backboard
    s. below-elbow cast
    S. bridge
    s. C-loop intraocular lens
    s. C-loop lens
    s. coarse bur
    s. fine bur
    s. Heaney retractor
    s. leg caliper brace
    s. leg cylinder cast
    s. leg nonwalking cast
    s. leg nonweightbearing cast
    s. leg plaster cast
    s. leg splint
    s. leg walker
    s. leg walking cast
    s. monorail imaging catheter
    s. monorail polyethylene imaging
     sheath
    s. needle
    s. occluder
    side-hole Judkins curve right 4 s.
    s. stent
    s. stretch bandage
    s. taper
    s. tooth forceps
    s. transition (ST)
    s. wooden backboard
Shortbent
    S. scissors
    S. stitch scissors
    S. suture scissors
short-bevel needle

short-bore magnet
Shorti
    S. limbal relaxing incision diamond knife
    S. LRI diamond knife
short-pulse laser
short-term
    flow-assisted s.-t. (FAST)
short-tip hemostatic bag
shot compressor
shotted suture
shoulder
    s. abduction immobilizer
    s. abduction pillow
    s. abduction positioner
    Bigliani/Flatow complete s.
    s. blade
    s. controller
    s. cuff
    s. disarticulation prosthesis
    s. Ease abduction support
    s. horn
    s. ladder
    s. orthosis
    s. prosthesis
    s. pulley
    s. ROM arc
    s. saddle sling
    s. subluxation inhibitor brace
    s. surface coil
    s. wheel
shoulder-elbow-wrist-hand orthosis
shoulderRAP postsurgical wound wrap
shovel
    Aesculap power s.
    Rosenwasser lamellar donor s.
shower
    s. chair
    Hot Tap portable hot s.
    Hydrokinetic Vichy s.
    Vichy s.
showerhead infiltrator
ShowerSafe
    S. protector material
    S. waterproof cast and bandage cover
    S. waterproof cast and bandage protector
Show'rbag cast and dressing cover
SH pop-off suture
Shrady saw
shrinker
    Juzo s.
Shuco-Myst nebulizer
Shug male contraceptive device
shunt
    Accura hydrocephalus s.
    adjustable pressure s.
    Al-Ghorab modification s.

Allen-Brown s.
Ames ventriculoperitoneal s.
angiographic portacaval s.
aqueous double-tubed valve s.
aqueous tube s.
Baerveldt s.
balloon s.
bidirectional s.
bidirectional Glenn s.
Blalock s.
Blalock-Taussig s.
Brener carotid s.
Brescia-Cimino s.
Brisman-Nova carotid endarterectomy s.
Burbank carotid s.
Buselmeier s.
capillary bed s.
cavernospongiosum s.
cerebrospinal fluid s.
Cimino arteriovenous s.
Cimino AV s.
Cimino dialysis s.
cisternal-peritoneal s.
cisternal-pleural s.
ClearView intracoronary s.
ClearView intravascular arteriotomy s.
Cobe AV s.
Codman Accu-Flow s.
congenital portacaval s.
Cordis-Hakim s.
coronary anastomotic s.
CSF T-tube s.
Delta s.
Denver s.
Denver ascites s.
Denver hydrocephalus s.
Denver peritoneovenous s.
Denver pleuroperitoneal s.
dialysis s.
Diamond valve flow-regulating s.
double-bubble ventriculoperitoneal s.
Drapanas mesocaval s.
Edwards-Barbaro T-shaped syringeal s.
endolymphatic-subarachnoid s.
Ex-PRESS mini glaucoma s.
extracardiac right-to-left s.
extracranial s.
extrahepatic s.
s. filter
Flo-Thru s.
Gibson inner ear s.
Glenn s.
Gore-Tex s.
Gott s.
Hakim s.
Hashmat s.

S

shunt *(continued)*
    Hashmat-Waterhouse s.
    hepatofugal portosystemic venous s.
    Heyer-Schulte hydrocephalus s.
    Holter s.
    House endolymphatic s.
    indwelling nonvascular s.
    Javid s.
    Javid carotid s.
    jejunoileal s.
    JI s.
    Kasai peritoneal venous s.
    s. kit
    LaVeen s.
    LeVeen s.
    LeVeen ascites s.
    LeVeen dialysis s.
    LeVeen peritoneal s.
    LeVeen peritoneovenous s.
    loop s.
    miniature glaucoma s.
    modified Blalock-Taussig s.
    neurosurgical s.
    Ommaya s.
    pentose phosphate s.
    1-piece s.
    portacaval s.
    portacaval H-graft s.
    portasystemic s.
    portosystemic s.
    Potts s.
    Pruitt-Inahara carotid s.
    Pruitt-Inahara vascular s.
    PTFE s.
    Pudenz s.
    Pudenz-Schulte s.
    Pudenz valve-flushing s.
    Quinton-Scribner s.
    radiologic portacaval s.
    Ramirez s.
    relative s.
    right-to-left intracardiac s.
    Rivetti-Levinson intraluminal s.
    Scribner s.
    single-reservoir, single-pump s.
    Spetzler lumbar-peritoneal s.
    spinal cord arteriovenous s.
    splenorenal bypass s.
    Sundt carotid endarterectomy s.
    syrinx s.
    T-AnastoFlo s.
    thecoperitoneal Pudenz-Schulte s.
    Thomas s.
    Thomas femoral s.
    Torkildsen s.
    tracheoesophageal s.
    tracheopharyngeal s.
    transhepatic portacaval s.

    transjugular intrahepatic
      portosystemic s.
    T-shaped Edwards-Barbaro
      syringeal s.
    s. tube
    s. tubing
    Uni-Shunt hydrocephalus s.
    Uresil Vascu-Flo carotid s.
    USCI s.
    VA s.
    valve-regulated s.
    Vascu-Flo carotid s.
    ventriculoperitoneal s.
    VP s.
    Warren s.
    Waterston s.
    Waterston-Cooley s.
    White glaucoma pump s.
    Winter s.
shunting circuit
Shur-Band self-closure elastic bandage
Shur-Clens wound cleanser
shutoff clamp
Shutt
    S. Aggressor forceps
    S. alligator forceps
    S. basket forceps
    S. B-scoop forceps
    S. grasping forceps
    S. Mantis retrograde forceps
    S. microscissors
    S. Mini-Aggressor forceps
    S. minibasket
    S. retrograde forceps
    S. scissors
    S. shovel-nosed forceps
    S. suction forceps
    S. suture punch system
shuttle
    S. balance trainer
    S. cardiomuscular conditioner
    Caspari s.
    S. MiniClinic resistance system
    S. MVP leg press
    S. Relay suture passer
**Shuttle-SL Flexor Tuohy Borst side-arm
   introducer set**
sialoendoscope
sialography needle
Siamese twin bracket
sick dermatome
sickle
    s. blade
    s. explorer
    s. knife
    s. scaler
    s. scissors
Sickle-Chex
Sickledex test

sickle-shaped Beaver blade
SICOR recording system
side
    s. biting clamp
    s. blade
    s. branch occlusion system
    s. lyer
    s. plate
side-arm
    s.-a. adapter
    s.-a. nebulizer
    s.-a. pressure port
side-biting
    s.-b. ostrum punch
    s.-b. spatula
    s.-b. Stammberger punch forceps
side-curved forceps
side-cut pin cutter
side-cutting
    s.-c. basket forceps
    s.-c. blade
    s.-c. bur
    s.-c. cannula
    s.-c. irrigating cystotome
    s.-c. rasp
    s.-c. rongeur
    s.-c. spatula
    s.-c. spatulated needle
    s.-c. Swanson bar
    s.-c. Swanson bur
sided
    4-s. cutting needle
side-exiting
    s.-e. coaxial needle system
    s.-e. coaxial system
    s. e. guide
side-fire
    s.-f. laser
    s.-f. reflecting dish
side-firing probe
side-flattened needle
side-grasping forceps
side-hole
    s.-h. cannulated probe
    s.-h. Judkins curve right 4 short
Sidekick foot support
side-lip forceps
side-lying hip abductor
side-opening laminar hook
sideplate
    sliding compression screw with s.
side-port
    s.-p. adapter
    s.-p. cannula
    s.-p. fixation knife
    s.-p. flat-bottomed Ommaya
      reservoir
SidePort AutoControl airway connector
Side Rester cushion

Sideris
    S. adjustable buttoned device
    S. buttoned device occluder
    S. clamp
sidestream capnometer
Sidestream high-efficiency nebulizer
Si detector
side-viewing
    s.-v. duodenoscope
    s.-v. endoscope
    s.-v. fiberscope
    s.-v. videoendoscope
sidewall
    s. holed needle
    s. infusion cannula
sidewinder
    s. aortic clamp
    s. diagnostic catheter
    s. percutaneous intra-aortic balloon
      catheter
Siegel
    S. otoscope
    S. pneumatic otoscope
    S. stent
Siegel-Cohen dilating catheter
Sieger insufflator
Siegle otoscope
Sielaff gastroscope
Siemens
    S. AG system
    S. biplane Neurostar digital
      subtraction angiography system
    S. couch
    S. DRH CT scanner
    S. Ecat EXACT HR+ CTI PET
      scanner
    S. ECAT 951/31R PET scanner
    S. Endo-P endodrectal transducer
    S. gamma camera
    S. HICOR/BICOR x-ray system
    S. Impact Expert MRI scanner
    S. Impact Expert Tesla scanner
    S. linear probe
    S. Lithostar
    S. Lithostar Plus
    S. Lithostar Plus System C
      lithotriptor
    S. Magnetom GBS II scanner
    S. Magnetom Harmony scanner
    S. Magnetom scanner
    S. Magnetom SP 4000 scanner
    S. Magnetom Vision scanner
    S. Magnetom Vision whole-body
      MR device
    S. Mammomat Novation DM full
      field digital mammography system
    S. Mevatron 74 linear accelerator
    S. MRI unit

S

Siemens *(continued)*
    S. Neurostar digital subtraction angiographic system
    S. One Tesla scanner
    S. open heart table
    S. Orbiter gamma camera
    S. Orbiter large field-of-view camera
    S. Orthoceph x-ray
    S. pacemaker
    S. Plus 4 Volume Zoom multidetector scanner
    S. Quantum 2000 Color Doppler
    S. Satellite CT evaluation console
    S. Servo ventilator
    S. Siecure implantable cardioverter-defibrillator
    S. SI ultrasound
    S. Somaform 512 CT scanner
    S. Somatom DR CT scanner
    S. Somatom DR2, DR3 whole-body scanner
    S. Somatom DRH CT analyzer
    S. Somatom DRH CT analyzer unit
    S. Somatom Plus
    S. Somatom Plus 4A scanner
    S. Somatom Plus CT scanner
    S. Somatom Plus-4 CT system
    S. Somatom Plus S computed tomographer
    S. Sonocur Basic extracorporeal shockwave therapy system
    S. Sonoline CD echograph
    S. Sonoline Elegra ultrasound
    S. Sonoline Elegra ultrasound scanner
    S. Sonoline Prima ultrasound
    S. Sonoline SI-400 ultrasound system
    S. Sonoline SL-2 echocardiograph
    S. Sonoline ultrasonography
    S. Symphony scanner
    S. system
    S. ventilator
    S. Vision scanner

Siemens-Elema
    S.-E. AB pulse transducer probe
    S.-E. AG bicycle ergometer
    S.-E. multiprogrammable pacemaker
    S.-E. Servo 900C ventilator
    S.-E. Servo ventilator

Siepser endocapsular controller
Sierra-Sheldon tracheotome
SieScape
    S. ultrasound
    S. ultrasound scanner

sieve
    s. graft

    Mobin-Uddin s.
    molecular s.

Sievers model 280 nitric oxide analyzer
Sievert unit
Sifoam padding
sigma
    S. II Dualplace hyperbaric chamber
    S. II Dualplace hyperbaric oxygen therapy system
    S. II hyperbaric system
    S. I monoplace hyperbaric therapy system
    S. 6000+ infusion pump
    S. 34 monoplace hyperbaric chamber
    S. Plus monoplace hyperbaric oxygen therapy system
    s. rectum pouch
    S. TMB assay kit
    unipolar Pisces S.

sigmoid
    s. anastomosis clamp
    s. notch retractor

sigmoidofiberscope
sigmoidoscope
    ACMI T-915, TX-915 fiberoptic s.
    adult s.
    Boehm s.
    Buie s.
    disposable sheathed flexible s.
    ESI fiberoptic s.
    fiberoptic s.
    flexible s.
    Fujinon ES-200ER s.
    Fujinon flexible s.
    Fujinon FS-100ER s.
    Fujinon SIG-E2 fiberoptic s.
    Hopkins s.
    Kelly s.
    KleenSpec fiberoptic disposable s.
    Lieberman s.
    s. light carrier
    Lloyd-Davies s.
    Montague s.
    Olympus CF-L series flexible s.
    Olympus CF-OSF series flexible s.
    Olympus CF100S s.
    Olympus fiberoptic s.
    Olympus OSF s.
    Olympus OSF flexible s.
    Pentax flexible s.
    Reichert fiberoptic s.
    Reichert flexible s.
    s. replacement lamp
    rigid s.
    sheathed flexible s.
    Strauss s.
    Vernon-David s.
    Vision System s.

VSI 2000 s.
Welch Allyn disposable s.
Welch Allyn fiberoptic s.
Welch Allyn flexible s.
Welch Allyn KleenSpec fiberoptic
disposable s.

sigmoscope
SIGN
Surgical Internet Generation Network
SIGN intramedullary nail
Signa
S. Advantage system
S. Excite system
S. Horizon LX MRI system
S. Horizon LX SR 77 gradients
MR scanner
S. Horizon X-Echo-Speed
S. imager
S. LX scanner
S. MR imaging system
S. MRI scanner
S. MR unit
S. OpenSpeed MR system
S. Ovation MR system
S. Pad
S. scanner
S. superconducting magnetic
resonance imaging scanner
S. VH/i3.0-T MR scanner
S. whole body imager/spectrometer
S. whole-body imager/spectrometer
SignaDress
S. sterile hydrocolloid
S. sterile hydrocolloid dressing
signal-averaged electrocardiograph
Signature Edition infusion system
Signet
S. disposable skin stapler
S. Optical lens
Signify ER drug screen test
Sigvaris
S. compression stocking
S. medical stocking
Siker mirror laryngoscope
silanated slide
silastic
s. ball
s. ball spacer prosthesis
s. band
s. bur hole cover
s. button
s. catheter
s. chin implant
s. chin prosthesis
s. closed-suction drain
s. collar-reinforced stoma
s. electrode casing
s. eustachian tube
s. foam dressing

s. Foley catheter
s. gel dressing
s. graft
s. grommet
s. HP tissue expander
s. indwelling ureteral stent
s. mammary prosthesis
s. medical adhesive
s. midfacial malar implant
s. mold
s. mushroom catheter
s. obstetrical vacuum cup
s. patch
s. penile implant
s. penile prosthesis
s. plate
s. poppet
s. ring
s. rod
s. scleral buckler implant
s. septal button
s. sheet
s. silicone rubber implant
s. sling
s. sphere
s. sponge
s. spring-loaded silo
s. stent
s. strain gauge
s. strap
s. subdermal implant
s. tape
s. testicular implant
s. testicular prosthesis
s. toe implant
s. tracheostomy tube
s. T tube
s. tube
s. tubing
s. wick
Silc extractor
Silent
S. Night diagnostic and screening
device
S. Nite alarm
S. Nite external nasal dilator
S. Speaker communication system
Silesian bandage
Silflex intramedullary prosthesis
Silhouette
S. endoscopic laser
S. IC implant
S. Laser-Lok implant
S. laser system
S. pedicle screw system
S. prosthetic foot
S. spinal system
S. therapeutic massage system

S

811

Silhouette *(continued)*
    S. therapeutic mattress
    S. therapeutic surface
silica contact lens
silicate cement
silicon diode dosimeter
silicone
    s. adhesive
    s. ball heart valve
    Biocell textured s.
    s. block
    s. brush back-flushed needle
    s. buckling implant
    s. button
    s. button eye implant
    s. cannula
    s. catheter
    Codman ventricular s.
    s. conformer
    s. diode dosimeter
    s. disc heart valve
    s. dressing
    s. elastomer
    s. elastomer band
    s. elastomer infusion catheter
    s. elastomer lens
    s. elastomer prosthesis
    s. elastomer ring
    s. elastomer rubber ball implant
    s. elastomer suspension implant
    s. epistaxis catheter
    s. eye sphere
    s. flexor rod
    s. gel
    s. gel breast implant
    s. gel prosthesis
    s. gel sheeting
    s. hemisphere
    s. hubless flat drain
    s. hydrogel contact lens
    s. insole
    s. intraocular lens
    s. introducer
    s. lead
    s. microimplant
    s. mold
    s. MP implant
    s. nasal strut implant
    s. pad
    s. pad eye implant
    s. plug
    s. Robinson catheter
    s. rod
    s. rod implant
    s. rod and sleeve forceps
    s. round drain
    s. rubber
    s. rubber Dacron-cuffed catheter
    s. self-expanding prosthesis

    s. sheet
    s. sizer
    s. sleeve eye implant
    s. spacer
    s. sponge
    s. sponge forceps
    s. sponge implant
    s. stent
    s. strip
    s. strip eye implant
    s. sump drain
    s. textured mammary implant
    s. thoracic drain
    s. tire
    s. tire eye implant
    tire-grooved s.
    s. toric IOL
    s. trapezium prosthesis
    s. T tube
    s. tube
    Wonderflex s.
silicone-coated metallic self-expanding stent
silicone-covered aspiration tip
silicone-filled
    s.-f. anatomical breast implant
    s.-f. mammary implant
    s.-f. round breast implant
silicone-lubricated endotracheal tube
silicone-spiked mat
silicone-treated surgical silk suture
Silicore foot pillow
Silimed implant
Silipos
    S. arthritic/diabetic gel sock
    S. digital pad
    S. Distal Dip prosthetic sheath/liner
    S. gel
    S. mesh cap
    S. mesh tubing
    S. silicone wonder cup
    S. soft walk gel sock
    S. suspension sleeve
Silitek
    S. ureteral stent
    S. Uropass stent
silk
    s. braided suture
    S. Bullet feeding tube
    s. guidewire
    s. jejunal tube
    S. Laser
    s. Mersilene suture
    s. nonabsorbable suture
    Owens s.
    S. Pill feeding tube
    s. pop-off suture
    s. screw
    S. Skin sheet

s. stay suture
s. suture
s. tie
S. Tip feeding tube
s. traction suture
virgin s.
SilkLaser
S. aesthetic CO_2 laser
S. aesthetic laser system
CO_2 FeatherTouch S.
EpiTouch Ruby S.
2040 erbium S.
FeatherTouch S.
Sharplan Erbium S.
Sharplan FeatherTouch S.
Sil-K OB barrier
SilkTouch
S. CO_2 laser
S. CO_2 laser scanner
S. laser
silkworm gut suture
silo
Prolene mesh s.
removal mesh s.
silastic spring-loaded s.
Si-Loc sacroiliac belt
SiloLiner gel liner
Silon
S. silicone elastomer sheeting
S. silicone thermoplastic splinting material
S. tent
S. wound dressing
Silopad
S. body sleeve
S. toe sleeve
Silosheath
S. gel
S. gel liner
S. sock
Siloskin dressing
Siloxane
S. graft
S. implant
S. prosthesis
SilqueClenz skin cleanser
Silsoft extended wear contact lens
Siltex
S. Becker 50 breast prosthesis
S. breast implant
S. mammary implant
silver
s. bead electrode
s. and cadexomer iodine-based wound dressing
S. cannula
s. catheter
s. clip
s. mylar roll

S. nasal osteotome
s. needle
s. nitrate stick
S. osteotome
s. probe
S. Speed hydrophilic guidewire
s. suture
s. thermal hat
s. wire suture
silver-coated
s.-c. catheter
s.-c. stent
SilverHawk
S. catheter
S. device
S. plaque excision system
silverized catgut suture
Silverman biopsy needle
silver-silver chloride electrode
Silverstein
S. facial nerve monitor
S. lateral venous sinus retractor
S. permanent aeration tube
S. stimulator probe
Silver-Thera
S.-T. stocking
S.-T. stocking electrode
Simaplast implant
SIM 2 catheter
Simcoe
S. anterior chamber capsule scrubber
S. anterior chamber receiving needle
S. anterior chamber retaining wire
S. cannula tip
S. capsular scraper
S. C-loop intraocular lens
S. connecting tubing
S. corneal marker
S. cortex extractor
S. cortex extractor aspiration cannula
S. double-barreled cannula
S. double-barreled irrigating/aspirating unit
S. double-end lens loupe
S. eye speculum
S. I&A system
S. II PC aspirating needle
S. II PC double cannula
S. II PC lens
S. II PC nucleus delivery loupe
S. interchangeable tip
S. intraocular lens implant
S. irrigating-positioning needle
S. lens-inserting forceps
S. lens-positioning set
S. notched irrigating spatula

Simcoe (*continued*)
S. nucleus delivery cannula
S. nucleus erysiphake
S. nucleus forceps
S. nucleus lens loupe
S. nucleus spatula
S. posterior capsule scrubber
S. posterior chamber forceps
S. reverse aperture cannula
S. reverse I&A cannula
S. scleral depressor
S. superior rectus forceps
S. suture needle
S. wire speculum
Simmons
S. catheter
S. II, III catheter
S. plate
S. plating system
S. sidewinder catheter
Simmons-type sidewinder catheter
Simon
S. bone curette
S. cup uterine curette
S. dermatome
S. fistula hook
S. fistula knife
S. nitinol inferior vena cava filter
S. nitinol IVC filter
S. vaginal retractor
Simonart
S. band
S. bar
Simplastic catheter
simple button patellar implant
Simplex P bone cement
Simplicity
S. adult disposable contoured undergarment liner system
S. spirometer
SimpliCT interventional guidance system
Simply Wet table
Simpson
S. atherectomy catheter
S. AtheroCath catheter
S. AtheroCath system
S. coronary AtheroCath
S. coronary AtheroCath catheter
S. Coronary AtheroCath system
S. directional atherectomy catheter
S. endoscope
S. forceps
S. lacrimal dilator
S. lacrimal probe
S. obstetrical forceps
S. peripheral AtheroCath
S. PET balloon
S. positron emission tomography balloon

S. uterine dilator
S. uterine sound
Simpson-Braun obstetrical forceps
Simpson-Luikart obstetrical forceps
Simpson-Robert
S.-R. ACS dilatation catheter
S.-R. catheter
S.-R. vascular dilation system
Simpulse
S. irrigation system
S. lavage system
S. pulsing lavage
S. S/I lavage
Sims
S. anoscope
S. cannula
S. nasal prongs
S. Per-fit percutaneous tracheostomy kit
S. rectal retractor
S. rectal speculum
S. sponge holder
S. suction tip
S. suture
S. uterine depressor
S. uterine dilator
S. uterine probe
S. uterine scissors
S. uterine sound
S. vaginal retractor
S. vaginal speculum
Sims-Maier sponge and dressing forceps
simulator
AcQsim CT s.
Baltimore Therapeutic Equipment Work S.
BTE work s.
Ergos work s.
flexible bronchoscopy s.
heartbeating s.
inanimate s.
Lido WorkSET work s.
Maxwell 3D field s.
MR s.
Nucletron s.
radiation s.
Spinal Physiotherapy S.
surgical s.
Tepper proprioceptor s.
Ultravoice speech s.
virtual reality s.
Work Seat driving s.
Ximatron s.
simultaneous multiple analyzer
Singer-Blom
S.-B. prosthesis
S.-B. tube
Singer needle

single
- s. chamber cardiac pacing system
- s. clamp
- s. cross-slot screwdriver
- s. hook
- s. lung PneuView stimulator
- s. occluder
- s. patient system
- s. photon emission computed tomography (SPECT)
- s. pigtail stent
- s. port
- s. reference point instrument
- s. running suture
- s. safe-sided chisel
- s. width bracket

single-action
- s.-a. pumping system
- s.-a. rongeur

single-armed suture

single-axis
- s.-a. ankle prosthesis
- s.-a. friction knee
- s.-a. locking knee
- s.-a. Syme DYCOR foot

single-base cane
single-beveled cutting instrument
single-bevel stylet
single-bladed Kurze microscissors
single-blade retractor

single-chamber
- s.-c. pacemaker
- s.-c. pulse generator

single-channel
- s.-c. analyzer
- s.-c. cochlear implant
- s.-c. colonoscope
- s.-c. electromyograph oscilloscope
- s.-c. fiberoptic bronchoscope
- s.-c. in vivo light dosimeter
- s.-c. wire-guided sphincterotome

single-crystal
- s.-c. endoprobe
- s.-c. gamma camera

single-curved Cobra catheter
single-cylinder penile prosthesis
single-day infuser

single-detector
- s.-d. helical scanner
- s.-d. row scanner

single-disc prosthesis
single/double occluder
single-energy x-ray absorptiometer
single-fiber EMG electrode
single-headed instrument
single-head rotating gamma camera
single-hole collimator
single-holed suction cannula

single-hook
- s.-h. Frazier skin hook
- s.-h. retractor

single-incision system
single-loop tourniquet

single-lumen
- s.-l. balloon stone extractor catheter
- s.-l. Broviac silicone catheter
- s.-l. cannula
- s.-l. infusion catheter

single-mirror goniolens
single-needle device
single-panel knee immobilizer

single-pass
- s.-p. lead
- s.-p. pacemaker

single-patient use manometer

single-photon
- s.-p. densitometer
- s.-p. electrospinal orthosis

single-piece
- s.-p. acrylic IOL
- s.-p. SN60AT IOL

single-plane instrument
single-prong broad acetabular retractor
single-reservoir, single-pump shunt
single-rod construct
single-running suture
single-sided bone saw

single-stage
- s.-s. catheter
- s.-s. screw implant
- s.-s. Straumann dental implant

single-stemmed silicone hemiprosthesis
single-stick system

single-tooth
- s.-t. forceps
- s.-t. subperiosteal implant
- s.-t. tenaculum

single-use
- s.-u. catheter
- s.-u. dermatome
- s.-u. device
- s.-u. electrode
- s.-u. instrument

single-vision lens
single-wall needle
single-wire electrode

Singley
- S. intestinal ring clamp
- S. tissue forceps

Singley-Tuttle
- S.-T. dressing forceps
- S.-T. intestinal forceps
- S.-T. tissue forceps

Singular Oval polypectomy snare
sinoatrial ball
SinoJect puncture set

Sinskey
  S. hook
  S. IOL manipulator
  S. iris hook
  S. J-loop intraocular lens
  S. lens-holding forceps
  S. lens hook
  S. lens implant
  S. lens manipulating hook
  S. lens manipulator
  S. needle holder
  S. nucleus spatula
  S. pick
sintered titanium mesh
Sinterlock
  S. implant
  S. implant metal prosthesis
Sinu-Knit dissolvable nasal dressing
SinuNEB sinus care system
sinus
  s. antral cannula
  s. balloon
  s. biopsy forceps
  s. bur
  s. chisel
  s. curette
  s. dilator
  s. irrigating cannula
  s. irrigator
  s. lift osteotome
  s. node pacemaker
  s. probe
  s. trephine
  s. tympani excavator
SinuScope
  S. rigid rod
  S. rigid rod lens optics
  S. scope
  S. system
sinuscope
  Panoview Plus s.
SinuSeal nasal packing
SinuSight ENT module
SinuSpacer turbinate stent
siphon suction tube
Sippy
  S. esophageal dilating set
  S. esophageal dilator piano-wire
    staff
Sirecust 404N neonatal monitoring
  system
Siremobil
  S. C-arm unit
  S. Iso-C3d isocentric C-arm
Sirocco evacuation chair
sirolimus-eluting
  s.-e. SMART nitinol stent
  s.-e. stent
SIR-Spheres radioactive sphere

SISCO spectrometer
Sisler punctum dilator
Sisson fracture reducing elevator
Sister Helen mustard table
sister-hook forceps
Sistron scissors
Sistrunk
  S. dissecting scissors
  S. retractor
  S. scissors
SiteGuard transparent dressing
Site-Rite II ultrasound system
SiteSelect percutaneous incisional breast
  biopsy system
SITEtrac spinal surgery system
sit/stand chair
Sit-Straight wheelchair cushion
sit-to-stand training parallel bar unit
sitz bath
Sitzmarks
  S. radiopaque marker
  S. radiopaque marker in gelatin
    capsule
six-shooter
  Saeed s.-s.
  Wilson-Cook s.-s.
sizer
  Björk-Shiley heart valve s.
  Brannock Device shoe s.
  breast s.
  Meadox graft s.
  silicone s.
  voice prosthesis s.
sizer-dissector
  Mizuho aneurysm s.-d.
sizing
  s. balloon
  s. clamp
  s. implant
  s. ring
SJM
  St. Jude Medical
  SJM Masters Series heart valve
  SJM mechanical heart valve
  SJM pericardial patch
  SJM Quattro mitral valve
  SJM Regent mechanical heart
    valve
  SJM Rosenkranz pediatric retractor
    system
  SJM Seguin annuloplasty ring
  SJM Tailor annuloplasty ring
  SJM X-Cell cardiac bioprosthesis
SkareKare silicon gel-filled cushion
skate
  arm s.
Skatron apparatus
SKBM microkeratome

Skeele
S. chalazion curette
S. corneal curette
S. curette
S. eye curette

Skeeter
S. otologic drill
S. otologic drill system

skeletal
s. bed
s. pin

skeleton
s. fine forceps
Teflon-coated wire s.

Skene
S. catheter
S. tenaculum forceps
S. uterine tenaculum
S. vulsellum
S. vulsellum forceps

ski
s. needle
walker s.

skiameter
skiascope
skid
bone s.
hip s.
MacAusland hip s.
Meyerding bone s.
Murphy s.
Murphy-Lane bone s.

SKI knee prosthesis
Skil-Care
S.-C. Alarm cushion
S.-C. cushion
S.-C. cushion grip
S.-C. reclining wheelchair

Skillbuilder half roll
Skillern
S. sinus curette
S. sphenoidal probe
S. sphenoid cannula

Skillman mosquito forceps
Skil saw
Skimmer
S. laryngeal blade
S. laryngeal blade tip

skin
Apligraf tissue-engineered s.
artificial s.
S. Care kit
CellSpray spray-on s.
s. clip
composite cultured s.
s. elevator
Epigard synthetic s.
s. flap retractor
s. forceps

s. graft expander mesh
s. graft mesher
s. hook
s. hook retractor
Integra artificial s.
s. marker
s. marking pen
s. punch
s. self-retaining retractor
S. Skribe marker
S. Skribe pen
s. splint
s. staple
S. Stretcher appliance
s. suture
S. Temp collagen

skin-contact instrumentation
skinfold calipers
SkinLaser system
Skinlight
S. erbium:YAG laser
S. erbium:YAG laser system for
skin resurfacing
S. erbium yttrium-aluminum-garnet
laser
S. Er:YAG laser

Skinny
S. balloon catheter
S. Chiba needle
S. dilatation catheter

Skin-Prep protective dressing
Skinscan device
Skinsense glove
SkinSleeves
Posey S.

SkinTech medical tattooing device
SkinTegrity
S. hydrogel dressing
S. impregnated gauze
S. wound cleanser

SkinTemp
S. biosynthetic collagen dressing
S. collagen skin dressing

Skirrow agar plate
skiving knife
Sklar
S. bone drill
S. bone saw
S. instrument polish
S. Kleen liquid
S. Kleen powder
S. ligature needle
S. lube
S. pin cutter
S. scrub
S. tonometer
S. wire tightener

Skoog nasal chisel

S

skull
> s. bur
> s. clamp
> s. elevator
> s. plate
> s. plate screwdriver
> s. punch
> s. traction drill
> s. traction tongs
> s. trephine

Sky-Boot stirrup system
Skylark TENS unit
SKYLight gantry-free nuclear medicine gamma camera
Skytron
> S. air-fluidized bed
> S. bed
> S. operating room table
> S. surgical table

SL1 sheath
slab
> 3D MRA s.

slab-off lens
Slade formed irrigation cannula
Slade-type adjustable aspirating LASIK speculum
Slalom
> S. balloon
> S. PTA balloon dilatation catheter
> S. PTA dilatation catheter

Slam'r wheelchair
slant
> foam s.
> S. haptic
> S. haptic intraocular lens
> s. hole collimator

slaphammer
Slatis fixation
SLA transducer
slatted plinth table
Slaughter saw
SL cage
sleds
> Penco Walker S.
> walker s.

sleep
> s. apnea monitor
> S. Guardian foam pad
> S. Sentry

Sleeper Gripper prosthetic device
Sleepscan
> S. airflow pressure transducer
> S. Traveler ambulatory polysomnography system
> S. Traveler home monitoring system

sleeve
> s. adapter

arthroscopic monopolar thermal stabilization forefoot compression s.
Assura irrigation s.
s. bag
Bard irrigation s.
BioCompression Pneumatic S.
biocompression pneumatic s.
Charles anterior segment s.
Charles infusion s.
Coloplast transparent irrigation s.
Cunningham-Cotton s.
delivery assistance s.
Dexterity pneumo s.
drill s.
drug infusion s.
Easy S.
Edwards-Levine s.
elbow s.
Electro-Mesh s.
epX suspension s.
excursion amplifier s.
forefoot compression s.
gel suspension s.
heel s.
Iceflex Endurance suction suspension s.
Iceross s.
s. implant
implant s.
Jobst s.
Knit-Rite suspension s.
Labtician oval s.
laparoscopic s.
LocalMed catheter infusion s.
malleolar gel s.
Mentor Foley catheter with comfort s.
neoprene elbow s.
Pedifix forefoot compression s.
phaco s.
pin s.
PMMA centering s.
pneumatic compression s.
Pneumo S.
Preclude IMA s.
primary hydroxyapatite-coated s.
Reid s.
retinal probe s.
s. selector
s. sensor
Silipos suspension s.
Silopad body s.
Silopad toe s.
Super Grip s.
Supramid eye muscle s.
Sur-Fit colostomy irrigation s.
Sur-Fit Natura irrigation s.
Surgiport trocar and s.

Ultra Duet Colostomy irrigating s.
Ultra Sleeve ultrasound s.
ultrasound s.
Watzke s.
Watzke silicone s.
sleeved nut
sleeveless phaco tip
sleeve-spreading forceps
sleuth
CO S.
ETO S.
HBT S.
SLE ventilator
Slick stylette endotracheal tube guide
slide
aminopropyltriethyoxysilane-coated
glass s.
ChemMate capillary gap s.
Colorfrost disposable microscope s.
Colormark s.
CytoRich cervical cytology s.
Fisher-plus s.
gelatin-subbed s.
Genta s.
s. hammer
Hemoccult Sensa s.
hydrogel-coated s.
muscle s.
Polaroid vectograph s.
silanated s.
Superfrost microscope s.
Superfrost Plus glass s.
Testsimplets prestained s.
triethylenethiophosphoramide
precoated s.
Ventana silanized capillary gap s.
slideboard
Activ s.
SlideMaker/Stainer (SMS)
Cell-Dyn S.
Slide-On EndoSheath
SlidePro slide heater
slider crank mechanism
sliding
s. AFO
s. barrel hook
s. compression screw with sideplate
s. hammer
s. laryngoscope
s. lock
slightly curved ear pick
Slik-Pak nonstick nasal pack
Slim
S. Fit flex clamp
S. Option shoe orthosis
slimcut blade
SlimLine
S. cast boot
S. disposable brief

S. fitted liner
S. peach sheet care pad
Slim-LOC anterior cervical plate system
Slimrest
Core S.
SlimSIGHT gastrointestinal videoscope
Slimthetics orthotic
sling
Advantage midurethral s.
Aldridge rectus fascia s.
AliMed hemi-arm s.
Ampoxen s.
Arjo loop s.
arm elevator s.
BioSling bioabsorbable urethral s.
Böhler-Braun leg s.
cardiac s.
clip-reinforced cotton s.
Cook Stratasis urethral s.
cradle arm s.
CVA S.
DLP cardiac s.
s. dressing
envelope arm s.
finger s.
Fits-All s.
FoamWrap finger s.
foot s.
FortaPerm surgical s.
s. frame
Givmohr upper extremity s.
Harris hemi-arm s.
Harris splint s.
head s.
Hemi s.
s. immobilizer
knee s.
Kodel s.
leg s.
Lynx midurethral s.
Mersilene mesh s.
Monarc transobturator s.
Murphy s.
muscle s.
muslin s.
Nada-Chair Back-Up portable
back s.
Perthes s.
Posey s.
pouch-type s.
pressure s.
pulmonary artery s.
Rauchfuss s.
Raz anterior vaginal wall s.
resting foot s.
Sabre s.
Salter s.
s. seat wheelchair
shoulder saddle s.

S

sling *(continued)*
   silastic s.
   static s.
   strap s.
   Stratasis urethral s.
   suburethral s.
   Supramid s.
   Suspend s.
   s. and swathe (S&S)
   temporalis s.
   tendon s.
   Thomas buckle s.
   transobturator s.
   triangular arm s.
   triple-tail fascia lata s.
   universal s.
   Velpeau s.
   Velpeau shoulder s.
   Vesica s.
   Vogue arm s.
   volar ulnar s.
   Weil pelvic s.
sling-and-swathe bandage
sling/mesh
   Surgisis s./m.
Slingshot shoulder immobilizer
Slip-Coat tip
slip-joint pliers
Slip-N-Snip scissors
slip-on finger splint
slipper
   Acu-Pressure s.
   s. cast
   PPCID s.
   WalkCare s.
slipper-tipped guidewire
slip-ring camera
slit
   s. blade
   s. blade knife
   s. collimator
   s. illuminator
slit-lamp, slitlamp *(See also* lamp)
   Bausch & Lomb-Thorpe s.-l.
   s.-l. biomicroscope
   Campbell s.-l.
   Canon RO-4000, -5000 s.-l.
   Coherent LaserLink s.-l.
   s.-l. cup
   s.-l. fluorophotometer
   Gullstrand s.-l.
   Haag-Streit s.-l.
   Haag-Streit Biomicroscope 900 s.-l.
   Heine HSL 100 handheld s.-l.
   Ishihara IV s.-l.
   Kowa handheld s.-l.
   Kowa Optimed s.-l.
   Lumenis 950 s.-l.

   Marco s.-l.
   s.-l. microscope
   Nikon zoom photo s.-l.
   Posner s.-l.
   Reichert s.-l.
   Rodenstock s.-l.
   Specular reflex s.-l.
   Thorpe s.-l.
   Topcon SL-E series s.-l.
   Universal s.-l.
   Zeiss carbon arc s.-l.
   Zeiss-Comberg s.-l.
SLM-8000 fluorescence spectrophotometer
Sloane
   S. Epi-Peeler
   S. flap repositor
   S. micro hoe
   S. trephine
Slocum meniscal clamp
Slo-Mo ball
Slot distraction device
slot-scanning detector
slotted
   s. anoscope
   s. bolt
   s. bone plate
   s. instrument
   s. intramedullary rod
   s. laryngoscope
   s. mallet
   s. nail
   s. needle
   s. nerve clamp
   s. obturator-cannula system
   s. tendon stripper
   s. tube articulated stent
   s. tube stent
   s. whisker
   s. wrench
slotting bur
slow palatal expander
10 SL/O Zeiss keratometer
SLP1000 diode laser system
SL-Plus stem
SLS
   SLS Chromos long-pulse ruby laser system
   SLS laser
SLT
   Surgical Laser Technologies
   SLT contact MTRL laser
   SLT laser cautery
Sluder
   S. retractor
   S. sphenoidal hook
   S. sphenoidal speculum
   S. tonsillar guillotine

Sluder-Ballenger
    S.-B. tonsillar punch forceps
    S.-B. tonsillectome
Sluder-Jansen mouthgag
Sluijter-Mehta SMK-C10 cannula
SLx
    Iris Medical OcuLight SLx
SMAC
    Sequential Multiple Analyzer Computer
small
    s. aperture Steri-Drape
    s. cup biopsy forceps
    s. egress cannula
    s. fragment screw
    s. lamina spreader
    s. LITT applicator
    s. nail spicule bur
    s. plate forceps
    s. rake retractor
    s. stature cervical plate (SSP)
    s. tissue retractor
    s. trapezoid (ST)
    s. vessel (SV)
small-aperture Steri-Drape drape
small-base quad cane
small-bore
    s.-b. cannula
    s.-b. needle
    s.-b. scanner
small-caliber
    s.-c. duodenovideoscope
    s.-c. needle
Small-Carrion
    S.-C. penile implant material
    S.-C. penile prosthesis
    S.-C. silastic rod for penile
       implant
small-diameter
    s.-d. endosonographic instrument
    s.-d. wire
SmallHand polypectomy snare
small-headed screw
small-loop electrode
small-particle aerosol generator
SmallPort needle
small-volume nebulizer
SMA portogram
SMART
    SMART Control self-expanding
       stent
    SMART nitinol self-expandable
       stent
    SMART self-expanding stent
    SMART stent
Smart
    S. Balance Master
    S. Balance Master system
    S. bile duct stent
    S. chalazion forceps

    S. enucleation scissors
    S. forceps
    S. Plug lacrimal plug
    S. position-sensing catheter
    S. Scope
    S. Screener infant hearing screener
    S. Splint
    S. System irrigation/suction system
    S. Tag triage tag
    S. Triage Pac
    S. Trigger
    S. Trigger Bear ventilator
    S. Trigger Bear 1000 ventilator
SmartBrace
    S. brace
    S. wrist splint
SmartCath esophageal balloon catheter
SmartCycler realtime PCR system
Smartdop Doppler
SmartDose infusion system
SmartFlow multiple-lesion device
SmartKard digital Holter system
SmartKnit seamless diabetic sock
SmartMist
    S. asthma management system
    S. respiratory management system
SmartNeedle needle
SmartPill pH.p capsule
SmartPin instrument set
SmartPin/PLLA pin
SmartPrep
    MR S.
SmartSet HV bone cement
SmartSite needleless system
SmartSPOT high-resolution digital
   imaging system
Smartstent
SmartSuction Harmony surgical suction
   device
SmartTack
    S. fixation
    S. tack
SmartWrap elbow brace
SMC-type collimator cone
Smec balloon catheter
Smedberg
    S. hand drill
    S. twist drill
Smedley dynamometer
SMEI
    SMEI ultrasound-assisted lipoplasty
      machine
    SMEI ultrasound device
Smellie
    S. obstetrical forceps
    S. obstetrical hook
    S. obstetrical perforator
    S. obstetrical scissors

S

Smeloff-Cutter
  S.-C. ball cage prosthetic valve
  S.-C. ball-valve prosthesis
Smeloff heart valve
SMI 3000, 5000 bed
SMIC
  SMIC rongeur
  SMIC surgical catgut
SmiLine abutment system
Smillie
  S. cartilage chisel
  S. cartilage knife
  S. knee joint retractor
  S. knee retractor
  S. meniscectomy chisel
  S. meniscotome
  S. pin
Smith
  S. anal retractor
  S. automatic perforated drill
  S. bandage scissors
  S. cartilage knife
  S. clip
  S. electrode
  S. expressor hook
  S. eye speculum
  S. genioplasty plate
  S. intraocular capsular amputator
  S. knife
  S. lens expressor
  S. lid-retracting hook
  S. & Nephew bracing and support
    system
  S. & Nephew ENT
    nasopharyngoscope
  S. & Nephew medium barbed
    staple
  S. & Nephew reflection acetabular
    cup implant component
  S. & Nephew Richards bipolar
    forceps
  S. & Nephew screw
  S. & Nephew small barbed staple
  S. orbital floor implant
  S. percutaneous endopyelotomy
    stent
  S. pessary
  S. separator
  S. speculum
  S. splitter
  S. STA-peg
  S. total ankle prosthesis
Smith-Buie rectal speculum
Smith-Fisher iris spatula
Smith-Green cataract knife
Smith-Hodge pessary
Smith-Leiske cross-action intraocular
  lens forceps

Smith-Petersen
  S.-P. chisel
  S.-P. cup
  S.-P. femoral neck nail
  S.-P. gooseneck gouge
  S.-P. impactor
  S.-P. intertrochanteric plate
  S.-P. nail
  S.-P. pin
  S.-P. straight osteotome
Smith-Richards instrumentation
Smithwick
  S. clip-applying forceps
  S. ganglion hook
  S. nerve hook
  S. retractor
  S. sympathectomy hook
smoke
  s. aspiration tip
  S. Controller device
  S. Control Porta-Pack aversive
    stimulator
  s. evacuator
  s. evacuator suction tube
  s. removal tube
SmokEvac trumpet valve
S-Monovette blood collection system
smooth
  s. cannula
  s. dressing forceps
  s. endoprosthesis
  s. grasping forceps
  s. jawed needle holder
  s. pin
  s. staple implant
  s. tissue forceps
  s. transfixion wire
smooth-tipped jeweler's forceps
smooth-walled tubing
SMS
  SlideMaker/Stainer
  Cell-Dyn SMS
SMZ-10A zoom stereo microscope
snail-headed catheter retriever
Snap
  S. fixation pin
  S. Lock wire/pin extractor
snap
  s. gauge
  s. gauge band
Snap-Gauge gauge
snap-lock brace
snap-off capability (SOC)
snap-on inserter plate
Snap-Pak
  Mitek GII S.-P.
snare
  AcuSnare s.
  Amplatz gooseneck s.

Amplatz retinal s.
automatic ratchet s.
Banner enucleation s.
barbed s.
Beck-Schenck tonsillar s.
BiSNARE bipolar polypectomy s.
Bruening ear s.
Bruening nasal s.
Bruening tonsillar s.
Captiflex polypectomy s.
Captivator polypectomy s.
Castroviejo enucleation s.
s. catheter
cautery s.
caval s.
coaxial s.
crescent s.
s. device
diathermal s.
diathermic s.
ear polyp s.
electrosurgery s.
enucleation wire s.
s. enucleator
Eves-Neivert tonsillar s.
Eves tonsillar s.
Förster enucleation s.
Foster enucleation s.
Frankfeldt diathermy s.
Frankfeldt rectal s.
frontalis s.
Glisson s.
gooseneck s.
Hobbs polypectomy s.
Hoyer s.
Jarvis s.
Krause ear polyp s.
Krause laryngeal s.
Krause nasal polyp s.
laryngeal s.
lasso s.
Lewis tonsillar s.
Marlex mesh s.
Martin s.
Mason-Allen s.
Meek s.
Microvena Amplatz goose neck s.
Nakao S. I, II
nasal s.
Needle's Eye s.
nitinol s.
Olympus SD-9L-1 s.
Olympus SD-5L semicircular s.
open electrocautery s.
Optimizer disposable
  polypectomy s.
oval s.
pelvic s.
pericardial s.

polypectomy s.
Posey s.
Profile pediatric polypectomy s.
ptosis s.
pulmonary arterial s.
Quire mechanical finger s.
rectal cautery s.
Reiner-Beck s.
rotatable polypectomy s.
Rotator polypectomy s.
self-opening rigid s.
Sensation Short Throw s.
Singular Oval polypectomy s.
SmallHand polypectomy s.
standard endoscopy polypectomy s.
surgical s.
tonsillar s.
transvenous nitinol s.
Tydings tonsil s.
UroSnare cystoscopic tumor s.
Wappler polypectomy s.
Weston rectal s.
Wilde ear polyp s.
Wilde nasal s.
Wilson-Cook polypectomy s.
s. wire
wire s.

Snellen
S. acuity chart
S. chart
S. conventional reform eye implant
S. conventional reform implant
S. entropion forceps
S. forceps
S. lens loupe
S. lens scoop
S. letter optotype
S. near-vision card
S. reform eye
S. soft contact lens
S. suture
S. vectis

Sniper
S. Elite hydrophilic guidewire
S. Elite hydrophilic Ni-Ti alloy
  guidewire
S. hydrophilic nitinol guidewire

Snoar appliance
snooze pillow
snore
s. guard
S. Guard mandibular repositioning
  device
S. Tec appliance
Snore-Ezzer oral appliance
Snorenomor device
SnoreSat sleep recorder
Snowden-Pencer
S.-P. insufflator

S

Snowden-Pencer *(continued)*
    S.-P. laparoscopic cholecystectomy instrument
    S.-P. Supercut scissors
snow plow rasp
SNPstream genotyping system
snub-nose diamond blade
Snug
    S. denture cushion
    S. seat
Snugfit eye patch
Snuggle Warm convective warming system
Snugs
    S. tapeless dressing
    S. tapeless wound care system
    S. wrap
Snyder
    S. corneal spring forceps
    S. deep surgery forceps
    S. drain
Soaker catheter
soap
    SoftCIDE-EC antimicrobial hand s.
    SoftCIDE hand s.
    SoftCIDE-NA plain hand s.
    TLC antiseptic s.
SOC
    snap-off capability
    SOC pin
sock
    active s.
    AFO brace s.
    s. aid
    arthritis s.
    Bio-Wick s.
    Carolon AFO s.
    Comfort Ag prosthetic s.
    Comfort n' Care Seamfree s.
    Creative diabetic s.
    Dero hole-in-1 prosthetic s.
    Dero hole-in-toe prosthetic s.
    diabetic s.
    edema s.
    electrode s.
    gel stump s.
    Kushyfoot s.
    molding s.
    polytetrafluoroethylene s.
    reflexology s.
    Regal Acrylic/Stretch prosthetic s.
    Rx Comfort s.
    Silipos arthritic/diabetic gel s.
    Silipos soft walk gel s.
    Silosheath s.
    SmartKnit seamless diabetic s.
    Soft Walk gel s.
    Strassburg s.
    STS molding s.

    stump s.
    Thorlo padded s.
    Venosan support s.
Sock-Assist device
socket
    adjustable postoperative protective prosthetic s.
    all-alumina s.
    all-polyethylene s.
    check s.
    Clearpro suction s.
    concave loading s.
    endoskeletal s.
    flexible s.
    Flo-Tech prosthetic s.
    hard s.
    Iceross silicone s.
    Icex s.
    intermediate s.
    ischial containment s.
    ischial-gluteal weightbearing s.
    metal-backed s.
    modular s.
    patellar tendon s.
    polyethylene s.
    preassembled metal-backed s.
    prosthetic s.
    Pump-It-Up pneumatic s.
    quadrilateral ischial weightbearing s.
    Sabolich s.
    standard s.
    supracondylar s.
    suspension-type s.
    temporary s.
    universal frame outer s.
    variable-circumference suprapatellar s.
    s. wrench
Socon spinal system
Socrates telementoring system
SOCS pad system
Sodas spheroidal oral drug absorption system
sodium
    s. acrylate and vinyl alcohol copolymer microsphere
    s. chloride-impregnated gauze
    s. detector
    s. dodecyl sulfate-polyacrylamide gradient slab gel
    s. hyaluronate-based bioresorbable membrane
    s. hyaluronate viscoelastic
    s. hyaluronate wound gel
    s. iodide detector
Soehendra
    S. catheter dilator
    S. catheter system
    S. dilator

S. endoscopic biliary stent system
S. graduated dilating catheter
S. stent extractor
S. stent retrieval device
S. stent retriever
S. Universal catheter

Sof
S. Airr insole
S. Matt pressure relieving mattress
S. Sole motion control orthotic

SofWire cable system

Sofamor
S. spinal device
S. spinal instrument
S. spinal instrumentation device

Sofamor-Danek component
Sof-Band bulky bandage
Sofban orthopaedic padding wool
Sof-Care
S.-C. chair cushion
S.-C. Plus cushion

Sofcare mattress
SofDraw safety syringe
Sofflex
S. mattress
S. mattress system

Sof-Flex pediatric double pigtail stent
Sof-Foam dressing
Sof-Form conforming gauze
Sof-Gel palm shield
Sof-Kling conforming bandage
SofLens66 toric contact lens
SofLens contact lens
SoFlex
S. intraocular lens
S. IOL
S. series lens

Sofnit
S. Birdseye reusable underpad
S. 300 reusable underpad

SofPort
S. AO aspheric lens
S. easy-load injector
S. easy-load lens delivery system
S. L161 AO lens

SofPulse device
Sofra-Tulle dressing
Sof-Rol
S.-R. cast pad
S.-R. dressing

Sofsilk
S. coated and braided suture
S. nonabsorbable silk suture

SofSole Airr insole
Sofsorb absorptive dressing
soft
s. acrylic IOL
s. ankle cushioned heel orthopaedic appliance

s. cataract aspirator
s. catheter
s. cervical collar
s. contact lens
s. copolymer foam
s. cosmetic cover
s. diverticuloscope
s. intraocular lens
s. IOL cutter
S. N' Dry Merocel sponge
s. palate retractor
S. Plug punctal plug
s. rubber curette
s. rubber drain
s. rubber string
S. Sack IV fluid warmer
s. scrub brush
S. & Secure spouted pouch system
S. Shield collagen corneal shield
S. & Silent diaper pant
S. & Silent vinyl pull-on brief
S. & Silent vinyl snap-on brief
s. silicone sponge
s. socket insert
S. Super Sport orthotic
S. Support Preforms orthotic
s. thoracoport
s. tissue blade retractor
s. tissue elevator
s. tissue expander
s. tissue shaving cannula
S. Torque uterine catheter
S. Touch hand exerciser
S. Touch lancet device
S. Touch stocking
S. Walk gel sock
s. wire loop
s. x-ray film

Sof-Tact
S.-T. diabetes glucose monitor
S.-T. diabetes management system
S.-T. glucose monitor
S.-T. test strip

Soft-Cell
S.-C. catheter
S.-C. eye spear
S.-C. permanent dual-lumen catheter

SoftCIDE-EC antimicrobial hand soap
SoftCIDE hand soap
SoftCIDE-NA plain hand soap
Softclamp
S. arterial return cannula
S. system

SoftCloth absorptive dressing
soft-cup extractor
Softech endotracheal tube
SofTec rigid brace
Softeze water pillow

SoftFlex
   S. computer glove
   S. wrist wear
Softflo fiberoptic probe
SoftForm
   S. collagen facial implant
   S. facial implant
   S. tube
SoftGrip pipette
SoftGUARD hand cream
Softie shoe
Softip
   S. catheter
   S. diagnostic catheter
   S. oxygen nasal cannula
SoftLight
   S. laser
   S. laser hair removal system
   S. laser/skin resurfacing process
soft-lined denture
Softopac intraoral film
Softouch
   S. cold/hot pack
   S. diagnostic catheter
   S. spinal angiography catheter
SofTouch vacuum erection device
Soft-Pass embryo transfer catheter
Softpatch
   Impress S.
SoftSITE high add aspheric multifocal contact lens
SoftSpec inflatable vaginal speculum
Softsplint foot splint
Soft-Tip catheter
soft-tipped
   s.-t. cannula
   s.-t. extrusion handpiece
soft-tissue Super Sport orthotic
Soft-Touch A-Probe
Soft-Vu
   S.-V. angiographic catheter
   S.-V. Omni flush catheter
Soft-Wand atraumatic tissue manipulator balloon
software-controlled internal hardware filter
Sof-Wick
   S.-W. drain
   S.-W. drain sponge
   S.-W. dressing
   S.-W. sponge
Sof'Wire
   S. cable
   S. cable system
   S. spinal fixation
SolAiris
   S. III oxygen concentrator
   S. III, V oxygen concentrator
Solanas cervicothoracic fixation system

Sola Optical USA Spectralite high-index lens
Solar
   S. Beam medical examination light
   S. pacemaker
Solcotrans
   S. autotransfusion system
   S. autotransfusion unit
   S. closed vacuum-drainage system
   S. drainage/reinfusion system
   S. orthopaedic drainage-refusion system
solder
   PF Universal s.
   tissue s.
soldering tweezers
sole
   Ambulator Bio-Rocker s.
   s. lift/heel drop
   plaster s.
   PodiAxis orthopaedic s.
   Poro-in-between s.
   shock-absorbent s.
   Texon s.
   Vibram s.
solenoid surface coil
Solera thrombectomy catheter
SOLEutions
   S. custom orthosis
   S. custom orthotic device
   S. Prefab orthotic device
   S. soft plus orthotic
   S. sport shell orthotic
Solfy ZX ultrasonic unit
solid
   s. ankle cushioned heel (SACH)
   s. ankle cushioned heel foot prosthesis
   s. buckling implant material
   s. carbon dioxide pencil
   s. copper head mallet
   s. hex bolt
   s. silicone buttock implant
   s. silicone exoplant implant material
   s. silicone orbital prosthesis
   s. silicone with Supramid mesh implant
solid-core needle with hollow tip
solid-phase
   s.-p. extraction chromatograph
   s.-p. extraction tube
solid-rod
   s.-r. rigid telescope
   s.-r. ureteroscope
solid-state
   s.-s. coagulator
   s.-s. dye laser
   s.-s. esophageal manometry catheter

s.-s. instrument
s.-s. manometry catheter
s.-s. nuclear track detector
solid-tip catheter
Solight forceps lighting system
Solitens
    S. TENS unit
    S. transcutaneous electrical nerve stimulation unit
Soll suture and incision marker
Solo
    S. balloon
    S. catheter
SoloPass
    S. catheter
    S. Percuflex biliary stent
Solos
    S. disposable cannula
    S. disposable trocar
SoloSite
    S. hydrogel dressing
    S. wound gel
SOLO-Surg Colorectal self-retaining retractor system
Solo-Tach resin
Solstice balloon
Solumbra 30+ SPF fabric
Solution
    S. prosthesis
    S. System acetabular cup
Soma
    S. Gonio system
    S. pulley system
    S. sacroiliac stabilization belt
Somanetics Invos 3100 cerebral oximeter
SomaSensor
    S. device
    S. pad
Somatics
    S. monitoring electrode
    S. mouth guard
Somatom
    S. DR CT scanner
    S. Plus S whole body scanner
    S. Volume Zoom computed tomography system
    S. Volume Zoom CT system
Somer uterine elevator
SOMI
    sternal occipital mandibular immobilizer
    SOMI brace
    SOMI Jr. brace
    SOMI orthosis
Somnoplasty system
SomnoStar apnea testing device
Somnus
    S. probe
    S. somnoplasty system

Sonablate
    S. 200 system
    S. transrectal probe
    S. 200 ultrasound system
Sonata imager
Sonde enteroscope
Sones
    S. catheter
    S. coronary catheter
    S. Hi-Flow catheter
    S. woven Dacron catheter
Songbird disposable hearing aid
Song covered duodenal stent
Songer
    S. cable
    S. cable system
sonic
    s. accelerated fracture healing system (SAFHS)
    S. Air 1500 device
    s. curette
    S. Hedgehog
Sonicaid System 8000
Sonicare Plus
Sonicath
    S. endoluminal ultrasound catheter
    S. imaging catheter
    S. intravascular ultrasound catheter
Sonicator portable ultrasound
Sonic-Care toothbrush
SonicWAVE phacoemulsification system
Sonifer sonicating system
Sonix 2000 ultrasonic nebulizer
Sonnenberg sump drain
Sonnenschein nasal speculum
Sonoace
    S. II ultrasound
    S. 6000 II ultrasound system
Sonoblate ablation device
Sonocath ultrasound probe
Sonoclot coagulation analyzer
Sonocur extracorporeal shockwave therapy system
Sonocut ultrasonic aspirator
Sonogage
    S. System Corneo-Gage center frequency transducer
    S. ultrasound pachymeter
sonographer
    Combison 530 3D s.
    Sonoline 400 2D s.
    Sonoline SL1 2D s.
    Trans-Scan pulsed Doppler s.
sonography unit
SonoHeart
    S. Elite ultrasound system
    S. handheld all digital echocardiography system
    S. scanner

Sonolayer ultrasound
Sonoline
   S. 400 2D sonographer
   S. Elegra ultrasound system
   S. Prima ultrasound
   S. Siemens ultrasound scanner
   S. Sienna ultrasound system
   S. Sierra ultrasound imaging device
   S. Sierra ultrasound imaging
     system
   S. SI-200/250 ultrasound imaging
     system
   S. SL1 2D sonographer
Sonolith
   S. 3000 lithotriptor
   S. Praktis portable lithotriptor
Sonomed
   S. A/B-Scan system
   S. 1500 A-scan instrument
   S. A-Scan system
   S. B-1500 system
sonometer
   clinical bone s.
   Omnisense 7000S bone s.
   Sahara clinical bone s.
   SoundScan 2000 bone s.
   SoundScan Compact bone s.
   UBIS quantitative ultrasound
     bone s.
   UBIS ultrasound bone s.
   ultrasound bone imaging s.
Sonometric Ocuscan
Sonoprobe endoscopic ultrasonography
  system
Sonopsy
   S. biopsy imaging system
   S. ultrasound-guided breast biopsy
     system
Sonos
   S. cardiovascular ultrasound
   S. 4500 echocardiography system
   S. imaging system
   S. 500 imaging system
   S. 1500, 2500 scanner
   S. ultrasonographic transducer
   S. 2000, 5500 ultrasound imager
   S. ultrasound unit
SonoSite
   S. digital ultrasound
   S. hand-carried ultrasound
   S. 180 hand-carried ultrasound
     device
   S. iLook 24 ultrasound
   S. MicroMaxx laptop ultrasound
   S. 180Plus ultrasound
   S. pulsed wave Doppler
   S. Titan ultrasound
   S. 180 ultrasound system
Sono-stat Plus EMG machine

Sonotrode lithotriptor
Sonotron electronic therapeutic device
SonoVue ultrasound contrast media
SonoVu US aspiration needle
SonoWand
   S. intraoperative imaging system
   S. ultrasound-based neuronavigation
     system
Sontac gel pad
Sontec pliers
Sony
   S. CCD/RGB color videocamera
   S. Promavica still capture device
   S. video recorder
Soothies glycerin gel breast pad
Sopha
   S. DSX1 camera
   S. Medical gamma camera
Sopher ovum forceps
Sophie mammography unit
Sophy
   S. adjustable pressure valve
   S. camera
   S. high-resolution collimator
   S. mini-programmable pressure
     valve
   S. programmable valve
Soprano
   S. cryoablation system
   S. cryotherapy unit
sorbent dialysis cartridge
Sorbex
   S. hydrocolloid wound dressing
   S. thin hydrocolloid dressing
Sorbie-Questor total elbow prosthesis
  system
Sorbothane
   S. antivibration glove
   S. heel cushion
   S. II heel cup
   S. insole
   S. recoil pad
   S. rice sheller roller
   S. wrap
Sorbsan
   S. alginate dressing
   S. alginate wound cover
Sorensen
   S. aspirator
   S. Transpac transducer
Soreson pressure transducer
Sorin
   S. Bicarbon bileaflet aortic valve
     prosthesis
   S. Carbostent stent
   S. heart valve
   S. lead
   S. mitral valve prosthesis

S. pacemaker
S. prosthetic valve
Sorrells hip arthroplasty retractor system
Sorrel-type snowboard boot
sorter
FACSVantage cell s.
fluorescence-activated cell s.
magnetically activated cell s.
Sorvall Discovery SE ultracentrifuge
SOS
SOS guidewire
SOS total hip system
SOS total knee system
Sos Pulse-Vu bloodless entry needle
Soules intrauterine insemination catheter
sound
Allport mastoid s.
Béniqué s.
bladder s.
bronchocele s.
Davis interlocking s.
Dittel s.
female s.
flexible s.
French steel s.
Greenwald s.
Guyon s.
Guyon urethral s.
interlocking s.
Jewett s.
Jewett urethral s.
Jewett uterine s.
Klebanoff common duct s.
Kocher bronchocele s.
lacrimal s.
LeFort s.
LeFort urethral s.
LeFort uterine s.
s. level meter
Mark-7 intrauterine s.
Martin uterine s.
McCrea infant s.
meatal s.
Mercier s.
metal s.
miniature s.
Otis s.
Pharmaseal disposable uterine s.
Pratt urethral s.
s. processor
radiolucent s.
rigid s.
Simpson uterine s.
Sims uterine s.
urethral s.
uterine s.
Van Buren canvas roll s.
Van Buren urethral s.

Walther s.
Walther urethral s.
Winternitz s.
Soundbridge
Symphonix Vibrant S.
Vibrant D, HF, P S.
sounder
mini-echo s.
pedicle s.
SoundScan
S. 2000 bone sonometer
S. Compact bone sonometer
Soundtec Direct system implant
source
cesium s.
diagnostic x-ray camera and imaging s.
dummy s.
ESI fiberoptic light s.
fiberoptic light s.
halogen dual light s.
halogen light s.
Heyman-Simon s.
Maxenon xenon light s.
Maxillume quartz halogen light s.
MX2-300 xenon quality light s.
Olympus CLV-U 20 endoscopic halogen light s.
PhotoDerm filtered flashlamp-pumped light s.
PhotoDerm VL light s.
Teclite fiberoptic light s.
xenon light s.
Zeiss Super Lux 40 light s.
SourceLink brachytherapy delivery system
Souter-Strathclyde elbow prosthesis
Souter Strathclyde total elbow system
Southern Eye Bank corneal cutting block
Souttar
S. cautery
S. tube
Sovereign
S. bifocal lens
S. Shield system
Sox
Champion Power S.
SP
suprapubic
SP Walker cast
SP-10 spirometer
SP6 camera
SP90 miniblade
Spa
S. Bed
S. Ready-To-Wear gradient pressure therapy hosiery
S. Touch hair removal device

S

space
> Barouk button s.
> s. retainer
> S. Saver volumetric pump

space-age wire
Spacehaler
Spacekeeper retractor
SpaceLabs Holter monitor
space-maintaining barrier
Spacemaker
> S. balloon dissector
> S. hernia balloon dissector
> S. II balloon
> S. II surgical balloon dissector
> S. surgical balloon dissector

Space-OR flexible internal retractor
spacer
> AlloCraft PL allograft s.
> Barouk s.
> Button S.
> ceramic vertebral s.
> dummy s.
> Ellipse compact s.
> eyelid s.
> GAIT s.
> Graftech cervical s.
> Graftech structural allograft
>   cervical s.
> Hourglass vertebral body s.
> s. inserter
> interbody s. (IBS)
> InterSpace hip s.
> InterSpace knee s.
> intraoral s.
> Kinemax s.
> methyl methacrylate s.
> Natural Selection PLIF wedge and
>   cervical s.
> OsteoStim cervical allograft s.
> Plexiglas s.
> proximal cement s.
> rubber s.
> silicone s.
> suture s.
> telescopic plate s.
> TraXis interbody s.
> TraXis Ti alloy s.
> TraXis Vue alloy s.

SpaceSEAL balloon tip cannula
Spadafora MemoryLens dialer
spaghetti drain
Spaide scleral depressor
Spaleck forceps
Spandage tubular stretch bandage
Spanish silk suture
spanner
> s. gauge
> s. wrench

spanning external fixator

SPARC sling system
spark-gap
> s.-g. apparatus
> s.-g. instrument
> s.-g. shock wave generator

Spark handheld dynamometer
Sparta
> S. microforceps
> S. micro-iris forceps

Spartacore 14 guidewire
SPART analyzer
Spartan jaw wire cutter
SpaTable
> Wet S.

SpaTouch PhotoEpilation System
spatula
> Alio-Rodriguez LASIK s.
> Allison lung s.
> angled iris s.
> angulated iris s.
> Ayers s.
> Aylesbury s.
> Ayre s.
> Banaji s.
> Bangerter angled iris s.
> Bangerter iris s.
> Barraquer cyclodialysis s.
> Barraquer iris s.
> Barraquer irrigator s.
> Berens s.
> brain s.
> Buratto contact lens spoon and s.
> s. cannula
> s. cannula tip
> capsule fragment s.
> Carones LASEK s.
> Castroviejo cyclodialysis s.
> Castroviejo synechia s.
> cement s.
> Children's Hospital brain s.
> Cleasby s.
> corneal fascia lata s.
> Culler iris s.
> curved tipped s.
> curved-tipped s.
> cyclodialysis s.
> Cytobrush s.
> Davis brain s.
> s. dissector
> double s.
> double-vector brain s.
> duck-billed anodized s.
> electrosurgical s.
> s. electrosurgical probe
> Elschnig cyclodialysis s.
> endarterectomy s.
> Fisher-Smith s.
> fishtail s.
> flat s.

s. forceps
Fox LASIK s.
Freer nasal s.
French hook s.
French lacrimal s.
French pattern s.
Fukasaku s.
Fukasaku-Lieberman
  phacoemulsification s.
Fukusaku s.
Fukushima malleable brain s.
Galin lens s.
Gills-Welsh s.
Girard synechia s.
Green lens s.
Guimaraes flap s.
Guimaraes ophthalmic s.
Guimaraes ophthalmic flap s.
Hersh LASIK retreatment s.
Hirschman s.
Hirschman iris s.
Hirschman lens s.
hook s.
s. hook
Hough s.
iridodialysis s.
iris s.
irrigating notched s.
Jaffe intraocular s.
Jaffe lens s.
Johnson s.
Kader intestinal s.
Katena iris s.
Kennerdell s.
Killian laryngeal s.
Kimura platinum s.
Kirby angulated iris s.
Knapp cyclodialysis s.
Knapp iris s.
Knolle lens cortex s.
Knolle lens nucleus s.
Kocher bladder s.
Kwitko lens s.
LASEK epithelial detaching s.
LASEK epithelial flap
  repositioning s.
lens s.
Leriche s.
Lewicky IOL s.
Lieppman s.
Lindner s.
Lindner cyclodialysis s.
Lindstrom LASIK s.
lingual s.
Lynch s.
MacRae flap flipper/retreatment s.
Maddox LASIK s.
malleable s.
Manhattan Eye & Ear s.

Masket phaco s.
Maumenee vitreous sweep s.
Mayfield malleable brain s.
McIntyre irrigating s.
McPherson s.
McPherson iris s.
McReynolds s.
McReynolds eye s.
Meller cyclodialysis s.
microvitreoretinal s.
Milex s.
Moran enhancement s.
Moran LASIK s.
s. needle
needle s.
nerve separator s.
nucleus s.
Obstbaum lens s.
Olivecrona brain s.
Olk retinal s.
Olk vitreoretinal s.
Pap-Perfect plastic s.
Paton s.
Paton double s.
Paton single s.
Paton transplant s.
plaster s.
platinum probe s.
probe s.
s. probe
Pucci-Seed s.
Rainin lens s.
rectangular brain s.
Rhein LASIK epithelial
  detaching s.
Rhein LASIK flap elevator and
  stromal s.
Rhein LASIK flap repositioning s.
Roux s.
Rowen s.
Sachs s.
Seibel double-ended LASIK flap
  lifter and s.
serrated T s.
Sheets lens s.
side-biting s.
side-cutting s.
Simcoe notched irrigating s.
Simcoe nucleus s.
Sinskey nucleus s.
Smith-Fisher iris s.
s. split needle
s. spoon
spoon s.
S-shaped brain s.
stainless s.
Steinert double-ended LASIK s.
surgical s.
suture pickup s.

spatula *(continued)*
    synechia s.
    Tan s.
    tapered brain s.
    Thomas s.
    Thornton malleable s.
    s. tip
    Troutman-Barraquer iris s.
    Tuffier abdominal s.
    ultrasound s.
    vaginal s.
    vitreous sweep s.
    wax-removing s.
    Wheeler cyclodialysis s.
    Wheeler iris s.
    Woodson s.
spatulated
    ASSI breast dissector s.
    s. half-circle needle
    s. needle
spatula-tip cannula
speaking
    s. tube
    s. valve
spear
    s. blade
    eye s.
    LASIK s.
    Merocel surgical s.
    Soft-Cell eye s.
    Ultracell LASIK s.
spear-ended chrome probe
Spears laser balloon
special
    s. Colles splint
    Heel Spur S.
specialized tissue aspirating resectoscope
Speci-Gard specimen transport bag
specimen
    s. forceps
    s. trap
Speck introducer
SPECT
    single photon emission computed
      tomography
      SPECT high-resolution brain system
spectacle-mounted
    s.-m. camera
    s.-m. telescope
spectacles
    bifocal s.
    bronchoscopic s.
    clerical s.
    compound s.
    decentered s.
    diver's s.
    divided s.
    Franklin s.
    half-eye s.

    half-glass s.
    Hallauer s.
    hemianopic s.
    industrial s.
    lid crutch s.
    Masselon s.
    orthoscopic s.
    pantoscopic s.
    periscopic s.
    photochromic s.
    prismatic s.
    protective s.
    pulpit s.
    safety s.
    stenopeic s.
    telescopic s.
    tinted s.
    wire frame s.
SPECT-CT
    Symbia TruePoint SPECT-CT
Spectra
    S. 400 extended surveillance and
      alert system
    S. pad
Spectra-Cath
Spectra-Diasonics ultrasound
spectral Doppler
Spectralite Transitions lens
SpectraMax spectrophotometer
Spectramed transducer
Spectranetics
    S. catheter
    S. C rapid-exchange laser catheter
    S. laser
    S. laser sheath
    S. Prima laser guidewire
    S. Statham transducer
Spectra-Physics
    S.-P. argon laser
    S.-P. microsurgical laser
Spectra-Pritchard photometer
Spectraprobe-Max probe
Spectraprobe-PLS laser angioplasty
   catheter
Spectra-System
    S.-S. abutment
    S.-S. implant
Spectrax
    S. bipolar pacemaker
    S. programmable Medtronic
      pacemaker
Spectris
    S. MR-compatible injector
    S. power injector
spectrocolorimeter
spectrofluorometer
spectrometer
    Amis 2000 respiratory mass s.
    atomic absorption s.

Bruker AMX 300 NMR s.
Burker Avance s.
Centronic 200 MGA respiratory
  mass s.
Compton suppression s.
Digilab FTS 40A s.
EDXRF s.
energy dispersive s.
gamma ray s.
gas isotope ratio mass s.
GE GN300 7.05-T/89-mm bore
  multinuclear s.
GE NMR s.
hard x-ray imaging s.
IBM NMR s.
InSpectra tissue s.
liquid scintillation s.
mass s.
Mossbauer s.
Nicolet NMR s.
NMR s.
nuclear magnetic resonance s.
scintillation s.
Shimadzu RF-5301 PC s.
SISCO s.
Varian Associates bore s.
Varian NMR s.
Varian Spectra s.
x-ray s.

Spectron
S. EF total hip system
S. prosthesis

Spectronic Genesys 5 spectrophotometer
spectrophotofluorometer
spectrophotometer
absorption s.
atomic absorbance s.
Beckman UV s.
Cary 118C s.
Cary 100 UV-Vis s.
digital imaging s. (DIS)
DU Series 500, DU 800
  UV/Vis s.
F-1200, -2000, -4500
  fluorescence s.
F-series fluorescence s.
Genetics Systems microplate
  reader s.
Hitachi s.
Hitachi F-2000 fluorescence s.
Hitachi F-series fluorescence s.
Hitachi U-2000 s.
liquid scintillation s.
mass s.
narrow band s.
Perkin-Elmer model 5000 atomic
  absorption s.
reflectance s.
SLM-8000 fluorescence s.

SpectraMax s.
Spectronic Genesys 5 s.
Uvidec-77 s.
UV-Vis s.
spectropolarimeter
Jasco s.
spectroradiometer
spectroscope
Auger electron s. (AES)
direct vision s.
near-infrared s.
PE2100 s.
2-wavelength near-infrared s.
spectroscopy
x-ray photoemission s.
spectroscopy-directed laser
Spectrum
S. color vision meter 712
  anomaloscope
S. Designs facial implant
S. Designs Medical facial implant
S. DG-P pediatric cradle
S. K1 laser
S. lens analysis system
S. ruby laser
S. silicone Foley catheter
S. stethoscope
S. tissue repair system
SpectRx glucose monitor
specular
s. attachment
s. microscope
s. reflection video-recording system
S. reflex slit-lamp
speculum, pl. **specula**
adolescent vaginal s.
Agrikola eye s.
Alfonso pediatric eyelid s.
Amko vaginal s.
anal s.
s. anoscope
aspirating lid s.
aural s.
Auvard weighted vaginal s.
Azar lid s.
Bárány s.
Barraquer-Colibri s.
Barraquer-Colibri eye s.
Barraquer eye s.
Barraquer solid s.
Barraquer wire s.
Barr rectal s.
Barr-Shuford s.
basket-style scleral supporter s.
Beckman nasal s.
Berens s.
Berlind-Auvard vaginal s.
Bionix nasal s.
bivalved anal s.

S

speculum *(continued)*
    blackened s.
    Boucheron ear s.
    Bozeman s.
    Brewer vaginal s.
    Brinkerhoff rectal s.
    Brown interchangeable lid s.
    Carpel s.
    Castroviejo s.
    Castroviejo eye s.
    Chelsea-Eaton anal s.
    Chevalier Jackson laryngeal s.
    Clark s.
    Clark eye s.
    Coakley nasal s.
    Collin vaginal s.
    Converse nasal s.
    Cook s.
    Cook eye s.
    Cook rectal s.
    Cottle nasal s.
    Cottle septal s.
    Cusco vaginal s.
    Cushing-Landolt transsphenoidal s.
    Czerny rectal s.
    David rectal s.
    Desmarres lid s.
    DeVilbiss-Stacy s.
    DeVilbiss vaginal s.
    Douvas-Barraquer s.
    Downes nasal s.
    Doyen vaginal s.
    duckbill s.
    Dudley-Smith rectal s.
    Duplay-Lynch nasal s.
    Duplay nasal s.
    ear s.
    Eisenhammer s.
    endaural s.
    Erhardt ear s.
    eye s.
    Fanta s.
    Farrior ear s.
    Farrior oval s.
    Feaster adjustable eyelid s.
    Fergusson tubular vaginal s.
    fiberoptic vaginal s.
    fine-wire s.
    Fishkind eye s.
    flat-bladed nasal s.
    Flint glass s.
    Floyd-Barraquer wire s.
    s. forceps
    Fox s.
    Fränkel s.
    Gaffee s.
    Garrigue weighted vaginal s.
    Gilbert-Graves s.
    Ginsberg eye s.
    Goligher s.
    Graefe eye s.
    Graves bivalve s.
    Graves open-side vaginal s.
    Gruber ear s.
    Guell LASIK s.
    Guell-type LASIK s.
    Guild-Pratt rectal s.
    Guist s.
    Guttmann vaginal s.
    Guyton-Park eye s.
    Halle infant nasal s.
    Halle-Tieck nasal s.
    1-hand s.
    Hardy s.
    Hardy bivalve s.
    Hartmann ear s.
    Hartmann nasal s.
    Hayes vaginal s.
    Helmholtz s.
    Henrotin weighted vaginal s.
    Hirschman s.
    Hirschman anoscope rectal s.
    s. holder
    Holinger infant esophageal s.
    House stapes s.
    Huffman adolescent s.
    Huffman-Graves vaginal s.
    Huffman vaginal s.
    illuminated vaginal s.
    s. illuminator transilluminator
    Ives rectal s.
    Jackson vaginal s.
    Katena s.
    Kelly rectal s.
    Kershner reversible eyelid s.
    Killian nasal s.
    Killian rectal s.
    Killian septal s.
    KleenSpec disposable vaginal s.
    Knapp eye s.
    Knolle lens s.
    Kogan endocervical s.
    Kogan urethra s.
    Kramer ear s.
    Kratz aspirating s.
    Kratz-Barraquer wire lid s.
    Kristeller vaginal s.
    Kyle nasal s.
    Lancaster eye s.
    Lancaster lid s.
    Lancaster-O'Connor s.
    Landau s.
    Lang eye s.
    Lawford s.
    LeeSpec disposable vaginal s.
    LeFort s.
    Lempert-Colver endaural s.
    Lester-Burch eye s.

lid s.
Lieberman aspirating s.
Lieberman K-wire s.
lighted s.
Lillie nasal s.
Lindstrom-Chu aspirating s.
Lucae ear s.
Luer eye s.
Machat adjustable aspirating
 wire s.
Machat-type adjustable aspirating
 LASIK s.
Mahoney intranasal antral s.
Manche LASIK s.
Markomanolakis aspirating wire s.
Martin rectal s.
Martin vaginal s.
Mathews rectal s.
Maumenee-Park eye s.
Mayer s.
McHugh oval s.
McKee s.
McKinney eye s.
McLaughlin s.
McPherson s.
McPherson eye s.
Mellinger s.
Mellinger-Axenfeld eye s.
Mellinger eye s.
Mellinger fenestrated blades s.
Merz-Vienna nasal s.
Metcher s.
Moria 1-piece s.
Mosher nasal s.
Mueller s.
Murdock eye s.
Murdock-Wiener eye s.
Myles nasal s.
nasal s.
nasal bivalve s.
nasopharyngeal s.
Nott vaginal s.
Omni-Park s.
open-side vaginal s.
O'Sullivan-O'Connor vaginal s.
otoscope s.
oval s.
Pannu-Kratz-Barraquer s.
Park s.
Park-Guyton s.
Park-Guyton-Callahan s.
Park-Guyton-Maumenee s.
Park-Maumenee s.
Pederson vaginal s.
pediatric lid s.
Pennington rectal s.
Pierse eye s.
plain wire s.
Politzer ear s.

Pratt rectal s.
Prima Series LEEP s.
4-prong finger s.
rectal s.
reversible lid s.
Rica vaginal s.
round s.
Sani-Spec vaginal s.
Sauer infant eye s.
Sawyer rectal s.
Schott lid s.
Seibel 3D s.
Serdarevic s.
Shea s.
shoehorn s.
Simcoe eye s.
Simcoe wire s.
Sims rectal s.
Sims vaginal s.
Slade-type adjustable aspirating
 LASIK s.
Sluder sphenoidal s.
Smith s.
Smith-Buie rectal s.
Smith eye s.
SoftSpec inflatable vaginal s.
Sonnenschein nasal s.
SRT vaginal s.
stapes s.
Steiner s.
Steiner-Auvard s.
stop s.
Thudichum nasal s.
Tieck-Halle infant nasal s.
Tieck nasal s.
Toynbee ear s.
transsphenoidal s.
Troeltsch ear s.
Universal s.
vaginal s.
Vernon-David rectal s.
Vienna Britetrac nasal s.
Voltolini nasal s.
Vu-Max vaginal s.
weighted vaginal s.
Weiss s.
Welch Allyn illuminated s.
Welch Allyn KleenSpec vaginal s.
Wiener eye s.
Williams eye s.
wire lid s.
Yankauer nasopharyngeal s.
Yankauer pharyngeal s.
Ziegler s.
Ziegler eye s.
speech aid
SpeechViewer
speed
 S. brace

speed *(continued)*
  S. hand splint
  S. Lok soft stent
  S. radius cap prosthesis
  s. vacuum concentrator
Speedband
  S. multiple-band ligator
  S. Superview ligator
Speedy-1 Auto refractometer
Spelcast car seat
Spence
  S. intervertebral disc rongeur
  S. rongeur forceps
Spencer
  S. biopsy forceps
  S. cannula
  S. chalazion forceps
  S. incontinence device
  S. labyrinth exploration probe
  S. plication forceps
  S. probe
  S. probe depth electrode
  S. scissors
  S. stitch scissors
  S. triangular adenoid punch
  S. triangular tip
  S. Universal adenoid punch tip
Spencer-Wells arterial forceps
Spenco
  S. arch support
  S. boot
  S. external breast form
  S. insole
  S. orthotic device
  S. shoe insert
  S. top cover
Sperma-Tex preshaped mesh
Sperm Select sperm recovery system
Spero forceps
Spetzler
  S. clip applier
  S. lumbar-peritoneal shunt
  S. MicroVac suction tube
  S. needle holder
  S. titanium aneurysm clip
SpF-PLUS spinal fusion stimulator
SpF spinal fusion stimulator
SpF-XL stimulator
sphenoidal
  s. bone punch
  s. bur
  s. cannula
  s. electrode
  s. probe
  s. punch forceps
sphenopalatine ganglion needle
sphenozygomatic suture
sphere
  AccuPoint targeting s.

  Carter s.
  Doherty s.
  s. implant
  infrared light-reflecting s.
  s. introducer
  Mules vitreous s.
  porous hydroxyapatite s.
  Pyrex eye s.
  resin s.
  silastic s.
  silicone eye s.
  SIR-Spheres radioactive s.
spherical
  s. bur
  s. eye implant
  s. implant
  s. IOL
  s. reamer
spheric lens
spherocentric knee prosthesis
spherocylinder
spherocylindrical lens
spherocylindric lens
Sphero Flex implant
spherometer
spheroprism
sphincter
  American Medical Systems
    urethral s.
  AMS 800 artificial urethral s.
  artificial s.
  AS-800 artificial s.
  s. dilator
  double-cuff urinary s.
  Hydroflex s.
  servomechanism s.
sphincteroscope
  Kelly s.
sphincterotome
  Autotome rotatable s.
  bipolar s.
  Bitome bipolar s.
  Cotton s.
  Cremer-Ikeda s.
  DASH s.
  Doubilet s.
  double-channel s.
  ERCP s.
  Fluorotome double-lumen s.
  long-nosed s.
  needle-tipped s.
  open s.
  single-channel wire-guided s.
  Ultratome double-lumen s.
  Ultratome XL triple-lumen s.
  Wilson-Cook double-channel s.
  Wilson-Cook modified wire-
    guided s.
  Wilson-Cook wire-guided s.

wire-guided s.
Zimmon s.
sphincterotomy basket
sphygmocorder
sphygmomanometer, sphygmometer
Ayers s.
Baumanometer standard mercury s.
s. cuff
cuff s.
Erlanger s.
Faught s.
Hader aneroid s.
Hawksley random zero mercury s.
Janeway s.
London School of Hygiene and Tropical Medicine s.
Mosso s.
Physio-Control Lifestat s.
random zero s.
Riva-Rocci s.
Tycos aneroid s.
sphygmoscope
Bishop s.
spica
s. bandage
s. cast
s. dressing
Formfit thumb s.
Freedom thumb s.
s. splint
s. table
TheraKool breathable neoprene thumb s.
thumb s.
spicule forceps
Spider
S. cervical plating system
S. embolic protection device
Spiegelberg intracranial pressure monitoring system
Spiegel-Wycis human apparatus
Spier elbow arthrodesis
Spiessel position screw
spike
cemental s.
Gaenslen s.
Gissane s.
Monoscopy locking trocar with Woodford s.
s. retractor
Spitzy s.
s. staple
sterile vent s.
s. washer implant
spiked
s. Darrach-type elevator
s. washer
SPI-Lite sleep position indicator

spinal
s. arthroscope
s. catheter
s. cord arteriovenous shunt
s. cord retractor
s. cord stimulator
s. disc prosthesis
s. fusion chisel
s. fusion curette
s. fusion device
s. fusion gouge
s. fusion system
s. needle
s. orthosis
s. perforating forceps
S. Physiotherapy Simulator
s. retractor blade
s. rod
s. rod cross-bracing
s. saw
s. screw and rod system
s. slip wrench
S. Technology bivalve TLSO brace
s. turning frame
ventral derotating s. (VDS)
s. wedge
SpinaLase Nd:YAG surgical laser system
SpinaLogic bone growth stimulator
SpinalPak
S. bone growth stimulator
S. spine fusion stimulator
SpinalSight spinal module
Spinal-Stim Lite
Spinchron DLX, 15 series centrifuge
spindle
muscle s.
spine
s. apparatus
s. board
S. Power pelvic stabilizer belt
SpineCATH
S. intradiscal catheter
SpineCor nonrigid brace
SpineLink-II independent intrasegmental spine fixation system
SpineLink system
SpineScope
Clarus S.
Spine-Six BioMotion spinal system
SpineStat side-directed discectomy probe
SpineWand
Cavity S.
Perc-DC S.
Perc-DLG S.
Perc-DLR S.
Spinhaler
S. inhaler
S. Turbo-Inhaler

S

Spinnaker Elite flow-directed microcatheter
spinner
    DiffSpin slide s.
spinning
    s. disc nebulizer
    s. probe
Spinocan Quincke bevel spinal needle
spinopelvic transiliac fixation system
spinous
    s. process spreader
    s. process wire
spiral
    s. bandage
    s. basket
    s. coil stent
    s. CT scanner
    s. CT, XCT scanner
    s. drill
    s. electrode
    s. endosteal implant
    s. filler
    S. Flute cranioblade
    s. fluted tungsten carbide bur
    s. forceps
    s. gallstone forceps
    intraprostatic s.
    S. Mark V portable ultrasonic drug inhaler
    s. probe
    s. reverse bandage
    s. stone dislodger
    s. trochanteric reamer
    s. vein stripper
    s. wound endotracheal tube
    s. XCT scanner
spiral-embedded tube
Spiralgold oxygenator
spiral-tipped
    s.-t. bougie
    s.-t. catheter
SpiraStent ureteral stent
Spirec drill
Spirette
    CCD S.
SpiroFlo bioabsorbable prostate stent
Spir-O-Flow peak flowmeter
SpiroFlow peak flow monitor
spirometer
    bedside s.
    Benedict-Roth s.
    Buhl s.
    Calculair s.
    closed-circuit s.
    Coach incentive s.
    Collins Survey s.
    Compact II desktop s.
    Datex Ultima s.
    Discovery handheld s.

    Eagle s.
    Eagle II survey s.
    Flash portable s.
    flow-sensing s.
    Gould Instrument Systems s.
    Horizon PFT s.
    incentive s.
    Inspiron incentive s.
    KoKo s.
    Krogh apparatus s.
    LifeSigns SP s.
    low-resistance rolling seal s.
    MasterLab Pro pneumotachograph s.
    MedicAIR Plus s.
    MicroLoop II handheld s.
    MicroPlus s.
    Pulmonet s.
    2120 Recording S.
    Respirex incentive s.
    Satellite s.
    Sensaire s.
    Simplicity s.
    SP-10 s.
    Spirometrics Micro s.
    SpiroVision-3+ s.
    Spirovit SP-1, -10 portable s.
    Stead-Wells water-seal type s.
    Timeter pocket s.
    Tissot s.
    Vitalograph handheld recording s.
    Vitalor incentive s.
    volume-displacement s.
    water-sealed s.
    wedge s.
    Welch Allyn Pneumocheck s.
    Wright s.
Spirometrics Micro spirometer
spirometry
SpiroSense
    S. flow sensor
    S. system
Spirosense system
Spiros inhalation system
SpiroVision-3+ spirometer
SpiroVision-3 spirometry system
Spirovit SP-1, -10 portable spirometer
Spitz-Holter
    S.-H. flushing device
    S.-H. valve
    S.-H. valve implant material
Spitzy
    S. button
    S. spike
Spivack axis marker
Spizziri cannula knife
splanchnic retractor
Splash-Shield
    endoscopic S.-S.
splaytooth forceps

splenorenal bypass shunt
Spline
    S. dental implant system
    S. Twist microtextured titanium
      implant
    S. Twist MTX implant
    S. Twist Ti implant
splint
    abduction finger s.
    abduction thumb s.
    abutment s.
    acrylic cap s.
    acrylic ear s.
    acrylic interocclusal s.
    acrylic palatal s.
    acrylic wafer temporomandibular
      joint s.
    acrylic wafer TMJ s.
    Adam and Eve rib belt s.
    adjustable s.
    Adjusta-Wrist s.
    A-Force dorsal night s.
    air s.
    AirFlex carpal tunnel s.
    airplane s.
    air pressure s.
    AliMed diabetic night s.
    AliMed turnbuckle elbow s.
    Alumafoam nasal s.
    aluminum finger cot s.
    alveolar arch acrylic s.
    anchor s.
    Anderson s.
    angle s.
    ankle s.
    ankle-foot orthotic s.
    ankle stirrup s.
    Aquaplast s.
    arm s.
    armchair s.
    banana finger extension s.
    baseball finger s.
    basic hand s.
    Basswood s.
    Bend-A-Boot foot s.
    Bennett basic hand s.
    Bilson fixable-removable cross arch
      bar s.
    bipolar traction s.
    birdcage s.
    Blue Line ThumbStay s.
    Blue Line Uno s.
    Blue Line wrist control s.
    board s.
    Böhler-Braun s.
    Böhler wire s.
    Boston thoracic s.
    boutonniere s.
    Bowlby arm s.
    bracketed s.
    Brady balanced suspension s.
    Breathe-Easy nasal s.
    bridge s.
    Brooke Army Hospital s.
    Browne s.
    buddy s.
    Budin hammertoe s.
    Budin toe s.
    Bunnell active hand and finger s.
    Bunnell finger extension s.
    Bunnell reverse knuckle-bender s.
    Bunnell safety-pin s.
    Bunny Boot foot s.
    Camo disposable dental s.
    cap s.
    Capener coil s.
    Capener finger s.
    Capner boutonniere s.
    Carpal Lock cock-up s.
    Carpal Lock cock-up wrist s.
    Carpal Lock wrist s.
    Carter intranasal s.
    cartilage elastic pullover kneecap s.
    clubfoot s.
    CMC s.
    coaptation s.
    cock-up arm s.
    Colles s.
    Comfort Cool thumb CMC
      restriction s.
    Comfort Cool wrist and thumb
      CMC restriction s.
    Comforter s.
    Comfy elbow s.
    composite spring elastic s.
    compression sleeve shin s.
    compressive plastic s.
    Comprifix ankle s.
    Cone s.
    constant tension s.
    cool Irom s.
    copper band-acrylic s.
    Cosmolon closure for s.
    counterrotational s.
    Craig abduction s.
    Cramer wire s.
    crib s.
    CTS Gripfit s.
    Darco foot s.
    Darco Medical-Surgical shoe and
      toe alignment s.
    Delbet s.
    Denis Browne s.
    Denis Browne clubfoot s.
    Denis Browne hip s.
    Denver nasal s.
    DePuy coaptation s.
    DePuy-Pott s.

S

splint *(continued)*
dermal interposition s.
derotator s.
DeRoyal LMB finger s.
digit s.
DonJoy knee s.
dorsal extension s.
dorsal wrist s.
dorsal wrist s. with outrigger
Dorsiwedge night s.
double-occlusal s.
Doyle bivalved airway s.
Doyle Combo nasal airway s.
Doyle Shark nasal s.
dropfoot s.
dynamic s.
Early Fit night s.
Easton cock-up s.
Easy Access foot s.
elastic plastic s.
Elastomull s.
elbow extension s.
elbow flexion s.
Engelmann thigh s.
Engen palmar wrist s.
Epitrain elbow s.
Erich maxillary s.
Erich nasal s.
Extend-It finger s.
Ezeform s.
Fasplint vacuum s.
fence s.
fiberglass s.
Fillauer night s.
finger s.
finger cot s.
finger flexion s.
Finger-Hugger s.
finger sled s.
folded aluminum ear s.
fold-over finger s.
footdrop night s.
Formatray mandibular s.
Fractomed s.
fracture s.
Framer s.
Freedom neutral position s.
Freedom omni progressive s.
Freedom Progressive Resting s.
Freedom SportsFit s.
Freedom ultimate grip s.
Frejka pillow s.
Friedman s.
frog s.
frog-leg s.
Froimson s.
Fruehevald s.
full hand s.
full occlusal s.

functional s.
functional resting position s.
Funsten supination s.
Futuro s.
gait lock s.
Gallows s.
Galveston s.
Ganley s.
Gilmer dental s.
Gilmer tooth s.
Goode nasal s.
Gordon s.
gutter s.
hairpin s.
half-ring leg s.
Hammond s.
Hammond orthodontic s.
hand cock-up s.
Hare compact traction s.
Haynes-Griffin mandibular s.
Heal Well night s.
Heel Free s.
Hexcelite sheet s.
hinged Thomas s.
HIPciser abduction s.
Hodgen hip s.
Hodgen leg s.
HV Nightsplint s.
HV Softsplint s.
Ilfeld s.
indexed s.
infant abduction s.
inflatable elbow s.
Innoboot s.
Inro surgical nail s.
interdental s.
intermediate s.
intranasal s.
intranasal bivalve s.
Irom bilateral s.
Irom Regal s.
Isoprene plastic s.
Jacoby heel s.
Jelenko s.
Jet-Air s.
Joint-Jack finger s.
Jones arm s.
Jones forearm s.
Jones metacarpal s.
Jones nasal s.
Jones traction s.
Joseph nasal s.
Joseph septal s.
Kanavel cock-up s.
Kazanjian nasal s.
Kenny-Howard s.
Kerr abduction s.
Keystone s.
kidney internal s.

Kingsley s.
Kirschner wire s.
Kleinert s.
Klenzak double-upright s.
knee s.
knee brace s.
knee immobilizer s.
Knuckle Bender s.
lace-lock ankle s.
leaf s.
Lewin baseball finger s.
Lewin finger s.
Lewin-Stern finger s.
Lewin-Stern thumb s.
Liberty One s.
s. liner
Link stack split s.
Link toe s.
Liston s.
live s.
LMB finger s.
LMB wire-foam economical
  resting s.
long arm s.
long leg posterior molded s.
Lorenz night s.
Love nasal s.
Lynch septal s.
Lynx wrist, hand, finger orthosis
  arm positioner s.
magnet s.
Magnuson abduction humeral s.
malleable s.
malleable metal finger s.
Malmö hip s.
Mason s.
Mason-Allen hand s.
Mayer nasal s.
McGee s.
McKie thumb s.
memory s.
Merocel s.
metal s.
modified Oppenheimer s.
Murphy s.
nasal s.
neutral position s.
New Mind Set toe s.
N'ice Stretch night s.
nose guard s.
OCL volar s.
OEC s.
O'Malley jaw fracture s.
Oppenheimer spring wire s.
Oppenheimer with reverse knuckle-
  bender s.
opponens s.
Orfit s.
Orfizip wrist s.

Ortho-Glass s.
Orthoglass s.
Orthomedics Stretch and Heel s.
Ortho-Mold s.
orthopaedic strap clavicle s.
Orthoplast s.
Orthoplast isoprene s.
outrigger s.
Oval-8 finger s.
Oval-8 ring s.
oyster s.
padded aluminum s.
padded board s.
s. padding
palmar wrist s.
s. pan netting
passive night stretch s.
Pavlik harness s.
PF Night Splint II s.
Phelps s.
Phoenix Outrigger s.
Pil-O-Splint elbow s.
Pil-O-Splint wrist s.
plantar fasciitis night s.
plaster of Paris s.
plaster slab s.
PneuGel posterior leg s.
pneumatic s.
PneuSplint s.
4-point IROM s.
polycentric hinged ulnar
  deviation s.
Polyform s.
polymethylmethacrylate ear s.
polymethylmethacrylate ear s.
polyvinyl alcohol s.
Pond adjustable s.
Pope night s.
Porzett s.
pressure s.
Pro-glide s.
Progress s.
4-prong finger s.
Pucci s.
Puth abduction s.
QualCraft s.
QuickCast s.
Quik s.
radial hinged ulnar deviation s.
radiolucent s.
ratchet flexor tenodesis s.
Redi-Around finger s.
replant s.
resting s.
resting pan s.
reverse knuckle-bender s.
rigid s.
Robert Jones s.

S

splint *(continued)*
Rolyan AquaForm wrist and thumb spica s.
Rolyan Gel Shell spica s.
Rosen s.
safety pin s.
Sager Combo-Pac adult/child and infant s.
Sager S304 bilateral s.
Sager S300 infant bilateral s.
Sager 2301 single s.
Sager traction s.
SAM s.
Sam s.
sandwich-type s.
Santa Barbara thumb s.
Saturn carpal tunnel s.
Schenck arcuate s.
Scott ankle s.
Scott Uniform tennis elbow s.
Seattle s.
Sheffield s.
short arm s.
short arm plaster s.
short arm posterior molded s.
short leg s.
skin s.
slip-on finger s.
Smart S.
SmartBrace wrist s.
Softsplint foot s.
special Colles s.
Speed hand s.
spica s.
spreading hand s.
spring cock-up s.
spring wire safety pin s.
stack s.
Stader s.
static s.
Stax fingertip s.
strap clavicle s.
Stretch and Heel night s.
Stubbs acromioclavicular s.
sugar-tong s.
surgical s.
suspension s.
swan-neck s.
synergistic wrist motion s.
Synergy s.
talipes hobble s.
Taylor s.
tennis elbow s.
tenodesis s.
therapeutic s.
thermoplastic s.
thermoplastic extension pan s.
Thomas full-ring s.
Thomas hinged s.
Thomas knee s.
Thomas leg s.
Thomas posterior s.
Thomas suspension s.
thumb spica s.
ThumSaver CMC long s.
ThumSaver CMC short s.
ThumSaver MP s.
ThumZ'Up functional thumb s.
Toad finger s.
Tobruk s.
Toronto s.
torsion bar s.
traction s.
trough s.
turnbuckle elbow s.
turnbuckle functional position s.
Ultraflex ankle dorsiflexion dynamic s.
Universal acromioclavicular s.
Universal support s.
Urias air s.
Urias pressure s.
U-splint s.
U-stirrup s.
vacuum s.
Van Rosen s.
VersaWrist wrist s.
volar s.
volar plaster s.
Volkmann s.
von Rosen s.
von Rosen abduction s.
Wanchik neutral position s.
well-padded s.
Wheaton bunion s.
wire s.
wire grip finger s.
wire grip toe s.
wrist s.
wrist positioning s.
Wrist Resist s.
Xomed s.
Xomed Doyle nasal airway s.
Zimfoam s.
Zimmer clavicular cross s.
Zucker s.

splinter forceps
splint/stent
kidney internal s./s.
split
s. beam
s. drape
s. overtube
s. Russell skeletal traction
s. screen
s. stirrup
split-beam coupler for TURP
split-cuff nipple

split-finger hook
split-sheath
    s.-s. catheter
    s.-s. introducer
splittable needle
splitter
    Akahoshi nucleus s.
    beam s.
    Brierley nucleus s.
    Goldberg side port s.
    Koch-Salz nucleus s.
    Kraff nucleus s.
    Lindstrom Trident ophthalmic s.
    Rosen phaco s.
    Salz nucleus s.
    Sharvelle side port s.
    Smith s.
    Zeiss small beam s.
split-thickness implant
splitting
    s. chisel
    s. forceps
S-P needle holder
SpO$_2$-5001 oximeter
spondylitic bar
spondylophyte
    s. anular dissector perforator
    s. impactor
spondylotic bar
sponge
    absorbable gelatin s.
    Accu-Sorb gauze s.
    Actifoam collagen s.
    Actifoam hemostat s.
    Adaptic s.
    Bernays s.
    Bicol collagen s.
    bronchoscopic s.
    buffing s.
    s. carrier
    cellulose surgical s.
    s. clamp
    collagen s.
    Collostat hemostatic s.
    cotton-ball s.
    Curity cover s.
    Curity disposable laparotomy s.
    Curity gauze s.
    Custodis s.
    cylindrical s.
    DeRoyal laparotomy s.
    s. dissector
    s. ear curette
    Endozime s.
    episcleral s.
    Excilon drain s.
    Excilon dressing s.
    Excilon IV s.
    Expandacell s.

    EZ Bend s.
    Fluftex gauze rolls and s.
    s. forceps
    gauze dissector s.
    gauze rosebud s.
    gelatin s.
    Gelfoam s.
    s. graft
    grooved silicone s.
    Helistat absorbable collagen
      hemostatic s.
    Helistat collagen matrix s.
    Heros chiropody s.
    Hibbs s.
    implant s.
    s. implant
    InductOs collagen s.
    Instat collagen s.
    Instat collagen matrix s.
    InstruSponge enzymatic s.
    Ivalon s.
    Ivalon embolic s.
    Johnson & Johnson gauze s.
    Kenwood laparotomy s.
    Kerlix laparotomy s.
    Kerlix packing s.
    Kerlix super s.
    King fluff rolls and s.
    Kling s.
    Krukenberg s.
    laminectomy wedge s.
    laparotomy s.
    Lapwall s.
    Lincoff lens s.
    lint-free s.
    Lisco s.
    Mediskin hemostatic s.
    Medline gauze s.
    Merocel s.
    Merocel lint-free s.
    Mesoft s.
    Microsponge Teardrop s.
    Miragel s.
    Mirasorb s.
    MultiPly s.
    nasal tampon s.
    neurological s.
    nonwoven s.
    Nu Gauze s.
    ophthalmic s.
    Optipore scrub s.
    Oto-Wick medicated ear s.
    peanut s.
    Pedic s.
    pledget s.
    polyvinyl s.
    polyvinyl alcohol s.
    Pope Oto-Wick medicated ear s.
    Protectaid contraceptive s.

S

sponge (*continued*)
 radial s.
 Ray-Tec x-ray detectable
  surgical s.
 Reston s.
 s. ring
 rubber s.
 silastic s.
 silicone s.
 s. silicone implant material
 Soft N' Dry Merocel s.
 soft silicone s.
 Sof-Wick s.
 Sof-Wick drain s.
 s. stick
 stippling s.
 strip and point s.
 surgical s.
 Teflon s.
 Telfa s.
 tonsillar s.
 Topper dressing s.
 tracheotomy s.
 Ultrafoam collagen s.
 Vaiser s.
 Versalon all-purpose s.
 VersaTool eye s.
 Visi-Spear eye s.
 Vistec x-ray detectable s.
 vitrectomy s.
 Weck s.
 Weck-cel s.
 x-ray detectable laparotomy s.
sponge-holding forceps
Spongel gelatin sponge particle
spongiosa bone graft
spontaneous timed (ST)
spoon
 Alfonso-McIntyre nucleus s.
 s. anastomosis clamp
 s. blade
 Bunge evisceration s.
 Castroviejo lens s.
 cataract s.
 Culler lens s.
 s. curette
 Cushing spatula s.
 Cutler lens s.
 Daviel s.
 Daviel cataract s.
 Daviel lens s.
 ear s.
 Elschnig s.
 enucleation s.
 evisceration s.
 Falk appendectomy s.
 Fisher s.
 Fisher eye s.
 s. forceps

 Graefe cataract s.
 graft carrier s.
 Gross ear s.
 Hardy pituitary s.
 Hess s.
 Hess lens s.
 Kalt eye s.
 Kirby intracapsular lens s.
 Knapp cataract s.
 Knapp lens s.
 s. knife
 Kocher brain s.
 LASIK aspiration s.
 lens s.
 Lindner cyclodialysis s.
 maroon s.
 meniscal s.
 s. needle
 needle s.
 pituitary s.
 plain ear s.
 s. retractor
 Rizzuti graft carrier s.
 Schepens s.
 Sellheim elevating s.
 spatula s.
 s. spatula
 Volkmann s.
 Wehner s.
 Wells enucleation s.
spoon-shaped forceps
S'port
 S. Max back support
 S. Max sacroiliac belt
 S. Max stabilization pad
 Posture S.
 Scully Hip S.
SportCord exercise and rehabilitation
 system
Sportelli system collimator mounted
 contact shield
Sporthotics orthotic
Sport Preforms orthotic
Sport-Rite
 S.-R. Olympian device
 S.-R. orthotic
 S.-R. Runner device
sports
 s. goggles
 s. tape
Sports-Caster I, II knee brace
Sports-Grip bar
Sports Plus II back belt
SportsRAC arm care system
Sportstape
 Leukotape P S.
Sportstim
 S. muscle stimulation electrode
 S. stimulator

Sport-Stirrup orthosis
SporTX
    S. pulsed direct-current stimulator
    S. stimulation device
spot
    s. compression paddle
    S. endoscopic marker
    s. face reamer
    s. film device
    s. retinoscope
    S. RT Monochrome Kodak KAI-
      2000 CCD digital camera
SpotCheck+ handheld pulse oximeter
spot-compression paddle
spotlight
    examining s.
    KDC-Healthdyne nonfluorescent s.
SPOT mobile 3D ultrasound system
Spotorno cementless hip arthroplasty
    stem
SPP color deficiency testing product
Spratt
    S. bone curette
    S. ear curette
    S. mastoid curette
spray
    AliCool splint s.
    s. bandage
    S. Band dressing
    Fisher Scientific Histo-freeze 2000
      freezing s.
    Prevacare Total Solution skin
      care s.
SprayGel adhesive barrier system
spreader
    Assistant Free calibrated femoral
      tibial s.
    Athens suture s.
    Bailey rib s.
    s. bar
    Beeson cast s.
    Beeson plaster s.
    Blount laminar s.
    Bobechko s.
    Burford-Finochietto rib s.
    Burford rib s.
    calcaneal s.
    Caspar disc space s.
    Caspar vertebral body s.
    cast s.
    Cloward s.
    conjunctiva s.
    Cox metatarsal s.
    DeBakey infant and child rib s.
    DeBakey rib s.
    Doyen rib s.
    Endotec s.
    Favaloro-Morse rib s.
    Finochietto-Burford rib s.

    Finochietto rib s.
    Finochietto-Stille rib s.
    Frederick sleeve s.
    s. graft
    gutta-percha s.
    Haglund s.
    Haglund-Stille plaster s.
    Haight pediatric rib s.
    Harken rib s.
    Harrington s.
    Henning cast s.
    Henning plaster s.
    incision s.
    Inge s.
    Inge laminar s.
    intervertebral s.
    Jarit 3-prong cast s.
    jaw s.
    Kirschner wire s.
    Kwitko conjunctival s.
    lamina s.
    laminar s.
    Landolt s.
    Lefferts rib s.
    Leksell sternal s.
    Lemmon sternal s.
    Lilienthal rib s.
    Lilienthal-Sauerbruch rib s.
    McGuire rib s.
    Medicon rib s.
    Millin bladder neck s.
    Miltex rib s.
    Mity s.
    Morse sternal s.
    M-Pact cast s.
    Nelson rib s.
    plaster s.
    Ramirez EndoForehead s.
    rib s.
    Rienhoff-Finochietto rib s.
    root canal s.
    small lamina s.
    spinous process s.
    sternal s.
    Suarez s.
    Texas Scottish Rite Hospital
      eyebolt s.
    Tudor-Edwards rib s.
    Tuffier rib s.
    Turner-Warwick bladder neck s.
    USA plaster s.
    Wakai s.
    Weinraub joint and calcaneal s.
    Wilder band s.
    Wölfe-Böhler plaster cast s.
spreading
    s. forceps
    s. hand splint

S

spring
- S. catheter
- s. clip
- s. cock-up splint
- s. coil
- coiled s.
- compression s.
- Gruca-Weiss s.
- s. hook
- internal fixation s.
- S. iris scissors
- Kesling tooth-spacing s.
- s. mechanism
- Mershon s.
- s. needle holder
- s. pin
- s. plate
- s. retractor
- Weiss s.
- s. wire loop
- s. wire safety pin splint

spring-assisted syringe

spring-eye needle

spring-handled
- s.-h. forceps
- s.-h. needle holder
- s.-h. scissors

spring-hook wire needle

Springlite
- S. Advantage DP
- S. G foot component
- S. II foot component
- S. II foot prosthesis
- S. lower limb prosthesis
- S. polyolefin BK cover
- S. polyurethane AK, BK conical cover
- S. super low profile Symes II
- S. toe filler

spring-loaded
- s.-l. automatic tack driver
- s.-l. biopsy gun
- s.-l. biopsy instrument
- s.-l. biopsy needle
- s.-l. nail
- s.-l. self-retaining retractor
- s.-l. vascular stent

spring-mounted electromagnet

spring-tipped guidewire

spring-wire retractor

Sprint
- S. Climber
- S. cross trainer
- S. fixed-detector research system
- S. Model 6942, 6943 tachyarrhythmia lead
- S. Runner

SPrint speech processor

Spri Xercise board

Sprotte
- S. epidural needle
- S. spinal needle

sprue pin

SPTL-1a laser

SPTL-1b vascular lesion laser

SPTL vascular lesion laser

S.P. 100 transcutaneous electrical neural stimulator

spud
- corneal s.
- curved needle s.
- Davis s.
- Davis foreign body s.
- Ellis foreign body s.
- Fisher s.
- flat needle s.
- foreign body s.
- Francis s.
- Goldstein golf-club s.
- golf club s.
- gouge s.
- Hosford s.
- Hosford foreign body s.
- knife s.
- LaForce golf club knife s.
- Levine s.
- Levine curetting s.
- Levine foreign body s.
- needle s.
- s. needle
- Nicati foreign body s.
- O'Brien s.
- Plange s.
- s. tool
- Walter corneal s.
- Walton s.

spur-crushing clamp

Spurling
- S. intervertebral disc forceps
- S. intervertebral disc rongeur
- S. laminectomy rongeur
- S. pituitary rongeur
- S. rongeur forceps

Spurling-Kerrison
- S.-K. laminectomy punch
- S.-K. rongeur forceps
- S.-K. upbiting and downbiting rongeur

Spurr resin

Sputnik Russian razor blade

sputum tube

Spyglass angiography catheter

Spy intraoperative imaging system

SpyroDerm

Spyrogel hydrogel wound dressing

square
- s. module seating system
- s. prism

rocker balance s.
s. specimen forceps
s. wire
square-ended
s.-e. distraction rod
s.-e. hook
square-end pliers
square-hole broach
squares of dressing
square-shaped occluder
square-tipped arterial dissector
squeegee capsule polisher
squeeze
s. ball
s. dynamometer
s. exerciser
squeeze-handle forceps
Squeeze-Mark surgical marker
squeezer
Squibb
S. system
S. urostomy pouch
squint hook
Squirt wound irrigation system
[89]Sr bracelet
SRI automated immunoassay analyzer
SR-Ivocap denture material
SR-IV programmed subjective refractor
[90]Sr-loaded eye applicator
S-ROM
S-ROM acetabular cup
S-ROM Arthropor I–III prosthesis
S-ROM Arthropor oblong prosthesis
S-ROM contained shell
S-ROM femoral stem prosthesis
S-ROM hip prosthesis
S-ROM hip replacement system
S-ROM modular femoral
component
S-ROM modular total knee system
S-ROM Poly-Dial insert
S-ROM proximally modular total
hip system
S-ROM super cup prosthesis
S-ROM ZZT I, II prosthesis
SRO x-ray tube
SRS/CRS cement
SRS injectable cement
SRT
SRT lead
SRT vaginal speculum
S&S
sling and swathe
S.S.
S.S. White clamp
S.S. White J-Notch surgical
handpiece bur
S.S. White 100 K surgical
handpiece bur

S-Scort
S.-S. New-Duet suction unit
S.-S. suction unit
S-Series sleep system
S-shaped
S-s. brain retractor
S-s. brain spatula
S-s. peripheral vascular clamp
SSI brace
S-Soles insole
SSP
small stature cervical plate
SSP system
SS suture
ST
short transition
small trapezoid
spontaneous timed
ST Mesh implant
St.
St. Clair-Thompson curette
St. Georg fully constrained
prosthesis
St. Georg sledge unicompartment
prosthesis
St. Jude bileaflet prosthetic valve
St. Jude cardiac device
St. Jude composite prosthetic
St.-Jude composite prosthetic valve
St.-Jude composite valve graft
St. Jude heart valve prosthesis
St. Jude Medical (SJM)
St. Jude Medical bileaflet tilting-
disc aortic valve
St. Jude Medical bioImplant valve
St. Jude medical heart valve
hemodynamic plus series
St. Jude Medical Port-Access
St. Jude Medical Port-Access
mechanical heart valve
St. Jude Medical valve prosthesis
St. Jude mitral valve prosthesis
St. Mark pudendal electrode
St. Martin eye forceps
St. Martin suturing forceps
St. Vincent tube clamp
St. Vincent tube-occluding forceps
ST3 amplified stethoscope
STA
STA analyzer
STA Compact hemostasis system
STA hemostasis system
STA Liatest D-DI
coagulation/inflammation test kit
Staar
S. AA 4207 lens
S. foldable intraocular lens
S. glaucoma wick
S. implantable contact lens

S

Staar *(continued)*
    S. intraocular lens
    S. IOL
    S. low-diopter IOL
    S. toric IOL
    S. toric lens
    S. 4203VF lens
    S. 4207VF lens
stab
    s. electrode
    s. incision angled blade
    s. needle
Stab-and-Grab screwdriver
Stabident system
Stabiliplan orthovolt applicator
Stability total hip system
stabilization plate
stabilizer
    Ace pelvic s.
    Agarwal nuclear manipulator
      globe s.
    ankle s.
    Axius vacuum 2 s.
    S. balanced performance guidewire
    Cohn cardiac s.
    Dynamic foot s.
    Embrace heart s.
    Flexsite heart s.
    foot s.
    Freedom thumb s.
    Goldstein Grasp atraumatic
      cervical s.
    Heel Hugger therapeutic heel s.
    Insall-Burstein posterior s.
    kneecap s.
    KT1000 foot s.
    Kwik Board IV and arterial
      line s.
    S. marker wire
    S. marker wire steerable guidewire
    Medline lateral s.
    Palumbo ankle s.
    S. Plus steerable guidewire
    Rousseau chin-lift s.
    Stamler corneal transplant s.
    subpectoral s.
    Verteflex arthrotonic s.
    S. XS extra-support steerable
      guidewire
    S. XS steerable guidewire
stabilizing
    s. bar
    s. guide pin
stab-in epicardial electrode
stable access cannula
Stablecut sawblade
Stableflex lens
Stableloc
    S. Colles fracture external fixator

S. external wrist fixation system
S. II external fixation
S. II external fixation system
S. II external fixator system
Stableyes capsular tension ring
Sta-Block head immobilizer
stab-wound drain
Stack
    S. autoperfusion balloon
    S. perfusion catheter
    S. perfusion coronary dilatation
      catheter
stacking cone
stack splint
Staclot protein S test kit
Stader splint
Stadie-Riggs microtome
stadiometer
    Harpenden s.
    Heightronic s.
    Holtain height s.
    neonatal s.
staff
    fiberglass s.
    Sippy esophageal dilator piano-
      wire s.
    Turner-Warwick urethral s.
    urethral s.
Sta-Fix tape
stage
    2-s. Sarns cannula
StageOne temporary hip prosthesis
  cement spacer mold
Stagnara gouge
Stahl calipers
stain
    Ventana ES s.
stainer
    Code-On Immunoslide s.
    Hematek 2000 slide s.
    Midas II automated s.
    Quick Slide automated s.
    Ventana Medical Systems Techmate
      automated s.
stainer/cytocentrifuge
    Aerospray acid-fast bacteria
      slide s./c.
    Aerospray hematology slide s./c.
stainless
    s. pellet
    s. spatula
    s. steel AO plate
    s. steel balloon expandable stent
    s. steel blade
    s. steel clamp
    s. steel crown
    s. steel cup
    s. steel flexible ruler
    s. steel guidewire

s. steel implant
s. steel mesh
s. steel mesh stent
s. steel screw
s. steel staple
s. steel wire
s. steel wire suture
stainless-steel Greenfield filter
stair chair
StairClimber assist device
StairMaster exercise system
Stallard dissector
stall bar
Staller
S. kit
S. point
Stallerpointe needle
Stamey
S. catheter
S. dorsal vein apical retractor
S. needle
S. open-tip ureteral catheter
S. percutaneous suprapubic catheter
Stamey-Malecot catheter
Stamler
S. corneal transplant stabilizer
S. side-port fixation hook
Stamm
S. bone-cutting forceps
S. gastrostomy tube
Stammberger
S. antral punch
S. punch forceps
stand
Atlas adjustable s.
Brown-Roberts-Wells floor s.
Cherf cast s.
Contraves s.
Grand Stand support s.
IMP turnstile casting s.
Keeler Lightsource s.
s. magnifier
Mayo s.
turnstile casting s.
Versa-Helper floor s.
Wilson Mayo s.
standard
s. above-elbow cast
s. arterial forceps
s. colonoscope
s. duodenoscope
s. endoscopy polypectomy snare
s. ERCP catheter
s. exchange wire
S. E-Z-On vest
s. fixed core guidewire
s. full-lumen esophagoscope
s. head halter
s. hook electrosurgical probe

s. implant
s. 2-inch blade retractor
s. 4-inch blade retractor
s. Jackson laryngoscope
s. Lehman catheter
s. LITT applicator
MapMarkers fluorescent DNA
sizing s.
s. needle
s. pattern mallet
s. pseudoisochromatic plates color
deficiency testing product
s. shell ankle-foot orthosis
s. silicone manometric assembly
s. socket
s. U patellar support
Uranyl S.
s. wire gauge
standardized constant bolus
standby pacemaker
stander
prone s.
standing frame orthosis
Stanford
S. bioptome
S. and Wheatstone stereoscope
Stangel modified Barraquer
microsurgical needle holder
Stanicor pacemaker
Stanmore
S. shoulder prosthesis
S. total knee
STAN S 21 fetal heart rate system
Staodyne EMS+2 neurostimulator
Staodyn Insight point locator
stapedectomy
s. footplate pick
s. forceps
s. knife
s. prosthesis
STA-peg
Smith STA-p.
STA-Pen writer pen
stapes
s. chisel
s. curette
s. dilator
s. elevator
s. excavator
s. forceps
s. hoe
s. hook
s. needle
s. pick
s. speculum
Staph-Chek
S.-C. pad
S.-C. Synergy fabric

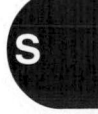

staphylorrhaphy
- s. elevator
- s. needle

staple
- Arthrotek meniscus s.
- bioabsorbable s.
- Biomet s.
- Blount epiphysial s.
- s. bone plate
- DePuy FRS standard s.
- Fastlok implantable s.
- s. forceps
- FRS standard s.
- GIA s.
- Hernandez-Ros bone s.
- Krackow HTO blade s.
- 3M s.
- mandibular transosseous s.
- memory compression s.
- meniscal s.
- metallic s.
- orthopaedic s.
- 5-pin s.
- 7-pin s.
- 7-pin s.
- polyglyconate s.
- Polysorb absorbable s.
- Richards fixation s.
- SD sorb s.
- skin s.
- Smith & Nephew medium barbed s.
- Smith & Nephew small barbed s.
- spike s.
- stainless steel s.
- stone s.
- surgical s.
- s. suture
- TA metallic s.
- titanium s.
- titanium mandibular s.
- Uni-Clip manual compression s.
- vitallium s.
- Wiberg fracture s.
- Zimaloy epiphyseal s.

stapler
- Androsov vascular s.
- Appose skin s.
- arcuate skin s.
- Auto Suture s.
- Auto Suture Multifire Endo GIA 30 s.
- Auto Suture Premium CEEA s.
- Auto Suture SFS s.
- Auto Suture surgical s.
- barbed s.
- Biologically Quiet s.
- CEEA s.
- circular s.
- circular intraluminal s.
- circular mechanical s.
- Closer s.
- Concorde disposable skin s.
- curved intraluminal s.
- disposable intraluminal s.
- s. doughnut
- EEA s.
- EEA Auto Suture s.
- end-end s.
- Endo Babcock s.
- Endo-Babcock s.
- Endo GIA s.
- Endo GIA 30, 60 s.
- Endo GIA suture s.
- Endo GIA 30 suture s.
- Endo Hernia s.
- Endopath 30, 60 s.
- Endopath EMS hernia s.
- Endopath endoscopic articulating s.
- Ethicon CDH29 s.
- Ethicon circular s.
- Ethicon Endopath EZ45 s.
- Ethicon TLH30 s.
- gastroplasty s.
- GIA s.
- GIA 60, 80 s.
- Graftac-S skin s.
- hernia s.
- ILS s.
- Imagyn surgical s.
- Insorb subcuticular skin s.
- intraluminal s.
- Lactomer copolymer absorbable s.
- laparoscopic s.
- ligating and dividing s.
- linear s.
- Multifire GIA-series s.
- Multifire TA-series s.
- PI-30 s.
- PKS-25 apparatus s.
- PLC-50 linear s.
- Poly GIA s.
- Polysorb 55 s.
- PPH s.
- Precise s.
- Precise disposable skin s.
- Premium s.
- Premium CEEA circular s.
- Premium Plus CEEA disposable s.
- ProTack s.
- Proximate disposable skin s.
- Proximate flexible linear s.
- Proximate II, III s.
- Proximate ILS curved intraluminal s.
- Proximate ILS SDH circular s.
- Proximate RH s.
- Reflex skin s.

roticulator 55 s.
Royal disposable skin s.
Signet disposable skin s.
TA-55 s.
TL90 Ethicon s.
UG-70 s.
United States Surgical circular s.
USSC s.
30-V-3 s.
vascular s.
VersaTack s.
Vista disposable skin s.
Wiberg fracture s.

stapling
s. device
expanding vascular s. (EVS)

Star
S. ankle joint prosthesis
S. biphasic AED
S. excimer laser
Lindstrom S.
S. S4 ActiveTrak 3D eye tracking
system
S. S3 ActiveTrak excimer laser
system
S. S4 excimer laser system
S. S2 SmoothScan excimer laser
system
S. ventilator
Visx S. S3

StarBurst
S. Flex RFA device
S. SDE RFA device
S. Semi-Flex RFA device
S. XLi-enhanced RFA device
S. XLi RFA device
S. XL RFA device

Starcam large field of view gamma camera
starch bandage
starch-based copolymer dressing
Starck dilator
StarClose vascular closure system
Stardox wrist brace
STARFlex device
Stargate falloposcopy catheter
STA-R hemostasis system
Starkey
S. hearing aid
S. stethoscope

Starlite
S. endodontic implant starter kit
S. Omni-AT bur
S. point

StarLock
S. multi-purpose submergible
threaded implant
S. press-fit cylinder implant

StarMed video otoscope

Starr
S. ball heart valve
S. fixation forceps

Starr-Edwards
S.-E. aortic valve prosthesis
S.-E. ball-and-cage valve
S.-E. ball valve prosthesis
S.-E. cardiac valve prosthesis
S.-E. cloth-covered metallic ball
heart valve
S.-E. disc valve prosthesis
S.-E. heart valve
S.-E. heart valve prosthesis
S.-E. mitral prosthesis
S.-E. pacemaker
S.-E. prosthetic aortic valve
S.-E. prosthetic mitral valve
S.-E. silastic valve
S.-E. silicone rubber ball valve

Starrett pin vise
STARRT falloposcopy system
STart-4 clot detection system
STart-8 clot detection system
starter
s. awl
s. broach
Brown pocket s.
Ritchie nail s.

StarTox 5 drugs of abuse screening test
Star/Vent 1-stage dental screw implant
Stat
S. aspirator
S. Profile pHOx blood gas
analyzer
S. 2 Pumpette
S. 2 Pumpette disposable IV pump
S. Scrub handwasher machine

Stat-60 centrifuge
Statak
S. anchor system
S. curette
S. soft tissue attachment device
S. suture
S. suture anchor
S. suturing device

state-of-the-art aberrometer
Statham
S. electromagnetic flow meter
S. external transducer
S. flowmeter
S. pressure transducer

static
s. air mattress
s. gray scale ultrasound equipment
s. magnet
s. orthosis
s. sling
s. splint

static (*continued*)
 s. testing frame
 s. topical occlusive hemostatic
 pressure device
station
 analog video acquisition s.
 Aquatrend water workout s.
 base s.
 Dicom acquisition s.
 LifeView care s.
 MedicAIR Plus spirometry s.
 oscilloscope tuning s.
 PlugStation earplug s.
 Stealth S.
stationary
 s. angle guide
 s. ankle flexible endoskeleton
Sta-Tite 2-ply elastic roll gauze
StatLock catheter securement device
statometer
**Stat-Shell disposable pulse oximeter
 sensor**
STAT-Site M Hgb test system
StatSpin
 S. Express 2 centrifuge
 S. MP centrifuge
 S. MP multipurpose centrifuge
**Stat-Temp II liquid crystal temperature
 monitor**
Status Cup Plus drug testing device
Status-X machine
Stax fingertip splint
stay
 s. plate
 s. wire
StayErec system
StayFuse implant
Stay-Put jejunal tube
StaySharp Supercut scissors
STC 900-series travel chair
Stead-Wells water-seal type spirometer
Stealth
 S. anchor
 S. angioplasty balloon catheter
 S. catheter balloon
 S. DBO diamond blade
 S. DBO freehand diamond knife
 S. frame
 S. image guided system
 S. knee brace
 S. Station
StealthStation
 S. image-guided system
 S. image-interactive system
 S. treatment guidance platform
steam
 s. box
 s. tent
steam-shaping mandrel

StediSpine collar
Stedman awl
steel
 austenitic stainless s.
 s. embolization coil
 martensitic stainless s.
 s. mesh suture
 s. ruler
 s. sole plate orthosis
Steele scaler
steel-slotted plastic bracket
steel-winged butterfly needle
Steeper powered Gripper
steerable
 s. angioplastic guidewire
 s. decapolar electrode catheter
 s. guidewire catheter
 s. guidewire system
 s. I/A
 s. nephroscope
steering catheter
Steerocath-A ablation catheter
Steerocath catheter
Steerocath-Dx
 S.-Dx octapolar and valve mapping
 catheter
 S.-Dx special procedure octa
 catheter
**Steerocath-T temperature ablation
 catheter**
Steers replicator
Steffee
 S. pedicle plate
 S. pedicle screw-plate system
 S. plate and screw
 S. screw plate
 S. spinal instrumentation
 S. variable spine plating system
Stegman-Tromovitch bandage
Steigmann-Goff
 S.-G. endoscopic ligator kit
 S.-G. endoscopic ligature overtube
Steinbach mallet
Steiner
 S. bracket
 S. electromechanical morcellator
 S. speculum
Steiner-Auvard speculum
Steinert
 S. double-ended claw chopper
 S. double-ended LASIK spatula
 S. II claw chopper
 S. laser-assisted intrastromal
 keratomileusis set
 S. LASIK set
Steinert-Deacon incision gauge
Steinhauser
 S. bone clamp

S. plate
S. screw

Steinmann
S. calibrated pin
S. extension nail
S. fixation pin
S. holder
S. pin
S. pin with ball bearing
S. tendon forceps
S. traction
S. traction tractor

Stelid II pacing lead
Stelix pacing lead
Stelkast Supass acetabular system
Stellant
S. D CT injector
S. Sx CT injector

Stellbrink fixation device
stem
Aequalis s.
APR I femoral s.
Bio-Groove HA hip s.
Biomet revision hip s.
calcar replacement s.
s. cell concentrator
CLS hip s.
collarless s.
s. component
Continuum hip s.
contoured femoral s. (CFS)
Corail HA-coated s.
CRM s.
Eon femoral s.
Exeter s.
Extend s.
s. extractor
femoral s.
fenestrated Moore-type femoral s.
F2L Multineck femoral s.
Howmedica hip fracture s.
hydroxyapatite-coated s.
Iowa s.
Kirschner s.
Kirschner II-C shoulder system s.
s. kit CD34+HPC enumeration
system
KMP femoral s.
Linear hip s.
Link microporous hip s.
Mallory-Head femoral s.
modular calcar replacement s.
Moore hip endoprosthesis system s.
Morse taper s.
Natural-Hip s.
Natural-Hip titanium hip s.
Omnifit Eon femoral s.
Omnifit HA hip s.
Osteonics Omnifit-C s.

Osteonics Omnifit-HA hip s.
PCA total hip s.
Perfecta femoral s.
Perfecta HA coated s.
Perfecta IMC s.
Perfecta PDA calcar replacement s.
Perfecta RS s.
s. pessary
PLR spine revision hip s.
Precision Osteolock s.
press-fit s.
Profix metaphysial tibial s.
quadrature surface coil system s.
Ranawat-Burstein porous s.
Reach revision s.
rectal snare insulated s.
revision hip s.
RIGS system s.
SL-Plus s.
s. spoon separator
Spotorno cementless hip
arthroplasty s.
Strata hip system s.
Taperloc femoral s.
Ultima calcar s.
Ultima Fx s.

stemmed tibial prosthesis
Stem-Trol control cell
stencil
stenopeic spectacles
stenosis clamp
Stenstrom rasp
stent
Aboulker s.
Absolute biliary self-expanding s.
absorbable s.
Acculink self-expanding s.
ACS Multi-Link coronary s.
ACS Multi-Link Duet s.
ACS Multi-Link Duet coronary s.
ACS Multi-Link RX Ultra s.
ACS Multi-Link Tristar s.
ACS Multi-Link Tristar coronary s.
ACS RX Multi-Link s.
activated balloon-expandable
intravascular s.
active MRI s.
ACT-One coronary s.
adherent s.
adjustable vaginal s.
Amsterdam biliary s.
AMS urethral s.
AneuRx s.
Angiomed blue s.
Angiomed Puroflex s.
angiopeptin-eluting s.
AngioStent s.
antegrade ureteral s.
antibiotic-coated s.

stent *(continued)*
antireflux double-J s.
antirestenotic s.
s. apposition
ASI prostatic s.
ASI Titan s.
aSpire covered s.
Assurant balloon-expanded s.
AVE s.
AVE Bridge flexible balloon-expanded s.
AVE Bridge SE self-expanding s.
AVE Bridge stainless steel balloon-expandable s.
AVE GFX coronary s.
AVE Micro s.
AVE Microstent II s.
AVE S540, S670 s.
balloon-expandable s.
balloon-expandable flexible coil s.
balloon-expandable intravascular s.
balloon-expandable metallic s.
balloon-expandable tracheal s.
Bard coil s.
Bard Memotherm colorectal s.
Bard Saxx s.
Bard soft double-pigtail s.
Bard XT coronary s.
bare-metal s.
Beamer injection s.
BeStent balloon-expandable s.
BeStent 2 coronary s.
BeStent Rival s.
bifurcated s.
biliary s.
biliopancreatic diversion with duodenal s.
biocompatible s.
biodegradable s.
BioDiamond F s.
BioDiamond Micro s.
BiodivYsio s.
BiodivYsio added support s.
BiodivYsio AS PC-coated s.
BiodivYsio OC over-the-wire s.
BiodivYsio open cell s.
BiodivYsio PC s.
BiodivYsio small vessel s.
BiodivYsio SV PC-coated s.
Biofix s.
bioresorbable s.
BioSorb resorbable urology s.
Biostent biliary s.
Black Beauty ureteral s.
Braun s.
Bx Sonic over-the-wire s.
Bx Velocity s.
Bx Velocity coronary artery s.
Carcon s.

CardioCoil self-expanding coronary s.
Carey-Coons biliary s.
Carey-Coons soft s.
carotid s.
Carson internal/external endopyelotomy s.
cell-coated s.
CellPlant s.
cell-seeded s.
C-flex s.
C-Flex Amsterdam s.
C-Flex ureteral s.
cobalt alloy s.
coil s.
coil vascular s.
colonic s.
compliance matching s.
composite polymer s.
Conformexx biliary s.
conventional s.
Cook s.
Cook FlexStent s.
Cook intracoronary s.
Cook Logic coronary s.
Cook ureteral s.
Cordis CrossFlex coronary s.
Cordis Palmaz Corinthian s.
Cordis Palmaz Schatz long medium s.
Cordis Smart nitinol s.
Cordis tantalum coil s.
Corinthian stainless steel balloon-expandable s.
Corvita s.
Cotton-Huibregtse double pigtail s.
Cotton-Leung biliary s.
covered s.
covered biliary metal s.
covered Gianturco s.
Cragg s.
Cragg Endopro System I s.
Cragg Endopro System I covered s.
CrossFlex coil s.
CrossFlex LC coronary artery s.
CrossFlex LC stainless steel laser-cut coronary s.
Crown s.
crutched stick-type biliary duct s.
s. cutter
Cypher sirolimus-eluting coronary s.
Cysto Flex s.
Dacron s.
Dacron-covered s.
s. delivery system (SDS)
s. deployment
detachable balloon-modified reducing s.

Diamond s.
diaphragm of s.
digestive-respiratory fistula s.
diversion s.
DNA-coated s.
Dobbhoff biliary s.
double-J s.
double-J indwelling catheter s.
double-J silicone s.
double-J ureteral s.
double-pigtail s.
DoubleStent biliary
  endoprosthesis s.
Doyle II silicone s.
s. dressing
Driver coronary s.
drug-coated s.
drug-eluting s.
drug-loaded biodegradable
  polymer s.
Dua antireflux s.
Duet coronary s.
Dumon endobronchial silicone s.
Dumon silicone s.
Dumon tracheobronchial s.
Easy Wallstent s.
Elastalloy esophageal s.
Elastalloy Ultraflex Strecker
  nitinol s.
electropolished s.
Eliminator biliary s.
Eliminator pancreatic s.
eluting s.
encrusted ureteral s.
Endeavor drug-eluting s.
endobiliary s.
endobronchial s.
Endocare nitinol s.
EndoCoil biliary s.
EndoCoil esophageal s.
endoesophageal s.
endoluminal s.
endovascular s.
Enforcer SDS coronary s.
EsophaCoil s.
EsophaCoil biliary s.
EsophaCoil self-expanding
  esophageal s.
esophageal s.
esophageal I s.
esophageal Strecker s.
esophageal Z stent with Dua
  antireflux s.
ev3 premounted balloon-
  expandable s.
ev3 self-expanding s.
ev3 unmounted balloon-
  expandable s.
expandable esophageal s.

expandable Gianturco metallic s.
expandable intrahepatic portacaval
  shunt s.
expandable metallic s.
expander s.
Express balloon-expanded s.
Express biliary LD s.
expulsion s.
Fabian s.
Fader Tip ureteral s.
Fair urethral s.
fibrin film s.
Firlit-Kluge urethral s.
Flamingo s.
flat wire coil s.
Flex s.
flexible coil s.
Flexima biliary s.
FlexStent s.
Flexx biliary s.
floating s.
Fluoro-4 silicone ureteral s.
foam rubber vaginal s.
FocalSeal-R neurosurgical s.
fork s.
Freedom s.
FreeFlo proximal nitinol s.
freestanding s.
Freitag s.
French s.
s. funnel
gauze s.
gelatin-covered mesh s.
Genesis s.
Genous bioengineered R s.
Genus s.
GFX Micro s. III
GFX over-the-wire coronary s.
Gianturco s.
Gianturco expandable self-expanding
  metallic biliary s.
Gianturco expanding metallic s.
Gianturco metal urethral s.
Gianturco-Rosch biliary s.
Gianturco-Roubin flexible coil s.
Gianturco-Roubin Flex II s.
Gianturco-Roubin FlexStent
  coronary s.
Gianturco-Roubin II s.
Gianturco zigzag s.
Gibbon indwelling ureteral s.
Global Therapeutics Freedom s.
Global Therapeutics V-Flex s.
gold-coated inflow coronary s.
gold-coated Inflow coronary s.
gold-marked s.
Greenen pancreatic s.
Greene renal transplant s.
Guidant Megalink peripheral s.

stent *(continued)*
heat-activated recoverable
  temporary s.
helical coil s.
helical ridged ureteral s.
Hemobahn s.
Hepacoat s.
heparin-coated Palmaz-Schatz s.
Hood stoma s.
Horizon prostatic s.
Horizon temporary s.
Huibregtse biliary s.
Hydroduct biliary plastic s.
hydromer-coated polyurethane s.
Hydro Plus s.
iCAST covered s.
Igaki-Tamai s.
ileal artery s.
iliac artery s.
indwelling s.
indwelling ureteral s.
InLay Optima ureteral s.
InStent EsophaCoil s.
InStent VascuCoil s.
internal biliary s.
internal ureteral s.
IntraCoil s.
IntraCoil nitinol s.
IntraCoil self-expanding s.
IntraCoil self-expanding nitinol s.
IntraCoil self-expanding
  peripheral s.
intracoronary s.
intraoral s.
intraprostatic s.
IntraStent balloon-expanded s.
IntraStent biliary s.
IntraStent DoubleStrut biliary s.
IntraStent DS balloon-expanded s.
IntraStent LD balloon-expanded s.
IntraStent LP balloon-expanded s.
intravascular s.
s. introducer
INX s.
iridium-192 s.
Iris coronary s.
Iris II s.
Isostent s.
J & J s.
JJIS s.
J-Maxx s.
Johnson & Johnson biliary s.
Johnson & Johnson coronary s.
Johnson & Johnson Interventional
  Systems s.
Jomed s.
Jomed Flexmaster s.
Jomed peripheral s.
Jostent coronary s.

Jostent covered s.
Jostent graft s.
Jostent SelfX nitinol s.
keel s.
kidney internal s.
Koken nasal s.
Koyle diaper s.
lacrimal s.
large-bore double-pigtail s.
laryngeal s.
LifeStent LP SDS biliary s.
LifeStent NT self-expanding
  biliary s.
LifeStent XL SDS biliary s.
lighted s.
Logic coronary s.
LP s.
Lubri-Flex s.
Lubri-Flex ureteral s.
Lubri-Flex urologic s.
luminal s.
Luminexx biliary s.
Luminexx self-expanding s.
Mac s.
Magic Wallstent s.
magnetic internal ureteral s.
main pancreatic duct s.
Mardis soft s.
Medex coronary C1 s.
Medivent self-expanding coronary s.
Medivent vascular s.
MedNova s.
Medtronic AVE S660 coronary s.
Medtronic BeStent s.
Medtronic 5670 coronary s.
Medtronic interventional vascular s.
Megalink biliary s.
membrane-covered s.
Memotherm s.
Memotherm colorectal s.
Memotherm endoscopic biliary s.
Memotherm Flexx biliary s.
Memotherm nitinol s.
Memotherm nitinol self-
  expandable s.
Mentor biliary s.
MeroGel nasal s.
MeroGel sinus s.
mesh s.
metal-coated s.
metallic s.
methyl methacrylate ear s.
Micro II s.
Microvasive s.
Miller double mushroom biliary s.
Mini Crown s.
ML-Ultra balloon s.
30-mm-long Palmaz s.
monocanalicular silicone s.

Monorail Wallstent self-expanding s.
MonoStent monocanalicular s.
Montgomery laryngeal s.
MPD s.
MS-CIS SV s.
multicellular s.
Multi-Flex s.
Multi-Link Ascent s.
Multi-Link Duet s.
Multi-Link Penta s.
Multi-Link Solo s.
Multi-Link Terra s.
nephroureterostomy s.
Neuroform s.
Neville s.
NexStent carotid s.
Nexus coronary s.
NIR s.
NIRflex coronary s.
NIR ON Ranger balloon-expandable s.
Niroyal Advance balloon-expandable s.
NIR Primo Monorail coronary s.
NIR Royal Advanced s.
Nissenkorn s.
Ni-Ti alloy s.
nitinol mesh s.
nitinol self-expandable s.
nitinol self-expanding coil s.
nitinol subglottic stenosis s.
nitinol Symphony s.
nitinol thermal memory s.
Niti-S s.
nuclear s.
Oasis s.
Omega s.
Omni Flex biliary s.
Omnilink biliary s.
Omnilink/Megalink balloon-expanded s.
OmniStent s.
Optima ureteral s.
Ostia s.
Palmaz s.
Palmaz 424, 784 s.
Palmaz Corinthian s.
Palmaz Genesis s.
Palmaz Genesis balloon-expanded s.
Palmaz large balloon-expanded s.
Palmaz medium balloon-expanded s.
Palmaz P564 s.
Palmaz P394 stainless steel balloon-expandable s.
Palmaz-Schatz s.
Palmaz-Schatz balloon-expandable s.
Palmaz-Schatz biliary s.
Palmaz-Schatz coronary s.

Palmaz-Schatz Crown s.
Palmaz-Schatz Crown balloon-expandable s.
Palmaz-Schatz long medium balloon-expanded s.
Palmaz-Schatz PS-204 s.
Palmaz vascular s.
pancreatic duct s.
Paragon Champion s.
Paragon coronary s.
Paragon nitinol s.
Paragon PAS s.
Passager nitinol self-expandable s.
patent s.
Percuflex s.
Percuflex Amsterdam s.
Percuflex biliary s.
Percuflex endopyelotomy s.
Percuflex flexible biliary s.
Percuflex Plus s.
Percuflex Plus ureteral s.
percutaneous s.
Perflex stainless steel s.
Perflex stainless steel balloon-expandable s.
Phytis s.
pigtail s.
pigtail biliary s.
Pixel coronary s.
plastic s.
platinum-marked s.
polyethylene s.
Polyflex s.
polymeric endoluminal paving s.
polyorganophosphazene-coated s.
polypropylene s.
polytetrafluoroethylene covered s.
polyurethane s.
polyurethane-covered metallic s.
porous metallic s.
Power Grip s.
^{32}P radioactive s.
Precise nitinol transhepatic biliary s.
Precise RX transhepatic biliary s.
Precise self-expanding s.
premounted s.
Prostacoil s.
Prostakath urethral s.
prostatic s.
Protg GPS s.
Protg self-expanding s.
Protégé self-expanding s.
PS 153 s.
PTFE s.
PTFE-covered Palmaz s.
Pura-Vario s.
Pura-Vario-A s.
Pura-Vario-AL s.

stent *(continued)*

Pura-Vario-AS s.
QuaDDS s.
QuaDDS-QP2 s.
Quadra-Coil ureteral s.
QuaDS drug-eluting s.
QueST s.
Racer over-the-wire biliary s.
radioactive s.
radioisotope s.
radiopaque nitinol s.
radiopaque tantalum s.
Radius self-expanding s.
Rains s.
reducing s.
[188]Re-labeled self-expanding
    nitinol s.
renovascular s.
Retromax endopyelotomy s.
ring biliary s.
rolling membrane Wallstent cobalt-
    based alloy balloon-expandable s.
R-Stent s.
Rusch s.
S670 s.
Salman FES s.
S7 AVE s.
Schatz-Palmaz intravascular s.
Schneider s.
Schneider enteral s.
Schneider Speedy s.
Scimed s.
S7 coronary s.
S660 coronary s.
S670 coronary s.
screw-thread s.
Seaquence s.
self-expandable s.
self-expandable metal s.
self-expandable metallic s.
self-expanding s.
self-expanding coil s.
self-expanding covered s.
self-expanding metallic s.
self-expanding open mesh s.
self-expanding stainless steel s.
self-retaining coil s.
SEM s.
S-F Precise s.
shape memory alloy s.
Shikani middle meatal
    antrostomy s.
short s.
Siegel s.
silastic s.
silastic indwelling ureteral s.
silicone s.
silicone-coated metallic self-
    expanding s.

Silitek ureteral s.
Silitek Uropass s.
silver-coated s.
single pigtail s.
SinuSpacer turbinate s.
sirolimus-eluting s.
sirolimus-eluting SMART nitinol s.
slotted tube s.
slotted tube articulated s.
SMART s.
Smart bile duct s.
SMART Control self-expanding s.
SMART nitinol self-expandable s.
SMART self-expanding s.
Smith percutaneous
    endopyelotomy s.
Sof-Flex pediatric double pigtail s.
SoloPass Percuflex biliary s.
Song covered duodenal s.
Sorin Carbostent s.
S670 over-the-wire coronary s.
Speed Lok soft s.
spiral coil s.
SpiraStent ureteral s.
SpiroFlo bioabsorbable prostate s.
spring-loaded vascular s.
S660 small vessel coronary s.
stainless steel balloon
    expandable s.
stainless steel mesh s.
straight s.
Strecker s.
Strecker balloon-expandable s.
Strecker balloon-expanded s.
Strecker esophageal s.
Strecker nitinol self-expandable s.
Strecker tantalum s.
Strecker tantalum balloon-
    expandable s.
s. strut
STS s.
Supra G s.
Supra G coronary s.
Supramid occluding s.
Surgitek Tractfinder ureteral s.
Surgitek Uropass s.
Symbiot covered s.
Symphony nitinol s.
Symphony nitinol self-expandable s.
Symphony self-expanding s.
synthetic s.
T s.
TAG Excluder s.
tandem s.
Tannenbaum s.
tantalum s.
tantalum balloon-expandable s.
tantalum wire s.
Tarkington urethral s.

Taxus Express s.
Teflon s.
Temp Tip ureteral s.
Tenax coronary s.
Tenax-XR Trinity s.
Terumo s.
thermal memory s.
thermoexpandable s.
thermoplastic s.
Titan s.
titanium urethral s.
tracheobronchial s.
transhepatic biliary s.
transpapillary cystopancreatic s.
T-tube s.
tubular slotted s.
T-Y s.
UltraCross s.
Ultraflex s.
Ultraflex Diamond s.
Ultraflex Microvasive s.
Ultraflex nitinol expandable
  esophageal s.
Ultraflex self-expanding s.
Ultraflex tracheobronchial s.
Ultrathane Amplatz ureteral s.
uncoated mesh s.
Universal s.
ureteral s.
UroCoil self-expanding s.
Uro-Guide s.
UroLume endoprosthesis s.
UroLume prostate s.
UroLume urethral s.
UroLume Wallstent s.
Urosoft s.
Urospiral urethral s.
U-tube s.
vaginal s.
VascuCoil peripheral vascular s.
vascular s.
vein graft s.
Velocity s.
s. and vent system
V-Flex FMJ s.
V-Flex Plus s.
Viabahn covered s.
Viabil s.
Vistaflex balloon-expanded s.
Vistaflex biliary s.
Wallgraft cobalt-based alloy
  balloon-expandable s.
Wallgraft covered s.
Wallstent s.
Wallstent-covered SEM s.
Wallstent expanding metallic s.
Wallstent flexible self-expanding
  wire-mesh s.

Wallstent Iliac RP self-
  expanding s.
Wallstent Magic s.
Wallstent RP self-expanding s.
Wallstent spring-loaded s.
Wavemax balloon-expandable
  transhepatic biliary s.
Westaby tracheobronchial silicone s.
whistle s.
Wiktor balloon-expandable
  coronary s.
Wiktor GX coronary s.
Wiktor-I implantable s.
Wilson-Cook French s.
wire mesh self-expandable s.
Xceed biliary s.
Xpert biliary s.
XT radiopaque coronary s.
Z s.
Zaontz urethral s.
Za-stent endoscopic biliary s.
Za-stent nitinol self-expandable s.
Zenith stainless steel self-
  expandable s.
zigzag s.
Zilver biliary self-expanding s.
Zilver self-expanding s.
Zilver vascular s.
Zimmon biliary s.

stent-anchoring device
stent-graft
AneuRx s.-g.
Cragg EndoPro s.-g.
Excluder s.-g.
FreeFlo s.-g.
Gore covered biliary s.-g.
Hemobahn s.-g.
Hemobahn endovascular
  prosthesis s.-g.
Hemobahn PTFE-covered s.-g.
Inoue endovascular s.-g.
Inoue triple-branched s.-g.
Jomed peripheral s.-g.
Jostent coronary s.-g.
Jostent peripheral s.-g.
Lifepath s.-g.
Medtronic AneuRx s.-g.
Opta balloon s.-g.
self-expanding s.-g.
transluminally placed endovascular
  branched s.-g.
transluminally placed Inoue
  endovascular s.-g.
Viatorr transjugular intrahepatic
  portosystemic shunt s.-g.
Wallgraft endoprosthesis s.-g.
stenting catheter

stentless
>s. porcine aortic valve
>s. porcine aortic valve prosthesis

stent-mounted
>s.-m. allograft valve
>s.-m. heterograft valve

stent-shunt
>transjugular intrahepatic portosystemic s.-s.

STENTube lacrimal intubation set

step
>CUBEx multifunctional s.
>S. device
>s. drill
>S. laparoscopic entry system
>S. laparoscopic trocar
>s. screw

step-down
>s.-d. cannula
>s.-d. drill

stepdown transformer

Stephan HF 300 respirator

Stephanie 8000 oscillator

Stephen-Slater valve

Stephens soft IOL-inserting forceps

Step-Knife diamond blade knife

stepper
>Diamondback 1100 recumbent s.
>Diamondback 100 upright s.
>NuStep total body recumbent s.

stepup transformer

stereocampimeter

stereo campimeter

stereoencephalotome

StereoGuide
>S. breast biopsy equipment
>Lorad S.
>S. needle
>S. stereotactic breast biopsy system

stereolithography cage

stereomicroscope

stereophantoscope

stereophorometer

stereophoroscope

stereoscope
>Stanford and Wheatstone s.

stereoscopic
>s. diagonal inverter
>s. fundus camera
>s. microscope

stereotactic
>s. apparatus
>s. atlas
>s. breast biopsy needle
>s. breast biopsy system
>s. device
>s. head frame
>s. instrument
>s. instrumentation

>s. localization frame
>s. needle
>s. retractor
>s. surgical guidance system
>s. vacuum-assisted biopsy device

stereotactic-assisted radiation therapy kit

stereotaxic
>s. device
>s. instrument
>s. laser
>s. positioning device

Stereotaxis magnetic surgery system

stereoviewer
>Donaldson s.

SteriCam endoscopic camera

Steri-Cath catheter

Steri-Clamp
>S.-C. clamp
>IMP S.-C.
>Innovative Medical Products S.-C.

Steri-Cuff
>S.-C. disposable tourniquet cuff
>S.-C. Plus

Steri-Dent dry heat sterilizer

Steri-Drape
>S.-D. drape
>3M small aperture S.-D.
>small aperture S.-D.

Steri-Drape 2

sterile
>s. adhesive bubble dressing
>s. calcium alginate swab
>s. compression dressing
>s. drape
>s. dry dressing
>s. electrodermatome blade
>s. field barrier
>s. forceps holder
>s. gauze dressing
>s. isolation bag
>s. sheet
>s. specimen trap
>s. stockinette
>s. transverse rod
>s. vent spike

sterilizer
>Anprolene s.
>autoclave s.
>s. box
>Cox rapid dry heat transfer s.
>Dry-Therm s.
>Esquire dental s.
>glass bead s.
>Harvey vapor s.
>hot salt s.
>Steri-Dent dry heat s.

sterilizing
>s. basket
>s. forceps

Steri-Oss
- S.-O. dental implant
- S.-O. dental implant device
- S.-O. endosteal dental implant
- S.-O. Hexlock implant
- S.-O. implant device

Steri-Pad gauze pad
Steris automatic reprocessor
Steriseal disposable cannula
Steri-Strips
- S.-S. bandage
- S.-S. skin closure

Steritek ICP mini monitor
Steritome microkeratome system
Sterivap cement gun
sternal
- s. approximator
- s. attachment component
- s. clip
- s. knife
- s. needle holder
- s. notch stethoscope
- s. occipital mandibular immobilizer (SOMI)
- s. punch forceps
- s. puncture needle
- s. retractor
- s. retractor blade
- s. saw
- s. shears
- s. spreader
- s. suture
- s. wire suture

sternal-occipital-manubrial immobilizer
Stern-Castroviejo locking forceps
Stern-McCarthy electrotome resectoscope
sternooccipital-mandibular immobilization brace
sternooccipital mandibular immobilizer orthosis
sternotomy retractor
sternum-perforating awl
sternum saw
steroid-eluting electrode
Stertzer brachial catheter
StethoDop
- S. Doppler stethoscope
- Imex S.

stethoscope
- Acoustascope esophageal s.
- Allen fetal s.
- Andries s.
- bell s.
- binaural s.
- Cammann s.
- Cardiocare s.
- Cardiology II s.
- Classic II s.
- DeLee fetal s.
- DeLee-Hillis fetal s.
- differential s.
- Doppler fetal s.
- Doppler ultrasound s.
- Doptone fetal s.
- electronic s.
- electronic amplified s.
- E-Scope electronic s.
- esophageal s.
- fetal s.
- First Beat ultrasound s.
- Harvey Elite s.
- Hillis fetal s.
- Labtron s.
- Leff s.
- Littmann Master Classic II s.
- MedaSonics first beat ultrasound s.
- MedaSonics ultrasound BF4A, BF5A s.
- oroesophageal s.
- pacing esophageal s.
- Pinard fetal s.
- Pocket-Dop fetal s.
- precordial s.
- Rappaport-Sprague s.
- Spectrum s.
- ST3 amplified s.
- Starkey s.
- sternal notch s.
- StethoDop Doppler s.
- Stethos electronic s.
- Tapscope esophageal pacing s.
- ultrasound s.

Stethos electronic stethoscope
Stevanovsky metal eye shield
Stevens
- S. eye scissors
- S. hook
- S. iris forceps
- S. muscle hook retractor
- S. needle holder
- S. tenotomy hook
- S. tenotomy scissors

Stevenson
- S. cupped-jaw forceps
- S. lacrimal sac retractor
- S. microsurgical forceps
- S. refractor
- S. retractor

Stewart
- S. cruciate ligament guide
- S. crypt hook
- S. rectal hook

stick
- Back Revolution S.
- bite s.
- dextrose s.
- dressing s.
- FMS Intracell s.

stick *(continued)*
> Grafco seizure s.
> Intracell Sprinter s.
> Johnson hockey s.
> percutaneous s.
> sharpening test s.
> silver nitrate s.
> sponge s.
> switching s.
> 1-s. system
> Universal indicator s.
> Vaxcel mini s.
> weighted walking s.

stick-on electrode
Sticky Thermoliner custom locking liner
Stieglitz splinter forceps
Stiegmann-Goff
> S.-G. Clearvue endoscopic ligator
> S.-G. variceal ligator

Stifcore
> S. aspiration needle
> S. biopsy injection needle
> S. transbronchial aspiration needle

stiffening wire
stiff guidewire
stiff-soled shoe
STIF system
stiletto knife
Stille
> S. bone biter
> S. bone chisel
> S. bone drill set
> S. bone gouge
> S. bone rongeur
> S. bur
> S. clamp
> S. conchotome
> S. dissecting scissors
> S. osteotome
> S. Super Cut scissors

Stille-Aesculap plaster shears
Stille-Björk forceps
Stille-Horsley
> S.-H. bone-cutting forceps
> S.-H. bone forceps
> S.-H. bone rongeur
> S.-H. rib forceps
> S.-H. shears

Stille-Liston
> S.-L. bone-cutting forceps
> S.-L. bone forceps
> S.-L. rib-cutting forceps
> S.-L. rongeur

Stille-Luer
> S.-L. angular duckbill rongeur
> S.-L. bone rongeur
> S.-L. duckbill rongeur
> S.-L. rongeur forceps

Stille-Luer-Echlin rongeur

Stille-pattern trephine and bone drill set
Stille-Ruskin bone rongeur
Stilling plate
Stim
> S. neuromuscular stimulation system
> S. Plus handheld microcurrent stimulator

STI Medical Products PneuSplint
Stimoceiver implant material
Stimprene
> S. electrotherapy brace
> S. wrap

Stimson
> S. dressing
> S. pedicle clamp

StIM system
Stim-Tech
stimulating
> s. catheter
> s. electrode

stimulation probe
stimulator
> Acupoint s.
> Acuscope microcurrent s.
> AcuTENS transcutaneous nerve s.
> Air Pulse sensory s.
> AME bone growth s.
> Amrex muscle s.
> Anustim electronic neuromuscular s.
> Arzco model 7 cardiac s.
> Atrostim phrenic nerve s.
> Back Hammer muscle s.
> Biolectron bone growth s.
> Bionicare s.
> BioStim Digital NMS muscle s.
> Bloom programmable s.
> bone growth s.
> Cam vision s.
> Cervical-Stim cervical bone growth s.
> 8-channel muscle s.
> cochlear s.
> constant current s.
> direct-current bone growth s.
> dorsal column s.
> DTU-215 cardiac digital s.
> EBI SpF-2 implantable bone s.
> EBI SpF-T implantable bone s.
> electrical brain s.
> electric nerve s.
> Electro-Acuscope s.
> Electro-Myopulse muscle s.
> electronic s.
> electronic muscle s.
> EMG s.
> EMS 2000 neuromuscular s.
> Endo Multi-Mode s.
> external functional neuromuscular s.

facial nerve s.
FastStart EMS neuromuscular s.
FastStart HVPC pulsed s.
Freedom Micro Pro s.
galvanic electrode s.
Ganzfeld s.
G5 Porta-Plus muscle s.
Grass model S9 s.
Grass S88 muscle s.
Hilger facial nerve s.
implantable gastric s.
implantable neural s.
Innova pelvic floor s.
InSync multisite cardiac s.
Intelect electric s.
Intelect Legend s.
Intelect 600MP microcurrent s.
interferential s.
magnetic s.
Magnum 100 s.
Magnum 101 Plus s.
Magstim 200 s.
Magstim Rapid magnetic s.
Master-Stim interferential s.
Maxima II transcutaneous electrical
  nerve s.
Medi-Stim s.
Mettler Trio neuromuscular
  electrical s.
microamperage electrical nerve s.
microcurrent electrical
  neuromuscular s. (MENS)
Micro-Z neuromuscular s.
monopolar cathodal s.
MS322 muscle s.
muscle s.
Myotest train-of-four nerve s.
nerve s.
neuromuscular electrical s. (NMES)
neuromuscular III s.
Neurosign 100 constant current s.
Nicolet SM-300 s.
Nuwave transcutaneous electrical
  nerve s.
oculogyric s.
Ojemann cortical s.
Optokinetic s.
Ortho DX electromedical s.
Orthofix Cervical-Stim s.
Orthofix Cervical-Stim bone
  growth s.
OrthoGen bone growth s.
OrthoLogic 1000 bone growth s.
OsteoStim implantable bone
  grown s.
percutaneous epidural nerve s.
PGS-3000 pulsed galvanic s.
photonic s.
Physio-Stim Lite bone growth s.

piezoelectrical s.
Precision spinal cord s.
Prizm Electro-Mesh Z-Stim II s.
Pulsatron II handheld nerve s.
pulsed galvanic s.
Quik-Coff electrical cough s.
Reese s.
single lung PneuView s.
Smoke Control Porta-Pack
  aversive s.
SpF-PLUS spinal fusion s.
SpF spinal fusion s.
SpF-XL s.
spinal cord s.
SpinaLogic bone growth s.
SpinalPak bone growth s.
SpinalPak spine fusion s.
Sportstim s.
SporTX pulsed direct-current s.
S.P. 100 transcutaneous electrical
  neural s.
Stim Plus handheld microcurrent s.
Stimuplex-S nerve s.
Super Stimm MF s.
surgical nerve s.
Surgi-Stim s.
SynchroSonic s.
SysStim muscle s.
SysStim 226 muscle s.
Theramini 1, 2 electrotherapy s.
Theratouch s.
ThermaStim muscle s.
Toennis ES stand-alone constant-
  current electrical s.
transcutaneous cranial electrical s.
transcutaneous electrical nerve s.
transcutaneous electrical
  neuromuscular s. (TENS)
transmural electrical s.
Trio-Stim neuromuscular s.
Ultratone electrical transcutaneous
  neuromuscular s.
URYS 800 nerve s.
vagus nerve s.
Vari-Stim III handheld nerve s.
Zimmer OsteoStim bone growth s.
Z-Stim microprocessor controlled s.

stimulator/ultrasound
  Intelect Combo s./u.
Stimulite
  S. honeycomb mattress overlay
  S. honeycomb seating pad
Stimuplex block needle
Stimuplex-S nerve stimulator
stinger
  Alio-Prats irrigating chopper s.
  S. M ablation catheter
  S. S ablation catheter
  S. SM ablation catheter

sting mat
stippling sponge
stirrup, pl. **stirrups**
     Aircast pneumatic air s.
     Allen s.
     Allen laparoscopic s.
     ankle air s.
     s. brace
     candy cane s.
     Comfort Cast s.
     Finochietto s.
     hanging s.
     Lloyd-Davies s.
     split s.
     Swivel-Strap ankle s.
     walking s.
     Yellowfin s.
stirrup-loop curette
stitch-removing knife
stitch scissors
Stiwer
     S. bone-holding forceps
     S. finger-ring saw
STKS automated cell counting instrument
S&T Lalonde hook forceps
Stocker needle
stockinette
     s. amputation bandage
     Bias s.
     Buck traction s.
     s. cap
     s. dressing
     impervious s.
     orthopaedic s.
     sterile s.
     Velpeau s.
stocking, pl. **stockings**
     adjustable thigh antiembolism s. (ATS)
     antiembolic s. (AES)
     antiembolism s.
     A-T antiembolism s.
     Atkins-Tucker antiembolism s.
     Bellavar medical support s.
     Camp-Sigvaris s.
     Carolon life support antiembolism s.
     CircAid elastic s.
     compression s.
     Compriform support s.
     Comtesse medical support s.
     dropfoot redression s.
     elastic s.
     Fast-Fit vascular s.
     Florex medical compression s.
     graduated compression s.
     Jobst Stride support s.
     Jobst Stridette support s.

     Jobst Vairox gradient compression vascular s.
     Jobst VPGS s.
     Juzo s.
     Juzo-Hostess 2-way stretch compression s.
     Kendall compression s.
     Linton elastic s.
     Medi Plus compression s.
     Medi-Strumpf s.
     Medi vascular s.
     Orthawear antiembolism s.
     Planostretch s.
     pneumatic antiembolic s.
     pneumatic compression s.
     SCD s.
     sequential compression s.
     Sigvaris compression s.
     Sigvaris medical s.
     Silver-Thera s.
     Soft Touch s.
     Stride support s.
     TED antiembolism s.
     thigh-high antiembolic s.
     thromboembolic disease s.
     True Form support s.
     Twee alternating cut-off compressor s.
     Vairox high-compression vascular s.
     VenES II Medical s.
     Venofit medical compression s.
     Venoflex medical compression s.
     venous pressure-gradient support s.
     Zimmer antiembolism s.
     Zimmer antiembolism support s.
     Zipzoc s.
Stokes
     S. basket
     S. lens
Stoller afferent nerve stimulation system (SANS)
Stolte capsulorrhexis forceps
stoma
     s. button
     s. cap microporous adhesive
     s. cone
     s. irrigator drain
     s. measuring device
     silastic collar-reinforced s.
stoma-centering guide
stomach
     s. brush
     s. clamp
     s. pump
     s. tube
Stomahesive
     S. powder
     S. sterile wafer
stomal bag

Stomate
>S. decompression tube
>S. extension tube
>S. low-profile gastrostomy kit

Stomeasure

stone
>artificial cystine s.
>s. basket
>s. basket screw-mounted handle
>S. clamp-locking device
>S. Cone
>S. Cone nitinol stone retrieval
>device
>s. crushing forceps
>s. dislodger
>s. extraction forceps
>s. grasping forceps
>S. intestinal clamp
>S. intestinal forceps
>pumice s.
>s. recognition system
>s. retriever
>s. searcher
>s. staple
>s. strainer
>S. tissue forceps

stone-retrieval
>s.-r. balloon
>s.-r. basket

StoneRisk diagnostic monitoring kit

stone-tissue
>s.-t. detection system
>s.-t. recognition system

Stookey
>S. cranial rongeur
>S. retractor

stool
>s. collector
>foot s.
>nested step s.
>Swedish support s.

STOP
>selective tubal occlusion procedure
>STOP nonsurgical permanent
>contraception device

stop
>s. action brace
>S. at Ring lead
>S. at Tip lead
>Bowman needle s.
>Castroviejo corneal scissors with
>inside s.
>s. cock
>s. collar telescope
>crimp s.
>Elite posterior adjustable s.
>Endo s.
>footdrop s.

>s. needle
>s. speculum

stopcock
>Accel s.
>Burron Discofix s.
>Discofix s.
>Luer-Lok s.
>3-s. manifold
>manometer s.
>Morse s.
>3-way s.

Storey clamp

Stormby brush

**Stormer OTW balloon dilatation
catheter**

Storz
>S. applicator
>S. arthroscope
>S. band
>S. biopsy forceps
>S. bronchoscope
>S. calipers
>S. capsule forceps
>S. cataract knife
>S. catheter adapter
>S. ceiling-mounted microscope
>system
>S. cholangiograsper
>S. choledochoscope-nephroscope
>S. cilia forceps
>S. continuous-flow rectoscope
>S. corneal bur
>S. corneal forceps
>S. corneal trephine
>S. corneoscleral punch
>S. curved forceps
>S. cystoscope
>S. diagnostic laparoscope
>S. disposable blade
>S. disposable cannula
>S. disposable fiberoptic light pipe
>S. disposable trocar
>S. ear knife handle
>S. ear knife set
>S. ear, nose and throat camera
>system
>S. endoscope
>S. esophagoscope
>S. esophagoscopic forceps
>S. face shield headband
>S. handpiece
>S. head holder
>S. hysteroscope
>S. infant bronchoscope
>S. infection ventilation laryngoscope
>S. keratome
>S. kidney stone forceps
>S. Laparocam camera
>S. Laparoflator

Storz *(continued)*
  S. laparoscope
  S. laser
  S. laser resectoscope
  S. light box
  S. magnet
  S. microscope
  S. microsurgical bipolar coagulator
  S. Microsystems drill bit
  S. Microsystems plate cutter
  S. Microsystems plate-holding
    forceps
  S. Microsystems pliers
  S. Microvit vitrector
  S. Millennium microsurgical system
  S. miniplate
  S. Modulith SL20 lithotriptor
  S. multifunction valve
    trocar/cannula system
  S. nasopharyngeal biopsy forceps
  S. needle cannula
  S. nephroscope
  S. operating laparoscope
  S. panendoscope
  S. plate
  S. Premiere Microvit
  S. resectoscope
  S. resectoscope electrode
  S. retractor
  S. rhinomanometer
  S. screw
  S. sheath
  S. Sine-U-View endoscope
  S. SK ureteroscope
  S. stitch scissors
  S. stone crushing forceps
  S. stone dislodger
  S. suction tube
  S. syringe
  S. Teflon forceps guard
  S. thoracoscope
  S. tonometer
  S. twisted snare wire
  S. twist hook
  S. urethrotome
  S. vent tube introducer
  S. wire-cutting scissors
Storz-Atlas hand eye magnet
Storz-Bonn suturing forceps
Storz-Bruening diagnostic head
Storz-DeKock 2-way bronchial catheter
Storz-Hopkins
  S.-H. laryngoscope
  S.-H. system
  S.-H. telescope
Storz-Walker retinal detachment unit
Stough punch
Stout continuous wiring
stout-neck curette

strabismometer
strabismus
  s. forceps
  s. hook
  s. needle
  s. scissors
strabotome
StraddleSitter seating aid
straight
  s. aneurysm clip
  s. bipolar pencil
  s. bistoury
  s. blade
  s. burnisher
  s. catheter guide
  s. chest tube
  s. chisel
  s. coagulating forceps
  s. compression plate
  s. connector
  s. curette
  s. end-hole catheter
  s. endoprosthesis
  s. explorer
  s. fissure bur
  s. flush percutaneous catheter
  s. forceps
  s. guidewire
  s. guiding sheath
  s. hex screwdriver
  s. inclined plane elevator
  s. iris scissors
  s. knot-tying forceps
  s. lacrimal cannula
  s. laryngeal mirror
  s. last shoe
  s. line bayonet forceps
  s. magnifying mirror
  s. Maryland forceps
  s. microbipolar forceps
  s. microscissors
  s. monopolar electrosurgical
    dissector
  s. mosquito clamp
  s. mosquito hemostat
  s. nerve hook
  s. nonirrigating Connor wand
  s. osteotome
  s. periosteal elevator
  s. rasp
  s. reamer
  s. retinal probe
  s. retractor
  s. ring curette
  s. sapphire knife
  s. shank bur
  s. sickle scaler
  s. side-hole catheter
  s. single tenaculum forceps

s. stem femoral component
s. stent
s. stylet
s. suturing needle
s. tenaculum
s. tenotomy scissors
s. tipped catheter
s. tube stylet
s. tying forceps
s. tympanoplasty knife
s. walker brace

straight-ahead bronchoscopic telescope
straight-blade
s.-b. electrode
s.-b. laryngoscope
straight-end cup forceps
straightener
external s.
septal s.
Walsham septal s.
straightening cannula
Straight-In
S.-I. male sling system
S.-I. surgical system
straight-leg immobilizer
straight-line bayonet forceps
straight-needle electrode
straight-point
s.-p. electrode
s.-p. needle
StraightShot
S. arterial cannula
S. Magnum handpiece
straight-tip
s.-t. bipolar forceps
s.-t. electrode
s.-t. jeweler's bipolar forceps
straight-wire electrode
strain
s. gauge
s. gauge transducer
strainer
stone s.
Strampelli lens
Strandell-Stille retractor
Strands
AcryDerm S.
FlexiGel S.
strap
Allen s.
API universal foam chin s.
Band-It tennis elbow s.
Bard catheter s.
Beta Pile II, III splint s.
buddy s.
Butterfly cushion with s.
catheter leg s.
chest s.
Cho-Pat Achilles tendon s.

Cho-Pat dual action knee s.
Cho-Pat elbow s.
Cho-Pat ITB s.
s. clavicle splint
Comfort Cool thumb abduction s.
comfort leg bag s.
control adjustment s.
Conveen leg bag s.
counterforce s.
deluxe leg bag s.
Dermicel Montgomery s.
distal over-shoulder s.
D-Ring s.
D-Ring wrist support s.
Eclipse Gel elbow s.
elastic back s.
extremity mobilization s.
fabric leg bag s.
figure-of-8 clavicle s.
Fitz-all fabric leg s.
FoamWrap ThumDuction s.
footdrop s.
forearm flexion control s.
fork s.
front support s.
Gel-Bank patellar s.
hook-and-loop fastener s.
infrapatellar s.
ischial s.
latex rubber tourniquet s.
Lema s.
S. Lok ankle brace
Matt Strap knee s.
McKie thumb supinator s.
medial T s.
Montgomery s.
Mueller jumper's knee s.
neoprene wrist s.
Nylatex s.
nylon s.
over-shoulder s.
Partridge s.
Pepper Medical Antidisconnect
Device s.
PIP/DIP s.
ProSys leg bag comfort s.
Pro-Tec patellar tendon s.
proximal over-shoulder s.
QualCraft s.
Scott elastic ankle s.
silastic s.
s. sling
stretch-out s.
suprapatellar s.
Synergistic suspension s.
ThumDuction s.
torso s.
tourniquet s.
valgus corrective ankle s.

strap (*continued*)
  varus corrective ankle s.
  Velcro s.
strap-on undergarment
strapping
  AliStrap Velcro-type s.
  loop and hook s.
  low-dye s.
Strasburger cell plate
Strassburg sock
Strata
  S. adjustable Delta valve
  S. hip system
  S. hip system stem
  S. shunt valve
Stratagene
  S. CastAway sequencing device
  S. SCS-96 thermocycler
  S. SCS-96 thermocycler cycle
Stratasis urethral sling
StrataSorb composite wound dressing
Stratis
  S. II MRI system
  S. ST ACL reconstruction system
Stratos orthotic
Stratte needle holder
Stratus
  S. II automatic analyzer
  S. impact-reducing pylon
  S. instrument
Straumann
  S. dental implant system
  S. Standard Plus implant
Straus curved retrobulbar needle
Strauss
  S. dental attachment
  S. sigmoidoscope
streak retinoscope
stream
  2-s. irrigating forceps
Strecker
  S. balloon-expandable stent
  S. balloon-expanded stent
  S. esophageal stent
  S. nitinol self-expandable stent
  S. stent
  S. tantalum balloon-expandable
    stent
  S. tantalum stent
Strelinger colon clamp
strengthening exerciser
Streptex rapid strep test
Stress Echo bed
Stress-Ray varus-valgus device
Stretch
  S. gauze roll
  S. and Heel night splint
  S. Net wound dressing

stretcher
  basket s.
  Brandy scalp s.
  flexible s.
  hamstring s.
  Lumex shower s.
  orthopaedic s.
  1-person s.
  2-person s.
  portable s.
  Reeves s.
  roll-in s.
  scoop s.
  shoe s.
  wheeled s.
stretch-out strap
Stretch-Rite exerciser system
Stretta
  S. catheter
  S. system
striascope
Strichman SME-810 camera
stricturotome
Stride
  S. Analyzer
  S. support stocking
string
  s. drawing board
  soft rubber s.
stringing peg
strip
  Accu-Chek Comfort Curve test s.
  Albustix reagent s.
  AlloDerm s.
  Ascensia Autodisc test s.
  Ascensia Elite test s.
  Bio-Gen urine test s.
  blood glucose reagent s.
  bovine pericardium s.
  boxing s.
  Breathe Right nasal s.
  cardiac monitor s.
  Cardiac Reader IQC test s.
  CarraGauze packing s.
  Chin-Up s.
  color bar Schirmer s.
  ColorpHast Indicator S.'s
  Cover-Strip wound closure s.
  demineralized flexible laminar
    bone s.
  DermAssist hydrogel packing s.
  DET fluorescein s.
  Dextrostix reagent s.
  DiaScreen 10 Reagent S.
  DisIntek reagent s.
  Excel GE electrochemical glucose
    monitoring test s.
  EyeClose adhesive s.
  felt s.

fibrillar collagen s.
flexible laminar bone s.
Flu-Glow s.
Fluorets fluorescein sodium s.
Focus test s.
FreeStyle test s.
Ful-Glo fluorescein s.
G-C polishing s.
Gore-Tex s.
Grafton DBM matrix s.
Hansamed s.
Hypoguard Advance test s.
Lacrytest s.
LC s.
leucocyte detection s.
MediSense Q.I.D. test s.
MediSense 2 test s.
Medline Packing s.
MicroFlo test s.
Nu-Hope skin barrier s.
OneTouch Ultra test s.
Pacific Coast flexible laminar
  bone s.
packing s.
pHydrion s.
plastic s.
s. and point sponge
polishing s.
s. posting
Precision Xtra test s.
Prestige Smart System test s.
PyloriTek reagent s.
QuickTek test s.
QuickVue UrinChek urine test s.
QuickVue UrinChek 10+ urine
  test s.
ReliOn test s.
Schirmer tear test s.
separating s.
silicone s.
Sof-Tact test s.
Supreme test s.
SureStep test s.
Suture Strip wound closure s.
tear s.
tear test s.
Telfa s.
Thera-Band s.
Titan III H cellulose acetate s.
UrinChek 10+ urine test s.

stripper

Acufex microsurgical tendon s.
Alexander rib s.
Bunnell tendon s.
Cannon-type s.
cartilage s.
Clark vein s.
Dorian rib s.
endonerve s.

external vein s.
fascia lata s.
Fischer s.
Fischer tendon s.
Furlong tendon s.
hydraulic vein s.
IM tendon s.
interchangeable vein s.
interproximal s.
Kurten vein s.
Linton vein s.
Martin endarterectomy s.
Masson fascial s.
Matson-Alexander rib s.
Matson-Mead periosteum s.
Matson rib s.
Mayo external vein s.
Nabatoff vein s.
Oesch perforation invagination s.
orthopaedic surgical s.
pigtail tendon s.
ramus s.
reusable vein s.
Rosenwasser irrigating endothelial s.
slotted tendon s.
spiral vein s.
surgical s.
tendon s.
thrombus s.
Trace hydraulic vein s.
Trace vein s.
vein s.
Wylie endarterectomy s.
Zollinger-Gilmore intraluminal
  vein s.

Strobe
Digital S.

stroboscope
Kay rhinolaryngeal s.

stroboscopic
s. disc
s. microscope

Stromgren ankle brace
Stronghands hand exerciser
strontium-90 ophthalmic beta-ray
  applicator
Stropko irrigator
Strow corneal forceps
Struble lid everter
structured coil electromagnet
Strulle scissors
Strully dissecting scissors
strut

Adkins s.
s. bar
s. bar hook
s. calipers
s. forceps
George Washington s.

S

strut *(continued)*
s. graft
Judet s.
Magnuson s.
s. measuring instrument
miniplate s.
s. pick
polyethylene s.
stent s.
sutured-in-place columellar s.
Teflon s.
tricuspid valve s.
valve outflow s.
wire loop s.
strut-type pin
Struycken turbinate forceps
StrykeFlow
S. PS suction irrigator
S. 2 suction irrigator
StrykeProbe
S. suction irrigator probe
S. suction irrigator tip
Stryker
S. arthrometer
S. arthroscope
S. autopsy saw
S. bed
S. BioZip suture anchor
S. blade
S. bur
S. cartilage knife
S. cast cutter
S. chip camera
S. chondrotome
S. CircOlectric bed
S. Conquest suture retriever
S. ConstaVac suction apparatus
S. CPM exerciser
S. device
S. drain
S. drill
S. Endoscopy radiofrequency
ablation system (SERFAS)
S. fracture table
S. frame
S. Hummer II
S. Inter-Lock screw and fixation
system
S. intracompartmental pressure
monitor system
S. knee joint laxity device
S. lag screw
S. leg exerciser
S. microdebrider
S. microirrigator
S. microshaver
S. Patriot disposable cannula
system
S. power instrumentation

S. resector
S. saw
S. screwdriver
S. shaver
S. suction irrigator
S. suture slider system
S. turning fracture frame
S. universal wedge screw
S. Xcel suture anchor
**Stryker-Leibinger Modular Internal
Distraction system**
STS
STS lithotripsy system
STS molding sock
STS stent
Stuart articulator
Stuart-Prower factor
Stubbs
S. acromioclavicular splint
S. elastic wrist support
S. 4-way clavicle brace
Stucker bile duct dilator
Studer pouch
Stulberg
S. hip positioner
S. Mark II leg positioner
stump sock
STx
STx lumbar traction device
STx Saunders lumbar disc device
Style S2 clear-loop lens
stylet, stylette
Bing s.
bipolar irrigating s.
Cook locking s.
endotracheal s.
Frazier s.
illuminating s.
S. internal esophageal MRI coil
Jelco intravenous s.
jet s.
K s.
L s.
Liberator locking s.
Liberator universal locking s.
lighted s.
locking s.
Malis irrigating forceps s.
malleable s.
retractable s.
single-bevel s.
straight s.
straight tube s.
surgical s.
TFX Medical catheter s.
Trachlight lighted intubating s.
transmyocardial pacing s.
transthoracic pacing s.
Universal curved-tube s.

Universal straight-tube s.
ureteral s.
wire s.
stylet-scope endoscope
Stylus suture needle
Suarez
S. continence ring
S. spreader
Sub-4
S.-4 Platinum Plus wire kit
S.-4 small vessel balloon dilatation catheter
subannular mattress suture
subarachnoid
s. drain
s. screw
subarticular screw
subclavian
s. apheresis catheter
s. approach for cardiac catheterization
s. cannula
s. dialysis catheter
s. hemodialysis catheter
s. peel-away sheath
s. Tegaderm dressing
s. vein access catheter
subconjunctival needle
subcostal trocar
subcutaneous
s. augmentation material (SAM)
s. morphine pump
s. patch electrode
s. peritoneal administration device
s. suture
s. tunneling device
subcuticular suture
subdermal implant
subdural
s. button
s. electrode array
s. grid electrode
s. strip electrode
subfascial gauze pack
subgaleal drain
subgingival explorer
subglottic forceps
sublaminar wire
subluxated crystalline lens
submammary dissector
submicroinfusion catheter
submucosal implant
submucous
s. chisel
s. curette
s. dissector
s. retractor
suboccipital Ommaya reservoir
subpectoral stabilizer

subperiosteal
s. glass bead inserter
s. implant
s. tissue expander
Sub-Q-Set subcutaneous continuous infusion device
Subramanian classic miniature aortic clamp
subretinal
s. aspiration cannula
s. fluid cannula
Subrini penile prosthesis
substitute
Accu-Flo dural s.
AlloCraft bone spacer s.
AlloMatrix injectable putty bone graft s.
bilayered skin s.
Biobrane experimental skin s.
Biobrane/HF skin s.
Biobrane skin s.
bone graft s. (BGS)
Boplant Surgibone bovine bone s.
Collagraft bone graft s.
Dermagraft dermal s.
Dermagraft skin s.
Dermagraft-TC temporary skin s.
dural s.
Gore Preclude MVP dura s.
Gore Preclude PDX dura s.
Healos bone graft s.
HemAssist blood s.
OsSatura BCP bone graft s.
OsSatura TCP bone graft s.
OsteoSet bone graft s.
OsteoStim resorbable bone graft s.
Preclude MVP dura s.
Preclude PDX dura s.
Pro Osteon 500 bone graft s.
protein-based bone graft s.
synthetic bone s.
TransCyte temporary skin s.
subtalar MBA implant
sub-Tenon anesthesia cannula
suburethral sling
SubVent implant system
sub-zero
Cincinnati S.-z. (CSZ)
sucker
s. apparatus
intracardiac s.
malleable s.
s. shaver
s. tip
sucrose pacifier
suction
s. adapter
s. apparatus
s. aspirator

S

suction *(continued)*
    autotransfusion s.
    s. biopsy needle
    s. biter
    Bowins s.
    S. Buster catheter
    s. cannula
    s. catheter
    s. cautery
    s. coagulator
    s. cup
    s. curette
    s. cylinder
    s. device
    s. drain
    ear forceps with s.
    s. elevator
    Ferguson s.
    s. forceps
    Frazier s.
    s. irrigator
    s. machine
    s. magnet
    s. nozzle
    s. ophthalmodynamometer
    S. oral brush
    s. polyp trap
    s. probe
    s. pump
    s. punch
    s. pyramid
    s. Regugauge regulator
    Res-Q-Vac handheld emergency s.
    s. ring
    s. suspension prosthesis
    s. tip
    s. tip curette
    s. tonsillar dissector
    Trach Care s.
    s. tube
    s. tube clip
    s. tube obturator
    Vactro perilimbal s.
    Wangensteen s.
    Yankauer s.
suction-coagulation tube
suction-irrigator
    Jako s.-i.
    Kurze s.-i.
    Nezhat-Dorsey s.-i.
Suetens-Gybels-Vandermeulen
  angiographic localizer
sugar-dipped pacifier
sugar-tong
    s.-t. cast
    s.-t. splint
Sugita
    S. aneurysm clip
    S. catheter

    S. clip
    S. cross-legged clip
    S. fork
    S. head clamp
    S. head holder
    S. headholder
    S. microsurgical table
    S. multipurpose head frame
    S. retractor
    S. temporary straight clip
suit
    anti-G s.
    antigravity s.
    antishock s.
    body exhaust s.
    Gladiator shock s.
    hot-water circulating s.
    Life S.
    MAST s.
    total body compression s.
Sukhtian-Hughes
    S.-H. fixation
    S.-H. fixation device
Sulcabrush
Sulfix-6 cement
Sullivan
    S. bubble cushion
    S. HumidAire heated humidifier
    S. III CPAP
    S. III nasal continuous positive air
      pressure device
    S. Mirage nasal mask
    S. nasal variable positive airway
      pressure unit
    S. nasal VPAP unit
    S. sinus rasp
    S. V Elite Real Time Clock
      CPAP machine
    S. VPAP II, III
Sully shoulder stabilizer brace
Sulzer
    S. Orthopaedics instrument
    S. prosthesis
SummaSketch III digitizing board
Summit
    S. Apex Plus excimer laser
    S. bone screw
    S. excimer laser
    S. Krumeich-Barraquer
      microkeratome
    S. occipito-cervico-thoracic spinal
      fixation system
    S. OmniMed excimer laser
    S. SI OCT spinal fixation system
    S. SVS Apex laser
    S. tapered hip system
    S. UV 200 ExciMed laser
sump
    Argyle silicone Salem s.

DLP pericardial s.
s. drain
s. drainage catheter
s. pump
s. pump catheter
Ring-MacLean s.
s. tube
Van Sonnenberg s.
ventricular s.

sun

s. lamp
S. SPARCstation system

SunBox light box
Sunday staphylorrhaphy elevator
Sundt

S. aneurysm clip-applier
S. AVM microclip system
S. booster clip
S. carotid endarterectomy shunt
S. cross-legged clip
S. slim-line aneurysm system
S. slim-line graft clip
S. slim-line mini-aneurysm clip
system
S. straddling clip
S. suction system

Sundt-Kees

S.-K. aneurysm clip
S.-K. booster clip
S.-K. encircling patch clip
S.-K. graft clip
S.-K. Slimline clip

Sung reverse nucleus chopper
Sunlight Omnisense ultrasound
Sunnex Tri-Star lamp
Sunrise LTK system
super

S. Angiorex model G DSA system
S. ArrowFlex catheterization sheath
S. 50 CP high-voltage generator
S. Cut laminectomy rongeur
S. Dopplex SDI vascular test unit
S. Eagle punctum plug
S. Field NC slit lamp lens
S. Flex punctum plug
S. Grip sleeve
S. Jock n' Jill store Superfeet
orthotic
s. long-pulse diode laser system
S. PFG tube
S. Pinky ball
S. Pinky device
S. punctum plug
S. Revo suture anchor
S. Stimm MF stimulator
s. syringe
S. Torque braided angiographic
catheter
S. Torque Plus catheter

s. wedge
s. wrap

Super-4 catheter ablation system
Super-9 guiding cardiac device
superabsorbent

s. polymer
s. polymer microsphere

super-absorptive polymer dressing
Superblade

S. blade
S. No. 75 blade
S. trapezoid

Super-Bright microsphere
supercam scintillation scanner
superconducting

s. magnet
s. open-magnet system
s. quantum interference device
s. quantum interference device
susceptometer

superconductive MR system
SuperCup acetabular cup prosthesis
SuperCut

S. blade
S. diamond bur

Supercut scissors
SuperEBA cement
Superfeet custom prefabricated orthotic
superfine fiberscope
Superform Contours orthotic
Superfrost

S. microscope slide
S. Plus glass slide

Superglue adhesive
superior

s. border plate
s. radial tenotomy scissors
s. rectus bridle suture
s. rectus forceps
s. thoracic pedicle screw

superpulsed laser
SuperQuad assistive device
Super-Sect

PK S.-S.

SuperSkin thin film dressing
Superstabilizer

S. cemented stem extender
S. press-fit stem extender

Superstat topical hemostatic wound pad
super-stiff guidewire
SuperStitch

S. closure device
S. device
Sutura S.

supervoltage generator
supine

s. C-Trax traction
s. C-Trax traction system

support
    Abee s.
    Accommodator arch s.
    Accu-Back back s.
    Achillotrain active Achilles
      tendon s.
    Acro ComforT shoulder s.
    Active Ankle s.
    Act joint s.
    Act knee s.
    advanced cardiac life s.
    advanced cardiovascular life s.
    advanced life s.
    advanced trauma life s.
    Airprene hinged knee s.
    AliMed-Freedom arthritis s.
    AliMed wrist/thumb s.
    Anna-Dote positioning s.
    arch s.
    Arizona universal leg s.
    Assistant Free foot/ankle s.
    Back-Huggar lumbar s.
    BackThing lumbar s.
    Band-It magnetic elbow s.
    Bauerfeind s.
    Bauerfeind OmoTrain active
      shoulder s.
    BetterBinder back s.
    BIOflex magnet back s.
    biomagnetic s.
    BioSkin DP wrist s.
    BioWrap lumbosacral/sacral s.
    Birkenstock Blue Footbed arch s.
    Birkenstock high-flange arch s.
    Body Gard neoprene s.
    Carabelt lower back s.
    cardiopulmonary s.
    Carpal-Lock wrist s.
    Castech extremity s.
    s. catheter
    cavus foot s.
    chin s.
    ChinUpps cervicofacial s.
    Chiroflow adjustable back s.
    Cho-Pat knitted compression s.
    cock-up wrist s.
    Comfort Cool neoprene s.
    Comprifix active ankle s.
    Compro Plus Knee s.
    Conve back s.
    Core Reflex wrist s.
    Core Universal elastic knee s.
    Core Universal elbow s.
    Core Universal rib s.
    Corfit System 7000-series
      lumbosacral s.
    Cryo/Cuff compression s.
    cutout knee s.
    Cybertech 1000 back s.

    Dale oxygen cannula s.
    Dale ventilator tubing s.
    DayTimer carpal tunnel s.
    Deltoid-Aid arm s.
    DePuy s.
    Desk-Rest arm s.
    3D worker's back s.
    elevated leg s.
    Epi-Lock elbow s.
    Epipoint elbow s.
    Epitrain active elbow s.
    Epitrain elastic elbow s.
    Epitrain knitted elbow s.
    Epitrain Viscoped s.
    Ergo Cush back s.
    Ergoflex Premiere back s.
    extracorporeal life s.
    Ezy Wrap lumbosacral s.
    facial s.
    firm D-ring wrist s.
    Fits-All s.
    flat brain spatula s.
    FlexLite hinged knee s.
    Flex-Rite lumbar s.
    Foot Hugger foot s.
    Freedom accommodator arch s.
    Freedom arthritis s.
    Freedom back s.
    Freedom elastic long wrist s.
    Futuro wrist s.
    Genutrain P3 active knee s.
    Genutrain P3 knee s.
    geriatric chair trunk s.
    Gynemesh PS polypropylene
      mesh s.
    Hand-Aid arterial wrist s.
    IMP-Capello arm s.
    Innovation Sports bracing s.
    Juzo s.
    Kallassy ankle s.
    Knee Sleeve knee s.
    lateral lumbar s.
    life s.
    Lo Bak spinal s.
    Loving Comfort maternity s.
    Loving Comfort postpartum s.
    Lumbotrain lumbosacral s.
    MalleoLoc ankle s.
    Malleo-Med soft ankle s.
    Malleotrain ankle s.
    ManuTrain active wrist s.
    Markwort ankle s.
    McKenzie AirBack inflatable
      back s.
    mechanical s.
    MKG knee s.
    Mold-In-Place back s.
    Morton toe s.
    Mother-To-Be abdominal s.

Mother-To-Be Support maternity s.
MouseMitt Keyboarders wrist s.
neck s.
neoprene ankle s.
neoprene back s.
Nightimer carpal tunnel s.
Night Splint s.
obese s.
Obus back s.
Omotrain active shoulder s.
Orion lumbar s.
Ortho-Pal body s.
OSI well leg s.
Palumbo knee s.
PattStrap knee s.
percutaneous cardiopulmonary
 bypass s.
Performance Wrap knee s.
Plastazote arch s.
Playmaker s.
postoperative mammary s.
Powerstep foot s.
ProFlex wrist s.
prosthetic s.
QualCraft ankle s.
QualCraft short elastic wrist s.
Rheuma wrist and thumb s.
Rolyan foot s.
Rolyan TakeOff thumb s.
sacral s.
Schick back s.
Scott double-strap ankle s.
Scott hinged knee s.
ShiatsuBACK back s.
shoulder Ease abduction s.
Sidekick foot s.
Spenco arch s.
S'port Max back s.
standard U patellar s.
Stubbs elastic wrist s.
SureStep ankle s.
TakeOff elbow s.
Tecnol ankle s.
Tecnol elbow s.
Tecnol knee s.
Tecnol wrist s.
Thera-Back back s.
therapeutic spinal s.
Thermoskin 4-way elastic knee s.
Thumboform s.
tibial fracture brace proximal s.
Titan thumb s.
urethrovesical angle s.
Valeo back s.
Viscoped S s.
ViscoSpot s.
wedge-shaped s.
well leg s.
Whitman arch s.

WorkAbout Carpal Mate wrist s.
WorkMod back s.
wrist-hand extension compression s.
WrisTimer CTS s.
WrisTimer PM carpal tunnel s.
Wrist Pro wrist s.

Supra
 S. G coronary stent
 S. G stent
 8000 S. Series auto refractometer
supraannular
 s. suture ring
supraanular valve (SAV)
supracondylar
 s. barrel/plate component
 s. cuff
 s. knee-ankle orthosis
 s. nail
 s. plate
 s. socket
Supracore 35 guidewire
SupraFOIL implant
SupraFoley
 S. catheter
 S. suprapubic introducer
suprahepatic caval clamp
Supralen
 S. cradle orthotic
 S. Schaefer orthotic
supramalleolar orthosis
Supramid
 S. bridle collagen suture
 S. Extra suture
 S. eye muscle sleeve
 S. graft
 S. implant
 S. lens implant suture
 S. occluding stent
 S. polyamide mesh
 S. sheet
 S. sling
 S. suture
Supramid-Allen implant
suprapatellar
 s. cannula
 s. cuff
 s. strap
suprapubic (SP)
 s. cannula
 s. catheter
 s. suction drain
 s. trocar
suprarenal Greenfield filter
Supratome microkeratome
Supreme
 S. electrophysiology catheter
 S. II blood glucose meter
 S. test strip
Suraci zygoma hook elevator

S

Surbaugh legholder
Sur-Catch NT stone retrieval basket
Sure
- S. Blot membrane
- S. Seal Golden Drain catheter
- S. Shot injection needle
- S. Sport pad
- S. Step ankle brace

SureBite biopsy forceps
SureCath port access catheter
Sure-Closure
- S.-C. device
- S.-C. skin closure system
- S.-C. skin stretching system

Surecut needle
!nSure fecal immunochemical test
Surefit AC 85J lens
Sure-Flex
- S.-F. III prosthetic foot
- S.-F. prosthesis

SureFlex nickel-titanium hand file
SureFold system
Sure-Gait folding walker
SureGrip breathing bag
SurePress
- S. absorbent padding
- S. high-compression bandage
- S. leg compression dressing

SureScan
- S. scanning handpiece
- S. system

Sureseal pressure bandage
SureSight
- S. autorefractor
- S. vision screener
- S. vision screening device

SureSite transparent film
SureStart
- S. contrast tracking
- S. imaging system

SureStep
- S. ankle support
- S. ankle support system
- S. Flexx professional blood glucose management system
- S. glucose meter
- S. glucose monitor
- S. Pro glucose analyzer
- S. test strip

Suretac
- S. bioabsorbable shoulder fixation device
- S. drill
- S. guidewire
- S. suture

SureTemp
- S. electronic thermometer
- S. 4 oral thermometer

SureTrans autotransfusion system

Surety Shield
Surevue contact lens
surface
- Advance Dynamicaire sleep s.
- Alpha Active pressure-relieving support s.
- Carmeda BioActive S.
- s. coil
- DeCube therapeutic s.
- s. electrode
- s. eye implant
- s. implant
- Silhouette therapeutic s.

Sur-Fast needle
Sur-Fit
- S.-F. auto-lock closed-end pouch with filter
- S.-F. colostomy bag
- S.-F. colostomy irrigation sleeve
- S.-F. flange cap
- S.-F. irrigation adapter faceplate
- S.-F. irrigation sleeve tail closure
- S.-F. loop
- S.-F. Natura closed-end pouch, opaque
- S.-F. Natura disposable convex insert
- S.-F. Natura flange cap
- S.-F. Natura flexible wafer and drainable pouch
- S.-F. Natura irrigation adapter face plate
- S.-F. Natura irrigation sleeve
- S.-F. Natura irrigation sleeve tail closure
- S.-F. Natura loop ostomy rod
- S.-F. Natura mini pouch
- S.-F. Natura night drainage container set
- S.-F. Natura night drainage container tubing
- S.-F. Natura opaque closed-end pouch with filter
- S.-F. Natura urostomy pouch
- S.-F. Natura Visi-Flow irrigation starter set
- S.-F. night drainage container set
- S.-F. urinary drainage bag

Surflo
- S. Teflon IV catheter
- S. winged infusion set

Surgairtome
- S. air drill
- S. II drill halo

Surgamid polyamide suture material
SurgAssist
- S. leg positioner
- S. surgical legholder

Surgenomic endoscope

surgery
  computer-assisted stereotactic s.
  (CASS)
Surg-E-Trol I/A System
Surgibone
  S. implant
  Unilab S.
Surgica K6 laser
surgical
  s. adhesive
  s. appliance
  s. appliance adhesive
  s. aspirator
  s. balloon
  s. bur
  s. cannula
  s. chromic suture
  s. clip
  s. clip applier
  s. compression garment
  s. contractor
  s. corset
  s. curette
  s. cutter
  s. drain
  s. drape
  s. dressing
  s. electrode
  s. exhaust apparatus
  s. file
  s. general rasp
  s. glue
  s. gouge
  s. gut suture
  s. hammer
  s. handle
  s. hood
  s. instrument guide
  s. instrument post
  S. Internet Generation Network
  (SIGN)
  s. keratometer
  s. laser
  S. Laser Technologies (SLT)
  s. leg pedestal
  s. linen suture
  s. loupe
  s. mallet
  s. marking pen
  s. mask
  s. mesh
  s. metallic mesh
  s. microscope
  s. microscope navigator system
  s. navigation system
  s. nerve stimulator
  S. Nu-Knit absorbable hemostatic
  material
  s. otoscope

S. Patient Arm shield
s. patient arm shield
s. pin driver
s. power magnet
s. retractor
s. rod
s. saw
s. saw blade
s. scissors
s. silk suture
S. Simplex P adhesive
S. Simplex P bone cement
S. Simplex P radiopaque bone
  cement
s. simulation virtual reality
  laboratory
s. simulator
s. skin graft expander
s. snare
s. spatula
s. splint
s. sponge
s. staple
s. stapling gun
s. steel gauze
s. steel suture
s. stripper
s. stylet
s. suction pump
s. tape
s. telescope
surgically implanted hemodialysis
  catheter
Surgicel
  S. fibrillar absorbable hemostat
  S. gauze
  S. Nu-Knit
  S. Nu-Knit absorbable hemostat
Surgicenter 40 CO$_2$ laser
Surgiclip
  Auto Suture S.
  S. clip
  McDermott S.
Surgicraft Copeland fetal scalp
  electrode
Surgicutt incision device
Surgidac suture
Surgi-Fine reusable cannula tip
Surgiflex
  S. elastic net
  S. Wave suction-irrigation device
  S. Wave XP suction/irrigation
  probe
Surgiflo hemostatic matrix
Surgifoam absorbable powder
Surgiguide template
Surgikos disposable drape
Surgilase
  S. CO$_2$ laser

Surgilase *(continued)*
- S. 150 high-powered CO_2 laser
- S. 150 laser
- S. Nd:YAG laser
- S. 55W laser

Surgilast tubular elastic dressing

Surgilav
- S. drain
- S. machine

Surgilene blue monofilament polypropylene suture

Surgilon braided nylon suture

Surg-I-Loop

Surgimedics/TMP multiperfusion set

Surgimed suture

Surgineedle pneumoperitoneum needle

Surgin hemorrhage occluder pin

Surgipad Combine dressing

Surgipath Decalcifier I, II

Surgi-PEG replacement gastrostomy feeding system

Surgiport
- S. disposable trocar
- S. trocar and sleeve

Surgipro
- S. hernia mesh
- S. mesh
- S. suture

Surgipulse XJ 150 CO_2 laser

SurgiPulse XJ laser

SurgiScope
- S. image-guided system
- Marco S.
- S. robotic microscope
- S. stereotactic system

Surgiscribe surgical marking pen

Surgisis sling/mesh

Surgi-Spec telescope

Surgistar
- S. corneal trephine
- S. ophthalmic blade

Surgi-Stim
- S.-S. postsurgical therapy system
- S.-S. stimulator

Surgitek
- S. button
- S. graduated cystocope GC-16
- S. handpiece
- S. mammary implant
- S. mammary prosthesis
- S. Tractfinder ureteral stent
- S. T-Span tissue expander
- S. Uropass stent

Surgitite ligating loop

Surgitron
- Ellman S.
- S. portable radiosurgical unit
- S. ultrasound-assisted lipoplasty machine

- S. 3000 ultrasound device
- S. unit

Surgitube
- S. tubing
- S. tubular gauze

Surgivac drain

Surgiview multi use disposable laparoscope

Surgi-Vision MRI coil

Surgiwip suture ligature

Surpasse balloon

Surpass PTCA perfusion catheter

Surveyor
- S. monitor
- S. recording device

susceptometer
- superconducting quantum interference device s.

suspended operating illuminator

Suspend sling

suspension
- s. apparatus
- DNAzole cell s.
- s. feeder
- s. laryngoscope
- s. splint

suspension-type socket

suspensory bandage

Sussman 4-mirror gonioscope

Sustain
- S. dental implant system
- S. HA-coated screw implant

sustainer
- Akahoshi nucleus ring s.

Sutcliffe laser shield and retracting instrument

Sutherland
- S. eye scissors
- S. lens
- S. rotatable microsurgery instrument
- S. scissors

Sutter
- S. device
- S. double-stem silicone implant prosthesis
- S. hinged great toe implant
- S. implant
- S. MCP finger joint prosthesis
- S. silicone metacarpophalangeal joint

Sutter-CPM knee device

Sutura SuperStitch

suture
- absorbable surgical s.
- Acier stainless steel s.
- Acufex bioabsorbable Suretac s.
- Acutrol s.
- Albert s.
- Albert-Lembert s.

Alcon s.
Allgöwer-Donati s.
already-threaded s.
American silk s.
Ancap braided silk s.
s. anchor
angiocatheter with looped
  polypropylene s.
antibody-coated s.
antitorque s.
Appolito s.
Arroyo encircling s.
Arruga encircling s.
arterial silk s.
S. Assistant endoscopic suturing
  device
S. Assistant instrument
Atraloc s.
Aureomycin s.
Auto S. (AS)
Barraquer silk s.
baseball s.
basting s.
Bell s.
bioabsorbable Dexon s.
Bio-FASTak s.
BioSorb s.
Biosyn synthetic monofilament s.
biparietal s.
black braided nylon s.
black braided silk s.
black silk bridle s.
black silk sling s.
blanket s.
blue-black monofilament s.
blue twisted cotton s.
bolster s.
Bondek absorbable s.
bone wax s.
braided Ethibond s.
braided Mersilene s.
braided Nurolon s.
braided nylon s.
braided polyamide s.
braided polyester s.
braided polyglactin s.
braided silk s.
braided Vicryl s.
braided wire s.
Bralon braided nylon s.
bridle s.
Brown-Sharp gauge s.
B&S gauge s.
Bunnell s.
Bunnell wire pull-out s.
s. button
capitonnage s.
caprolactam s.
Caprosyn monofilament s.

cardinal s.
Cardioflon s.
Cardionyl s.
s. carrier
catgut s.
cervical s.
Chinese fingertrap s.
chromated catgut s.
chromic s.
chromic blue dyed s.
chromic catgut s.
chromic collagen s.
chromic gut s.
chromicized catgut s.
circular s.
circumcisional s.
s. clamp
s. clip forceps
coated polyester s.
coated Vicryl s.
coated Vicryl Rapide s.
collagen absorbable s.
compound s.
concha-mastoid s.
Connell s.
Cooley U s.
cotton s.
cotton nonabsorbable s.
cottony Dacron hollow s.
CT1 s.
Cushing s.
Custodis s.
Cutalon nylon polyamide
  surgical s.
s. cutter
Czerny s.
Czerny-Lembert s.
Dacron bolstered s.
Dacron traction s.
Dafilon s.
Dagrofil s.
Davis-Geck s.
Deklene II cardiovascular s.
Deklene polypropylene s.
Deknatel silk s.
dermal s.
Dermalene polyethylene s.
Dermalon cuticular s.
Dexon s.
Dexon absorbable synthetic
  polyglycolic acid s.
Dexon II s.
Dexon Plus s.
DG Softgut s.
double-armed wire s.
double right-angle s.
double-running penetrating
  keratoplasty s.
Dulox s.

suture *(continued)*
EEA Auto S.
Endoknot s.
Endoloop s.
end-to-end s.
end-to-side s.
EPTFE vascular s.
Ethibond polybutilate-coated
  polyester s.
Ethicon s.
Ethicon-Atraloc s.
Ethicon micropoint s.
Ethicon Sabreloc s.
Ethicon silk s.
Ethiflex s.
Ethiflex retention s.
Ethilon s.
Ethilon nylon s.
Ethi-pack s.
everting mattress s.
extrachromic s.
eyelid crease s.
Faden s.
FiberWire s.
figure-of-8 s.
filament s.
fine chromic s.
fine silk s.
fingertrap s.
Flaxedil s.
Flexitone s.
Flexon steel s.
formaldehyde catgut s.
Foster s.
Fothergill s.
Frost s.
Gaillard-Arlt s.
Gambee s.
gastrointestinal surgical gut s.
gastrointestinal surgical linen s.
gastrointestinal surgical silk s.
Gély s.
general closure s.
Gillies horizontal dermal s.
GI pop-off silk s.
glue-in s.
Gore-Tex s.
gossamer silk s.
Gould s.
green braided s.
green Mersilene s.
green monofilament
  polyglyconate s.
groove s.
s. guide
Gussenbauer s.
gut s.
guy s.
guy-steading s.

Halsted mattress s.
harmonic s.
Heaney s.
heavy-gauge s.
heavy monofilament s.
heavy retention s.
heavy silk retention s.
heavy wire s.
helical s.
hemostatic s.
s. holder
Horsley s.
Hu-Friedy PermaSharp s.
India rubber s.
interrupted pledgeted s.
intraluminal s.
Investa s.
iodine catgut s.
Ivalon s.
Kelly s.
Kessler s.
Kessler-Kleinert s.
Kirschner s.
Krackow s.
Küstner s.
L-25 absorbable surgical s.
s. lancet
lancet s.
Lang s.
Lapra-Ty s.
large-caliber nonabsorbable s.
lateral trap s.
lead s.
Le Fort s.
Linatrix s.
Lindner corneoscleral s.
linen s.
Linvatec meniscal BioStinger
  anchor s.
s. lock
lockout s.
Look s.
Lukens catgut s.
malar periosteum-SMAS flap
  fixation s.
Mannis s.
Marlex s.
mattress s.
Maxon absorbable s.
Mayo linen s.
McCannel s.
McLean s.
Meigs s.
Mersilene braided nonabsorbable s.
Mersilk black silk s.
mesh s.
metal band s.
metallic s.
Micrins microsurgical s.

Micro-Glide corneal s.
MicroMite anchor s.
micropoint s.
Miralene s.
modified Frost s.
Monocryl s.
monofilament absorbable s.
monofilament clear s.
monofilament green s.
monofilament nonabsorbable s.
monofilament nylon s.
monofilament polypropylene s.
monofilament skin s.
monofilament steel s.
monofilament wire s.
multifilament steel s.
multistrand s.
nasofrontal s.
natural s.
Needle-Less S.
nerve s.
neurosurgical s.
nonabsorbable surgical s.
Novafil s.
Nurolon s.
nylon s.
nylon 66 s.
nylon monofilament s.
nylon retention s.
oiled silk s.
opaque wire s.
Panacryl s.
Panalok absorbable s.
Pancoast s.
s. passer
PDS II s.
PDS II Endoloop s.
PDS Vicryl s.
Perlon s.
Perma-Hand braided silk s.
PermaSharp PGA s.
PGA synthetic absorbable s.
s. pickup hook
s. pickup spatula
pickup spatula s.
pin s.
pink twisted cotton s.
plain catgut s.
plain collagen s.
plain gut s.
plastic s.
pledget s.
pledgeted Ethibond s.
pledgeted mattress s.
poliglecaprone 25 s.
polyamide s.
polybutester s.
Polydek s.
polydioxanone s. (PDS)

polyester fiber s.
polyethylene s.
polyfilament s.
polygalactic acid s.
polyglactin s.
polyglactin 910 s.
polyglecaprone 25 s.
polyglycolate s.
polyglycolic acid s.
polyglyconate s.
polypropylene s.
polypropylene button s.
Polysorb s.
polytetrafluoroethylene s.
pop-off s.
PremiCron nonabsorbable s.
Prolene s.
Prolene polypropylene s.
Pronova s.
Proxi-Strip s.
Pulvertaft weave s.
Quickert s.
Rapide wound s.
reabsorbable s.
releasable compression s.
s. ring
rip-cord s.
rubber s.
Safil synthetic absorbable
  surgical s.
s. scissors
self-adjusting s.
Serralnyl s.
Serralsilk s.
serrated s.
seton s.
Sharpoint ophthalmic
  microsurgical s.
Sharpoint Ultra-Glide corneal
  transplant s.
Sharpoint Ultra-Glide ophthalmic
  transplant s.
Shirodkar s.
Shoch s.
shotted s.
SH pop-off s.
silicone-treated surgical silk s.
silk s.
silk braided s.
silk Mersilene s.
silk nonabsorbable s.
silk pop-off s.
silk stay s.
silk traction s.
silkworm gut s.
silver s.
silverized catgut s.
silver wire s.
Sims s.

S

suture *(continued)*
single-armed s.
single-running s.
single running s.
skin s.
s. slider system
Snellen s.
Sofsilk coated and braided s.
Sofsilk nonabsorbable silk s.
s. spacer
Spanish silk s.
sphenozygomatic s.
SS s.
stainless steel wire s.
staple s.
Statak s.
steel mesh s.
sternal s.
sternal wire s.
S. Strip Plus
S. Strip Plus wound closure
S. Strip wound closure strip
subannular mattress s.
subcutaneous s.
subcuticular s.
superior rectus bridle s.
Supramid s.
Supramid bridle collagen s.
Supramid Extra s.
Supramid lens implant s.
Suretac s.
surgical chromic s.
surgical gut s.
surgical linen s.
surgical silk s.
surgical steel s.
Surgidac s.
Surgilene blue monofilament
  polypropylene s.
Surgilon braided nylon s.
Surgimed s.
Surgipro s.
swaged s.
swaged-on s.
Swiss silk s.
synthetic absorbable s.
Synthofil s.
s. tag forceps
Tapercut s.
Teflon-coated s.
Teflon-pledgeted s.
s. tension adjustment reel
tension-requiring s.
tentalum wire tension s.
Tevdek s.
Tevdek pledgeted s.
Thiersch s.
through-and-through continuous s.
through-and-through reabsorbable s.

through-the-wall mattress s.
Ti-Cron s.
tiger gut s.
TigerWire s.
traction s.
S. Tram
S. Tram instrument
transfixion s.
transosseous s.
transscleral s.
twisted virgin silk s.
s. tying platform forceps
tympanomastoid s.
umbilical tape s.
unabsorbable s.
undyed s.
Verhoeff s.
Vicryl s.
Vicryl pop-off s.
Vicryl Rapide s.
Vicryl SH s.
violet monofilament s.
virgin silk s.
white braided silk s.
white nylon s.
white twisted s.
wing s.
s. wire
s. wire-cutting scissors
Worst s.
ZF s.
Zimmer Statak s.
sutured-in-place columellar strut
sutured plaque electrode
SutureGroove
S. gold eyelid weight
S. gold eye weight
S. gold eye weight implant
SutureLasso
Arthrex Banana S.
Banana S.
Suturelassos
micro S.
sutureless
s. biofragmentable ring
s. pacemaker electrode
Suture-Mate
Suture-Self dressing
suturing
s. forceps
s. instrument
s. needle
temporary keratoprosthesis s.
**SuturTek 360-degree fascia closure
  device**
SV
small vessel
SV guidewire
SVAB device

SVC lead
Sven-Johansson
    S.-J. extractor
    S.-J. femoral neck nail
swab
    calcium alginate s.
    Chamois s.
    eye s.
    Koenig tonsillar s.
    Mesoft s.
    Persist skin prep s.
    Phenol EZ s.
    Puritan s.
    sterile calcium alginate s.
    wooden s.
    wound s.
swaged
    s. arthroscopic needle
    s. needle
    s. suture
swaged-on
    s.-o. needle
    s.-o. suture
swager
    wax s.
Swan
    S. aortic clamp
    S. knife needle
    S. lancet
Swan-Ganz
    S.-G. balloon catheter
    S.-G. balloon flotation catheter
    S.-G. bipolar pacing catheter
    S.-G. catheter
    S.-G. flow-directed catheter
    S.-G. guidewire TD catheter
    S.-G. pacing TD catheter
    S.-G. pulmonary artery catheter
    S.-G. thermodilution catheter
    S.-G. tube
swan-neck
    s.-n. clamp
    s.-n. Missouri catheter
    s.-n. pediatric Coil-Cath catheter
    s.-n. splint
Swann-Morton surgical blade
Swanson
    S. carpal lunate implant
    S. carpal scaphoid implant
    S. elevator
    S. finger joint implant
    S. finger joint prosthesis
    S. great toe implant
    S. great toe prosthesis
    S. Grip-X hand exerciser
    S. lunate awl
    S. mallet
    S. metacarpal prosthesis
    S. metacarpophalangeal implant

    S. metatarsal broach
    S. metatarsal prosthesis
    S. osteotome
    S. radial head implant
    S. reamer
    S. scaphoid awl
    S. silastic implant
    S. small joint implant
    S. trapezium implant
    S. wrist joint implant
    S. wrist prosthesis
swathe
    arm s.
    sling and s. (S&S)
Sweat-Chek conductivity analyzer
Swede-O
    S.-O. Ankle Lok brace
    S.-O. Arch Lok
    S.-O. Universal brace
    S.-O. Universal orthosis
Swede-Vent TL self-tapping external hex implant
Swedish
    S. Adjustable Gastric Band
    S. Helparm
    S. Helparm device
    S. knee cage
    S. support stool
Sween-A-Peel wound dressing
sweep
    Barraquer s.
    The Cell S.
sweeper
Sweet
    S. clip-applying forceps
    S. esophageal scissors
    S. locator
    S. original magnet
    S. Tip bipolar lead
    S. Tip Rx pacing lead
sweetened pacifier
sweetheart retractor
Swenson
    S. papillotome
    S. wire-guided
    papillotome/sphincterotome
Swets goniotomy knife cannula
Swift
    S. dynamic anterior cervical plate
    S. dynamic anterior cervical plate system
swift-cut phaco incision knife
SwimEx
    S. aquatic therapy BodyCushion
    S. hydrotherapy system
    S. pool
swimmer's goggles
swing
    Vestibulator II roll s.

S

SwingAlong walker caddy
Swinger car bed
Swiss
    S. Balance orthotic
    S. ball
    S. blade
    S. Lithoclast lithotriptor
    S. Lithoclast Master device
    S. Lithoclast pneumatic lithotripsy
      probe
    S. OrthoClast
    S. pack
    S. Precision cannula system
    S. silk suture
    S. Therapy eye mask
SwissBlade
    S. diamond surgical knife
    S. disposable surgical knife
SwissPlus 1-stage implant
Swissray scanner
switch
    s. box
    internal reed s.
    optical s.
    Prescott wireless foot s.
switchable coil
switching stick
swivel
    s. adapter
    s. clamp
    s. knife
    Universal s.
    s. utensil
    s. walker
swivel-arm system
Swivel-Strap
    Aircast S.-S.
    S.-S. ankle brace
    S.-S. ankle stirrup
sword knife
Swyrls swim mold
Syed
    S. template
    S. template implant
Syed-Neblett
    S.-N. dedicated vulvar plastic
      template
    S.-N. implant
    S.-N. template
Syed-Puthawala-Hedger esophageal
    applicator
Sykes Endobrowlift instrument set
Sylva I&A unit
Symbia
    S. TruePoint SPECT-CT
    S. TruePoint SPECT-CT scanner
Symbicort Turbuhaler
Symbion
    S. cardiac device

    S. Jarvik-7 artificial heart
    S. J-7 70-mL ventricle total
      artificial heart
    S. pneumatic assist device
    S. total artificial heart
Symbios 7006 pacemaker
Symbiot covered stent
symblepharon ring
Syme
    S. amputation prosthesis
    S. Dycor prosthetic foot
    S. foot prosthesis
Symes
    Springlite super low profile S. II
symmetrical
    s. sacral plate
    s. thoracic vertebral plate
Symmetry
    S. angioplasty balloon
    S. bypass system aortic connector
    S. endobipolar generator
sympathectomy hook
Symphonix
    S. Vibrant Soundbridge
    S. Vibrant Soundbridge hearing
      device
Symphony
    S. graft delivery system
    S. I/C graft chamber
    Magnetom S.
    S. MR imaging system
    S. MR unit
    S. nitinol self-expandable stent
    S. nitinol stent
    S. patient monitoring system
    S. platelet concentrate system
    S. self-expanding stent
Syms tractor
Synaptic 2000 pain management system
Synchro
    S. microfabricated nitinol guidewire
    S. neurovascular guidewire
SynchroMed
    S. implantable pump
    S. infusion system
    S. infusion system intraspinal
      catheter
    S. programmable pump
Synchron
    S. CX9 ALX clinical system
    S. CX clinical chemistry system
    S. CX-5, CX-7 automated analyzer
    S. CX4, CX5, CX9, CX500,
      CX1000 PRO clinical system
    S. CX3, CX4, CX5 Delta clinical
      system
    S. CX4, CX5, CX7 Super clinical
      system
    S. LX clinical chemistry system

S. LX20 clinical system
S. LX4201 clinical system
S. LXi 725 clinical system
S. LX20, LX2000 PRO clinical system
S. LX20 pro chemical analyzer

synchronizer
CardioSync cardiac s.

synchronous mode pacemaker

Synchrony
S. Dual Optic Accommodating IOL
S. II, III DDDR pulse generator

SynchroSonic
S. stimulator
S. ultrasound/stimulator

syndesmotic screw

synechia spatula

synechotome

Synectics
S. 6000 digital pH-meter meter
S. PC Polygraf 16HR
S. visceral stimulator electronic barostat

Synectics-Dantec
S.-D. Flo-Lab II uroflowmeter
S.-D. uroflowmeter

Synergetics
S. Awh serrated pick
S. DDMS
S. directional laser probe
S. endo illuminator

synergistic
S. suspension strap
s. wrist motion splint

Synergist vacuum erection device

SynerGraft
S. implant
S. pulmonary heart valve
S. tissue-engineered heart valve

synergy
Esteem s.
S. flexible splinting material
S. hinge system
S. neurostimulation system
S. Plus
S. posterior titanium spinal system
S. spine rehab system
S. splint
S. ultrasound
S. ultrasound system
S. Versitrel neurostimulator

Synergyst
S. DDD pacemaker
S. II pacemaker

Synevac vacuum curettage system

synoptoscope

Synovator arthroscopic blade

synovectomy
s. blade
s. rongeur

synovial
s. dissector
s. separator

synovium biopsy forceps

Synox fractal pacemaker lead

Syntel latex-free embolectomy catheter

Synthaderm foam

Synthes
S. AO reconstruction plate
S. CerviFix system
S. compression hip screw
S. dorsal distal radius plate
S. drill
S. facial curette
S. fixation system
S. guide pin
S. ligament washer
S. maxillofacial locking reconstruction plate
S. maxillofacial titanium plate
S. Microsystems drill bit
S. Microsystems plate cutter
S. Microsystems plate-holding forceps
S. Microsystems pliers
S. mini-depth gauge
S. mini L-plate
S. Schuhli implant system
S. stainless steel minifragment plate
S. titanium elastic nail
S. titanium mesh screen
S. titanium minifragment plate
S. transbuccal trocar
S. Universal spinal system
S. universal spinal system

synthesizer
deoxyribonucleic acid s.

synthetic
s. absorbable suture
s. bone implant
s. bone substitute
s. cancellous bone void filler
s. 5-channel water-perfused motility catheter
s. cortical bone void filler
s. hygroscopic cervical dilator
s. implant
s. intervertebral disc
s. mesh
s. sapphire tip
s. stent
s. zipper

Synthetics dual-channel solid-state Digitrapper

Synthofil suture

Syracuse anterior I-plate
Syrex syringe
Syrijet Mark II needleless injector
syringe
Accuguide s.
anaerobic Pulsator s.
Anel s.
Arnold-Bruening s.
Arrow Raulerson s.
Arrow Raulerson introducer s.
Asepto bulb s.
aspirating s.
Auto S.
Autoblock safety s.
bulb s.
bulbous-tip ear s.
Canyons irrigation s.
s. cap
Carpuject s.
Centrix-type s.
C-R s.
D s.
Davidson s.
DeVilbiss s.
ear s.
electric s.
E-Z s.
Fink-Weinstein 2-way s.
Fluorescite s.
FNA-21 s.
Fortuna s.
Fuchs retinal detachment s.
Fuchs 2-way s.
Fuchs 2-way eye s.
Gabriel s.
Gas-Lyte ABG s.
G-C s.
Gemini s.
GlideCath s.
glycerine s.
Goldstein anterior chamber s.
Goldstein lacrimal s.
Hamilton s.
impression material s.
intraligamentary s.
Irrivac s.
Isovue prefilled s.
Isovue-370 prefilled s.
laryngeal s.
LeVeen inflation s.
Lewy s.
Ligmajet s.
Luer s.
Luer-Lok s.
Luer-Lok B-D s.
Luer-type s.
Lyo-Ject s.
Max-I-Probe endodontic irrigation s.
Namic angiographic s.

Neisser s.
Omnican Piston s.
Osciflator balloon inflation s.
PDL intraligamentary s.
PermaRidge delivery s.
Pitkin s.
Politzer air s.
Pomeroy ear s.
Pulsator s.
Pulsator anaerobic s.
s. pump
Raulerson introducer s.
retinal detachment s.
Roughton-Scholander s.
SofDraw safety s.
spring-assisted s.
Storz s.
super s.
Syrex s.
tapered-tip ear s.
Terumo s.
Terumo insulin s.
tonsillar s.
Toomey s.
tuberculin s.
Tubex metal s.
Ultraject contrast medium s.
Ultraject prefilled s.
VanishPoint s.
Vibraject injection s.
VisionBlue s.
Visitec s.
2-way s.
Wolff s.
Yale Luer-Lok s.
syringe-driven system
syringe-type infusion pump
syrinx shunt
Sysmex
S. CA-6000 coagulation instrument
S. HS-330 robotic hematology system
S. NE-8000 CBC analyzer
S. NE8000 cell counter
S. R-1000 reticulocyte counter
S. SE-9500 machine
S. XE-2100 hematology analyzer
S. XT-2000i automated hematology analyzer
SysStim
S. muscle stimulator
S. 226 muscle stimulator
Systec-like system
System-1
Topographic Modeling S.-1
System-2
Topographic Modeling S.-2
system
Aastrom Replicell S.

ABaer infant hearing screening s.
ABBI s.
Abbott LifeCare PCA Plus II
 infusion s.
Abbott Lifeshield needleless s.
ABC anterior cervical plating s.
ABC cervical plating s.
ABG cement-free hip s.
ABI model 373, 377 sequencing
 gel s.
Abiomed biventricular support s.
ABI vest airway clearance s.
ABL 625 s.
Ablatherm HIFU s.
ABL520 blood gas measurement s.
AbMap electrophysiologic
 imaging s.
above-knee suction enhancement s.
Absolute biliary self-expanding
 stent s.
Accents s.
Access 2 immunoassay s.
Access MV s.
Acclaim total elbow s.
Accu-Chek Advantage non-wipe
 blood glucose monitoring s.
Accu-Chek Complete blood glucose
 monitoring s.
Accu-Chek Complete glucose
 meter s.
Accu-Chek InstantPlus s.
Accu-Cut osteotomy guide s.
accuDEXA bone mineral density
 assessment s.
Accugraft ALIF allograft s.
AccuMeter cholesterol test s.
Accunet embolic protection s.
AccuProbe s.
Accurus vitreoretinal surgical s.
AccuSway balance measurement s.
Ace self-drilling bone screw s.
acetabular prosthesis s.
Ace titanium large fragment s.
Ace TK2 hip screw s.
Achieve off-pump s.
Acist contrast delivery injection s.
ACIT s.
Acra-clip s.
Acragun s.
AcroMed VSP fixation s.
Acryl-X orthopaedic cement
 removal s.
ACS Concorde over-the-wire
 catheter s.
ACS Multi-Link coronary s.
ACS Multi-Link RX Ultra
 coronary stent s.
ACS 180 SE automated
 chemiluminescent immunoassay s.

Action traction s.
Activa Parkinson control s.
Activa tremor control s.
Active Can defibrillator lead s.
Active Life Flushaway 1-piece
 flushable closed-end pouch s.
Act MicroCoil delivery s.
Acucair continuous airflow s.
Acufex microsurgical rear-entry to
 front-entry femoral guide s.
AcuFix anterior cervical plate s.
AcuMatch integrated hip s.
Acumed great toe s.
Acuson cardiovascular s.
Acuson imaging s.
Acuson XP-128
 echocardiographic s.
Acuson 128XP ultrasound s.
Acustar I neurosurgical
 localization s.
Acustar surgical navigation s.
Acutrak bone fixation s.
Acutrak fusion s.
Acutrak screw s.
Acutrak small bone fixation s.
Add-On Bucky digital x-ray image
 acquisition s.
Add-On Bucky image acquisition s.
Adeza TLi fetal fibronectin
 analysis s.
adhesive s.
Adjustaback wheelchair backrest s.
Adolph Gasser camera s.
ADS PLIF broach s.
Advanced Cardiovascular S. (ACS)
advanced visual instrument s.
Advance PS total knee s.
Advantim revision knee s.
Advantim total knee s.
Advantx digital s.
Advantx-E Legacy s.
Advantx LC+ cardiovascular
 imaging s.
Advantx LC/LP cardiac biplane s.
Advia 120 hematology s.
Aegis ICD s.
Aegis sonography management s.
Aequalis s.
AeroNOx nitric oxide transport s.
Aeroset clinical chemistry s.
AeroView optical intubation s.
AERx diabetes management s.
AERx pain management s.
AERx pulmonary drug delivery s.
Aesculap ABC cervical plating s.
Aesculap-Meditec MEL60 s.
Aesop Hermes-Ready s.
Affinity anterior cervical cage s.

S

system *(continued)*

Affirm VP microbial
identification s.
Affymetrix GeneChip s.
AGC Biomet total knee s.
AGC knee replacement s.
Agee carpal tunnel release s.
Agee WristJack fracture
reduction s.
Agfa ADC 70 storage phosphor s.
Agfa CR, PACS s.
Agility total ankle s.
AI 5200 diagnostic ultrasound s.
AIM femoral nail s.
Air-Back spinal s.
Aircast knee s.
AirFlo alternating pressure s.
Airis II MRI s.
AirSep OxiScan oximetry recording,
reporting, and archiving s.
Airtrac ambulatory cervical/lumbar
traction s.
AI 5200 S Open Color Doppler
imaging s.
AI 5200 S open color Doppler
imaging s.
Aladdin infant flow s.
Aladdin nasal CPAP s.
AlaSTAT allergy immunoassay s.
Albert Grass Heritage digital
EEG s.
Albert Grass Heritage digital
PSG s.
Albert Grass Heritage EEG s.
Albert Grass neurodata s.
Alcon Closure S. (ACS)
Alcon EyeMap EH-290 corneal
topography s.
Alcon Infiniti s.
AlereNet s.
Alexa 1000 s.
Alexa 1000 breast diagnostic s.
AlgoMed infusion s.
Alice4 sleep diagnostic s.
alimentary s.
All Access laser s.
Allegretto Wave excimer laser s.
Allen shoulder/wrist arthroscopy
traction s.
Allen traction s.
Alliance integrated inflation s.
Alliance rehabilitation s.
Alloclassic hip s.
Allofit acetabular cup s.
AlloMune s.
Allo-Pro hip s.
Aloka color Doppler s.
Aloka SD ultrasound s.
Aloka SSD ultrasound s.

Alpha Dx point-of-need test s.
Alphatec mini lag-screw s.
Alphatec small fragment s.
Alta modular trauma s.
ALT ultrasound s.
Alveolus stent technology s.
Ambi compression hip screw s.
ambulatory measurement s.
American Medical S.'s (AMS)
Amersham International ECL gene
detection s.
A2 MicroArray s.
AMK fixed bearing knee s.
AMK total knee s.
AMO Prestige advanced cataract
extraction s.
AMO Prestige phaco s.
AMO Sovereign compact
WhiteStar s.
Amplatz anchor s.
Amplatz TractMaster s.
Amset anterior locking plate s.
Amset R-F fixation s.
AMS ProstaJect ethanol injection s.
Anaconda device and delivery s.
Analyze s.
anatomic medullary locking hip s.
Anchorlok soft tissue suture
anchor s.
Anchron biodegradable anchor s.
ANCOR imaging s.
Ancure s.
Ancure endograft s.
AneuRx bifurcated stent-graft s.
AneuRx IDS delivery s.
AneuRx stent graft s.
AngeCool RF catheter ablation s.
Anger gamma camera s.
Angioflow meter s.
AngioJet rapid thrombectomy s.
AngioJet rheolytic thrombectomy s.
Angiomat 3000, 6000 contrast
delivery s.
Angiomat Illumena contrast
delivery s.
Angiomat Illumena injector s.
AngioRad afterloader s.
AngioRad radiation s.
Angio-Seal s.
Angio-Seal hemostasis s.
AngioSURF s.
AnkleTough ankle rehabilitation s.
AnnuloFlo annuloplasty ring s.
Anspach 65K instrument s.
Anspach 65K Universal
instrument s.
Answer hip s.
anterior cervical plate s.

anterior cervical plate fixation s. (ACFS)
anterior eye segment analysis s.
anterior locking plate s. (ALPS)
anterior vented gas forced fusion s.
AO/ASIF titanium craniofacial s.
AO mandibular s.
Aortic Connector s.
Apex Modular femoral stem s.
Apogee CX100, CX200 echocardiography s.
Apogee RX400 diagnostic ultrasound s.
Apogee 800 ultrasound s.
Apogee vaginal vault prolapse repair s.
Apollo DXA bone densitometry s.
Apollo 95E tooth-whitening and curing s.
Apollo hip s.
Apollo knee prosthesis s.
Apollo Light S.'s
Apollo total knee s.
Aqua-Cel heating pad s.
Aquaciser hydrodynamic measurement s.
Aquaciser 100R underwater treadmill s.
AquaLase cataract removal s.
Aquanex hydrodynamic measurement s.
AquaSens FMS 1000 fluid monitoring s.
Aqua Spray wet nail débridement s.
arc guidance s.
archival s.
Arcitumomab diagnostic imaging s.
arc-quadrant stereotactic s.
Arctic Sun temperature management s.
ArF excimer laser s.
Argyle-Turkel safety thoracentesis s.
Aria CPAP s.
Aria LX CPAP s.
Ariel computerized exercise s.
Arndorfer capillary perfusion s.
Arndorfer pneumohydraulic capillary infusion s.
Arnett-TMP s.
Array 360, 360CE/CE-AL protein/drug/serology s.
arrhythmia mapping s.
Arrow UserGard injection cap s.
arterial port catheter s.
Arthrex instruments and s.'s
Arthrex TransFix ACL reconstruction s.

ArthroCare arthroscopic s.
ArthroCare Coblation-based cosmetic surgery s.
ArthroCare multielectrode s.
Arthro-Flo arthroscopic irrigation s.
Arthro-Flo powered irrigation s.
ArthroProbe laser s.
ArthroSew suturing s.
Artisan cement s.
Artoscan MRI s.
Arx ceramic spinal spacer s.
Asap biopsy s.
Asap Stacker automated multisample biopsy s.
Ascensia Breeze blood glucose monitoring s.
Ascensia DEX2 diabetes care s.
Ascensia Elite blood glucose monitoring s.
Ascensia Elite XL diabetes care s.
Ascent total knee s.
Asnis 3 cannulated screw s.
Asnis 2 guided-screw s.
Aspen digital ultrasound s.
Aspen echocardiography s.
Aspen ultrasound s.
AspenVac smoke evacuation s.
Aspire continuous imaging s.
aSpire controlled release delivery s.
Assistant Free self-retaining hip surgery retractor s.
Assure blood glucose monitoring s.
Aston cartilage reduction s.
Astra Tech dental implant s.
Astro-Med Albert Grass Heritage digital EEG s.
Atakr s.
Atavi atraumatic spine fusion s.
Atavi atraumatic spine surgery s.
Atavi TiTLE rod fixation s.
Atec TriMark marker s.
Athena high frequency mammography s.
Atlantis anterior cervical plate s.
Atlantis cervical plate s.
Atlantis Vision anterior cervical plate s.
Atlas cable s.
Atlas 2.0 diagnostic ultrasound s.
AtLast blood glucose monitoring s.
ATL HDI 3000, 3500, 4000, 5000 ultrasound s.
ATL UltraMark 9 ultrasound s.
ATL ultrasound s.
A-Trac atraumatic clamping s.
atrial septal defect occlusion s.
atrial septum defect occluder s.
Atridox drug delivery s.
Atrigel drug delivery s.

S

system *(continued)*

Atrioverter s.
Atrium blood recovery s.
ATS 500/1500 tourniquet s.
AuRA cemented total hip s.
Aura Laser s.
Aurora dedicated breast MRI s.
Aurora diode-based dental laser s.
Aurora MR breast imaging s.
AutoCapture pacing s.
AutoCyte Image Analysis s.
AutoCyte Prep s.
autofluorescent endsocopic s.
autoLog autotransfusion s.
autologous blood management s.
automated angle encoder s.
automated cellular imaging s.
Automated Quantification of After-Cataract automated analysis s.
automatic positioning s.
AutoPap 300 QC s.
AutoPulse resuscitation s.
Autoread centrifuge hematology s.
AutoSet Portable II CPAP s.
Auto Suture ABBI s.
Autotrans s.
autotransfusion s.
Autovac autotransfusion s.
Autovac LF autotransfusion s.
Autovac TC orthopaedic autotransfusion s.
Avera breast imaging s.
avidin-biotin complex immunodetection s.
Avi lens s.
A-V Impulse s.
Aviva mammography s.
AVS spinal s.
Axcis percutaneous myocardial revascularization s.
Axcis PMR s.
Axiom modular knee s.
Axiom total knee s.
Axis 360-degree stabilization s.
Axis fixation s.
AxyaWeld bone anchor s.
AxyaWeld J-tip suture welding s.
BABE OB ultrasound reporting s.
BacFix s.
Back Bull lumbar support s.
Back Revolution S.
Back Trainer spinal exercise s.
BacT/Alert automated blood culture s.
BacT/Alert automated microbial detection s.
BacT/Alert microbial detection s.
Bactec automated blood culture s.
Bactec blood culture s.

Bactec blood culturing s.
Bactec 9000 MB s.
Bactiseal antimicrobial-impregnated catheter s.
Badal stimulus s.
Bad Wildungen Metz spine s.
Baha s.
Bair Hugger patient warming s.
BakVista radiolucent interbody fusion s.
BAK/C interbody fusion s.
BAK interbody fusion s.
BAK-1 interbody fusion s.
BAK/T thoracic interbody fusion s.
Balanced Knee s.
Balance Master-training and assessment s.
Balance Master training and assessment s.
Balloon-on-a-Wire dilatation s.
BAPS ankle s.
Bard CPS s.
Bard EndoCinch endoscopic suturing s.
Bard flexible endoscopic injection s.
Bard percutaneous cardiopulmonary support s.
Bard rotary atherectomy s. (BRAS)
Bard Urolase fiber laser s.
basolateral membrane transport s.
Bateman UPF II bipolar knee s.
Batson vertebral brain s.
Baxter Interline IV s.
Bayer AG II chemistry analyzer s.
Baylor autologous transfusion s.
BClear s.
BD BBL CultureSwab Plus collection and transport s.
BD Beaver safety knife s.
BD Phoenix automated microbiology s.
BD ProbeTec ET s.
Beamer injection stent s.
Beaver clear cornea incision s.
Becker orthopaedic spinal s. (BOSS)
Becker orthopaedic thermoformablc ankle s.
Becker-Rojas Sub-Sonic surgical s.
Becker vibrating cannula s.
Beckman ICS Nephelometer s.
Bedbugg sleep apnea s.
bedside sterile drainage collection s.
Benephit CV infusion s.
Benephit HF infusion s.
Benephit PV infusion s.
Bennett contour mammography s.

Bentley autotransfusion s.
Benzaquen-Chajchir
  extraction/reinjection s.
BeStent Rival coronary stent s.
BeStent 2 with Discrete
  Technology coronary stent s.
Beta-Cath s.
Betaseron needle-free delivery s.
Bevalac s.
BIAcore s.
Biad SPECT imaging s.
Biax total wrist s.
BIB s.
Bident electrosurgical s.
Bigliani/Flatow shoulder s.
bilateral variable screw
  placement s.
BiliBed phototherapy s.
BiliBlanket Plus phototherapy s.
BiliCheck battery-powered s.
bioartificial liver support s.
BioBarrier membrane-guided tissue
  regeneration s.
Biodex S.
Biodex Balance s.
Biodex Unweighing Support S.
BioDIMENSIONAL s.
BioDisc spinal disc repair s.
Bio-Esthetic abutment s.
Bio-Fit total hip s.
Bio Flote air flotation s.
Biogel Reveal puncture
  indication s.
biograph molecular imaging s.
Bio-Groove HA hip s.
Biojector 2000 needle-free injection
  management s.
Bio-1000 knee brace s.
Biolase TwiLite laser s.
BioLogic-DT s.
BioLogic-DTPF s.
BioLogic-HT s.
biomechanical ankle platform s.
BioMerieux Vitek s.
Biomet Ascent total knee s.
Biomet Finn salvage/oncology knee
  reconstruction s.
Biomet Genus uni knee s.
Biomet M2A metal-on-metal
  articulation for hip replacement s.
Biomet Maxim knee s.
Biomet Maxim total knee s.
Biomet revision knee s.
Biomet Ultra-Drive ultrasonic
  revision s.
BIOM noncontact panoramic
  viewing s.
BIOM noncontact wide-angle
  viewing s.

Bio-Modular total shoulder s.
Bionicare 1000 stimulator s.
Bio-Optics Bambi cell analysis s.
Bio-Optics Bambi image analysis s.
Bioplate screw fixation s.
bioptic amorphic lens s.
Bio-Rad Model 5000 titanium s.
bioresorbable drug delivery s.
Biosense NOGA catheter-based
  endocardial mapping s.
Biosound AU3, AU4, AU5 s.
Biosound Genesis II scanning s.
BioSpec MR imaging s.
BioStinger fixation s.
biotelemetry s.
BioZ s.
BioZ hemodynamic monitoring s.
BioZ noninvasive cardiac function
  monitoring s.
BioZ.pc s.
BiPAP Duet LX CPAP s.
BiPAP S/T-D 30 s.
BiPAP S/T-D ventilatory support s.
BiPAP Vision s.
biphasic s.
biplane s.
biplane image intensifier s.
Birmingham Hip resurfacing s.
Bispectral Index S.
Bitome bipolar s.
BKS refractive s.
Blade-Vent implant s.
BMP cabling and plating s.
body logic rehabilitation s.
Body Masters MD 510 hi-lo
  pulley s.
Body Response s.
Boehringer Autovac
  autotransfusion s.
Bolin wedge filter s.
bone staple s.
bone tack s.
Bonopty needle s.
Bookwalter retractor s.
Bosker TMI reconstruction s.
Boston brace s.
Boston elbow s.
2-bottle thoracic drainage s.
Bottoms-Up posture s.
Bracco s.
BrachyVision brachytherapy
  planning s.
Brackmann II EMG s.
BrainLAB VectorVision
  neuronavigation s.
BrainSCAN computer planning s.
Brånemark implant s.
Bravo Catheter-Free pH testing s.
Breast Cancer S. 2100

system (continued)
BreastScan IR s.
Breeze E150 ventilation s.
Bremer halo s.
Bremer halo crown s.
Bridge Assurant biliary stent delivery s.
Bridge extra-support over-the-wire renal stent s.
Bridge Hip s.
Bridge X3 renal stent s.
Bristol-Myers s.
BriteSmile laser tooth-whitening s.
Broselow-Hinkle pediatric emergency s.
Broselow-Luten pediatric s.
Browlift bone bridge s.
Brown-Roberts-Wells stereotactic s.
Bruker Biospec s.
Bruker CSI Omega MR s.
Bruker S 200 MR s.
BRW stereotactic s.
Bryan cervical disc s.
BTA S-2000 biofeedback s.
Budde halo retractor s.
Buechel-Pappas integrated hip replacement s.
Buechel-Pappas total ankle replacement s.
Burette multiple patient delivery s.
BVS-5000 biventricular support s.
BWM spine s.
Bx Velocity stent with Raptor OTW delivery s.
Bx Velocity with Hepacoat on Raptor stent s.
CAAS QCA s.
Cable-Ready cable grip s.
CADD-Prizm pain control s.
CADD-TPN ambulatory infusion s.
Cadence tiered therapy defibrillator s.
CADx SecondLook s.
Calandruccio external fixation s.
Calasept medicament delivery s.
Calcitek implant s.
Caldwell needle/cannula Quick-Tap paracentesis s.
Calvitron hair replacement s.
6-camera Vicon motion capture s.
Camino intracranial pressure monitoring s.
Canal Finder s.
candela videoimaging s.
Cannulated Plus screw s.
Can-Opt dual-lumen ERCP s.
Capasee diagnostic ultrasound s.
Capless polyaxial pedicle screw s.
CapnoProbe sublingual CO_2 s.

Caps-Lock shoulder cannula s.
capsule applier s.
carbon dioxide laser scanner s.
cardiac conduction s.
CardiArc cardiac SPECT s.
Cardica PAS-Port s.
Cardioblate BP, RF surgical ablation s.
Cardioblate surgical ablation s.
CardioCamera imaging s.
CardioGenesis PMR s.
CardioGenesis TMR s.
CardioLab 2000 single monitor EP s.
cardiopulmonary support s.
cardioscope U s.
CardioSEAL septal occlusion s.
CardioTek electrophysiologic tracer s.
Cardiovascular Angiography Analysis S.
Cardiovit AT-10 ECG/spirometry combination s.
C-arm DSA s.
Carolon multi-layer stocking s.
Carpuject syringe s.
Carter-Thomason CloseSure S.
cartesian reference coordinate s.
Carto EP navigation s.
Cascade Up and About s.
CASE computerized exercise ECG s.
Case 16 exercise s.
CASS whole-brain mapping s.
Catarex cataract removal s.
Cathcor LX hemodynamic recording s.
catheter-tip micromanometer s.
Cath-Finder catheter tracking s.
CathScanner ultrasound imaging s.
CathTrack catheter locator s.
CatsEye digital camera s.
Cavi-Endo ultrasonic s.
Cavitron irrigation/aspiration s.
Cavitron-Kelman irrigation/aspiration s.
Cavitron ultrasonic s.
CB MercuRay maxillofacial imaging s.
CD Horizon Eclipse spinal s.
CD Horizon Legacy spinal s.
CD Horizon Sextant s.
CD Horizon Sextant percutaneous screw-rod s.
CDI 2000 blood gas monitoring s.
CDO s.
CDRPan digital x-ray s.
Ceegraph 128 EEG s.
Celay s.

cell analysis s.
CellFIT acquisition s.
CellPrep sample preparation s.
Cell Recovery S.
Cell Saver autologous blood
   recovery s.
Cell Saver Haemonetics
   autotransfusion s.
Cell Saver Haemonetics
   Autotransfusion s.
Cell Soft s.
Cellvizio-GI endoscopic imaging s.
Celsius Control intravascular
   cooling catheter s.
Cemax/Icon PACS s.
Cemex s.
Cencit imaging s.
Cenflex central monitoring s.
CenSlide 2000 urinalysis s.
Centauri Er:YAG dental laser s.
CenterPointLock 2-piece ostomy s.
central DXA bone densitometry s.
Centrax bipolar s.
Centrica rotational core biopsy s.
Ceprate SC stem cell
   concentration s.
CEQ 8000, 8800 genetic
   analysis s.
Ceralas PDT 633 diode laser s.
CeraOne implant s.
CerviFix s.
Cervive anterior cervical plating s.
CFC BioScanner s.
CGR biplane angiographic s.
ChamberLift 2000 patient lift s.
Champion stent s.
Champy miniplate rigid fixation s.
chandelier illumination s.
2-channel Badal optical s.
2-channel phased-array RF receiver
   coil s.
Charité artificial disc s.
Charnley-Howorth Exflow s.
Chattanooga Balance s.
Checkmate s.
Checkmate gamma brachytherapy s.
Checkmate gamma radiation s.
ChemoBloc vial venting s.
Chemo-Port vascular access s.
CHEMXpress s.
CHI s.
Chilli cooled ablation s.
C-2 hip s.
Chirotech x-ray s.
chirped-pulse amplification s.
Christensen TMJ prosthesis s.
Chromos imager s.
ChromoVision video s.
Ciba TearSaver punctal gauging s.

Cinch bladder neck suspension
   anchor s.
Cineloop image review
   ultrasound s.
CineView Plus Freeland s.
CipherGen Express software
   biomarker analysis s.
CircPlus bandage/wrap s.
Circulaire aerosol drug delivery s.
Circul'Air shoe process s.
Circulator boot s.
CKS knee s.
Clarion CII Bionic Ear s.
Clarion cochlear implant s.
Clarity multiparameter monitoring s.
Clark hemoperfusion s.
CLAVE needleless s.
Clave needleless s.
ClearChart digital acuity s.
CLeaRS cardiac lead removal s.
Clinac 600SR stereotactic radiation
   treatment s.
Clinical HandMaster s.
Clini-Care low-air-loss s.
Clini.Float flotation therapy bed s.
closed-circuit television vision
   enhancement s.
closed-loop s.
closed-loop infrared video
   tracking s.
CloseSure S.
CLS hip s.
CMA 600 neuromonitoring s.
CMI vacuum delivery s.
CMS AccuProbe 450 s.
CMSI warming s.
CoaguChek aPTT testing s.
CoaguChek Pro/DM s.
Cobe 2991 computerized
   centrifuge s.
Cobe Spectra apheresis s.
Coblation-based spinal surgery s.
Coblation spinal surgery s.
Coblator II surgery s.
Coburn irrigation/aspiration s.
Codman ACP s.
Codman anterior cervical plating s.
Codman Bactiseal antimicrobial
   impregnated catheter s.
Codman neurological headrest s.
Codman Ti-frame posterior
   fixation s.
COER-24 delivery s.
Cofield 2 total shoulder s.
Cohort anterior plate s.
Co₂ject s.
Coleman microinfiltration s.
CollectFirst s.
ColonoSight s.

system *(continued)*

Colorado 2 spinal s.
ColorZone Management s.
Colour-Quad-System imaging s.
Coltene direct inlay s.
Coltene inlay s.
Combi 40+ cochlear implant s.
Combiline S.
combined magnetic field s.
Comfort Care bed s.
Comfort Cast casting s.
ComfortScan s.
ComfortWalk foot s.
Command hip instrumentation s.
Command joint replacement
  instrument s.
compact plating s. (CPS)
CompAire Elite compressor
  nebulizer s.
Companion 314, 318 nasal
  CPAP s.
Compass arc-quadrant stereotactic s.
Compass frame-based stereotactic s.
Compass stereotactic s.
Complement C31 desArg Biotrack
  RIA s.
Complete Ophthalmic Analysis S.
complete pacemaker patient
  testing s.
compliant prestress s.
Compton suppression s.
Compumedics P-series sleep
  monitoring s.
Computed Anatomy Corneal
  Modeling S.
computer-assisted neurosurgical
  navigational s.
computer-controlled neurological
  stimulation s.
computerized bedside transfusion
  identification s.
computerized image analysis s.
computerized morphometric s.
computerized sleep analysis s.
computer navigation s.
Concentrix dual aspiration pump s.
Conceptus fallopian tube
  catheterization s.
Concise compression hip screw s.
Concorde implant and implement s.
condom catheter collecting s.
Conforma 3000 proton beam
  treatment s.
ConQuest incontinence s.
Conserve hip s.
ConstaVac autoreinfusion s.
Contact SPH cups s.
contact-tip laser s.
Contak CD CRTD Easytrak s.

Contak Renewal 3 CRTD s.
ContiCath catheter s.
continuous insulin delivery s.
  (CIDS)
continuous-wave high-frequency
  Doppler ultrasound s.
continuous-wave laser s.
Continuum knee s.
Contour Genesis UAL s.
Contour Genesis ultrasonic-assisted
  lipoplasty s.
Contour Meniscus Arrow
  bioresorbable repair s.
Contour spine s.
Contour tilting compression
  mammography s.
Contrajet ERCP contrast delivery s.
Control cable and wire s.
Converge porous acetabular s.
Convertible trocar s.
CoolGlide aesthetic laser s.
Cool-tip RF s.
CoolTouch 1320nm laser s.
Coombs bone biopsy s.
Coonrad/Morrey total elbow s.
Coordinate complete revision
  knee s.
CO_2 powered gun s.
Corail hip s.
Cordis endovascular s.
Cordis LC multipurpose stent s.
Cordis Mini stent s.
Core-Vent implant s.
Corin hip arthroplasty s.
Corkscrew rotator cuff repair s.
corneal topography s. (CTS)
CorneaSparing LTK s.
Corometrics Medical Systems Inc.
  fetal monitoring s.
coronary angiography analysis s.
Coroskop Plus cardiac
  angiography s.
CorRestore s.
Cosgrove-Edwards annuloplasty s.
Cosman ICP Tele-Sensor s.
Cosman-Roberts-Wells stereotactic s.
COSTART s.
Cotrcl-Dubousset s.
Cotrel-Dubousset distraction s.
Cotrel-Dubousset screw-rod s.
Coulter reticONE s.
CoumaCare Coumadin
  management s.
CozMore insulin technology s.
CPD Commander combined
  air/fluid exchange and silicone oil
  delivery s.
CPS s.
CPT hip s.

Cragg Endopro s.
cranial osteosynthesis s.
cranial plating s.
craniomaxillofacial plating s.
CritiCore monitoring s.
CRM s.
Crock-Yamagishi s.
Crosslink plate spinal s.
Crossover cross-connector s.
Crown mattress s.
CRS tibial torsion s.
CRW stereotactic s.
Cryocare cardiac surgical s.
Cryocare cryoablation s.
CryoCor cryoablation s.
Cryo/Cuff knee compression
dressing s.
CryoGuide ultrasound guidance s.
CryoHit tumor ablation s.
Cryomedical Sciences AccuProbe
450 s.
Cryomedics electrosurgery s.
CryoSeal fibrin sealant s.
CryoSeal FS s.
Cryo-Surg cryosurgical s.
cryotherapy s.
Cryo-Vac-A cryostat vacuum s.
CrystalEyes endoscopic video s.
CS-5 cryosurgical s.
CSM Stretta s.
CTDx electrostimulation s.
C-Tek anterior cervical plate s.
C-Trak surgical guidance s.
Curix Capacity Plus film
processing s.
CurvTek s.
CUSA CEM s.
Cusp-Lok cuspid traction s.
CustomCornea wavefront s.
CustomCornea wavefront
measurement s.
C-Vest radiation detector s.
CVIS information s.
CyberKnife planning s.
CyberKnife robotic radiosurgery s.
CyberKnife SRS image-guided
stereotactic radiosurgery precision
radiotherapy s.
CyberKnife stereotactic
radiosurgery s.
CyberKnife stereotactic
radiosurgery/radiotherapy s.
Cyberware 3D scanning s.
Cybex I, II+ exercise s.
Cybex 340 isokinetic rehabilitation
and testing s.
Cybex training s.
Cygnet Laboratories fetal
monitoring s.

Cygnus PFS image-guided s.
Cytomics FC 500 series flow
cytometry s.
CytoRich cervical cytology
monolayer s.
Dako fast red substrate s.
Dall-Miles cable/crimp cerclage s.
Dall-Miles cable grip s.
Dansac irrigation s.
Dantec 12-channel Urocolor
video s.
Dantec Menuet s.
DAR breathing s.
Dascor disc arthroplasty s.
DASH s.
data-acquisition s.
data collection s.
DataHand s.
daughter endoscopic retrograde
cholangiopancreatoscopy s.
da Vinci robotic surgical s.
da Vinci surgical s.
Davol irrigation s.
DCI-S automated coronary
analysis s.
Debioclip single-dose delivery s.
dedicated mammography s.
DeepLight glaucoma treatment s.
Deknatel orthopaedic
autotransfusion s.
Delm imaging s.
Delta CTA reverse shoulder s.
Delta 32 digital stereotactic s.
DELTAmanager MedImage s.
Delta 32 TACT 3-dimensional
breast imaging s.
Deltoid-Aid arm counterbalance s.
DentiCAD s.
DentiPatch lidocaine transoral
delivery s.
Dentsleeve pneumohydraulic
perfusion s.
Dentsply implant s.
Denver hydrocephalus shunt s.
DePuy Acclaim total elbow s.
DePuy Ace TiMAX Pe.R.I. small
fragment lower extremity plate s.
DePuy Biax total wrist s.
DePuy Casting FRC s.
DePuy Control cable and wire s.
DePuy Endurance all-polyethylene
acetabular cup s.
DePuy fusion and reconstruction s.
DePuy Global FX shoulder
fracture s.
DePuy Mitek Rigidfix anterior
cruciate ligament cross-pin s.
DePuy Pinnacle acetabular cup s.

S

system *(continued)*

DePuy Preservation unicompartmental knee s.
DePuy Prodigy total hip s.
DePuy Replica total hip s.
DePuy Summit tapered hip s.
DePuy total hip s.
Derma K laser s.
Dermalase laser s.
Derma 20 laser s.
Dermaphot s.
DermMaster first macroabrasion s.
Desai VectorCath mapping s.
Desilets introducer s.
detector s.
Devex spinal s.
DFS 2 mattress replacement s.
Diab-A-Foot protection s.
Dialock hemodialysis access s.
dichroic filter s.
Difco ESP testing s.
Digi-Flex exercise s.
Digi Grip traction s.
digital Add-On Bucky image acquisition imaging s.
Digital Cardiac Imaging s.
digital chest imaging s.
digital flat-panel amorphous silicon detector-radiography s.
digital holography s.
digital mammographic s.
digital mammography s.
digital selenium-based chest imaging s.
Digital Traumex s.
Digitrace home sleep s.
Digitrapper Mark II pH monitoring s.
Digitron digital subtraction imaging s.
dilator-sheath s.
2-dimensional linear plating s.
3-dimensional plating s.
Dinamap s.
Dingman oral retraction s.
DioLite 532 laser s.
Director Guidewire s.
DirectView CR 900 imaging s.
Discovery elbow s.
Discovery II DDD pacing s.
Discovery II DR pacing s.
Discovery II SR pacing s.
Discovery II SSI pacing s.
Discovery LS imaging s.
Disposa-Shield dental barrier s.
Disten-U-Flo fluid s.
DL2000 data management s.
2D linear plating s.

DNA-Prep workstation & reagent s.
DNA sequencing s.
DOBI s.
Doc ventral cervical stabilization s.
Dodick laser photolysis s.
Dodick photolysis s.
Dogbone anterior cervical plate fixation s.
Dolphin hysteroscopic fluid management s.
Doppler Quantum color-flow s.
DORC fast freeze cryosurgical s.
DORC Hexon Illumination S.
Dornhoffer Hapex implant s.
Dornier MPL 9000 electrohydraulic lithotriptor ultrasound focusing s.
double-detector Vertex s.
DPAP interactive airway management s.
3D plating s.
Drake-Willock automatic delivery s.
Drake-Willock delivery s.
DryView laser imaging s.
DS-60 diode laser s.
DSX automated ELISA s.
DTU-one UltraSure imaging s.
dual aspiration pump s.
dual-head coincidence detection s.
dual-lock total hip replacement s.
Dual-Port s.
Dual Quattrode spinal cord stimulation s.
Dual Range Limiter S.
Duct-Occlud s.
Duet s.
Dumbach mandibular reconstruction s.
Dumon-Gilliard endoprosthesis s.
Dunlap cold compression wrap s.
Duoloid impression s.
Duovisc viscoelastic s.
Dupel drug delivery s.
DuPont distal humeral plate s.
Duracon PS total knee s.
Duraloc acetabular cup s.
Duraloc Option ceramic hip s.
Dur-A-Sil silicone impression s.
Durasul head s.
Durasul large diameter head s.
Durette s.
DxI 800 immunoassay s.
Dymer excimer delivery s.
Dyna-Care pressure pad s.
DynaFix external fixation s.
Dyna-Flex multilayer compression s.
Dynal CELLection s.

S

Dynalink biliary self-expanding stent s.
Dyna-Lok plating s.
dynamic optical breast imaging s.
Dynamite mattress s.
DynaRad portable imaging s.
DynaRad portable x-ray s.
Dynasplint shoulder s.
Dynasty delivery s.
DynaSurg I, II electric irrigation s.
Dynesys dynamic stabilization s.
Dyonics Dyosite office arthroscopy s.
Dyonics 25 fluid management s.
Dyonics InteliJet fluid management s.
Eagle portable ventilation s.
Eagle rigid anterior cervical plate s.
ears education and retraining s.
EAS-1000 anterior eye segment analysis s.
EasyGuide Neuro image-guided surgery s.
Easy Introduction s.
EasyOne spirometry s.
Easyspine pedicle screw and rod s.
EBI Array spinal s.
EBI bone healing s.
EBI Omega21 spinal fixation s.
EBI XFix DynaFix s.
E.CAM dual-head emission imaging s.
ECAT Reveal PET/CT imaging s.
Eccocee CS ultrasound s.
Eccocee ultrasound s.
Eccovision acoustic reflection imaging s.
Eccovision acoustic rhinometry s.
echocardiographic scoring s.
EchoEye 3D ultrasound imaging s.
EchoEye ultrasound imaging s.
EchoFlow blood velocity meter s.
Echovar Doppler s.
Eckardt vitrectomy s.
Eclipse infusion s.
Eclipse MR s.
Eclipse PTMR s.
Eclipse spinal s.
ECT internal fracture fixation s.
Ectra s.
EdenTrace sleep s.
EDG s.
Edwards LifeStent LP SDS biliary stent s.
Edwards LifeStent NT self-expanding biliary stent s.
Edwards LifeStent XL SDS biliary stent s.

Edwards MC^3 annuloplasty s.
Edwards modular s.
Edwards Thrombex PMT s.
e10 electrosurgery s.
Efos Lite curing s.
Eklund breast positioning s.
Elan-E electronic motor s.
ElastaTrac home lumbar traction s.
Elecsys troponin T immunoassay s.
Electra 1400C, 1800C coagulation s.
Electri-Cool cold therapy s.
electroanatomical mapping s.
electrode positioning s.
Electronic HouseCall s.
electronic patient care reporting s.
electronic PCR s.
electroshield monitoring s.
electrotherapy s.
ELISA-Light Chemiluminescent Detection s.
Elite hip s.
Ellman pressform s.
Elscint Prestige MRI s.
Embol-X arterial cannula and filter s.
Emboshield embolic protection s.
Emerald implantation s.
Emergence Profile implant s.
emergency life support s.
EMG biofeedback s.
EMI digital imaging s.
EnAbl thermal ablation s.
ENAC ultrasonic instrument s.
Encode restorative s.
Encore ceramic hip and knee joint replacement s.'s
Endermologie adipose destruction s.
Endermologie LPG s.
Endius endoscopic access s.
Endius TriFix thoracolumbar pedicle screw s.
Endobag laparoscopic specimen retrieval s.
EndoButton CL BTB fixation s.
endocavitary applicator s.
EndoCinch suturing s.
Endodirect s.
Endo-Dop transendoscopic Doppler catheter probe s.
Endo-Flo irrigation s.
Endolite transtibial s.
EndoLumina II transillumination s.
Endopore dental implant s.
Endoprothetik CSL-Plus cemented-hip s.
Endosaph vein harvest s.
endoscopic carpal tunnel release s.
EndoSheath s.

system *(continued)*
EndoSheath endoscopy s.
Endotak lead s.
Endotek urodynamics s.
Endotrac blade s.
Endotrac carpal tunnel release s.
Endotrac endoscopic carpal tunnel
 release s.
EndoVasix EPAR laser s.
Endurance all-polyethylene
 acetabular cup s.
Enfant pediatric vision testing s.
EnPulse pacing s.
EnRhythm pacing s.
EnSite 3000 s.
EnSite 3000 imaging s.
EnSite NavX intracardiac
 nonfluoroscopic navigation s.
ENTec Coblator plasma s.
ENTec surgery s.
Enterra Therapy implantable
 neurostimulation s.
Entree II trocar and cannula s.
Entree Plus trocar and cannula s.
EntriStar gastrostomy s.
Envision anterior cervical plate s.
EnVision non-avidin-biotin
 detection s.
Envoy middle ear implantable s.
Envoy totally implantable hearing
 restoration s.
EPAR laser s.
EP2000 electrophysiology
 imaging s.
Epics Altra cell sorting s.
Epics XL, XLMCL flow
 cytometer s.
EpiFLO SD transdermal sustained
 oxygen delivery s.
EpiLaser s.
EpiLaser laser-based hair
 removal s.
EpiLift epikeratome s.
EpiLight hair removal s.
EpiStar diode laser s.
EpiTouch Alex laser hair
 removal s.
EpiTouch Ruby SilkLaser hair
 removal s.
EPT-1000 XP cardiac ablation s.
Equation spinal s.
Equinox digital EEG s.
Equinox EEG neuromonitoring s.
Equinoxe shoulder s.
Equinox occlusion balloon s.
erbium:YAG laser s.
ErecAid vacuum s.
ErgoTec vitreoretinal instrument s.
ESA s.

Eska modular hip s.
ESP II s.
ESSential shaver s.
EsteLux s.
esthetic laser s.
etch s.
EUB-405 ultrasound s.
EuroPeel s.
eVent Inspiration ventilator s.
Evis 140 endoscope reprocessing s.
Evis Exera video s.
EVS vascular closure s.
ExAblate 2000 ultrasound s.
Exactech Equinoxe shoulder s.
Exactech hip s.
Exact-Fit broaching s.
Exact-Touch Saccomanno Pap
 smear collection s.
Exakt cutting/grinding s.
Excel fracture s.
Excell DXA bone densitometry s.
excimer laser s.
EX-FI-RE external fixation s.
Exogen 2000+ low-intensity
 ultrasound fracture healing s.
Exogen 2000 sonic accelerated
 fracture healing s.
Exonix ultrasonic surgical s.
Expedium anterior spine s.
Explorer common bile duct
 exploration s.
Explorer X70 intraoral
 radiography s.
Express seeding cartridge s.
Extend total hip s.
extracorporeal membrane
 oxygenation s.
EyeCap ophthalmic image
 capture s.
eyeFix speculum s.
EyeMap EH-290 corneal
 topography s.
EyeSys corneal analysis s.
EyeSys 2000 corneal topographic
 mapping s.
EyeSys surface topography s.
eye-tracking s.
EZ-EM Bio-Gun automated
 biopsy s.
E-Z Flap cranial flap fixation s.
E-Z Flap titanium miniplate s.
EZ-On traction belt s.
E-Z Tac soft-tissue reattachment s.
facet screw s.
Fanal Finder s.
FASTak suture anchor s.
Fast-Flap cranial flap fixation s.
FastGrind lens s.
FAST 1 intraosseous infusion s.

FastPack blood analyzer s.
FastTake blood glucose monitoring s.
Feather-Lite Pouching S.
FeatherTouch SilkLaser s.
fecal containment s.
feedback s.
FemoStop femoral compression s.
femtosecond laser s.
Fenlin total shoulder s.
Ferno AquaCiser underwater treadmill s.
FiberLase beam delivery s.
FiberLase flexible fiberoptic delivery s.
fiberoptic catheter delivery s.
Fillauer endoskeletal alignment s.
Fillauer modular shuttle lock s.
FilmFax teleradiology s.
FilterWire EX embolic protection s.
FiltraCheck-UTI colorimetric filtration s.
FiltraCheck-UTI disposable colorimetric bacteriuria detection s.
filtration s.
Finger Phantom pulse oximeter testing s.
Finn knee s.
Finn knee revision s.
FirstQ departure alert s.
Fischer modular stereotaxic s.
Fitnet joint testing s.
Fixateur Interne fixation s.
FlapMaker microkeratome s.
Fletcher-Suit-Delclos s.
flexible over-wire s.
Flexi-Cut directional debulking s.
Flexiflo gastrostomy tube enteral delivery s.
Flexiflo top-fill enteral nutrition s.
Flexi-Therm liquid crystal s.
Flex 4 microwave surgical ablation s.
Flex 10 microwave surgical ablation s.
F. L. Fischer modular stereotaxy s.
FL3095 fluorescence spectrometer s.
Flo-Stat fluid management s.
Flowplus therapeutic pneumatic compression s.
Flowtron DVT external pneumatic compression s.
Flowtron DVT pump s.
Flowtron Excel DVI prophylaxis s.
Flowtron pneumatic compression system BioCryo s.
FluoroNav virtual fluoroscopy s.

FluoroPlus Cardiac digital imaging s.
FluoroPlus real-time digital imaging s.
FluoroPlus Roadmapper digital fluoroscopy s.
fluoroptic thermometry s.
FluoroScan imaging s.
FluoroTrak fluoroscopy-based surgical navigation s.
flying spot excimer laser s.
F-MAT screening s.
FMP acetabular s.
Foamart foot impression s.
FoamCare cleansing s.
Focus glucose monitoring s.
Fonar Standing Ovation MRI s.
Fonix 6500-CX hearing aid test s.
Force GSU argon-enhanced electrosurgery s.
foreign body retrieval s.
Foundation total hip s.
Foundation total knee s.
Foundation total knee and hip s.
FP5000 pump s.
FPS s.
fracture computer-aided surgery s.
frame-based radiosurgical s.
frameless air support therapy s.
frameless stereotaxy s.
Frank ECG lead placement s.
Frank EKG lead placement s.
Frank XYZ orthogonal lead s.
FRC s.
Freedom leg bag collection s.
Freehand neuroprosthetic s.
Freehand prosthesis s.
Free-Lock femoral fixation s.
freestanding tissue retraction bridge s.
FreeStyle blood glucose monitoring s.
Freezor CryoAblation s.
French Pharmacovigilance s.
Fresenius volumetric dialysate balancing s.
Frialit-2 dental implant s.
F-Scan foot force and gait analysis s.
F-Scan in-shoe s.
F-Scan pressure measurement s.
Fuji AC2 storage phosphor computed radiology s.
Fujinon SP-501 sonoprobe s.
full-field digital mammography s.
fusion and reconstruction s. (FRS)
Galaxy IVUS imaging s.
Galen teleradiology s.
Galileo intravascular radiotherapy s.

S

system *(continued)*
Gambro hemofiltration s.
gamma radiation therapy s.
GaSampler collection s.
gasless laparoscopic s.
GastrographH ambulatory pH
  monitoring s.
gastrointestinal therapeutic s.
Gatekeeper reflux repair s.
GDLH posterior spinal s.
GE Advantx s.
GE 9800 CT s.
GE CT Advantage high-speed
  CT s.
GE CT HiSpeed Advantage CT s.
GE Electric Advantx s.
Gemini laser s.
Gem 21S enhanced tissue
  regeneration s.
Gem SensiCath blood gas
  monitoring s.
GemStar infusion s.
Gem total knee s.
General Electric Advantx s.
Generation 6 integrated
  radiotherapy s.
generator s.
GenESA s.
GenESA closed-loop delivery s.
Genesis II foot s.
Genesis II foot/ankle s.
Genesis II total knee s.
Genesis neurostimulation s.
Genic coronary stent delivery s.
GenomeLab SNPstream
  genotyping s.
Genotropin s.
GentleLASE Plus laser s.
GentlePeel skin exfoliation s.
Gentle Touch loop ostomy s.
Genucom ACL laxity analysis s.
Genucom knee flexion analysis s.
GERDcheck ambulatory esophageal
  pH monitoring s.
GE Senographe 2000D digital
  mammography s.
GE Signa MR s.
GE Signa MRI s.
GE single-axis SR-230
  echoplanar s.
GE Voluson 730 4D ultrasound s.
GFX 2 coronary stent s.
Gillette double-flexure ankle
  joint s.
Given diagnostic imaging s.
Given videocapsule s.
GliaSite radiation therapy s.
GliaSite radiation therapy RTS s.
GliaSite radiotherapy s.

GliaSite RTS s.
Glider II patient transfer s.
Global Fx shoulder fracture s.
Global total shoulder arthroplasty s.
Glucometer DEX diabetes care s.
Glucometer II home glucose
  monitoring s.
GlucoWatch G2 Biographer
  diabetes monitoring s.
GlyMed Camouflage s.
Goldenberg implant s.
Gold Series bone drilling s.
Golf exercise s.
GoodKnight 418A, 418G, 418P
  CPAP s.
Gore Tag endoprosthesis s.
Graf stabilization s.
graft containment s.
graft delivery s. (GDS)
Granberg cervical traction s.
GRASS s.
gravity extension locking s.
Gray revision instrument s.
Greenberg retracting s.
Greenberg retractor mounting s.
Greenfield vena cava filter s.
GreenLight PV laser s.
Grieshaber power injector s.
Grote 2000 ossicular replacement s.
GSI balloon dissector s.
GS Modular pulmonary testing s.
GTS great toe s.
GTS 2-piece implant s.
Guardian DNA s.
Guardian limb salvage s.
Guardian 2-piece ostomy s.
Guardwire angioplasty s.
Guardwire embolus containment s.
GuardWire Plus s.
GuardWire temporary occlusion and
  aspiration s.
Guglielmi detachable coil s.
Guidant Heart Rhythm
  Technologies Linear Ablation s.
Guidant Multi-Link Tetra coronary
  stent s.
Guidant Triad 3-electrode energy
  defibrillation s.
Guidant TRIAD three-electrode
  energy defibrillation s.
guided trephine s. (GTS)
Gynecare Monitorr urodynamic
  measurement s.
Gynecare Monitorr urodynamic
  measuring s.
Gynecare Thermachoice uterine
  balloon therapy s.
Gynecare TVT obturator s.
Gynecare TVT support s.

Gynecare Veristat fluid management s.
Gynecare Versascope hysteroscopy s.
Gyroscan HP Philips 15S whole-body s.
Gyrus endourology s.
Haemolite autologous blood recovery s.
Haemonetics Cell Saver s.
Haid UBP s.
Haid Universal bone plate s.
Hakim programmable valve s.
Halifax interlaminar clamp s.
Hall mandibular implant s.
Hall modular acetabular reamer s.
Hallu Fix MTP fusion s.
halo cervical traction s.
halo retractor s.
Halo Sleep S.
Hamilton repeating pipette dispenser s.
HandPort s.
Hands Free knee retractor s.
Harrington rod and hook s.
Hartmann-Shack wavefront sensor s.
Hausmann Work-Well work hardening s.
HDI 1000, 3000, 3500, 4000, 5000 ultrasound imaging s.
3-head gamma camera-based SPECT s.
headless bone screw s.
HeartMate implantable pneumatic left ventricular assist s.
HeartMate vented electric left ventricular assist s.
Heartport catheter s.
Heartport Port-Access s.
Heartstring proximal seal s.
Heartwave EP s.
Heelbo L-Bow arm restraint s.
Helix multihead nuclear imaging s.
Hemasure r\LS red blood cell filtration s.
Hematome s.
HemiCAP resurfacing s.
HemoCue blood glucose s.
HemoCue blood hemoglobin s.
HemoCue hemoglobin test s.
hemoglobin-based therapeutic s.
hemoglobin glutamer-250[bovine] oxygen-based therapeutic s.
Hemopump cardiac assist s.
Hemopure oxygen-based therapeutic s.
heparin-induced extracorporeal lipoprotein precipitation s.
HepatAssist bioartificial liver s.

HepatAssist liver support s.
HEPAtech air purification s.
Herbert bone screw s.
Herbert-Whipple cannulated screw s.
Hercules Nd:YAG laser s.
Herculite XRV Lab s.
Heritage hip s.
Hermes Evolution tricompartmental knee s.
Hermes total knee s.
Hermetic external ventricular drainage s.
Hermetic II drainage management s.
Her Option uterine cryoablation therapy s.
Hewlett-Packard IVUS imaging s.
Hewlett-Packard 5 MHz phased-array TEE s.
Hewlett-Packard phased-array ultrasound imaging s.
Hewlett-Packard Sonos 1000, 1500, 2500 ultrasound s.
Hexcel total condylar knee s.
Hex-Fix s.
Hexon illumination s.
Hi-Care closed suction and pulmonary hygiene s.
Hicor s.
high-field s.
high-force Sundt clip s.
high-resolution brain SPECT s.
high-speed drill s.
s. high-speed microdrill
Hind-SITE 20/20 s.
Hipokrat bimodular shoulder s.
Hi-Star MRI s.
Histofreezer cryosurgical s.
Hitachi Altaire Open MRI s.
Hitachi EUB-555 diagnostic ultrasound s.
Hitachi EUB 405 imaging s.
Hitachi 4-head s.
Hitachi Open MRI s.
Hitachi PCT-3600W PET s.
Hitachi rotating detector array s.
Hitachi UB 420 digital ultrasound s.
HmX H20 hematology s.
Hoffman external fixation s.
Hoffmann external fixation s.
Holter external drainage s.
Holter hydrocephalus shunt s.
Homepump infusion s.
HomMed monitoring s.
homonuclear spin s.
hook probe s.

S

system *(continued)*

Hopkins angle-view 30-degree optical s.
Hopkins II optical s.
Hopkins rod-lens s.
Hopkins straight-view optical s.
Horizon AutoAdjust CPAP s.
Horizon Eclipse spinal s.
Horizon Legacy spinal s.
Horizon LT CPAP s.
Horizon nasal CPAP s.
Hot/Ice S. III
Housecall transtelephonic monitoring s.
House grading s.
Howmedica HNR s.
Howmedica pediatric osteotomy s.
Howmedica total ankle s.
Howmedica Unitrax hip fracture s.
Howmedica VSF fixation s.
HP7754 pneumohydraulic capillary infusion s.
HP Sonos 5500 ultrasound echocardiography s.
HP Sonos 5500 ultrasound imaging s.
Huene biaxial elbow s.
Humphrey Atlas Eclipse corneal topography s.
Humphrey Mastervue corneal topography s.
Hunsaker Mon-Jet tube anesthesia s.
Hunstad tumescent liposuction s.
Hybrid Capture s.
HybridFit total hip s.
HybridFit total knee s.
Hybriwix probe s.
HydraClear endoscopic cleansing s.
Hydradjust urology s.
hydraulic capillary infusion s.
Hydra Vision Es urological imaging s.
Hydra Vision IV urology s.
Hydra Vision Plus DR, ES, HP urological imaging s.
Hydra Vision Plus DR urological imaging s.
Hydra Vision Plus urologic s.
HydroCoil embolization s. (HES)
HydroDot neuromonitoring s.
hydrodynamic thrombectomy s.
HydroFlex arthroscopy irrigating s.
HydroThermAblator endometrial ablation s.
HydroTrack underwater treadmill s.
Hyperion LTK s.
HyperPACS teleradiology s.
Hypobaric transfemoral s.

Hypobaric transtibial s.
Hy-Tec automated allergy diagnostic s.
I&A s.
IBP elbow s.
i-CAT cone beam 3D dental imaging s.
ID-Micro typing s.
IDXrad radiology information s.
Igloo Heatshield s.
3i Implant Innovations implant s.
iiRAD DR1000C digital radiographic s.
IL 1640 blood gas/electrolyte s.
Ilizarov limb-lengthening s.
Illumina Pro Series CO_2 surgical laser s.
iLook 15 handheld ultrasound s.
image analysis s.
Imagecast imaging s.
ImageChecker CT CAD software s.
IMAGEnet 2000 series digital imaging s.
ImageView s.
Imatron s.
Imelab vascular diagnostic s.
Immage immunochemistry s.
Immediate Implant Impression s.
immediate response mobile analysis blood analysis s.
Immulite 1000, 2000, 2500 immunoassay s.
Immulite 2500 SMS immunoassay s.
Immunomedics s.
ImmunoPrep reagent s.
Impact lithotriptor s.
Impact modular total hip s.
Impact on-site drug and alcohol test s.
Impax PACS s.
ImplaMed implant s.
implantable internal s.
implantable neuromodulation s.
Implatome dental tomography s.
IMx PSA s.
IMZ implant s.
INCA s.
Incardia valve s.
InCare pelvic floor therapy office s.
InCare PRES 9300 s.
In Charge diabetes control s.
incident command s.
InCompass thoracolumbar fixation s.
Indiana Tome carpal tunnel release s.

Indiana Tome carpal tunnel syndrome release s.
Indigo LaserOptic treatment s.
Indigo Optima laser s.
InDuo s.
Infant Flow nCPAP s.
Infant Flow noninvasive nasal CPAP s.
infant resuscitation s.
In-Fast bone screw s.
Infinia Hawkeye nuclear medicine s.
Infiniti catheter introducer s.
Infinity hip s.
InFix interbody fusion s.
Infravision imaging s.
Infuse-a-Port vascular access s.
Infuset T fluid delivery s.
Inion GTR biodegradable membrane s.
Inion S-1 biodegradable anterior cervical s.
InjecAid s.
InnerVasc expandable vascular access s.
InnerVue diagnostic scope s.
Innomed arthroplasty measuring s.
Innova feminine incontinence treatment s.
Innova 4100 flat-panel x-ray s.
Innova home incontinence therapy s.
Innovative COR/T implant s.
INOvent delivery s.
INR home anticoagulation blood monitoring s.
Insall-Burstein II modular total knee s.
Insight knee positioning and alignment s.
InSIGHT manometry s.
Insignia Ultra DR, SR pacing s.
Inspiration ventilator s.
InstaTrak ENT image-guidance s.
Instrumentation Laboratory s.
In-Tac bone-anchoring s.
Integral hip s.
Integra skin replacement s.
integrated automatic stone-tissue detection s.
integrated clinical information s.
Integrated Core s.
integrated lead s.
Integre 532 delivery s.
Integris cardiac imaging s.
Integris H5000 digital x-ray imaging s.
Integris III-V DSA s.

Integris V 3000 digital subtraction s.
Integris V3000 digital subtraction s.
Integrity AFx AutoCapture pacing s.
InteliJET fluid management s.
intensified radiographic imaging s.
Inteq small joint suturing s.
Interax total knee s.
interbody fusion cage s.
Intercept platelet s.
Inter-Lock screw and fixation s.
Intermate infusion s.
Intermedics natural hip s.
International 10-20 s.
International Biomedical Mode 745-100 microcapillary infusion s.
International compression s.
Interpore IMZ implant s.
interprobe s.
Intrabeam intraoperative radiotherapy s.
IntraLuminal Safe-Steer s.
intramedullary skeletal kinetic distractor s.
Intra-Op autotransfusion s.
intraspinal drug infusion s.
IntraStent DoubleStrut ParaMount premounted stent-biliary s.
IntraStent DoubleStrut ParaMount XS premounted stent-biliary s.
intrauterine contraceptive progesterone s.
Invacare Venture HomeFill complete home oxygen s.
Inverter vitrectomy s.
INVISx cranial fixation s.
Invos 3100, 3100A cerebral oximeter monitoring s.
Ionic spine spacer s.
iON intraoperative navigation s.
ipos arch support s.
IPS total hip s.
Iris Medical OcuLight green laser s.
Iris Medical OcuLight infrared laser s.
Iris OcuLight SLx indirect ophthalmoscope delivery s.
IRMA blood gas analysis s.
Irri-Cath suction s.
irrigation s.
Irrijet DS irrigation s.
IS1000 gel documentation imaging s.
ISG Wand navigation s.
ISKD s.
Isocam scintillation imaging s.

system *(continued)*

Isocam SPECT imaging s.
Isogard s.
Isola fixation s.
Isola spinal implant s.
Isola spinal instrumentation s.
Isolator blood culture s.
Isolator endoscopic ablation s.
Isolex 300i magnetic stem cell
 selection s.
IsoMed constant-flow infusion s.
Isotechnologies B-200 back testing
 and rehabilitation s.
i-STAT s.
ITI dental implant s.
I-TRAC Plus transfusion s.
Itrel II, III spinal cord
 stimulation s.
IVAC needleless IV s.
3i wide-diameter dental implant s.
Jace continuous passive motion
 ankle s.
Jackson staging s.
Jaguar lumbar I/F cage s.
Java arthrodesis s.
Jay Care wheelchair seating s.
Jimmy John colonic irrigation s.
Jinotti closed suctioning s.
Jobst athrombic pump s.
Johnson & Johnson PFC Sigma s.
joint activated s. (JAS)
Joyce-Loebl Magiscan image
 analysis s.
JS Quick-fill s.
Julstro Self-Treatment s.
Jurgan pin ball s.
JustVision diagnostic ultrasound s.
J-Vac closed wound drainage s.
Kaltenborn joint mobilization s.
Kaneda anterior scoliosis s.
Kaneda anterior spinal s.
Kaneda anterior spinal/scoliosis s.
Kaneda SR spinal s.
Kaneda SR threaded rod s.
Kaplan PenduLaser 115 laser s.
Kappa CTD finishing s.
Kappa 700, 900 pacing s.
Kappa SP lens finishing s.
Karl Storz D-Light AF
 autofluorescence s.
Karl Storz D-LIGHT AF
 autofluorescence s.
Karl Storz pediatric
 bronchoscopy s.
Kartush Hapex implant s.
Katena quick switch I/A s.
KaVo oral surgery s.
K-Centrum anterior spinal
 fixation s.

Keithly DAS-500 series data-
 acquisition s.
Kellan capsular sparing s.
Kelly-Goerss Compass
 stereotactic s.
Kelly stereotactic s.
Kendall A-V impulse s.
Kendall Ventex wound dressing s.
Keramos ceramic/ceramic total
 hip s.
keratinocyte fibroblast coculture s.
Keratograph corneal topography s.
Keratome excimer laser s.
Keratron Scout topography s.
K-Fix fixator s.
K2 hemi toe implant s.
Kinamed Exact-Fit ATH s.
Kin-Con isokinetic exercise s.
Kinematic II condylar and
 stabilizer total knee s.
Kinematic II rotating-hinge knee s.
Kinemax modular condylar and
 stabilizer total knee s.
Kinemax Plus total knee s.
Kinetik great toe implant s.
King double umbrella closure s.
Kirschner hip replacement s.
Kirschner II-C shoulder s.
Kirschner integrated shoulder s.
Kirschner Medical Dimension hip
 replacement s.
Kleen Needle s.
KLS-Martin modular
 osteosynthesis s.
Knee Signature S.
KnightStar 335 respiratory-
 support s.
Koby Isogard surgical treatment s.
Koeller illumination s.
Koenig MPJ implant and
 arthroplasty s.
KOH colpotomizer s.
Kolibri ENT image-guided s.
Komet K-wire/Steinman pin and
 delivery tray s.
Komet Medical/Brasseler USA XK-
 95 high-speed drill s.
Konan SP8000 image analysis s.
Kostuik-Harrington anterior
 distraction s.
Kostuik-Harrington distraction s.
Kostuik internal spine fixation s.
Kowa fluorescein s.
Kretz ultrasound s.
KTP/532 laser s.
KTP/Nd:YAG XP surgical laser s.
KTP/532 surgical laser s.
KTP/YAG surgical laser s.
Kulzer inlay s.

laboratory automation s.
LabraFix s.
Lact-Aid nursing trainer s.
LactoSorb craniofacial plate
  fixation s.
LactoSorb craniomaxillofacial
  fixation s.
LactoSorb resorbable fixation s.
LactoSorb trauma plating s.
LADARTracker closed-loop
  tracking s.
LADARVision excimer laser s.
LADARVision 4000 excimer
  laser s.
LADARWave CustomCornea
  wavefront s.
Ladd fiberoptic s.
LaFaci surgical s.
LAGB s.
Laitinen CT guidance s.
Laitinen stereotactic s.
Lambda Plus PDL 1, 2 laser s.
Lambotte exhaust s.
laminar flow s.
LaminOss implant s.
Lamis infusion s.
LandmarX s.
Langerman diamond knife s.
Lanier clinical reporting s.
Laparolift s.
Laparomed cholangiogram
  vacuum s.
laparoscopic retraction s.
Laparoshield laparoscopic smoke
  filtration s.
Lap-Band adjustable gastric
  banding s.
LaseAway ruby laser s.
laser s.
Laser CHRP rigid fiberscope s.
LaserLite s.
LaserScan LSX excimer laser s.
LaTIS endovascular laser s.
LazerSmile tooth-whitening s.
LCS mobile bearing knee s.
LCS total knee s.
LDD delivery s.
lead extraction s.
Learning retinal implant s.
left ventricular assist s.
Legacy cannulated implant s.
Legacy cataract surgical s.
Legacy spinal s.
Legend high-speed pneumatic s.
Leibinger/Karlis intermaxillary
  fixation screw s.
Leibinger locking s.
Leibinger miniplate s.
Leibinger plating s.

Leibinger Profyle hand s.
Leibinger titanium mini Würzburg
  implant s.
Leibinger titanium Würzburg
  mandibular reconstruction s.
Leitz image analysis s.
Leksell micro-stereotactic s.
Leksell stereotactic s.
Lens Comfort ultrasound cleaning
  and disinfecting s.
Lens Opacities Classification S. II
Leukotrap RC storage s.
Leukotrap red cell storage s.
Level Anchorage s.
Level I normothermic irrigating s.
Levulin PDT s.
Liberty spinal s.
Lido Active Multijoint s.
Lidoback isokinetic dynamometry s.
Lido Passive Multijoint s.
Liebel-Flarsheim CT 9000 contrast
  delivery s.
Life-Air 1000 hypothermic
  therapy s.
Lifecore Restore wide-diameter
  implant s.
LifeGuide s.
Lifeline Wall Gym 2000 fitness s.
LIFE-Lung s.
Lifepath AAA endovascular graft s.
LifeScan blood glucose
  monitoring s.
LifeShirt ambulatory monitoring s.
LifeSite hemodialysis access s.
LifeSync wireless ECG s.
LigaSure vessel sealing s.
LightCycler s.
LightSheer diode laser s.
LightSheer SC laser hair
  removal s.
LightSpeed Ultra CT s.
limb preservation s. (LPS)
LINAC s.
LINAC-based radiosurgical s.
linear accelerator s.
Linear total hip s.
Link custom partial pelvis
  replacement s.
Link Endo-Model rotational knee s.
Link Lubinus AP hip s.
Link Lubinus SP II hip
  replacement s.
Link Lubinus SP II total hip
  replacement s.
Link Saddle Prosthesis Endo-Model
  hip replacement s.
Lipoprint cholesterol subfraction
  test s.
Liposorber LA-15 s.

system *(continued)*

Liquid Embolic s.
Lithostar multiline lithotripsy s.
Lithostar Plus electromagnetic lithotriptor bidimensional x-ray focusing s.
Lithovac master suction s.
LocaLisa cardiac navigation s.
LoCon-T distal radial plating s.
LogiCal pressure transducer s.
Logic mandibular distraction s.
Lone Star retractor s.
Lorad full-field digital mammography s.
Lorad StereoGuide prone breast biopsy s.
Lorad StereoGuide stereotactic breast biopsy s.
Lordex lumbar spine s.
Lorenz Micro-Power dense bone drilling and cutting s.
Lorenz osteosynthesis s.
Lorenz plating s.
Lorenz temporomandibular prosthetic joint s.
low-compliance perfusion s.
low-field MRI s.
low-vision enhancement s. (LVES)
LPI excimer laser s.
LP^2 stainless steel delivery s.
LS 6500 liquid scintillation counting s.
LTK s.
LTX3000 lumbar rehabilitation s.
Lubinus AP hip s.
Lubinus SP II anatomically adapted hip s.
Luhr maxillofacial fixation s.
Luhr microfixation s.
Luhr pan fixation s.
Luma cervical imaging s.
Lumax Pro cystometry s.
Lumbo 90 home care traction s.
Lumex PT fiberoptic cystometry s.
Luque II fixation s.
Luxtec fiberoptic s.
LX4201 clinical s.
LX EchoSpeed CV/i, NVi MR s.
LXi 725 clinical s.
LX20, LX200, LX2000 PRO clinical s.
LymphoScan nuclear imaging s.
Lynco biomechanical orthotic s.
Lyra-i laser s.
Lyra laser s.
LySonix 2000 Micro ultrasonic surgical s.
LySonix Post-Operative patient s.
LySonix Series 250 operative s.

LySonix 2000 standard ultrasonic surgical s.
LySonix TTD cannula s.
LySonix 2000 ultrasonic surgical s.
Mackool s.
Macroduct collecting s.
MacroPore fixation s.
MacroPore OS spinal s.
MadaJet XL jet-injection anesthesia s.
MadaJet XL local anesthesia s.
Maestro s.
Maestro surgical drill s.
Maestro wrist joint replacement s.
Magellan electromagnetic navigation s.
Magerl hook-plate s.
Magerl plate-screw s.
Magna-Fx cannulated screw fixation s.
Magna-Site locating s.
Magnes biomagnetometer s.
Magnetic Surgery s.
Magnetom Open s.
MagnetomSonata MR s.
Magnetom Sonata 1.5T MR s.
Magnetom Trio unlimited MRI s.
Magnetom Vision MR s.
Magnetom Vision MR imaging s.
Magnex Alpha MR s.
Malcolm-Lynn radiolucent spinal retraction s.
Malcolm-Rand radiolucent headrest and retraction s.
Malis bipolar coagulating/cutting s.
Malis CMC-III electrosurgical s.
Mallinckrodt Hi-Care Pulmonary Hygiene s.
Mallinckrodt sensor s.
Mallory-Head modular calcar s.
mammalian olfactory s.
Mammex TR computer-aided mammography diagnosis s.
Mammomat C3 mammography s.
Mammo Plus mammography s.
MammoReader computer-aided detection s.
MammoReader mammography s.
MammoScan digital imaging s.
MammoSite radiation therapy s.
Mammotest Plus breast biopsy s.
Mammotome biopsy s.
Mammotome breast biopsy s.
Mammotome ultrasound s.
Manchester LDR implant s.
Mandelkorn gauge/dilator s.
M-2 anterior plate s.
manual gun s.
Mapleson D breathing s.

Maramed Miami fracture brace s.
Marex MRI s.
Marion oxygen resuscitation s.
Mark III halo s.
Mark II Sorrells hip arthroplasty
  retractor s.
Mark V ProVis injection s.
Marlen UltraLite s.
Marquette Case-12
  electrocardiographic s.
Marquette Case-12 exercise s.
Marx bridging plate s.
Mason-Likar 12-lead ECG s.
Mastel compass-guided arcuate
  keratotomy s.
matrix seating s.
mattress s.
Mattrix spinal cord stimulation s.
Maturna bra s.
Mauch GaitMaster s.
maxillofacial plating s.
Maxim modular knee s.
Maxi-Myst nebulizer s.
MaxLock plate and screw s.
maxwellian view optical s.
Mayfield surgical headrest s.
McCain TMJ arthroscopic s.
McGuire I&A s.
McGuire screw s.
McIntyre coaxial I&A s.
McIntyre III nucleus removal s.
M/D 4 defibrillator s.
MDS s.
mechanical assist s.
Mectra I&A s.
Mectra irrigation/aspiration s.
Meddars cardiac catheterization
  analysis s.
Medex Secure s.
MedGraphics Cardio O2 s.
Medical Graphics Cardiopulmonary
  Exercise S. 2001
Medical Support S.'s, Inc.
medication monitoring event s.
MediClenze hygiene and water
  therapy s.
Medi-Duct ocular fluid
  management s.
Medi-Facts s.
Mediflex MD-7 endoscopic
  video s.
Medi-Ject needle-free insulin
  injection s.
Medi-Jector Choice needle-free
  insulin injection s.
Medipad drug delivery s.
Medisorb drug delivery s.
Meditech catheter s.
Meditech ureteral stent s.

Medi-Vac suction canister s.
MedNova NeuroShield cerebral
  protection s.
Medos mechanical circulatory
  support s.
Medspec MR imaging s.
Medstone IRIS s.
Medstone STS lithotripsy s.
Med Tec Vac Loc
  immobilization s.
Medtronic Hemopump s.
Medtronic interactive tachycardia
  terminating s.
Medtronic InterStim sacral nerve
  stimulation s.
Medtronic Micro Jewel
  cardioverter-defibrillator s.
Medtronic Midas Rex Legend s.
Medtronic Octopus 2+ tissue
  stabilizing s.
Medtronic Sequestra 1000
  autotransfusion s.
Medtronic spinal cord
  stimulation s.
Medtronics Sequestra 1000
  autotransfusion s.
Medtronic Transvene endocardial
  lead s.
Medweb clinical reporting s.
Med-Wick medication delivery s.
MEGA-Pouch laparoscopic
  retrieval s.
MEG head-based coordinate s.
MEI s.
Meier-Magnum s.
MEMS 6 TrackCap Monitor
  medication monitoring s.
Meniscus Mender II s.
Mentor Contour Genesis ultrasonic
  assisted lipoplasty s.
Mesa spinal s.
MetaFluor s.
Metalift crown and bridge
  removal s.
Metasul metal-on-metal hip
  prosthesis s.
Metrix atrial defibrillation s.
METRx s.
METRx X-Tube retraction s.
MG II total knee s.
Miami Modular Orthopaedic
  Spinal S.
MIBB breast biopsy s.
Micro-Aire facial plating s.
Micro-Aire pulse lavage s.
Micro-Aire surgical instrument s.
MicroChoice electric powered
  surgical s.
microdebrider s. (MDS)

S

system *(continued)*
Micro Delta/Max Delta s.
microdilution s.
microelectromechanical s.
MicroGas 7650 transcutaneous
monitoring s.
MicroGuide microelectrode
recording s.
MicroLap Gold s.
MicroLux videocamera s.
micromanometer catheter s.
Micro-Mill knee instrument s.
micromultileaf collimator s.
MicroPhor iontophoretic drug
delivery s.
Micro Plus plating s.
Microprobe integrated laser and
endoscope s.
microSelectron rapid delivery s.
MicroShape keratome s.
Micros infusion s.
MicroSpan microhysterescopy s.
Microsponge delivery s.
Microsponge drug delivery s.
Microsulis microwave endometrial
ablation s.
Microvasive biliary stent s.
Microvasive Ultraflex esophageal
stent s.
Micro-Vent implant s.
Microvit probe s.
microwave cardiac ablation s.
MicroWick s.
Midas Rex instrumentation s.
Midas Rex Legend s.
Midas Rex Quick-Connect s.
MIDCAB s.
middle ear implantable s.
Millennium CX, LX
microsurgical s.
Millennium microsurgical s.
Millennium transconjunctival
standard vitrectomy s.
Millennium VG SPECT s.
Miller-Galante I condylar total
knee s.
Miller-Galante revision knee s.
Miller-Galante total knee s.
Milli-Q water purification s.
Mimix bone replacement s.
Minerva s.
mini Acutrak small bone
fixation s.
mini Hoffmann external fixation s.
mini lag screw s.
MiniMed continuous glucose
monitoring s.
MiniMite suture anchor s.
Mini-Revo suture anchor s.

mini Vidas automated
immunoassay s.
mini Würzburg Flexplates
craniomaxillofacial plating s.
mini Würzburg implant s.
mini Würzburg standard
craniomaxillofacial plating s.
Mirage nasal ventilation mask s.
Mirage spinal s.
mirror optical s.
M.I.S. multi-port illumination s.
Mitek Exojet fluid-jet resection s.
Mitek GII suture anchor s.
Mitek Vapr tissue removal s.
mitochondrial ethanol oxidase s.
Mityvac vacuum delivery s.
MK-2000 keratome s.
Mobetron electron beam s.
Mobetron intraoperative radiation
therapy treatment s.
MobilExcimer laser s.
modular acetabular revision s.
(MARS)
modular implant s.
modular internal distraction s.
modular S-ROM total hip s.
Modulus CD anesthesia s.
Mojave cataract extraction s.
molecular adsorbents recirculating s.
Monaldi drainage s.
Monarch IOL delivery s.
Monarch spinal s.
Monitorr urodynamic measuring s.
Monotube external fixator s.
Montgomery thyroplasty implant s.
Monticelli-Spinelli circular external
fixation s.
Moore hip endoprosthesis s.
MOP-Videoplan morphometric s.
Morganstern aspiration/injection s.
morphology s. CAS-200
Moss fixation s.
Moss-Miami spinal s.
Most Options s.
mother-baby endoscope s.
mother-baby-scope s.
mother endoscopic retrograde
cholangiopancreatoscopy s.
motion artifact rejection s.
Mport foldable lens placement s.
Mport lens insertion s.
MRI-compatible plate and screw s.
MT-100 ECG Holter s.
Mui Scientific pressurized capillary
infusion s.
Mulholland growth guidance s.
Mullins sheath s.
multidetector s.

Multidex chronic wound
treatment s.
multileaf collimating s.
MultiLight s.
Multi-Link coronary stent s.
Multi-Link Frontier coronary
stent s.
Multi-Link Penta coronary stent s.
Multi-Link Pixel coronary stent s.
Multi-Link Pixel stent s.
Multi-Link Tetra coronary stent s.
Multi-Link Zeta coronary stent s.
multiple-electrode probe s.
multiple side-hole infusion s.
Multi Podus boot s.
Multi Podus foot s.
Multistar Top Plus DSA s.
Multitak SS s.
Multitak suture snap s.
Multitest cell-mediated immunity s.
muscle tone inhibitor s.
MW 2000 microwave delivery s.
M3-X extremity fixation s.
myeloperoxidase-H2O2-halide s.
Myobock s.
myocardial protection s.
MyoSight dedicated nuclear
cardiology camera s.
MyoSight imaging s.
MYOtherm XP cardioplegia
delivery s.
Nanoduct neonatal sweat
analysis s.
nasal CPAP s.
Natchez Mobil-Trac s.
Natural-Hip s.
Natural-Knee II s.
Natural Profile abutment s.
Navi Ball guidance s.
navigation s.
Navigus cranial electrode s.
Navitrack computer-assisted
surgery s.
NCP s.
NC-stat nerve conduction s.
Nd:YAG laser s.
needle trephination s.
Neer II shoulder s.
Neer II total knee s.
Nellcor N-400/FS s.
Nellcor Symphony blood pressure
monitoring s.
NeoControl pelvic floor therapy s.
NeoCure cryoablation s.
neodymium:yttrium-aluminum-garnet
laser s.
neon occipitocervical s.
Neoprobe 1000 radioisotope
detection s.

Neosonic P-5 SPM super-powered
mini retroprep/endo s.
NeoSoniX s.
Neotrend s.
nephroureteral stent s.
NeuroCybernetic prosthesis s.
Neuroform microdelivery stent s.
Neuroform3 microdelivery stent s.
NeuroLink II EEG data
acquisition s.
NeuroMap s.
Neuropak 8 s.
neuroprobe pain management s.
Neuro-Sat frameless isocentric
stereotactic s.
Neurosector ultrasound s.
Neurosign 100 s.
Neurotrend continuous
multiparameter s.
Neuroview integrated
visualization s.
Newport hip s.
Newport total hip orthosis s.
New Vision magnification s.
NexGen complete knee s.
NexGen complete knee
replacement s.
Nex-Link implant s.
Nex-Link spinal fixation s.
NexPill SmartCap medication
monitoring s.
Nexus wheelchair seating s.
Niamtu video imaging s.
Nicolet Viking II
electrophysiologic s.
Nidek combo laser s.
Nidek EC-5000 excimer laser s.
Nidek EC-5000 refractive laser s.
Nidek MK-2000 keratome s.
Niox nitric oxide breath test s.
Niox nitric oxide monitoring s.
NIR Elite Monorail s.
NIR Elite OTW stent s.
Nobelpharma implant s.
Node Seeker surgical radiation
detection s.
Noga XP cardiac navigation s.
nondilated s.
nonthoracotomy defibrillation
lead s.
Norian skeletal repair s.
Norland XR-46 central DXA bone
densitometry s.
Norm testing and rehabilitation s.
Norwegian s.
No-Touch delivery and mounting s.
Novacor Diasys left ventricular
assist s.
Novacor left ventricular assist s.

system *(continued)*

Novacor mechanical circulatory support s.
Nova Microsonics ImageVue s.
NovaPulse laser s.
NovaSure impedance controlled endometrial ablation s.
Novoste Beta-Cath delivery s.
Novum s.
NS2000 bipolar generator s.
Nucleus C124M cochlear implant s.
Nucleus 24 Contour cochlear implant s.
NuMe microdermabrasion and exfoliation s.
Nu-Trake Weiss emergency airway s.
Nuvolase 660 laser s.
Oasis pusher tube s.
Oasis thrombectomy s.
Obtura II gutta percha s.
Ocelot stackable cage s.
OctaFix cervical fixation s.
OctaFix occipital fixation s.
OCT comprehensive s.
OctreoScan s.
ocular magnification s.
Oculex drug delivery s.
Oculus BIOM noncontact lens s.
Ocutech vision enhancing s.
Odyssey phacoemulsification s.
OEC-Diasonics 9400 fluoroscopy C-arm s.
OEC Mini 6600 imaging s.
OEC series 9600 cardiac s.
Ogden plate s.
Ogden tissue reattachment mini s.
OIS image digitizing s.
OIS WinStation 5000 ophthalmic imaging s.
Oklahoma cable s.
Olerud PSF fixation s.
Olson calibrated cornea trephine s.
Olympic Vac positioning s.
Olympus endoscopy s.
Olympus EU-M30 s.
Olympus EVIS color computer chip s.
Olympus GF-UM3, -UM20 s.
Olympus MAJ363 FNA needle s.
Olympus OSP fluorescence measuring s.
Olympus videourology procedure s.
Omega AcuBase s.
OmniCell supply s.
Omnifit HA hip s.
Omnifit Plus enhanced offset cemented hip s.
Omnifit Plus hip s.
Omni-Flow 4000 Plus medical management s.
Omni-LapoTract support s.
Omniloc dental s.
OmniSight EXcel image-guided surgery s.
Omni-Tract s.
Oncor Inform HER2/neu gene amplification detection s.
One Action Stent Introduction S.
OneTouch II hospital blood glucose monitoring s.
On-Q C-bloc continuous nerve block s.
On-Q PainBuster postoperative pain relief s.
On-Q pain management infusion s.
OnTrack s.
Onyx liquid embolic s.
Opdima digital mammography s.
OPD-Scan diagnostic s.
OPD-Scan optical path difference scanning s.
OpenGene automated DNA sequencing s.
open-loop insulin delivery s.
open MRI s.
OpenPACS s.
Opera s.
ophthalmic YAG laser s.
Ophtho-Burr foreign body removal s.
Opmilas laser s.
Opmilas 144 Plus laser s.
Opmi Vario/NC 33 s.
Optetrak comprehensive knee s.
Optetrak total knee replacement s.
Opthascan Mini B s.
optical biopsy s.
optical multichannel analyzer s.
Optical Sensors stand-alone arterial blood gas monitoring s.
optical tracking s.
OptiCor digital cardiac communication and storage s.
Opti-Fix total hip s.
OptiHaler drug delivery s.
OptiMax immunostaining s.
Option hip s.
Optistar MR contrast delivery s.
Optivac vacuum mixing s.
Optotrak motion-analysis s.
Optotrak motion measurement s.
Optotrak motion and position measurement s.
Oracle delivery s.
Oral Scan computer imaging s.
Oral Scan videoimaging s.

Orascoptic acuity s.
Orbasone s.
Orbscan s.
Orbscan II corneal diagnostic s.
Orbscan II corneal topography s.
Orbscan II diagnostic s.
Orbscan II multidimensional
  diagnostic s.
Orbscan II topography s.
Orbscan topography analysis s.
Orca robot s.
OR1 electronic s.
OR-340 imaging s.
Orion laser s.
Orth-evac postoperative
  transfusion s.
OrthoClast joint revision s.
Orthodoc presurgical planning s.
Ortho Dx electrotherapy s.
Orthogenesis LPS limb preservation
  prosthesis s.
Ortho-Ice Multipaks s.
Ortholoc Advantim revision knee s.
Ortholoc Advantim total knee s.
Orthomerica TC AFO s.
Orthomet Axiom total knee s.
Orthomet Perfecta total hip s.
OrthOneXT dedicated MRI s.
orthopaedic trauma plating s.
  (OTPS)
OrthoPak bone growth stimulator s.
OrthoPAT s.
OrthoPAT blood salvage s.
OrthoPAT orthopaedic perioperative
  autotransfusion s.
Orthopedic S.'s Inc. (OSI)
Orthotec pressurized fluid
  irrigation s.
Osada ENAC-W10 quartz
  piezoelectric ultrasonic s.
Osada portable electric
  handpiece s.
Osada portable handpiece s.
Osada XL-S30 electric handpiece s.
Oscar ultrasonic bone cement
  removal s.
OSI modular table s.
OssaTron shock wave therapy s.
Osseofix dental implant s.
osseous Coagulum Trap
  collecting s.
osteochondral autograft transfer s.
Osteo-Clage cerclage cable s.
Osteonics Scorpio posterior cruciate
  retaining total knee s.
Osteonics spinal s.
OsteoView 2000 s.
OsteoView desktop hand x-ray s.
OsteoView 2000 digital imaging s.

OsteoView 2000 imaging s.
Ostreg spinal marker s.
OSV II Smart Valve s.
OtoScan ear aeration s.
OTPS mesh s.
Otto Bock Mobis mobility s.
Oulu neuronavigator s.
Ovation falloposcopy s.
Oxford meniscal unicompartmental
  knee s.
OxiFirst fetal monitoring s.
OxiScan oximetry recording and
  reporting s.
Oxydome oxygen therapy s.
oxygen-based therapeutic s.
oxylate dentin bonding s.
Oxylator positive pressure
  resuscitation and inhalation s.
Oxylite ambulatory oxygen s.
Oxymax aeration s.
Paceart complete pacemaker patient
  testing s.
P/ACE MDQ series capillary
  electrophoresis s.
Packard Merlin life-monitoring s.
Packard radioimmunoassay s.
PadKit sample collection s.
PainBuster postoperative pain
  relief s.
Palco enuretic alarm s.
Palmaz Corinthian biliary stent and
  delivery s.
PalmVue s.
Palomar SLP1000 diode laser s.
Panasol II home phototherapy s.
PapNet automated cervical
  cystology s.
PapNet testing s.
Pap-Perfect supply s.
Parabath paraffin heat treatment s.
Par 5 acetabular reconstruction s.
PARAflow circulatory support s.
Paragon CZE 2000 capillary
  electrophoresis s.
Paragon laser s.
Paragon single-stage dental
  implant s.
Paramax ACL guide s.
paranasal sinus shaver s.
Parastep I s.
Paratrend 7 intravenous blood gas
  monitoring s.
PAR CTS corneal topography s.
Paris ultrasound s.
Park-O-Tron drill s.
Partnership s.
PAS Port s.
PAS Port proximal anastomosis s.
Pasys ST cardiac pacing s.

system *(continued)*

PathFinder pedicle screw s.
PathFinder percutaneous pedicle fixation s.
Patil stereotactic s. I, II
Patriot disposable cannula s.
Paulus trocar s.
PCA s.
PCA modular total knee s.
PCD Transvene implantable cardioverter-defibrillator s.
P-700 Color Velocity Imaging s.
PDB preperitoneal distention balloon s.
PDT laser s.
Peak anterior compression plate s.
Peak fixation s.
Peak Motus motion measurement s.
Peak polyaxial anterior cervical fixation s.
PEC modular total knee s.
PEC total hip s.
Pedar in-shoe measurement s.
Pedar pressure insole s.
Pedar pressure measurement s.
pediatric circle s.
Pediatric LifeShirt s.
PE-400 ERG/VEP s.
Pegasus Airwave pressure relief s.
Pelorus stereotactic s.
Pelorus surgical s.
pelvic floor therapy s.
PelviLace TO biourethral support s.
PelviLace transobturator biourethral support s.
PenChant coronary stent delivery s.
PenRad mammography clinical reporting s.
Pentax-Hitachi FG32UA endosonographic s.
Perclose vascular surgical closure s.
PercuGuide lesion marking s.
percutaneous mechanical thrombectomy s.
Perfecta total hip s.
PerfectCapsule s.
Perfectprep Plasmid 96 VAC direct bind purification s.
PerFixation s.
Perflex delivery s.
Perflex stainless steel stent and delivery s.
Performa acoustic imaging s.
Performa diagnostic ultrasound imaging s.
Performa mammography s.
Performance modular total knee s.

Performance unicompartmental knee s.
Performa ultrasound s.
Perigee prolapse repair s.
Perigee vaginal vault s.
Perimed PeriFlux Doppler probe s.
Perimount Theon mitral replacement s.
periodontal attachment s.
perioperative autotransfusion s.
Periotest s.
peripheral access s. (PAS)
peripheral AngioJet s.
peripheral atherectomy s.
Pe.R.I. plate s.
Permark micropigmentation s.
permucosal implant s.
peroral pancreatoscope s.
PerQ SANS s.
Personal Scanner TM 18 bedside real-time ultrasonography s.
Perspective dental imaging s.
PFA-100 s.
PFC modular total knee s.
PFC Sigma knee s.
PFC Sigma total knee s.
PFC TC3 modular knee s.
PFC total hip replacement s.
PF-8P peroral pancreatoscope s.
phacoemulsification s.
Phacojack phaco s.
PharmChek sweat patch drug detection s.
phased-array color-flow ultrasound s.
PHD personal hemodialysis s.
Philips DVI 1 s.
Philips EasyGuide navigation s.
Philips Integris 5000 digital subtraction angiography s.
PHILOS fixation s.
Phoenix fifth ventricle s.
Phoresor II iontophoretic drug delivery s.
Phoresor PM900 iontophoresis s.
PhorMax CR desktop workstation s.
phosphonated dimethacrylate/phosphated bis-GMA s.
PhosphorImager s.
photocatalytic air filtration s.
PhotoDerm bright light delivery s.
PhotoDerm MultiLight s.
PhotoDerm VL/PL hair removal s.
photodynamic therapy laser s.
PhotoGenica laser s.
PhotoGenica T laser s.
PhotoGenica T^{10} tattoo removal s.

photon-activated drug delivery s.
photonic radiosurgical s.
Photon ocular surgery s.
photon radiosurgery s.
Photopic Imaging ultrasound s.
Phototome s.
Physios CTM 01 noninvasive cardiac transplant monitoring s.
Picker s.
Picker Vistar image analysis s.
Picker Voxel image analysis s.
picture archival communication s.
picture archiving and communication s.
Pie Medical CAAS II analysis s.
Pie Medical ultrasound s.
Pillar palatal implant s.
Pillo-Pump alternating pressure s.
pin ball s.
Pinch Gauge and Jackson Strength Evaluation S.
pin-index safety s.
Pinnacle acetabular cup s.
Pinn-ACL guide s.
Pinn anterior cruciate ligament guide s.
Pinwheel S.
Pipeline access s.
Pisces spinal cord stimulation s.
Pittman IMA retractor s.
pivot link universal s. (PLUS)
Pivot MIS system posterior stabilization s.
PixCell II laser capture microdissection s.
Placido disc videokeratoscopy s.
Planoscan treatment s.
PlastiCast adjustable joint cast s.
plastic endosurgical s.
plastic Vortex Port s.
Plast-O-Fit thermoplastic bandage s.
platelet concentrate s. (PCS)
PlateTrak automated microplate processing s.
Pleur-evac autotransfusion s.
Plexis bone void filling s.
PLI-100 pico-injector pipette s.
PlumeSafe Whisper 602 smoke evacuation s.
PMT halo s.
PMT robotic fulcrumless tomographic s.
PneuMicro small bone power s.
pneumohydraulic capillary infusion s.
PneuView ventilator testing and training s.
PolarCath peripheral dilatation s.
polar coordinate s.

Polaris camera s.
Polaris CPAP s.
Polaroid HealthCam s.
Polarus Plus humeral fixation s.
Polarus positional humeral fixation s.
polyaxial s.
Poly-Chem automated chemistry-immunoassay s.
PolyMax resorbable fixation s.
Porex drainage s.
portable perfused manometric s.
Port-A-Cath implantable catheter s.
PortaFlo urine collection s.
PortalVision radiation oncology s.
port-catheter s.
4-in-1 positioning block s.
posterior rod s.
Pouchkins pediatric ostomy s.
Powerbelt exercise s.
PowerGrip stent delivery s.
Powerlink endoluminal graft s.
PowerProxi Sonic interdental toothbrush s.
PPT insole s.
Precision hip s.
Precisionist Thirty Thousand cataract removal s.
Precision office TUNA s.
Precision Osteolock femoral component s.
Precision QID glucose monitoring s.
Precision SpeedTac transvaginal anchor s.
Precision Strata hip s.
Precision Tack transvaginal anchor s.
Precision Twist transvaginal anchor s.
Precision Xtra advanced diabetes management s.
PreClean soak s.
Premier anterior cervical plate s.
Preservation unicompartmental knee s.
press-fit total condylar knee s.
press-in bone anchor s.
pressure-gradient wire s.
Pressure Sentinel intramedullary reaming s.
pressure transducer-monitor s.
pressurizing s. (PS)
Prestige advanced cataract extraction s.
Presto-Flash spirometry s.
Presto spirometry s.
pretarget filtration s.
PreVue III digitizing s.

system *(continued)*
    Price corneal transplant s.
    Primaloc cementless hip s.
    Prima total occlusion s.
    Prime ECG mapping s.
    PrinceStar electrophysiologic imaging study s.
    Prism 3-head s.
    ProAire portable rotation s.
    Procera s.
    ProComp Infiniti s.
    Prodigy total hip s.
    Profile anterior plate s.
    Profile mammography s.
    Profile total hip s.
    Profix total knee replacement s.
    Profore bandage s.
    Profore Four-Layer bandage s.
    programmable implantable medication s.
    programmable VariGrip II prosthetic control s.
    Prolene hernia s.
    Prolieve microwave therapy s.
    Prolieve thermodilation s.
    Promise pad and pant s.
    Promos modular shoulder s.
    Proscan ultrasound imaging s.
    ProSeries laparoscopic laser s.
    ProstaJect ethanol injection s.
    Prostalase laser s.
    ProstaLund CoreTherm s.
    Prostar percutaneous vascular surgery s.
    ProstaScint s.
    Prostathermer prostatic hyperthermia s.
    Prostatron microwave s.
    Protg GPS self-expanding Nitinol stent-biliary s.
    Protector meniscus suturing s.
    protein characterization s.
    ProteinChip Biomarker DU, PA s.
    ProteinChip System Series 4000 biomarker/assay s.
    ProteomeLab DU, PA 800 protein characterization s.
    ProteomeLab PF 2D protein fractionation s.
    ProteomeLab XL-A, XL-I protein characterization s.
    ProTime microcoagulation s.
    ProTime prothrombin time test s.
    ProTrac cruciate reconstruction s.
    Providence scoliosis s.
    ProVis injection s.
    Provisional Fixation TC-100 plating s.
    Proxiderm wound closure s.

    proximal humerus internal locking s. (PHILOS)
    PSA stationary oxygen s.
    P-Series sleep monitoring s.
    PSI chromosome analysis s.
    Puddu osteotomy s.
    Pulsar Max II DR pacing s.
    Pulsar Max II SR pacing s.
    Pulsavac III wound débridement s.
    Pulsavac Plus wound debridement s.
    PulseDose portable compressed oxygen s.
    2010 Pulse Holter s.
    PulseSpray infusion s.
    Pulse-Spray pulsed infusion s.
    Pump It Up pneumatic socket volume management s.
    Pump-Vac III s.
    punch myringotomy s.
    Puno-Winter-Byrd s.
    Puregene DNA extraction s.
    Puros Accugraft ALIF allograft s.
    Pursuit s.
    PWB transpedicular spine fixation s.
    Pylon intramedullary nail s.
    Q-cath catheterization recording s.
    QCT bone densitometry s.
    Qlicksmart scalpel blade removal s.
    Q-Prep s.
    QRS pulsating magnetic field s.
    Quadracut ACL shaver s.
    quadrature surface coil MRI s.
    Quantimet 500 analyzing s.
    quantitative sweat measurement s.
    Quantrex Sweep 650 ultrasonic cleansing s.
    Quantronic resonance s.
    Quartet s.
    Quest MPS myocardial protection s.
    Quick-Core biopsy s.
    Quick-Fix maxillomandibular fixation s.
    QuickFlow DPS distal perfusion s.
    QuickRinse automated instrument rinse s.
    QuickSeal femoral arterial closure s.
    Quick-Sil silicone s.
    Quickswitch irrigation/aspiration ophthalmic s.
    QuickTack periosteal fixation s.
    Quick-Tap paracentesis s.
    Quik-Stitch endoscopic suturing s.
    Quimby implant s.
    Quinton Synergy cardiac information management s.

Quips genetic imaging s.
Racer over-the-wire biliary stent s.
radiation therapy s. (RTS)
radiation therapy planning s.
radiation treatment s.
radiofrequency interstitial tissue ablation s.
radiofrequency needle electrode s.
radiographic image processing s.
radiographic imaging s.
radiolucent wrist fixation s.
Radionics articulated arm s.
radionuclide carrier s.
RadiStop radial compression s.
RadNet radiology information s.
RAMP biological test s.
Ranawat-Burstein total hip s.
Rancho Cube s.
Rancho external fixation s.
Rapidlab 800 Critical Care s.
Rapid One single dipstick s.
Rasor blood pumping s.
RatioVision digital fluorescent imaging s.
rature surface coil s.
RDX coronary radiation catheter delivery s.
Reach revision s.
Readit SNP genotyping s.
real-time 2-dimensional Doppler flow-imaging s.
real-time 4D ultrasound imaging s.
real-time position management tracking s.
Red s.
RED II s.
Redi-Vacette wound drainage s.
Redi-Vu teleradiology s.
Redi+Wash cleansing s.
Redy hemodialysis s.
Redy 2000 hemodialysis s.
Redy sorbent dialysis s.
Reebok Slide s.
Reebok Step s.
reference coordinate s.
Refinity Coblation s.
Reflection ceramic acetabular s.
ReFlexion first MPJ implant s.
Refractec ViewPoint CK S.
Regulus frameless stereotactic s.
Reichert stereotaxy s.
Rekow s.
Relay suture delivery s.
ReLume s.
Remac s.
Remedy sleep therapy s.
remote afterloading s.
REMstar CPAP s.
Renaissance crown s.

Renaissance spirometry s.
renal kallikrein-kinin s.
Renatron II dialyzer reprocessing s.
Renessa stress urinary incontinence s.
Renew spinal cord stimulation s.
renin-angiotensin s.
Replace implant s.
Replica total hip replacement s.
Repose s.
resorbable copolymer PGA/PLLA-Lactosorb miniplate fixation s.
resorbable graft containment s.
Res-Q-Vac emergency suction s.
Restoration acetabular s.
Restoration-HA hip s.
Restore ACL guide s.
Restore close tolerance dental implant s.
Restore neurostimulation s.
reticONE s.
RetinaLyze s.
RetroScrew s.
Retzius s.
ReUnite resorbable orthopaedic fixation s.
Reuter suprapubic trocar and cannula s.
revascularization s.
Reveal XVI PET/CT imaging s.
Revelation hip s.
revised Salzburg lag screw s.
revised Würzburg mandibular reconstruction s.
ReVision nail s.
Revo rotator cuff repair s.
RF ablation s.
RF needle electrode s.
RF vacuum ablation s.
rHead implant s.
Rhein blade cleaning s.
Rhinoline endoscopic sinus surgery s.
RiboPrinter microbial characterization s.
Richards fixator s.
Richards hip endoprosthesis s.
Richards modular hip s.
Richards Solcotrans orthopaedic drainage-reinfusion s.
Richards Solcotrans Plus drainage s.
Richard Wolf nasal epistaxis s.
Riechert-Mundinger stereotactic s.
rigid external distraction s.
Rigidfix anterior cruciate ligament cross-pin s.
RigiScan Plus rigidity assessment s.

S

system *(continued)*
    RIGS s.
    ring-type imaging s.
    RinoFlow nasal wash and sinus s.
    RITA s.
    Robodoc s.
    Roche Septi-Chek blood culture s.
    Roche Sysmex hematology s.
    Rodenstock s.
    rod-lens s.
    Rod TAG suture anchor s.
    Rogan teleradiology s.
    Roger s.
    Rogozinski screw s.
    Rogozinski spinal rod s.
    Roho pediatric seating s.
    Rolyan Reach-N-Range pulley s.
    Romano curved drilling s.
    Romano surgical curved drilling s.
    Romhilt-Estes point scoring s.
    Rotablator s.
    Rotacs s.
    Rotaglide total knee s.
    Rotograph Plus imaging s.
    Rotograph Plus panoramic dental
      tomography imaging s.
    Royal Marsden Hospital staging s.
    RPM tracking s.
    R-Port implantable vascular
      access s.
    RUMI uterine manipulation s.
    Russell-Taylor femoral interlocking
      nail s.
    RX Acculink carotid stent s.
    Rx5000 cardiac pacing s.
    RxFISH DNA probe and
      analysis s.
    RX Herculink 14 biliary stent s.
    RX Herculink Plus biliary stent s.
    RX Multilink coronary stent s.
    Rx90 smooth femoral s.
    RX stent delivery s.
    RZ mandibular matrix s.
    Saber lumbar I/F cage s.
    Sabolich above-knee socket s.
    SabreSource realtime imaging
      guidance s.
    Sacks-Vine PEG s.
    Safeset blood sampling s.
    Safe-Steer s.
    Safestretch incontinence s.
    SAFHS 2000 sonic accelerated
      fracture healing s.
    Safsite IV therapy s.
    Saf-T-Intima intravenous catheter
      safety s.
    SalEst preterm labor test s.
    Salute fixation s.
    SAM s.

SAMBA imaging s.
Sanders Venturi injector s.
Sandhill esophageal motility s.
Sandman s.
SaphLITE saphenous vein s.
SAPHtrak balloon dissection s.
Savant imaging s.
Save-A-Tooth tooth preserving s.
S-1 biodegradable anterior
  cervical s.
SBI Universal Hand S.
SC-AcuFix anterior cervical
  plate s.
Scanditronix MLC s.
Scanmaster DX s.
scanned-slot detector s.
scanning beam digital s.
scattering s.
Scepter s.
Schatzker fracture classification s.
Schmidt optics s.
Schneider-Meier-Magnum s.
Scintiview nuclear computer s.
Scintron IV nuclear computer s.
ScleroLaser laser s.
ScleroPlus HP laser s.
ScleroPlus LongPulse dye laser s.
S660 coronary stent s.
Scorpio total knee s.
Scotchcast length splinting s.
Scott chronic wound care s.
Screw-Vent implant s.
SDI-BIOM wide angle viewing s.
Secca radiofrequency s.
Second Look CAD s.
Secor s.
SecureStrand cervical fusion s.
Secure Yet Gentle surgical
  dressing s.
Security clip enclosed carpal tunnel
  release s.
SeedNet s.
SeedNet cryotherapy s.
segmental spinal correction s.
segmented orthopaedic system total
  hip and knee s.
Selby I, II fixation s.
Selecta Duet combination laser s.
Selecta Duet glaucoma laser s.
Selecta Duo ophthalmic laser s.
Selecta 7000 glaucoma laser s.
Selecta II glaucoma laser s.
Selecta Trio glaucoma laser s.
Select GT blood glucose s.
selective tubal occlusion
  procedure s.
Selectron s.
Selenia imaging s.
selenium-based digital chest s.

selenium-drum-detector s.
Self-Cath closed catheterization s.
SenDx 100 blood gas and electrolyte analysis s.
Senographe 2000D digital mammography s.
Senographe 2000D mammography s.
Senographe DMRt mammography s.
Senographe DS mammography s.
SenoScan full-field digital imaging s.
SenoScan full-field digital mammography s.
SenoScan mammography s.
Sens-A-Ray dental imaging s.
Sens-A-Ray 2000 dental imaging s.
Sens-A-Ray digital dental imaging s.
SensiCath s.
SensiCath blood gas measurement s.
SensoScan mammography s.
Septi-Chek blood culture s.
Sequel compression s.
Sequenza immunostaining s.
Sequestra 1000 s.
Sequestra 1000 blood processing s.
Sequoia Acuson s.
Sequoia echocardiography s.
Sequoia ultrasound s.
SERFAS endoscopic s.
SeroJet needle-free injection s.
Seroma-Cath s.
Seroma-Cath wound drainage s.
Sextant II surgical instrumentation s.
Shadow-Line ACF spine retractor s.
Shape Maker s.
Sharplan sight s.
SharpShooter tissue repair s.
sheath and dilator s.
Sherlock bone screw suture/anchor s.
Sherman remote podiatric vacuum s.
Shiley catheter distention s.
Shimadzu HeadTome s.
Shimadzu ultrasound s.
Shuttle MiniClinic resistance s.
Shutt suture punch s.
SICOR recording s.
side branch occlusion s.
side-exiting coaxial s.
side-exiting coaxial needle s.
Siemens s.
Siemens AG s.

Siemens biplane Neurostar digital subtraction angiography s.
Siemens HICOR/BICOR x-ray s.
Siemens Mammomat Novation DM full field digital mammography s.
Siemens Neurostar digital subtraction angiographic s.
Siemens Somatom Plus-4 CT s.
Siemens Sonocur Basic extracorporeal shockwave therapy s.
Siemens Sonoline SI-400 ultrasound s.
Sigma II Dualplace hyperbaric oxygen therapy s.
Sigma II hyperbaric s.
Sigma I monoplace hyperbaric therapy s.
Sigma Plus monoplace hyperbaric oxygen therapy s.
Signa Advantage s.
Signa Excite s.
Signa Horizon LX MRI s.
Signa MR imaging s.
Signa OpenSpeed MR s.
Signa Ovation MR s.
Signature Edition infusion s.
Silent Speaker communication s.
Silhouette laser s.
Silhouette pedicle screw s.
Silhouette spinal s.
Silhouette therapeutic massage s.
SilkLaser aesthetic laser s.
SilverHawk plaque excision s.
Simcoe I&A s.
Simmons plating s.
Simplicity adult disposable contoured undergarment liner s.
SimpliCT interventional guidance s.
Simpson AtheroCath s.
Simpson Coronary AtheroCath s.
Simpson-Robert vascular dilation s.
Simpulse irrigation s.
Simpulse lavage s.
single-action pumping s.
single chamber cardiac pacing s.
single-incision s.
single patient s.
single-stick s.
SinuNEB sinus care s.
SinuScope s.
Sirecust 404N neonatal monitoring s.
Site-Rite II ultrasound s.
SiteSelect percutaneous incisional breast biopsy s.
SITEtrac spinal surgery s.
SJM Rosenkranz pediatric retractor s.

system *(continued)*

Skeeter otologic drill s.
SkinLaser s.
Sky-Boot stirrup s.
Sleepscan Traveler ambulatory
 polysomnography s.
Sleepscan Traveler home
 monitoring s.
Slim-LOC anterior cervical plate s.
slotted obturator-cannula s.
SLP1000 diode laser s.
SLS Chromos long-pulse ruby
 laser s.
Smart Balance Master s.
SmartCycler realtime PCR s.
SmartDose infusion s.
SmartKard digital Holter s.
SmartMist asthma management s.
SmartMist respiratory
 management s.
SmartSite needleless s.
SmartSPOT high-resolution digital
 imaging s.
Smart System irrigation/suction s.
SmiLine abutment s.
Smith & Nephew bracing and
 support s.
S-Monovette blood collection s.
SNPstream genotyping s.
Snuggle Warm convective
 warming s.
Snugs tapeless wound care s.
Socon spinal s.
Socrates telementoring s.
SOCS pad s.
Sodas spheroidal oral drug
 absorption s.
Soehendra catheter s.
Soehendra endoscopic biliary
 stent s.
SofWire cable s.
Sofflex mattress s.
SofPort easy-load lens delivery s.
Sof-Tact diabetes management s.
Softclamp s.
SoftLight laser hair removal s.
Soft & Secure spouted pouch s.
Sof'Wire cable s.
Solanas cervicothoracic fixation s.
Solcotrans autotransfusion s.
Solcotrans closed vacuum-
 drainage s.
Solcotrans drainage/reinfusion s.
Solcotrans orthopaedic drainage-
 refusion s.
Solight forceps lighting s.
SOLO-Surg Colorectal self-retaining
 retractor s.
Soma Gonio s.

Soma pulley s.
Somatom Volume Zoom computed
 tomography s.
Somatom Volume Zoom CT s.
Somnoplasty s.
Somnus somnoplasty s.
Sonablate 200 s.
Sonablate 200 ultrasound s.
Songer cable s.
sonic accelerated fracture healing s.
 (SAFHS)
Sonicaid S. 8000
SonicWAVE phacoemulsification s.
Sonifer sonicating s.
Sonoace 6000 II ultrasound s.
Sonocur extracorporeal shockwave
 therapy s.
SonoHeart Elite ultrasound s.
SonoHeart handheld all digital
 echocardiography s.
Sonoline Elegra ultrasound s.
Sonoline Sienna ultrasound s.
Sonoline Sierra ultrasound
 imaging s.
Sonoline SI-200/250 ultrasound
 imaging s.
Sonomed A/B-Scan s.
Sonomed A-Scan s.
Sonomed B-1500 s.
Sonoprobe endoscopic
 ultrasonography s.
Sonopsy biopsy imaging s.
Sonopsy ultrasound-guided breast
 biopsy s.
Sonos 4500 echocardiography s.
Sonos imaging s.
Sonos 500 imaging s.
SonoSite 180 ultrasound s.
SonoWand intraoperative imaging s.
SonoWand ultrasound-based
 neuronavigation s.
Soprano cryoablation s.
Sorbie-Questor total elbow
 prosthesis s.
Sorrells hip arthroplasty retractor s.
SOS total hip s.
SOS total knee s.
SourceLink brachytherapy
 delivery s.
Souter Strathclyde total elbow s.
Sovereign Shield s.
SPARC sling s.
SpaTouch PhotoEpilation S.
SPECT high-resolution brain s.
Spectra 400 extended surveillance
 and alert s.
Spectron EF total hip s.
Spectrum lens analysis s.
Spectrum tissue repair s.

specular reflection video-recording s.
Sperm Select sperm recovery s.
Spider cervical plating s.
Spiegelberg intracranial pressure monitoring s.
SpinaLase Nd:YAG surgical laser s.
spinal fusion s.
spinal screw and rod s.
SpineLink s.
SpineLink-II independent intrasegmental spine fixation s.
Spine-Six BioMotion spinal s.
spinopelvic transiliac fixation s.
SpiroSense s.
Spirosense s.
Spiros inhalation s.
SpiroVision-3 spirometry s.
Spline dental implant s.
SportCord exercise and rehabilitation s.
SportsRAC arm care s.
SPOT mobile 3D ultrasound s.
SprayGel adhesive barrier s.
Sprint fixed-detector research s.
Spy intraoperative imaging s.
square module seating s.
Squibb s.
Squirt wound irrigation s.
S-ROM hip replacement s.
S-ROM modular total knee s.
S-ROM proximally modular total hip s.
S-Series sleep s.
SSP s.
Stabident s.
Stability total hip s.
Stableloc external wrist fixation s.
Stableloc II external fixation s.
Stableloc II external fixator s.
STA Compact hemostasis s.
STA hemostasis s.
StairMaster exercise s.
STAN S 21 fetal heart rate s.
StarClose vascular closure s.
STA-R hemostasis s.
STARRT falloposcopy s.
Star S4 ActiveTrak 3D eye tracking s.
Star S3 ActiveTrak excimer laser s.
Star S4 excimer laser s.
Star S2 SmoothScan excimer laser s.
STart-4 clot detection s.
STart-8 clot detection s.
Statak anchor s.
STAT-Site M Hgb test s.

StayErec s.
Stealth image guided s.
StealthStation image-guided s.
StealthStation image-interactive s.
steerable guidewire s.
Steffee pedicle screw-plate s.
Steffee variable spine plating s.
Stelkast Supass acetabular s.
stem kit CD34+HPC enumeration s.
stent delivery s. (SDS)
stent and vent s.
Step laparoscopic entry s.
StereoGuide stereotactic breast biopsy s.
stereotactic breast biopsy s.
stereotactic surgical guidance s.
Stereotaxis magnetic surgery s.
Steritome microkeratome s.
1-stick s.
STIF s.
StIM s.
Stim neuromuscular stimulation s.
Stoller afferent nerve stimulation s. (SANS)
stone recognition s.
stone-tissue detection s.
stone-tissue recognition s.
Storz ceiling-mounted microscope s.
Storz ear, nose and throat camera s.
Storz-Hopkins s.
Storz Millennium microsurgical s.
Storz multifunction valve trocar/cannula s.
Straight-In male sling s.
Straight-In surgical s.
Strata hip s.
Stratis II MRI s.
Stratis ST ACL reconstruction s.
Straumann dental implant s.
Stretch-Rite exerciser s.
Stretta s.
Stryker Endoscopy radiofrequency ablation s. (SERFAS)
Stryker Inter-Lock screw and fixation s.
Stryker intracompartmental pressure monitor s.
Stryker-Leibinger Modular Internal Distraction s.
Stryker Patriot disposable cannula s.
Stryker suture slider s.
STS lithotripsy s.
SubVent implant s.
Summit occipito-cervico-thoracic spinal fixation s.
Summit SI OCT spinal fixation s.

S

system *(continued)*

Summit tapered hip s.
Sundt AVM microclip s.
Sundt slim-line aneurysm s.
Sundt slim-line mini-aneurysm clip s.
Sundt suction s.
Sunrise LTK s.
Sun SPARCstation s.
Super Angiorex model G DSA s.
Super-4 catheter ablation s.
superconducting open-magnet s.
superconductive MR s.
super long-pulse diode laser s.
supine C-Trax traction s.
Sure-Closure skin closure s.
Sure-Closure skin stretching s.
SureFold s.
SureScan s.
SureStart imaging s.
SureStep ankle support s.
SureStep Flexx professional blood glucose management s.
SureTrans autotransfusion s.
Surg-E-Trol I/A S.
surgical microscope navigator s.
surgical navigation s.
Surgi-PEG replacement gastrostomy feeding s.
SurgiScope image-guided s.
SurgiScope stereotactic s.
Surgi-Stim postsurgical therapy s.
Sustain dental implant s.
suture slider s.
Swift dynamic anterior cervical plate s.
SwimEx hydrotherapy s.
Swiss Precision cannula s.
S660 with Discrete Technology coronary stent s.
S670 with Discrete Technology coronary stent s.
swivel-arm s.
Symphony graft delivery s.
Symphony MR imaging s.
Symphony patient monitoring s.
Symphony platelet concentrate s.
Synaptic 2000 pain management s.
SynchroMed infusion s.
Synchron CX9 ALX clinical s.
Synchron CX clinical chemistry s.
Synchron CX4, CX5, CX9, CX500, CX1000 PRO clinical s.
Synchron CX3, CX4, CX5 Delta clinical s.
Synchron CX4, CX5, CX7 Super clinical s.
Synchron LX20 clinical s.
Synchron LX4201 clinical s.

Synchron LX clinical chemistry s.
Synchron LXi 725 clinical s.
Synchron LX20, LX2000 PRO clinical s.
Synergy hinge s.
Synergy neurostimulation s.
Synergy posterior titanium spinal s.
Synergy spine rehab s.
Synergy ultrasound s.
Synevac vacuum curettage s.
Synthes CerviFix s.
Synthes fixation s.
Synthes Schuhli implant s.
Synthes Universal spinal s.
Synthes universal spinal s.
syringe-driven s.
Sysmex HS-330 robotic hematology s.
Systec-like s.
System Alloclassic hip s.
TAG anchor s.
Talairach bicommissural reference s.
Talairach stereotactic s.
Talairach-Tournoux s.
Talent LPS endoluminal stent-graft s.
Talos stent delivery s.
Tamarack flexure joint s.
Tango SLT/YAG combination laser s.
Targis microwave catheter-based s.
Tarsys tilt and recline seating s.
TBird ventilator s.
TCD100M digital transcranial Doppler s.
TCI HeartMate left ventricular assist s.
TCI Heartmate mechanical circulatory support s.
TD Glucose Monitoring s.
TD glucose monitoring s.
Tebbetts EndoPlastic instrument s.
TEC atherectomy s.
Tech-Attach connection s.
TechMate 500 automated immunohistochemical s.
Techmedica CAD/CAM total temporomandibular joint reconstruction s.
Technolas 217 excimer laser s.
Technos ultrasound s.
Techstar percutaneous vascular surgery s.
Techstar XL percutaneous vascular surgery s.
Techstar XL percutaneous vascular surgical s.
Techstar XL PVS s.
TEC interface s.

Tecmag Libra-S16 s.
TEGwire ST s.
Telefactor beehive s.
telemanipulator s.
Telescale CHF patient home
  monitoring s.
Telescopic Plate Spacer spinal s.
Telocin diagnostic ultrasound s.
TempFix spanning knee external
  fixation s.
temporolimbic s.
temporomandibular joint metal-on-
  metal total joint replacement
  prosthesis s.
TenderWet s.
Terry-Schanzlin astigmatome s.
Terumo telescoping catheter s.
tesla s.
Testoderm testosterone
  transdermal s.
tetraONE s.
Tetrax interactive balance s.
Tewameter TM 210 open loop s.
Texas Scottish Rite Hospital hook-
  rod s.
Texas Scottish Rite Hospital screw-
  rod s.
ThAIRapy vest airway clearance s.
The Healthy Back S.
Theon mitral replacement s.
Therabath paraffin heat therapy s.
TheraBite jaw motion
  rehabilitation s.
Thera Cool cold therapy s.
Therakos UVAR s.
TheraPEP positive expiratory
  pressure therapy s.
Therasonics lithotripsy s.
TheraTest Laboratories EL-RF test
  kit s.
Thera-turn rotational s.
Thera-Wedge s.
Thermachoice uterine balloon
  therapy s.
thermal balloon s.
thermal dosimetry s.
ThermoChem-HT s.
ThermoFlex s.
ThermoFlo s.
TherOx Aqueous Oxygen s.
The Wave phacoemulsion s.
ThinPRep imaging s.
Thoracoport trocar s.
Thora-Klex chest drainage s.
Thoraseal chest tube drainage s.
Thoratec VAD s.
THORP s.
Thrombex PMT s.
Thumper CPR s.

Thumper 1007 CPR s.
tibial torsion s.
time-of-flight PET imaging s.
TiMesh craniofacial s.
TiMesh craniomaxillofacial
  plating s.
TiMesh LP cranial miniplate and
  screw s.
TiMesh midface and cranial s.
TiMesh rigid fixation bone
  plating s.
TiMesh titanium bone plating s.
TiMX low back s.
tissue anchor guide s.
titanium alloy screw and rod s.
titanium hollow screw plate s.
titanium micro s.
titanium Vortex Port s.
TMJ Concepts patient-fitted TMJ
  prosthesis s.
TMJ metal-on-metal total joint
  replacement prosthesis s.
TMS 3-dimensional radiation
  therapy treatment planning s.
TMS 1000 tachyarrhythmia
  monitoring s.
TMx-2000 BPH thermotherapy s.
Tomey topographic modeling s.
Tomey topography s.
Tomolex tomographic s.
Tomomatic 2-slice SPECT
  imaging s.
Tomomatic 3-slice SPECT
  imaging s.
Tomomatic 5-slice SPECT
  imaging s.
TomoTherapy Hi-ART s.
TomTec Imaging S.'s
Toomey tip s.
Topcon CM-1000 corneal
  mapping s.
Topcon IMAGEnet digital
  imaging s.
top-loading screw and rod s.
Top Notch automated biopsy s.
topographic scanning s.
TopSS/AngioScan s.
TopSS topographic scanning s.
Torus external fixation s.
Total Condylar Knee s.
total facet arthroplasty s. (TFAS)
Total O_2 delivery s.
Total O_2/Oxilite oxygen s.
Total O_2 supplementary oxygen s.
Total Recall digital imaging s.
Total Synchrony s.
Trake-Fit s.
Tranquility Auto CPAP s.
Tranquility bilevel s.

system *(continued)*

Tranquility Quest CPAP s.
transesophageal pacing s.
TransFix ACL s.
TransFix ACL reconstruction s.
transluminal lysing s.
Transonics s.
TransScan electrical impedance breast scanning s.
TransScan electrical impedance scanning s.
transtelephonic ambulatory monitoring s.
Trap cardiovascular filtration s.
Trap neurovascular filtration s.
Trap vascular filtration s.
trauma care s.
TraumaJet wound debridement s.
Traveler portable oxygen s.
Trex digital mammography s.
TriActiv balloon-protected flush extraction s.
TriActiv embolic protection s.
Triad defibrillator s.
Triad SPECT imaging s.
Triage cardiac s.
Triage cardiac rapid diagnostic test s.
triangle blade s.
Triax monotube external fixation s.
tricomponent coaxial s.
Trident ceramic hip s.
Trilogy AB acetabular s.
Trilogy acetabular cup s.
Trilogy image-guided radiation therapy s.
Trilogy image-guided radiosurgery s.
Trim-It screw s.
Tri-Motion knee s.
Trinity polyaxial pedicle screw s.
Trio medialized rod s.
triple-lumen perfused catheter s.
TriTis tibial fixation s.
TriVex s.
trocar-cannula s.
TroGARD electrosurgical blunt trocar s.
TRON 3 VACI cardiac imaging s.
True/Fit femoral intramedullary rod s.
True/Flex intramedullary rod s.
True-Lok external fixator s.
TrueMax metabolic measuring s.
Trufill n-BCA liquid embolic s.
TruPulse CO2 laser s.
TruTrak data sampling s.
TS s.
TSRH fixation s.
TSRH screw-rod s.
T-Tac s.
Tulip syringe s.
TUNA s.
turbine-powered ICU ventilator s.
Turbo 7000 s.
TurnAide therapeutic s.
Tylok high-tension cable s.
Tylok high-tension cerclage cabling s.
UBP s.
UlcerJet high-pressure fluid jet s.
Ulson fixator s.
Ultima hip replacement s.
Ultima II refrigerator s.
Ultima mammography s.
Ultima OPCAB s.
Ultima total hip s.
Ultimax distal femoral intramedullary rod s.
Ultimax Haig II nail s.
Ultrabag dialysis s.
Ultra-Drive bone cement removal s.
Ultra-Drive ultrasonic revision s.
UltraFine erbium laser s.
UltraFix MiniMite suture anchor s.
UltraFix RC suture anchor s.
UltraFix rotator cuff suture anchor s.
Ultraflex esophageal stent s.
Ultraflex stent delivery s.
Ultra-Guard FS hip bracing s.
Ultra-Guard hip orthosis s.
UltraLite headlight s.
UltraLite One-Piece convex-disposable s.
Ultramark ultrasound s.
UltraPACS diagnostic imaging s.
UltraPak enteral closed feeding s.
UltraPower basic drill s.
UltraPower bur guard drill s.
UltraPower drill s.
UltraPower revision drill s.
UltraPulse SurgiTouch CO2 laser s.
Ultraseed s.
ultrasonic retroprep s.
ultrasound s.
ultrasound biomicroscope s.
UltraSTAR computer-based ultrasound reporting s.
UltraSure DTR-1 imaging ultrasound s.
Ultra Twin bag s.
UltraVent radioaerosol delivery s.
Ultra-X external fixation s.
Ultra Y-set s.
UMC-I microwave delivery s.
underwater drainage s.

Unfolder Sapphire implantation s.
unicompartmental knee s.
Uniflex nailing s.
Uni-frame patient immobilization s.
Unilink s.
Unilink hand surgery s.
UniPlast Imaging and Archiving s.
Uniportal fascial release s.
UniPulse surgical CO_2 laser s.
Uni-Shunt hydrocephalus shunt s.
Unistep Plus delivery s.
UniSyn modular hip s.
United Sonics J shock phaco
  fragmentor s.
Unitek I convoluted innerspring
  mattress s.
Uni-Thread versatile thoracolumbar
  spinal s.
Unitrax unipolar s.
Universal bone plate s.
Universal bone screw
  insertion/extraction s.
Universal cannulated screw s.
Universal F breathing s.
Universal Hand S.
Universal Plus instrument s.
Universal sheath s.
Universal Spine S.
Univision echocardiographic s.
Unopette s.
Up and About s.
uPACS picture archiving s.
UPlink point-of-care sample
  testing s.
Uretex self-anchoring urethral
  support s.
Uretex TO urethral support s.
Uriscreen bacteriuria detection s.
Urocyte diagnostic cytometry s.
urodynamic measurement s.
Uro-jet delivery s.
Urolab Janus S. III
Uro-Pak s.
Urotract x-ray s.
Urovision ultrasound imaging s.
UroVive self-contained balloon s.
USCI Probe balloon-on-a-wire
  dilatation s.
UVAR photophoresis s.
Uvar photophoresis s.
VAC Freedom s.
Vac-Lok patient immobilization s.
Vacutainer s.
vacuum-assisted venous return s.
vacuum cassette s.
Valleylab CUSA CEM s.
Valleylab REM s.
Valley Vac smoke evacuation s.
Vanguard M unicondylar s.

Vanguard PFR s.
Vapor-Phase heated
  humidification s.
Vapotherm oxygen delivery s.
Vapr s.
Varian brachytherapy s.
Varian MLC s.
VariCare pulsed lavage s.
VariGrip spine fixation s.
Vari-Lase endovenous laser s.
VasoView balloon dissection s.
VasoView Uniport endoscopic
  saphenous vein harvesting s.
VAX 4100 s.
V-beam pulsed dye laser s.
VDD pacing s.
Vector II guide s.
Vector low back analysis s.
VectorVision image-guided
  surgery s.
VectorVision surgical tracking s.
VectorVision Uni-Knee s.
Vectra Genisys laser s.
Velocity-U digital imaging s.
VenaFlow compression s.
VenaFlow DVT prophylaxis s.
Venodyne compression s.
Venodyne external pneumatic
  compression s.
Ventak Prizm 2 s.
Ventak PRx defibrillation s.
Ventak PRx III/Endotak s.
Ventex wound dressing s.
ventilator s.
Ventritex TVL s.
Ventrix tunnelable ventricular
  intracranial pressure monitoring s.
VentTrak monitoring s.
Venturi-Flo valve s.
Venus-i laser s.
Veris III s.
Veristat fluid management s.
Verruca-Freeze freezing s.
Versaback back s.
Versa-Fx femoral hip fixation s.
Versajet hydrosurgery s.
Versalok low back fixation s.
Versapoint s.
Versaport trocar s.
Versascope hysteroscopy s.
VersaStep laparoscopy s.
Versatone perioperative Doppler s.
VerSys hip s.
VertAlign spinal support s.
vertebral artery s.
Vertetrac ambulatory traction s.
Vertex reconstruction s.
Vesica press-in suture anchor s.
vesicular transport s.

system *(continued)*

vessel occlusion s.
VestaBlate s.
Vet-Co vacuum s.
ViaCath computer-assisted robotic
  endoluminal s.
Viagraph ECG s.
Viatronix virtual colonoscopy s.
Vicon 3-dimensional gait
  analysis s.
VidaMed TUNA s.
VID 1 color microcamera s.
video imaging s.
ViewPoint CK s.
view shadow projection
  microtomographic s.
Vigilance monitoring s.
Vilex bone staple s.
Vilex cannulated screw s.
Vilex CHI s.
Vingmed CFM echocardiographic s.
Vingmed CFM ultrasound s.
Vingmed Sound CFM ultrasound s.
ViraType in situ s.
Viridia telemetry s.
Viridis laser s.
ViroSeq HIV-1 genotyping s.
virtual biopsy s.
virtual retinal display s.
Virtuoso imaging s.
Virtuoso LX Smart CPAP s.
Virtuoso portable 3D imaging s.
Visage cosmetic surgery s.
Visa Iris s.
Visica treatment s.
Vision blood cardioplegia s.
Vision Master excimer laser s.
Vision MR imaging s.
Vision Sciences flexible
  sigmoidoscope s.
Visitec surgical vitrectomy s.
Vista radiolucentinterbody fusion s.
visual-evoked response imaging s.
Visupac digital s.
Visx 20/20 s.
Visx Star 3 excimer laser s.
Visx Star II stromal
  photoablation s.
Visx Star S2 excimer laser s.
Visx Twenty/Twenty s.
Visx Wavefront s.
Visx WaveScan wavefront s.
VitalStim Therapy electrical
  stimulation s.
Vitatron pacing s.
Vitek-Kent hemi TMJ
  replacement s.
Vitek-Kent total TMJ
  replacement s.

Vitrea 3D s.
Vivonex Acutrol enteral feeding s.
VNUS closure s.
Vocare bladder s.
voice restoration s.
Voluson ultrasound s.
Vornado air quality s.
Vortex port s.
Vortex stabilization s.
VoxelView s.
VPAP II ST ventilatory support s.
VPI nonadhesive colostomy s.
VPI nonadhesive ileostomy s.
VPI nonadhesive urostomy s.
VSF fixation s.
V-sign single-ear sensory s.
V-tunnel drill s.
VueLock anterior cervical spine s.
VuePASS portal access surgical s.
Wagner revision hip s.
WalkAide s.
Wallaby II phototherapy s.
Wallach ophthalmic cryosurgery s.
Wallstent endoprosthesis with
  Unistep Plus delivery s.
Wampole Isolater blood culture s.
WarmTouch patient warming s.
Warm-Up active wound therapy s.
Warm-Up wound care s.
water-based tinting s.
Waterlase Millennium laser s.
WaveMap intracoronary blood
  pressure measurement s.
Wave nucleic acid fragment
  analysis s.
WaveScan Wavefront s.
WaveWire intracoronary blood
  pressure measurement s.
WavSTAT optical biopsy s.
Wedge TAG suture anchor s.
Welch Allyn ear wash s.
Welch Allyn/Schiller AT-10
  Exercise Testing s.
Wheeler cyclodialysis s.
White s.
WhiteStar power modulation s.
whole-body MR imaging s.
W&H surgical s.
Wiktor GX Hepamed coated
  coronary stent s.
Wiktor GX Hepamed coronary
  stent s.
Wiktor Prime coronary stent s.
Wiltse pedicle screw fixation s.
Wingspan self-expanding stent s.
Winquist tibial/femoral extraction s.
Wisconsin spinal fracture s.
Wolf aspiration/injection s.
Wolf delivery s.

Wound Stick measuring s.
Wrightlock posterior fixation s.
Wrightlock spinal fixation s.
WrisTimer carpal tunnel support s.
Würzburg fracture s.
Würzburg maxillofacial plating s.
Würzburg reconstruction s.
WuScope s.
Xact ACL graft fixation s.
xenon illumination s.
Xerox dental radiographic
  imaging s.
Xia hook s.
Xia hook/spinal s.
Xia spinal s.
Xillix LIFE-GI fluorescence
  endoscopy s.
Xillix LIFE-Lung s.
Xillix LIFE-Lung fluorescence
  endoscopy s.
XKnife stereotactic radiosurgery s.
Xplorer digital imaging s.
X-PRESS vascular closure s.
XPS 3000 powered ENT s.
XPS shaver s.
XPS Straightshot s.
x-ray shadow projection
  microtomographic s.
Xsensor pressure mapping s.
X-Sizer single-use catheter s.
X-Spine Capless polyaxial pedicle
  screw s.
X-Stop IPD s.
Xtrac laser s.
X-Tube retraction s.
XYZ lead s.
YAGLazr s.
Yellow IRIS s.
Y-knot tying s.
Y-set s.
ZAAG bone anchoring s.
ZAAG implant s.
Zaldivar limbal-relaxing incision s.

Zassi bowel management s.
Zeiss DAS-1 hydrophobic s.
Zeiss fiberoptic illumination s.
Zeiss fluorescein filter s.
Zeiss stereotactic tool navigator s.
Zenith AAA endovascular graft s.
Zenith abdominal aortic aneurysm
  endovascular graft s.
Zenith electrotherapy ultrasound s.
Zephir anterior cervical plate s.
Zeppelin micromotor s.
Zest Anchor Advanced Generation
  bone anchoring s.
Zeus s.
Zeus computer-controlled robotic s.
Zeus voice-controlled robotic s.
Zimmer anatomic hip s.
Zimmer anatomic hip prosthesis s.
Zimmer collarless polished taper
  hip s.
Zimmer CPT hip s.
Zimmer crossover instrumentation s.
Zimmer hip implant s.
Zimmer Pulsavac wound
  débridement s.
Zimmer Tharies surface
  arthroplasty s.
ZMR hip s.
Zone Specific II meniscal repair s.
Z stent esophageal
  endoprosthesis s.
Zuni exercise s.
Zweymuller hip s.
Zyoptix excimer laser s.
system/catheter
  RPM tracking s./c.
systemic arterial catheter
System-Loc back brace
SyvekPatch
Syvek Patch closure device
Szabo-Berci needle driver
Szulc orbital implant material

S

T

tonometer
T adapter
T band
T bandage
T bar
T clamp
T connector
T drain
T lens
T stent
T tube

T2-weighted scan

TA

TA II loading unit
TA metallic staple
TA stapling device

T&A

tonsillectomy and adenoidectomy

TA-55 stapler

tab

T. Grabber
vitrectomy prism lens t.

Tabb crura tissue forceps

table

Adapta physical therapy t.
Advocate electric flexion
 distraction t.
Air-Drop chiropractic t.
Air-Flex chiropractic t.
Akron tilt t.
Allen hand/arm surgery t.
AlphaStar operating room t.
American Chiropractic College of
 Radiology adjusting t.
American Sterilizer operating t.
AMIS extension t.
AM-MI orthopaedic t.
Anatomotor traction/massage t.
Andrews spinal surgery t.
Andrews SST-3000 spinal
 surgery t.
Apollo TM electric flexion t.
APS Hi-Lo electric lift t.
ATT-300 LAT traction t.
back t.
Back Specialist chiropractic t.
Back Specialist electric t.
Back Specialist manual t.
bariatric mat t.
t. binding
body t.
bracket t.
chemonucleolysis t.
Chick CLT operating t.

Chick-Langren t.
Chick surgical t.
Chiro-Manis chiropractic t.
chiropractic t.
circumductor t.
craniosacral t.
crank t.
Crystal adjusting t.
cutout t.
cystoscopy t.
DC-101 chiropractic t.
DDP t.
DeLorme t.
DePuy graft preparation t.
Diamond biomechanical t.
Dornier Urotract cystoscopy t.
drop-piece t.
dual lookup t.
Ergo style flexion t.
Eurotech Diamond t.
Eurotech Emerald t.
Eurotech Platinum t.
Eurotech Sapphire t.
EX-OP operating t.
EZ Lift t.
EZ-Up inversion t.
flexion-distraction chiropractic t.
floating t.
fracture t.
friction-reduced examination t.
friction-reduced segmented t.
Galaxy 900HS adjusting t.
Galaxy McManis hylo t.
Gemini chiropractic t.
Gerhardt t.
harmonic attenuation t.
Hawley t.
t. heating pad
Hercules TM drop-adjusting t.
Hessco 300, 500 series
 hydrotherapy t.
Hill Air-Drop HA90C t.
Hill Air-Flex t.
hi lo t.
HiLo MultiPro t.
HLT-405 instrument adjusting t.
horseshoe therapy t.
Hydradjust IV t.
hydromassage t.
intersegmental traction
 chiropractic t.
Jackson spinal surgery and
 imaging t.
Jackson spine t.
knavel t.

T

table *(continued)*
    Leander chiropractic t.
    Leander motorized flexion t.
    Legend Hy-Lo adjusting t.
    lithotripsy t.
    Lloyd chiropractic t.
    Lloyd flexion distraction t.
    long axis traction chiropractic t.
    Magnum 101 Plus t.
    Maquet operating t.
    Massage Time Pro hydromassage t.
    mat t.
    Mayo instrument t.
    McKee t.
    McKenzie Repex t.
    Meridian intersegmental t.
    Midland tilt t.
    MobiTrak automated t.
    MobiTrak moving t.
    Multi-Lock hand operating t.
    MultiPro t.
    music vibration t.
    Orthostar surgical t.
    over-bed t.
    Paris manual therapy t.
    passive traction t.
    pedestal massage t.
    PET/Eurotech Generation 2000 t.
    physical therapy t.
    pivoting t.
    Platinum stationary t.
    Powermatic t.
    Protege manual flexion
      distraction t.
    PRO traction t.
    PT tilt t.
    Rath treatment t.
    Re-Lax-O chiropractic t.
    resistive exercise t.
    Roto Rest delta kinetic therapy
      treatment t.
    Sapphire t.
    Siemens open heart t.
    Simply Wet t.
    Sister Helen mustard t.
    Skytron operating room t.
    Skytron surgical t.
    slatted plinth t.
    spica t.
    Stryker fracture t.
    Sugita microsurgical t.
    Telos fracture t.
    t. tie
    tilt t.
    Titan Apollo electric flexion t.
    Titan Meridian Intersegmental
      Traction t.
    Titan Nova manual flexion-
      extension multi flex t.
    Titan Nova manual flexion-
      extension multiflex t.
    Topaz manual flexion t.
    traction t.
    traction t.
    treatment t.
    Tri W-G t.
    T-shaped Edwards-Barbaro syringeal
      shunt t.
    Urodiagnost x-ray t.
    VAX-D therapy t.
    Verteflex intersegmental traction t.
    Williams t.
    Williams Advantage t.
    Winco folding treatment t.
    600XLE mobile surgery t.
    Zenith ACS t.
    Zenith chiropractic t.
    Zenith-Cox flexion/distraction t.
    Zenith Hylos t.
    Zenith stationary t.
    Zenith Thompson t.
    Zenith Verti-Lift t.
    Zodiac TM manual flexion-
      distraction t.
table-fixed retractor
tabletop
    auxiliary CT t.
Tabs Elite mobility monitor
Tab-Strap knee immobilizer
Tachdjian orthosis
Tach-EZ dental attachment
tachistoscope
tachycardia
    atrioventricular t. (AVT)
tachycardia-terminating pacemaker
Tacit threaded anchor
tack
    Ace bone screw t.
    Bankart t.
    biodegradable surgical t.
    Graftac absorbable skin t.
    membrane t.
    SmartTack t.
    titanium t.
    titanium retinal t.
tack-and-pin forceps
Tacker
    Origin T.
Tacoma sacral plate
Tactaid
    T. hearing aid
    T. I vibrotactile aid
Tacticon
    T. peripheral neuropathy kit
    T. peripheral neuropathy screening
      device
tactile probe
Tactyl 1 glove

TADcath temporary transvenous
  defibrillation catheter
TAG
    tissue anchor guide
        TAG anchor system
        TAG Excluder stent
        TAG instrumentation
tag
        Gore-Tex t.
        H-shaped tilt t.
        Smart Tag triage t.
Tagarno 3SD cineangiography projector
Tago diagnostic kit
Tahoe Surgical Instruments ligature
taiki magnet
4-tailed
        4-t. bandage
        4-t. dressing
Takahashi
        T. cutting forceps
        T. ethmoidal forceps
        T. iris retractor forceps
        T. nasal forceps
Takara
        T. Biomedicals One-Step RNA
          PCR kit
        T. Biomedicals Suprec tube
Takata laser
take-apart
        t.-a. forceps
        t.-a. instrument
        t.-a. scissors
TakeOff elbow support
Take-Out Extractor
Talairach
        T. bicommissural reference system
        T. stereotactic frame
        T. stereotactic system
Talairach-Tournoux system
Talent
        T. bifurcated abdominal aortic stent
          graft
        T. bifurcated endograft
        T. LPS endoluminal stent-graft
          system
        T. stent graft
talipes hobble splint
Tall-ette toilet seat
Talon
        T. balloon dilatation catheter
        T. compression hip screw
Talos stent delivery system
Tamarack
        T. flexure joint
        T. flexure joint system
tamp
        bone t.
        CPT revision t.
        inflatable bone t. (IBT)

        interbody graft t.
        Kiene bone t.
        KyphX Xpander inflatable bone t.
        Richards t.
tamper
        McIntyre suture t.
tampon
        Corner t.
        t. forceps
        Merocel t.
        nasal t.
        Trendelenburg t.
tamponade
        balloon t.
        cardiac t.
        esophageal balloon t.
        nasal t.
        postnasal balloon t.
        vaselinized nasal t.
T-AnastoFlo shunt
tandem
        t. applicator
        T. cardiac device
        t. connector
        Fletcher-Suit afterloading t.
        Fletcher-Suit-Delclos t.
        t. and ovoid
        t. scanning confocal microscope
        t. scanning microscope
        t. stent
        T. thin-shaft transureteroscopic
          balloon dilatation catheter
        T. XL triple-lumen ERCP cannula
TandemHeart pVAD
Tandem-R
        T.-R assay kit
        T.-R Ostase osteoporosis test
tangent
        T. posterior impacted instrument
          set
        t. screen
        T. spinal instrumentation
tangential
        t. forceps
        t. occlusion clamp
        t. port
Tango SLT/YAG combination laser
  system
Tang retractor
Tanita professional body composition
  analyzer
tank
        Hubbard t.
        Hubbard hydrotherapy t.
        oxygen t.
        therapy t.
Tanne corneal punch
Tannenbaum stent

Tanner
   T. mesher
   T. mesher device
Tanner-Vandeput mesh dermatome
Tano
   T. device
   T. diamond-dusted needle
   T. double-mirror peripheral
     vitrectomy lens
   T. eraser
   T. membrane scraper
   T. microserrated forceps
   T. ring
   T. scraper
Tan spatula
tantalum
   t. ball marker
   t. balloon-expandable stent
   t. clip
   t. gauze
   t. hemostasis clip
   t. mesh
   t. mesh eye implant
   t. mesh implant
   t. O ring
   t. plate
   t. ring
   t. stent
   t. wire
   t. wire stent
tantalum-178 generator
tantalum-ball marker
tap
   t. drill
   T. N' Tones
   screw t.
   4-t. screw
   t. water wet dressing
tape
   Aquasorb Border with Covaderm t.
   Aris transobturator t.
   Blenderm t.
   t. board
   Broselow t.
   Broselow emergency t.
   Broselow pediatric resuscitative t.
   brow t.
   Cath-Secure t.
   Coban t.
   CollaTape t.
   ColorZone t.
   Dacron retraction t.
   Deknatel wound t.
   Deknatel wound closure t.
   Delta-Lite casting t.
   Dermicare hypoallergenic paper t.
   Dermicel t.
   Dermicel hypoallergenic cloth t.
   Dermicel hypoallergenic knitted t.

Dermiclear t.
Dermiform hypoallergenic knitted t.
Dermiview hypoallergenic
  transparent t.
Dissolve-A-Way t.
DynaSport athletic t.
Elastikon elastic t.
EnduraFIX t.
EnduraSPORTS t.
EnduraTape t.
fiberglass-free cast t.
foam t.
Gulick II t.
Haelan t.
Hypafix retention t.
Hy-Tape latex-free surgical t.
Hy-Tape surgical t.
Hy-Tape waterproof adhesive t.
instrument coding t.
Johnson & Johnson waterproof t.
lap t.
LeMaitre Glow 'N Tell t.
Leukotape P sports t.
Leukotape sports t.
t. marker
Medipore H soft cloth surgical t.
Medipore H surgical t.
Mefix adhesive t.
Megazinc Pink adhesive t.
Mepitac soft silicone t.
Mersilene t.
Micropore t.
3M matrix t.
3M Micropore surgical t.
Omnifix t.
Original Pink Tape waterproof
  adhesive t.
Polyderm border with Covaderm t.
Powerflex t.
Ramirez EndoPlastic t.
Scanpor t.
Scanpor surgical t.
Scotchcast 2 cast t.
silastic t.
sports t.
Sta-Fix t.
surgical t.
tension-free vaginal t.
Transpore eye t.
TufStuf II cast t.
twill t.
umbilical t.
vascular t.
Zonas porous t.

taper
   collarless polished t.
   Eurotaper 12/14 t.
   fiber metal t.
   funnelform t.

t. hand file
laser t.
Morse t.
t. needle
short t.
VerSys fiber metal t.

Tapercut
T. needle
T. suture
taper-cut needle
tapered
t. blade
t. brain spatula
t. catheter
t. core guidewire
t. fissure bur
t. Micro-Vent implant
t. needle
t. pin
t. reamer
tapered-shaft punctum plug
tapered-spring needle holder
tapered-tip
t.-t. dilator
t.-t. ear syringe
t.-t. guidewire
t.-t. hydrophilic-coated push catheter
Tapered Torque guidewire
taper-jaw
t.-j. forceps
t.-j. rongeur
Taperloc
T. femoral component
T. femoral stem
Taper-Lock external hex implant
taper-point suture needle
Taperseal hemostatic device
taping
low-dye t.
prophylactic t.
tapper
3-I t.
round t.
tapping hammer
Tapscope esophageal pacing stethoscope
Taq
T. DyeDeoxy Terminator Cycle Sequencing kit
T. extender
T. Master Mix kit
TAR-200 dual-channel electronystagmograph
TARA total hip prosthesis
Tarbell-Loeffler-Cosman frame
Tardy osteotome
Targa+ image capture board
target
Air Force test grid t.
T. prosthesis

T. Therapeutics Stealth angioplasty balloon
von Graefe t.
targeted cryoablation device
targeter
bone screw t.
IMP bone screw t.
targeting drill guide
Targis microwave catheter-based system
Tarkington urethral stent
Tarnier
T. axis traction forceps
T. cephalotribe
T. cranioclast
T. obstetrical forceps
tarsal bar
tarsoconjunctival composite graft
Tarsys tilt and recline seating system
Tasserit shoulder attachment
tattoo
Derma-Tattoo surgical t.
t. needle
tattooing needle
Taub minute stain kit
Taut
T. capillary drain
T. cholangiographic catheter
T. cystic duct catheter
T. M55, M56, M57 catheter
T. percutaneous introducer
Taveras injector
tax double needle
Taxus Express stent
Taylor
T. brain scissors
T. Britetrac retractor
T. catheter holder
T. dissecting forceps
T. dural scissors
T. gastric balloon
T. gastroscope
T. percussion hammer
T. reflex hammer
T. spinal frame
T. spinal retractor
T. spinal retractor blade
T. spine brace
T. splint
T. thoracolumbosacral orthosis
T. tissue forceps
Taylor-Knight brace
T-bar
T-b. immobilization device
T-b. retractor
T-Bar trigger point massager
T-binder
TBird
T. ventilator
T. ventilator system

931

T-buttress plate
T-C
>T-C needle holder
>T-C pin cutter
>T-C ring-handle pin and wire extractor

TC62
>oligonucleotide probe T.

TC7 adhesion barrier
TCCK unconstrained knee prosthesis
TC CO₂ monitor
TCD
>transcranial Doppler
>Multigon 500M non-contrast-enhanced TCD

TCD100M digital transcranial Doppler system
TCFO placement wand
TCI
>TCI HeartMate left ventricular assist system
>TCI Heartmate mechanical circulatory support system
>TCI OcuLook saliva ovulation tester kit
>TCI OvuLook ovulation tester

TCM30 transcutaneous oxygen monitor
TCOM
>transcutaneous oxygen monitor

TCR Vgamma9 test
TCT900S helical CT scanner
TD
>TD Glucose meter
>TD Glucose Monitoring system
>TD glucose monitoring system

TDX analyzer
TDxFlx analyzer
Teale
>T. tenaculum forceps
>T. uterine forceps
>T. vulsellum forceps

tear
>t. duct tube
>t. strip
>t. test strip
>t. trough-style implant

tear-away introducer sheath
teardrop dissector
TearSaver punctum plug
Tearscope
>Keeler T.
>T. Plus photographer
>T. Plus tear film kit

tear-strength eugenol-based sealer
Teaser device
teaspoon
>nylon t.

Tebbetts
>T. EndoPlastic instrument system

>T. rhinoplasty set
>T. ribbon retractor

TEC
>TEC atherectomy device
>TEC atherectomy system
>TEC extraction catheter
>TEC guide catheter
>TEC interface system
>TEC liner

TEC-2100 postioning laser
Teca Sapphire EMG machine
TECA-TD20 EMG machine
TEC-guide catheter
Tech-Attach connection system
TechLite lancet
TechMate
>T. 500 automated immunohistochemical system
>T. 500 automatic immunostaining device
>T. 1000 immunostainer

Techmedica
>T. CAD/CAM total temporomandibular joint reconstruction system
>T. implant
>T. prosthesis

TechneScan MAG-3
technetium H2 autoanalyzer
technetium-99m generator
technical biomaterial
Technicare
>T. camera
>T. Delta 2020 scanner

Techni-Care wound cleanser
TechnoGel insole
Technolas
>T. 217 excimer laser
>T. 217 excimer laser system
>T. 217 laser
>T. 217z excimer laser

technology
>Kumetrix microneedle t.
>Surgical Laser T.'s (SLT)
>virtual reality t.

Technomed
>T. C-Scan
>T. C-scan videokeratoscope

Technos ultrasound system
Technovit
>T. acrylic resin
>T. 7210 VLC contact glue

Techstar
>T. device
>T. percutaneous closure device
>T. percutaneous vascular surgery system
>T. suturing closure device

T. XL percutaneous vascular
surgery system
T. XL percutaneous vascular
surgical system
T. XL PVS system
Teclite fiberoptic light source
Tecmag
T. Libra-S16 system
T. Libra-S16 system scanner
Tecnis
T. acrylic IOL
T. foldable intraocular lens
T. foldable IOL
T. Z9000 lens
Tecnol
T. ankle support
T. elbow support
T. knee support
T. wrist support
tectal plate
Tectonic magnet
TED
TED antiembolism stocking
TED hose
Tedlar bag
Tefcat intrauterine insemination catheter
TefGen-FD
T.-FD guided tissue regeneration
membrane
T.-FD plastic membrane
TefGen regenerative membrane
Teflon
T. Bardic plug
T. block
T. catheter
T. clip
T. collar button
T. dilator
T. fascial dilator
T. felt
T. felt bolster
T. felt patch
T. graft
T. guiding catheter
T. implant
T. injection catheter
T. injector
T. intracardiac patch
T. iris retractor
T. liner
T. mesh
T. mesh implant
T. mold
T. needle catheter
T. orbital floor implant
T. piston
T. plate
T. pledget
T. pledget suture buttress

T. plug
T. probe
T. pyeloureteral catheter
T. sheath
T. sheet
T. sponge
T. stent
T. strut
T. trileaflet prosthesis
woven T.
T. woven prosthesis
Teflon-coated
T.-c. driver
T.-c. guidewire
T.-c. hollow-bore needle
T.-c. needle
T.-c. suture
T.-c. wire
T.-c. wire skeleton
Teflon-covered needle
Teflon-pledgeted suture
Teflon-Proplast TMJ implant
Teflon-tipped catheter
Tegaderm
T. dressing
T. HP transparent film
T. occlusive dressing
T. semipermeable dressing
T. semipermeable occlusive dressing
T. transparent dressing
T. transparent dressing with
absorbent pad
Tegagel
T. hydrogel
T. hydrogel dressing
T. hydrogel sheet
Tegagen
T. HG, HI alginate wound cover
T. HG, HI alginate wound
dressing
Tegam microprocessor thermometer
Tegapore contact layer sheet
Tegasorb
T. dressing
T. occlusive dressing
T. Thin hydrocolloid
T. Thin hydrocolloid dressing
T. ulcer dressing
Tegress endoscopic urethral implant
TEGwire
T. balloon
T. ST system
Tel-Shin
Tek-Clear accommodating intraocular lens
Tekscan in-shoe monitoring device
Tektronix
T. digital oscilloscope

933

Tektronix *(continued)*
    T. digital phonometer
    T. 2214 oscilloscope
Tel-A-Fever forehead thermometer
Telangitron device
telebinocular
telecentric fundus camera
Telectronics
    T. Accufix pacing lead
    T. ATP implantable cardioverter-
      defibrillator
    T. Guardian ATP 4210 device
    T. Guardian ATP II ICD
    T. pacemaker
Teledyne Water Pik misting massage
Telefactor beehive system
telemanipulator system
telemeter
telemetric intracranial pressure sensor
telemonitor
    Physios CTM 01 noninvasive t.
TelePACS
telephone probe
**Telescale CHF patient home monitoring
system**
telescope
    ACMI microlens Foroblique t.
    angled t.
    biopsy t.
    bioptic t.
    bronchoscopic t.
    catheterizing Foroblique t.
    convertible t.
    30-degree t.
    70-degree t.
    direct-vision t.
    endoscopic t.
    Eschenbach monocular t.
    examining t.
    fiberoptic right-angle t.
    foroblique bronchoscopic t.
    High-Vision surgical t.
    Hopkins t.
    Hopkins direct-vision t.
    Hopkins forward oblique t.
    Hopkins lateral t.
    Hopkins nasal endoscopy t.
    Hopkins pediatric t.
    Hopkins retrospective t.
    Hopkins rigid t.
    Hopkins rod-lens t.
    implantable miniature t.
    implantable miniaturized t.
    infant t.
    Keeler panoramic surgical t.
    Kramer direct-vision t.
    laryngeal-bronchial t.
    lateral microlens t.
    Lumina operating t.

    Luxtec illuminated surgical t.
    McCarthy foroblique operating t.
    McCarthy miniature t.
    Microlens foroblique t.
    nasal t.
    nasal endoscopic t.
    pediatric t.
    retrospective bronchoscopic t.
    right-angle bronchoscopic t.
    right-angle examining t.
    solid-rod rigid t.
    spectacle-mounted t.
    stop collar t.
    Storz-Hopkins t.
    straight-ahead bronchoscopic t.
    surgical t.
    Surgi-Spec t.
    transilluminating t.
    Zeiss binocular prism t.
telescopic
    t. aerial dilator
    t. bougie set
    t. plate spacer
    T. Plate Spacer spinal system
    t. spectacles
    t. view guide
telescoping
    t. brace
    t. guide
    t. plugged catheter
    t. rod
    t. tubular device
Telestill photo adapter
Telethermometer
    YSI T.
Telfa
    T. adhesive pad
    T. bolster
    T. Clear contact layer sheet
    T. Clear nonadherent wound
      dressing
    T. composite dressing
    T. gauze
    T. gauze dressing
    T. island dressing
    T. plastic film dressing
    T. Plus barrier island dressing
    T. sponge
    T. strip
    T. 4 x 4 bandage
    T. Xtra barrier island dressing
Telfamax absorptive dressing
TeliCam intraoral camera
Teller acuity card
Telocin diagnostic ultrasound system
Telos
    T. fracture table
    T. radiographic stress device

Temno
- T. biopsy needle
- T. II cutting needle

TEMoo mode beam laser

Temp
- T. Tip drainage catheter
- T. Tip ureteral stent

Tempa-DOT single-use clinical thermometer

Temp-a-dot thermometer

Temper
- T. Foam cube
- T. Foam cushion
- T. foam sheet

temperature
- t. exchange apparatus
- t. and galvanic skin response biofeedback device
- t. probe

temperature-controlled isolette

temperature-sensing pacemaker

Temperlite saw blade

TempFix spanning knee external fixation system

template
- Charnley t.
- dermal regeneration t.
- DNA t.
- Integra dermal regeneration t.
- Jacobsen t.
- Kuske breast t.
- Mallory-Head modular acetabular t.
- Martinez universal perineal interstitial t.
- Mick prostate t.
- rod t.
- Surgiguide t.
- Syed t.
- Syed-Neblett t.
- Syed-Neblett dedicated vulvar plastic t.
- thermoplastic t.
- tissue expander t.
- tissue sizer t.
- total toe t.

temple
- Venturi adjusted t.

Temple-Fay laminectomy retractor

Tempo
- T. denture liner
- T. diagnostic catheter
- T. selective and flush catheter

Tempofilter vena cava filter

Tempo+ modular ear-level speech processor

temporal
- t. bone holder
- t. electrode

temporalis
- t. sling
- t. transfer clamp

temporary
- t. dental cement
- t. endoprosthetic device
- t. keratoprosthesis suturing
- t. pacemaker
- t. pacing catheter
- t. percutaneous SCS electrode
- t. pervenous lead
- t. prosthesis
- t. socket
- t. transvenous pacemaker
- t. vascular clip
- t. vessel clip

temporolimbic system

temporomandibular
- t. joint (TMJ)
- t. joint fossa eminence prosthesis
- t. joint metal-on-metal total joint replacement prosthesis system

temporomandibular joint (TMJ)

TempTouch home infrared temperature probe

Tempur-Med
- T.-M. hospital replacement mattress
- T.-M. seat wedge
- T.-M. wheelchair cushion
- T.-M. x-ray table pad

Tempur-Pedic
- T.-P. mattress
- T.-P. pressure-relieving Swedish mattress
- T.-P. pressure-relieving Swedish pillow

tenacular clamp

tenaculum
- Adair breast t.
- Barrett uterine t.
- Braun-Schroeder single-tooth t.
- breast t.
- cervical t.
- Coakley t.
- Cottle single-prong t.
- double-tooth t.
- t. forceps
- t. hook
- t. hook loop
- Hulka uterine t.
- Jacobs uterine t.
- Jarcho uterine t.
- Joseph t.
- Kahn traction t.
- Kelly uterine t.
- Küstner t.
- Lahey goiter t.
- lion jaw t.
- Martin t.

T

tenaculum *(continued)*
>   nasal t.
>   Pozzi t.
>   t. reducing forceps
>   Ritchie cleft palate t.
>   Schroeder uterine t.
>   single-tooth t.
>   Skene uterine t.
>   straight t.
>   thyroid t.
>   toothed t.
>   tracheal t.
>   traction t.
>   uterine t.
>   White t.

Tena pouch
Tenax coronary stent
Tenax-XR
>   T.-XR Complete
>   T.-XR Trinity stent

Ten balloon
Tenckhoff
>   T. catheter
>   T. 2-cuff catheter
>   T. peritoneal dialysis catheter
>   T. renal dialysis catheter

Tender
>   T. subcutaneous infusion set
>   T. Touch extractor
>   T. Touch vacuum birthing cup

Tenderlett
>   T. device
>   T. Jr. lancing device
>   T. Plus fingerstick blood collection
>   device
>   T. Toddler lancing device

Tendersorb
>   T. ABD absorptive dressing
>   T. ABD pad

TenderWet system
Tenderwrap
>   T. leg compression dressing
>   T. Unna boot

tendon
>   t. carrier
>   t. forceps
>   t. gouge
>   t. grabber
>   t. harvester
>   t. hook
>   t. implant
>   t. knife
>   t. leader
>   t. needle
>   t. passer
>   t. plate
>   t. prosthesis
>   t. sheath

>   t. sling
>   t. stripper
>   t. tucker
>   t. tunneler

tendon-holding forceps
tendon-passing forceps
tendon-pulling forceps
tendon-retrieving forceps
tendon-seizing forceps
Tendril
>   T. DX implantable pacing lead
>   T. DX steroid-eluting active-fixation
>   pacing lead
>   T. SDX model 1688 active-fixation
>   pacing lead

Tennant
>   T. Anchorflex AC lens
>   T. eye needle holder
>   T. implant
>   T. intraocular lens forceps
>   T. lens forceps
>   T. nuclear ball rotator
>   T. thumb-ring needle holder
>   T. titanium suturing forceps
>   T. tying forceps

Tennant-Colibri corneal forceps
Tennant-Troutman superior rectus
forceps
Tenner lacrimal cannula
tennis
>   t. elbow arm band
>   t. elbow splint

tenodesis
>   t. orthosis
>   t. splint

tenotome
tenotomy
>   t. hook
>   t. scissors

TENS
>   transcutaneous electrical neuromuscular
>   stimulator
>   TENS machine
>   TENS pad
>   TENS unit

ten-shooter
>   Saeed t.-s.

Tensilon implant
tensiometer
>   Acufex t.

tension
>   t. clamp
>   t. collar
>   t. isometer

tensioner
>   Arthrotek graft t.

tension-free vaginal tape
tension-requiring suture

Tensor
    T. elastic bandage roll
    T. elastic dressing
tensor
    V-Stat variable soft tissue
    alignment t.
tensostat
Tensys T-line blood pressure monitor
tent
    croup t.
    Croupette child t.
    hydrophilic t.
    laminaria cervical t.
    mist t.
    oxygen t.
    Silon t.
    steam t.
tentalum wire tension suture
Ten-Ten duodecapolar diagnostic catheter
Tenzel
    T. bipolar forceps
    T. calipers
    T. elevator
Tepper proprioceptor simulator
Teq-Trode electrode
teres knife
Terino
    T. anatomical chin implant
    T. facial implant retractor
    T. implant
    T. malar shell
terminal
    t. device
    t. electrode
    t. electrode adapter
    t. extensor mechanism
Terox RV lead
Terrmocork diabetic shoe
Terry
    T. astigmatome
    T. keratometer
    T. nail
    T. silicone capsule polisher
Terry-Mayo needle
Terry-Schanzlin
    T.-S. astigmatome
    T.-S. astigmatome system
Terson
    T. capsular forceps
    T. capsule forceps
    T. extracapsular forceps
Terumo
    T. AV fistula needle
    T. Crosswire PTCA guidewire
    T. dental needle
    T. dialyzer
    T. Doppler fetal heart rate monitor
    T. Glidewire

    T. guidewire
    T. hydrophilic guidewire
    T. hypodermic needle
    T. insulin syringe
    T. Pinnacle R/OII radiopaque marker introducer sheath
    T. Pinnacle sheath
    T. Radifocus Glidewire
    T. Radiofocus sheath
    T. SP coaxial catheter
    T. SP hydrophilic polymer-coated microcatheter
    T. stent
    T. syringe
    T. telescoping catheter system
    T. transducer protector
Terumo-Clirans dialyzer
Terumo/Meditech guidewire
Terumo-Radiofocus hydrophilic polymer-coated guidewire
TES belt
Tesberg esophagoscope
Tesio catheter
tesla
    t. GE Signa whole-body scanner
    t. magnet
    t. magnetic resonance imager
    t. Signa magnetic resonance imager
    t. Signa MR imager
    t. superconductive magnet unit
    t. system
Teslar watch
Tessier
    T. bone bender
    T. craniofacial instrument
    T. disimpaction device forceps
    T. dislodger
    T. elevator
    T. osteomicrotome
    T. osteotome
    T. rib-contouring forceps
TEST
test
    Acaderm patch t.
    AccuStat hCG pregnancy t.
    Actalyke activated clotting time t.
    Activin AB free beta-HCG ELISA t.
    AneuVysion Assay prenatal genetic t.
    Arloing-Courmont t.
    ASPIRINcheck urine t.
    Aware AccuMeter rapid HIV t.
    AxSYM free PSA t.
    Babystart ovulation t.
    BiliCheck t.
    Binax Now *Legionella* urine antigen t.

T

test *(continued)*

Binax Now *Streptococcus pneumoniae* antigen t.
Binax Now urinary antigen t.
Biosafe TSH t.
BreathTek UBT *H. pylori* t.
Cambridge Biotech HIV-1 urine Western blot t.
Cardiac STATus CK-MB t.
¹⁴C-glycocholate breath t.
ChemTrak AccuMeter theophylline t.
ClearView C. Diff A t.
color bar Schirmer tear t.
ColorPAC toxin A t.
Concise Plus hCG urine t.
C-urea breath t.
Diatest diabetes breath t.
Dynatron 2000 muscle t.
Eitest MONO P-II t.
Elecsys total PSA t.
EquiTest motor coordination t.
EquiTest sensory organization t.
ExacTech blood glucose meter t.
Eyecuity wireless visual acuity t.
EZ-HP *Helicobacter pylori* t.
FertilMARQ fertility screening t.
FIBROSpec t.
GenESA system for radionuclide imaging stress t.
Haidinger brush t.
t. handle instrument
HealthCheck One-Step One Minute pregnancy t.
Heartscan heart attack prediction t.
Helicobacter pylori gII t.
Hemifield glaucoma t.
Hemoccult II t.
HemoCue glucose t.
HemoCue hemoglobin t.
HER-2/neu serum t.
Holladay contrast acuity t.
HRR pseudoisochromatic t.
Hybrid Capture 2 HPV DNA t.
Hypan t.
IBD First Step t.
Icon 25 hCG t.
IDI-Strep B t.
IgA HIV antibody t.
ImmunoCyt cytopathology recurrent bladder cancer t.
ImmunoDip urinary albumin t.
influenza t.
Jackson compression t.
KidneyScreen At·Home mail-in t.
Kodak Surecell Chlamydia t.
lysoPC diagnostic ovarian cancer t.
menopause home t.

Mentor B-VAT II BVS contour circles distance stereoacuity t.
Mentor B-VAT II BVS random dot E distance stereoacuity t.
MicroTrac direct specimen t.
Monospot t.
NMR LipoProfile t.
O'Connor tweezer dexterity t.
One-Step hCG combo t.
Optec 3000 contrast sensitivity t.
OralScreen 4 substance abuse t.
OraQuick rapid HIV-1 antibody t.
PACE-2C DNA probe t.
t. paper
Pease-Allen Color t.
PLAC coronary heart disease t.
Pre-Gen 26 colorectal cancer t.
Pro-PredictRx diagnostic t.
ProteinChip t.
Q-Stress treadmill stress t.
QuantiFERON-TB t.
QuickVue Advance *Gardnerella vaginalis* t.
QuickVue *Chlamydia* t.
QuickVue *H. pylori* gII t.
QuickVue In-Line One-Step Strep A t.
QuickVue one-step hCG-Combo pregnancy t.
QuPID pregnancy t.
RAMP myoglobin t.
Randot Stereo Smile t.
rapid urease t.
SAS Rota t.
Semi-Q hCG combo t.
Sero-Strip HIV t.
Sickledex t.
Signify ER drug screen t.
StarTox 5 drugs of abuse screening t.
Streptex rapid strep t.
!nSure fecal immunochemical t.
Tandem-R Ostase osteoporosis t.
TCR Vgamma9 t.
Thrombostat platelet function t.
Triage BNP t.
T.R.U.E. t.
UroVysion bladder cancer recurrence t.
Vgamma9 t.
Vitalor screening pulmonary function t.
West Nile virus IgM capture t.
X-Scribe stress t.

tester

Accu-Measure personal body fat t.
Analytic Technology pulp t.
Artscan 200 arthroscopic cartilage stiffness t.

Green Endo-Ice pulp t.
GripTrack Commander strength t.
IRMA SL blood glucose strip t.
Ismat manual muscle t.
Komet medical battery t.
Mentor B-VAT II video acuity t.
Miller-Nadler glare t.
Neosono Ultima apex
  locator/pulp t.
Nicholas manual muscle t.
Novapath HIV-1 immunoblot t.
Polar Electro sport t.
Prio video display terminal
  vision t.
Quik-Chek external pacer t.
TCI OvuLook ovulation t.
Tinius Olsen stiffness t.
Topcon vision t.
Vistech Multivision contrast t.
West nerve t.
testicular implant
testing
Baylor-Video Acuity T.
t. drum knife
filter glasses for color t.
Testoderm
T. patch
T. testosterone transdermal system
Testsimplets prestained slide
Test-Size orchidometer
tethered catheter
Tetko nylon mesh filter
tetracaine pledget
tetraONE system
tetrapolar esophageal catheter
Tetrax interactive balance system
Teurlings wrist brace
Tevdek
T. implant
T. pledgeted suture
T. prosthesis
T. suture
Tewameter TM 210 open loop system
Tew cranial retractor
Texas
T. cannula tip
T. condom catheter
T. Goodstein sharp tip
T. Scottish Rite Hospital (TSRH)
T. Scottish Rite Hospital buttressed
  laminar hook
T. Scottish Rite Hospital circular
  laminar hook
T. Scottish Rite Hospital corkscrew
  device
T. Scottish Rite Hospital crosslink
T. Scottish Rite Hospital double-
  rod construct

T. Scottish Rite Hospital eyebolt
  spreader
T. Scottish Rite Hospital hook
  holder
T. Scottish Rite Hospital hook
  inserter
T. Scottish Rite Hospital hook-rod
  system
T. Scottish Rite Hospital I-bolt
T. Scottish Rite Hospital mini-
  corkscrew device
T. Scottish Rite Hospital pedicle
  hook
T. Scottish Rite Hospital pedicle
  screw
T. Scottish Rite Hospital screw-rod
  system
T. Scottish Rite Hospital trial
  hook
T. Scottish Rite Hospital wrench
Texas-style 2-piece catheter
Texon sole
TFAS
total facet arthroplasty system
T-fastener
Brown-Mueller T-f.
T-f. delivery needle
T-f. device
TFE-coated wire guide
T-file
engine T-f.
T-Fix absorbable meniscal repair device
TFN
trochanteric fixation nail
TFN trochanteric fixation nail
T-Foam
T-F. bed pad
T-F. cushion
T-F. mattress
T-F. pillow
TFX Medical catheter stylet
TG140 needle
T-Gel cushion
TG Osseotite single-stage procedure
  implant
Thackray hip prosthesis
ThAIRapy
T. vest
T. vest airway clearance system
thallium-201
Thal-Quick chest tube
T-handle
T-h. bone awl
T-h. curette
T-h. elevator
T-h. Jacob chuck
T-h. nut wrench
ratcheting T-h.

T-handle *(continued)*
  T-h. reamer
  T-h. screw wrench
T-handled
  T-h. awl
  T-h. cup curette
  T-h. nut wrench
  T-h. screw wrench
Tharies
  T. femoral resurfacing component
  T. hip component
  T. hip replacement prosthesis
THC:YAG laser
The
  T. Asta-Cath female catheter guide
  T. Backstroke
  T. Beachcomber prosthetic foot
  T. Cell Sweep
  T. Closer arterial puncture site
    closure device
  T. Corner cushion
  T. Dale tracheostomy tube holder
  T. Deluxe Button Bag
  T. Edge coated blade
  T. Feminal female urinal
  T. Foot screw set
  T. Healthy Back System
  T. Heeler inflatable heel protector
  T. Jacknobber II
  T. MMG Golden drain
  T. Original Backknobber muscle
    massager
  T. Original Backnobber massage
    tool
  T. Original Index Knobber II
    massage tool
  T. Original Jacknobber massage
    tool
  T. Painless One acupuncture needle
  T. Pigment Peel Plus
  T. Richie brace
  T. Rope stretch-and-traction device
  T. Rope stretching device
  T. Sports Breather
  T. Summit HeNe aiming beam
  T. Unloader
  T. VAC Vacuum Assisted Closure
  T. Wave phacoemulsion system
  T. Wedge bioresorbable interference
    fit implant
  T. Wedge bioresorbable
    interference-fit implant
  T. Woodpecker
thecoperitoneal Pudenz-Schulte shunt
Theis
  T. rib retractor
  T. self-retaining retractor
Theken
Theobald sinus probe

Theon mitral replacement system
Thera
  T. cane
  T. Cane massager
  T. Cane shoulder exerciser
  T. Cool cold therapy system
Thera-Back back support
Thera-Band
  T.-B. Aqua Belt
  T.-B. assist
  T.-B. Assist exerciser
  T.-B. exercise ball
  T.-B. hand exerciser
  T.-B. handle
  T.-B. Max
  T.-B. Max band
  T.-B. Max resistive exercise
  T.-B. progressive weight
  T.-B. resistive exerciser
  T.-B. strip
  T.-B. therapy band
  T.-B. therapy device
  T.-B. tubing
Therabath paraffin heat therapy system
TheraBeads microwaveable moist heat
  pack
TheraBite
  T. jaw exerciser
  T. jaw motion rehabilitation system
  T. mobilizer
Thera-Boot
  T.-B. bandage
  T.-B. compression dressing
  T.-B. compression wrap
  T.-B. leg compression dressing
Theracloud pillow
Theraflex wrist exerciser
Therafoam padding
Thera-Gesic cream
Theragloves
TheraGym exercise ball
Ther-A-Hoop exerciser
TheraKair mattress
TheraKnit electrode glove
TheraKool breathable neoprene thumb
  spica
Therakos UVAR system
Thera-Loop exerciser
Thera-Med cold pack
Thera-Medic shoe
Theramini 1, 2 electrotherapy
  stimulator
TheraPEP positive expiratory pressure
  therapy system
therapeutic
  t. appliance
  t. endoscope
  t. shoe
  t. side-viewing duodenoscope

t. spinal support
t. splint
Therapeutica sleeping pillow
Thera-P exercise bar
Thera-Plast putty
Therap-Loop
T.-L. door anchor
T.-L. door handle
Thera-Pos elbow orthosis
TheraPress
T. DUO
T. DUO Lite
Therapress pressure point release tool
TheraPulse pulsating air suspension bed
Thera-Putty
T.-P. CTS exerciser
T.-P. exercise putty
T.-P. therapy device
therapy
t. ball
T. Carrot Finger Orthosis
photodynamic t. (PDT)
T. Putty
t. roll
t. tank
TherArc pillow
TheraRest mattress
TheraSeed implant
Therasense
T. FreeStyle
T. subcutaneous glucose sensor
Ther-A-Shapes positioner
Therasleep cervical pillow
TheraSnore
T. device
T. oral appliance
Therasonics
T. lithotripsy system
T. lithotriptor
Therasound transducer
TheraSphere
Thera-SR pacemaker
TheraTest Laboratories EL-RF test kit system
TheraTogs
Theratouch stimulator
Thera-turn rotational system
Thera-Wedge system
Therevac Plus
Therevac-SB
TheriLok bone void filler
Therma
T. Jaw disposable hot biopsy forceps
T. Jaw hot urologic forceps
Thermachoice
T. catheter
T. uterine balloon
T. uterine balloon therapy system

ThermaCool TC radiofrequency device
Thermafil
T. plastic carrier
T. Plus obturator
thermal
t. balloon system
t. conductivity detector
t. cycler
t. dosimetry system
t. energy analyzer
t. knife
t. memory stent
t. pack
t. plastic wrap
t. space blanket
thermalator
Whitehall t.
Thermalator heating unit
Thermalon heat-cold pad
ThermalSoft hot & cold packs
Thermapad pad
Thermasonic gel warmer
Thermasplint heating bath
Thermassage
Aqua T.
ThermaStim
T. muscle stimulator
T. muscle warming device
TherMatric hyperthermia device
TherMatrx TMx-2000 device
Thermedics
T. cardiac device
T. left ventricular assist device
Thermex
Direx T.
Thermex-II transurethral prostate heating device
thermistor
t. catheter
t. electrode
t. needle
nostril t.
t. probe
t. rectal thermometer
t. thermometer
Thermo
T. Cardiosystems left ventricular assist device
T. hand comforter
T. HK/Rohadur orthotic
T. HK/Tepefom orthotic
T. knee comforter
Thermocardiosystems left ventricular assist device
ThermoChem-HT system
thermocoagulator
Olympus CD-Z-series heat probe t.
ThermoCork orthotic

thermocouple
  Chromel-Alumel t.
  copper-constantan t.
  t. device
  low-impedance t.
  Mon-a-Therm t.
  needle t.
thermocoupler
thermocycler
  GeneAmp PCR System 9600 t.
  Perkin-Elmer Cetus 480, 9600
    DNA t.
  Stratagene SCS-96 t.
  Touchdown t.
thermodilution
  t. balloon catheter
  t. cardiac output computer
  t. catheter
  t. catheter introducer kit
  t. Swan-Ganz catheter
thermodisinfector
  endoscopic t.
thermoexpandable stent
ThermoFlex
  Maramed T.
  T. system
  T. thermotherapy unit
ThermoFlo
  T. humidifier
  T. system
ThermoFlow ETC unit
ThermoFX
  T. mesh
  T. mesh bioabsorbable fixation
    plate
thermographic scanner
Thermograph temperature monitor
Thermold heat moldable shoe lining
thermoluminescence
  t. detector
  t. dosimeter
thermoluminescent
  t. dosimeter
  t. dosimeter rod
thermometer
  Acuprobe t.
  aural t.
  basal body t.
  Braun tympanic t.
  Celsius t.
  centigrade t.
  Core-Check tympanic t.
  Coretemp deep tissue t.
  disposable t.
  electronic t.
  Fahrenheit flat bath t.
  FirstTemp Genius tympanic t.
  First Temp Genius tympanic t.
  glass t.

infrared t.
Instant Fever Tester t.
IVAC Temp Plus II t.
LighTouch Neonate t.
Ototemp 3000 ear t.
Philips SensorTouch temple t.
Quik-Temp t.
SureTemp electronic t.
SureTemp 4 oral t.
Tegam microprocessor t.
Tel-A-Fever forehead t.
Temp-a-dot t.
Tempa-DOT single-use clinical t.
thermistor t.
thermistor rectal t.
Thermoscan Pro-1 instant t.
Thermoscan Pro-1 tympanic
  instant t.
Thermoscan tympanic instant t.
tympanic membrane t.
Thermophore
  T. bandage
  T. hot pack
  T. moist heat pad
thermoplastic
  DynaPrene splinting t.
  t. elastomer (TPE)
  t. extension pan splint
  t. head mask
  t. heating unit
  t. splint
  t. stent
  t. template
Thermoprep heating oven
Thermoscan
  T. Pro-1 instant thermometer
  T. Pro-1 tympanic instant
    thermometer
  T. tympanic instant thermometer
Thermoskin
  T. arthritic knee wrap
  T. back wrap
  T. brace
  T. heat retainer
  T. shoulder wrap
  T. U wrist wrap
  T. 4-way elastic knee support
ThermoSKY orthotic material
thermotherapy
  laser-induced t.
  transurethral microwave t. (TUMT)
  Urowave t.
Thermovac tissue pulverizer
**Thermovent heat and moisture
  exchanger**
Thero-Skin gel padding
TherOx
  T. Aqueous Oxygen system
  T. infusion guidewire

thick-septa collimator
thick-walled Dacron-backed implant
Thiersch
    T. graft
    T. suture
    T. wire
thigh
    T. Thing pump holder
    t. tourniquet
thigh-high antiembolic stocking
Thin
    Hydrocol T.
thin
    t. acupuncture needle
    t. disposable cannula
    t. film dressing
    t. glenoid retractor
THI needle
thin-layer
    t.-l. chromatograph
    T.-l. Rapid-Use Transcutaneous
    (T.R.U.E.)
ThinLine
    T. EZ bipolar pacemaker lead
    T. EZ pacing lead
Thinline uncovered orthotic
ThinPRep imaging system
ThinPrep 2000 processor
ThinProfile eyelid implant
thin-septa collimator
thin-shaft nasal scissors
THINSite
    T. dressing
    T. hydrogel sheet
    T. topical wound dressing
thin-walled
    t.-w. catheter
    t.-w. guiding needle
    t.-w. needle
thin-wall introducer catheter
thin-wire Ilizarov fixator
thiopurine methyltransferase (TPMT)
third-generation lithotriptor
third-order Butterworth filter
Thomas
    T. brush
    T. buckle sling
    T. cervical collar brace
    T. collar cervical orthosis
    T. cryoextractor
    T. cryoprobe
    T. cryoptor
    T. endotracheal tube holder
    T. femoral shunt
    T. fixation forceps
    T. fixator
    T. fracture frame
    T. full-ring splint
    T. heel

    T. heel orthosis
    T. hinged splint
    T. hyperextension frame
    T. I&A cannula
    T. knee splint
    T. leg splint
    T. long-term endotracheal tube
    holder
    T. LT endotracheal tube holder
    T. needle
    T. posterior splint
    T. Quick Block endotracheal tube
    holder
    T. retractor
    T. rigid collar
    T. scissors
    T. shunt
    T. spatula
    T. splint with Pearson attachment
    T. subretinal instrument set II
    T. suspension splint
    T. traction
    T. uterine curette
    T. walking brace
Thompson
    T. dowel
    T. endoprosthesis
    T. femoral head prosthesis
    T. femoral neck prosthesis
    T. lithotrite
    T. nail
    T. rasp
    T. retractor
    T. stem rasp
Thompson-Parkridge-Richards (TPR)
Thoms-Allis
    T.-A. tissue forceps
    T.-A. vulsellum
Thoms-Gaylor
    T.-G. biopsy punch
    T.-G. uterine forceps
Thomson adenoidal punch
Thoms tissue forceps
ThoraCath catheter
thoracentesis needle
thoracic
    t. artery forceps
    t. cage
    t. catheter
    t. clamp
    t. drain
    t. extension component
    t. orthosis
    t. scissors
    t. tissue forceps
    t. trocar
thoracolumbar
    t. pedicle screw
    t. standing orthosis brace

T

thoracolumbosacral
  t. orthosis (TLSO)
  t. plate
  t. spinal orthosis
thoracolumbosacroiliac implant system thread
Thoracoport
  T. single-use trocar
  T. trocar system
thoracoport
  soft t.
thoracoscope
  Boutin t.
  Storz t.
thoracostomy tube
thoracotome
  Bettman-Fovash t.
Thora-Drain III chest drainage
Thora-Klex
  T.-K. chest drainage system
  T.-K. chest tube
Thoramat
Thora-Port port
Thoraseal chest tube drainage system
Thora-Seal III chest drainage unit
Thoratec
  T. biventricular assist device
  T. cardiac device
  T. implantable vascular access device
  T. IVAD
  T. pump
  T. right ventricular assist device
  T. VAD system
  T. ventricular assist device
Thoravision selenium x-ray detector
Thoreau filter
Thorek
  T. gallbladder aspirator
  T. thoracic scissors
Thorlo padded sock
Thornton
  T. anterior positioner
  T. arcuate blade
  T. double corneal ruler
  T. globe fixation ring
  T. K3-7991 360-degree arcuate marker
  T. limbal fixation ring
  T. limbal incision ruler
  T. low-profile marker
  T. malleable spatula
  T. nail
  T. needle
  T. plate
  T. triple micrometer knife
  T. tri-square blade
Thornton-Fine ring

Thorpe
  T. calipers
  T. conjunctival forceps
  T. corneal forceps
  T. flowmeter
  T. 4-mirror goniolaser
  T. 4-mirror goniolaser lens
  T. 4-mirror goniolens
  T. 4-mirror vitreous fundus laser lens
  T. plastic lens
  T. scissors
  T. slit-lamp
  T. surgical gonioscope
Thorpe-Castroviejo
  T.-C. goniolens
  T.-C. vitreous foreign body forceps
Thorpe-Westcott scissors
THORP system
THORP-type mandibular reconstruction plate
Thorton
  T. globe fixation ring
  T. optic zone marker
Thrasher lens implant forceps
thread
  polyene t.
  thoracolumbosacroiliac implant system t.
threaded
  t. cortical dowel
  t. eye needle
  t. fusion cage
  t. guide pin
  t. interbody fusion cage
  t. mandrel
  t. rod
  t. sheath
  t. titanium acetabular prosthesis
threader
  cannulated wire t.
  wire t.
ThreadLoc
  T. driver mount screw
  T. implant
  T. retaining screw
thread-locking device
threadwire saw
three-quarter
  t.-q. circle electrode
  t.-q. pigtail plastic endoprosthesis
Threshold
  T. inspiratory muscle trainer device
  T. PEP device
  T. positive expiratory pressure device
ThRevo suture anchor

throat
    ears, nose, t. (ENT)
    t. forceps
thrombectomy catheter
Thrombex PMT system
ThrombiGel bandage
thrombin-soaked Gelfoam
Thrombix bandage
thromboelastograph
thromboembolic
    t. disease hose
    t. disease stocking
Thrombolizer catheter
Thrombostat platelet function test
thrombosuction catheter
thrombus stripper
through-and-through
    t.-a.-t. continuous suture
    t.-a.-t. reabsorbable suture
through-cutting
    t.-c. forceps tip
    t.-c. sinus surgery forceps
through-the-balloon ultrasound
through-the-needle catheter
through-the-scope (TTS)
    t.-t.-s. balloon
    t.-t.-s. bougie
    t.-t.-s. catheter probe
    t.-t.-s. dilator
    t.-t.-s. injection needle
through-the-wall mattress suture
thrust plate prosthesis (TPP)
Thudichum nasal speculum
thulium-holmium-chromium:yttrium-
    aluminum-garnet laser
thulium-holmium:YAG laser
thumb
    t. forceps
    t. interphalangeal extension assist
    t. retractor
    t. spica
    t. spica bandage
    t. spica cast
    t. spica splint
    t. tissue forceps
thumbkeeper
    Freedom t.
Thumboform support
Thumb-Saver introducer clamp
ThumDuction strap
Thumper
    T. CPR system
    T. 1007 CPR system
    T. device
ThumSaver
    T. CMC long splint
    T. CMC short splint
    T. MP splint

ThumSling
    Action T.
ThumWrap
    FoamWrap T.
ThumZ'Up functional thumb splint
Thurmond
    T. iris retractor
    T. nucleus-irrigating cannula
    T. pachymetry marker
thymus retractor
ThyRex timer
thyroid
    t. drain
    t. forceps
    t. retractor
    t. shield
    t. tenaculum
    t. uptake probe
Ti
    Ti alloy screw
    Ti rotor
Ti-Bac
    T.-B. acetabular component
    T.-B. II hip prosthesis
Tibbs
    T. arterial cannula
    T. semiautomatic suturing device
tibial
    t. aligner
    t. augmentation block
    t. bolt
    t. broach
    t. cutter guide
    t. cutting block
    t. drill guide
    t. endoprosthesis
    t. fracture brace proximal support
    t. guide pin
    t. head screw
    t. plate
    t. plateau prosthesis
    t. resector
    t. retractor
    t. torsion system
Tib-Transformer orthosis
Ti-Cron suture
Tidal
    T. Wave handheld capnograph
    T. Wave Sp capnometer/pulse
      oximeter
tie
    cable t.
    silk t.
    table t.
Tieck-Halle infant nasal speculum
Tieck nasal speculum
Tielle
    T. absorptive dressing
    T. Plus hydropolymer dressing

T

Tiemann
>T. bullet forceps
>T. coudé catheter

Tiemann-Foley catheter

tie-on needle

tie-over
>t.-o. bolster
>t.-o. bolster dressing
>t.-o. dressing
>t.-o. Sellotape dressing

tier
>Adson knot t.
>Harris wire t.
>knot t.

tiered-therapy
>t.-t. antiarrhythmic device
>t.-t. implantable cardioverter-
>defibrillator

Tierney otoplasty dressing

tiger
>T. blade
>t. gut suture

TigerTail ureteral catheter

tiger-tip cannula

TigerWire suture

tightener
>Charnley wire t.
>Harris wire t.
>Kirschner t.
>Kirschner wire t.
>Nordt knot t.
>Sklar wire t.
>wire t.

**tight-to-shaft Aire-Cuf tracheostomy
tube**

TIJ lead

Tilastin hip prosthesis

Tilley-Henckel forceps

Tilley nasal dressing forceps

Tillyer bifocal lens

tilt
>t. board
>T. System wheelchair
>t. table
>T. and Turn Paragon bed

tilt-board
>Vari-Tilt adjustable t.-b.

tilting
>t. disc aortic valve prosthesis
>t. disc heart valve

tilting-frame wheelchair

TiMAX titanium captured hip screw

Timberlake
>T. obturator
>T. obturator resectoscope

time
>t. gain compensator

time-based counter

time-cycled ventilator

timed
>spontaneous t. (ST)

time-of-flight
>t.-o.-f. PET imaging system
>t.-o.-f. positron emission
>tomographic camera

timer
>Apgar t.
>Medela Apgar t.
>Medtronic automated coagulation t.
>ThyRex t.
>video t.

TiMesh
>T. cranial mesh
>T. craniofacial system
>T. craniomaxillofacial plating
>system
>T. emergency screw
>T. hardware
>T. LP cranial miniplate and screw
>system
>T. mandibular crib
>T. midface and cranial system
>T. orbital mesh
>T. orthognathic strap plate
>T. patient configured titanium
>craniomaxillofacial implant
>T. rigid fixation bone plating
>system
>T. screw
>T. titanium bone plating system
>T. titanium mesh

Timeter pocket spirometer

time-to-pulse height converter

Timex TMX optical eyewear

timing circuit

Timo headrest

TiMX low back system

TINA monitor

tin-bullet probe

T-incision marker

tined
>t. lead pacemaker
>t. ventricular electrode

Tinius Olsen stiffness tester

tinnitus relief device (TRD)

tinted
>t. lens
>t. spectacles

Tiny-Tef ventilation tube

Tiny Tytan ventilation tube

TiOblast dental implant

tip
>accelerator t.
>ACMI cystoscopic t.
>acromionizer t.
>aerosol barrier pipette t.
>Andrews suction t.
>atraumatic t.

Bard t.
Batt t.
beavertail t.
Becker flat dissector t.
Becker round dissector t.
Becker twist dissector t.
Binkhorst t.
bipolar diathermy forceps t.
buccal fat extractor t.
Burnett power t.
cannula t.
catheter t.
chisel t.
t. cleaner caddie
Cloward cervical drill t.
Cobra+ cannula t.
Cobra K+ cannula t.
Colorado electrocautery t.
Combitip Plus pipette t.
coned heparin t.
conical inserter t.
Corometrics Gold Quik Connect
  spiral electrode t.
coronary perfusion t.
curved slim-diameter t.
CUSA laparoscopic t.
custom t.
diathermy t.
disposable cannula t.
disposable Keratoplast t.
dissecting t.
exit t.
extended wear self-adhering urinary
  external catheter with
  removable t.
E-Z Clean cautery t.
Fell sucker t.
fiberoptic t.
flap t.
flared ABS t.
Flexoreamer Batt t.
Fournier t.
fragmatome t.
Frazier suction t.
furcation slim-diameter t.
Gasparotti bevel t.
Girard irrigating t.
grasping forceps t.
t. guard
guillotine cutting t.
Henke punch forceps t.
2-hole standard t.
3-hole standard t.
hydrodissection t.
Illouz modified t.
Illouz standard t.
Implantech SE-100 smoke
  aspiration t.
irrigating t.

Japanese suction t.
Kahler double-action t.
Keeler lancet t.
Keeler micro round t.
Keeler micro spear t.
Keeler puncture t.
Keeler razor t.
Keeler triple facet t.
Kelman t.
Kelman-Mackool flare t.
Keratoplast t.
K-Flexofile Batt t.
Killian cutting forceps t.
Killian double articulated forceps t.
Klein cannula t.
Klein 1-hole infiltrator t.
Klein multihole infiltrator t.
Krause oval punch t.
Krause punch forceps t.
Krause square basket t.
Leon cobra t.
Luer syringe t.
Marlow Primus t.
Mayo coronary perfusion t.
Medtronic t.
MegaDyne E-Z clean cautery t.
Mercedes t.
Microprobe t.
microtip phaco t.
Mitchell viscoelastic removal I/A t.
modified submental retractor
  flared t.
nonaspirating ultrasonic phaco
  chopper t.
Nu-Tip disposable scissor t.
oblique mucosectomy device t.
Omni laser t.
open-end flow-through radiopaque t.
OtoClear disposable t.
overprojecting nasal t.
phaco t.
Pinto dissector t.
pointed cystotome t.
pole t.
policeman t.
2-port radial t.
3-port radial t.
pyramidal t.
pyramid Toomey t.
Radovan tissue expander t.
rectal t.
retroprep t.
Roane bullet t.
Rosenberg dissector t.
rubber acorn t.
Savary-Gilliard t.
Saverburger irrigation/aspiration t.
Sensor PTFE-nitinol guidewire with
  hydrophilic t.

T

tip *(continued)*
    sharp-edged t.
    silicone-covered aspiration t.
    Simcoe cannula t.
    Simcoe interchangeable t.
    Sims suction t.
    Skimmer laryngeal blade t.
    sleeveless phaco t.
    Slip-Coat t.
    smoke aspiration t.
    solid-core needle with hollow t.
    spatula t.
    spatula cannula t.
    Spencer triangular t.
    Spencer Universal adenoid punch t.
    StrykeProbe suction irrigator t.
    sucker t.
    suction t.
    Surgi-Fine reusable cannula t.
    synthetic sapphire t.
    Texas cannula t.
    Texas Goodstein sharp t.
    through-cutting forceps t.
    Tischler-Morgan t.
    Toledo flap dissector t.
    Toledo standard dissector t.
    Toledo V-dissector t.
    Trevisani t.
    Trevisani cannula t.
    Tricut laryngeal blade t.
    TriEye t.
    triple-bend t.
    triport t.
    TT t.
    tulip t.
    tungsten t.
    Unitri t.
    Universal adenoid punch t.
    Universal handle with nasal-
      cutting t.
    water-cooled t.
    weighted t.
    Yankauer suction t.
    Yankauer tonsil suction t.
tip-deflecting
    t.-d. catheter
    t.-d. guidewire
    t.-d. wire
tire
    276 t.
    implant t.
    t. implant
    silicone t.
    Watzke t.
tire-grooved silicone
TIRR foot-ankle orthosis
Tischler
    T. cervical biopsy forceps

    T. cervical biopsy punch
    T. cervical biopsy punch forceps
Tischler-Morgan
    T.-M. biopsy punch
    T.-M. tip
    T.-M. uterine biopsy forceps
Tisseel
    T. biologic fibrogen adhesive
    T. fibrin glue
    T. fibrin sealant
    T. surgical glue
    T. VH kit
**Tissomat application device and spray
set**
Tissot spirometer
Tissucol fibrin sealant
tissue
    t. adhesive
    AlloDerm t.
    t. anchor guide (TAG)
    t. anchor guide system
    t. culture flask
    t. desiccation needle
    t. desiccation needle electrode
    t. dilator
    t. drain
    t. expander
    t. expander template
    FasLata allograft t.
    t. forceps
    t. glue
    t. graft press
    t. grasping forceps
    t. holding forceps
    human allograft t.
    t. lifter
    t. link floating ball
    t. mandrel implant material
    t. morcellator
    t. occlusion clamp
    Ogura t.
    t. plane dissector
    t. protector
    t. reflectance oximeter
    t. retractor
    t. scissors
    t. sizer template
    t. solder
    t. spectrum analyzer TS-200
    t. spreading forceps
    T. Technologies TruPulse laser
    T. Tek-II cryostat
    tissue-engineered meniscal t.
    Tutoplast t.
tissue-engineered
    t.-e. construct
    t.-e. meniscal tissue
    t.-e. polymer device
tissue-equivalent detector

Tissue-Guard bovine pericardial patch
TissueMend soft tissue repair matrix
TissueTak corkscrew implant
Tis-U-Sol
Tis-U-Trap endometrial suction catheter
Titan
- T. Apollo electric flexion table
- T. endoprosthesis
- T. hip cup
- T. III H cellulose acetate strip
- T. Mega XL PTCA dilatation catheter
- T. Meridian Intersegmental Traction table
- T. Nova manual flexion-extension multi flex table
- T. Nova manual flexion-extension multiflex table
- T. scaler
- T. slow-speed handpiece
- T. stent
- T. thumb support

titanium
- t. alloy implant
- t. alloy needle
- t. alloy screw and rod system
- t. aneurysm clip
- t. AO plate
- t. cable
- t. cage
- t. cancellous bone screw
- t. clip
- t. construct
- t. elastic nail
- t. fixation device
- t. flexible humeral nail
- t. foil
- t. Greenfield filter
- t. half pin
- t. hollow osseointegrated reconstruction plate
- t. hollow osseointegrating reconstruction plate
- t. hollow-screw osseointegrated reconstruction plate
- t. hollow screw plate system
- t. implant material
- t. mandibular plate
- t. mandibular staple
- t. mesh
- t. mesh cage
- t. mesh screen
- t. mesh tray
- t. microsurgical bipolar forceps
- t. micro system
- t. mini bur hole cover
- t. miniplate
- t. nail
- t. needle
- t. plasma sprayed dental implant
- t. plate
- t. prosthesis
- t. retinal tack
- t. screw
- t. spiked washer
- t. staple
- t. tack
- t. urethral stent
- t. VasPort port
- t. vocal fold medialization implant
- t. Vortex Port system
- T. Wedge electrosurgical resection device
- t. wire
- t. wound retractor

titanium:sapphire laser
titanium-sprayed IMZ implant
Titer
- Image T.

titrator
Titus venoclysis needle
TiUnite dental implant
TJF-100, -130 large-channel duodenoscope
TKS laser
TL90 Ethicon stapler
TLA needle
TLC
- TLC antiseptic soap
- TLC Baxter balloon catheter

TLC-II portable VAD driver
T-lens therapeutic contact lens
TLS
- TLS suction drain
- TLS surgical drain
- TLS surgical marker

TLSO
- thoracolumbosacral orthosis
- Boa Duel TLSO
- DonJoy Boa Duel TLSO

TMC needle
TMI implant
TMJ
- temporomandibular joint
- TMJ acrylic
- TMJ Concepts patient-fitted TMJ prosthesis system
- TMJ fossa eminence prosthesis
- TMJ fossa-eminence prosthesis
- TMJ halter
- TMJ head positioner
- TMJ metal-on-metal total joint replacement prosthesis system

T-model endaural retractor
TMS
- TMS 3-dimensional radiation therapy treatment planning system

TMS *(continued)*
 TMS 1000 tachyarrhythmia
 monitoring system
TMS-1
 TMS-1, -2 videokeratoscope
 TMS-1 videokeratoscope GTS
TMS-2
 TMS-2 computer-assisted
 videokeratoscope
 TMS-2 computerized corneal
 topographer
TMx-2000 BPH thermotherapy system
TO
 transobturator
Toad finger splint
Tobey
 T. ear forceps
 T. ear rongeur
Tobold
 T. laryngeal forceps
 T. laryngoscopic apparatus
 T. tongue depressor
TobraDex-soaked Gelfoam
tobramycin-impregnated PMMA implant
Tobruk splint
Tocantins bone marrow biopsy needle
tocodynamometer
 guard-ring t.
 Nihon t.
tocotonometer
tocotransducer
Todd
 T. bur hole button
 T. cautery
 T. electrocautery
 T. gouge
Todd-Wells
 T.-W. apparatus
 T.-W. guide
 T.-W. stereotactic frame
toe
 t. comb
 t. loop
 t. plate
 Primus flexible great t.
 t. prosthesis
 t. protector
 t. wedge
Toe-Aid dressing
toedrop brace
Toennis
 T. dissecting scissors
 T. dissector
 T. ES stand-alone constant-current
 electrical stimulator
 T. needle holder
 T. retractor
 T. tumor forceps

Toennis-Adson
 T.-A. dissector
 T.-A. dural scissors
 T.-A. forceps
ToeOFF orthosis
Tofflemire
 T. matrix band
 T. retainer
toggle
 screw t.
Toitu MT-810 cardiographic monitor
Tokos monitor
Toledo
 T. dissector
 T. flap dissector tip
 T. roller
 T. standard dissector tip
 T. V-dissector cannula
 T. V-dissector tip
Tolentino
 T. prism lens
 T. ring
 T. vitrectomy lens
 T. vitreous cutter
Tolman micrometer
Tomac
 T. catheter
 T. clip
Tomac-Nélaton catheter
Tomas
 T. iris hook
 T. suture hook
Tomcat PTCA guidewire
tome
 Laschal precision suture t.
Tomenius gastroscope
Tomey
 T. autorefractor
 T. autotopographer
 T. ConfoScan confocal microscope
 T. retinal function analyzer
 T. TMS-1 photokeratoscope
 T. topographic modeling system
 T. topography system
 T. trabeculectomy punch
Tommy trapeze bar
tomograph
 ECAT III positron t.
 Heidelberg retina t.
 Heidelberg retina t. II
tomographer
 Siemens Somatom Plus S
 computed t.
tomographic
 t. multiplane scanner
 t. skull immobilizer
tomography
 computed t. (CT)
 positron emission t. (PET)

single photon emission computed t. (SPECT)

t. wedge

Tomolex tomographic system

Tomomatic

T. 2-slice SPECT imaging system

T. 3-slice SPECT imaging system

T. 5-slice SPECT imaging system

Tomoscan

T. AVEU spiral CT scanner

Philips T.

T. SR 7000 scanner

tomoscanner

TomoTherapy Hi-ART system

TomTec

T. cell harvester

T. echo platform

T. Imaging Systems

tone-reducing ankle-foot orthosis

Tones

Tap N' T.

tongs

adjustable skull traction t.

Böhler t.

Cherry traction t.

Crutchfield skeletal traction t.

DePuy Ace Pe.R.I. t.

Edmonton extension t.

Gardner-Wells t.

Gardner-Wells traction t.

Pe.R.I. t.

Raney-Crutchfield skull t.

skull traction t.

traction t.

Trippi-Wells t.

Vinke t.

tongue

t. depressor

t. forceps

t. plate

t. plate electrode

t. retainer

t. retractor

t. retractor blade

tongue-locking device

tongue-retaining device

Tonkaflo pump

tonofilm

Schiötz t.

tonograph

Tonomat applanation tonometer

tonometer (T)

air-puff t.

Alcon t.

Allen-Schiötz plunger retractor t.

AO Reichert Instruments applanation t.

applanation t.

Bailliart t.

Barraquer applanation t.

Barraquer operating room t.

Berens t.

Carl Zeiss t.

Challenger digital applanation t.

Coburn t.

CT-10 computerized t.

Digilab t.

Draeger t.

Gärtner t.

Goldman t.

Goldman applanation t.

Harrington t.

hollow visceral t.

impression t.

indentation t.

Intermedics intraocular t.

Keeler Pulsair t.

Keeler Pulsair noncontact t.

Linear KGT t.

Lombart t.

low-weight t.

Mack t.

MacKay-Marg t.

McLean t.

Mueller electronic t.

noncontact t.

OBF t.

Pach-Pen XL t.

Perkins applanation t.

pneumatic t.

portable PT100 noncontact t.

pressure phosphene t.

ProTon portable t.

Pulsair t.

Recklinghausen t.

Reichert noncontact t.

Rosner t.

Schiötz t.

Sklar t.

Storz t.

Tonomat applanation t.

Tono-Pen t.

Tono-Pen XL t.

tonometric blood pressure monitor

Tono-Pen

Oculab T.-P.

T.-P. tonometer

T.-P. XL

T.-P. XL tonometer

tonsil

t. clamp

t. forceps

t. guillotine

tonsillar

t. abscess forceps

t. artery forceps

t. calipers

t. clamp

T

tonsillar *(continued)*
    t. coblation
    t. compressor
    t. curette
    t. dissector
    t. electrode
    t. expressor
    t. guillotine
    t. hemostatic forceps
    t. hook
    t. knife
    t. loop
    t. pillar grasping forceps
    t. pillar retractor
    t. punch
    t. punch forceps
    t. scissors
    t. screw
    t. snare
    t. snare wire
    t. sponge
    t. suction tube
    t. suture needle
    t. syringe

tonsillectome
    hemostatic t.
    LaForce hemostatic t.
    Mack lingual tonsillar t.
    Sluder-Ballenger t.

tonsillectomy
    t. and adenoidectomy (T&A)
    t. loop

tonsil-tip catheter

Tooke
    T. angled corneal knife
    T. blade

tool
    Acuforce 7.0 therapy t.
    AcuPressor myotherapy t.
    ArthroWand t.
    Backnobber II massage t.
    Bates-Jensen pressure ulcer status t.
    blend t.
    copy t.
    Cybon surgical navigation t.
    Index Knobber II massage t.
    lapping t.
    lens simulation sales t.
    Lillie-Koffler t.
    LIMA-Lift t.
    LIMA-Loop t.
    Magnassager massage t.
    MMS-900 balancing t.
    Original Backnobber massage t.
    Original Index Knobber II
      massage t.
    OsteoStat disposable power t.
    policeman transfer t.
    pressure sore status t.

    Quant-X color quantification
      imaging t.
    Rampart EMS clinical support t.
    Rolz massage t.
    spud t.
    The Original Backnobber
      massage t.
    The Original Index Knobber II
      massage t.
    The Original Jacknobber massage t.
    Therapress pressure point release t.

Toomey
    T. angled cannula
    T. evacuator
    T. G-bevel cannula
    T. standard cannula
    T. surgical steel instrument set
    T. syringe
    T. syringe kit
    T. tip system

tooth
    t. band
    t. cement
    t. guard

tooth-borne distraction device

Toothbrush
    Biotene Ultra Soft T.

toothbrush
    DexTBrush t.
    Sonic-Care t.
    Waterpik t.

tooth-colored abutment

toothed
    t. forceps
    2-t. forceps
    t. pickup
    t. retractor
    t. tenaculum
    t. thumb forceps
    t. tissue forceps

tooth-extracting forceps

toothless forceps

Top
    Bicor T.
    T. Notch automated biopsy system

Topaz
    T. CO_2 laser
    T. manual flexion table
    T. MicroDebrider
    T. microdebrider

Topcon
    T. aspheric lens
    T. chart projector
    T. CM-1000 corneal mapping
      system
    T. 50IA camera
    T. IMAGEnet digital imaging
      system
    T. keratometer

T. KR-7000P auto-kerato-refractometer
T. LM P5 digital lensometer
T. refractor
T. RM-A2300 auto refractometer
T. RM8000B table-mounted autorefractor
T. Screenoscope
T. SL-45 camera
T. SL-E series slit-lamp
T. SP-series noncontact specular microscope
T. TRC-501A fundus camera
T. TRC-50IX ICG-capable fundus camera
T. TRC-SS2 stereoscopic fundus camera
T. TRC-50VT retinal camera
T. TRC-50X retinal camera
T. TRV-50VT fundus camera
T. vision tester

Top-Count microplate scintillation counter
Topel
T. endoscopic cyst aspirator
T. endoscopic cyst aspirator set
top-entry hook
Topex fluoride tray
Top-Fill enteral feeding bag
Top-Hat supraanular aortic valve
TopiFoam silicone gel adhesive foam pad
top-loading screw and rod system
topogometer
topographer
AstraMax stereo t.
Atlas 995 t.
Atlas corneal t.
computerized corneal t.
CT 200 corneal t.
Dicon CT 200 corneal t.
Keratron corneal t.
Keratron scout t.
Medmont E300 t.
TMS-2 computerized corneal t.
topographic
T. Modeling System-1
T. Modeling System-2
t. scanning/indocyanine green angiography combination instrument
t. scanning system
topolyzer
Allegretto wave t.
topometer
C-Scan color-ellipsoid t.
toposcopic catheter

Topper
T. dressing sponge
T. nonadherent gauze
TopSS
T. scanning laser ophthalmoscope
T. topographic scanning system
TopSS/AngioScan system
Torbot cement
Torcon
T. blue catheter
T. NB Advantage coronary angiographic catheter
T. NB selective angiographic catheter
toric
t. intraocular lens
t. lens
Toric-Optima series lens
Torkildsen shunt
Tornado embolization coil
Tornambe infusion cannula
Toronto
T. Medical CPM exerciser
T. parapodium
T. parapodium orthosis
T. splint
T. SPV aortic valve
T. SPV bioprosthesis
T. SPV stentless porcine heart valve
Toronto-Western catheter
TORP
total ossicular replacement prosthesis
TORP ossicular prosthesis
Plastiport TORP
TORP prosthesis
torpedo
Gelfoam t.
Torpin automatic uterine gauze packer
Torq-Flex wire guide
torque
t. attenuating diameter wire
t. catheter
t. control balloon catheter
t. depressor
t. ratchet wrench
t. transducer
t. tube catheter
t. vise
t. wire
torqueable guidewire
torque-control balloon catheter
torqued slot bracket
torque-meter
Compudriver digital t.-m.
torquer
Clip On t.
torque-type prosthesis
torsiometer

torsion
- t. bar splint
- t. forceps
- t. unit

torsionometer

torso
- t. phased-array coil
- t. strap

Torus external fixation system

Toshiba
- T. biplane transesophageal transducer
- T. brain scanner
- T. echocardiograph machine
- T. electrocardiography machine
- T. ERVF 1A video floppy recorder
- T. GGA 9300 camera
- T. helical CT scanner
- T. microendoscope
- T. MR scanner
- T. Sal real-time ultrasonography
- T. scanner
- T. 900S helical CT scanner
- T. Sonolayer transrectal ultrasonography
- T. Sonolayer ultrasound
- T. 900S/XII scanner
- T. TCE-M series colonoscope
- T. TCT-80 CT scanner
- T. ultrasound
- T. videoendoscope
- T. Xpress SX helical CT scanner
- T. X-Vigor scanner
- T. Xvision scanner

total
- T. Abscession drainage catheter
- t. alloplastic TMJ reconstruction prosthesis
- t. anatomical hinge knee brace
- t. articular replacement arthroplasty
- t. artificial heart
- t. body compression suit
- T. Concept ankle/foot prosthesis
- t. condylar III fully constrained prosthesis
- T. Condylar Knee system
- t. contact bivalve ankle-foot orthosis
- t. contact cast
- t. contact orthosis
- t. contact shell ankle-foot orthotic
- T. Cross balloon catheter
- t. facet arthroplasty system (TFAS)
- T. Gym
- t. hip stabilization orthosis
- T. Knee for Children
- t. knee implant
- T. Knee 2100 prosthetic knee

- T. O₂ delivery system
- T. O₂/Oxilite oxygen system
- t. ossicular prosthesis
- t. ossicular reconstruction implant
- t. ossicular replacement prosthesis (TORP)
- T. O₂ supplementary oxygen system
- t. parenteral nutrition line
- t. range of motion (TROM)
- T. Recall digital imaging system
- T. Shock prosthesis
- T. Synchrony system
- t. toe template

TotalBond 4-Meta cement

Totallift-II lifter

totally
- t. implantable access port
- t. implantable catheter
- t. implantable lengthening device

Toti trephine drill

Tott ring remover

TouchAmerica BodyTable

Touchdown thermocycler

Touchlite zoom lens

Touch-Test sensory evaluator

TouchTrak glucose sensor

Touma dissector

Touma-type tube

Tourguide guiding catheter

Tourni-Cot
- T.-C. elastic ring
- T.-C. exsanguinating tourniquet

tourniquet
- Accuflate t.
- automatic t.
- t. band
- Bodenstab t.
- Campbell-Boyd t.
- cotton-covered t.
- t. cuff
- Digikit finger t.
- double-loop t.
- Drake t.
- Esmarch t.
- Field t.
- forearm t.
- Gill renal t.
- Grafco t.
- horseshoe t.
- Johnson & Johnson t.
- Kidde t.
- Linton t.
- Löfqvist t.
- nonpneumatic t.
- Petit t.
- pneumatic t.
- pneumatic ankle t.
- Profex arthroscopic t.

ratchet t.
Robbins automatic t.
Rumel-Belmont t.
Rumel cardiovascular t.
Shenstone t.
single-loop t.
t. strap
thigh t.
Tourni-cot exsanguinating t.
Universal t.
U.S. Army t.
Velcro t.
Wright pneumatic t.

Tovell tube
towel
t. clamp
t. clip
DisCide disinfecting t.
t. drape
fat t.
Kaycel t.
Mambo polishing t.
wound t.

towelette
mini Hype-Wipe bleach t.

tower
ARC surgical wrist traction t.
Linvatec wrist arthroscopy
traction t.

Townley
T. bone graft screw
T. calipers
T. horizontal platform prosthesis
T. implant

Townsend
T. biopsy punch
T. endocervical biopsy curette
T. knee brace
T. Rebel convertible brace

toxemia curette
Toynbee
T. diagnostic tube
T. ear speculum
T. otoscope

TPE
thermoplastic elastomer
TPE ankle-foot orthosis
TPE biomechanical foot orthosis

T-piece
Ayers T-p.

T-plate
dorsal T-p.
palmar T-p.

TPMT
thiopurine methyltransferase
Pro-PredictRx TPMT

TPP
thrust plate prosthesis
TPP hip endoprosthesis

TPR
Thompson-Parkridge-Richards
TPR ankle prosthesis

TPS-coated
T.-c. cylinder
T.-c. screw

trabeculectomy
Pearce t.

trabeculotome
Harms t.
McPherson t.

trabeculotomy probe
Trabucco double balloon catheter
Trac
T. II knee implant
T. II knee prosthesis

trace
T. hydraulic vein stripper
T. vein stripper

tracer
T. blood glucose micromonitor
t. catheter
frequency t.
Gothic arch t.
T. hybrid wire guide
T. microcatheter
T. ST wire

Tracey aberrometer
trach
tracheostomy
t. Care suction
t. plate

TrachCare
Neonatal Y T.

tracheal
t. band
t. button
t. cannula
t. catheter
t. dilator
t. fenestrator
t. forceps
t. hook
t. retractor
t. tenaculum
t. tube
t. tube brush
t. tube changer
t. tube cuff

tracheobronchial
t. stent
t. Z-stent

tracheoesophageal
t. puncture dilator
t. shunt

Tracheolife HME
tracheopharyngeal shunt
tracheoscope
Jackson t.

TracheoSoft XLT tracheostomy tube
tracheostoma valve
tracheostomy (trach)
    t. anatomical model
    t. button
    t. cannula
    t. collar
    t. hook
    Montgomery t.
    t. plate
    t. TOM anatomical model
    t. tube
    t. tube flange
tracheotome
    Sierra-Sheldon t.
tracheotomy
    t. cannula
    t. hook
    t. sponge
Trach-Eze closed suction catheter
Trachlight lighted intubating stylet
Trach-Mist aerosol drainage bay
trachoma forceps
Trach-Talk
    Olympic T.-T.
    T.-T. trachesostomy tube
tracing
    Narco Bio-Systems physiograph t.
Track
    T. Plus
    T. Plus distractor
TrackEASE glucose monitor
tracker
    Breath T.
    T. 10 catheter
    T. Excel catheter
    T. Excel microcatheter
    T. infusion catheter
    T. knee brace
    T. microcatheter
    T. 10 microcatheter
    Palumbo patella t.
    patella t.
    Polaris position t.
    Purkinje image t.
    T. Soft Stream sidehole
      microinfusion catheter
Tracker-18
    T.-18 Soft Stream sidehole
      microinfusion catheter
    T.-18 Unibody catheter
tracker-assisted PRK laser
tracking
    SureStart contrast t.
Trackmaster treadmill
traction
    Ace Trippi-Wells tong cervical t.
    Ace Universal tong cervical t.
    t. anchor

AOA halo cervical t.
t. apparatus
balanced suspension t.
t. bar
t. belt
t. bow
t. bow nut
Bremer halo cervical t.
Bremer halo crown t.
Bryant t.
Buck t.
cervical AOA halo t.
C-Flex supine cervical t.
Chattanooga t.
Cotrel t.
Crutchfield skeletal t.
t. device
device for transverse t.
Dunlop elbow t.
Econo-Cerv supine cervical t.
Econo 90 lumbar home t.
ElastaTrac lumbar t.
t. forceps
Frejka t.
Georgiade visor cervical t.
Hamilton-Russell t.
t. handle
Handy-Buck t.
head halter cervical t.
t. helmet
Holter t.
HomeStretch lumbar t.
t. hook
Houston halo cervical t.
Jones suspension t.
Kirschner skeletal t.
Kirschner wire t.
leg t.
t. legging
lumbosacral support pelvic t.
McBride tripod pin t.
Miami acute collar cervical t.
Miami J collar cervical t.
Neufeld roller t.
Perkins t.
Philadelphia collar cervical t.
Pronex home t.
Pronex pneumatic cervical t.
Quantum t.
Saunders t.
Saunders cervical HomeTrac t.
Sayre suspension t.
t. splint
split Russell skeletal t.
Steinmann t.
supine C-Trax t.
t. suture
t. table
t. table

t. tenaculum
Thomas t.
t. tongs
t. tongs screw
transfer t.
Watson-Jones t.
tractograph
MOM t.
tractor
Böhler t.
Exo-Bed t.
Fisk t.
halo t.
Kirschner wire t.
Lowsley t.
Lowsley prostatic t.
Lowsley suprapubic t.
Lyman-Smith t.
prostatic t.
Pugh t.
Steinmann traction t.
Syms t.
Young prostatic t.
traditional IOL
TRAFO orthosis
tragus House hook
Trailblazer screw guide
trainer
Biodex gait t.
Biodex target balance t.
computer-aided fluency
  establishment t.
dynamic stabilization t.
impulse inertial exercise t.
Monark rehab t.
Personal EMG t.
positional feedback stimulation t.
Posture Pump spine t.
Regain home EMG t.
Shuttle balance t.
Sprint cross t.
training
CDBR respiratory muscle t.
trajectory
Trak Back pullback device
Trake-Fit
T.-F. system
T.-F. tracheal tube holder
T.-F. tracheostomy tube
Trakstar balloon catheter
Tram
Suture T.
Tramscope 12
Tranquility
T. Auto
T. Auto CPAP system
T. Bilevel airway patency
  maintenance device
T. Bilevel CPAP unit

T. Bilevel positive airway pressure
  therapy device
T. bilevel system
T. Quest
T. Quest CPAP
T. Quest CPAP device
T. Quest CPAP system
transabdominal transducer
TransAct intraaortic balloon pump
transanal catheter
transarticular screw
transaxillary needle
TransBleph implant
transbuccal trocar
transcallosal band
transcatheter
t. device
t. intravascular ring platform
t. patch
t. umbrella
t. umbrella implant material
transcervical
t. Foley catheter
t. tubal access catheter
transconjunctival retractor
transcranial
t. Doppler (TCD)
t. Doppler probe
t. imaging transducer
transcutaneous
t. bilirubinometer
t. blood gas monitor
t. broadband sector transducer
t. carbon dioxide monitor
t. cranial electrical stimulator
t. electrical nerve stimulator
t. electrical neuromuscular
  stimulator (TENS)
t. extraction catheter
t. jaundice meter
t. lead
t. oxygen monitor (TCOM)
t. pacemaker
Thin-Layer Rapid-Use T. (T.R.U.E.)
TransCyte
T. skin substitute graft
T. temporary skin substitute
transdermal fentanyl device
transducer
Acuson t.
Acuson linear array t.
Acuson V5M multiplane TEE t.
Acuson V5M multiplane
  transesophageal
  echocardiographic t.
Aloka t.
anular array t.
Array ultrasound t.
ART t.

transducer *(continued)*
arterial line t.
ATL UltraMark IV linear-array t.
Bentley t.
bifocal multiplane rectal t.
biplanar t.
biplane TEE t.
bite force t.
blood pressure t.
Brüel & Kjaer axial t.
t. catheter
catheter-borne sector t.
Combitrans t.
curved-array t.
Dantec Etude uroflow t.
Deltran disposable t.
Diasonics t.
differential variable reluctance t.
Dräger MTC t.
electromagnetic flow t.
Elema-Siemens AB pressure t.
end-fire t.
endovaginal t.
epicardial Doppler flow sector t.
external pressure t.
fluid-filled pressure t.
force t.
forced displacement t.
Gaeltec catheter-tip pressure t.
Gould pressure t.
Gould-Statham pressure t.
Hall-effect strain t.
high-resolution linear-array t.
HP Sonos t.
in-shoe t.
intracavitary t.
linear t.
linear-array t.
linear-array B-mode ultrasound t.
linear-variable-differential t.
Logic MR t.
LSC curved-array t.
magnetic motion t.
magnetic resonance imaging-guided focused ultrasound sector t.
Medex t.
microtip pressure t.
Mikro-Tip t.
Millar catheter-tip t.
Millar Mikro-Tip catheter pressure t.
M-mode sector t.
Mountain View t.
multifrequency t.
multiplanar t.
multiplane t.
nasal cannula pressure t.
Nellcor Durasensor adult oxygen t.
Neuroguard pulsed wave t.

Ocuscan t.
Olympus intracavity t.
Oxisensor t.
Oxisensor oxygen t.
phased-array sector t.
piezoelectric t.
piezoelectric ultrasound t.
piezo-resistive t.
pressure t.
pressure t.
pulsed-wave Doppler t.
puncture t.
quartz t.
radial-sector scan t.
range-gated t.
rectal multiplane t.
rotatory variable-differential t.
SensorMedics pressure t.
Siemens Endo-P endodrectal t.
SLA t.
Sleepscan airflow pressure t.
Sonogage System Corneo-Gage center frequency t.
Sonos ultrasonographic t.
Sorensen Transpac t.
Soreson pressure t.
Spectramed t.
Spectranetics Statham t.
Statham external t.
Statham pressure t.
strain gauge t.
Therasound t.
torque t.
Toshiba biplane transesophageal t.
transabdominal t.
transcranial imaging t.
transcutaneous broadband sector t.
Transpac disposable pressure t.
Transpac IV pressure t.
transrectal multiplane 3-dimensional t.
TruWave disposable pressure t.
UBM t.
Ultramark 8 t.
ultrasound t.
Unisensor strain-gauge t.
variomatrix t.
Vingmed CFM t.
Voluson sector t.
transducer-tipped catheter
Transeal
T. transparent film
T. transparent wound dressing
transection hook
transendoscopic
t. ultrasound
Transend steerable guidewire
transensor
Ommaya reservoir t.

transesophageal
    t. echocardiography probe
    t. echo probe
    t. pacing system
transfemoral
    t. endoaortic occlusion catheter
    t. modular prosthesis
transfer
    t. board
    t. forceps
    T. Handle support handle
    t. traction
TransFix
    T. ACL reconstruction system
    T. ACL system
    T. ACL system fixation
    T. bio-interference screw
transfixing screw
transfixion
    t. bolt
    t. screw
    t. suture
transform
    fast Fourier t.
transformer
    Coolidge t.
    distribution t.
    doughnut t.
    filament t.
    high-voltage t.
    linear variable differential t.
    stepdown t.
    stepup t.
transgastric esophageal bougienage
transgrow bottle
transhepatic
    t. biliary stent
    t. catheter
    t. portacaval shunt
TransiGel
    T. hydrogel-impregnated gauze
    T. impregnated gauze
    T. woven gauze dressing
transilluminating telescope
transillumination
transilluminator
    Finnoff t.
    Finnoff sinus t.
    hooded t.
    Jako t.
    Lancaster ocular t.
    National opal glass t.
    rotating t.
    speculum illuminator t.
    UV t.
    Welch Allyn t.
transistor
    field-effect t.
    insulated gate field-effect t.

ion-sensitive field-effect t.
    junction field-effect t.
    metal oxide semiconductor field-
      effect t.
transition
    t. lens
    short t. (ST)
transit time flowmeter
transjugular
    t. intrahepatic portosystemic shunt
    t. intrahepatic portosystemic stent-
      shunt
translaminar facet screw
translin-associated factor X (TRAX)
translocation needle
translucent
    t. drain tube
    t. myringotomy tube
    t. silicone tube
translumbar inferior vena cava catheter
transluminal
    t. angioplasty catheter
    t. balloon
    t. endarterectomy catheter
    t. lysing system
transluminally
    t. placed endovascular branched
      stent-graft
    t. placed Inoue endovascular stent-
      graft
transmandibular implant
transmaxillary screw
transmission electron microscope
transmit-receive coil
transmitter
    chest-band t.
    false neurochemical t.
    miniature ultrasound t.
transmitter-receiver
    Itrel programmed t.-r.
transmural
    t. antitachycardia pacemaker
    t. electrical stimulator
transmyocardial pacing stylet
transnasal
    t. intraduodenal feeding catheter
    t. pancreaticobiliary drain
    t. videoesophagoscope
    t. videogastroscope
transobturator (TO)
    t. sling
Transonic flow probe
Transonics
    T. flowmeter
    T. Flow probe
    T. laser Doppler flowmeter
    T. laser Doppler perfusion monitor
    T. system
    T. Systems flow probe

transoral
  t. catheter
  t. retractor
Transorbent
  T. dressing
  T. hydrogel sheet
  T. topical wound dressing
Transorb wound dressing
transosseous
  t. implant
  t. post
  t. suture
transosteal pin implant
Transpac
  T. disposable pressure transducer
  T. IV pressure transducer
transpapillary
  t. cystopancreatic stent
  t. drain
  t. endoscope
  t. endoscopic endoprosthesis
transparent
  t. adhesive film dressing
  t. drape
  t. elastic band ligating device
  t. film dressing
transpedicular
  t. cannulated screw
  t. drill guide
  t. screw
transpedicularly implanted anterior spinal support device
transpericardial pacemaker
Transpire wrist orthosis
transplant
  osteochondral t. (OCT)
  t. trephine
Transpore
  T. eye tape
  T. surgical tape dressing
transport
  air medical t.
  T. dilation balloon catheter
  T. drug delivery catheter
  fixed-wing t.
  Monte Carlo photon t.
  t. vehicle
transporter
  Dura-Temp specimen t.
transpubic needle
transpupillary laser
transpyloric feeding tube
transrectal
  t. multiplane 3-dimensional transducer
  t. probe
TransScan
  T. electrical impedance breast scanning system

  T. electrical impedance scanning system
Trans-Scan
  T.-S. noninvasive physiological monitor
  T.-S. pulsed Doppler sonographer
transscleral suture
transseptal
  t. cannula
  t. catheter
  t. needle
  t. sheath
transsphenoidal
  t. bipolar forceps
  t. curette
  t. dissector
  t. enucleator
  t. speculum
transtelephonic
  t. ambulatory monitoring system
  t. exercise monitor
transthoracic
  t. catheter
  t. pacemaker
  t. pacing stylet
transthoracically implanted ICD
transtracheal oxygen catheter
transurethral
  t. catheter
  t. microwave thermotherapy (TUMT)
  t. needle ablation (TUNA)
  t. resection of prostate (TURP)
transvaginal
  t. bone anchor
  t. ultrasound
Transvene
  T. nonthoracotomy implantable cardioverter-defibrillator
  T. tripolar electrode
transvenous
  t. defibrillator lead
  t. electrode
  t. implantable defibrillator
  t. nitinol snare
  t. pacemaker catheter
  t. ventricular demand pacemaker
transventricular dilator
transverse
  t. connector
  t. gradient coil
Transwell membrane
transzonular vitreal injection cannula
trap
  Allergenco MK-3 spore t.
  Burkard spore t.
  T. cardiovascular filtration system collection t.
  Endodynamics suction polyp t.

extraction t.
filtered specimen t.
Hirst spore t.
inline t.
Kramer-Collins spore t.
laser t.
Lukens t.
Luki specimen t.
T. neurovascular filtration system
osseous coagulum t.
specimen t.
sterile specimen t.
suction polyp t.
T. vascular filtration system

TrapEase
T. inferior vena cava filter
T. permanent IVC filter
T. permanent vena cava filter
T. vena cava filter

trapeze bar
trapeziometacarpal joint replacement prosthesis
trapezium implant
trapezoid
t. angled CVD diamond knife
t. blade
large t. (LT)
small t. (ST)
Superblade t.

trapezoidal metal cage
trapezoidal-28 prosthesis
trapper
T. catheter exchange device
FoamWrap finger t.

Traquair periosteal elevator
trauma
cardiac t.
t. care system

TraumaJet wound debridement system
traumatic grasping forceps
Trautmann chisel
Traveler
T. portable oxygen system
Pulmo-Aide T.

Travenol
T. biopsy needle
T. infuser
T. infusion pump
T. Infusor pump

TRAX
translin-associated factor X
TRAX catheter

TraXis
T. interbody spacer
T. Ti alloy spacer
T. Vue alloy spacer

tray
Bard universal Foley catheter
sterile insertion t.

Bard urethral catheter sterile t.
Curity irrigation t.
Dacron t.
Davol sterile irrigation t.
EZ-EM PercuSet amniocentesis t.
Henry instrument t.
HSG t.
I-tech cannula t.
lock pericardiocentesis set and t.
Mayo instrument t.
mobile dilator storage t.
Monoject laceration irrigation t.
Müller t.
One Time sharp debridement t.
orthodontic impression t.
Papanicolaou smear t.
PFC offset tibial t.
ProTech instrument protection t.
Russell gastrostomy t.
titanium mesh t.
Topex fluoride t.
Unimar HSG t.
urethral intermittent catheter and t.
Urine Meter Foley t.
vacuum-formed resin impression t.
Weck microsurgical t.

TRD
tinnitus relief device

treadmill
Aquaciser underwater t.
AquaGaiter t.
arm ergometry t.
Cateye t.
exercise t.
HydroTrack underwater t.
Lifestride t.
Marquette t.
Orbiter t.
Q-Stress t.
Trackmaster t.
Woodway t.

treatment
t. port
t. table
Wartner over-the-counter wart
removal t.

Tredex
T. powered bicycle
Universal T.

tree
BTE assembly t.
finger blocking t.
pinch t.
pipe t.

trefoil
t. balloon catheter
t. Schneider balloon

Trelex natural mesh
Trelles metal scleral shield

Trendelenburg
  T. cannula
  T. tampon
trepan
trephine
  Arroyo t.
  Arruga lacrimal t.
  automated t.
  automatic t.
  Bard-Parker t.
  Barraquer t.
  Barron disposable t.
  Barron epikeratophakia t.
  Barron-Hessburg corneal t.
  Barron radial vacuum t.
  t. blade
  Boston t.
  Caldwell suction t.
  cam-guided t.
  Castroviejo corneal transplant t.
  chalazion t.
  t. core biopsy needle
  corneal prosthesis t.
  Cross scleral t.
  Davis t.
  disposable t.
  t. drill
  Elliot corneal t.
  Elschnig t.
  epithelial t.
  Franceschetti corneal t.
  Galt skull t.
  Gradle corneal t.
  Grieshaber calibrated t.
  Grieshaber corneal t.
  Guyton corneal transplant t.
  hand t.
  handheld t.
  Hanna t.
  Hessburg-Barron disposable
    vacuum t.
  Hessburg vacuum t.
  Horsley t.
  Katena t.
  Katzin t.
  Keyes cutaneous t.
  King corneal t.
  lacrimal t.
  Lahey Clinic skull t.
  LASEK alcohol well and
    epithelial t.
  Leksell t.
  Lichtenberg corneal t.
  t. marker
  Martinez disposable corneal t.
  M-Brace corneal t.
  Michele vertebral t.
  mini t.
  Moria t.

  Mueller electric corneal t.
  Olson calibrated cornea t.
  Ophtec t.
  Oto-Flex t.
  Paton corneal t.
  Paufique corneal t.
  Pharmacia corneal t.
  punch t.
  razor blade t.
  Rochester bone t.
  Searcy chalazion t.
  sinus t.
  skull t.
  Sloane t.
  Storz corneal t.
  Surgistar corneal t.
  transplant t.
  Troutman tenotomy t.
  Turkel t.
  Von Hippel mechanical t.
  Walker t.
  Walker corneal t.
  Weck t.
Trerotola thrombectomy device
Trestle prostatic bridge
Trevisani
  T. cannula
  T. cannula tip
  T. tip
Trex digital mammography system
TriActiv
  T. balloon-protected flush extraction
    system
  T. embolic protection system
triad
  T. defibrillator system
  T. hydrocolloid
  T. hydrocolloid dressing
  T. hydrophilic wound dressing
  T. SPECT imaging system
  Widal-Abrami-Lermoyez t.
TriaDyne
  T. bed
Triage
  T. BNP test
  T. cardiac rapid diagnostic test
    system
  T. cardiac system
  T. MeterPlus
trial
  t. acetabular cup
  t. component
  t. contact lens
  t. driver
  t. fracture frame
  t. frame
  t. implant
  t. lens
  t. prosthesis

triangle
t. blade system
T. gelatin-sealed sling material
IMP knee-positioning t.
Kager t.
knee-positioning t.
Tri-Angle shoulder abduction brace
triangle-tipped knife
triangular
t. ankle fusion frame
t. arm sling
t. bandage
t. bone reamer
t. dressing
t. encompassing clip
t. punch forceps
t. rasp
triangulated pedicle screw
triaxial
t. accelerometer
t. prosthesis
t. semiconstrained elbow prosthesis
Triax monotube external fixation system
Tri-Beeled trapezoidal keratome
tricalcium
trichoesthesiometer
trichoscope
TriClip endoscopic clipping device
Tricodur
T. compression support bandage
T. Epi compression bandage
T. Omos compression bandage
T. Talus compression bandage
tricomponent coaxial system
Tri-Con component
Tricon-M
T.-M cruciate-sparing prosthesis
T.-M patellar prosthesis
Tricoplast adhesive elastic bandage
Tri-Core cervical support pillow
TricOs T bone void filler
tricuspid
t. aortic valve
t. valve strut
Tricut
T. blade
T. laryngeal blade tip
Trident ceramic hip system
triethylenethiophosphoramide precoated slide
Tri-Ex triple-lumen extraction balloon
TriEye
T. cannula
T. tip
trifacet
t. blade
t. diamond knife
Tri-Flex auxiliary suspension belt

Tri-Float pressure reduction mattress
trifocal
executive t.
t. glasses
t. lens
trigeminal
t. electrode
t. knife
t. scissors
trigeminus cannula
trigger
t. cannula
t. finger release knife
Smart T.
triggered
atrial t. (AAT)
ventricular t. (VVT)
ventricular, atrial, t. (VAT)
TriggerWheel
T. device
T. wand
trigonotome
trilaminate cushion
trileaflet prosthesis
Tri-Lock
T.-L. acetabular cup
T.-L. press-fit prosthesis
Trilogy
T. AB acetabular system
T. acetabular cup
T. acetabular cup system
T. DC, DR, SR pulse generator
T. DC+ pacemaker
T. I hearing aid
T. image-guided radiation therapy system
T. image-guided radiosurgery system
T. low-profile balloon dilatation catheter
T. prosthesis
T. SR+ single-chamber pacemaker
Trilon multilayered material
Trilucent breast implant
trimandibular plate
Trimedyne
T. Flex MAX fiber
T. holmium laser
T. Optilase device
Trim-It screw system
Trimline knee immobilizer
trimmer
Mallory-Head Interlok calcar t.
Tri-Motion knee system
Trinion meniscus screw
Trinity polyaxial pedicle screw system
Trinkle
T. bone drill
T. chuck

Trinkle *(continued)*
   T. chuck adapter
   T. screwdriver
   T. socket wrench
Trio
   T. arthroscope
   T. medialized rod system
triode tube
Trionix
   T. camera
   T. scanner
Trionix-Triad camera
Trio-Stim neuromuscular stimulator
trip
   T. tonometry catheter
   t. wire
tri-panel knee immobilizer
Triphasix generator
triplanar
   t. protractor
   t. protractor apparatus
triplane construct
triple
   t. hook
triple-bend tip
triple-edge diamond-blade knife
triple-frequency probe
triple-head gamma camera
triple-injection
   t.-i. cine arthrogram
   t.-i. cinearthrography
triple-lumen
   t.-l. Arrow catheter
   t.-l. balloon flotation thermistor catheter
   t.-l. biliary manometry catheter
   t.-l. catheter
   t.-l. central catheter
   t.-l. implant
   t.-l. manometry catheter
   t.-l. needle
   t.-l. perfused catheter system
   t.-l. sump drain
   t.-l. tube
triple-tail fascia lata sling
triple-thermistor coronary sinus catheter
tripod
   t. grasper
   t. grasping forceps
   t. intraocular lens
tripolar
   t. Damato curved catheter
   t. defibrillation coil electrode
   t. electrode catheter
   t. lead
   t. nerve cuff electrode
   t. with Damato curve catheter
triport
   t. cannula

   t. sub-Tenon anesthesia cannula
   t. tip
TriPort hemostasis introducer sheath kit
Trippi-Wells tongs
Tripter
   Direx T.
triradial resector blade
tris-acryl gelatin microsphere
trisector
   Alfonso nucleus t.
   Alfonso nucleus ophthalmic t.
TriSpan
   T. aneurysm neck-bridge device
   T. detachable coil
Tri-Spike acetabular component
TriStander
Tristar blunt-tip trocar
TriTis tibial fixation system
triton reciprocating saw
TriTrac-R3D accelerometer
TriVex system
Tri W-G table
TRIzol
   T. RNA extractor
trocar
   abdominal t.
   AMS disposable t.
   antral t.
   Argyle t.
   Axiom thoracic t.
   BD Potain thoracic t.
   Beardsley cecostomy t.
   beveled t.
   blunt t.
   Bluntport disposable t.
   brain t.
   Bülau t.
   Cabot t.
   Circon-ACMI t.
   Coakley antral t.
   Cook urological t.
   Core Dynamics disposable t.
   Curschmann t.
   Davidson thoracic t.
   Dexide disposable t.
   Diamond-Flex t.
   disposable t.
   Douglas antral t.
   Duchenne t.
   Duke t.
   Endopath bladeless t.
   Endopath dilating tip t.
   Endopath TriStar t.
   Endopath Xcel bladeless t.
   Endopath Xcel blunt-tip t.
   ensheathing t.
   Entree II t.
   Entree thoracoscopy t.

Ethicon t.
Ethicon disposable t.
Flexipath flexible surgical
  thoracic t.
Hasson t.
Hasson laparoscopic t.
hollow stainless steel t.
Hunt angiographic t.
Ingram t.
intercostal t.
intestinal decompression t.
Jarit disposable t.
Johannson-Stille cystotomy t.
Judd t.
Kidd t.
Krause antral t.
Landau t.
large-bore t.
laryngeal t.
Lichtwitz abdominal t.
Lichtwitz antral t.
Lillie antral t.
Marlow disposable t.
Mayo-Ochsner t.
Monoscopy locking t.
Neal catheter t.
t. needle
nested t.
Olympus disposable t.
Optiview t.
Origin t.
Pierce antral t.
plain vesical t.
Poole t.
pyramidal tip t.
rectal t.
Saber BT blunt-tip surgical t.
sharp t.
Solos disposable t.
Step laparoscopic t.
Storz disposable t.
subcostal t.
suprapubic t.
Surgiport disposable t.
Synthes transbuccal t.
thoracic t.
Thoracoport single-use t.
transbuccal t.
Tristar blunt-tip t.
Universal abdominal t.
Van Alyea antral t.
Visiport optical t.
Weck disposable t.
Wisap disposable t.
Wolf disposable t.
Wolf needle t.
Xcel blunt-tip t.
Ximed disposable t.
trocar-cannula system

trocar-point Kirschner wire
Trocath peritoneal dialysis catheter
trochanter holder
trochanter-holding clamp
trochanteric
    t. bolt
    t. fixation nail (TFN)
    t. pin
    t. plate
    t. wire
Troeltsch
    T. dressing forceps
    T. ear forceps
    T. ear speculum
Troemner percussion hammer
TroGARD electrosurgical blunt trocar
  system
Trokel lens
trolley
    Bolero lift bath t.
TROM
    total range of motion
    TROM knee brace
Troncoso
    T. gonioscope
    T. tubular lens
TRON 3 VACI cardiac imaging system
Tronzo
    T. elevator
    T. prosthesis
Trooper floppy moderate-support guide
  wire
tropometer
troposcope
trough splint
trousers
    air t.
    MAST t.
    military antishock t. (MAST)
Trousseau
    T. dilating forceps
    T. mouthgag
    T. tracheal dilator
Trousseau-Jackson
    T.-J. esophageal dilator
    T.-J. tracheal dilator
Troutman
    T. alpha-chymotrypsin cannula
    T. blade
    T. bladebreaker
    T. blade holder
    T. cannula
    T. conjunctival scissors
    T. corneal forceps
    T. corneal knife
    T. eye implant
    T. implant
    T. lens loupe
    T. microsurgery forceps

T

965

Troutman *(continued)*
    T. microsurgical scissors
    T. needle
    T. needle holder
    T. nonincisional lamellar dissector
    T. punch
    T. rectus forceps
    T. superior rectus forceps
    T. suture scissors
    T. tenotomy trephine
    T. tying forceps
Troutman-Barraquer
    T.-B. corneal fixation forceps
    T.-B. iris forceps
    T.-B. iris spatula
    T.-B. miniblade breaker
    T.-B. needle holder
Troutman-Barraquer-Colibri forceps
Troutman-Castroviejo corneal section scissors
Troutman-Katzin corneal transplant scissors
Troutman-Llobera fixation forceps
Trowbridge
    T. TerraRound all-terrain prosthesis
    T. TerraRound foot
    T. TerraRound sports limb
Truarch wire
Tru-Area Determination wound measuring device
TruBlock
    T. BGS block
    T. BGS block implant
Tru-Canal hearing aid
Tru-Cut
    T.-C. biopsy needle
    T.-C. biopsy needle holder
    T.-C. needle
    T.-C. needle biopsy
T.R.U.E.
    Thin-Layer Rapid-Use Transcutaneous T.R.U.E. test
True
    T. Blue exercise band
    T. Form support stocking
    T. separator
    T. Sheathless intraaortic balloon catheter
    T. test kit
True/Fit femoral intramedullary rod system
True/Flex
    T. intramedullary nail
    T. intramedullary rod system
True-Lok
    T.-L. external fixation
    T.-L. external fixator system
TrueMax metabolic measuring system
TrueTorque wire guide

Trufill n-BCA liquid embolic system
TruFill n-BCA surgical glue
TruFit
    T. BGS plug
    T. BGS plug implant
Tru-Fit
    T.-F. brace
    T.-F. custom-molded shoe
TruGraft BGS granule
TruKor site preparation kit
Trulife silicone breast form
TruLine forceps
Tru-Mold shoe
trumpet
    t. cannula
    Iowa t.
    nasal t.
    t. needle guide
truncated NMR probe
truncus clamp
trunk-hip-knee-ankle-foot orthosis
trunnion
trunnion-bearing hip prosthesis
Trupower aspherical lens
TruPro lacrimal cannula
TruPulse
    T. carbon dioxide laser
    T. CO2 laser system
    T. CO_2 skin resurfacing laser
    T. laser
truss
    t. element
    Kansas City band t.
    Nu-Form t.
    scrotal t.
Tru-Stain acrylic powder
TruStep foot prosthesis
Tru-Support
    T.-S. EW bandage
    T.-S. SA bandage
Tru Taper Ethalloy needle
TruTone artificial larynx
TruTrak data sampling system
TruWave disposable pressure transducer
TruWedge
    T. BGS osteotomy wedge
    T. osteotomy wedge
TruZone
    T. asthma action plan wallet card
    T. peak flowmeter
    T. PFM
TS-200
T-Scan 2000
T-shaped
    T-s. AO plate
    T-s. constriction ring
    T-s. Edwards-Barbaro syringeal shunt

T-s. Edwards-Barbaro syringeal shunt table
T-s. forceps
T-Sling
T-Span tissue expander
TSRH
Texas Scottish Rite Hospital
TSRH buttressed laminar hook
TSRH circular laminar hook
TSRH corkscrew device
TSRH crosslink
TSRH double-rod construct
TSRH 3D spinal instrumentation
TSRH fixation system
Galveston fixation with TSRH
TSRH hook holder
TSRH hook inserter
TSRH hook-rod
TSRH I-bolt
TSRH instrumentation
TSRH mini-corkscrew device
TSRH pedicle hook
TSRH pedicle screw
TSRH pedicle screw-laminar claw construct
TSRH screw-rod system
TSRH trial hook
TSRH wrench
TS system
T-Stick adhesive
T-strap
Tsunami laser
Tsuneoka irrigating chopper
TT
T. Pylon prosthesis
T. tip
TT-3 needle
T-Tac system
TTAP-ST acetabular prosthesis
TTS
through-the-scope
TTS Aire-Cuf endotracheal tube
TTS Aire-Cuf tracheostomy tube
TTS catheter
TTS dilator
Rigiflex esophageal TTS
T-tube
T-t. catheter
T-t. drain
T-t. round suction tube
T-t. stent
T-type
T-t. dental implant
T-t. matrix band
T-t. myringotomy tube
tub
hydrotherapy t.
tubal
t. hook

t. insufflation cannula
t. scissors
Tubbs
T. aortic dilator
T. mitral valve dilator
tube
Abbott t.
Abbott-Rawson gastrointestinal double-lumen t.
AccuMark calibrated infant feeding t.
Activent antimicrobial ventilation t.
Activent ear t.
Adson suction t.
Ahmed glaucoma drainage t.
Ahmed glaucoma valve t.
Ahmed shunt t.
Aire-Cuf endotracheal t.
Aire-Cuf tracheostomy t.
All-Silicone Side-Eye EPT feeding t.
American tracheotomy t.
Amersham J t.
Anderson gastric t.
Andrews-Pynchon suction t.
Angio-Seal carrier t.
angled pleural t.
angled suction t.
anode t.
Anthony mastoid suction t.
Arm-a-Med endotracheal t.
Armstrong t.
Armstrong ventilation t.
Aromamist steam t.
aspiration t.
Aspisafe nasogastric t.
Atkins-Cannard tracheal t.
Atkinson t.
t. attachment device
auditory t.
Baerveldt glaucoma implant t.
Baerveldt shunt t.
Baggish injection t.
bag-valve device to tracheostomy t.
Baker jejunostomy t.
Baker self-sumping t.
Baldwin butterfly ventilation t.
Bard gastrostomy feeding t.
Bard PEG t.
Baron-Frazier suction t.
Baron suction t.
Baylor cardiovascular sump t.
Benjamin t.
Ben-Jet t.
bicanalicular silicone t.
bilateral pleural t.
Bilbao-Dotter t.
Biolite ventilation t.
Biosystems feeding t.

tube *(continued)*

Bivona Fome-Cuf t.
Bivona Medical Technologies customized tracheostomy t.
Bivona tracheostomy t.
Bivona TTS tracheostomy t.
Blakemore-Sengstaken t.
Blue Line cuffed endotracheal t.
blunt suction t.
bobbin myringotomy t.
Bouchut laryngeal t.
Bourdon t.
Bower PEG t.
Bowman t.
bronchial t.
Broncho-Cath double-lumen endotracheal t.
bronchoscopy disposable suction t.
Buie rectal suction t.
button-type G t.
Buyes air-vent suction t.
Caluso PEG gastrostomy t.
calyx t.
Cantor intestinal t.
capillary t.
Carabelli t.
Carden bronchoscopy t.
Carlen double-lumen endotracheal t.
carrier t.
cathode ray t. (CRT)
Cattell T t.
Celestin t.
Celestin esophageal t.
t. changer
Chaoul voltage x-ray t.
Chaussier t.
chest t.
Chinese fingertrap t.
cholecystostomy t.
ClearCRIT microhematocrit t.
Clerf laryngectomy t.
closed suction t.
coagulation aspirator t.
coagulation suction t.
Cobed t.
Cole endotracheal t.
Cole orotracheal t.
Cole uncuffed endotracheal t.
collecting t.
Combitube endotracheal t.
Comfit endotracheal t.
conical centrifuge t.
t. connector
continuous suction t.
Cooley graft suction t.
Cooley sump t.
Coolidge x-ray t.
Cope loop nephrostomy t.
Corflo enteral feeding t.

Corflo PEG t.
corneal t.
Corpak weighted-tip self-lubricating t.
Corvac integrated serum separator t.
Council-tip t.
Coupland nasal suction t.
Craigie t.
Crawford t.
Crookes-Hittorf t.
cryovial t.
cuffed endotracheal t.
cuffed ET t.
cuffed tracheostomy t.
cul-de-sac irrigation T t.
Dale-Schwartz t.
Dandy suction t.
Davol colon t.
Davol feeding t.
Dawson-Yuhl suction t.
DeBakey-Adson suction t.
Debove t.
decompressive chest t.
Dennis colorectal t.
DePaul t.
t. device
Devine-Millard-Frazier fiberoptic suction t.
diagnostic t.
Diamond t.
DIC tracheostomy t.
digestive t.
digit t.
direct percutaneous jejunostomy t.
discharge t.
disposable Yankauer aspirating t.
disposable Yankauer suction t.
Dobbhoff feeding t.
Dobbhoff gastrectomy feeding t.
Dobbhoff gastric decompression t.
Dobbhoff nasogastric feeding t.
Dobbhoff PEG t.
Donaldson t.
Dotter t.
double-cannula tracheostomy t.
double-focus t.
double-lumen endobronchial t.
double-lumen endotracheal t.
double-lumen suction irrigation t.
double setup endotracheal t.
t. dressing
dual-lumen sump nasogastric t.
dual percutaneous gastrostomy t.
Dundas-Grant t.
Duo-Tube feeding t.
Durham tracheostomy t.
Dynamic digit extensor t.
EDTA-Vacutainer t.

electron multiplier t.
endobrachial double-lumen t.
endobronchial t.
endoesophageal t.
EndoFlex endotracheal t.
Endosoft reinforced cuffed t.
endothelin-1 platinum Dacron
  microcoil endotracheal t.
endotracheal t.
Endotrol endotracheal t.
Endotrol tracheal t.
Endo-Tube nasojejunal feeding t.
EnteraFlo feeding t.
enteroclysis t.
EntriStar feeding t.
EntriStar polyurethane PEG t.
Eppendorf t.
Esmarch t.
esophagotracheal combination t.
ET t.
Ethox feeding t.
ETView endotracheal t.
eustachian t.
Ewald t.
Exerband Pak bilateral t.
Exerband Pak unilateral t.
extension t.
feeding t.
fenestrated t.
fenestrated tracheostomy t.
Ferguson-Frazier suction t.
fermentation t.
Feuerstein split ventilation t.
fiberoptic suction t.
field emission t.
Finsterer suction t.
Fitzpatrick suction t.
flanged Teflon t.
Flex DIC tracheostomy t.
Flexiflo enteral feeding t.
Flexiflo Inverta-PEG t.
Flexiflo Sacks-Vine t.
Flexiflo stoma-creator t.
Flexiflo Stomate low-profile
  gastrostomy t.
Flexiflo suction feeding t.
Flexiflo tungsten weighted
  feeding t.
Flexiflo Versa-PEG t.
flow regulated suction t.
flow-regulated suction t.
Flow-Thru feeding t.
fluffy-cuffed t.
t. foam
Foley t.
follicle aspiration t.
Fome-Cuf endotracheal t.
Fome-Cuf pediatric tracheostomy t.
Fome-Cuf tracheostomy t.

Franco triflange ventilation t.
Frazier aspirating t.
Frazier brain suction t.
Frazier Britetrac nasal suction t.
Frazier-Ferguson aspirating t.
Frazier-Ferguson ear suction t.
Frazier fiberoptic suction t.
Frazier nasal suction t.
Frazier-Paparella mastoid suction t.
Frazier suction t.
Frederick-Miller t.
French nasogastric t.
French T t.
frontal sinus wash t.
gastric t.
gastric lavage t.
gastrojejunostomy t.
Gastro-Port II feeding t.
gastrostomy t.
gastrostomy feeding t.
Geiger-Müller t.
Gillquist-Stille arthroplasty
  suction t.
Gilman-Abrams gastric t.
glow modular t.
glutaraldehyde-tanned bovine
  collagen t.
Gomco suction t.
Goode T t.
Goode T-tube ventilating t.
Goodhill-Pynchon tonsillar
  suction t.
Gore-Tex t.
Gott t.
Gowen decompression t.
t. graft
graft suction t.
Great Ormond Street pediatric
  tracheostomy t.
Greiling gastroduodenal t.
Greiner Vacuette coagulation
  plastic t.
grommet t.
grommet drain t.
grommet myringotomy t.
grommet ventilating t.
Guibor silastic t.
Guilford-Wright suction t.
Haldane t.
Haldane-Priestley t.
Hamamatsu high-sensitivity
  photomultiplier t.
Hardy suction t.
Harris t.
Heimlich t.
Helsper tracheostomy vent t.
Hemagard collection t.
Hemochron glass-activated ACT t.
Hemovac suction t.

tube *(continued)*

Herring t.
high heat-capacity x-ray t.
high-pressure connecting t.
Hi-Lo Evac endotracheal t.
Hi-Lo Jet tracheal t.
Holter t.
hot cathode x-ray t.
House-Baron suction t.
House endolymphatic shunt t.
Houser cul-de-sac irrigator t.
Houser cul-de-sac irrigator T t.
House suction t.
House-Urban t.
Hunsaker jet ventilation t.
Hyperflex tracheostomy t.
image intensifier t.
image Orthicon t.
infusion t.
intracardiac suction t.
intracardiac sump t.
intratracheal t.
intubation t.
Isolator lysis-centrifugation t.
Jackson aspirating t.
Jackson cone-shaped tracheal t.
Jackson laryngectomy t.
Jackson-Pratt suction t.
Jackson-Rees endotracheal t.
Jackson silver tracheostomy t.
Jako laryngeal suction t.
Javid bypass t.
jejunal feeding t.
jejunostomy t.
Jiffy t.
Johnson coagulation suction t.
Johnson intestinal t.
Jones Pyrex t.
Jones tear duct t.
J-shaped t.
K t.
Kamen-Wilkinson endotracheal t.
Kam Vac suction t.
Kangaroo gastrostomy t.
Kangaroo gastrostomy feeding t.
Kangaroo silicone gastrostomy feeding t.
Kehr gallbladder t.
Kehr T t.
Kelly t.
Kelly inflatable T t.
Keofeed t.
Keofeed II feeding t.
KeyMed esophageal t.
Kidd U t.
Killian t.
Klein ventilation t.
Kozlowski t.
Kuhn t.

Kuhn endotracheal t.
Kurze suction t.
lacrimal duct T t.
Lahey Y t.
Lanz endotracheal t.
Lanz low-pressure cuff endotracheal t.
Lanz tracheostomy t.
large-bore aspiration t.
large-bore chest t.
large-caliber t.
large-caliber chest t.
Laryngoflex reinforced endotracheal t.
laser t.
Laser-Shield XII wrapped endotracheal t.
Lasertubus tracheal t.
Lenard ray t.
Lester Jones bypass t.
Levin t.
Levin duodenal t.
Lewis laryngectomy t.
lifesaving t.
Lindeman-Silverstein Arrow t.
Lindeman-Silverstein ventilation t.
Lindholm tracheal t.
Linton t.
Linton esophageal t.
Linton-Nachlas t.
LipoClear reagent t.
Lo-Pro tracheal t.
Lore-Lawrence trachea t.
Lore suction t.
Luer t.
Luer speaking t.
Luer tracheal t.
Lukens collecting t.
Luki aspirating t.
Lymphoprep t.
Lyon t.
Mackler t.
Magill Safety Clear endotracheal t.
Maingot gallbladder t.
Malecot t.
Malecot nephrostomy t.
malleable multipore suction t.
Mallinckrodt endotracheal t.
Mallinckrodt Laser-Flex t.
Martin laryngectomy t.
Martin tracheostomy t.
Mason suction t.
Massie sliding nail t.
mastoid suction t.
Mead Johnson t.
mediastinal t.
Medina t.
Medoc-Celestin t.
Methodist vascular suction t.

Mic bolus gastrostomy t.
Mic gastroenteric t.
Mic gastrostomy t.
Mic jejunal t.
Mic jejunostomy t.
Mic-Key gastrostomy t.
Mic-Key low-profile transgastric-jejunal feeding t.
microbore Tygon t.
microfocal direct magnification in vitro x-ray t.
microfuge t.
Microgel surface-enhanced ventilation t.
Mic-TJ transgastric jejunal t.
Mic transgastric jejunal feeding t.
Miller-Abbott double-lumen intestinal t.
Minnesota t.
Miser t.
Mitrofanoff t.
modified suction t.
Molteno shunt t.
molybdenum rotating anode x-ray t.
molybdenum target t.
Momberg t.
Montgomery salivary bypass t.
Montgomery T t.
Montgomery tracheal t.
Montgomery tracheal T t.
Mosher lifesaving tracheal suction t.
Moss t.
Moss balloon triple-lumen gastrostomy t.
Moss feeding t.
Moss gastric decompression t.
Moss gastrostomy t.
Moss Mark IV t.
Moss nasal t.
Moss Suction Buster t.
muscular t.
mycobacteria growth indicator t.
myringotomy t.
Nachlas gastrointestinal t.
nasal suction t.
nasobiliary t.
nasocystic drainage t.
nasoendotracheal t.
nasoenteric feeding t.
nasogastric t.
nasogastric feeding t.
nasojejunal t.
nasotracheal t.
nephrostomy t.
neural t.
New speaking t.
Newvicon camera t.

NG t.
NG feeding t.
Nishizaki-Wakabayashi suction t.
Norton endotracheal t.
Nuport PEG t.
Nutriflex t.
obstructed shunt t.
O'Dwyer t.
Olshevsky t.
Olympus One-Step Button t.
Olympus one-step button gastrostomy t.
Ommaya ventricular t.
opaque myringotomy t.
open-end aspirating t.
oral endotracheal t.
oral esophageal t.
oroendotracheal t.
orogastric t.
orogastric Ewald t.
orogastric feeding t.
orotracheal t.
overcouch t.
Panda gastrostomy feeding t.
Panda nasoenteric feeding t.
Paparella myringotomy t.
Paparella type II ventilation t.
Paparella ventilation t. type II
Paul-Mixter t.
pear-shaped extension t.
Pedi PEG t.
Pee Wee low-profile gastrostomy t.
PEG t.
PEG-400 t.
Penrose t.
percutaneous endoscopic gastrostomy tube
percutaneous nephrostomy t.
Per-Lee ventilation t.
Perspex t.
Pezzer t.
pharyngotympanic t.
photoelectric multiplier t.
photomultiplier t.
pickup t.
pigtail nephrostomy t.
Pitot t.
Pitt talking tracheostomy t.
plastic-cuffed tracheostomy t.
pleural t.
Pleur-evac suction t.
plexiglas t.
polyethylene t.
polyethylene feeding t.
polyethylene T t.
polyvinyl chloride endotracheal t.
Ponsky-Gauderer gastrostomy t.
Ponsky PEG t.
Poole abdominal suction t.

T

tube *(continued)*

Poole suction t.
Poppen suction t.
Portex Blue Line tracheostomy t.
Portex Per-fit tracheostomy t.
Portex preformed blue line
  tracheal t.
Porto-Vac suction t.
postpyloric feeding t.
pressure equalization t.
primordial catheter t.
Pudenz t.
pull-type gastrostomy t.
pus t.
pusher t.
Pynchon suction t.
Pyrex glass t.
Pyrex T t.
Questek laser t.
Quinton t.
Radius enteral feeding t.
RAE endotracheal t.
rectal t.
rectifier t.
red rubber endotracheal t.
Rehfuss duodenal t.
Rehfuss stomach t.
reinforced tracheostomy t.
Replogle sump t.
Reuter t.
Reuter-Bobbin t.
Rhoton-Merz suction t.
Rica mastoid suction t.
right-angle chest t.
Ring-McLean sump t.
Robertshaw t.
roentgen t.
Rosen suction t.
rotating anode t.
Rubin t.
Ruschelit polyvinyl chloride
  endotracheal t.
Rusch laryngectomy t.
Rusch red rubber rectal t.
Ryle t.
Sacks-Vine PEG t.
SafeCrit microhematocrit t.
Safetex t.
Safety Clear Plus endotracheal t.
Salem sump t.
Salem sump double-lumen
  polyvinyl t.
salivary bypass t.
Sandoz balloon replacement t.
Sandoz balloon replacement t.
Sandoz Caluso PEG gastrostomy t.
Sandoz feeding/suction t.
Sandoz nasogastric feeding t.
Sandoz suction/feeding t.

Sarns intracardiac suction t.
Saticon vacuum chamber pickup t.
scavenging t.
Schachowa spiral t.
Schuknecht suction t.
sediment t.
sedimentation t.
self-quenched counter t.
Sengstaken-Blakemore t.
Sengstaken-Blakemore
  esophagogastric tamponade t.
Sengstaken nasogastric t.
Sensiv endotracheal t.
separator t.
Seroma-Cath drainage t.
Seroma-Cath feeding t.
Shah permanent t.
Sheehy collar button ventilating t.
Shepard grommet ventilation t.
Shiley cuffless fenestrated t.
Shiley cuffless tracheostomy t.
Shiley disposable cannula low-
  pressure cuffed tracheostomy t.
Shiley extra-length single-cannula
  tracheostomy t.
Shiley fenestrated low-pressure
  cuffed tracheostomy t.
Shiley laryngectomy t.
Shiley neonatal tracheostomy t.
Shiley pediatric tracheostomy t.
Shiley single-cannula cuffed
  tracheostomy t.
Shiley TracheoSoft XLT
  tracheostomy t.
Shiley tracheostomy t.
Shiner radiopaque t.
shunt t.
silastic t.
silastic eustachian t.
silastic T t.
silastic tracheostomy t.
silicone t.
silicone-lubricated endotracheal t.
silicone T t.
Silk Bullet feeding t.
silk jejunal t.
Silk Pill feeding t.
Silk Tip feeding t.
Silverstein permanent aeration t.
Singer-Blom t.
siphon suction t.
smoke evacuator suction t.
smoke removal t.
Softech endotracheal t.
SoftForm t.
solid-phase extraction t.
Souttar t.
speaking t.
Spetzler MicroVac suction t.

spiral-embedded t.
spiral wound endotracheal t.
sputum t.
SRO x-ray t.
Stamm gastrostomy t.
Stay-Put jejunal t.
stomach t.
Stomate decompression t.
Stomate extension t.
Storz suction t.
straight chest t.
suction t.
suction-coagulation t.
sump t.
Super PEG t.
Swan-Ganz t.
T t.
Takara Biomedicals Suprec t.
tear duct t.
Thal-Quick chest t.
thoracostomy t.
Thora-Klex chest t.
tight-to-shaft Aire-Cuf
    tracheostomy t.
Tiny-Tef ventilation t.
Tiny Tytan ventilation t.
tonsillar suction t.
Touma-type t.
Tovell t.
Toynbee diagnostic t.
tracheal t.
TracheoSoft XLT tracheostomy t.
trachcostomy t.
Trach-Talk trachesostomy t.
Trake-Fit tracheostomy t.
translucent drain t.
translucent myringotomy t.
translucent silicone t.
transpyloric feeding t.
triode t.
triple-lumen t.
TTS Aire-Cuf endotracheal t.
TTS Aire-Cuf tracheostomy t.
T-tube round suction t.
T-type myringotomy t.
Tucker aspirating t.
Tucker tracheal t.
Turkel t.
twist-in drain t.
tympanostomy t.
uncuffed endotracheal t.
underwater-seal suction t.
Univent endotracheal t.
Unopette t.
urinary drainage t.
uterine t.
UTTS endotracheal t.
Vacuette blood sample t.
Vacutainer t.

Vacutainer collection t.
Vacutainer vacuum t.
valve t.
Veillon t.
velvet-eye aspirating t.
ventilation t.
ventilatory support t.
Venturi t.
Vidicon camera t.
Vidicon vacuum chamber pickup t.
vinyl t.
vinyl T t.
Vivonex gastrostomy t.
Vivonex Moss t.
Von Eichen antral wash t.
Vortex tracheotomy t.
Wangensteen duodenal t.
waterseal chest t.
Webster infusion t.
Welch Allyn suction t.
Wendl t.
Williams esophageal t.
Wilson-Cook nasobiliary t.
Wilson-Cook NJFT-series feeding t.
wire-guided J t.
wire-wound endotracheal t.
Wolf suction t.
Woodbridge t.
woven Dacron t.
Wullstein microsuction t.
Xomed endotracheal t.
Xomed plastic and rubber
    endotracheal t.
Xomed straight-shank t.
Xomed Treace ventilation t.
x-ray t.
Y t.
Yankauer aspirating t.
Yankauer suction t.
Yasargil microsuction t.
Yasargil suction t.
Young-Dees t.
Z-wave t.

**TubeChek esophageal intubation
    detector**
TubeGauz
    T. bandage
    T. elastic net
    T. seamless tubular knitted cotton
        bandage
tubeless lithotriptor
tube-occluding
    t.-o. clamp
    t.-o. forceps
tuberculin syringe
Tubex
    T. gauze dressing
    T. injector
    T. metal syringe

TubiFast bandage
Tubigrip
    T. bandage
    T. circumferential elastic bandage
    T. dressing
    T. elastic support bandage
    T. glove
tubing
    t. adapter
    Bard extension t.
    t. clamp
    clear sterile premium t.
    connecting t.
    dialysate t.
    dialysis t.
    elastic t.
    evacuator t.
    Exerband t.
    Fit-Lastic therapy t.
    fluted spiral t.
    foam t.
    gel t.
    t. hand roller
    Hi Vac t.
    insufflation t.
    Intramedic polyethylene t.
    t. introducer forceps
    K-Tube hypodermic needle t.
    Lifemed blood t.
    Mini-Med t.
    Nezhat irrigation t.
    Nu-Hope t.
    polyethylene t.
    polyvinyl t.
    PVC t.
    ribbed sterile t.
    shunt t.
    silastic t.
    Silipos mesh t.
    Simcoe connecting t.
    smooth-walled t.
    Sur-Fit Natura night drainage
      container t.
    Surgitube t.
    Thera-Band t.
    Tygon t.
    Vacutainer t.
    viscodissector t.
    X-span t.
    Y-connecting t.
Tubipad bandage
tuboplasty surgical kit
Tubsider kneeling seat
tubular
    t. dressing
    t. elastic bandage
    t. forceps
    t. Gore material
    t. magnet

    t. plate
    t. slotted stent
Tubulitec cavity liner
Tuckables underpad
tucker
    T. anterior commissure
      laryngoscope
    T. aspirating tube
    Bishop tendon t.
    T. bougie
    Burch-Greenwood tendon t.
    T. esophagoscope
    Green strabismus t.
    T. hallux forceps
    ligature t.
    McGuire tendon t.
    T. mediastinoscope
    T. retrograde bougie
    T. staple forceps
    T. tack-and-pin forceps
    tendon t.
    T. tracheal tube
    T. vertebrated guide
    T. vertebrated lumen finder
    Vilex wire t.
    wire t.
Tucker-McLane
    T.-M. axis traction forceps
    T.-M. forceps
    T.-M. obstetrical forceps
Tucker-McLane-Luikart forceps
Tudor-Edwards
    T.-E. bone-cutting forceps
    T.-E. rib shears
    T.-E. rib spreader
Tuffier
    T. abdominal retractor
    T. abdominal spatula
    T. arterial forceps
    T. rib retractor
    T. rib spreader
Tuf Nex neck exerciser
Tuf-Skin tape adherent
TufStuf II cast tape
Tuke saw
Tulevech lacrimal cannula
Tuli
    T. heel cup
    T. Pro heel cup
    T. rubber heel cup
tulip
    T. cannula
    t. pedicle screw
    t. probe
    t. sheath
    T. syringe system
    t. tip
tulle gras dressing

Tumble
- T. Forms feeder
- T. Forms feeder seat
- T. Forms roll

tumbling
- t. E chart
- t. E cube

tumescent
- t. absorbent bandage
- t. infiltrator cannula

tumor
- t. forceps
- t. probe
- t. replacement endoprosthesis

tumor-grasping forceps

TUMT
- transurethral microwave thermotherapy
- 30-minute TUMT

TUNA
- transurethral needle ablation
- TUNA system

tunable
- t. dye laser
- t. laser with Hexascan
- t. notch filter
- t. pulsed-dye laser

tungsten
- t. carbide bur
- t. eye shield
- t. microdissection needle
- t. microelectrode
- t. syringe shield
- t. tip

tungsten-halogen lamp

tunic
- Bichat t.

tuning fork

Tun-L-Kath epidural catheter

tunnel
- t. drill guide
- t. graft

tunneled
- t. catheter
- t. eye implant
- t. implant

tunneler
- crescent scleral t.
- Davol t.
- DeBakey femoral bypass t.
- Diethrich-Jackson femoral graft t.
- Jackson t.
- SatinCrescent t.
- tendon t.
- vascular access t.

Tunneloc bone mulch screw

tunnel-type implant material

Tunturi
- T. bicycle ergometer
- T. hand exerciser

Tuohy
- T. aortography needle
- T. catheter
- T. lumbar puncture needle
- T. needle
- T. spinal needle

Tuohy-Borst
- T.-B. adapter
- T.-B. connector
- T.-B. introducer

Tupper
- T. handholder
- T. handholder and retractor

Turapy device

turbinate
- t. electrode
- t. forceps
- t. scissors

turbinectomy scissors

turbine-powered ICU ventilator system

turbo
- t. file
- T. 7000 system
- T. Tracker catheter

Turbo-Inhaler
- Spinhaler T.-I.

turbo-tip of phacoemulsification unit

Turbuhaler
- T. inhaler
- Pulmicort T.
- Symbicort T.

TUR-Cue photometer

Turkel
- T. bone biopsy trephine set
- T. needle
- T. punch
- T. trephine
- T. tube

turkey-claw clamp

turn
- 2-t. epicardial lead
- 3-t. epicardial lead

TurnAide therapeutic system

turnbuckle
- t. ankle brace
- t. distractor
- t. elbow splint
- t. functional position splint
- Giannestras t.
- t. knee brace
- t. wrist orthosis

Turn-Easy transfer aid

3-turn epicardial lead

turner
- T. biopsy needle
- T. cystoscopic fulgurating electrode
- T. dilator
- T. pin
- T. prosthesis

T

turner *(continued)*
    rotating t.
    T. spinal gouge
Turner-Warwick
    T.-W. adult retractor ring
    T.-W. bladder neck spreader
    T.-W. blade
    T.-W. diathermy scissors
    T.-W. needle
    T.-W. needle holder
    T.-W. stone forceps
    T.-W. urethral staff
turnout gear
turn-Q-plus
turnstile casting stand
TURP
    transurethral resection of prostate
        direct-beam coupler for TURP
        split-beam coupler for TURP
Turrell rectal biopsy forceps
turret
    5-position t.
Tutofix cortical pin
Tutoplast
    T. auditory ossicle
    T. bone
    T. Dura
    T. Dura patch
    T. processed allograft
    T. tissue
Tuttle
    T. proctoscope
    T. thoracic forceps
    T. thumb forceps
    T. tissue forceps
Tuxedo collar
Twee alternating cut-off compressor stocking
tweezers
    Dumont t.
    jeweler's t.
    Kaprelian easy-access t.
    laser t.
    optic t.
    soldering t.
twig
    nerve t.
TwiLite laser
twill
    t. dressing
    t. tape
twin
    Bennett t.
    t. edgewise bracket
    t. Flash scanner
    T. Jet nebulizer
    t. knife
    VersaLab APM2 for T.'s
twin-coil dialyzer

Twinheads shock wave lithotriptor
twin-pattern chisel
Twisk microscissors
twist
    t. drill
    t. fixation hook
    t. hook
    T. MTX implant
    T. Ti implant
twisted
    t. plate
    t. virgin silk suture
    t. wire snare loop
twister
    Axel wire t.
    Batzdorf cervical wire t.
    cerclage wire t.
    Cooley-Baumgarten wire t.
    Corwin wire t.
    DMP wire t.
    Miltex wire t.
    Ochsner wire t.
    orthotic coiled spring t.
    wire t.
twist-in
    t.-i. drain tube
    t.-i. drain tube inserter
TwistLock
    T. Cath-Gard
    Hands-Off infusion port heparin-coated thermodilution catheter with T.
Twist-Lock drill guard
twist-off screw
twist-release coil
Tycos
    T. aneroid sphygmomanometer
    T. gauge
    T. manometer
    T. pressure infusion line
Tydings
    T. tonsillar forceps
    T. tonsil snare
Tygon
    T. catheter
    T. esophageal prosthesis
    T. tubing
tying forceps
tying/stitch removal forceps
Tylok
    T. high-tension cable system
    T. high-tension cerclage cabling system
tympanic membrane thermometer
tympanomastoid suture
tympanometer
    diagnostic t.
    MicroTymp2 handheld t.

Welch Allyn MicroTymp
   impedance t.
tympanoplasty
   t. forceps
   t. knife
tympanoscope
tympanostomy tube
tympanum perforator
Typhoon
   T. cutter blade
   T. microdebrider blade

Tyrrell
   T. iris hook
   T. skin hook
   T. tympanic membrane hook
Tyshak
   T. balloon
   T. balloon valvuloplasty catheter
   T. catheter
T-Y stent

U

U clip
U Luque vertebral rod
U rod
U sheet
U wrench
U X-Acto gouge

U6 riboprobe
UA

urinalysis

UAL
UAM universal fixation driver
UBIS

ultrasound bone imaging scanner
UBIS quantitative ultrasound bone sonometer
UBIS ultrasound bone sonometer

UBM

ultrasound biomicroscopy
UBM transducer

UBP

Universal bone plate
U. system

UCBL

University of California Biomechanics Laboratory
U. prosthesis

UCI

University of California-Irvine
UCI unconstrained prosthesis

UCI-Barnard aortic valve
UCLA

University of California at Los Angeles
UCLA functional long leg brace

U-clip

nitinol U-c.

UCOheal orthotic
UCOlite

U. orthosis
U. orthotic

Uebe applicator
uEEG ProSystem 5000
UFO

Universal plantar fasciitis orthosis
Orthomerica UFO

UG-70 stapler
UGI

upper gastrointestinal
UGI endoscope
UGI endoscopy

uHead

u. ulnar head implant
u. ulnar head prosthesis

UHMWPE

ultrahigh molecular weight polyethylene
UHMWPE prosthesis

UHR locking ring mechanism
UJV AMS high-frequency jet ventilator
ulcer

u. dressing
u. marker

UlcerJet high-pressure fluid jet system
Ulcosan Unna boot with inelastic zinc plaster bandage
Uldall

U. subclavian hemodialysis cannula
U. subclavian hemodialysis catheter

Ullrich

U. drill guard
U. self-retaining laminectomy retractor

ulnar

u. nerve motor/sensory electromyogram
u. rasp
u. ruler

ULP

ultralow profile
ULP catheter

Ulramax knitted double velour vascular graft
Ulrich

U. bone-holding clamp
U. bone-holding forceps

Ulrich-St. Gallen forceps
Ulson fixator system
Ultamet metal-on-metal articulation
Ultec

U. hydrocolloid
U. hydrocolloid dressing
U. Pro alginate hydrocolloid dressing
U. thin dressing

Ultex

U. lens
U. lens implant
U. Thin extra-thin hydrocolloid dressing

Ultima

U. calcar stem
U. C femoral component
U. Fx stem
U. hip replacement system
U. II refrigerator system
U. mammography system
U. OPCAB system
U. photocoagulator
U. total hip system

Ultimate
- U. Cold N' Hot Pack
- U. knee
- U. knee prosthesis
- U. nasal mask
- U. Seal CPAP mask seal
- U. Seal gel interface

Ultimatics demineralized cortical bone powder

Ultimax
- U. distal femoral intramedullary rod system
- U. Haig II nail system

Ultimum hemostasis introducer

ultra
- U. 8 balloon catheter
- U. Dream Ride car bed
- U. Duet Colostomy
- U. Duet Colostomy irrigating sleeve
- u. high-resolution parallel-hole collimator
- U. ICE catheter
- LifeScan U.
- u. low-profile fixed-wire balloon dilation catheter
- u. low-resistance voice prosthesis
- U. mag lens
- U. pacemaker
- U. Scent diffuser
- U. Sleeve ultrasound sleeve
- U. Stim silver electrode
- U. Twin bag system
- U. ultrasonic aspirator
- U. View SP slit-lamp lens
- U. vision rapid screen
- U. Voice speech aid
- U. Y-set system

Ultrabag dialysis system

UltrAblator electrode

Ultrabrace
- U. brace
- U. knee orthosis

Ultracell LASIK spear

ultracentrifuge
- Airfuge u.
- Discovery SE u.
- Optima preparative u.
- Sorvall Discovery SE u.

UltraCision
- U. harmonic laparoscopic cutting shears
- U. harmonic scalpel
- U. ultrasonic knife

Ultracranio T

UltraCross
- U. profile imaging catheter
- U. stent

Ultra-Cut
- U.-C. Cobb curette
- U.-C. Cobb spinal instrument
- U.-C. Hoke osteotome
- U.-C. instrument

Ultra-Drive
- U.-D. bone cement removal system
- U.-D. plug puller
- U.-D. ultrasonic revision system

UltraEase ultrasound pad

UltraEdge keratome blade

ultrafast
- u. computed tomographic scanner
- u. computed tomography scanner
- u. CT scanner

Ultrafera wound dressing

ultrafiltration membrane

UltraFine
- U. erbium laser
- U. erbium laser system

Ultra-Fit brief

UltraFix
- U. anchor
- U. MicroMite suture anchor
- U. MiniMite suture anchor
- U. MiniMite suture anchor system
- U. RC implant
- U. RC suture anchor
- U. RC suture anchor system
- U. rotator cuff repair implant
- U. rotator cuff suture anchor system

Ultraflex
- U. ankle dorsiflexion dynamic splint
- U. Diamond stent
- U. esophageal prosthesis
- U. esophageal stent system
- U. Microvasive stent
- U. nitinol expandable esophageal stent
- U. self-adhering male external catheter
- U. self-expanding stent
- U. stent
- U. stent delivery system
- U. tracheobronchial stent

Ultrafoam collagen sponge

UltraForm
- U. mattress overlay
- U. therapeutic mattress

UltraFuse
- U. balloon
- U. infusion catheter

Ultra-Guard
- U.-G. FS hip bracing system
- U.-G. hip orthosis system

ultrahigh molecular weight polyethylene (UHMWPE)

Ultra-Image A-scan
Ultraject
    U. contrast medium syringe
    U. prefilled syringe
UltraKlenz wound cleanser
Ultra-Lase
UltraLine
    U. fiber
    U. laser
    Lasersonic ACMI U.
    U. Nd:YAG laser fiber
UltraLite
    U. flow-directed microcatheter
    U. headlight system
    U. One-Piece convex-disposable
       system
Ultra-Lite portable aspirator
ultra-low
ultralow profile (ULP)
Ultramark
    U. 9 echocardiograph
    U. 9 HDI ultrasound
    U. scanner
    U. 8 transducer
    U. 4 ultrasound
    U. ultrasound system
Ultramatic
    U. Project-O-Chart
    U. Rx Master phoroptor
    U. Rx Master phoroptor retractor
Ultramer catheter
ultramicrotome
    Reichert-Jung Ultracut u.
Ultra-Neb nebulizer
UltraPACS diagnostic imaging system
UltraPak enteral closed feeding system
UltraPower
    U. basic drill system
    U. bur guard
    U. bur guard drill system
    U. drill system
    U. revision drill system
Ultra-Precision ultrasonic probe
Ultrapro mesh
UltraPulse
    U. CO_2 laser
    U. laser
    U. surgical laser
    U. SurgiTouch CO2 laser system
Ultra-Retractor device
Ultrascan Digital contact ultrasound A-scan
Ultraseed system
Ultra-Select nitinol PTCA guidewire
UltraShaper keratome
Ultrasharp round blade microknife
UltraSling
ultrasmall incision implant
ultrasmall-shafted balloon

UltraSoft GDC
ultrasonic
    u. aspirating device
    u. aspirator and dissector
    u. biomicroscope
    u. bone-cutting instrument
    u. cannula
    u. cataract-removal lancet
    u. cataract-removal lancet needle
    u. cell disrupter
    u. cleaner basket
    u. dissector
    u. electrode
    u. endoscope
    u. flow director
    u. harmonic scalpel
    u. lancet
    u. lithotriptor
    u. lithotriptor probe
    u. micrometer
    u. microscope
    u. mobility aid
    u. nebulizer
    u. oscillating bur
    u. pachymeter
    u. piezoelectric scaler
    u. probe
    u. retroprep system
    u. retrotip
    u. scaler
    u. scalpel
    u. stone crusher
    u. suction scalpel
    u. surgical aspirator
    u. tactile sensor
ultrasonically activated scalpel
ultrasonogram
    A-scan u.
    B-scan u.
    gray-scale u.
ultrasonography
    contact B-scan u.
    Doppler u.
    endoscopic color Doppler u.
    intraportal endovascular u.
    power Doppler u.
    Siemens Sonoline u.
    Toshiba Sal real-time u.
    Toshiba Sonolayer transrectal u.
    Voluvision 3-dimensional u.
ultrasonometer
    Achilles+ u.
    QUS-2 calcaneal u.
ultrasonoscope
    Acuson u.
UltraSorb suture anchor
ultrasound
    u. ablation catheter
    Acuson u.

U

ultrasound *(continued)*

Acuson Doppler u.
ADR Ultramark 4 u.
Advantage u.
AI diagnostic u.
Alcon Digital B u.
Aloka u.
Aloka CL u.
Aloka linear u.
Aloka OB/GYN u.
Aloka sector u.
Amrex therapeutic u.
Ansaldo u.
Aspen digital u.
ATL real-time u.
ATL Ultramark u.
Axisonic II u.
u. biomicroscope system
u. biomicroscopy (UBM)
Biosound high-resolution u.
BladderScan u.
B-mode u.
u. bone analyzer
u. bone imaging scanner (UBIS)
u. bone imaging sonometer
Brüel & Kjaer u.
u. catheter probe
catheter probe u.
Cineloop u.
color Doppler u.
colorvascular Doppler u.
CooperVision u.
Diasonics u.
3D i-Scan ophthalmic u.
Doppler u.
Doppler pulsed u.
duplex u.
Dynatron u.
Eccocee u.
EchoEye u.
u. electrotherapy
Elscint u.
endoanal u.
Endosound endoscopic u.
Exogen noninvasive u.
GE Advantage II u.
u. gel
u. generator
HDI u.
Hewlett-Packard u.
high-intensity focus u.
Hitachi u.
Hitachi digital u.
u. inhaler
u. intercom
InterTherapy intravascular u.
intraductal u.
intraluminal u.
intravascular u. (IVUS)

Irex Exemplar u.
LeFort urethral u.
Maggi disposable biopsy needle
  guide for u.
u. monitor
Mysono portable u.
Neurosector u.
Nicolet Elite Doppler u.
Olympus endoscopic u.
u. pachymeter
u. pachymeter-KMI
u. pad
Performa u.
Pie Medical u.
power Doppler u.
PowerVision u.
u. probe
ProSound u.
pulsed Doppler u.
real-time u.
Rich-Mar external u.
RT u.
RT Advantage u.
Shimadzu cardiac u.
Shimadzu IIQ u.
Siemens SI u.
Siemens Sonoline Elegra u.
Siemens Sonoline Prima u.
SieScape u.
u. sleeve
Sonicator portable u.
SonoAce II u.
Sonolayer u.
Sonoline Prima u.
Sonos cardiovascular u.
SonoSite digital u.
SonoSite hand-carried u.
SonoSite iLook 24 u.
SonoSite MicroMaxx laptop u.
SonoSite 180Plus u.
SonoSite Titan u.
u. spatula
Spectra-Diasonics u.
u. stethoscope
Sunlight Omnisense u.
Synergy u.
u. system
through-the-balloon u.
Toshiba u.
Toshiba Sonolayer u.
u. transducer
transendoscopic u.
transvaginal u.
Ultramark 4 u.
Ultramark 9 HDI u.
vaginal probe u.
Vingmed u.
Vingmed System Five u.

ultrasound-assisted PEG placement

ultrasound-guided laser
ultrasound/stimulator
    SynchroSonic u./s.
ultrasound-tipped catheter
UltraSTAR computer-based ultrasound
   reporting system
UltraStep orthotic
ultrastiff wire
UltraSure
    U. DTR-1 imaging ultrasound
      system
    U. DTU-1 ultrasound scanner
Ultrata capsulorrhexis forceps
UltraTag RBC kit
Ultrathane Amplatz ureteral stent
ultrathin
    U. balloon catheter
    U. Diamond balloon
    u. endoscope
    u. needle brachytherapy-style
      delivery renal application
    u. pancreatoscope
    u. surgical blade
ultrathin-walled 2-stage (UTTS)
UltraTLC adjustable lancing device
ultratome
    U. double-lumen sphincterotome
    Microvasive u.
    U. XL triple-lumen sphincterotome
Ultratone electrical transcutaneous
   neuromuscular stimulator
UltraVent radioaerosol delivery system
ultraviolet (UV)
    u. A (UVA)
    u. A light
    u. autoblood radiation (UVAR)
    u. B (UVB)
    u. detector
    u. lamp
    u. laser
    u. light
    u. light-polymerized resin
    u. radiation (UVR)
ultraviolet-blocking intraocular lens
Ultravoice speech simulator
Ultra-Vue amniocentesis needle
Ultra-X external fixation system
Ultraxx nephrostomy balloon
Ultrex
    U. cylinder
    U. Plus penile prosthesis
    U. wound dressing
Ultroid
umbilical
    u. artery catheter
    u. clamp
    u. clip
    u. cord clamp
    u. scissors

    u. tape
    u. tape drain
    u. tape suture
    u. vein catheter
    u. venous catheter
Umbilicutter
umbrella
    ASDOS u.
    Bard Clamshell septal u.
    Bard PDA U.
    clamshell septal u.
    u. dissector
    u. filter
    PDA u.
    u. punctum plug
    Rashkind u.
    u. retractor
    transcatheter u.
umbrella-type prosthesis
UMC-I microwave delivery system
UMI
    Universal Medical Instruments
    UMI catheter
    UMI transseptal Cath-Seal catheter
    introducer
U-Mid-O$_2$ Jet Set
UM 4 real-time sector scanner
unabsorbable suture
unclassified air cleaner
uncoated mesh stent
unconstrained prosthesis
uncuffed endotracheal tube
undergarment
    Attends beltless u.
    Dignity Plus Briefmates beltless u.
    First Quality belted u.
    MaxiCare adult disposable u.
    Protection Plus belted u.
    Safe & Dry u.
    strap-on u.
underpad
    Attends u.
    Chamois u.
    Dignity Plus u.
    Dri-flo u.
    Excel Plus u.
    Excel quilted u.
    First Quality high-performance and
      nighttime u.
    Harmonie u.
    MaxiCare disposable u.
    Maxiflo breathable disposable u.
    PatientGuard reusable u.
    Pinnacle reusable u.
    PrimeTime disposable u.
    Protection Plus disposable u.
    Provide u.
    reusable and washable u.
    Safe & Dry u.

U

underpad *(continued)*
Sahara super-absorbent reusable u.
Sofnit Birdseye reusable u.
Sofnit 300 reusable u.
Tuckables u.

underwater
u. Bovie
u. drainage system
u. electrode

underwater-seal
u.-s. drainage
u.-s. suction tube

underwear
HipSaver protective u.
Prevail protective u.

undyed suture

unfilled resin

Unfolder Sapphire implantation system

uniaxial
u. accelerometer
u. strain gauge

unibevel chisel

unicare breast pump

Unicat diamond knife

Uni-Clip manual compression staple

unicompartmental
u. knee implant
u. knee system

unicondylar prosthesis

Uni-Cor biopsy needle

unicortical
u. interosseus wire
u. screw

unidirectional
u. airflow ball tracheostomy
speaking valve
u. block

unifascicular block

Unifile
Burns U.

Uni-Flate penile prosthesis

Uniflex
U. calibrated step drill
U. distal targeting awl
U. dressing
U. drill bushing
U. humeral nail
U. intramedullary nail
U. nailing system

Unifold shelter

Uni-frame patient immobilization system

Uni-Fuse infusion catheter

Uni-Gard piggyback connector

Unigraft bone graft material

UniHeart IV universal nebulizer

Unilab
U. Surgibone

U. Surgibone bone replacement
material
U. Surgibone surgical implant

Unilase CO_2 laser

unilateral
u. bar
u. calcaneal brace
u. removable partial denture

Unilink
U. anastomotic device
U. hand surgery system
U. system

Unimar
U. HSG tray
U. Pipelle
U. Pipelle curette

UniMax laser micromanipulator

union
u. broach retention drill
u. broach retention pin
Osteotron stimulator for bone u.

uniplanar intraocular lens

uniplanar-style PC II lens

Uniplane rocker

Uniplant contraceptive implant

UniPlast
U. Imaging and Archiving system

unipolar
u. atrial pacemaker
u. atrioventricular pacemaker
u. bearing
u. cautery
u. cutting loop
u. defibrillation coil electrode
u. electrode
u. glass electrode
u. hand-switching needlepoint
electrocautery forceps
u. J-tined passive fixation lead
u. Pisces Sigma
u. precordial lead
u. sequential pacemaker
u. static magnet

Uniportal fascial release system

Unipost implant

UniPuls electrostimulation instrument

UniPulse surgical CO_2 laser system

Unisensor strain-gauge transducer

UniShaper single-use keratome

Uni-Shunt
U.-S. catheter passer
U.-S. hydrocephalus shunt
U.-S. hydrocephalus shunt system
U.-S. right-angle clip
U.-S. with elliptical reservoir
U.-S. with reservoir introducer

Uni-Silicone lead

Unistat bilirubinometer

Unistep
    U. Plus delivery system
    U. Plus Permalume covered biliary
      Wallstent
UniSyn modular hip system
unit
    Accu-o-Matic TENS u.
    Acu-Ray x-ray u.
    AdvanTeq II TENS u.
    Alcon cryosurgical u.
    Alcon Legacy u.
    Alcon Master u.
    Alcon phacoemulsification u.
    AME microcurrent TENS u.
    3-u. anterior bridge
    AO Reichert Instruments Ful-Vue
      diagnostic u.
    Aqua-Seal chest drainage u.
    Arrow-Trerotola rotator drive u.
    Asepticator u.
    Aspen sonography u.
    Autocon electrosurgical u.
    Autoflex II continuous passive
      motion u.
    Back Bubble gravity traction u.
    Back Revolution traction/exercise u.
    bag-valve u.
    Baird Electric System Power Plus
      electrosurgical u.
    Bair Hugger convective warming u.
    Bair Hugger patient heating u.
    Bart abdominoperineal u.
    BCD Plus cardioplegic u.
    BICAP u.
    BiLAP bipolar cautery u.
    BiliBed phototherapy u.
    BioMed TENS u.
    Biosound II ultrasound u.
    Biosound ultrasound u.
    BiPAP u.
    biplane DSA u.
    bipolar electrosurgical u.
    body cooling u.
    bone marrow transplant u.
    Bovie u.
    Bovie electrocautery u.
    Bovie electrosurgical u.
    Bovie retinal detachment u.
    Brymill CryAc cryosurgical u.
    Brymill 30 cryosurgical u.
    Cal-20 central dialysate
      preparation u.
    calf compression u.
    Cameron electrosurgical u.
    Cameron-Miller electrocoagulation u.
    C-arm fluoroscopy u.
    C-arm portable x-ray u.
    Cavitron phacoemulsification u.
    Celay milling u.

    Centry dialysis u.
    Century bicarbonate dialysis
      control u.
    Clinitron Elexis air-fluidized
      therapy u.
    Clinitron II air-fluidized therapy u.
    Clinitron uplift air-fluidized
      therapy u.
    Conmed Aspen Excalibur-Plus
      electrosurgical u.
    Contimed II measuring u.
    Cooper irrigating/aspirating u.
    CooperVision irrigation/aspiration u.
    Cox sterilizer and incinerator u.
    critical care u.
    cryosurgical u.
    Cryo-Surg liquid nitrogen spray u.
    CSV Bovie electrosurgical u.
    Cybex torso rotation testing and
      rehabilitation u.
    Cybex trunk extension flexion u.
    Dent-X intraoral x-ray u.
    DeVilbiss I&A u.
    Diasonics DRF ultrasound u.
    diathermy u.
    dry heat sterilizer and
      incinerator u.
    DynaLator ultrasound u.
    Dynasplint knee extension u.
    ECG triggering u.
    Eclipse TENS u.
    Econo 90 traction u.
    EEA disposable loading u.
    E-2 hydrocollator heating u.
    ElastaTrac home lumbar traction u.
    Electricator electrosurgical u.
    electrosurgical u. (ESU)
    Elypse control u.
    EMG retrainer biofeedback u.
    EMI u.
    Empac-Cavitron I&A u.
    enhanced external
      counterpulsation u.
    Erbe electrocautery u.
    Exakt cutting/grinding u.
    Exo-Bed traction u.
    Exo-Overhead traction u.
    fast motor u.
    fingertip u.
    fixed suction u.
    Flexercell strain u.
    Flexicair eclipse low-air-loss
      therapy u.
    Fleximatic massage/percussion u.
    Flowtron DVT prophylactic deep
      venous thrombosis u.
    Fox irrigating/aspirating u.
    Freedom dental u.
    FreeDop portable Doppler u.

U

unit *(continued)*

Frigitronics cryosurgical u.
Gass irrigating/aspirating u.
Gaymar Thermacare warming u.
Geiger electrocautery u.
GIA II loading u.
Gibson irrigating/aspirating u.
Girard ultrasonic u.
Grass stimulation isolation u.
Gymmy exercise u.
Gyroscan ACS-NT MR u.
Hampton electrosurgical u.
Hercules mobile x-ray u.
Hewlett-Packard ultrasound u.
Hyde irrigator/aspirator u.
hydrocollator heating u.
Iceman continuous cold therapy u.
image-processing u.
inhalation breath u.
Intelect Legend Combo stimulator
  and ultrasound u.
Intermedics phaco I/A u.
intrapleural sealed drainage u.
Irvine irrigating/aspirating u.
Jace hand continuous passive
  motion u.
Keeler cryosurgical u.
Kelman-Cavitron I&A u.
Kelman cryosurgical u.
Kelman irrigating/aspirating u.
Kelman phacoemulsification u.
KeyMed u.
King-Armstrong u.
Kreiselman u.
Kreiselman resuscitation u.
LAD-01 ER:YAG lightweight
  portable laser u.
laminar air flow u.
Leksell gamma u.
Leksell stereotactic gamma u.
Life SoftPac AED companion
  oxygen u.
linear accelerator u.
Lithostar lithotripsy u.
liver dialysis u.
Living Air u.
Log-a-Rhythm signal acquisition u.
low-grade suction u.
Magnatherm pulsed therapy high-
  frequency u.
Magnatherm SSP electromagnetic
  therapy u.
Magnetom Espree open MRI u.
Magnetom Vision MR u.
Malis electrocoagulation u.
Maxima II TENS u.
Mayfield radiolucent base u.
McKesson suction bottle u.
Meda 2500 TENS u.

MENS u.
microamps TENS u.
microcautery u.
Mira u.
mobile eye u.
mobile response u.
Moblvac suction u.
Multi Dopplex MDI vascular
  test u.
Multistar angiographic u.
Neosonic piezo ultrasonic u.
Neuropulse u.
N_2O cryosurgical u.
Nytone enuretic control u.
Ocoee scalp cleansing u.
ocutome vitrectomy u.
Odelca camera u.
Ohmeda intermittent suction u.
Olympus heater probe u.
OneTouch electrolysis u.
Optiplanimat automated u.
Orbix x-ray u.
Orthoceph x-ray u.
Orthodyne Enhancer u.
Orthopantomograph panoramic
  digital radiography u.
OSMO reverse osmosis u.
over-the-door traction u.
Peczon I&A u.
Permark Enhancer III
  pigmenting u.
phaco emulsifier Cavitron u.
photodisplay u.
Picker Eclipse MR u.
Pierce I&A u.
Plasma ICP-AES u.
Premier I&A u.
Proscan ultrasound u.
Pulmonex dynamic air therapy u.
Pulsar obstetrical 2-channel
  TENS u.
Pulsatron u.
QAD-1 sonography u.
Radionics bipolar coagulation u.
real-time sonographic u.
reflectometer tuning u.
Restcue CC dynamic air
  therapy u.
RinoFlow ENT wash u.
Ritter-Bantam Bovie
  electrosurgical u.
Ritter coagulator electrosurgical u.
Rollet irrigating/aspirating u.
Root ZX ultrasonic u.
Schepens retinal detachment u.
Sentinel Seal pleural drainage u.
Sharpx needle destruction u.
Sheffield gamma u.
Siemens MRI u.

Siemens Somatom DRH CT analyzer u.
Sievert u.
Signa MR u.
Simcoe double-barreled irrigating/aspirating u.
Siremobil C-arm u.
sit-to-stand training parallel bar u.
Skylark TENS u.
Solcotrans autotransfusion u.
Solfy ZX ultrasonic u.
Solitens TENS u.
Solitens transcutaneous electrical nerve stimulation u.
sonography u.
Sonos ultrasound u.
Sophie mammography u.
Soprano cryotherapy u.
u. spinal rod
S-Scort New-Duet suction u.
S-Scort suction u.
Storz-Walker retinal detachment u.
Sullivan nasal variable positive airway pressure u.
Sullivan nasal VPAP u.
Super Dopplex SDI vascular test u.
Surgitron u.
Surgitron portable radiosurgical u.
Sylva I&A u.
Symphony MR u.
TA II loading u.
TENS u.
tesla superconductive magnet u.
Thermalator heating u.
ThermoFlex thermotherapy u.
ThermoFlow ETC u.
thermoplastic heating u.
Thora-Seal III chest drainage u.
torsion u.
Tranquility Bilevel CPAP u.
turbo-tip of phacoemulsification u.
UroCystom u.
vacuum polymerization u.
Valleylab cautery u.
Vari-Stim u.
Vibramatic massage/percussion u.
Visio Beta vacuum polymerization u.
Visitec aspiration u.
Visitec vitrectomy u.
Wangensteen suction u.
whole-body u.
wrist flexion u.
X-Cel dental x-ray u.
Yoshida dental x-ray u.

Unitech
U. cannula series

U. instrument
U. Toomey cannula
United
U. Sonics J shock phaco fragmentor system
U. States of America (USA)
U. States Catheter & Instruments Company (USCI)
U. States Marine Corps (USMC)
U. States Surgical circular stapler
Unitek
U. appliance
U. I convoluted innerspring mattress system
Uni-Thread versatile thoracolumbar spinal system
UniTrack shaft
Unitrax unipolar system
Unitri
U. cannula
U. tip
Unitron Esteem CIC hearing aid
Uni-Vent Eagle portable ventilator
Univent endotracheal tube
universal
U. abdominal trocar
U. acromioclavicular splint
U. adenoid punch tip
U. AerobiCycle
u. aerosol cloud enhancer
U. appliance
U. aspirator
U. bone grafting/impacting forceps
U. bone plate (UBP)
U. bone plate system
U. bone screw insertion/extraction system
U. cannula
U. cannula series
U. cannulated screw system
u. canvas body restraint
U. catheter access port
U. chuck handle
U. clip remover
U. conformer
U. connector
U. curved-tube stylet
U. drainage catheter
u. dressing
U. drill point
U. electron microscope
U. esophagoscope
U. eye shield
U. F breathing system
U. Fitstep
U. fixation screw
u. frame outer socket
U. gastroscope
U. goniometer

U

universal *(continued)*
    U. handle with nasal-cutting tip
    U. Hand System
    U. head holder
    U. hex screwdriver
    U. II forceps
    U. I, II prosthesis
    U. implant
    U. indicator stick
    U. ISH detection kit
    U. joint device
    U. Kerrison rongeur
    U. knee positioner
    U. laminectomy set
    U. lateral positioner
    U. lens-folding forceps
    u. Luer-Lok
    U. Medical Instruments (UMI)
    U. modular femoral hip component extractor
    U. nasal instrument handle
    U. nasal saw blade
    U. nerve hook
    U. Pathfinder knife
    U. pelvic traction belt
    U. phaco chopper/manipulator
    U. plantar fasciitis orthosis (UFO)
    U. plantar fasciitis orthotic
    U. Plus instrument system
    U. reducer cap
    U. retractor
    U. sheath
    U. sheath system
    u. sling
    U. sling and swathe shoulder immobilizer
    U. slit-lamp
    U. soft-tip cannulated sliding extrusion needle
    U. speculum
    U. 2-speed hand drill
    U. Spine System
    U. stent
    U. straight-tube stylet
    U. support splint
    U. swivel
    U. T adapter
    U. tourniquet
    U. Tredex
    u. tri-panel knee immobilizer
    U. vaginal probe
    u. wedge screw
    U. wire clamp
    U. wire scissors
University
    U. of California at Los Angeles (UCLA)
    U. of California Biomechanics Laboratory (UCBL)
    U. of California Biomechanics Laboratory heel cup
    U. of California-Irvine (UCI)
    U. of Florida linear accelerator
    U. of Illinois biopsy needle
    U. of Illinois marrow needle
    U. of Illinois sternal puncture needle
    U. Plate spinal attachment
    U. of Southern California (USC)
Univision
    U. echocardiographic system
    U. low-vision microscopic lens
Unloader
    U. ADJ unloader brace
    U. Bi-ComPF knee brace
    U. Express unloader brace
    U. Select unloader brace
    U. Spirit knee brace
    The U.
unmodified zinc oxide-eugenol cement
Unna
    U. boot
    U. boot bandage
    U. boot dressing
    U. boot wrap
    U. comedo extractor
    U. expressor
Unna-Flex
    U.-F. compression wrap
    U.-F. elastic Unna boot
    U.-F. leg compression dressing
    U.-F. Plus dressing
    U.-F. Plus venous ulcer convenience pack
    U.-F. Plus venous ulcer kit
Unna-Pak leg compression dressing
Uno nasal prongs
Unopette
    U. pipette
    U. system
    U. tube
unpegged hydroxyapatite implant
unsegmented bar
unstented
    u. pulmonary homograft heart valve
    u. xenograft valve
unzipper
    Katzen flap u.
UP7 film
Up and About system
uPACS picture archiving system
up-angled curette
up-angle hook
upbiting
    u. biopsy forceps
    u. cup forceps

u. forceps
u. peapod
up-cupped forceps
upcurved basket forceps
updraft handheld nebulizer
UP*link* point-of-care sample testing system
upper
u. body cycle
u. body dressing
u. body ergometer
u. cervical spine anterior construct
u. cervical spine posterior construct
u. esophagoscope
u. extremity myoelectric prosthesis
u. gastrointestinal (UGI)
U. Hands retractor
U. Hands self-retaining retractor
u. lateral exposing retractor
u. lateral scissors
u. limb orthosis
u. limb prosthesis
u. occlusive clamp
Uppsala screw
upright
u. Bucky
u. compression spot film
upturned forceps
upward-cutting triangular knife
Ura-1 flexible fiberoptic nasopharyngoscope
URAM E2 compact MicroProbe laser
Uranyl Standard
Urban
U. microscope
U. microsurgery closed-circuit color TV camera
U. Walkers
U. Walkers shoe
Uresil
U. biliary catheter
U. embolectomy-thrombectomy catheter
U. irrigation catheter
U. occlusion balloon catheter
U. radiopaque silicone-band vessel loop
U. Vascu-Flo carotid shunt
ureteral
u. basket stone dislodger
u. brush biopsy kit
u. catheter forceps
u. catheter obturator
u. clamp
u. dilation catheter
u. implant
u. isolation forceps
u. meatotomy electrode
u. occlusion balloon catheter

u. occlusion catheter
u. stent
u. stone basket
u. stone dilator
u. stone extractor
u. stone forceps
u. stone retriever
u. stylet
u. visualization instrument
ureteric retrieval net
ureteropyeloscope
Karl Storz flexible u.
ureterorenoscope procedure sheath
ureteroscope
Circon-ACMI u.
flexible u.
FlexVision flexible u.
Gautier u.
Laser Tripter u.
Micro-6 u.
Olympus URF-type P2 flexible u.
Panoview rod-lens u.
solid-rod u.
Storz SK u.
Wolf u.
Wolf rigid u.
ureterotome
optical u.
Otis u.
Uretex
U. self-anchoring urethral support system
U. TO urethral support system
urethane
Poron cellular u.
urethral
u. barrier device
u. candle
u. catheter
u. female dilator
u. instillation cannula
u. intermittent catheter and tray
u. male dilator
u. meatus dilator
u. sound
u. staff
urethrographic
u. cannula
u. cannula clamp
u. catheter
urethroplasty needle
urethroscope
Judd u.
Lowsley u.
urethrotome
u. blade
Hertel bougie u.
infant u.
Maisonneuve u.

U

urethrotome *(continued)*
>Otis u.
>Storz u.

urethrovesical angle support
Uri-Aid
Urias
>U. air splint
>U. pressure splint

Uribe orbital implant
Uri-Drain
>U.-D. leg bag
>U.-D. male incontinence device

Urihesive expandable adhesive
Uri-Kit culture kit
urinacidometer
urinal
>condom u.
>Feminal u.
>Millie female u.
>The Feminal female u.
>Uro-Tex McGuire male u.
>Ursec u.

urinalysis (UA)
urinary
>u. catheter
>u. control urethral insert
>u. drainage bag and urine meter
>u. drainage tube
>u. incontinence clamp
>u. incontinence prosthesis
>u. leg bag
>u. night drainage bottle

UrinChek 10+ urine test strip
urine
>u. collection device
>U. Meter Foley tray

Uriscreen bacteriuria detection system
Urisheath
>Conveen self-sealing U.

Urisys urine analyzer
Uri-Three urine culture kit
Uri-Two petri dish
Uro-Bond II brush-on silicone adhesive
Urocam videocamera
Urocare
>U. Foley catheter
>U. latex reusable leg bag

Urocath
>U. external catheter
>U. molded latex male external catheter

UroCoil self-expanding stent
UroCystom unit
Urocyte diagnostic cytometry system
Urodiagnost x-ray table
urodynamic catheter
urodynamic measurement system
uroflowmeter, uroflometer
>Dantec Urodyn u.

>Drake u.
>Etude cystometer u.
>FloPoint u.
>Synectics-Dantec u.
>Synectics-Dantec Flo-Lab II u.

UroForce ureteral balloon dilator
urogram
>intravenous u.

urograph
>Disa u.

urography
>excretory u.
>retrograde u.

Uro-Guide stent
Uro-jet delivery system
Urolab Janus System III
Urolase
>Bard U.
>U. CO_2 laser
>CR Bard U.
>U. fiber laser
>U. laser
>U. neodymium:YAG laser fiber

urological catheter
Uroloop
>U. electrode
>U. instrument

UroLume
>U. endoprosthesis
>U. endoprosthesis stent
>U. endourethral Wallstent prosthesis
>U. prostate stent
>U. urethral prosthesis
>U. urethral stent
>U. Wallstent
>U. Wallstent stent

UroMax II high-pressure balloon catheter
Uro-Pak system
Uro-Safe vinyl disposable leg bag
Uro-San Plus external catheter
UROS infuser
UroSnare cystoscopic tumor snare
Urosoft stent
Urospiral urethral stent
Uro-Tex McGuire male urinal
Urotract x-ray system
Urovac bladder evacuator
UroVision bladder cancer recurrence kit
Urovision ultrasound imaging system
UroVive self-contained balloon system
UroVysion
>U. bladder cancer kit
>U. bladder cancer recurrence test
>U. test kit

Urowave
>U. device
>U. thermotherapy

Urrets-Zavalia
  U.-Z. localizer
  U.-Z. retinal surgical lens
Ursec urinal
URYS 800 nerve stimulator
U.S.
  U.S. Army bone chisel
  U.S. Army double-ended retractor
  U.S. Army gauze scissors
  U.S. Army gouge
  U.S. Army osteotome
  U.S. Army tourniquet
  U.S. Army umbilical scissors
US-2000 echo scan
USA
  United States of America
  USA Elite System GYN rotating
    continuous flow resectoscope
  USA plaster spreader
  USA Series Distortion Free Hydro
    laparoscope
usage
  heroin u.
  ventilator u.
USC
  University of Southern California
  USC marker
  USC scleral planer
  USC scleral shaver
USCI
  United States Catheter & Instruments
    Company
  USCI Bard catheter
  USCI cannula
  USCI catheter
  USCI Goetz bipolar electrode
  USCI guiding catheter
  USCI introducer
  USCI Mini-Profile balloon
    dilatation catheter
  USCI NBIH bipolar electrode
  USCI pacing electrode
  USCI PET balloon
  USCI Positrol coronary catheter
  USCI probe
  USCI Probe balloon-on-a-wire
    dilatation system
  USCI shunt
U-shaped
  U-s. cannula
  U-s. forceps
  U-s. retractor
Usher Marlex mesh implant material
Uslenghi drill guide
USMC
  United States Marine Corps
  USMC luxury liner
  USMC multiaxis ankle
  USMC stance locking safety knee

U-splint splint
USSC stapler
Ussing chamber
U-stirrup splint
US uroflow meter
Utah
  U. arm electronic prosthesis
  U. artificial arm
  U. total artificial heart
Utas electroretinography instrument
utensil
  Good Grips u.
  swivel u.
uterine
  u. activity monitor
  u. artery forceps
  u. aspirator
  u. biopsy curette
  u. biopsy punch
  u. biopsy punch forceps
  u. clamp
  u. cornual access catheter
  u. curette
  u. dilator
  u. dressing forceps
  u. elevating forceps
  u. elevator
  u. evacuator
  U. Explora Curette endometrial
    sampling device
  u. grasping forceps
  u. holding forceps
  u. injector
  u. irrigating curette
  u. manipulating forceps
  u. manipulator
  u. needle
  u. ostial access catheter
  u. packing forceps
  u. polyp forceps
  u. probe
  u. scissors
  u. scoop
  u. self-retaining cannula
  u. sound
  u. specimen forceps
  u. suction curette
  u. tenaculum
  u. tenaculum forceps
  u. tube
  u. vacuum cannula
  u. vulsellum forceps
Uterobrush endometrial sample collector
utility
  u. bandage scissors
  u. forceps
  u. scissors
  u. shears

U

Utrata
  U. capsulorrhexis forceps
  U. foldable lens cutter
  U. forceps
  U. retriever
Utrata-Kershner capsulorrhexis cystotome forceps
UTTS
  ultrathin-walled 2-stage
  UTTS endotracheal tube
U-tube
  U-t. drain
  U-t. stent
U-type dental implant
UV
  ultraviolet
  UV biometer
  UV blocking filter
  UV transilluminator
UVA
  ultraviolet A
  UVA lamp

UV-absorbing IOL
UVAR
  ultraviolet autoblood radiation
  UVAR photophoresis system
Uvar photophoresis system
UVB
  ultraviolet B
  UVB lamp
  UVB phototherapy
uvea-fixated intraocular lens
uvea-supported intraocular lens
Uvex
  U. lens
  U. mask
UV-Flash ultraviolet germicidal exchange device
Uvidec-77 spectrophotometer
UVR
  ultraviolet radiation
uvular retractor
UV-Vis spectrophotometer

V

V blade plate
V clip
V medullary nail
V nail plate

VA

Veterans Administration
VA shunt

Vabra

V. aspirator
V. cannula
V. catheter
V. cervical aspirator
V. suction curette

VAC

vacuum-assisted closure
VAC Freedom system
VAC GranuFoam heel dressing
Wound VAC

Vac

Sani V.
vaper V. II

Vaccaria press seed

Vac-Lok

V.-L. bag immobilizer
V.-L. cushion
V.-L. immobilization cushion
V.-L. patient immobilization system

Vac-Pac

V.-P. pad
V.-P. positioner

Vac-Pak-II ultra-lite portable aspirator
Vactro perilimbal suction
Vacu-Aide

V.-A. home-use aspirator
V.-A. portable suction device

Vacuette blood sample tube
Vacu-Irrigator

Lap V.-I.
Vozzle V.-I.

Vaculance

V. lancing device
Microlet V.

Vacumix vacuum pump
Vac-Up
Vac-U-Port suction canister
Vacurette

Berkeley V.
V. suction curette

Vacutainer

V. collection tube
V. drain
EDTA-anticoagulated V.
V. holder
V. needle

V. system
V. tube
V. tubing
V. vacuum tube

Vacutron suction regulator
vacuum

v. apparatus
v. aspiration catheter
v. aspirator
v. beanbag positioner
v. cannula
v. cassette system
v. centering guide
v. clitoral therapy device
v. constriction device (VCD)
v. controller
v. cup
v. curette
v. disc
v. drain
Egnell v.
v. entrapment device
ErecAid v.
v. erection device (VED)
v. extraction device
v. extractor
v. fixation device
v. fixation ring
M-Pact cast v.
v. pillow
v. polymerization unit
Rainbow v.
v. retractor
v. splint
v. tube apparatus
v. tube voltmeter
v. tumescence constrictor device
v. tumescence device
v. uterine cannula
Venturi-type live v.
VTU-1 v. erection device

vacuum-assisted

v.-a. closure (VAC)
v.-a. closure device
v.-a. closure dressing
v.-a. venous return system

vacuum-based pump
vacuum-formed resin impression tray
vacuuming needle
vacuum-operated viscous restraint
VAD

vascular access device
venous access device
ventricular assist device

VAD *(continued)*
    DeBakey VAD
    HeartSaver VAD
vagal
vaginal
    v. candle
    v. contraceptive film
    v. cuff
    v. cuff clamp
    v. cylinder
    v. dilator
    v. hysterectomy forceps
    v. packing
    v. pessary
    v. pouch
    v. probe ultrasound
    v. prolapse prosthesis
    v. retractor
    v. ring
    v. spatula
    v. speculum
    v. speculum loop
    v. stent
vaginometer
vaginoscope
    Cameron-Myers v.
    Huffman v.
vagotomy retractor
vagus nerve stimulator
Vairox high-compression vascular
  stocking
Vaiser-Cibis muscle retractor
Vaiser sponge
valence
    electron v.
Valenti arthroereisis device
Valeo back support
valgus
    v. bar
    v. corrective ankle strap
    v. knee control pad
Valilab electrocautery
Valle hysteroscope
Valleylab
    V. ball electrode
    V. cautery
    V. cautery unit
    V. CUSA CEM system
    V. electrocautery
    V. Force 2 electrosurgical device
    V. Force IC electrosurgical
      generator
    V. generator
    V. II generator
    V. laparoscopic instrument
    V. loop electrode
    V. pencil
    V. REM system
Valley Vac smoke evacuation system

Valls hip prosthesis
Valtrac
    V. absorbable biofragmentable
      anastomosis ring
    V. anastomosis device
    V. anastomosis ring
    V. BAR
Valtzhev uterine manipulator
Value Walker brace
valve
    Abrams-Lucas flap heart v.
    absent pulmonary v.
    Access-9 large-bore hemostasis v.
    Aesculap-Miethke v.
    Ahmed glaucoma v.
    Ahmed glaucoma artificial v.
    Ahmed glaucoma biplate v.
    Ambu-E v.
    Angell-Shiley bioprosthetic v.
    Angell-Shiley bioprosthetic heart v.
    Angell-Shiley xenograft
      prosthetic v.
    Angiocor prosthetic v.
    antisiphon v.
    aortic bioprosthetic v.
    Argyle antireflux v.
    Argyle-Salem sump antireflux v.
    ATS Open Pivot heart v.
    BacStop dental antiretraction
      check v.
    Ball v.
    ball heart v.
    Beall v.
    Beall disc heart v.
    Beall prosthetic v.
    Beall-Surgitool ball-cage
      prosthetic v.
    Beall-Surgitool disc prosthetic v.
    Benchekroun hydraulic ileal v.
    Béraud v.
    Beverly referential v.
    Bianchi v.
    Bicarbon Sorin v.
    Bicer-Val prosthetic v.
    bileaflet tilting-disc prosthetic v.
    Biocor porcine v.
    Biocor porcine stented aortic v.
    biological aortic v.
    biological tissue v.
    bioprosthetic heart v.
    Bio-Vascular prosthetic v.
    Björk-Shiley convexoconcave disc
      prosthetic v.
    Björk-Shiley mitral v.
    Björk-Shiley monostrut v.
    bleed-back v.
    Blom-Singer v.
    bovine heart v.
    bovine pericardial v.

Braunwald-Cutter v.
Braunwald heart v.
bulb and thumb screw v.
butterfly heart v.
caged ball heart v.
CarboMedics bileaflet prosthetic
    heart v.
CarboMedics Top-Hat
    supraannular v.
Carpentier-Edwards bioprosthetic v.
Carpentier-Edwards mitral
    annuloplasty v.
Carpentier-Edwards pericardial v.
Carpentier-Edwards Perimount
    mitral v.
Carpentier-Edwards porcine
    prosthetic v.
Carpentier-Edwards porcine
    supraannular v.
Carpentier-Edwards SAV aortic
    porcine bioprosthesis v.
Carpentier pericardial v.
central caged ball occluder v.
central caged disc occluder v.
CirKuit-Guard pressure relief v.
Codman Hakim programmable v.
Codman Medos programmable v.
convexoconcave heart v.
Cooley-Bloodwell-Cutter v.
Cooley-Cutter disc prosthetic v.
Copilot bleed-back control v.
CPHV OptiForm mitral v.
Cribier-Edwards aortic percutaneous
    heart v.
Cross-Jones disc prosthetic v.
Cross-Jones mitral v.
CRx Diamond v.
CryoLife-O'Brien v.
cryopreserved homograft v.
Cutter-Smeloff disc v.
Cutter-Smeloff mitral v.
DeBakey prosthetic v.
DeBakey-Surgitool prosthetic v.
Delrin disc heart v.
Delrin heart v.
Delta v.
Denver v.
Diamond v.
diastolic fluttering aortic v.
differential pressure v.
v. dilator
Double Play large-bore double-Y
    hemostasis v.
double-spring ball v.
dual-switch v.
Duostat rotating hemostatic v.
Duromedics bileaflet mitral v.
Duromedics mitral v.
dysplastic v.

early opening v.
eccentric monocuspid disc v.
eccentric monocuspid tilting disc
    prosthetic v.
echodense v.
Edmark mitral v.
Edwards-Duromedics bileaflet
    heart v.
Edwards heart v.
Edwards seamless heart v.
Epic v.
Equi-Flow v.
esophageal Z stent with Dua
    antireflux v.
expiratory v.
fascia lata heart v.
Fink v.
flexible cardiac v.
floating-disc heart v.
flow-controlled v.
flushing v.
Freestyle bioprosthetic heart v.
Freestyle stentless aortic heart v.
Frumin v.
Georgia v.
glutaraldehyde-tanned bovine
    heart v.
glutaraldehyde-tanned porcine
    heart v.
Gott butterfly heart v.
Groningen v.
Guangzhou GD-1 prosthetic v.
Hakim high-pressure v.
Hakim precision v.
Hall-Kaster heart v.
Hall prosthetic heart v.
Hammersmith heart v.
Hancock bioprosthetic heart v.
Hancock heterograft heart v.
Hancock II tissue v.
Hancock modified orifice v.
Hancock MO II bioprosthesis
    porcine v.
Hancock porcine v.
Hans Rudolph 3-way v.
Harken v.
Harken ball v.
Harken ball heart v.
Harken prosthetic v.
Hasner v.
heart v.
Heimlich chest drainage v.
Heimlich heart v.
Heister v.
Heyer-Pudenz v.
Heyer-Schulte v.
v. holder
hollow silastic disc heart v.
Holter elliptical v.

V

valve *(continued)*

Holter-Hausner v.
Holter high-pressure v.
Holter medium-pressure v.
Holter mini-elliptical v.
Holter straight v.
Hood speaking v.
Hufnagel prosthetic v.
impedance threshold v.
Inspector large-bore inline
  hemostasis v.
Intact xenograft v.
intussuscepted nipple v.
Ionescu-Shiley artificial cardiac v.
Ionescu-Shiley pericardial v.
Ionescu trileaflet v.
Kay-Shiley heart v.
Kay-Suzuki heart v.
Kistner speaking v.
Kock nipple v.
Krupin-Denver v.
Krupin-Denver eye v.
Lanz pressure-regulating v.
4-legged cage v.
3-legged cage heart v.
4-legged cage heart v.
lens mitral heart v.
LeVeen v.
Lifemed heterologous heart v.
Lillehei-Kaster pivoting-disc
  prosthetic v.
Liotta-BioImplant low-profile
  bioprosthesis prosthetic v.
Lopez enteral v.
low-profile mitral heart v.
Magovern-Cromie ball-cage
  prosthetic v.
Malteno glaucoma artificial v.
V. Mapper Steerocath-Dx mapping
  catheter
Masters series mechanical heart v.
MBA hemostasis v.
Medos Hakim programmable v.
Medtronic-Hall monocuspid tilting-
  disc v.
Medtronic-Hall prosthetic heart v.
Medtronic Hancock II tissue v.
Medtronic Intact bioprosthetic v.
Medtronic Mosaic bioprosthetic v.
Medtronic prosthetic v.
Miethke dual-switch v.
Mishler dual-chamber v.
Mishler flushing v.
Mitrofanoff v.
Mitroflow pericardial prosthetic v.
Mitroflow Synergy PC stented
  pericardial v.
monocuspid tilting-disc v.
Monostrut Bjödork-Shiley v.

Monostrut heart v.
Montgomery speaking v.
Mosaic porcine bioprosthetic
  heart v.
multipurpose v.
Nezhat-Dorsey trumpet v.
nonrebreathing v.
Olympic speaking v.
Omnicarbon prosthetic heart v.
Omniscience v.
Omniscience tilting disc v.
On-X mechanical bi-leaflet
  prosthetic heart v.
Open Pivot heart v.
Orbis-Sigma cerebrospinal fluid
  shunt v.
v. outflow strut
Panje v.
Passage hemostasis v.
Passy-Muir v.
Passy-Muir tracheostomy
  speaking v.
PASV v.
pedi-gravity assisted v.
PEEP v.
Phoenix ancillary v.
Phoenix cruciform v.
Phonate speaking v.
PlegiaGuard pressure relief v.
PMV v.
PMV speaking v.
pop-off v.
porcine v.
porcine heart v.
pressure-activated safety v.
pressure relief v.
programmable v.
programmable ventricular shunt v.
prosthetic ball v.
prosthetic heart v.
Provox speaking v.
Provox tracheoesophageal
  speaking v.
PS Medical Flow Control v.
Puig-Massana-Shiley anuloplasty v.
pulmonary autograft v.
quadricusp stentless mitral
  bioprosthetic v.
Quadtro cushion with Isoflap v.
Quinton single-port scissor v.
Regent mechanical heart v.
Ross pulmonary porcine v.
rotating hemostatic v.
Rudolph 1-way respiratory v.
Safsite v.
Setguard antireflux v.
Shikani-French speaking v.
Shiley convexoconcave heart v.

Shiley low-pressure cuffed tracheostomy tube with pressure relief v.
Shiley monostrut heart v.
Shiley Phonate speaking v.
silicone ball heart v.
silicone disc heart v.
SJM Masters Series heart v.
SJM mechanical heart v.
SJM Quattro mitral v.
SJM Regent mechanical heart v.
Smeloff-Cutter ball cage prosthetic v.
Smeloff heart v.
SmokEvac trumpet v.
Sophy adjustable pressure v.
Sophy mini-programmable pressure v.
Sophy programmable v.
Sorin heart v.
Sorin prosthetic v.
speaking v.
Spitz-Holter v.
Starr ball heart v.
Starr-Edwards ball-and-cage v.
Starr-Edwards cloth-covered metallic ball heart v.
Starr-Edwards heart v.
Starr-Edwards prosthetic aortic v.
Starr-Edwards prosthetic mitral v.
Starr-Edwards silastic v.
Starr-Edwards silicone rubber ball v.
stentless porcine aortic v.
stent-mounted allograft v.
stent-mounted heterograft v.
Stephen-Slater v.
St. Jude bileaflet prosthetic v.
St. Jude composite prosthetic v.
St. Jude Medical bileaflet tilting-disc aortic v.
St. Jude Medical bioImplant v.
St. Jude Medical Port-Access mechanical heart v.
Strata adjustable Delta v.
Strata shunt v.
supraanular v. (SAV)
SynerGraft pulmonary heart v.
SynerGraft tissue-engineered heart v.
tilting disc heart v.
Top-Hat supraanular aortic v.
Toronto SPV aortic v.
Toronto SPV stentless porcine heart v.
tracheostoma v.
tricuspid aortic v.
v. tube
UCI-Barnard aortic v.

unidirectional airflow ball tracheostomy speaking v.
unstented pulmonary homograft heart v.
unstented xenograft v.
Vascor porcine prosthetic v.
ventilator speaking v.
3-way Hans Rudolph v.
Wessex prosthetic v.
Xenotech prosthetic v.

valved
v. holding chamber (VHC)
v. voice prosthesis
valve-ended catheter
valve-regulated shunt
valvuloplasty balloon catheter
valvulotome
angioscopic v.
expandable LeMaitre v.
Hall v.
Harken v.
Leather retrograde v.
Mills v.
retrograde v.

VAMP
Baxter VAMP
Van
V. Alyea antral trocar
V. Alyea frontal sinus cannula
V. Aman pulmonary pigtail catheter
V. Buren bone-holding forceps
V. Buren canvas roll sound
V. Buren catheter
V. Buren catheter guide
V. Buren dilator
V. Buren sequestrum forceps
V. Buren urethral sound
V. catheter
V. de Graaf generator
V. der Bend chamber
V. Herick filtration
V. Praagh loop rule
V. Rosen splint
V. Slyke apparatus
V. Sonnenberg chest drain set
V. Sonnenberg gallbladder catheter
V. Sonnenberg sump
V. Sonnenberg sump catheter
V. Sonnenberg sump drain
V. Tassel catheter
van
v. Andel dilating catheter
v. den Berg stray-light meter
Vancaillie uterine cannula
Vancenase Pockethaler
Vance prostatic aspiration cannula
Vanguard
V. device

V

Vanguard *(continued)*
    V. endograft
    V. III endovascular aortic graft
    V. M unicondylar system
    V. PFR system
    V. Uni unicompartmental knee
      replacement
VanishPoint syringe
Vannas
    V. capsulotomy scissors
    V. corneal scissors
    V. iridocapsulotomy scissors
VanSonnenberg biopsy needle
Vantage
    V. ophthalmoscope
    V. Performance monitor
    V. tube-occluding forceps
Vantex central venous catheter
VAPC
    Veterans Administration Prosthetics
    Center
    VAPC dorsiflexion assist orthosis
vaper
    V. Cut loop
    v. Vac II
Vapor Cut loop
vaporization
    contact laser v.
    photoselective v. (PV)
vaporizer
    cool mist v. (CMV)
    draw-over v.
    flow-over v.
    Fluotec v.
    Goldman v.
    Maxi-Myst v.
    Penlon v.
    water v.
vaporizing rust inhibitor
vapor-permeable dressing
Vapor-Phase heated humidification system
vapor pressure osmometer
VaporTome resection electrode
VaporTrode roller electrode
Vapotherm oxygen delivery system
Vapr
    V. coagulation and cautery device
    V. system
Vapro vapor pressure osmometer
Varady phlebectomy hook
Varco
    V. dissecting clamp
    V. thoracic forceps
variable
    v. positive airway pressure (VPAP)
    v. screw placement (VSP)
    v. spinal plating (VSP)
variable-angle gamma camera

variable-axis knee
variable-circumference suprapatellar socket
variable-flow insufflator
variable-focus scope
variable-power cross-cylinder lens set
variable-rate pacemaker
variable-stiffness
    v.-s. endoscope
    v.-s. enteroscope
    v.-s. guidewire
    v.-s. wire guide
Varia laser
Varian
    V. accelerator
    V. Associates bore spectrometer
    V. brachytherapy system
    V. CT scanner
    V. gas chromatograph
    V. LINAC
    V. MLC system
    V. NMR spectrometer
    V. Spectra spectrometer
Vari-Angle
    V.-A. clip
    V.-A. clip applier
    V.-A. screw
vari-balance board set
VariCare pulsed lavage system
variceal pressure measuring device
Varicoscreen
Vari-Duct hip and knee orthosis
Vari-Firm Medicine Ball
VariFix spinal implant device
Variflex catheter
Vari-Flex prosthetic foot
Varigray lens
VariGrip
    V. spinal implant device
    V. spine fixation system
Variject needle
Vari-Lase
    V.-L. endovenous laser procedure kit
    V.-L. endovenous laser system
VariLock socket lock
Varilux
    V. Infinity lens
    V. lens implant
    V. Pangamic thin plastic lens
    V. Plus lens
Vari-Mix II amalgamator
Vari/Moist wound dressing
variomatrix transducer
Vario microscope
Vari-Stim
    V.-S. III handheld nerve stimulator
    V.-S. unit
Vari-Tilt adjustable tilt-board

VariTone
Varivas
    V. loop graft
    V. R vein graft
varus
    v. corrective ankle strap
    v. knee control pad
vas
    v. clamp
    v. hook
Vas-Cath catheter
Vasceze vascular access flush device
Vasclip alternative to vasectomy
Vasco-Posada orbital retractor
Vascor porcine prosthetic valve
VascuClamp
    V. minibulldog vessel clamp
    V. vascular clamp
VascuCoil peripheral vascular stent
Vascu-Flo carotid shunt
Vascugel device
vascular
    v. access catheter
    v. access device (VAD)
    v. access flush device
    v. access safety kit
    v. access tunneler
    v. bulldog
    v. clamp
    v. clip
    v. clip applier
    v. dilator
    v. dissector
    v. graft prosthesis
    v. hemostatic device (VHD)
    v. loop
    v. needle holder
    v. ring
    v. scissors
    v. sealing device
    v. sheath
    v. stapler
    v. stent
    v. tape
    v. tissue forceps
    v. volume of distribution (VVD)
VascuLink vascular access graft
Vascutek
    V. Gelseal vascular graft
    V. knitted vascular graft
    V. vascular prosthesis
    V. woven vascular graft
vasectomy
    v. forceps
    Vasclip alternative to v.
Vaseline
    V. gauze dressing
    V. petrolatum pack
Vaseline-coated gauze

Vaseline-impregnated gauze
vaselinized nasal tamponade
vasodilator
vasoepididymostomy
    ASSI end-to-end v.
    Goldstein Microspike approximator
    clamp for v.
Vasoscope 3 Doppler probe
VasoSeal
    V. closure device
    V. diagnostic device
    V. Elite
    V. Elite vascular closure
    V. ES, VHD arterial puncture site
    closure device
    V. therapeutic device
    V. vascular hemostasis device
    V. VHD
Vasotrax handheld monitor
vasovasostomy
    v. clamp
    Goldstein Microspike approximator
    clamp for v.
VasoView
    V. balloon dissection device
    V. balloon dissection system
    V. Uniport endoscopic saphenous
    vein harvesting system
VAT
    ventricular, atrial, triggered
    VAT pacemaker
Vaughan abscess knife
Vaxcel
    V. catheter
    V. dialysis catheter
    V. mini stick
    V. peripherally inserted catheter
    V. peripherally inserted central
    catheter
    V. PICC
    V. Plus chronic dialysis catheter
VAX-D
    vertebral axial decompression
    VAX-D therapy table
VAX 4100 system
V510B
Vbeam
V-beam
    V-b. pulsed dye laser
    V-b. pulsed dye laser system
    V-b. vascular laser
VBH
    Vogele-Bale-Hohner
    VBH head holder
V-brace support garment
VC2 atrial caval cannula
V-Cath catheter
VCD
    vacuum constriction device

V

VCD *(continued)*
 Dacomed Catalyst VCD
 Mentor-Piston VCD
 Mentor Response VCD
 Mentor-Touch VCD
 Mission VCD
 Osbon ErecAid VCD
 Pos-T-Vac VCD

VCUG
 voiding cystourethrogram

VDD
 ventricular depolarization duration
 VDD pacemaker
 VDD pacing system

VDS
 ventral derotating spinal
 VDS compression rod
 VDS hex nut
 VDS screw
 VDS screwdriver
 VDS wrench

Veau elevator

Vectastain Elite ABC kit

vectis
 Anis irrigating v.
 anterior chamber irrigating v.
 v. blade
 Drews-Knolle reverse irrigating v.
 irrigating/aspirating v.
 Knolle-Pearce v.
 Look irrigating v.
 v. loop
 Peczon I&A v.
 Pierce I&A v.
 plastic disposable irrigating v.
 Sheets irrigating v.
 Snellen v.

vector
 V. Elite Reagent
 V. II guide system
 V. intertrochanteric nail
 V. low back analysis system
 v. phased-array ultrasound tipped
 catheter

VectorVision
 V. image-guided surgery system
 V. surgical tracking system
 V. Uni-Knee system

VectorVision₂

VectorVision₂Fluoro

Vector-X coronary guiding catheter

Vectra
 V. Genisys laser system
 V. Genisys laser system device

VED
 vacuum erection device
 Mission VED

Veda-scope

vehicle
 transport v.

veil
 Conformant 2 nonadherent
 transparent wound v.

Veillon tube

vein
 v. dilator
 v. graft cannula
 v. graft ring marker
 v. graft stent
 v. hook retractor
 Krukenberg v.
 Kuhnt postcentral v.
 opticociliary shunt v.
 portal v.
 v. retractor
 v. stripper

Veirs cannula

Velband orthopaedic padding wool

Velcro
 V. fastener dressing
 V. Hand Exerboard
 V. immobilizer
 V. strap
 V. strap immobilizer
 V. tourniquet

Velegrakis piston

velocimeter
 Doppler v.
 Doppler laser v.
 FloMap v.
 laser Doppler v.
 optical Doppler v.

velocimetry
 Doppler v.

Velocity stent

Velocity-U digital imaging system

velolaryngeal endoscope

velour collar graft

Velpeau
 V. axillary radiograph
 V. bandage
 V. cast
 V. shoulder immobilizer
 V. shoulder sling
 V. sling
 V. stockinette
 V. wrap

Velstretch/Velcro headgear

velvet-eye aspirating tube

vena
 v. cava cannula
 v. cava clamp
 v. cava clip
 v. cava filter
 v. cava forceps
 V. Tech dual vena cava filter
 V. Tech filter

V. Tech LGM filter
V. Tech LGM vena cava filter
V. Tech low-profile filter
V. Tech LP vena cava filter

Venaflo
V. needle
V. vascular graft

VenaFlow
V. compression system
V. DVT prophylaxis system

Venaport coronary sinus guiding catheter
veneer retention wire
VenES II Medical stocking
Venflon
V. cannula
V. needle

Veni-Gard stabilization dressing
venipuncture needle
venoclysis cannula
Venodyne
V. boot
V. compression system
V. external pneumatic compression system
V. pneumatic compressive device

Venofit medical compression stocking
Venoflex medical compression stocking
Venosan
V. support hose
V. support sock

venoscope
Landry vein light v.

venous
v. access device (VAD)
v. access port
v. cannula
v. catheter
v. irrigation catheter
v. needle
v. plethysmograph
v. pressure-gradient support stocking
v. thrombectomy catheter
v. Y adapter
v. Y connector

venous/arterial management protection
vent
Heartport endopulmonary v.
Yung percutaneous mastoid v.

Ventak
V. AICD
V. AICD pacemaker
V. A-V III DR automatic implantable cardioverter-defibrillator
V. ECD
V. ECD pacemaker
V. Mini II AICD

V. Mini II and III automatic implantable cardioverter-defibrillator
V. Mini III implantable defibrillator
V. Prizm 2 automatic implantable cardioverter-defibrillator
V. Prizm AVT cardioverter device
V. Prizm dual-chamber implantable defibrillator
V. Prizm implantable defibrillator
V. Prizm 2 system
V. PRx cardioverter-defibrillator
V. PRx defibrillation system
V. PRx III/Endotak system
V. PRx pacemaker

Ventana
V. alkaline phosphatase blue detection kit
V. automated immunostainer
V. ES slide processor machine
V. ES stain
V. immuno-automated machine
V. Medical Systems Techmate automated stainer
V. NexES immunostainer
V. silanized capillary gap slide
V. TechMate immunostainer

VentCheck handheld respiratory monitor
vented-electric HeartMate LVAD
Ventex
V. composite dressing
V. dressing
V. wound dressing system

ventilated
v. incontinence pad
v. mask

ventilation
v. adapter
v. bronchoscope
high-frequency oscillatory v.
mask v.
v. mask
v. tube
v. tube inserter

ventilator (*See also* respirator)
Acutronic AMS automatic jet v.
Acutronic Mistral v.
Acutronic Monsoon v.
Adult Star ultra-high-frequency v.
Aequitron v.
Amadeus v.
Amsterdam v.
automatic transport v.
Avian transport v.
BABYbird II v.
babyPAC v.
Bear v.
Bear 1, 2 adult volume v.

V

ventilator *(continued)*
  Bear Cub infant v.
  Bennett v.
  Bio-Med pediatric v.
  Bird Ascension v.
  blow-by v.
  Bourns-Bear I v.
  Bourns infant v.
  Breas v.
  CPAP v.
  critical care v.
  cuirass v.
  Datex-Ohmeda v.
  Dräger v.
  E-150 Breeze v.
  Emerson postoperative v.
  Esprit v.
  flow-cycled v.
  Galileo v.
  Hamilton v.
  Healthdyne v.
  high-frequency jet v.
  high-frequency oscillation v.
  high-frequency oscillatory v.
  high-oscillation v.
  humidification v.
  Impact Uni-Vent v.
  Infant Star v.
  Infant Star high-frequency v.
  infant Star high-frequency v.
  IVAC v.
  jet v.
  Lifecare v.
  Life Pulse high-frequency jet v.
  manual jet v.
  Maquet Servo-i v.
  Max v.
  mechanical v.
  MicroVent v.
  Mistral v.
  Monaghan v.
  Monsoon v.
  nebulization v.
  Nellcor Puritan Bennett v.
  Newport v.
  Newport Wave v.
  noninvasive extrathoracic v.
  PEEP v.
  Pneupac v.
  pneuPAC v.
  portable volume v.
  Porta-Lung noninvasive
    extrathoracic v.
  positive support v.
  pressure v.
  pressure-cycled v.
  v. pressure manometer
  pressure-preset v.
  pressure support v. (PSV)

  Pulmo-Aid v.
  Pulmo-Aide v.
  Puritan Bennett v.
  Puritan Bennett KnightStar v.
  Quantum PSV v.
  Respironics BIPAP bilevel v.
  Sechrist hyperbaric v.
  Sechrist infant v.
  Sechrist neonatal v.
  SensorMedics v.
  Servo v.
  Servo v.
  Servo-i v.
  Siemens v.
  Siemens-Elema Servo v.
  Siemens-Elema Servo 900C v.
  Siemens Servo v.
  SLE v.
  Smart Trigger Bear v.
  Smart Trigger Bear 1000 v.
  v. speaking valve
  Star v.
  v. system
  TBird v.
  time-cycled v.
  UJV AMS high-frequency jet v.
  Uni-Vent Eagle portable v.
  v. usage
  Venturi v.
  VIP Bird neonatal v.
  Vix infant v.
  volume v.
  volume-cycled v.
  volume-limited v.
  Wave v.
ventilatory support tube
Ventimask
venting catheter
Ventolin Rotacaps
vent-plate implant
Ventra catheter
VenTrak respiratory mechanics monitor
ventral derotating spinal (VDS)
Ventralex hernia patch
VentrAssist heart pump
ventricle impedance adapter (VIA)
ventricle impedance adapter (VIA)
ventricle-paced, ventrical-sensed
  inhibited, rate-responsive (VVIR)
ventricular
  v. assist device (VAD)
  v. asynchronous (VOO)
  v. asynchronous pacemaker
  v. cannula
  v. catheter
  v. catheter introducer
  v. demand-inhibited pacemaker
  v. demand pacemaker
  v. demand pulse generator

v. demand-triggered pacemaker
v. depolarization duration (VDD)
v. function curve (VFC)
v. implantable cardioverter-defibrillator
v. inhibited (VVI)
v. inhibited, atrial inhibited (VVI/AAI)
left v. (LV)
v. needle
v. sump
v. triggered (VVT)
v. triggered pacemaker
ventricular, atrial, triggered (VAT)
ventriculoatrial
v. shunt catheter
ventriculogram retractor
ventriculography catheter
ventriculoperitoneal (VP)
v. shunt
ventriculoscope
4-channel Aesculap v.
rigid v.
ventriculosubarachnoid (VS)
Ventritex
V. Angstrom MD implantable cardioverter-defibrillator
V. Cadence device
V. Cadence ICD
V. Cadence implantable cardioverter-defibrillator
V. Contour
V. generator
V. TVL system
Ventrix tunnelable ventricular intracranial pressure monitoring system
ventroposterolateral (VPL)
Vent-Trach
Montgomery V.-T.
VentTrak monitoring system
Venture demand oxygen delivery device
Venturi
V. adjusted temple
V. apparatus
V. aspiration vitrectomy device
V. exhalation assist
V. jet adapter
V. mask
V. meter
V. pump
V. tube
V. ventilation adapter
V. ventilator
Venturi-Flo valve system
Venturi-type live vacuum
Venturi Venti-mask Mark 2
Venus-i laser system

VEPTR
vertical expandable prosthetic titanium rib
VEPTR device
Vera-Lift
Verbrugge
V. bone clamp
V. bone-holding clamp
V. bone-holding forceps
Verbrugge-Hohmann bone retractor
Verbrugge-Mueller bone lever
Verdict-II drug screening device
Veress
V. laparoscopic cannula
V. needle
V. pneumoperitoneum needle
V. spring-loaded laparoscopic needle
Verhoeff
V. capsule forceps
V. lens expressor
V. scissors
V. suture
Veriflex cardiac device
Verifuse ambulatory infusion pump
Veripath peripheral guiding catheter
Veris III system
Veristat fluid management system
Verisyse phakic IOL
Verlow brace
Vermont
V. spinal fixator (VSF)
V. spinal fixator clamp
Vernier
V. caliber gauge
V. calipers
V. optometer
Vernon-David
V.-D. proctoscope
V.-D. rectal speculum
V.-D. sigmoidoscope
Verruca-Freeze freezing system
Versaback back system
VersaBond medium-viscosity bone cement
VersaClimber RX exercise machine
Versadopp ultrasonic Doppler probe
Versafil tissue expander
VersaFlex tubing kit
Versaflow peristatic pump
Versa-Fx femoral hip fixation system
Versa-Helper floor stand
Versajet hydrosurgery system
VersaLab
V. APM2 portable antepartum monitor
V. APM2 for Twins
VersaLap

V

VersaLight
> V. laser
> Lübke-Berci V.

Versalok
> V. low back fixation device
> V. low back fixation system

Versalon all-purpose sponge
VersaNail tibial nail
Versa-PEG gastrostomy kit
Versapoint system
Versaport trocar system
VersaPulse
> V. holmium laser
> V. laser
> V. PowerSuite dual-wavelength laser
> V. PowerSuite holmium laser
> V. Select laser
> V. variable pulse-width green laser

Versascope hysteroscopy system
VersaStep laparoscopy system
VersaTack stapler
Versatone
> V. perioperative Doppler
> V. perioperative Doppler system

VersaTool eye sponge
Versa-Trainer exerciser
Versatrax
> V. cardiac pacemaker
> V. II 7000A pacemaker

VersaWrist wrist splint
Versi-Splint carry bag
Versitrel neurostimulator
VerSys
> V. Beaded FullCoat Plus hip prosthesis
> V. fiber metal taper
> V. hip system
> V. prosthesis

VertAlign spinal support system
vertebra axial decompression
vertebral
> v. artery system
> v. axial decompression (VAX-D)
> v. body impactor

vertebrated
> v. catheter
> v. probe

Verteflex
> V. arthrotonic stabilizer
> V. intersegmental traction table

Vertetrac ambulatory traction system
Vertex
> V. camera
> V. reconstruction system

vertical
> v. expandable prosthetic titanium rib (VEPTR)
> v. forceps

> v. ring curette
> v. self-retaining bone retractor
> v. shock pylon
> v. spreading scissors

VertiGraft textured allograft bone graft
vertometer
Vesica
> V. percutaneous bladder neck suspension kit
> V. press-in suture anchor system
> V. sling
> V. Sling kit

vesical retractor
vesicular transport system
Vespore disinfectant
Vess chair
vessel
> v. band
> v. clamp
> v. clip
> v. dilator
> v. forceps
> v. hook
> v. knife
> v. loop
> nondominant v.
> v. occlusion system
> v. punch
> v. retractor
> small v. (SV)

vessel-occluding clamp
Vesseloops rubber band
vessel-sizing catheter
VEST
> VEST ambulatory nuclear detector
> VEST ambulatory ventricular function monitor

vest
> Breast V.
> Bremer AirFlo v.
> Bremer AirFlo halo v.
> E-Z-On v.
> halo v.
> immobilizing v.
> Little cargo v.
> Mark VII cooling v.
> Minerva v.
> Orthotrac pneumatic v.
> Standard E-Z-On v.
> ThAIRapy v.
> weighted v.

VestaBlate
> V. system
> V. system balloon device

vestibular
> v. ball
> v. board
> v. clamp
> v. oral plate

Vestibulator
> V. II roll swing
> V. positioning tumble form

vest-type
> v.-t. backboard
> v.-t. extrication device

Vet-Co vacuum system

Veterans
> V. Administration (VA)
> V. Administration Prosthetics
> Center (VAPC)

VFC
> ventricular function curve
> Actis V.

V-Flex
> V-F. FMJ stent
> V-F. Plus stent

Vgamma9 test

VHC
> valved holding chamber
> AeroChamber VHC

VHD
> vascular hemostatic device
> VHD closure device
> VasoSeal VHD

VIA
> ventricle impedance adapter

Via
> V. arterial blood gas and
> chemistry monitor
> V. silicone surgical wound drain

Viabahn
> V. covered stent
> V. endoprosthesis

Viabil
> V. biliary endoprosthesis
> V. stent

ViaCath computer-assisted robotic endoluminal system

Viadur implant

Viagraph ECG system

vial
> multiple-dose v.
> Nickerson BiGGY v.
> Port-A-Germ anaerobic transport v.

Viamonte-Hobbs dye injector

Viasorb
> V. composite dressing
> V. dressing
> V. occlusive film dressing
> V. wound dressing

Viatorr
> V. endoprosthesis
> V. transjugular intrahepatic
> portosystemic shunt stent-graft

Viatrac 14 Plus peripheral dilation catheter

Viatronix virtual colonoscopy system

Vibracare percussor

Vibraject injection syringe

Vibramat

Vibramatic massage/percussion unit

Vibram sole

Vibrant
> V. D, HF, P Soundbridge
> V. Soundbridge implantable middle
> ear hearing device

vibrating-reed electrometer

vibrating scissors

vibration glove

Vibratome

vibrator
> Magic Wand v.

vibrometer

Vicat needle

Vi-Cell series cell viability analyzer

Vichy shower

Vickers
> V. forceps
> V. isolator
> V. microdensitometer
> V. needle holder
> V. ring-tip forceps
> V. Ventimask Mark 2 mask

Vicon 3-dimensional gait analysis system

vicrosurgery

Vicryl
> V. mesh
> V. pop-off suture
> V. Rapide suture
> V. SH suture
> V. suture

Victoreen
> V. digital densitometer
> V. dosimeter

Victorian collar dressing

VID
> videodensitometry
> VID 1 color microcamera system

Vidal-Adrey modified Hoffmann external fixation device

Vidal device

VidaMed TUNA system

Vidar scanner

Vidaurri
> V. double irrigation cannula
> V. irrigator
> V. LASIK cannula

video
> v. densitometer
> v. disc
> v. display camera
> v. image processor
> v. imaging system
> v. monitor
> v. otoscope
> v. pill camera

V

video *(continued)*
    v. push enteroscope
    v. recorder
    v. specular microscope
    v. timer
videoarthroscopic shaver
videobronchoscope
videocamera
    charge-coupled device v.
    Circon v.
    DyoCam arthroscopic v.
    endoscope v.
    5 lux color v.
    MedCam Pro Plus v.
    Sony CCD/RGB color v.
    Urocam v.
videocapsule
    Given M2A endoscopic v.
videocholangioscope
videocolonoscope
    EVE Fujinon v.
    Fujinon v.
    Olympus v.
    Olympus Evis v.
videoconverter
videodensitometric
videodensitometry (VID)
videoduodenoscope
    Fujinon v.
    Olympus v.
    Olympus JF-V series v.
videoelectroscope
    Fujinon v.
videoendoscope
    3-dimensional v.
    double-channel v.
    fiberoptic v.
    Fujinon v.
    infrared v.
    Olympus double-channel
      therapeutic v.
    Olympus Evis v.
    Olympus GIF-T series v.
    Pentax v.
    Pentax EG-series v.
    side-viewing v.
    Toshiba v.
    Welch Allyn v.
videoendoscopy
    zoom v.
videoenteroscope
    Olympus v.
videoesophagoscope
    transnasal v.
videofluoroscope
videofluoroscopic imaging chair
videofluoroscopy
videogastroscope
    Fujinon super-image v.

    Olympus v.
    Pentax v.
    transnasal v.
videoinstrument
    XQ v.
videokeratograph
    EyeSys v.
videokeratographer
    Humphrey v.
videokeratoscope
    computer-assisted v.
    EyeSys v.
    Keratron v.
    Technomed C-scan v.
    TMS-1, -2 v.
    TMS-2 computer-assisted v.
videolaparoscope
    flexible v.
videolaryngoscope
    Kantor-Berci v.
videooculography
videoprocessor
    real-time v.
**video-rate laser 2-photon scanning
  microscope**
videoresectoscope
    Richard Wolf v.
videoscope
    Cabot Medical Corporation v.
    CV-1 v.
    oral v.
    SlimSIGHT gastrointestinal v.
videosigmoidoscope
videothorascopic (VTC)
Vidicon
    V. camera tube
    V. vacuum chamber pickup tube
Vi-Drape
    V-D. bowel bag
    V-D. drape
    V-D. dressing
    Ioban V-D.
Vielle menopause home test kit
Vienna Britetrac nasal speculum
Vieth-Mueller horopter
Vietnam catheter
viewbox
    virtual reality v.
viewer
    cephalometric v.
    Mammo Mask dedicated v.
viewing wand
ViewPoint CK system
**view shadow projection
  microtomographic system**
Viggo Spectramed catheter
VigiFOAM dressing
Vigilance monitoring system

Vigilon
- V. drain
- V. dressing
- V. gel dressing
- V. hydrogel sheet
- V. primary wound dressing
- V. semipermeable nonocclusive dressing
- V. synthetic occlusive dressing

Vigor DR pacemaker
vigorimeter
- Martin v.

Viking
- V. Bard catheter
- V. coronary guiding catheter
- V. II EMG system electromyograph
- V. II nerve monitoring device
- V. postoperative shoe

Viladot
- V. arthroereisis device
- V. prosthesis

Vilex
- V. bone estimator
- V. bone staple system
- V. cannulated screw
- V. cannulated screw system
- V. CHI system
- V. F-Series dual-thread screw
- V. Ouchless Hook
- V. plastic surgery instrument
- V. wire tucker

Villalta retractor
Villasenor-Navarro fixation ring
Villasensor ultrasonic pachymeter
vimentin filament
Vim-Silverman biopsy needle
Vingmed
- V. CFM echocardiographic system
- V. CFM transducer
- V. CFM ultrasound system
- V. Sound CFM ultrasound system
- V. System Five ultrasound
- V. ultrasound

Vinke tongs
vinyl
- v. alternating air mattress
- v. gloves
- v. palatal appliance
- v. T tube
- v. tube

violet monofilament suture
VIP
- VIP Bird neonatal ventilator
- VIP Bird volume monitor

Viper suture passer
Virag injector

ViraType
- V. probe
- V. in situ system

Virchow
- V. brain knife
- V. chisel

Viresolve ultrafiltration membrane
virgin
- v. silk
- v. silk suture

Virginia needle
Viridia telemetry system
Viridis
- V. laser system
- V. Lite photocoagulator
- V. photocoagulator
- V. pulsed laser

Viringe vascular access flush device
ViroSeq HIV-1 genotyping system
Virtis blender
virtual
- v. biopsy system
- v. colonoscopy side fire APC probe
- V. distortion-product otoacoustic emission device
- V. hip joint
- v. reality head-mouthed display
- v. reality simulator
- v. reality technology
- v. reality viewbox
- v. retinal display system
- v. retinol display
- V. Vision
- V. Vision audiovisual system for EGD and colonoscopy

Virtuoso
- V. imaging system
- V. LX Smart CPAP system
- V. portable 3D imaging system

Virtus splinter forceps
Visa
- V. II ST PTCA balloon catheter
- V. Iris system

Visage cosmetic surgery system
Visante OCT
viscera-holding forceps
visceral forceps
viscera retainer
Viscoat viscoelastic
viscocanalostomy cannula
viscodissector
- v. tubing
- vitreoretinal v.

viscoelastic
- CoEase v.
- v. heel insert
- v. product

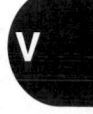

viscoelastic *(continued)*
  sodium hyaluronate v.
  Viscoat v.
Viscoflow cannula
Viscoheel
  V. K heel cushion
  V. K, N orthosis
  V. K, N prosthesis
  V. N cushion
  V. SofSpot orthosis
  V. SofSpot prosthesis
  V. SofSpot viscoelastic heel
  cushion
Viscolas orthosis
Viscolens lens
viscometer
  Brookfield v.
Viscopaste PB7 zinc paste bandage
Viscoped
  V. S insole
  V. S support
viscosimeter
  capillary tube plasma v.
viscosity
  gentamicin high v. (G-HV)
  high v. (HV)
ViscoSpot
  V. heel cushion
  V. support
viscosurgical device
viscous fluid controller
vise
  allograft bone v.
  pin v.
  Starrett pin v.
  torque v.
vise-grip pliers
Visian
  V. implantable collamer lens
  V. IOL
Visicath endoscope
Visica treatment system
Visidex II
Visi-Drape
Visidrape drape
Visiflex drape
Visi-Flow
  V.-F. irrigation starter set
  V.-F. stoma cone
Visijet HydroKeratome
Visilex polypropylene mesh
Visio Beta vacuum polymerization unit
Visioform light-curing resin
Vision
  V. acetabular component
  V. analyzer
  V. blood cardioplegia system
  V. camera
  V. Curvette curette

V. Epic wheelchair
V. Master excimer laser system
V. MR imaging system
V. PTCA catheter
V. Sciences flexible sigmoidoscope
  system
V. Sciences Inc. (VSI)
V. Siemens MRI scanner
V. System EndoSheath
V. System sigmoidoscope
V. Tech lens
V. Ten V-scan scanner
Virtual V.
VisionBlue syringe
VisionLAB
VisionSaver lab lamp
Visipitch digital tape recorder
Visiport
  V. device
  V. optical trocar
Visiprep solid-phase extraction vacuum manifold
Visi-Spear eye sponge
Visitec
  V. angled lens hook
  V. anterior chamber cannula
  V. aspiration unit
  V. capsule polisher curette
  V. Company lens
  V. corneal shield
  V. corneal suture manipulating
    hook
  V. cortex extractor
  V. crescent knife
  V. double-cutting cystotome
  V. EdgeAhead phaco slit knife
  V. I&A cannula
  V. intraocular lens dialer
  V. iris retractor
  V. irrigating/aspirating cannula
  V. lens pusher
  V. manipulator
  V. micro double-iris hook
  V. microhook
  V. microiris hook
  V. nucleus removal loupe
  V. retrobulbar needle
  V. RK zone marker
  V. stiletto knife
  V. straight lens hook
  V. surgical vitrectomy system
  V. syringe
  V. vitrectomy unit
Vismark surgical skin marker
Visometer
  Lotmar V.
visor
  Georgiade v.
  v. halo fixation device

Vista
 Blue V.
 V. Brite Tip guiding catheter
 V. Brite Tip IG introducer guide
 V. Brite Tip large-lumen guiding
  catheter
 V. disposable skin stapler
 V. radiolucent interbody fusion
  system
 V. TRS pacemaker
Vistaflex
 V. balloon-expanded stent
 V. biliary stent
Vistakon contact lens
Vistech
 V. Multivision contrast tester
 V. wall chart
Vistec x-ray detectable sponge
visual
 v. endoscopically controlled laser
 v. hemostatic forceps
 v. obturator
visual-evoked response imaging system
Visual-Tech machine
Visucam
 V. C fundus camera
 V. nonmydriatic fundus camera
Visulas
 V. argon C laser
 V. argon/YAG laser
 V. Combi 532/YAG laser
 V. 532 laser
 V. Nd:YAG laser
 V. 690s PDT laser
 V. 690s photodynamic therapy
  laser
 V. YAG C, E, S laser
 V. YAG II plus laser
VisuMed MEL60 laser
Visupac digital system
Visuscope
 V. motor
 V. ophthalmoscope
Visx
 V. 20/20 excimer laser
 V. refractive planner
 V. S2, S3 excimer laser
 V. Star 3 excimer laser system
 V. Star II stromal photoablation
  system
 V. Star Reticule aiming beam
 V. Star S3
 V. Star S3 ActiveTrak laser
 V. Star S2 excimer laser system
 V. Star S2 laser
 V. 20/20 system
 V. Twenty/Twenty system
 V. Wavefront system

 V. WaveScan
 V. WaveScan wavefront system
VitaCuff
 V. cuff
 V. device
 V. dressing
 V. infection control device
 V. tissue interface barrier
Vitadur Alpha porcelain
Vitadur-N porcelain powder
Vitagel surgical hemostat
Vitagraft vascular graft
VitaGuard
 V. event recorder
 V. monitor
**Vitalab ViVa clinical chemistry
analyzer**
VitaLase Er:YAG laser
VitalCare monitor
Vitalcor cardioplegia infusion cannula
Vital French eye needle holder
Vital-Heaney needle holder
vitallium
 v. alloy
 v. clip
 v. cup
 v. device
 v. eye implant
 v. implant
 v. implant material
 v. Luhr plate
 v. mesh component
 v. miniplate
 v. Moore self-locking prosthesis
 v. nail
 v. plate
 v. screw
 v. staple
Vital-Metzenbaum scissors
Vitalock
 V. cluster acetabular component
 V. solid-back acetabular component
Vitalograph
 V. bacterial/viral filter
 V. BreathCO monitor
 V. handheld recording spirometer
 V. pulmonary monitor
Vitalor
 V. incentive spirometer
 V. screening pulmonary function
  test
Vital-Port Infusion Pal
Vital-Ryder microvascular needle holder
**VitalStim Therapy electrical stimulation
system**
Vitatron
 V. catheter electrode
 V. Diamond ICD

V

Vitatron *(continued)*
  V. Diamond II pacemaker
  V. pacing system
Vitek
  V. GPI
  V. interpositional implant
Vitek-Kent
  V.-K. hemi TMJ replacement
  system
  V.-K. total TMJ replacement
  system
Vitesse
  V. Cos laser
  V. Cos laser catheter
  V. E2 rapid-exchange catheter
Vitoss
  V. Scaffold foam bone void filler
  V. Scaffold synthetic cancellous
  bone void filler
  V. synthetic bone
Vitox femoral head
Vitrasert
  V. implant
  V. intraocular device
  V. intraocular implant
  V. intravitreal implant
Vitrathene jacket
Vitrea 3D system
Vitrebond cement
vitrectomy
  v. prism lens tab
  v. sponge
vitrector
  Alcon v.
  automated v.
  CooperVision v.
  Frigitronics v.
  guillotine v.
  Kaufman type II v.
  mechanical v.
  Microvit v.
  ocutome v.
  v. probe
  Storz Microvit v.
vitreophage
  Kaufman v.
vitreoretinal
  v. infusion cutter
  v. micropick
  v. viscodissector
vitreous
  v. aspirating cannula
  v. aspirating needle
  v. foreign body forceps
  v. grasping forceps
  v. infusion suction cutter
  v. microextractor
  v. pencil
  v. strand scissors

  v. sweep spatula
  v. transplant needle
vitreous-aspirating
  v.-a. cannula
  v.-a. needle
Vitros
  V. analyzer
  V. HBsAg confirmatory kit
  V. Immunodiagnostic Products anti-
  HBc calibrator
  V. Immunodiagnostic Products anti-
  HBc reagent pack
  V. Immunodiagnostic Products
  HBsAg Confirmatory Kit
  V. Immunodiagnostic Products
  HBsAg Reagent Pack and
  Calibrator
Viva
  Air V.
  V. Primo balloon catheter
ViVa binocular infrared vision analyzer
Vivacare TPS probe
Vivatek ultimate healing machine
Vivonex
  V. Acutrol enteral feeding system
  V. gastrostomy tube
  V. jejunostomy catheter
  V. Moss tube
Vix infant ventilator
VixOne small-volume nebulizer
**ViziLite oral abnormality detection
  device**
**V-Lace real-time digital video
  enhancement**
V-lance
  V-l. blade
  V-l. eye knife
V-Lok disposable blood pressure cuff
V-Max roller bar electrode
VNUS
  VNUS Closure catheter
  VNUS Closure
  catheter/radiofrequency generator
  VNUS closure system
  VNUS radiofrequency generator
  VNUS Restore catheter
Vocalogen collagen
Vocare bladder system
Vogele-Bale-Hohner (VBH)
  V.-B.-H. head holder
Vogue arm sling
voice
  v. button
  v. prosthesis
  v. prosthesis sizer
  v. restoration system
VoiceMaster indwelling voice prosthesis
Void-Ease urine collection bag
voiding cystourethrogram (VCUG)

volar
- v. buttress plate
- v. plaster splint
- v. plate
- v. splint
- v. ulnar sling

Volk
- V. aspheric lens
- V. coronoid lens
- V. G-Series lens
- V. high-resolution aspherical lens
- V. 3-mirror ANF+ lens
- V. panretinal lens
- V. QuadrAspheric fundal lens
- V. retinal scale adapter
- V. SuperMacula 2.2 focal laser lens
- V. SuperPupil NC lens
- V. SuperQuad 160 contact lens
- V. SuperQuad 160 panretinal lens
- V. Transequator lens
- V. Ultra Field aspherical lens adapter
- V. yellow filter adapter

Volkmann
- V. bone curette
- V. bone hook
- V. finger retractor
- V. oval curette
- V. rake retractor
- V. scoop
- V. splint
- V. spoon

Volkov-Oganesian external fixation device
Volkov-Oganesian-Povarov hinged distraction apparatus
Voll machine
volt
- electron v.
- kiloelectron v.

voltage amplifier
voltametry
- adsorptive v.

voltmeter
- digital v.
- electronic v.
- vacuum tube v.

Voltolini nasal speculum
volume
- v. controller
- v. thickness index (VTI)
- v. ventilator
- v. zoom

volume-cycled ventilator
volume-displacement spirometer
volume-limited ventilator
volumeter
- Ableware v.

- Dräger v.
- foot v.
- hand v.
- v. set

volumetric
- v. diffusive respirator
- v. infusion pump

voluntary control 4-bar knee
Voluson
- V. sector transducer
- V. ultrasound system

Voluvision 3-dimensional ultrasonography
volvulus
- gastric v.

vomerine gouge
vomer septal forceps
Von
- V. Eichen antral cannula
- V. Eichen antral wash tube
- V. Hippel mechanical trephine

von
- v. Graefe cataract knife
- v. Graefe cautery
- v. Graefe cystotome
- v. Graefe electrocautery
- v. Graefe fixation forceps
- v. Graefe iris forceps
- v. Graefe knife needle
- v. Graefe muscle hook
- v. Graefe strabismus hook
- v. Graefe target
- v. Graefe tissue forceps
- v. Helmholtz eye model
- v. Petz clamp
- v. Petz forceps
- v. Petz intestinal clamp
- v. Petz suture clip
- v. Rosen abduction splint
- v. Rosen splint

VOO
- ventricular asynchronous
- VOO pacemaker

Voorhees
- V. bag
- V. needle

Vornado air quality system
Vorse-Webster clamp
Vortex
- V. Clear-Flow port
- V. port system
- V. router
- V. stabilization system
- V. tracheotomy tube

vortex effect catheter
VortX vascular occlusion coil
VortXX coil
Voxar Plug n View 3D imager
VoxelView system

V

Voyager aortic IntraClusion device
Vozzle Vacu-Irrigator
VP
    ventriculoperitoneal
        VP shunt
VPAP
    variable positive airway pressure
        VPAP III ST bilevel device
        VPAP II ST-A bilevel flow
        generator
        VPAP II ST ventilatory support
        system
        Sullivan VPAP II, III
VPI
        Coloscreen VPI
        VPI nonadhesive colostomy system
        VPI nonadhesive condom catheter
        VPI nonadhesive ileostomy system
        VPI nonadhesive urostomy system
        VPI stone basket
        VPI urinary leg bag
VPL
    ventroposterolateral
VS
    ventriculosubarachnoid
VSF
    Vermont spinal fixator
        VSF clamp
        VSF fixation system
        VSF rod
        VSF screw
VSI
    Vision Sciences Inc.
        VSI 2000 sigmoidoscope
V-sign single-ear sensory system
V-slit lamp
VSP
    variable screw placement
    variable spinal plating
        VSP plate
V-Stat variable soft tissue alignment
    tensor
VTC
    videothorascopic
        VTC biliary catheter
VTI
    volume thickness index

VTI oxygen monitor with
    disposable polarographic oxygen
    sensor
VT Mercury Vac organic mercury
    vacuum cleaner
V-tunnel drill system
VueLock anterior cervical spine system
VuePASS portal access surgical system
Vueport balloon-occlusion guiding
    catheter
Vuero meter
vulcanite
    v. bur
    v. chisel
vulsellum
    v. clamp
    v. forceps
    Jacobs v.
    Kelly v.
    Schroeder v.
    Skene v.
    Thoms-Allis v.
vulvar algesiometer
Vu-Max vaginal speculum
VuRyser monitor lift
V-Vac suction apparatus
VVD
    vascular volume of distribution
        VVD mode pacemaker
VVI
    ventricular inhibited
        VVI pacemaker
VVI/AAI
    ventricular inhibited, atrial inhibited
        VVI/AAI pacemaker
VVIR
    ventricle-paced, ventrical-sensed
    inhibited, rate-responsive
        VVIR single-chamber rate-adaptive
        pacemaker
VVT
    ventricular triggered
        VVT pacemaker
V33W high-density endocavity probe
Vygantas-Wilder retinal drainage probe
Vysis probe

WACH
    wedge adjustable cushioned heel
        WACH shoe
Wachenfeldt
    W. clip-applying forceps
    W. suture clip
Wackenheim clivus canal line
Wacker Sil-Gel 604 silicone cement
Wadia elevator
Wadsworth lid clamp
Wadsworth-Todd eye cautery
wafer
    acrylic bite w.
    BCNU-impregnated polymer w.
    carmustine w.
    Coloplast w.
    Curagel w.
    Gliadel w.
    Little Ones Sur-Fit flexible w.
    polyanhydride biodegradable
        polymer w.
    Stomahesive sterile w.
    wax bite w.
Waffle seating cushion
Wagner
    W. apparatus
    W. distraction device
    W. distractor
    W. epiretinal membrane dissector
    W. external fixation device
    W. fixation
    W. fixer
    W. leg-lengthening distraction
        device
    W. resurface prosthesis
    W. revision hip system
    W. rongeur
Wagner-Schanz screw device
wagon
    dumbbell w.
waist
    w. belt
    w. of catheter
    w. immobilizer
    W. It pump holder
Wakai spreader
Wako NEFA test kit
Waldeau fixation forceps
Walden-Aufrecht nasal retractor
Waldman episiotomy scissors
Waldmann UV5000 cabinet
Wales
    W. rectal bougie
    W. rectal dilator

WALK
    weight-activated locking knee
Walkabout
    W. oxygen conserver
    W. walker
WalkAide system
Walk-A-Matic walker
WalkCare slipper
walker
    air w.
    Aircast pneumatic w.
    W. articulator
    W. aspirator
    ATO w.
    w. basket
    Body Armor short leg w.
    Cam Walker ankle w.
    Castaway leg w.
    W. cautery
    Charcot restraint orthotic w.
    W. coagulator
    Comfy w.
    W. corneal scissors
    W. corneal trephine
    Darco Body Armor short leg w.
    Delta w.
    DH pressure relief w.
    EasyStep pressure relief w.
    W. electrode
    Equalizer air w.
    W. forceps
    front-wheeled w.
    Guardian Red Dot w.
    Hi-Top II adjustable w.
    W. lid everter
    low-profile w.
    Lumex w.
    W. magnet
    Merry W.
    W. micro pin
    Moon W.
    Nextep Contour lower leg w.
    obese w.
    Orlau swivel w.
    pneumatic w.
    4-point w.
    ProROM w.
    W. retractor
    Roll-A-Bout 4-wheel w.
    Rollator Nova w.
    rubber sole cast w.
    W. ruptured disc curette
    Sabel cast w.
    W. scissors
    short leg w.

W

walker *(continued)*
    w. ski
    w. sleds
    W. submucous elevator
    W. suction tonsillar dissector
    Sure-Gait folding w.
    swivel w.
    W. trephine
    Urban W.'s
    Walkabout w.
    Walk-A-Matic w.
    3-wheel w.
    Zimmer w.
Walker-Apple scissors
Walker-Atkinson scissors
Walker-Lee sclerotome
walking
    w. aid
    w. brace
    w. heel
    w. heel cast
    w. pole
    w. stirrup
WalkMed
    W. patient-controlled analgesia
    W. PCA
Walk-'n-Tone exerciser
Walk-Rite device
Wallaby II phototherapy system
Wallace Flexihub central venous pressure cannula
Wallach
    W. cryosurgery freezer
    W. cryosurgical pencil
    W. Endocell device
    W. Endocell endometrial cell sampler
    W. freezer cryosurgical device
    W. LL100 cryosurgical cryogun
    W. ophthalmic cryosurgery system
    W. pencil cryosurgical device
    W. ZoomStar colposcope
Wallach-Papette disposable cervical cell collector
Wallgraft
    W. cobalt-based alloy balloon-expandable stent
    W. covered stent
    W. endoprosthesis
    W. endoprosthesis stent-graft
    W. tracheobronchial endoprosthesis
Wallner interstitial prostate implanter
Wallstent
    W. biliary endoprosthesis
    W. delivery device
    W. endoprosthesis
    W. endoprosthesis with Unistep Plus delivery system
    W. esophageal prosthesis

    W. expanding metallic stent
    W. flexible self-expanding wire-mesh stent
    W. Iliac RP self-expanding stent
    Magic W.
    Magic S/P W.
    W. Magic stent
    W. RP self-expanding stent
    Schneider W.
    Schneider esophageal W.
    self-expanding Easy W.
    W. spring-loaded stent
    W. stent
    Unistep Plus Permalume covered biliary W.
    UroLume W.
Wallstent-covered SEM stent
Wallstent-I
Wal-Pil-O neck pillow
Walser
    W. corneoscleral punch
    W. matrix
Walsh
    W. dermal curette
    W. pressure ring
Walsham
    W. forceps
    W. nasal forceps
    W. septal forceps
    W. septal straightener
    W. septum-straightening forceps
Walter
    W. corneal spud
    W. nasal retractor
    W. Reed implant
    W. splinter forceps
Walter-Liston forceps
Walther
    W. female catheter
    W. sound
    W. urethral dilator
    W. urethral sound
Walton
    W. cartilage clamp
    W. comedo extractor
    W. corneoscleral punch
    W. expressor
    W. extractor
    W. foreign body gouge
    W. punch
    W. scissors
    W. spud
    W. wire-pulling forceps
Walton-Ruskin forceps
Waltz endoscopic lithotriptor
Wampole Isolater blood culture system
Wanchik
    W. neutral position splint
    W. writer

wand
    angled Connor w.
    ArthroCare w.
    ArthroCare thermal w.
    ArthroWand disposable surgical w.
    CLO Cool W.
    CollagENT w.
    Connor w.
    Connor angled w.
    Connor curved w.
    Connor straight irrigating w.
    Connor straight nonirrigating w.
    curved Connor w.
    disposable ReFlex w.
    Elekta viewing w.
    Essential Energy whole house w.
    EVac 70 suction w.
    EVac T&A suction w.
    flexible w.
    Hummingbird w.
    InstruSponge flexible plastic w.
    ISG viewing w.
    light w.
    Powell w.
    programmer w.
    programming w.
    ReFlex Ultra 45, 55 channeling w.
    straight nonirrigating Connor w.
    TCFO placement w.
    TriggerWheel w.
    viewing w.
wandering atrial pacemaker
Wang
    W. applicator
    W. lens
    W. needle
    W. transbronchial needle
Wang-Binford edge detector
Wangensteen
    W. anastomosis clamp
    W. apparatus
    W. dissector
    W. drain
    W. duodenal tube
    W. intestinal needle
    W. needle holder
    W. patent ductus clamp
    W. suction
    W. suction unit
    W. tissue forceps
    W. tissue inverter
Wanger leg-lengthening device
Wappler
    W. cystoscope
    W. cystoscope with microlens
      optics
    W. microlens cystourethroscope
    W. polypectomy snare
    W. resectoscope

Warburg apparatus
Ward
    W. nasal osteotome
    W. periosteal elevator
Warm
    W. 'n' Form lumbosacral corset
    W. Springs brace
    W. Springs crutch
warm-and-form insert
Warmatowel
warmer
    Alton Dean blood/fluid w.
    Bair Hugger forced-air w.
    Echowarm gel w.
    fluid w.
    gel w.
    Hamilton fluid w.
    high-capacity fluid w.
    Hotline blood and fluid w.
    hypothermia oxygen w.
    Kreiselman infant w.
    Ohio w.
    radiant w.
    radiant heat w.
    Resuscitaire birthing room w.
    Soft Sack IV fluid w.
    Thermasonic gel w.
WarmTouch patient warming system
Warm-Up
    W.-U. active wound therapy
      system
    W.-U. wound care system
Warren shunt
Warsaw hip prosthesis
Wartenberg pinwheel
**Wartner over-the-counter wart removal
treatment**
Warwick James elevator
Wasca aberrometer
wash
    ENT w.
    w. mitt
    Zila Pro-Wash antiseptic hand w.
washer
    anchor w.
    barbed plastic w.
    biconcave w.
    connector with lock w.
    contoured w.
    female w.
    Gravlee jet w.
    w. holder
    male w.
    narrow w.
    Olympus Europe ETD automated
      endoscope w.
    plate-spacer w.
    rotation-stop w.
    Salzburg biconcave w.

W

washer *(continued)*
    spiked w.
    Synthes ligament w.
    titanium spiked w.
    wide w.
WasherLoc device
washing catheter
washout cannula
Wasserstein
    W. fixation
    W. fixation device
Watanabe
    W. apparatus
    W. arthroscope
    W. catheter
    W. pin
watch
    Pulse Pro heart rate monitor w.
    Teslar w.
    Yperwatch gamma control w.
watchmaker forceps
Watco knee immobilizer
water
    w. bed
    w. bottle
    w. cushion lithotriptor
    w. displacing balloon
    w. dressing
    w. gauge
    w. magnet
    w. pacifier
    w. probe
    w. scalpel
    w. vaporizer
water-based tinting system
water-cooled
    w.-c. power bur
    w.-c. tip
Waterfield needle
water-filled balloon sheath
**water-impermeable nonsilicone-based
  occlusive dressing**
**water-infusion esophageal manometry
  catheter**
Water-Jel burn dressing
Waterlase Millennium laser system
Waterman sump drain
water-perfused manometry catheter
Waterpik
    W. irrigator
    W. lavage
    W. toothbrush
Waterpillow
Waters
    W. M-440 fixed wavelength
      detector
    W. positioner
waterseal
    w. chest tube

    w. drain
    w. drainage
water-sealed spirometer
Waterston-Cooley shunt
Waterston shunt
watertight seal
watertrap drain
Watson
    W. angular rate sensor
    W. capsule
    W. duckbill forceps
    W. heart valve holder
    W. knife
    W. skin graft knife
Watson-Jones
    W.-J. bone gouge
    W.-J. dressing
    W.-J. frame
    W.-J. nail
    W.-J. traction
Watson-Williams
    W.-W. conchotome
    W.-W. ethmoidal punch
    W.-W. intervertebral disc rongeur
    W.-W. nasal forceps
    W.-W. needle
    W.-W. polyp forceps
    W.-W. sinus rasp
Watt stave bender
Watzke
    W. band
    W. forceps
    W. silicone sleeve
    W. sleeve
    W. tire
Waugh
    W. dissection forceps
    W. dressing forceps
    W. tissue forceps
wave
    w. guide catheter
    w. keyboard
    W. nucleic acid fragment analysis
      system
    W. ventilator
wave-edge knife
waveform
    CO_2 w.
    w. generator
    rectilinear biphasic w.
wavefront-corrected IOL
wavelength
    2-w. near-infrared spectroscope
**WaveMap intracoronary blood pressure
  measurement system**
**Wavemax balloon-expandable
  transhepatic biliary stent**

WaveScan
  Visx W.
  W. Wavefront system
wave-tooth forceps
WaveWire
  W. angioplasty guidewire
  W. intracoronary blood pressure
    measurement system
Wavicide disinfectant
WavSTAT optical biopsy system
wax
  Aluwax impression w.
  w. bite wafer
  Bite Wafer denture bite w.
  bone w.
  w. bougie
  w. curette
  dental w.
  Flex-E-Z w.
  Horsley bone w.
  Kwik w.
  w. swager
wax-removing spatula
1-way valved silicone voice prosthesis
2-way
  2-w. cataract aspirating cannula
  2-w. catheter
  2-w. syringe
  2-w. towel clip
3-way
  3-w. bridge
  3-w. Foley catheter
  3-w. Hans Rudolph valve
  3-w. irrigating catheter
  3-w. stopcock
Wayfarer modifiable foot prosthesis
weapon
  bone w.
wear
  Design Veronique compression w.
  protective sports eye w.
  Rainey Ultra-Flex compression w.
  SoftFlex wrist w.
wearable
  w. cardioverter-defibrillator
  w. cardioverter-defibrillator device
  w. speech processor
Weathertech EMS 3-in-1 systems jacket
Weavenit
  W. patch graft
  W. prosthesis
Weaver
  W. chalazion forceps
  W. trocar introducer
Webb
  W. bolt nail
  W. cannula
  W. pin
  W. retractor

Weber
  W. antiglide plate
  W. aortic clamp
  W. colonic insufflator
  W. hip implant
  W. human genome screening set
  W. knife
  W. lens scoop
  W. Permalock
  W. rectal catheter
  W. winged catheter
Weber-Elschnig lens loupe
Webril
  W. bandage
  W. cotton padding
  W. dressing
Webster
  W. coronary sinus catheter
  W. halo catheter
  W. infusion tube
  W. meniscectomy scissors
  W. needle holder
  W. orthogonal electrode catheter
Weck
  W. blade
  W. clamp
  W. clip
  W. clip applier
  W. dermatome
  W. disposable cannula
  W. disposable trocar
  W. electrosurgery pencil
  W. eye shield
  W. Hemoclip clip
  W. High-Flow laparoflator
  W. hysterectomy forceps
  W. iris scissors
  W. knife
  W. microscope
  W. microsurgical tray
  W. microsuture cutting scissors
  W. shears
  W. sponge
  W. trephine
  W. uterine biopsy forceps
Weck-cel
  W.-c. dressing
  W.-c. implant
  W.-c. microsponge
  W.-c. sponge
Wecker iris scissors
Weck-Prep blade
Wedeen wire passer
wedge
  abduction w.
  w. adjustable cushioned heel
    (WACH)
  w. adjustable cushioned heel shoe
  ball w.

W

wedge *(continued)*
    bone w.
    bumper w.
    45-degree spinal w.
    disconnect w.
    Duo-Cline Dual Support contoured
        bed w.
    W. electrosurgical resection device
    w. filter
    Good 'N Bed w.
    Hapad heel w.
    inner heel w.
    knee w.
    Livingston peribulbar w.
    W. loop
    medial heel w.
    medial heel-and-sole w.
    medial sole w.
    Medline w.
    Medpor biomaterial w.
    membrane delamination w.
    Positex knee w.
    w. and post forceps
    w. posting
    w. pressure balloon catheter
    w. resection clamp
    roof w.
    Saunders mobilization w.
    self-adhering varus/valgus w.
    spinal w.
    w. spirometer
    super w.
    W. TAG suture anchor system
    Tempur-Med seat w.
    toe w.
    tomography w.
    TruWedge BGS osteotomy w.
    TruWedge osteotomy w.
    Yancy cast w.
wedge-line needle
wedge-shaped
    w.-s. platform
    w.-s. support
WeeFIM instrument
Weeks needle
Weerda
    W. distending operating
        laryngoscope
    W. endoscope
    W. laparoscope
Wehner spoon
Wehrs incus prosthesis
Weider tongue depressor
weight
    ankle w.
    Blinkeze eyelid external lid w.
    w. boot
    EyeClose external eyelid w.
    Femina vaginal w.

    FemTone vaginal w.
    gold w.
    SutureGroove gold eye w.
    SutureGroove gold eyelid w.
    Thera-Band progressive w.
weight-activated locking knee (WALK)
weightbearing brace
weighted
    w. glove
    w. pen
    w. posterior retractor
    w. tip
    w. vaginal speculum
    w. vest
    w. walking stick
weight-relieving orthosis
Weil
    W. ear forceps
    W. implant
    W. lacrimal cannula
    W. modified Swanson implant
    W. pelvic sling
    W. pituitary rongeur
Weil-Blakesley
    W.-B. conchotome
    W.-B. ethmoidal forceps
    W.-B. intervertebral disc rongeur
**Weil-type Swanson-design hammertoe
    implant**
Weimert epistaxis packing
Weinberg
    W. blade
    W. vagotomy retractor
Weiner spatially varying filter
Weingartner alligator ear forceps
Weinraub joint and calcaneal spreader
Weinstein
    W. fixation ring
    W. fixation ring and flap lifter
Weiss
    W. amputation saw
    W. forceps
    W. needle
    W. speculum
    W. spring
Weitlaner
    W. brain retractor
    W. hinged retractor
    W. microsurgery retractor
    W. retractor
    W. self-retaining retractor
Welch
    W. Allyn anal biopsy forceps
    W. Allyn anoscope
    W. Allyn AudioPath Platform
        hearing acuity instrument
    W. Allyn AudioScope
    W. Allyn disposable sigmoidoscope
    W. Allyn dual-purpose otoscope

W. Allyn ear wash system
W. Allyn fiberoptic sigmoidoscope
W. Allyn flexible sigmoidoscope
W. Allyn halogen penlight
W. Allyn hook
W. Allyn illuminated speculum
W. Allyn KleenSpec fiberoptic disposable sigmoidoscope
W. Allyn KleenSpec vaginal speculum
W. Allyn laryngoscope
W. Allyn laryngoscope blade
W. Allyn LumiView portable binocular microscope
W. Allyn MicroTymp impedance tympanometer
W. Allyn operating otoscope
W. Allyn ophthalmoscope
W. Allyn Pneumocheck spirometer
W. Allyn pocket scope
W. Allyn proctoscope
W. Allyn rectal probe
W. Allyn/Schiller AT-1 3-channel ECG
W. Allyn/Schiller AT-10 Exercise Testing system
W. Allyn/Schiller AT-2 full-size ECG
W. Allyn/Schiller AT-10 hospital grade ECG
W. Allyn/Schiller AT-10 hospital-grade ECG
W. Allyn/Schiller AT-2*plus* full-size ECG
W. Allyn/Schiller MS-3 pocket size ECG
W. Allyn single-fiber illumination headlight
W. Allyn Solarc headlight
W. Allyn standard retinoscope
W. Allyn streak retinoscope
W. Allyn suction tube
W. Allyn SureSight autorefractor
W. Allyn SureSight eye chart
W. Allyn transilluminator
W. Allyn video colonoscope
W. Allyn videoendoscope

welding
chromophore-enhanced laser w.

well
alcohol w.
LASEK alcohol w.
w. leg holder
w. leg support
96-w. scanning fluorometer

well-centered IOL

Weller
W. cartilage forceps
W. cartilage scissors

W. meniscal forceps
W. total hip joint prosthesis

well-padded splint

Wells
W. enucleation scoop
W. enucleation spoon
W. forceps
W. Johnson cannula
W. Johnson pump
W. Johnson transfer device
W. pedicle clamp
W. stereotactic apparatus

well-type ionization chamber

Welsh
W. cortex extractor
W. cortex stripper cannula
W. flat olive-tip double cannula
W. iris retractor
W. pupil-spreader forceps

Wendl tube

Werb
W. right-angle probe
W. scissors

Wertheim
W. deep surgery scissors
W. hysterectomy forceps
W. kidney pedicle clamp
W. needle holder
W. uterine forceps
W. vaginal forceps

Wertheim-Cullen
W.-C. compression forceps
W.-C. hysterectomy forceps
W.-C. kidney pedicle clamp
W.-C. kidney pedicle forceps

Wescor Sweat-Chek conductivity analyzer

Wesley-Jessen lens

Wessex prosthetic valve

Wesson mouthgag

West
W. blunt dissector
W. bone chisel
W. bone gouge
W. cannula
W. gouge
W. hand dissector
W. lacrimal cannula
W. lacrimal chisel
W. nasal chisel
W. nasal dressing forceps
W. nasal gouge
W. nerve tester
W. Nile virus IgM capture test
W. osteotome
W. Point axillary lateral radiograph

Westaby tracheobronchial silicone stent

Westcott
W. biopsy needle

W

Westcott *(continued)*
- W. conjunctival scissors
- W. double-end scissors
- W. micro scissors
- W. needle
- W. stitch scissors
- W. tenotomy scissors
- W. utility scissors

Western Electric artificial larynx
Weston rectal snare
wet
- w. bandage
- w. cup
- w. dressing
- w. sheet
- W. SpaTable

wet-field
- w.-f. cautery
- w.-f. coagulator
- w.-f. electrocautery

wet-to-dry dressing
Wexler
- W. abdominal retractor
- W. deep spreader blade abdominal retractor
- W. large-frame abdominal retractor
- W. lateral side-blade abdominal retractor
- W. malleable-blade abdominal retractor
- W. retractor
- W. self-retaining retractor
- W. vaginal retractor

Wexler-Bantam retractor
W&H
- W&H Endodontic Contra Angle
- W&H handpiece
- W&H surgical system

whalebone filiform catheter
Whaledent Parapost
Wharton jelly
Whatman
- W. filter paper
- W. 3MM
- W. No. 1 qualitative-type filter paper
- W. paper

Wheaton
- W. bunion splint
- W. Pavlik harness
- W. Pavlik harness brace
- W. tissue homogenizer

wheel
- w. bur
- Carborundum grinding w.
- OsteoGraft bone grafting w.
- pin w.
- shoulder w.
- 3-w. walker

wheelchair
- Action Jr. w.
- Amigo mechanical w.
- antitipper w.
- Applause Super-Hemi w.
- W. Buddy
- w. chain
- w. cushion
- electric w.
- Epic w.
- folding-frame w.
- Gendron bariatric w.
- Hoveround programmable w.
- Invacare manual w.
- Jay J2 w.
- Kid-Kart w.
- Kuschkin Ace w.
- Landeez all-terrain w.
- Lumex lightweight w.
- Lumex Tilt-in-Space reclining w.
- manual w.
- Navigator power w.
- Nitro w.
- w. pad
- power w.
- Quickie Carbon w.
- Quickie EX w.
- Quickie GPS w.
- Quickie GP Swing-Away w.
- Quickie GPV w.
- Quickie Kidz w.
- Quickie Recliner w.
- Quickie Ti w.
- reclining-frame w.
- rigid-frame w.
- w. seating component
- self-propelling w.
- Shark pediatric w.
- Skil-Care reclining w.
- Slam'r w.
- sling seat w.
- tilting-frame w.
- Tilt System w.
- Vision Epic w.
- Zippie 2 w.

wheeled stretcher
Wheeler
- W. cyclodialysis spatula
- W. cyclodialysis system
- W. cystotome
- W. discission knife
- W. eye sphere implant
- W. iris spatula

whip bougie
Whip-Mix articulator
whirlybird
whisker
- slotted w.

Whisper Mist humidifier

whistle
Bárány noise apparatus w.
Galton ear w.
peak flow w.
w. stent
whistle-tip
w.-t. catheter
w.-t. Foley catheter
w.-t. ureteral catheter
Whitacre spinal needle
Whitaker hook
White
W. bone chisel
W. clamp
W. glaucoma pump shunt
W. LuMax guiding catheter
W. mallet
W. scissors
W. screwdriver
W. system
W. tenaculum
W. tonsillar forceps
W. vessel sizing catheter
white
w. braided silk suture
w. laser
w. nylon suture
w. twisted suture
Whitehall
W. Glacier Pack
W. thermalator
Whitehead mouthgag
white-light
w.-l. bronchoscope
w.-l. tandem-scanning confocal
microscope
Whitesides total knee prosthesis
WhiteStar power modulation system
Whiting mastoid rongeur
Whitman
W. arch support
W. fracture appliance
W. fracture frame
W. frame
W. plate
Whitney
W. single-use plastic curette
W. superior rectus forceps
Whitten fixation ring
WHO
World Health Organization
WHO probe
whole-body
w.-b. counter
w.-b. digital scanner
w.-b. MR imaging system
w.-b. MRI system scanner
w.-b. Siemens Vision scanner

w.-b. Tesla scanner
w.-b. unit
whole-cell patch clamp
whole-head neuromagnetometer
Wholey
W. balloon occlusion catheter
W. Hi-Torque Floppy guidewire
W. Hi-Torque modified J
guidewire
W. Hi-Torque standard guidewire
W. wire
Wiberg
W. fracture staple
W. fracture stapler
W. periosteal elevator
Wichman retractor
wick
Bone-Dri femoral surgical w.
w. catheter
w. dressing
gauze w.
glaucoma w.
Pope w.
silastic w.
Staar glaucoma w.
Wickham retractor
wicking
w. catheter
w. glue patch
Widal-Abrami-Lermoyez triad
wide
w. periosteal elevator
w. washer
wide-base quad cane
wide-blade laminar hook
wide-diameter abutment
wide-field eyepiece
wide-seal diaphragm
Widex listening device
Wieder
W. dental retractor
W. pillar retractor
W. retractor
Wiener
W. antral rasp
W. corneal hook
W. eye needle
W. eye speculum
W. filter
W. hysterectomy forceps
W. keratome
W. MRI filter
W. nasal rasp
W. scleral hook
Wies chalazion forceps
Wiet
W. cup forceps
W. graft-measuring instrument

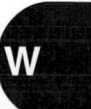

Wiet (*continued*)
W. otologic scissors
W. retractor
Wigmore plaster saw
Wikco ankle machine
Wikström
W. arterial forceps
W. gallbladder clamp
Wikström-Stilgust clamp
Wiktor
W. balloon-expandable coronary stent
W. GX coronary stent
W. GX Hepamed coated coronary stent system
W. GX Hepamed coronary stent system
W. Prime coronary stent system
Wiktor-I implantable stent
Wilco ankle exerciser
Wild
W. laser
W. lens
W. microscope
W. operating microscope
Wildcat orthodontic wire
Wilde
W. ear forceps
W. ear polyp snare
W. ethmoidal exenteration forceps
W. ethmoid forceps
W. forceps
W. intervertebral disc forceps
W. intervertebral disc rongeur
W. nasal dressing forceps
W. nasal punch
W. nasal snare
W. rongeur forceps
W. septal forceps
Wilde-Blakesley ethmoidal forceps
Wilder
W. band spreader
W. cystotome
W. cystotome knife
W. dilating forceps
W. foreign body hook
W. lacrimal dilator
W. lens loupe
W. lens scoop
W. scleral depressor
W. scleral self-retaining retractor
W. scoop
Wiles prosthesis
Wilke
W. boot
W. boot brace
Wilkerson intraocular lens insertion forceps
Wilkes self-retaining retractor

Wilkinson
W. ring-frame abdominal retractor
W. self-retaining abdominal retractor
Wilkinson-Deaver blade abdominal retractor
Willauer
W. intrathoracic forceps
W. thoracic scissors
Willauer-Allis
W.-A. thoracic forceps
W.-A. tissue forceps
Willett
W. clamp
W. placenta previa forceps
W. scalp flap forceps
William
W. Harvey arterial blood filter
W. Harvey cardiotomy reservoir
Williams
W. Advantage table
W. back brace
W. clamp
W. cystoscopic needle
W. discectomy forceps
W. esophageal tube
W. eye speculum
W. interlocking Y nail
W. intestinal forceps
W. lacrimal dilator
W. lacrimal probe
W. microclip
W. microlumbar retractor
W. nail
W. needle
W. orthosis
W. perforator
W. probe
W. rod
W. screwdriver
W. splinter forceps
W. table
W. tissue forceps
W. varix injection overtube
Williamson-Noble scissors
Williger
W. bone curette
W. bone mallet
W. hammer
W. periosteal elevator
W. rasp
Wills
W. eye lacrimal retractor
W. Hospital eye cautery
W. Hospital ophthalmic forceps
W. utility forceps
Willscher catheter
Wilmer
W. conjunctival scissors

W. conjunctival and utility scissors
W. cryosurgical iris retractor
W. iris forceps
W. iris scissors

Wilmington
W. arthroscopic portal
W. orthosis
W. plastic jacket
W. scoliosis brace

Wilson
W. bimetric arch
W. bolt
W. clamp
W. convex frame
W. fracture appliance
W. intraocular scissors
W. lead
W. Mayo stand
W. spinal frame
W. spinal fusion plate
W. vitreous foreign body forceps

Wilson-Cook
W.-C. bronchoscope biopsy forceps
W.-C. Carey capsule set
W.-C. coagulation electrode
W.-C. colonoscope biopsy forceps
W.-C. cytology brush
W.-C. dilating balloon
W.-C. double-channel sphincterotome
W.-C. electrode needle
W.-C. endoprosthesis
W.-C. esophageal balloon prosthesis
W.-C. esophageal Z-stent
W.-C. feeding tube kit
W.-C. fine-needle aspiration catheter
W.-C. French stent
W.-C. gastric balloon
W.-C. gastroscope biopsy forceps
W.-C. grasping forceps
W.-C. hot biopsy forceps
W.-C. low-profile esophageal prosthesis set
W.-C. metal reinforcement
W.-C. modified wire-guided sphincterotome
W.-C. nasobiliary tube
W.-C. NJFT-series feeding tube
W.-C. papillotome
W.-C. plastic prosthesis
W.-C. polypectomy snare
W.-C. prosthesis repositioner
W.-C. Protector guidewire
W.-C. Quantum TTC esophageal balloon dilatation catheter
W.-C. retrieval forceps
W.-C. six-shooter
W.-C. standard wire guide

W.-C. stone basket
W.-C. THSF-series guidewire
W.-C. Tracer guidewire
W.-C. tripod retrieval forceps
W.-C. 8-wire basket stone extractor
W.-C. wire-guided sphincterotome

Wiltek papillotome
Wiltmoser optical arm
Wilton
W. Webster coronary sinus thermodilution catheter
W. Webster thermodilution flow and pacing catheter

Wiltse
W. fixator
W. pedicle screw
W. pedicle screw fixation system
W. screw-rod
W. system cross-bracing
W. system double-rod construct
W. system H construct
W. system single-rod construct
W. system spinal rod

Winco
W. adjusting bench
W. folding treatment table

Wincor enucleation scissors
window
bone w.
w. clip
Hanning w.
w. rasp
w. rasp marker

windowed esophageal balloon
wing
w. clip
2-w. Malecot drain
w. suture

4-wing
4-w. Malecot drain
4-w. Malecot retention catheter

winged
w. catheter
w. steel needle

Wingspan self-expanding stent system
Winquist tibial/femoral extraction system
Winston cervical clamp
Winter
W. arch bar
W. elevator
W. facial fracture appliance
W. Helping Hand
W. ovum forceps
W. placental forceps
W. shunt

Winternitz sound
wipe
AllKare protective barrier w.

W

wipe *(continued)*
Kimwipes w.
Microclens w.
Sani-Cloth HB disposable w.
Sani-Cloth Plus germicidal
  disposable w.

wire *(See also* guidewire)
ACS microglide w.
all track w. (ATW)
Amplatz exchange length w.
Amplatz tapered movable core w.
Amplatz torque w.
w. appliance
atrial pacing w.
ATW core w.
Australian Special Plus w.
Babcock stainless steel w.
bayonet-point w.
bead-loaded w.
Bentson exchange length w.
biventricular pacing w.
bone fixation w.
braided w.
brass w.
Brooker w.
central core w.
cerclage w.
cesium-137 w.
chisel-tip w.
Choice PT exchange w.
Choice PT plus w.
circumdental w.
w. closure forceps
coffin-type transpalatal w.
Compere fixation w.
control w.
Cope w.
coronary w.
crenulated tantalum w.
w. crimper
w. crimping forceps
crossed Kirschner w.
curved J exchange w.
w. cutter
Dall-Miles cerclage w.
delivery w.
Dentaflex w.
diamond tip w.
diathermy w.
Doppler velocity w.
double keyhole loop w.
double-looped cerclage w.
w. drill
w. driver
ear snare w.
Eder-Puestow w.
w. electrode
endocardial w.
Eve-Neivert tonsillar w.

extraflexible w.
extra-stiff Amplatz w.
Fast Dasher 14 w.
w. fixation bolt
flexible spiral w.
flow w.
Force w.
w. frame collar
w. frame spectacles
Gilmer w.
w. grip finger splint
w. grip toe splint
w. guide
Hancock temporary cardiac
  pacing w.
heavy-duty standard exchange w.
high-torque w.
Hi-Per Flex exchange w.
Hi-Torque balance middleweight
  universal guide w.
House w.
hydrophilic w.
intermaxillary w.
interosseous w.
intracoronary Doppler flow w.
^{192}Ir w.
Isola w.
Ivy w.
Jagwire w.
J exchange w.
Johnson canaliculus w.
J retention w.
J-tipped w.
K w.
Katzen infusion w.
Kirschner w. (K-wire)
Kirschner boring w.
lead w.
Lengemann w.
w. lid speculum
ligature tie w.
lingual w.
Linx extension w.
w. loop
w. loop connector
w. loop strut
Lunderquist coat hanger w.
Lunderquist exchange w.
Luque cerclage w.
Luque sublaminar w.
magnet w.
w. mandrin
Markley orthodontic w.
Meditech w.
w. mesh eye implant
w. mesh implant
w. mesh self-expandable stent
monofilament snare w.
Mullan w.

nasal snare w.
needle-knife w.
nitinol w.
nitinol shape-memory alloy w.
olive w.
olive-tipped Magnum w.
w. osteosynthesis
outrigger w.
over-tying w.
pacing w.
w. passer
Pathfinder w.
piston w.
platinum w.
pressure guide pressure w.
w. probe
w. prosthesis crimping forceps
prosthesis smooth w.
protector plus w.
pusher w.
Quadcat w.
Radifocus w.
Radi pressure w.
rectal cautery w.
rectangular w.
Respond w.
Roadrunner w.
Rosen w.
Rotablator w.
w. saw
w. scissors
Sentalloy w.
w. side blade
Simcoe anterior chamber
  retaining w.
small-diameter w.
smooth transfixion w.
snare w.
w. snare
space-age w.
spinous process w.
6-w. spiral-tip Segura basket
w. splint
square w.
Stabilizer marker w.
stainless steel w.
standard exchange w.
w. stapes prosthesis
stay w.
stiffening w.
Storz twisted snare w.
w. stylet
w. stylet catheter
sublaminar w.
suture w.
tantalum w.
Teflon-coated w.
Thiersch w.
w. threader

w. tightener
tip-deflecting w.
titanium w.
tonsillar snare w.
torque w.
torque attenuating diameter w.
Tracer ST w.
trip w.
trocar-point Kirschner w.
trochanteric w.
Trooper floppy moderate support
  guide w.
Truarch w.
w. tucker
w. twister
ultrastiff w.
unicortical interosseus w.
veneer retention w.
Wholey w.
Wildcat orthodontic w.
Wisconsin button w.
Wisconsin interspinous w.
Wisconsin spinous w.
wire-cutting
  w.-c. forceps
  w.-c. scissors
  w.-c. suture scissors
wire-extracting forceps
wire-fat ear prosthesis
wire-fixation buckle
wire-foam
Wirefoam orthotic
Wire-Gelfoam prosthesis
wire-guided
  w.-g. hydrostatic balloon
  w.-g. J tube
  w.-g. metal spiral retrieval device
  w.-g. papillotome
  w.-g. polyvinyl bougie
  w.-g. sphincterotome
wire-holding forceps
wireless
  w. capsule endoscope
  w. handheld Web pad
wire-loop keratoscope
wire-passing
  w.-p. awl
  w.-p. bur
wire-pulling forceps
wire-tightening
  w.-t. clamp
  w.-t. forceps
wire-twisting forceps
wire-vein prosthesis
wire-wound endotracheal tube
Wire-Wrap
wiring
  w. retractor
  Stout continuous w.

W

Wirsung dilation
Wisap
    W. disposable cannula
    W. disposable trocar
Wisconsin
    W. blade
    W. button
    W. button wire
    W. interspinous wire
    W. laryngoscope
    W. laryngoscope blade
    W. spinal fracture system
    W. spinous wire
Wise
    W. iridotomy laser lens
    W. iridotomy-sphincterotomy laser lens
    W. sphincterotomy laser lens
Wiseguide guide catheter
Wishbone
    W. Omni-Track retractor
    W. retractor
    W. table-mounted retractor
Wishbook adjustable frame
Wissinger
    W. rod
    W. set
Wister wire/pin cutter
Witherspoon vertical scissors
Wittmann patch artificial bur
Wittner
    W. biopsy punch
    W. cervical biopsy punch
    W. uterine biopsy forceps
Witzel pneumatic dilator
Wixson hip positioner
Wizard
    W. disposable inflation device
    W. gamma counter
    W. MagneSil PCR cleanup
    W. MagneSil sequencing cleanup
    W. microdebrider
    W. plasmid purification
Wizdom ST steerable guidewire
wobble
    w. board
    Wooden W.
woggle device
Wolf
    W. arthroscope
    W. aspiration/injection system
    W. biopsy forceps
    W. curved basket forceps
    W. delivery system
    W. disposable cannula
    W. disposable trocar
    W. drainage cannula
    W. endoscope
    W. graft

    W. implant
    W. insufflation laparoscope
    W. laparoscope
    W. lithotrite
    W. needle trocar
    W. nephrostomy catheter
    W. percutaneous universal nephroscope
    W. Piezolith lithotripsy device
    W. Piezolith lithotriptor
    W. prosthesis
    W. rigid panendoscope
    W. rigid ureteroscope
    W. Sonolith lithotriptor
    W. suction tube
    W. ureteroscope
Wolf-Castroviejo needle holder
Wolfe
    W. eye forceps
    W. forceps
    W. miniscope
Wölfe-Böhler
    W.-B. cast breaker
    W.-B. cast remover
    W.-B. plaster cast spreader
Wölfe-Krause
    W.-K. graft
    W.-K. implant
Wolff
    W. dermal curette
    W. syringe
Wolf-Henning gastroscope
Wolf-Knittlingen gastroscope
Wolfram needle electrode
Wolf-Schindler gastroscope
Wolfson
    W. forceps
    W. frame
    W. intestinal clamp
Wolf-Veress needle
Wollaston doublet
Wolvek
    W. fixation device
    W. sternal approximator
Wonder-Cup heel cup
Wonderflex silicone
Wonder-Spur heel cup
Wong-Stall scissors
wood
    W. glasses
    W. lamp
    W. lens
    W. light
    W. screw
    w. tongue depressor
Woodbridge tube
wooden
    w. postoperative clog
    w. swab

W. Wobble
W. Wobble balance ball
Woodpecker
The W.
Woodruff
W. screw
W. screwdriver
Woods Concept lens
Woodson
W. dental periosteal elevator
W. dural separator
W. elevator
W. plug
W. probe
W. spatula
Woodward
W. antral rasp
W. forceps
W. retractor
Woodway treadmill
wool
w. pledget
Sofban orthopaedic padding w.
Velband orthopaedic padding w.
Woolley tibia punch
Worcester instrument holder
Word Bartholin gland catheter
WorkAbout Carpal Mate wrist support
WorkHorse percutaneous transluminal
  angioplasty balloon catheter
WorkMod back support
Work Seat driving simulator
World Health Organization (WHO)
Worst
W. Claw lens
W. double-ended pigtail probe
W. implantation forceps
W. Medallion lens
W. needle
W. pigtail probe
W. suture
Worth
W. advancement forceps
W. amblyoscope
W. cystotome
W. strabismus forceps
wound
w. cleanser
w. clip
w. clip forceps
w. drain
w. drainage collector
w. drainage reservoir
w. dressing
w. forceps
w. measuring guide
w. packing
W. Stick measuring system
w. swab

w. towel
W. VAC
Wound-Evac drain
Woun'Dres
W. collagen
W. hydrogel dressing
W. natural collagen hydrogel
  wound dressing
Wound-Span
woven
w. cotton gauze
w. Dacron catheter
w. Dacron fabric graft
w. Dacron tube
w. Dacron tube graft
w. elastic bandage
w. Teflon
w. Teflon prosthesis
WovenFlexie diagnostic catheter
woven-tube vascular graft prosthesis
wrap
Ace w.
Action elbow w.
Action wrist w.
ankleRAP postsurgical wound w.
backRAP postsurgical wound w.
bias w.
BodyIce w.
BodyIce cold pack w.
Champ CTS cold therapy w.
CircPlus w.
Circulon w.
Coban w.
Coflex adherent w.
Coflex flexible w.
Comprilan w.
cryotherapy w.
digit w.
Dura-Kold reusable compression
  ice w.
Dura-Soft soft compression reusable
  ice or heat w.
Dyna-Flex w.
Elasto-Gel hot/cold w.
Electro-Link joint w.
Fabco w.
Flex-Wrap self-adherent w.
FoamWrap Final Flexion w.
gel w.
Gelocast Unna boot
  compression w.
Goode w.
Heat Plus Massage lower body w.
hipRAP postsurgical wound w.
Ice Wedge hot/cold therapy w.
Kerlix w.
Kling w.
kneeRAP w.
Kold w.

W

wrap *(continued)*
    loop-over w.
    magnetic w.
    3M Coban LF self-adherent w.
    mummy w.
    Nylatex w.
    Ocu-Guard ophthalmic w.
    orthoRaps postsurgical wound w.
    PneuGel ankle w.
    PneuGel shoulder w.
    primer compression w.
    Scott wrist w.
    shoulderRAP postsurgical wound w.
    Snugs w.
    Sorbothane w.
    Stimprene w.
    super w.
    Thera-Boot compression w.
    thermal plastic w.
    Thermoskin arthritic knee w.
    Thermoskin back w.
    Thermoskin shoulder w.
    Thermoskin U wrist w.
    Unna boot w.
    Unna-Flex compression w.
    Velpeau w.
    wristRAP postsurgical wound w.
    Zipzoc compression w.
wraparound dressing
wrap-a-round eye shield
wrapping
    nerve w.
Wratten filter
wrench
    Allen w.
    Cloward spanner w.
    conical nut w.
    DynaTorq w.
    Hagie w.
    hexagonal w.
    hex socket w.
    slotted w.
    socket w.
    spanner w.
    spinal slip w.
    Texas Scottish Rite Hospital w.
    T-handled nut w.
    T-handled screw w.
    T-handle nut w.
    T-handle screw w.
    torque ratchet w.
    Trinkle socket w.
    TSRH w.
    U w.
    VDS w.
Wright
    W. fascia needle
    W. knee plate
    W. knee prosthesis
    W. Medical bone anchor
    W. monoblock titanium implant
    W. nebulizer
    W. needle
    W. ophthalmic needle
    W. peak flowmeter
    W. pneumatic tourniquet
    W. ptosis needle
    W. respirometer
    W. spirometer
    W. titanium prosthesis
Wright-Guilford
Wrightlock
    W. posterior fixation system
    W. spinal fixation system
Wrigley forceps
wrinkle filler
Wrist
    W. Pro wrist support
    W. Pro wrist support device
    W. Resist splint
    W. Restore brace
wrist
    w. flexion unit
    w. positioning splint
    w. quadrature phased-array surface
      coil
    w. splint
wristband
    Sea-Band acupressure w.
wrist-driven
    w.-d. lateral prehension orthosis
    w.-d. prehension orthosis
    w.-d. wrist-hand orthosis
wrist-hand
    w.-h. extension compression support
    w.-h. orthosis
Wristiciser exerciser
WrisTimer
    W. carpal tunnel support system
    W. CTS support
    W. PM carpal tunnel support
wristlet
    Freedom USA w.
wristRAP postsurgical wound wrap
wristwatch
    QT-Watch messaging w.
writer
    Wanchik w.
W-shaped ileoneobladder
W-shape forceps
W-stapled urinary reservoir
Wullstein
    W. contraangle handpiece
    W. ear forceps
    W. ear scissors
    W. microsuction tube
    W. retractor

W. self-retaining ear retractor
W. tympanoplasty forceps
Würzburg
W. fracture system
W. maxillofacial plating system
W. plate
W. reconstruction system
W. screw
WuScope system
W. W. Walker appliance

Wyeth bifurcated needle
Wylie
W. carotid artery clamp
W. endarterectomy set
W. endarterectomy stripper
W. J clamp
W. renal vein retractor
W. uterine dilator
W. uterine forceps

W

X

X clamp
X knife
translin-associated factor X (TRAX)

X-Act

X-A. cutaneous x-ray marker
X-A. podiatric marker

Xact

X. ACL graft fixation system
X. positioning cushion

X-Acto

X-A. blade
X-A. gouge
X-A. knife
X-A. utility knife

Xanar

X. 20 Ambulase CO_2 laser
X. laser adapter

Xceed biliary stent

Xcel

X. blunt-tip trocar
X. suture anchor

X-Cel dental x-ray unit

X-Cell cardiac bioprosthesis

Xcelon nylon

X-Echo-Speed

Signa Horizon X-E.-S.

XeCl excimer laser

XenoDerm graft

xenogeneic graft

xenograft

Ionescu-Shiley pericardial x.

xenon

x. arc
x. arc coagulator
x. arc lamp
x. arc photocoagulator
x. chloride excimer laser
x. cold-light fountain
x. flash lamp
x. illumination system
x. lamp
x. light source

Xenophor femoral prosthesis

Xenotech prosthetic valve

Xercise

X. band
X. band exercise device
X. tube resistive device

Xeroflo dressing

Xeroform

X. dressing
X. gauze
X. gauze dressing

xeroradiography

Xerox dental radiographic imaging system

Xertube

XGIF-MR30

nonferromagnetic MR

Xia

X. hook/spinal system
X. hook system
X. spinal system

Xillix

X. LIFE-GI fluorescence endoscopy system
X. LIFE-Lung fluorescence endoscopy system
X. LIFE-Lung system

Ximatron simulator

Ximed

X. disposable cannula
X. disposable trocar

XiScan

X. fluoroscope
X. mini-C-arm

Xi-scan

Linde X.-s.

XKnife

X. knife
X. stereotactic radiosurgery system

XL

extra large
Carter-Thomason CloseSure System XL
CloseSure System XL
XL illuminator
Jung Autostainer XL
Tono-Pen XL

XLS

Polysorb meniscal stapler XLS

X-Omat AR film

Xomed

X. Audiant bone conductor
X. Doyle nasal airway splint
X. drill
X. dual-chamber balloon
X. endotracheal tube
X. intraoral artificial larynx
X. Kartush tympanic membrane patcher
X. micro-oscillating saw
X. plastic and rubber endotracheal tube
X. rectal probe
X. sinus irrigation kit
X. sinus secretion collector
X. skimmer shaver
X. splint

X

Xomed *(continued)*
- X. straight-shank tube
- X. Treace nerve integrity monitor
- X. Treace ventilation tube
- X. XPS motor and handpiece

XO soft sole orthotic
Xpeedior catheter
XPE foot orthosis
Xpert biliary stent
Xplorer 1000 digital imaging system
X-Port
- X-P. Duo dual-lumen implantable port
- X-P. Inline implantable port

Xpose 3 access device
Xpouch emergency kit
XP peritympanic hearing instrument
Xpress 100 disposable perforator bur hole drill
X-Press suture-mediated closure device
Xpress/SW helical CT scanner
Xpress/SX helical CT scanner
X-PRESS vascular closure system
XPS
- XPS 3000 powered ENT system
- XPS shaver system
- XPS Straightshot system

XQ videoinstrument
x-ray
- x-r. calipers
- x-r. detectable laparotomy sponge
- x-r. film
- x-r. generator
- Infinix DP-i vascular x-r.
- Infinix NB-i vascular x-r.
- Infinix VC-i vascular x-r.
- x-r. microscope
- x-r. overlay
- x-r. photoemission spectroscopy
- Precision digital x-r.
- real-time low-intensity x-r.
- scanning-beam digital x-r.
- x-r. shadow projection microtomographic system
- Siemens Orthoceph x-r.
- x-r. spectrometer
- x-r. tomographic microscope
- x-r. tube
- x-r. tube housing

X-Scribe stress test
Xsensibles shoe
Xsensor pressure mapping system
x-shaped
- x-s. guidewire
- x-s. plate

X-Sizer single-use catheter system
Xsorb punctal plug
X-span tubing
X-Spine Capless polyaxial pedicle screw system
X-Static silver fiber shoe lining fiber
X-Stop IPD system
XTB knee extension device
X-tend back protector
Xtra
- X. Depth shoe
- Medisense Precision X.

Xtrac laser system
X-Tract tissue morcellator
XT radiopaque coronary stent
Xtrax DNA commercial extraction kit
X-Tube retraction system
X-Vigor CT scanner
XWire biliary guidewire
Xylocaine jelly
xylol pulse indicator
X-Y plotter
Xyrel pacemaker
XYZ lead system

Y

Y adapter
Y bandage
Y bone plate
Y connector
Y drain
Y hook
Y piece
Y tube
Y wave pressure on right atrial catheterization

Yaeger plate

YAG

yttrium-aluminum-garnet
YAG laser

Yaghouti LASIK polisher

YAGLazr system

Yale

Y. brace
Y. Luer-Lok
Y. Luer-Lok needle
Y. Luer-Lok syringe

Yamagishi viscocanalostomy cannula

Yamanda myelotomy knife

Yancy cast wedge

Yang needle

Yankauer

Y. aspirating tube
Y. bronchoscope
Y. catheter
Y. curette
Y. ear curette
Y. esophagoscope
Y. ethmoid-cutting forceps
Y. eustachian catheter
Y. laryngoscope
Y. nasopharyngeal speculum
Y. periosteal elevator
Y. pharyngeal speculum
Y. punch
Y. scissors
Y. suction
Y. suction tip
Y. suction tube
Y. tonsil suction tip
Y. tonsil-tip suction catheter

Yannuzzi fundus laser lens

Yasargil

Y. aneurysm clip applier
Y. angled forceps
Y. applying forceps
Y. bayonet needle holder
Y. bayonet scissors
Y. bipolar forceps
Y. carotid clamp

Y. clip applier
Y. cross-legged clip
Y. curette
Y. dissector
Y. elevator
Y. flat serrated ring forceps
Y. Leyla retractor arm
Y. ligature carrier
Y. ligature guide
Y. microclip
Y. microneedle holder
Y. microrasp
Y. microscissors
Y. microsuction tube
Y. microvascular bayonet scissors
Y. microvessel clip-applying forceps
Y. needle holder
Y. neurosurgical bipolar forceps
Y. retractor
Y. scoop
Y. spring hook
Y. straight forceps
Y. suction tube
Y. tissue lifter
Y. titanium aneurysm clip

Yasargil-Aesculap

Y.-A. instrument
Y.-A. spring clip

Yasargil-Leyla brain retractor z-gradient coil

Yashica Dental Eye II camera

Y-bandage dressing

Y-connecting tubing

Yellen clamp

yellow

y. dye laser
Y. IRIS system
Y. Springs Instrument (YSI)
Y. Springs probe

yellow-eyed dilating bougie

Yellowfin stirrup

yellow-tip aspirator

Yeoman

Y. biopsy punch
Y. forceps

Yesavage depression instrument

Y-jaws

Y-knot tying system

yoga mat

yoke

y. block
y. hanger

Yoon ring

Yoshida dental x-ray unit

Y

You-Bend hemodialysis catheterization kit
Youens lens
Youlten nasal inspiratory peak flowmeter
Young
    Y. anterior prostatic retractor
    Y. bifid retractor
    Y. bladder retractor
    Y. boomerang needle holder
    Y. bulb retractor
    Y. cystoscope
    Y. enucleator
    Y. hinged knee prosthesis
    Y. lateral prostatic retractor
    Y. lobe forceps
    Y. needle holder
    Y. pediatric rectal dilator
    Y. prostatectomy forceps
    Y. prostatic forceps
    Y. prostatic retractor
    Y. prostatic tractor
    Y. renal pedicle clamp
    Y. rubber dam fracture frame
    Y. tongue forceps
    Y. urological dissector

Young-Dees tube
Younger-Good scaler
Yperwatch gamma control watch
Y-port connector
Y-set system
Y-shaped plate
YSI
    Yellow Springs Instrument
        YSI Foley probe
        YSI neonatal temperature probe
        YSI STAT glucose and lactate analyzer
        YSI Telethermometer
Y-stent
    dynamic Y-s.
Y-strap knee immobilizer
yttrium-90
yttrium-aluminum-garnet (YAG)
    y.-a.-g. laser
Yudkoff-Okun periodontal instrument set
Yueh centesis needle
Yu-Holtgrewe
    Y.-H. malleable blade
    Y.-H. prostatic retractor
Yung percutaneous mastoid vent

Z

Z cardiac catheter
Z clamp
Z disc
Z fixation nail
Z pin
Z plate
Z retractor
Z sampler endometrial sampling device
Z stent
Z stent esophageal endoprosthesis system
Z1, Z2 series Coulter counter
ZAAG
Zest Anchor Advanced Generation
ZAAG abutment
ZAAG bone anchoring system
ZAAG guide and pin
ZAAG implant anchor
ZAAG implant system
Zachary-Cope clamp
Zaldivar
Z. degree gauge
Z. iridectomy forceps
Z. iridectomy scissors
Z. knife
Z. limbal-relaxing incision system
Z. LRI marker
Z. microacrylic lens implantation forceps
Z. reverse capsulorrhexis forceps
Zalkind-Balfour center-blade retractor
Zalkind lung retractor
Z-alpha lens
Zander apparatus
Zang
Z. metatarsal cap
Z. metatarsal cap implant
Zaontz urethral stent
ZAP diamond knife
Zapit resin
Zassi bowel management system
Za-stent
Z.-s. endoscopic biliary stent
Z.-s. nitinol self-expandable stent
Zaufel-Jansen bone rongeur
Zavala lung biopsy needle
ZCI
Zyderm collagen implant
ZCI collagen
Z-clamp hysterectomy forceps
Zebra exchange guidewire
Zeichner implant

Zeiss
Z. aspheric lens
Z. Axiophot fluorescent microscope
Z. Axiophot microscope
Z. Axioskop microscope
Z. Axiovert microscope
Z. binocular prism telescope
Z. carbon arc slit-lamp
Z. cine adapter
Z. coagulator
Z. colposcope
Z. DAS-1 hydrophobic system
Z. electron microscope
Z. EndoLive endoscope
Z. fiberoptic illumination system
Z. fluorescein filter system
Z. fundus camera
Z. goniolens
Z. gonioscope
Z. IDO3 phase-contrast microscope
Z. IIIRS photomicroscope
Z. IOL Master laser interferometer
Z. lens loupe
Z. LSM-10 laser microscope
Z. MD laser
Z. operating camera
Z. operating field loupe
Z. operating microscope
Z. operating microscope
Z. ophthalmoscope
Z. Opmi-6 FR microscope
Z. Opmilas surgical laser
Z. Opmi Neuro/NC4 surgical microscope
Z. osteotome
Z. photocoagulator
Z. projection Lensmeter
Z. small beam splitter
Z. stereotactic tool navigator system
Z. STN surgical tool navigator
Z. Super Lux 40 light source
Z. transmission electron microscope
Z. ureteral stone dislodger
Z. vertex refractometer
Z. Visulas 532, 532s laser
Z. Visulas YAG II laser
Z. xenon arc photocoagulator
Zeiss-Barraquer
Z.-B. cine microscope
Z.-B. surgical microscope
Zeiss-Comberg slit-lamp
Zeiss-Gullstrand
Z.-G. lens
Z.-G. loupe

Zeiss-Humphrey UBM scanner
Zeiss/Jena surgical microscope
Zeiss-Nordenson fundus camera
Zelicof orthopaedic awl
Zelsmyr cytobrush
Zenith
    Z. AAA endovascular graft
    Z. AAA endovascular graft system
    Z. abdominal aortic aneurysm
       endovascular graft system
    Z. ACS table
    Z. chiropractic table
    Z. electrotherapy ultrasound system
    Z. Hylos table
    Z. stainless steel self-expandable
       stent
    Z. stationary table
    Z. Thompson table
    Z. Verti-Lift table
Zenith-Cox flexion/distraction table
Zenker
    Z. forceps
    Z. retractor
Zenotech
    Z. graft material
    Z. synthetic ligament
Zephir anterior cervical plate system
Zeppelin
    Z. clamp
    Z. micromotor system
    Z. S vaginal hysterectomy clamp
zero-degree
ZeroRad MRI scan
Zest
    Z. Anchor Advanced Generation
       (ZAAG)
    Z. Anchor Advanced Generation
       bone anchoring system
    Z. implant
    Z. implant anchor
    Z. subperiosteal implant
Zetafuge
Zeta probe nylon filter
Zeus
    Z. computer-controlled robotic
       system
    Z. robot
    Z. system
    Z. voice-controlled robotic system
ZF
   zygomaticofrontal
    ZF suture
z-gradient coil
Zickel
    Z. nail
    Z. nail fixation
    Z. subtrochanteric fracture fixation
    Z. supracondylar rod

Ziegler
    Z. blade
    Z. cautery
    Z. cautery electrode
    Z. cilia forceps
    Z. electrocautery
    Z. eye speculum
    Z. iris knife
    Z. knife
    Z. lacrimal dilator
    Z. probe
    Z. speculum
Zielke
    Z. distraction device
    Z. gouge
    Z. instrumentation for scoliosis
       spinal fusion
    Z. pedicular instrumentation
    Z. rod
    Z. screw
zigzag stent
Zila
    Z. Pro-Scrub
    Z. Pro-Wash antiseptic hand wash
Zilver
    Z. biliary self-expanding stent
    Z. self-expanding stent
    Z. vascular stent
Zilverstent
Zimaloy
    Z. epiphyseal staple
    Z. femoral head prosthesis
Zimfoam
    Z. head halter
    Z. pad
    Z. pad and patient positioner
    Z. splint
Zimmer
    Z. anatomic hip prosthesis system
    Z. anatomic hip system
    Z. antiembolism stocking
    Z. antiembolism support stocking
    Z. arthroscope
    Z. bone cement
    Z. bur
    Z. Cebotome bone cement drill
    Z. Centralign Precoat hip prosthesis
    Z. clavicular cross splint
    Z. clip
    Z. collarless polished taper hip
       system
    Z. continuous anatomical passive
       exerciser
    Z. CPT hip system
    Z. crossover instrumentation system
    Z. dermatome
    Z. electrical stimulation device
    Z. fracture frame
    Z. Gigli saw blade

Z. goniometer
Z. gouge
Z. hand drill
Z. head halter
Z. hip implant system
Z. hip prosthesis
Z. knee immobilizer
Z. low-viscosity adhesive
Z. Micro-E fixation drill
Z. Micro 100 reciprocating saw
Z. microsaw
Z. M/L taper hip prosthesis
Z. modular revision (ZMR)
Z. NexGen LPS knee femoral component
Z. Orthair ream driver
Z. orthopaedic device
Z. OsteoStim bone growth stimulator
Z. pin
Z. PMMA precoat process
Z. postoperative shoe
Z. protractor
Z. Pulsavac wound débridement system
Z. screw
Z. screwdriver
Z. shoulder prosthesis
Z. skin graft mesher
Z. Statak suture
Z. Statak suturing device
Z. telescoping nail
Z. Tharies surface arthroplasty system
Z. tibial bolt
Z. tibial prosthesis
Z. walker

Zimmer-Hall drill
Zimmerman-Walton expressor
Zimmer-Statak anchor
Zimmon
Z. biliary stent
Z. catheter
Z. endoscopic biliary stent set
Z. endoscopic pancreatic stent set
Z. esophagogastric balloon tamponade set
Z. papillotome
Z. papillotome/sphincterotome
Z. sphincterotome

zinc
z. ball electrode
z. oxide bandage
z. phosphate cement

zinc-free
z.-f. plastic bag
z.-f. plastic specimen cup

Zinco
Z. Air Cam brace

Z. Airprene brace
Z. ankle orthosis
Z. Cam Walker brace
Z. Castaway D brace
Z. Hi-Top brace
Z. Minerva cervical brace
Z. Multi-Lig knee brace
Z. Pin Cam Walker brace
Z. thumb-wrist immobilizer

Zinnanti
Z. clamp
Z. uterine manipulator/injector (ZUMI)

zipper
abdominal z.
Z. antidisconnect device
z. cast
fascial z.
Z. Medical tracheostomy tube neck band
z. ring
synthetic z.

Zippie 2 wheelchair
Zipser
Z. meatal clamp
Z. penile clamp

Zipzoc
Z. compression wrap
Z. stocking
Z. stocking leg compression dressing

Ziramic
Z. femoral head
Z. femoral head prosthesis

zirconia
z. femoral head prosthesis
z. orthopaedic prosthesis
z. orthopaedic prosthetic head

zirconium oxide ceramic prosthesis
Z-Med balloon catheter
ZMR
Zimmer modular revision
ZMR hip system

Zodiac TM manual flexion-distraction table
Zohar shoe
Zoladex implant
Zoll
Z. M series critical care transport defibrillator
Z. M-series defibrillator monitor pacemaker
Z. noninvasive pacemaker

Zollinger-Gilmore intraluminal vein stripper
Zollner rasp
zona drilling pipette

Zonas
    Z. porous adhesive tape dressing
    Z. porous tape
zone
    Z. Specific II meniscal repair system
zoom
    overhead z. (OZM)
    Z. and Sniper sports goggles
    z. videoendoscopy
    volume z.
ZoomScope colposcope
Zorbacel shock-absorbing material
Zoroc plaster
Z-Sampler endometrial suction curette
Z-Scissors hysterectomy scissors
Z-shaped plate
ZstatFlu test kit
Z-stent
    colonic Z-s.
    covered Z-s.
    Gianturco Z-s.
    Gianturco biliary Z-s.
    Gianturco-Rosch biliary Z-s.
    Gianturco-Rosch self-expandable Z-s.
    Gianturco-Rosch self-expandable biliary Z-s.
    metal Z-s.
    modified Z-s.
    Z-s. prosthesis
    tracheobronchial Z-s.
    Wilson-Cook esophageal Z-s.
Z-Stim IF 100, 250 microprocessor controlled stimulator
Z-Touch
    Z-T. ENT laser pointer
    Z-T. laser device
    Z-Touch laser pointer
ZTT
    ZTT acetabular cup

    ZTT I, II acetabular cup prosthesis
    ZTT I, II cup
Zucker
    Z. cardiac catheter
    Z. splint
Zuelzer hook plate
Zuma guiding catheter
ZUMI
    Zinnanti uterine manipulator/injector
    ZUMI uterine manipulator
Zuni
    Z. exercise system
    Z. gym
    Z. harness
Zurich suturing forceps
Z-View aberrometer
Zwanck pessary
Z-wave tube
Zweymuller
    Z. cementless hip prosthesis
    Z. hip prosthesis
    Z. hip system
Zyderm collagen implant (ZCI)
zygoma
    z. elevator
    z. fixture
    z. hook
zygomaticofrontal (ZF)
zygomaticus implant
Zylik-Joseph hook
Zymderm collagen implant
zymography
Zynergy Zolution electrophysiology catheter
Zyoptix
    Z. excimer laser system
    Z. Infinity laser
Zyplast collagen implant
Zyranox femoral head
Zywave II aberrometer

Contents: The Appendices

Appendix 1
Illustrations

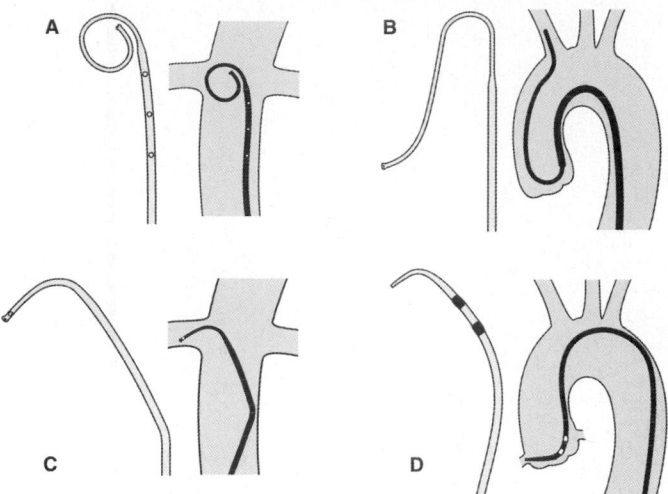

Figure 1. Angiographic catheters: (A) aortic catheter with side holes; (B) side-bending cerebral catheter (sidewinder); (C) side-bending catheter for selective viewing of visceral vessels; (D) Judkins coronary catheter.

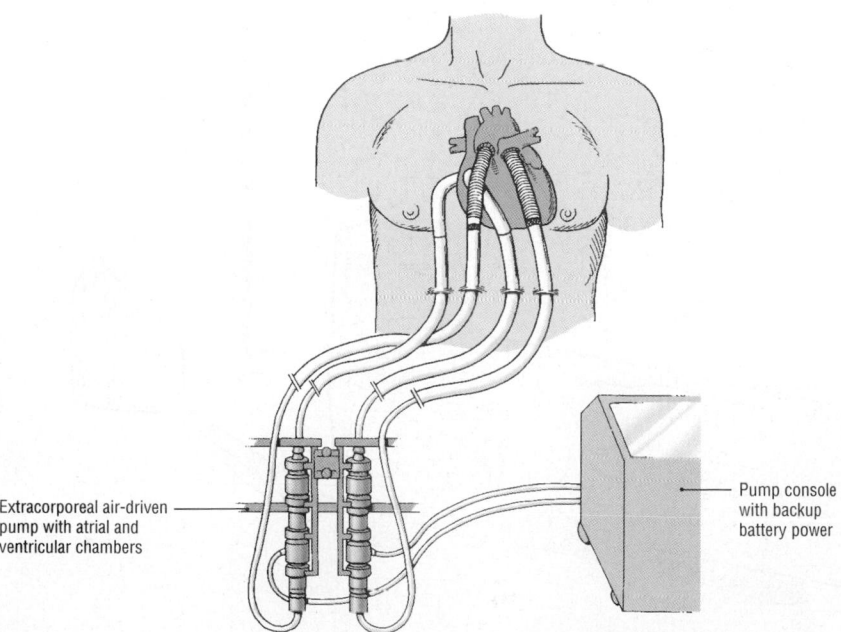

Extracorporeal air-driven pump with atrial and ventricular chambers

Pump console with backup battery power

Figure 2. Abiomed BVS-5000 biventricular support system.

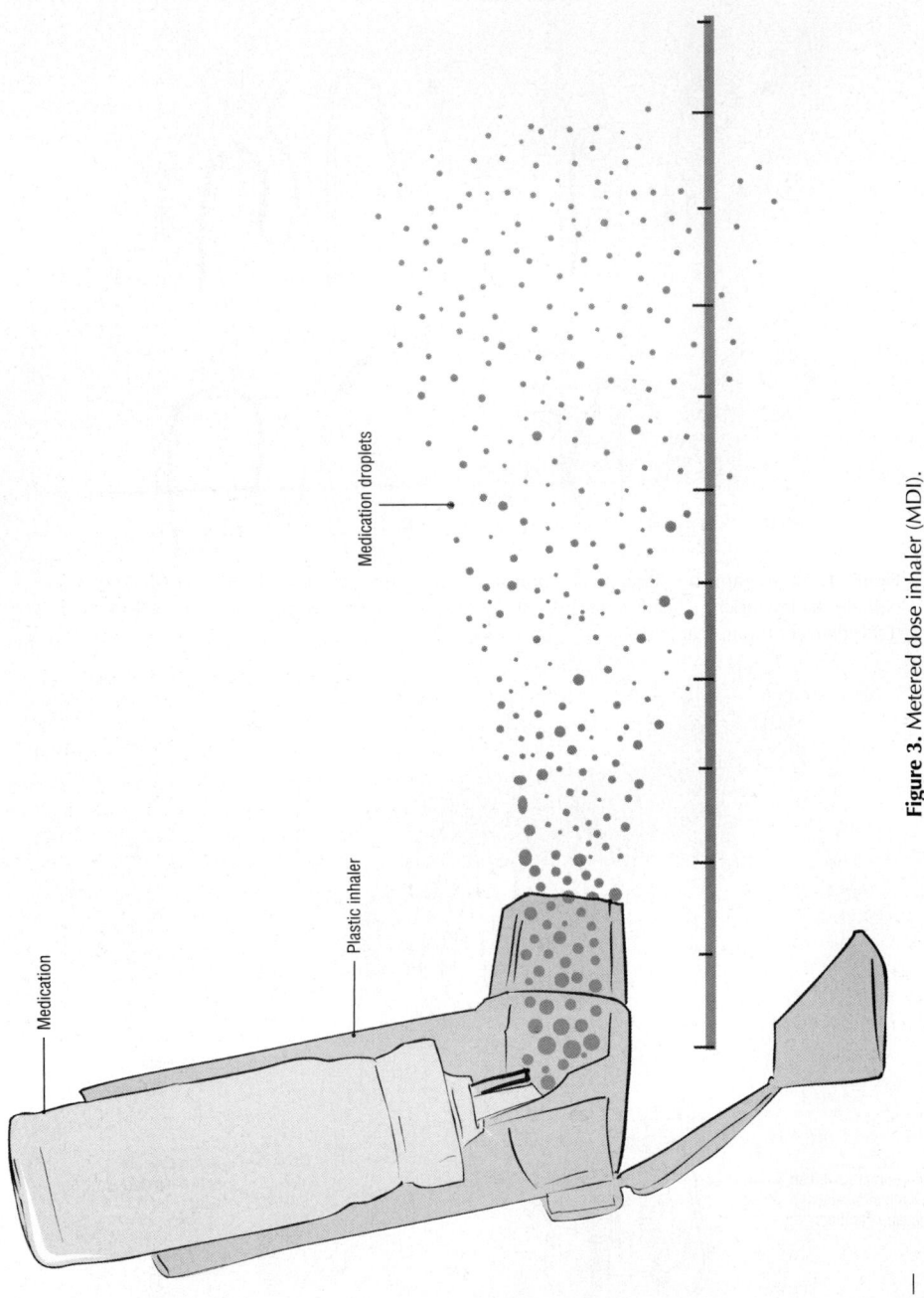

Figure 3. Metered dose inhaler (MDI).

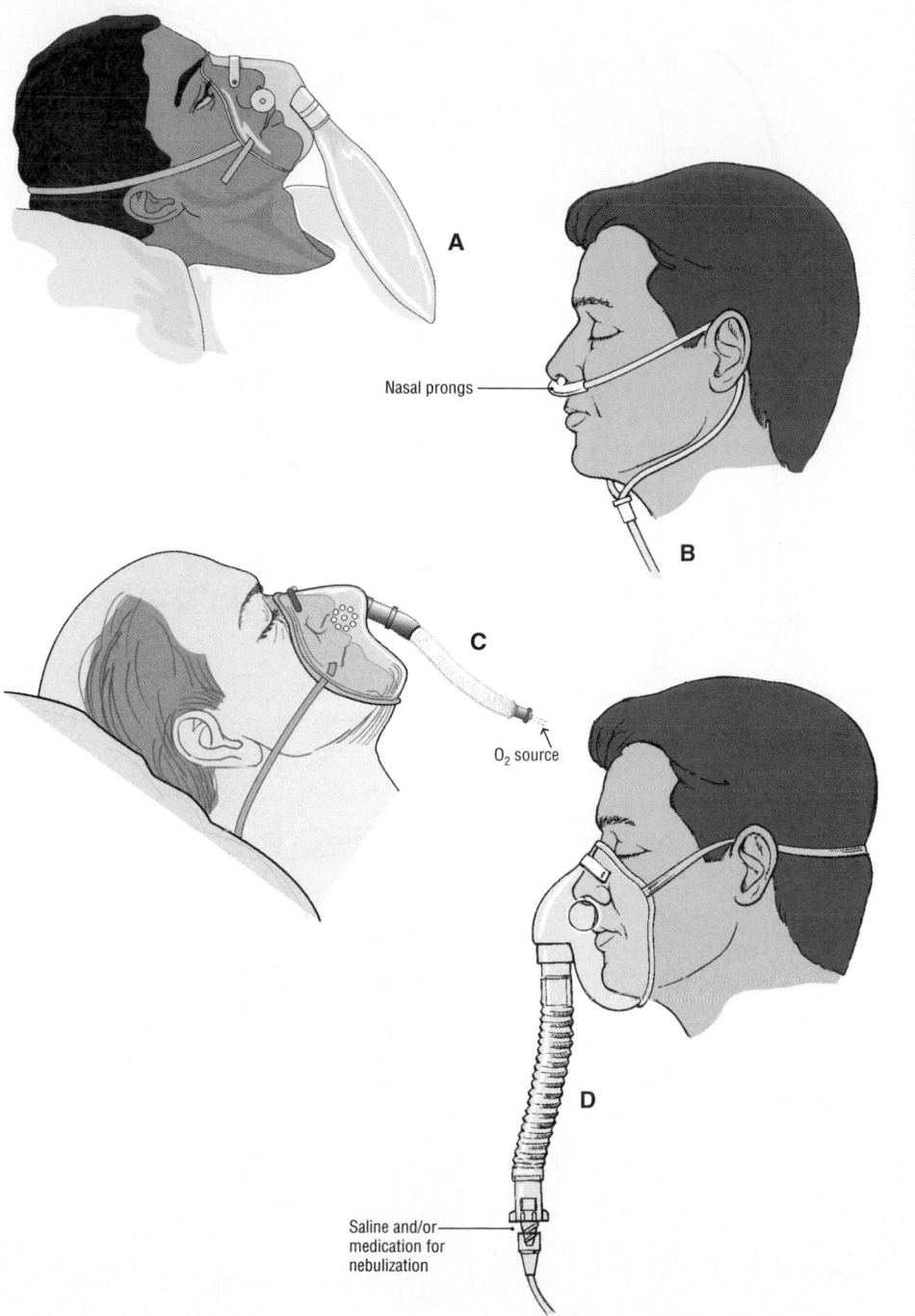

Figure 4. (A) Nonrebreathing mask; (B) nasal oxygen cannula; (C) Venti mask; (D) Venturi mask with nebulizer.

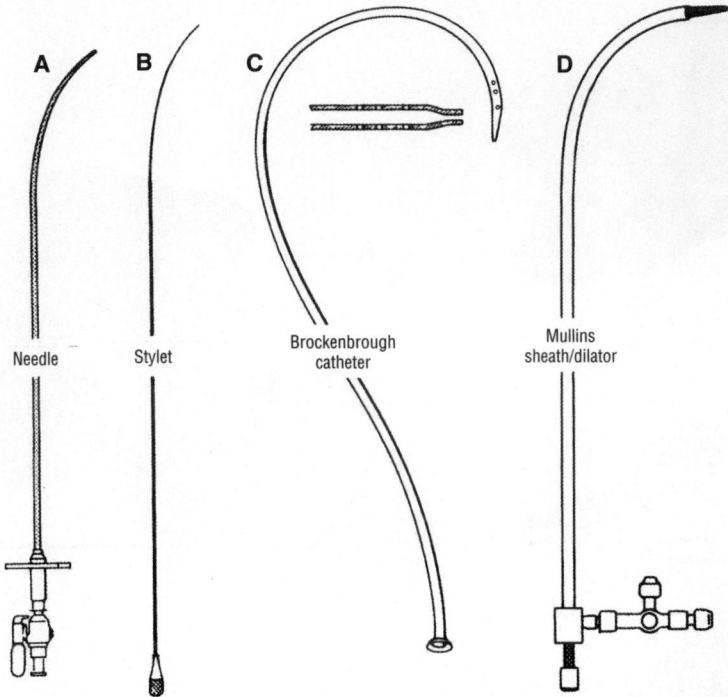

Figure 5. (A) Brockenbrough needle; (B) Bing stylet used in conjunction with the following: (C) Brockenbrough catheter; (D) Mullins sheath/dilator system.

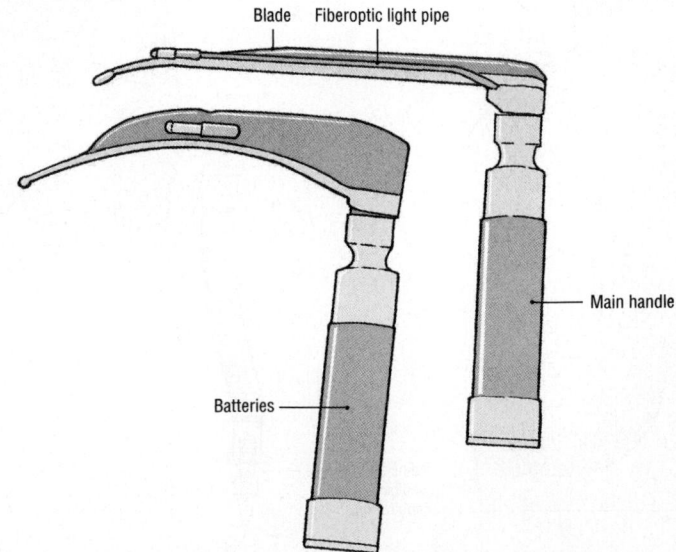

Figure 6. MacIntosh laryngoscope.

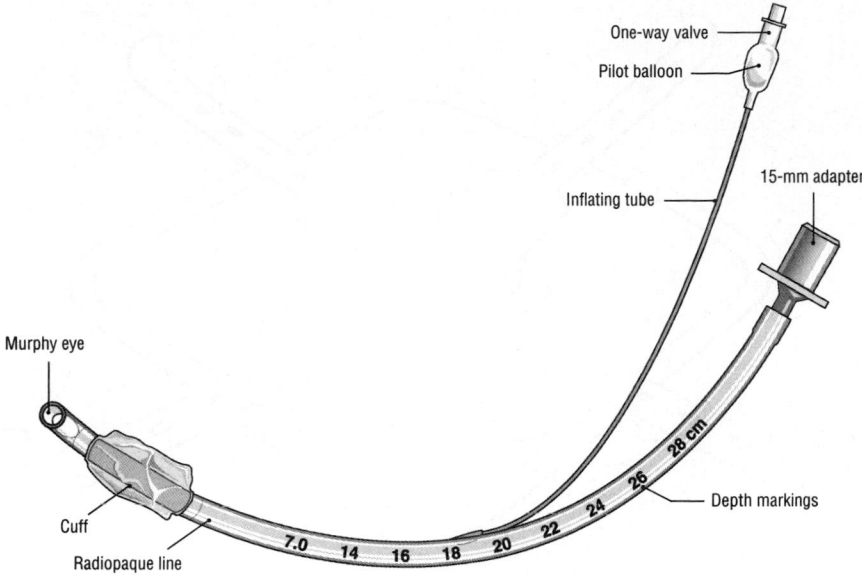

Figure 7. Parts of an endotracheal tube.

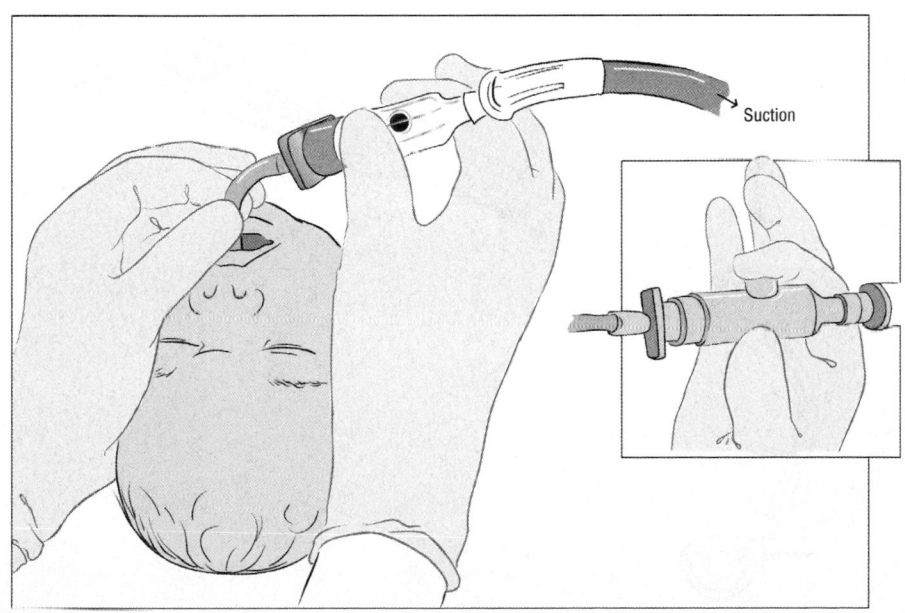

Figure 8. Meconium aspirator.

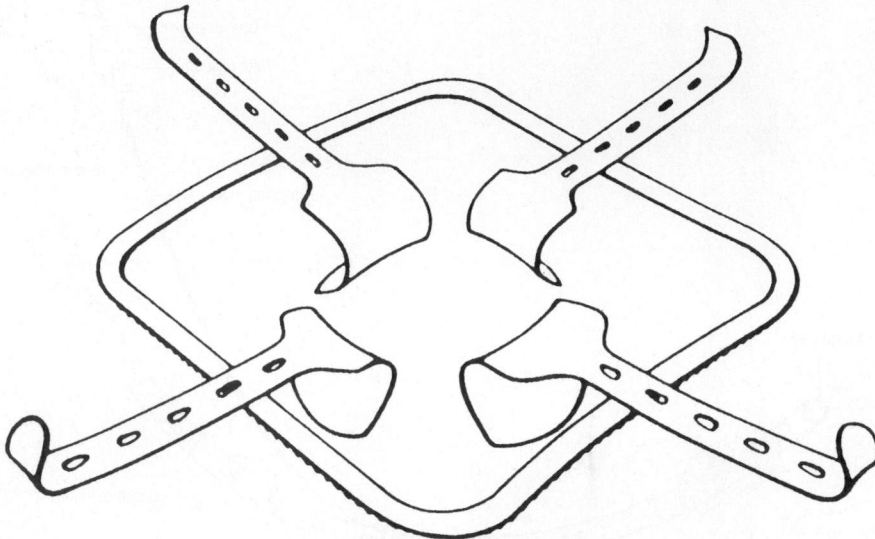

Figure 9. Kirschner abdominal retractor.

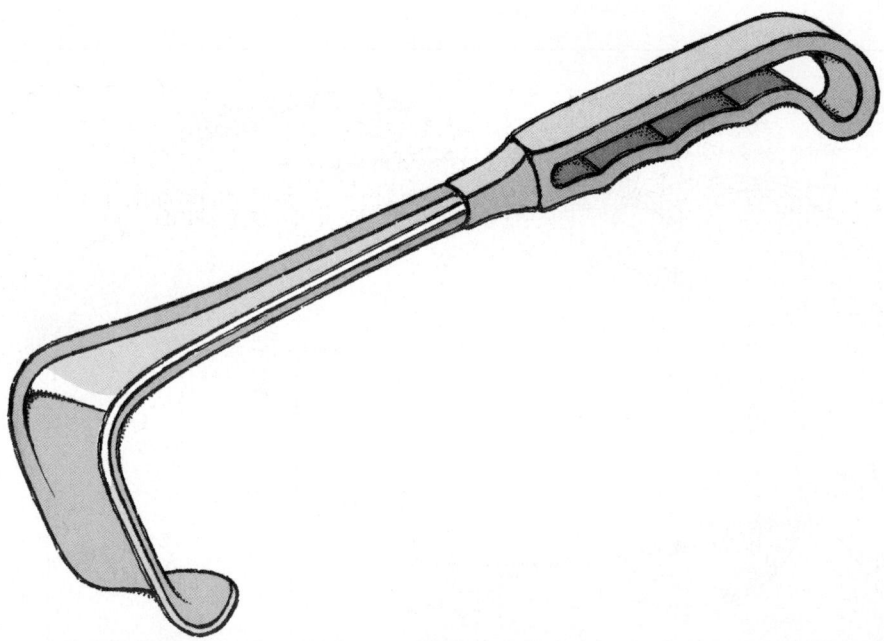

Figure 10. Abdominal retractor.

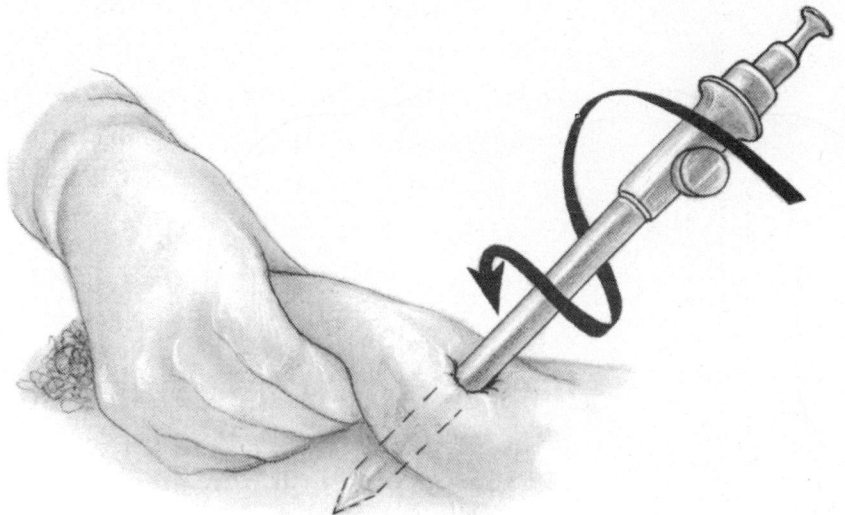

Figure 11. Trocar.

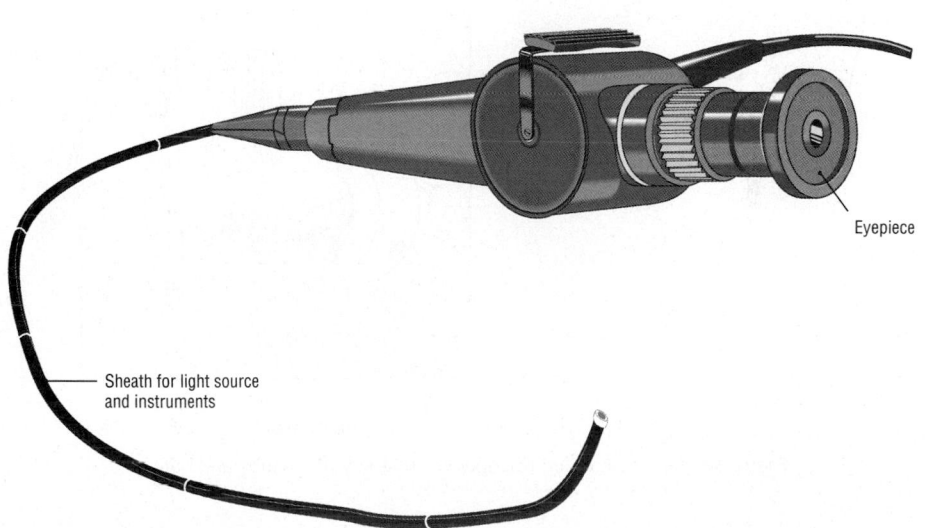

Eyepiece

Sheath for light source
and instruments

Figure 12. Endoscope.

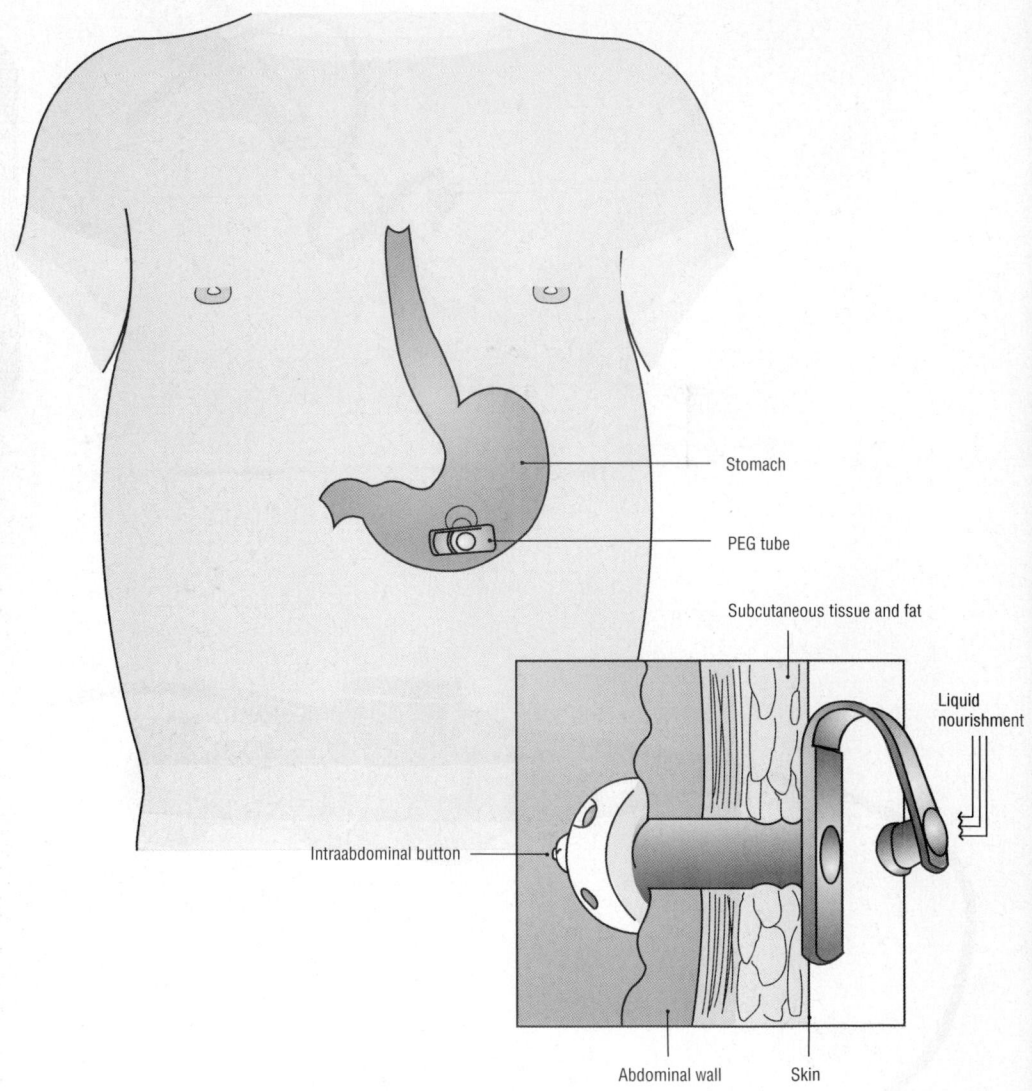

Figure 13. Percutaneous endoscopic gastrostomy (PEG) tube and button.

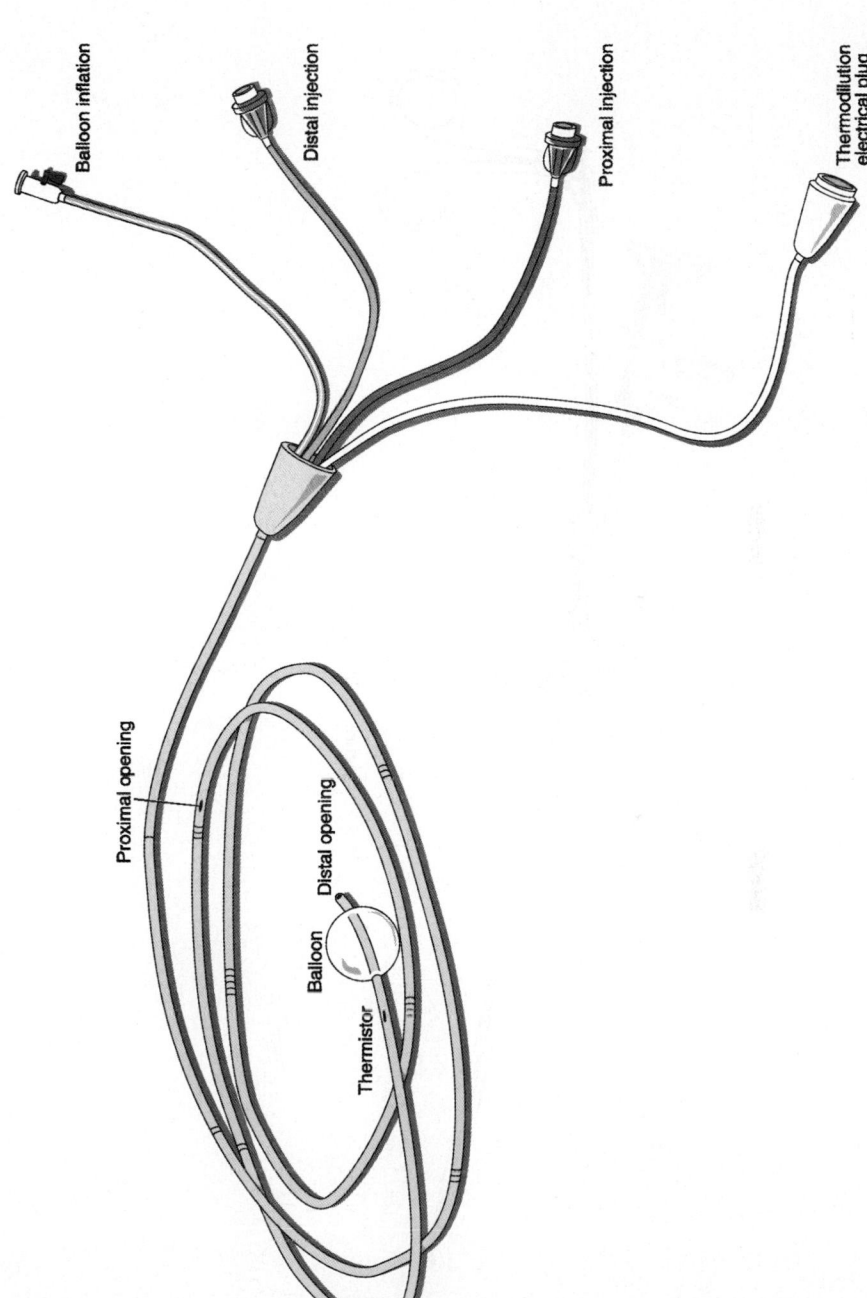

Balloon inflation

Distal injection

Proximal injection

Thermodilution
electrical plug

Proximal opening

Distal opening

Balloon

Thermistor

Figure 14. Swan-Ganz thermodilution catheter.

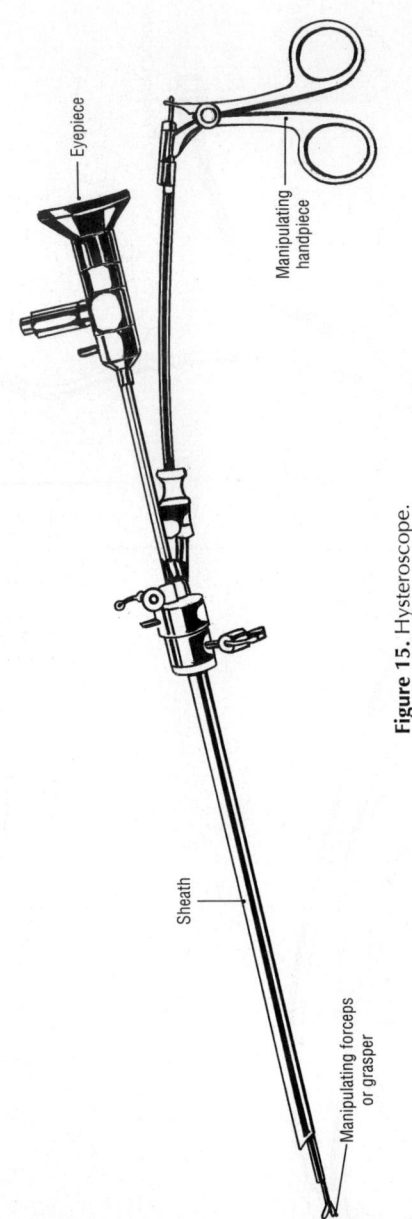

Figure 15. Hysteroscope.

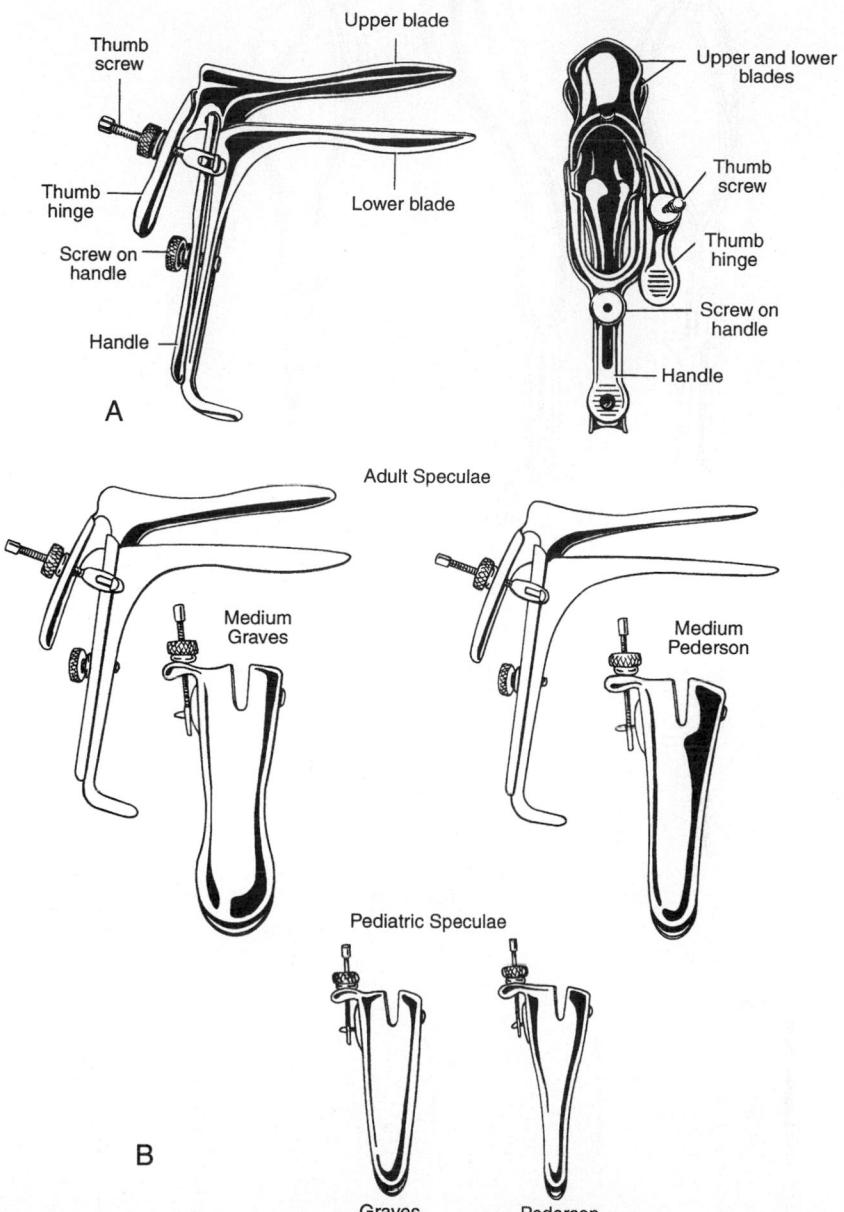

Figure 16. The vaginal speculum. (A) Parts of the vaginal speculum. (B) Types of vaginal specula.

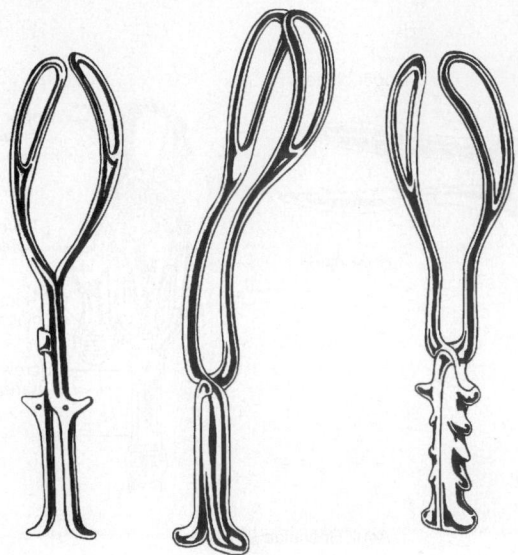

Figure 17. Obstetrical forceps: (A) Kjelland; (B) Piper; (C) Simpson.

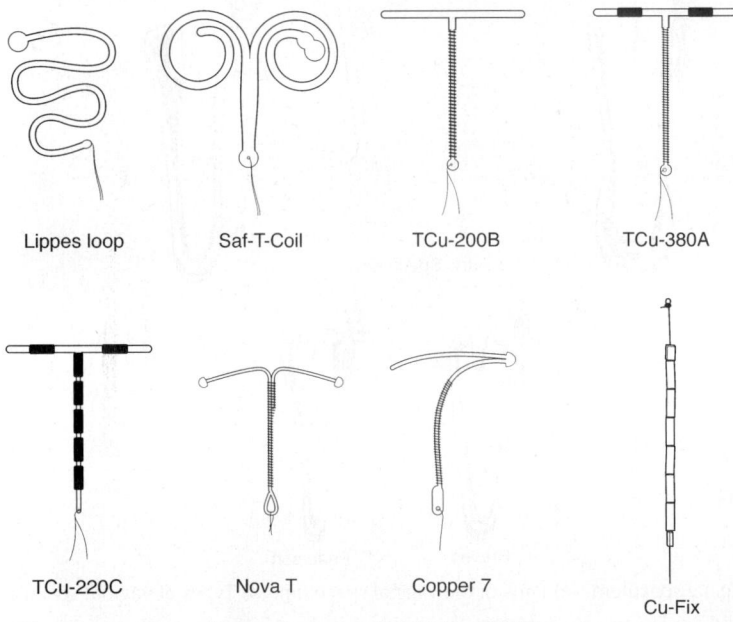

Lippes loop	Saf-T-Coil	TCu-200B	TCu-380A

TCu-220C	Nova T	Copper 7	Cu-Fix

Figure 18. Intrauterine devices (IUDs).

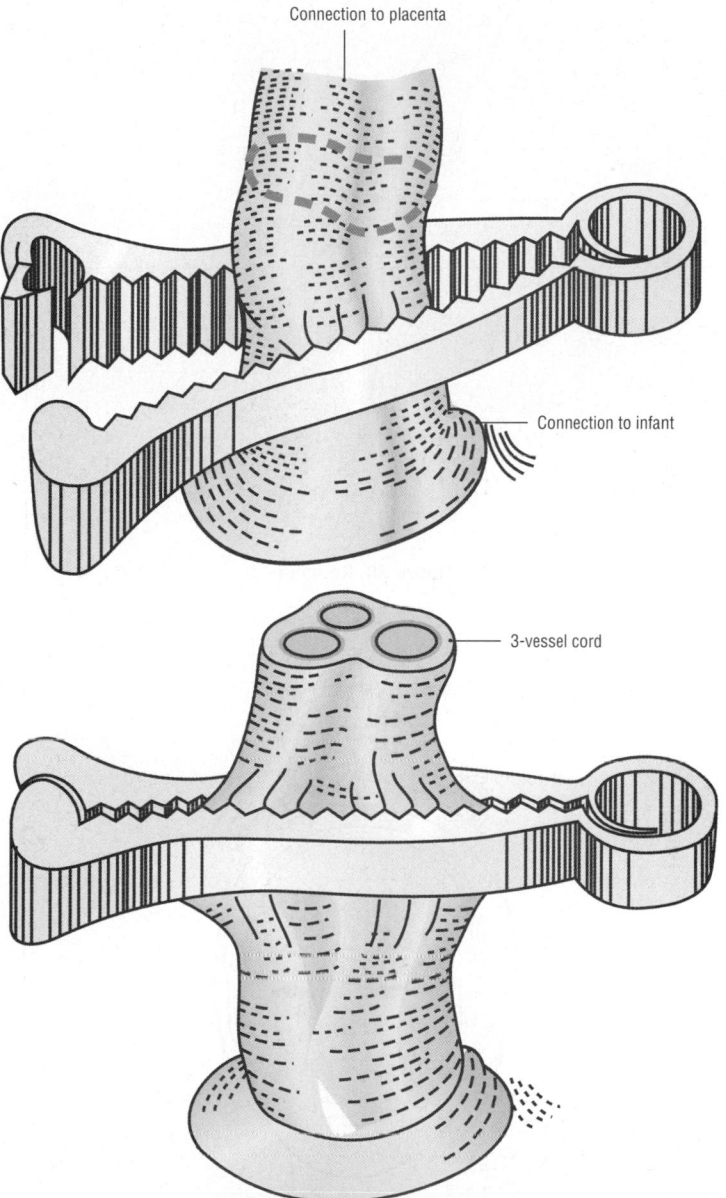

Figure 19. Umbilical cord clamp.

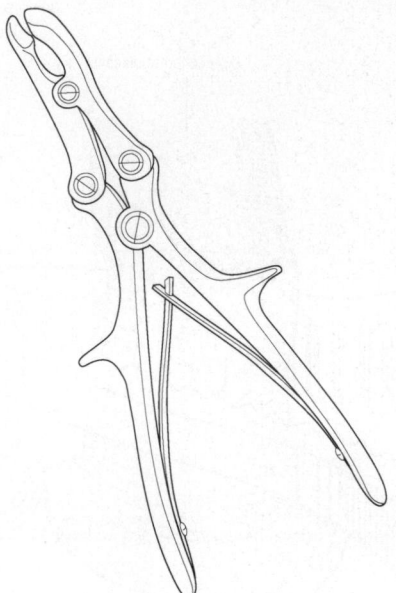

Figure 20. Rongeur.

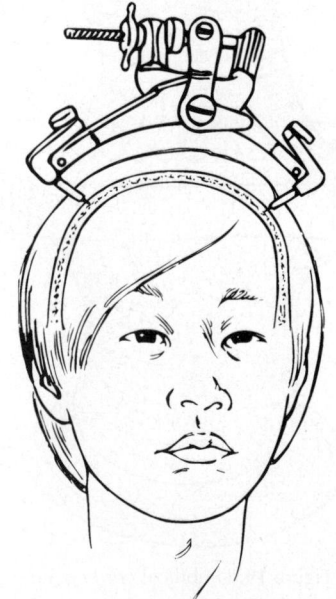

Figure 21. Crutchfield-Raney skull tongs.

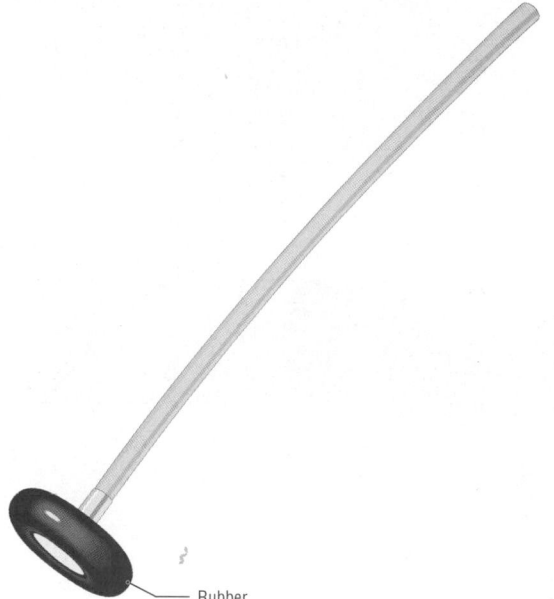

Rubber

Figure 22. Babinski percussion hammer.

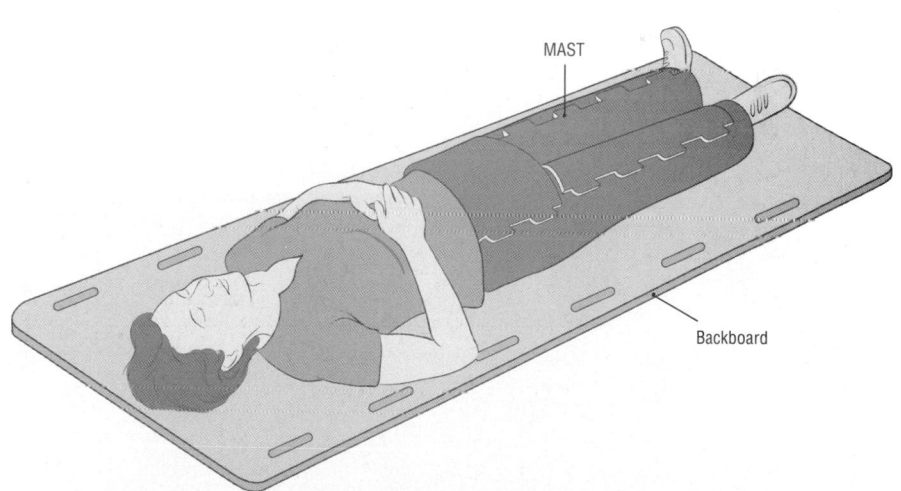

MAST

Backboard

Figure 23. Military antishock trousers (MAST).

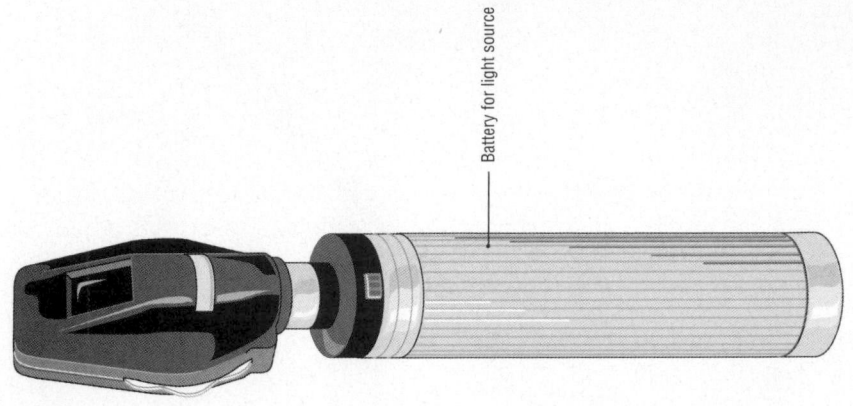

Battery for light source

Figure 25. Ophthalmoscope.

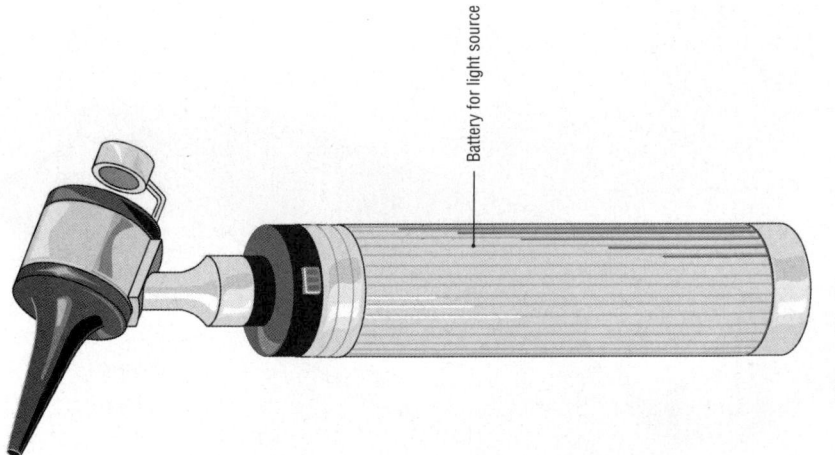

Battery for light source

Figure 24. Otoscope.

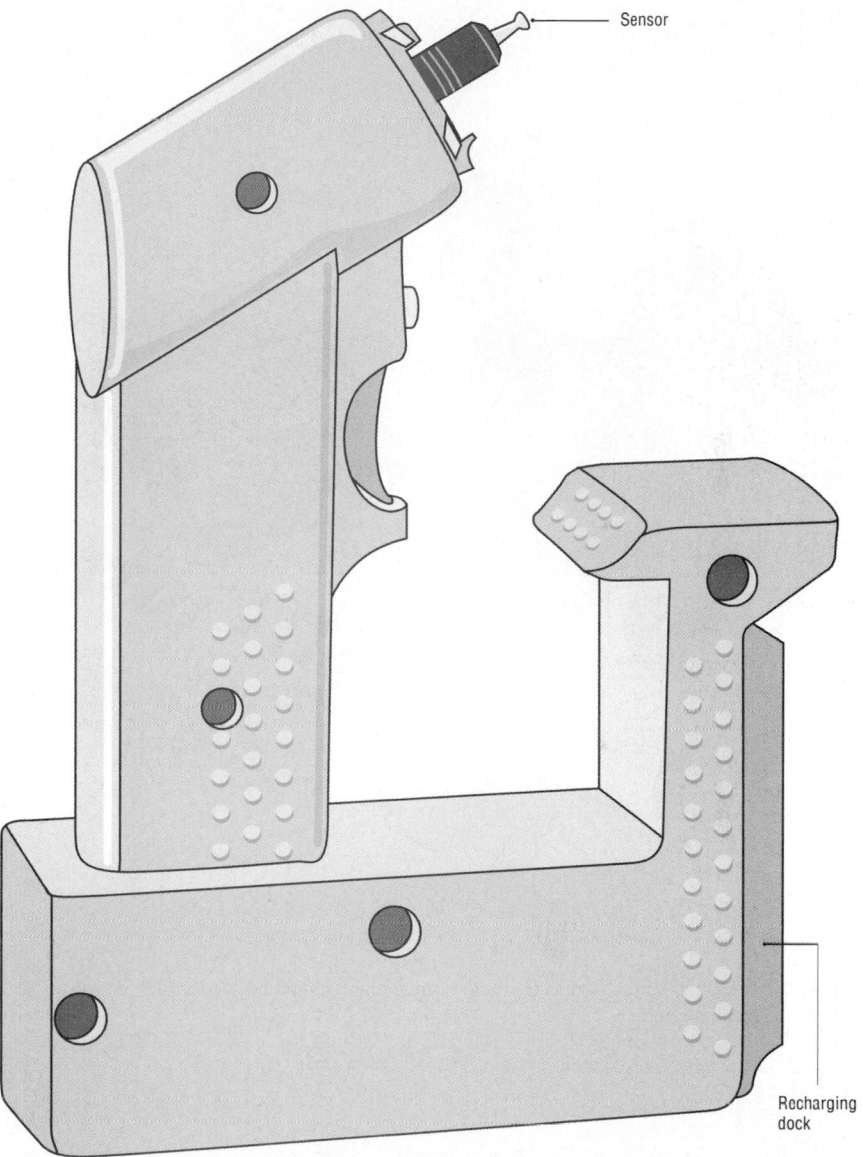

Sensor

Recharging
dock

Figure 26. Tympanic membrane thermometer.

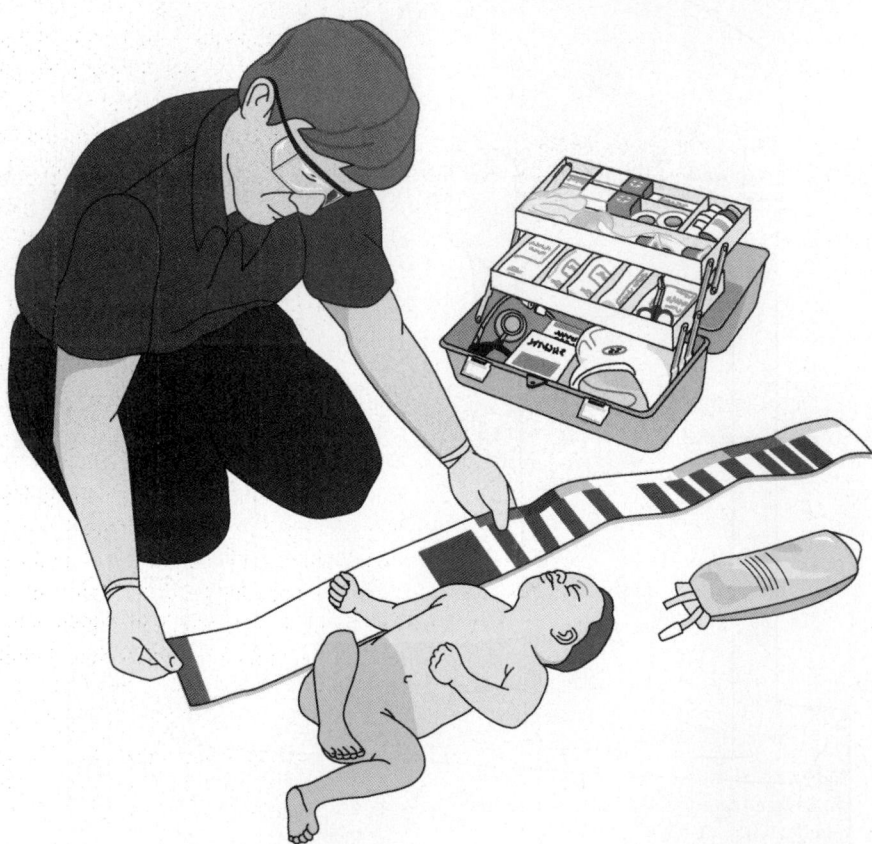

Figure 27. Broselow tape. Used to estimate body weight and tracheal tube size based on body length in small children.

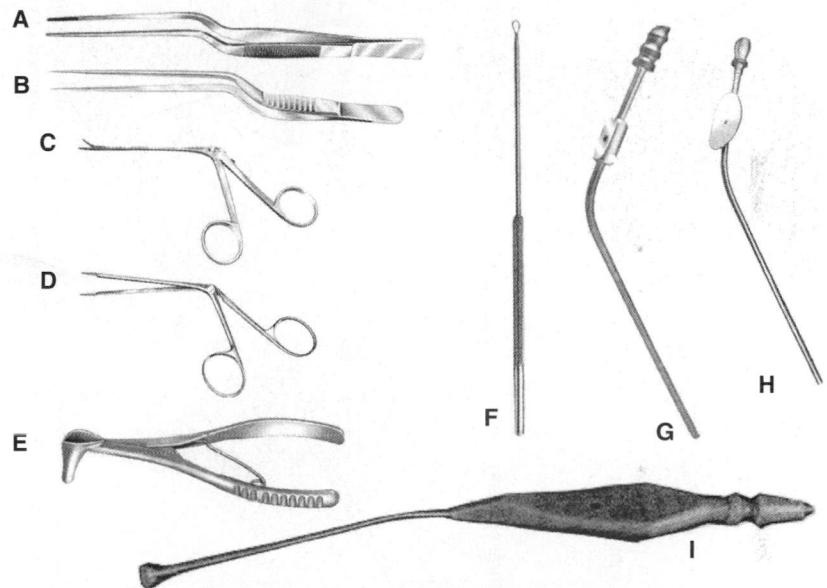

Figure 28. Selected instruments used for foreign-body removal. (A) Foreign body forceps; (B) Bayonet forceps; (C) Alligator forceps; (D) Hartmann forceps; (E) Nasal speculum; (F) Ear curette; (G) Frazier suction tube; (H) Barnes suction tube; (I) Schuknecht foreign-body remover.

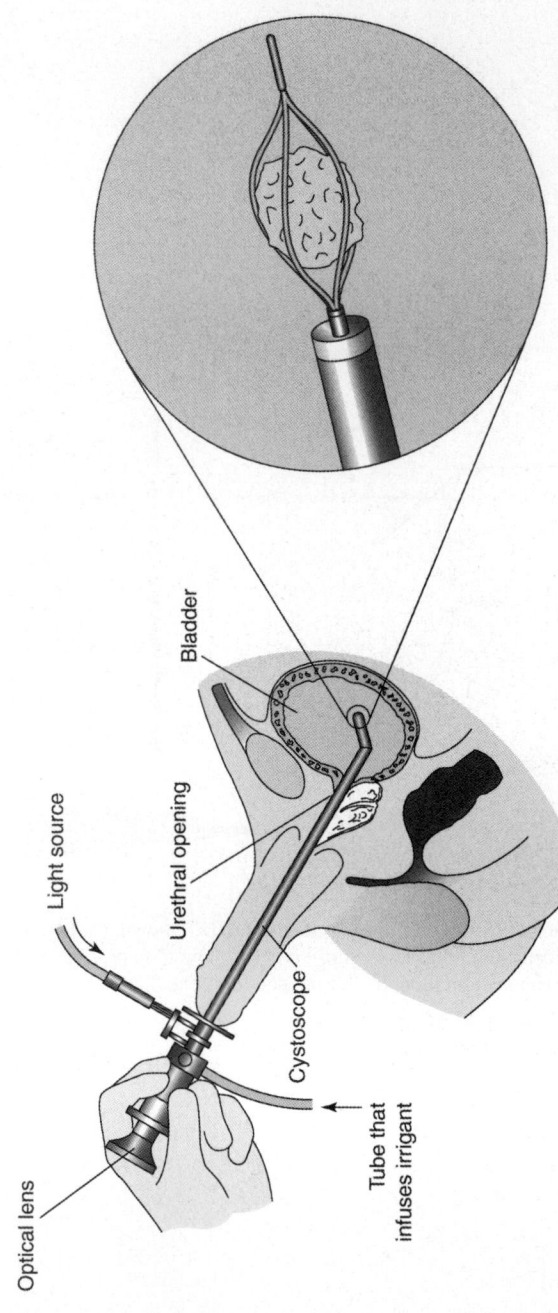

Figure 29. Cystoscopy. During a cystoscopy, which is used for removing small renal stones located close to the bladder, a ureteroscope is inserted into the ureter to visualize the stone. The stone is then fragmented or captured and removed.

Light source

Urethral opening

Bladder

Cystoscope

Optical lens

Tube that infuses irrigant

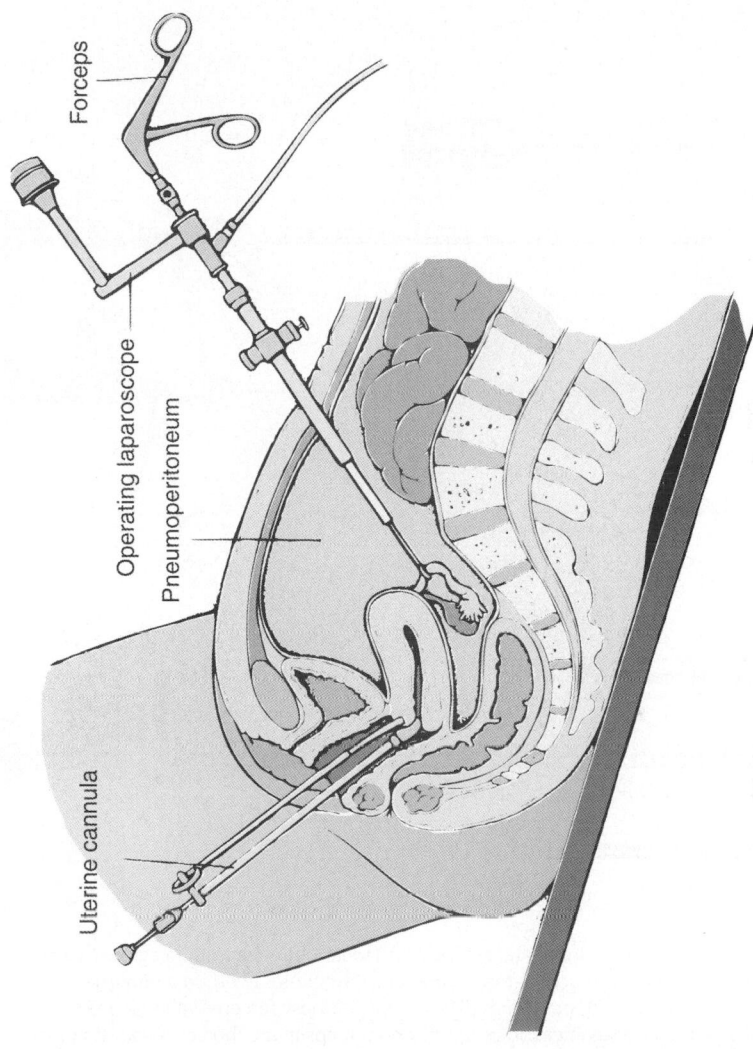

Forceps

Operating laparoscope

Pneumoperitoneum

Uterine cannula

Figure 30. Laparoscopy. The laparoscope (right) is inserted through a small incision in the abdomen. A forceps is inserted through the scope to grasp the fallopian tube. To improve the view, a uterine cannula (left) is inserted into the vagina to push the uterus upward. Insufflation of gas creates an air pocket (pneumoperitoneum), and the pelvis is elevated (note the angle), which forces the intestines higher in the abdomen.

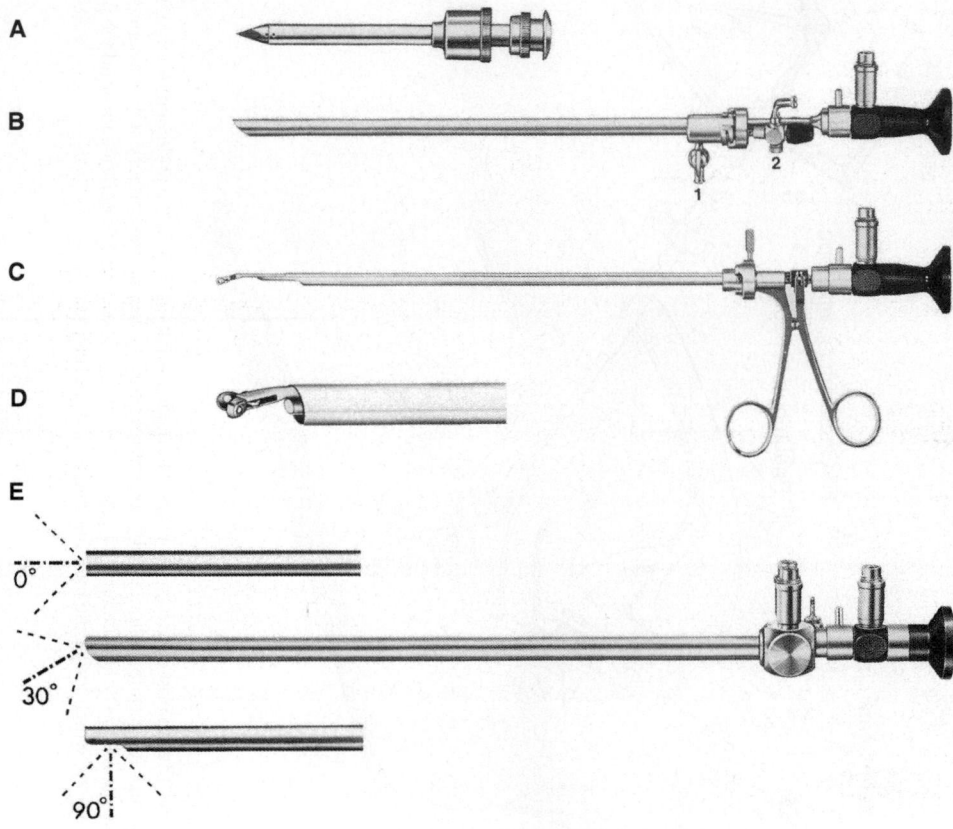

A

B

C

D

E

0°

30°

90°

Figure 31. Thoracoscopy (basic instrumental set for). (A) Trocar obturator with integrated valve and sharp internal cannula of 7-, 9-, or 11-mm diameter for single- or two-port technique. (B) Single incision thoracoscope (9- or 11-mm diameter). (C) Biopsy forceps with integrated 0 degrees-optical system. (D) Magnification of optics and forceps in the thoracoscope shaft ready for biopsy. (E) Various straight and angled vision telescopes for the single-entry technique, with adapted photograph light shaft.

Appendix 2

Sample Reports

DUAL-CHAMBER PACEMAKER INSERTION

PREOPERATIVE DIAGNOSIS: Sick sinus syndrome.

POSTOPERATIVE DIAGNOSIS: Sick sinus syndrome.

OPERATION PERFORMED: Insertion of dual-chamber pacemaker.

INDICATIONS: This pleasant 88-year-old lady had weakness and an irregular heart rate with a Holter monitor showing a heart rate down in the 20s.

FINDINGS: The most striking finding with this patient was that the instant the ventricular lead touched the endocardium during the insertion, she developed this profound heart block and became for all intents and purposes completely pacemaker dependent.

DESCRIPTION OF PROCEDURE: With the patient under local anesthesia with intravenous sedation and using the C-arm fluoroscope, a small incision was made in the upper outer left chest. The deltopectoral groove was explored and the cephalic vein was dissected up and ligated distally. It was then hemisected, and an introducer guidewire was passed into the central venous system. A ventricular lead was passed along side this wire, and it was positioned in the right ventricle, revealing an R-wave of 10.4 mV and resistance of 649 ohms, and the threshold showing a loss of capture at 0.2 V was achieved. The current was 0.3 mA at 0.3 V. The peel-away sheath of the introducer set was then introduced over the guidewire, and the dilator and wire were removed. The atrial lead was inserted into the right heart, and it was secured in place in the right atrium. This showed a P-wave of 1.9 mV and resistance of 586 ohms, and the threshold showed a loss of capture at 0.7 V. The current was 1.6 mA at 0.8 V.

The leads were sutured in place at the pectoralis fascia with a 3-0 Prolene, and then the leads were hooked to a Medtronic Adapta L generator. The generator was then implanted in a bluntly created pouch in the upper outer left chest, and then the wound was closed in two layers of 3-0 and 4-0 Vicryl. The skin was closed with Steri-Strips and an occlusive pressure dressing. The patient tolerated the procedure well, and there were no complications.

Sample Reports

ELASTIC INTRAMEDULLARY WIRE FIXATION (NANCY NAILS)

PREOPERATIVE DIAGNOSIS: Fracture, left femur.

POSTOPERATIVE DIAGNOSIS: Fracture, left femur.

OPERATION PERFORMED: Elastic intramedullary wire fixation (Nancy nails).

CLINICAL HISTORY: This very pleasant young lad was snowboarding. After coming out of a jump, he hit a tree. He was seen in the emergency room, had no other injuries and was subsequently referred to me for operative intervention.

The risks of surgery were explained to the family today, including the risks and benefits of antegrade nailing versus elastic retrograde nailing. They have consented.

PROCEDURE: The patient was brought to the operating suite and administered a general anesthetic without complication. The patient was placed on the traction table with the left foot placed in the traction boot and well padded. The unaffected right leg was placed in flexion, abduction and external rotation. The fracture was reduced under fluoroscopic guidance, and the limb was prepped and draped in the usual fashion.

Utilizing 2 focal incisions on the medial and lateral aspects of the femur, both approximately 2 cm above the growth plate, a drill was utilized to gain entry into the metaphyseal region. The drill was then angled, and this was followed by placement of a 4.0 Nancy nail. This was done bilaterally. This was a very difficult fracture to reduce, and we were only able to gain 1 guidewire through the fracture site. For that reason, it necessitated an open aspect over the fracture site, and this allowed us to put bone clamps onto the fracture and reduce it. Once this was performed, both nails were placed across the fracture site, and under fluoroscopic guidance their position was identified both on AP and lateral. The Nancy nails were introduced to the proximal aspect of the femur and to the junction between the greater and lesser trochanter. These were then subsequently pulled back and cut and then reintroduced with a tamp mallet.

The Nancy nails were extruding approximately 2 cm from the bone and not palpable on the skin. Closure consisted of #1 Polysorb for the open aspect of the fracture site, 2-0 Polysorb for the iliotibial band, and staples were applied to the skin. Staples were utilized for the 2 insertion incisions for the distal femur. Appropriate dressings were applied. A Tensor bandage and a posterior splint were applied at the end of the case. Fluoroscopic images were utilized to ensure the near anatomic fixation of the femur.

Instrument, needle, and sponge counts were correct.

ESTIMATED BLOOD LOSS: 600 mL.

COMPLICATIONS: Difficult reduction requiring mini-open procedure.

FOUR-CORNER PARTIAL CARPAL FUSION

PREOPERATIVE DIAGNOSIS: Osteoarthritis stage III to IV right wrist, secondary to scapholunate disruption.

POSTOPERATIVE DIAGNOSIS: Osteoarthritis stage III to IV right wrist, secondary to scapholunate disruption.

PROCEDURE PERFORMED: Four-corner partial carpal fusion, right wrist, with excision of proximal pole of scaphoid.

CLINICAL HISTORY: This is a 50-year-old man with a past history of carcinoma of the prostate who has had a long history of right-greater-than-left wrist arthritis. He has had 2 previous arthroscopies of the right wrist with temporary relief. X-rays show stage III to stage IV ostearthritis of the right wrist secondary to scapholunate ligament disruption. There is some contact of the capitate on the distal radius, but there is still a fairly good lunate facet on the distal radius. The plan is for a 4-corner fusion to unload the wrist radially.

PROCEDURE: The patient was given a spinal anesthetic. A pneumatic tourniquet was elevated to 250 mmHg. A standard 8-cm dorsal approach to the right wrist was used. The interval between the 2nd and 4th extensor compartments was used, removing the EPL tendon from harm's way. A direct dorsal arthrotomy was performed. The joint was completely filled with noninflammatory synovial tissue, and the anatomy was quite distorted. The wrist was quite shortened and radially deviated.

The patient had complete splaying between the scaphoid and the lunate, and the capitate was almost touching the distal radius and had migrated proximally. The scaphoid was quite unstable, and I removed the part that was impinging on the radial styloid with a small osteotome. I removed about a 1- x 1-cm x 5-mm portion of bone. This dealt with the radial carpal impingement, particularly with radial deviation of the wrist.

With distraction, I removed the articular cartilage from the joints between the capitate and the lunate, between the lunate and the hamate, and between the triquetrum and the hamate in particular. The articulation between the hamate and the capitate seemed quite good, as well as between the triquetrum and the lunate, so I did not specifically take these joints apart since they seemed to be so strong ligamentously.

He had enough instability in the wrist without me making the wrist even more unstable. I morselized a portion of the proximal scaphoid that I had excised and packed it between the bony surfaces and then supplemented this with 1 mL of Allomatrix bone putty. Then in compression, I inserted 4 K-wires; 2 in a retrograde fashion from the capitate and hamate into the lunate and triquetrum bones and 1 from the radial side, 1 from the ulnar side, and transversely across the proximal carpal row. Good overall stability was achieved clinically. X-rays confirmed good position of the K-wires and good overall position of the wrist. I tried to correct the deformity and correct the radial deviation. The K-wires were all bent 1 cm from the skin and left protruding. They were manipulated around the extensor tendons so that there was no impingement in particular, and the EPL tendon was spared the K-wire impingement.

The wound was closed with interrupted 2-0 Vicryl suture for the capsule of the wrist, interrupted 2-0 Vicryl for the fascia around the tendon sheaths, interrupted 3-0 Vicryl for subcutaneous and the skin with staples. The wound was dressed with Sofratulle gauze, sterile toppers, and then a below-elbow volar thumb spica splint was applied and held with Kling. Tourniquet time was 105 minutes.

HYBRID EXETER TOTAL HIP ARTHROPLASTY

PREOPERATIVE DIAGNOSIS: Advanced osteoarthritis, right hip.

POSTOPERATIVE DIAGNOSIS: Advanced osteoarthritis, right hip.

PROCEDURE PERFORMED: Right hybrid Exeter total hip arthroplasty.

INDICATIONS: This patient presents with advanced osteoarthritis involving the right hip. She has contralateral disease as well.

PROCEDURE: The patient was anesthetized with a spinal anesthetic. She was on her side, and the leg was prepped and draped. We made a posterior incision and went down through the skin and subcutaneous tissue. Bleeding points were controlled with cautery as they were encountered. We went through the gluteus maximus. The short external rotators were tagged and swept posteriorly. We dislocated the hip. We amputated the femoral head. On the acetabular side, we reamed it. We put in a Trident cup with 2 screws. A polyethylene liner was then snapped into place. On the femoral side, we put in a distal bone plug. The cement was pressure injected. We put in a #0 stem and 28-mm head. This hip was reduced and was found to be very stable.

The patient tolerated this well. She was returned to the recovery room in good condition.

LEFT TOTAL HIP ARTHROPLASTY

PREOPERATIVE DIAGNOSIS: Avascular necrosis, left hip.

POSTOPERATIVE DIAGNOSIS: Avascular necrosis, left hip.

PROCEDURE PERFORMED: Left total hip arthroplasty.

APPROACH: Anterolateral.

DEVICES USED: Stryker, Exeter #4, 44-mm offset cemented stem, 54-mm Trident PSL solid cup with standard neutral polyethylene.

PROCEDURE: The patient was brought to the operating room, and spinal anesthetic was applied. The patient was moved into the right lateral decubitus position and supported on the Montreal frame. Sterile prep and free drape was performed on the left hip, leg, and buttock. A lateral incision was made, and dissection was carried down to the subcutaneous tissues and through the iliotibial band and tensor fascia lata. The anterior third of the abductors was elevated using electrocautery. Then a capsulotomy was performed, and the hip was dislocated. This was quite a deformed head with avascular collapse. A femoral neck cut was made. A retractor was placed on the acetabulum. Acetabular tissues were excised. The acetabulum was then reamed up to 54 considering that we did not overly medialize. A #54 solid cup was impacted with good fit, and a neutral liner was put into position. We then brought the leg over to the side of the table in the leg bag and approached the proximal femur with a box osteotome and a T-handled awl, followed by a rasp up to a #4, 44 offset. Trial reduction with a standard head revealed good soft tissue tension and stability. After dislocating, the box osteotome was removed. A large cement restrictor was placed at 18 cm from the tip of the trochanter. The canal was irrigated with cold saline and packed with gauze.

Three packs of Simplex cement with antibiotics were vacuum mixed. The canal was then dried, and, at approximately 4 minutes' time, the cement was injected into the canal and pressurized. A prosthesis was passed into the canal at approximately 6 minutes' time and held in position until the cement was hard. All excess cement was removed. Trial reduction with a +4 head revealed the hip to be quite tight. We dislocated, and we placed a standard 28-mm head onto the Morse taper and reduced the hip. We had good range of motion and stability. The hip was irrigated and closed by re-apposition of the abductors on the greater trochanter in anatomic fashion using #2 Tycron through soft tissues. The hip had been infiltrated with local anesthetic and Toradol. We closed the iliotibial band and fascia lata with #1 Vicryl, the subcutaneous layer with 2-0 Vicryl, and the skin with staples. The wound was dressed with Coverlet, reinforcing gauze and Cover-Roll.

The patient was taken from the operating room to the postanesthetic recovery room without difficulty. He will be transferred back to the floor when stable. He will be mobilized and weightbearing as tolerated. He will be started on DVT prophylaxis and will continue on infection prophylaxis, of which he received one dose preoperatively.

OPEN REDUCTION PLATING AND WIRING, LEFT FEMORAL FRACTURE, TYPE 2 PERIPROSTHETIC FRACTURE

PREOPERATIVE DIAGNOSIS: Periprosthetic femoral fracture, left midshaft femur.

POSTOPERATIVE DIAGNOSIS: Periprosthetic femoral fracture, left midshaft femur.

PROCEDURE PERFORMED: Open reduction plating and wiring, left femoral fracture, type 2 periprosthetic fracture.

CLINICAL HISTORY: This is a 76-year-old man with numerous medical problems, including a recent coronary artery bypass, Parkinson disease, and left total hip replacement 4 years ago. Late yesterday he fell injuring his left hip. He was kept in the cast room until beds were available. He was subsequently admitted and prepared for surgery in the trauma room. I was asked to take over care because I was the trauma room surgeon today. X-rays show a well-cemented Exeter-type total hip replacement. He had a fracture starting at the tip and extending distally in a spiral; a type 2 or 3 periprosthetic fracture.

PROCEDURE: The patient was given a spinal anesthetic and converted to a general anesthetic by the anesthesiologist. Anatomy of the patient was difficult.

The patient was rolled into the decubitus position, left side up. He was extremely stiff from his Parkinson disease, and he had a lot of swelling in the leg. After prepping and draping, a standard 30-cm lateral approach to the femur was used. Dissection was difficult because of his large leg and his stiffness, and he bled throughout the procedure. Ultimately, the fracture was cleared of debris. The cement restrictor was removed since it was somewhat protuberant. Ultimately, with a lot of effort, I was able to get the fracture reduced anatomically with bone clamps and my assistant nurse helping. I used 2 interfragmentary screws, applied a 10-inch Howmedica Dall-Miles cable plate and then fixed it distally with 4 screws; 1 to 2 screws in the interfragmentary area and then proximally with 3 wires. Anatomical reduction was achieved and maintained with good stable fixation. The patient continued to bleed throughout the procedure. I would estimate the blood loss to be about 2000 mL. He received 2 units of cross-matched blood intraoperatively and received 2 units postoperatively.

The wound was closed with interrupted and continuous 0 Vicryl suture in 2 layers, interrupted 2-0 Vicryl to subcutaneous, and skin with staples. The wound was dressed with Sofratulle, gauze, sterile toppers, and Cover-Roll. The leg lengths were equal at the end of the procedure.

POLYETHYLENE CUP REVISION, PLACEMENT OF FEMORAL STEM

PREOPERATIVE DIAGNOSIS: Loose stem and worn patellar cup, right total hip arthroplasty.

POSTOPERATIVE DIAGNOSIS: Loose stem and worn patellar cup, right total hip arthroplasty.

OPERATION PERFORMED: Revision of polyethylene cup and placement of femoral stem, right total hip arthroplasty.

PROCEDURE: This 68 year-old lady was taken to the operating room with a preoperative diagnosis of loose stem and worn patellar cup, right total hip arthroplasty.

The patient was anesthetized, was placed in the left lateral position, and the right hip was prepped and draped. Dissection was carried down to the greater trochanter, and the pseudojoint capsule was excised posteriorly. The loose femoral stem was removed. Then the acetabular component was removed and replaced with a new 62-mm outer diameter, 28-mm inner diameter shell. Cleansing and débridement of the femoral canal was carried out. Then methyl methacrylate was pressure injected into the femur and the Exeter stem placed. Trial was made with different necks, and the +4 long neck was applied. This provided satisfactory stability with some increase in length. Range of motion was stable.

The wound was irrigated with vancomycin and saline solution and then closed in layers with Vicryl and staples to the skin. A sterile bandage was applied with a pressure bandage and a knee splint to that leg.

The patient was sent to the recovery room in satisfactory condition.

REVISION TOTAL KNEE ARTHROPLASTY, LEFT

PREOPERATIVE DIAGNOSIS: Aseptic loosening, total knee arthroplasty, left.

POSTOPERATIVE DIAGNOSIS: Aseptic loosening, total knee arthroplasty, left.

OPERATION PERFORMED: Revision total knee arthroplasty, left.

APPROACH: Medial parapatellar with quadriceps turn down.

DEVICES USED: Scorpio TS #5 stemmed femoral component with distal 5-mm augments and lateral posterior 5-mm augment, 18-mm polyethylene constrained, #5 stemmed tibial component cemented with a 10-mm full augmentation block.

PROCEDURE: Spinal anesthetic was applied. Sterile prep and drape was performed on the left knee. A midline incision was made along the existing scar under tourniquet control. Dissection was carried down to subcutaneous tissue. This knee only flexed to about 35 degrees. We did a medial parapatellar arthrotomy. The tissues were very tight, so I decided to proceed with a quadriceps turn down. This was performed. We then dissected into the joint and resected chronic granulation tissue, which was black in color from wear. We did a full synovectomy. We were then able to remove the polyethylene. Following this we were able to remove the femoral component, which was loose and came out easily without any bone loss. We were then able to flex the knee and remove the tibial component, again without difficulty. I proceeded to remove all remaining cement. There was significant bone loss on the tibia. We reamed up the tibial canal to 12. We then put our cutting guide in position and took off minimal bone, but to get good adequate bone we did have to lower the joint line considerably. We then proceeded to size the tibia for #5 and used a 4-mm offset to make the stem fit.

We then went to the femur and reamed up the femoral canal and placed our Mancini block and set the appropriate rotation, and we used a 4-mm offset as well. We then set our flexion and extension, bringing the leg into extension and into flexion and adjusting the distal femoral component to size the polyethylene. With the 21-polyethylene in, we had roughly equal flexion and extension gaps, so we therefore decided to go with a full block augment on the tibia. The appropriate cuts were made for the femur using the Mancini block with distal 5-mm augments and a posterolateral 5-mm augment. Trial components were removed. Some bone graft was morselized from the bank. We had one femoral head. This bone graft was placed in the distal femur where there were some constrained defects. There was a defect in the posteromedial tibia, and some bone graft was placed in this area. We then thoroughly completed our débridement. There were no signs of infection, and tissue was sent for culture.

We then prepared the components as previously mentioned on the back table. Two packages of Simplex cement with antibiotics were mixed. The tibial component was cemented in place. We did not cement the stem. We then cemented the femoral component, snapped in the trial polyethylene and brought the leg into extension. Excess cement was removed. Once the cement was hard, we once again examined the knee for flexion and extension, and it was equal as we anticipated, but we did go up to an

18-mm poly. This was put into position. The patella was stable, and we did not revise the patella. We had to do a lateral release, and then at this point we recognized there was some partial avulsion of the insertion of the patellar tendon. This reduction though was prior to cementing, and we placed two #5 Ethibond through the bone at that level. We then passed the suture up along the tendon to help secure it in position.

We then proceeded to close by re-apposing the quadriceps turn down with #2 Tycron. The remainder of the arthrotomy was closed with #1 Vicryl. The knee was infiltrated with local anesthetic and Toradol. The subcutaneous layer was closed with 2-0 Vicryl and the skin with staples. Total tourniquet time was 135 minutes. This was in 2 blocks, roughly equal, with about half an hour in between when the tourniquet was down. The wound was dressed with Coverlet, reinforcing gauze, abdominal lap pad, and Tensor.

The patient was taken to the postanesthetic recovery room without difficulty. She will be mobilized, partial weightbearing. She will be started on early range of motion. At the end of the procedure, we had flexion up to about 95 degrees and full extension. Estimated blood loss was approximately 500 mL.

RIGHT TOTAL HIP ARTHROPLASTY

PREOPERATIVE DIAGNOSIS: Advanced osteoarthritis, possible avascular necrosis, right hip.

POSTOPERATIVE DIAGNOSIS: Advanced osteoarthritis, possible avascular necrosis, right hip.

PROCEDURE PERFORMED: Right total hip arthroplasty.

APPROACH: Anterolateral.

DEVICES USED: Stryker Exeter #1, 50 mm offset cemented stem, 62-mm Trident cluster PSL cup with 3 screws and a Crossfire liner 36-mm internal diameter and +5, 36-mm head.

PROCEDURE: The patient was brought to the operating room, and a general anesthetic was applied in the supine position. The patient was moved into the left lateral decubitus position and supported with a Montreal frame. Sterile prep and free drape was performed on the right hip, leg, and buttock. A lateral incision was made. Dissection was carried down to subcutaneous tissues into the iliotibial band and tensor fascia lata. The anterior third of the abductors was elevated using electrocautery, and then a capsulectomy was performed. The hip was dislocated, and a femoral neck cut was made. This was a grossly deformed femoral head. We then placed retractors around the acetabulum and excised periacetabular and foveal tissues. We then reamed the acetabulum up to 62. There was some posterior and superior deficiency where there has been excessive wear from the head, but overall there was over 80% circumferential coverage. We then impacted a #62 cluster PSL cup and secured it with 3 screws with good purchase. A Crossfire liner with 36 mm internal diameter was applied. We then brought the leg over to the side of the table in the leg bag and approached the proximal femur with a box osteotome and a T-handled awl followed by a rasp. We were able to see the #1, 15-mm offset stent. I had templated the patient for at least #50 offset. We then did a trial reduction with a standard head, and we had reasonable soft tissue tension and stability. We therefore dislocated the hip and removed the broach. The canal was irrigated with cold saline after placing a cement restrictor. The canal was packed with gauze.

Two packages of Simplex cement with antibiotics were vacuum mixed. In approximately 4.5 minutes' time, the cement was injected into the dried canal and then pressurized. At approximately 5.5 minutes' time, the prosthesis was passed into the canal into appropriate position. It did seat a little deeper than the trial. It was held in position until the cement was hard. We then did a trial reduction of the +5 head. This allowed good soft tissue tension and stability. We therefore dislocated the hip and applied the +5, 36-mm head. The hip was atraumatically reduced after irrigating.

We then proceeded to close by re-apposing the abductors onto the trochanter which we débrided, and we then used #2 Tycron through bone to repair the abductors. The hip was infiltrated with local anesthetic and Toradol. We repaired the iliotibial band and tensor fascia lata with #1 Vicryl, the subcutaneous layer with 2-0 Vicryl, and the skin with staples. The wound was dressed with Coverlet, reinforcing gauze, and Cover-Roll.

The patient was reversed from anesthetic and transferred to the postanesthetic recovery room without difficulty. He will be transferred back to the floor when stable. He will be mobilized, weightbearing as tolerated. He will be started on DVT prophylaxis and will continue on infection prophylaxis, of which he received one dose preoperatively.

RIGHT TOTAL HIP ARTHROPLASTY - 2

PREOPERATIVE DIAGNOSIS: Osteoarthritis, right hip.

POSTOPERATIVE DIAGNOSIS: Osteoarthritis, right hip.

PROCEDURE PERFORMED: Right total hip arthroplasty.

APPROACH: Anterolateral.

DEVICES USED: Stryker Secur-Fit HA #8 uncemented stem, -2.5 ceramic alumina head, 52-mm Trident PSL solid cup with neutral ceramic alumina liner.

PROCEDURE: The patient was brought to the operating room, and a spinal anesthetic was applied. The patient was moved into the left lateral decubitus position and supported with the Montreal frame. Sterile prep and free drape was performed on the right hip, leg, and buttock. A lateral incision was made, and dissection was carried down to the subcutaneous tissues and through the iliotibial band and tensor fascia lata. The anterior third of the abductors was elevated using electrocautery. Capsulectomy was performed, and the hip was dislocated. A femoral neck cut was made. Retractors were placed around the acetabulum. Acetabular tissues were excised. The acetabulum was then reamed up to 52. There was a superior cyst, which was filled with some bone reamings. A 52 solid Trident cup was impacted with good fit. A neutral ceramic liner was then applied without difficulty.

The leg was brought over to the side of the table in a leg bag. The proximal femur was approached using a box osteotome, a T-handled awl, and followed by rasps, starting with the smallest up to a #8 which seated well. Trial reduction revealed the hip to be a little tight. The hip was dislocated, and the rasp was seated another 2 to 3 mm. The rasp was then removed. We irrigated the canal. We then took a #8 Secur-Fit HA stem and passed it into the proximal femur, and it seated quite well, although a little bit proud. I could not advance it after a significant amount of tapping. We then did trial reduction of -2.5, and the hip was a little tight but certainly acceptable. We dislocated the hip and placed a -2.5 alumina head and reduced the hip atraumatically. The hip had good range of motion and was stable. We had removed some osteophytes inferior and posterior around the acetabulum.

The hip was irrigated and closed by re-opposing the abductors on the trochanter in an anatomic fashion using #2 Tycron. This was done through soft tissue and through bone. The hip was infiltrated with local anesthetic and Toradol. The iliotibial band and tensor fascia lata were closed with #1 Vicryl, subcutaneous layer with 2-0 Vicryl, and skin with staples. The wound was dressed with Coverlets, reinforcing gauze, and Cover-Roll.

The patient was taken from the operating room to the postanesthetic recovery room without difficulty. She will be transferred back to the floor when stable. She will be mobilized, partial weightbearing. She will be started on DVT prophylaxis and will continue on infection prophylaxis, of which she received one dose preoperatively.

TOTAL HIP ARTHROPLASTY, RIGHT

PREOPERATIVE DIAGNOSES: Developmental dysplasia, right hip with subsequent degenerative changes.

POSTOPERATIVE DIAGNOSES: Developmental dysplasia, right hip with subsequent degenerative changes.

OPERATION PERFORMED: Total hip arthroplasty, right.

CLINICAL HISTORY: This very pleasant lady has been suffering from endstage arthritic changes. She had what appeared to be a Crowe 1/Crowe 2 DDH hip with subsequent degenerative changes. The risks of surgery were explained to her. Certainly the biggest risk was that of requirement for revision, as she is a very young lady. She was understanding and arrives to the operating suite in stable condition.

INSTRUMENTATION

1. Longevity crosslink polyethylene liner (36-mm inside diameter, 3.5-mm offset).

2. Bone screw x 2.

3. Trabecular metal modular acetabular system, 50-mm outside diameter (multi-hole porous).

4. VerSys Hip System femoral head, 12/14 taper, 36-mm diameter (plus 0).

5. ZMR Hip System femoral body, 12/14 taper, standard 40-mm neck offset, cone body, size AA, 35-mm build up.

6. ZMR Hip System femoral stem revision, 12-mm diameter, 115-mm stem length, straight porous.

PROCEDURE: The patient was brought to the operating suite and administered general anesthetic without complication. Ancef 1 g was given, and the patient was placed in the left lateral decubitus position with the right hip uppermost. This position was held in place with a Montreal frame. All bony prominences were protected. The planned posterolateral skin incision was marked with a marker, and the limb was prepped and draped in the usual fashion.

Utilizing a posterolateral skin incision, the skin and subcutaneous tissues were dissected. The iliotibial band was identified and dissected in line with the skin incision. The bursa off the greater trochanter was released. All visible bleeders were identified and coagulated. The sciatic nerve was identified and a vessel loop placed around it for identification throughout the case. The piriformis and the external rotators were identified, dissected, and tagged for closure at the end of the case. A separate posterior capsule layer was identified, dissected, and tagged for closure at the end of the case. An inferior capsulectomy and a superior capsulectomy were performed. The labrum was removed, and the hip was dislocated. Osteotomy of the femoral head was performed approximately 1.5 cm above the lesser trochanter. The head was significantly deformed.

Our attention then turned to visualization of the acetabulum, and an appropriate retractor was utilized to allow removal of soft tissue. The teardrop was identified, and soft tissue was removed. All interfering overhanging soft tissue was also removed from the acetabulum. As per preoperative templating, we started small and reached to 50 mm reaming of the acetabulum. This showed good coverage, and a trial window was placed in this with a nice snug fit. For this reason, a trabecular metal cup was introduced and seated very well with a nice tight fit. One screw was placed into the safe zone, and a temporary liner was placed in the acetabulum.

Our attention then turned to the femoral component, and a box osteotome was followed by placement of the starter reamer followed by sequential reaming. As per preoperative templating, we got significantly good chatter at approximately 11 mm, and at the planned 12 mm there was a nice snug fit. It should be noted that the neck in this DDH situation was relatively retroverted, and thus it was felt that a cone body would be required. For that reason, the proximal body was reamed, and a cone body with a 115-mm straight temporary stem was placed down and a -3.5, 36-mm ball trialed. This in fact was very snug.

Ranawat sign appeared normal indicating that we had achieved appropriate combined anteversion. Thornhill shuck test was normal indicating that we had good soft tissue tension. At zero degrees flexion, the hip could not be reduced to internal rotation. At 90 degrees of flexion and zero degrees adduction, the hip was seen to dislocate at approximately 90 degrees internal rotation. At slight adduction (10 degrees) and 90 degrees of flexion, the hip was dislocated at 85 degrees internal rotation. This was very stable. A routine intraoperative x-ray was performed while thorough irrigation was placed in the wound. Assessment of this demonstrated good anteversion and good fit and fill of the component. Temporary components were removed, and one further acetabular screw was placed in the safe zone followed by placement of the crosslink polyethylene, which was introduced and seated without complication.

Our attention was then turned to placing the femoral component together, and this was done on the back table and then introduced with a nice snug fit. It sat down slightly more than the trial, and thus we trialed a +0 ball, and this correlated with the previously mentioned areas of stability. The femoral ball was placed on, and the hip was reduced and was found to be very stable.

Thorough irrigation was placed in the wound, and closure consisted of piriformis and external rotation closure to soft tissue followed by closure of the posterior capsule through drill holes into the greater trochanter. The iliotibial band was closed with heavy nonabsorbable stitch, 2-0 Polysorb was utilized subcutaneously and staples were applied to the skin. A drain was utilized and introduced through a separate stab hole and sutured in place. Appropriate dressings were applied, and the patient was placed on her back and an abduction pillow placed prior to transfer to her hospital bed. She was returned to the recovery room in stable condition for routine recovery room x-ray. Instrument, needle, and sponge counts were correct.

ESTIMATED BLOOD LOSS: 800 mL.

PLAN: This patient will be partial weightbearing. We will progress her as we can, pending clinical and radiographic correlation.

URETEROSCOPIC STONE EXTRACTION AND PLACEMENT OF DOUBLE-J STENT

PREOPERATIVE DIAGNOSIS: Left renal colic with impacted large calculus, distal left ureter.

POSTOPERATIVE DIAGNOSIS: Left renal colic with impacted large calculus, distal left ureter.

OPERATION PERFORMED: Ureteroscopic stone extraction and placement of double-J stent.

CLINICAL HISTORY: The patient is a 71-year-old gentleman who was admitted to the hospital through the emergency room when he presented with an acute renal colic. A CT scan confirmed the presence of a 7-mm calculus in the distal ureter, and there was a question about other little stones, although in the reports that he had with him that was not reported. A plain film of the abdomen in the emergency room showed a big stone at the distal left ureter and a possible other little calculus in the upper part of the left kidney, but it was difficult to know if it was in the bowel or in the kidney itself. So he obviously needed attention to the stone in the distal left ureter.

PROCEDURE: He was taken to the operating room, and under satisfactory general anesthesia in the lithotomy position he was prepped and draped. A #21 scope was introduced into the bladder. He was found to have discrete trilobar prostatic hypertrophy and a lot of residual urine which was sent for C&S. He had at least 500 mL. He apparently had gone to the washroom just before he came down, and that is significant, as he thought he had been voiding very well. The left ureter was somewhat edematous, and attempts to pass by the calculus with an extra stiff Amplatz guidewire proved to be extremely difficult. So we tried an extra slippery guidewire, and again we could not do it. So we put a balloon dilator in the distal ureter, so we could then dilate the distal ureter enough to be able to put a #8 ureteroscope into the ureter.

We could actually see the stone, and just behind the stone there was the lumen of the ureter. In an attempt to put the guidewire through before that, we made a couple of little false passages in the ureter, so it was important to leave in a stent for at least a couple of weeks to make sure that the ureter heals well. The stone was removed. This was a big jagged stone, and little fragments were removed, and we could not see any stones in the upper tract, but we will be repeating x-rays tomorrow. We left a double-J stent #6, 24-cm long in the left collecting system. This will provide him with drainage, and we will make sure that his bladder empties completely by doing an ultrasound scan in the next day or two to make sure that he really gets rid of all the urine; if not he will have to be tried on medical management.

The procedure was really very well tolerated. On the rectal exam, the prostate is well circumscribed, maybe 25 to 30 g, bilobar in nature and benign in consistency. It is anticipated he will have an entirely uneventful recovery.

Appendix 3
Common Terms by Procedure

Dual-Chamber Pacemaker Insertion
3-0 Prolene
4-0 Vicryl
anesthesia
atrial lead
atrium
C-arm fluoroscope
cephalic vein
deltopectoral groove
dilator
dual-chamber pacemaker
endocardium
guidewire
heart block
hemisect
Holter monitor
intravenous sedation
introducer guidewire
ligate
Medtronic Adapta L generator
pectoralis fascia
peel-away sheath
pressure dressing
P-wave
resistance
right ventricle
R-wave
sick sinus syndrome.
Steri-Strips
ventricular lead

Elastic Intramedullary Wire Fixation (Nancy Nails)
#1 Polysorb
2-0 Polysorb
4.0 Nancy nail

anatomic fixation
anesthetic
antegrade nailing
bone clamp
drill
elastic intramedullary wire fixation
elastic retrograde nailing
femur
fluoroscopic guidance
fluoroscopic image
fracture
guidewire
iliotibial band
metaphyseal
Nancy nail
posterior splint
staple
tamp mallet
Tensor bandage
traction boot
traction table

Four-Corner Partial Carpal Fusion
4-corner fusion
Allomatrix bone putty
arthroscopy
articular cartilage
capitate
carpal fusion
carpal impingement
deformity
distal radius
dorsal arthrotomy
EPL tendon
extensor compartment
extensor tendon

hamate
interrupted 2-0 Vicryl suture
interrupted 3-0 Vicryl
Kling
K-wire
lunate
lunate facet
osteoarthritis
osteotome
pneumatic tourniquet
proximal scaphoid
radial deviation
radial styloid
retrograde
scaphoid
scapholunate disruption
scapholunate ligament
Sofratulle gauze
spica splint
spinal anesthetic
staple
sterile topper
subcutaneous
synovial tissue
tourniquet
triquetrum

Hybrid Exeter Total Hip Arthroplasty
#0 stem
28-mm head
acetabular
bleeding point
cautery
cement
contralateral disease
distal bone plug
external rotator
femoral head
gluteus maximus
hybrid Exeter total hip arthroplasty
osteoarthritis

polyethylene liner
pressure inject
screw
skin
spinal anesthetic
subcutaneous tissue
Trident cup

Left Total Hip Arthroplasty
#1 Vicryl
#2 Tycron
#54 solid cup
2-0 Vicryl
28-mm head
44-mm offset cemented stem
54-mm Trident PSL solid cup
abductor
acetabulum
anatomic fashion
apposition
avascular collapse
avascular necrosis
box osteotome
capsulotomy
cement restrictor
cold saline
Coverlet
Cover-Roll
dissection
DVT prophylaxis
electrocautery
Exeter #4
fascia lata
femoral neck
free drape
gauze
greater trochanter
iliotibial band
infection prophylaxis
right lateral decubitus position
leg bag
local anesthetic

Montreal frame
Morse taper
neutral liner
polyethylene
prosthesis
proximal femur
range of motion
rasp
reduction
reinforcing gauze
retractor
Simplex cement with antibiotics
soft tissue tension
spinal anesthetic
stability
staple
sterile prep
Stryker
subcutaneous tissue
tensor fascia lata
T-handled awl
Toradol
total hip arthroplasty
trochanter
vacuum mixed

Open Reduction Plating and Wiring, Left Femoral Fracture, Type 2 Periprosthetic Fracture

0 Vicryl suture
2-0 Vicryl
30-cm lateral approach
anatomical reduction
bone clamp
cement restrictor
Cover-Roll
cross-matched blood
decubitus position
Exeter-type total hip replacement
femoral fracture
femur
gauze

general anesthetic
Howmedica Dall-Miles cable plate
interfragmentary area
interfragmentary screw
midshaft femur
open reduction
periprosthetic fracture
plating
Sofratulle
spinal anesthetic
spiral
stable fixation
staple
sterile topper
subcutaneous
wire
wiring

Polyethylene Cup Revision, Placement of Femoral Stem

+4 long neck
acetabular component
débridement
dissection
Exeter stem
femoral canal
femoral stem
femur
greater trochanter
knee splint
left lateral position
loose stem
methyl methacrylate
polyethylene cup
pressure bandage
pseudojoint capsule
range of motion
saline solution
shell
stability
staple
sterile bandage

total hip arthroplasty.
vancomycin
Vicryl
worn patellar cup

Revision Total Knee Arthroplasty, Left
#1 Vicryl
#2 Tycron
#5 Ethibond
#5 stemmed tibial component
18-mm poly
18-mm polyethylene
2-0 Vicryl
21-polyethylene
4-mm offset
5-mm augment
abdominal lap pad
arthrotomy
aseptic loosening
bank
bone graft
cement
chronic granulation tissue
Coverlet
cutting guide
débridement
dissection
extension gap
femoral canal
femoral component
femoral head
femur
flexion gap
full augmentation block
full block augment
joint line
lateral release
local anesthetic
Mancini block
medial parapatellar arthrotomy
midline incision

parapatellar
partial avulsion
partial weightbearing
patella
patellar tendon
polyethylene
posteromedial tibia
quadriceps turn down
range of motion
reduction
reinforcing gauze
revision
Scorpio TS #5 stemmed femoral
    component
Simplex cement with antibiotics
spinal anesthetic
staple
stem
sterile prep and drape
subcutaneous layer
subcutaneous tissue
suture
synovectomy
tendon
Tensor
tibia
tibial canal
tibial component
Toradol
total knee arthroplasty
tourniquet control
tourniquet time
trial component
trial polyethylene

Right Total Hip Arthroplasty
#1 Vicryl
#2 Tycron
#50 offset
#62 cluster PSL cup
+5 head
+5, 36-mm head

2-0 Vicryl
50-mm offset cemented stem
62-mm Trident cluster PSL cup
abductor
acetabulum
avascular necrosis
box osteotome
canal
capsulectomy
cement
cement restrictor
circumferential coverage
cold saline
Coverlet
Cover-Roll
Crossfire liner
dissection
DVT prophylaxis
electrocautery
femoral head
femoral neck cut
foveal tissue
free drape
gauze
general anesthetic
iliotibial band
infection prophylaxis
left lateral decubitus position
leg bag
local anesthetic
Montreal frame
offset stent
osteoarthritis
periacetabular tissue
prosthesis
proximal femur
rasp
reinforcing gauze
retractor
screw
Simplex cement with antibiotics
soft tissue tension and stability
standard head

staple
sterile prep
Stryker Exeter #1
subcutaneous layer
supine position
tensor fascia lata
T-handled awl
Toradol
total hip arthroplasty
trial reduction
trochanter
vacuum mixed
weightbearing

Right Total Hip Arthroplasty - 2

#1 Vicryl
#2 Tycron
#8 Secur-Fit HA stem
-2.5 ceramic alumina head
2-0 Vicryl
52 solid Trident cup
52-mm Trident PSL solid cup
abductor
acetabular tissue
acetabulum
alumina head
anatomic fashion
anterolateral
bone reamings
box osteotome
canal
capsulectomy
ceramic liner
Coverlets
Cover-Roll
dissection
DVT prophylaxis
electrocautery
femoral neck cut
free drape
iliotibial band

infection prophylaxis
left lateral decubitus position
leg bag
local anesthetic
Montreal frame
neutral ceramic alumina liner
osteoarthritis
osteophyte
partial weightbearing
proximal femur
range of motion
rasp
reinforcing gauze
retractor
spinal anesthetic
staple
sterile prep
Stryker Secur-Fit HA #8 uncemented
  stem
subcutaneous tissue
tensor fascia lata
T-handled awl
Toradol
total hip arthroplasty
trial reduction

Total Hip Arthroplasty, Right

+0 ball
12/14 taper
2-0 Polysorb
abduction pillow
acetabular screw
acetabulum
adduction
Ancef
anteversion
bleeders
bone screw
bony prominence
box osteotome
bursa
chatter

coagulate
cone body
crosslink polyethylene
Crowe 1/Crowe 2 DDH hip
DDH (developmental dislocation of the
  hip)
degenerative change
developmental dysplasia
dissect
drain
drill hole
endstage arthritic change
external rotator
femoral ball
femoral body
femoral head
flexion
general anesthetic
greater trochanter
iliotibial band
inferior capsulectomy
internal rotation
intraoperative x-ray
irrigation
labrum
left lateral decubitus position
lesser trochanter
longevity crosslink polyethylene liner
marker
Montreal frame
multihole porous
nonabsorbable stitch
osteotomy
partial weightbearing
piriformis
posterior capsule
posterior capsule layer
posterolateral skin incision
preoperative template
proximal body
Ranawat sign
recovery room x-ray
retractor

safe zone
sciatic nerve
screw
soft tissue tension
stab hole
standard 40-mm neck offset
staple
starter reamer
straight temporary stem
subcutaneous tissue
superior capsulectomy
teardrop
temporary liner
Thornhill shuck test
total hip arthroplasty
trabecular metal cup
trabecular metal modular acetabular
  system
trial window
VerSys Hip System femoral head
vessel loop
ZMR Hip System
ZMR Hip System femoral stem revision

Ureteroscopic Stone Extraction and Placement of Double-J Stent

#21 scope
#8 ureteroscope

acute renal colic
Amplatz guidewire
balloon dilator
benign
bilobar
bladder
bowel
calculus
collecting system
CT scan
distal ureter
double-J stent
drainage
edematous
general anesthesia
kidney
lithotomy position
lumen
medical management
prostate
rectal exam
stent
stone
plain film
trilobar prostatic hypertrophy
ultrasound scan
ureter
ureteroscopic stone extraction
urine
x-ray

Common Manufacturers and Web Sites

Note: Mergers, acquisitions, and new entrants in the medical and scientific equipment industry contribute to this collection.

Manufacturer	Web Site
Abbott Laboratories	www.abbott.com
ABCO Dealers, Inc.	www.goetzedental.com/abco.html
Accurate Surgical & Scientific Instrument Corp. (ASSI)	www.accuratesurgical.com
Accuscope	www.accu-scope.com
Accutome	www.accutome.com
Achilles USA	www.achillesusa.com
ACI Medical	www.acimedical.com
Ackrad Laboratories, Inc.	www.ackrad.com
Acme United Corp., Medical Division	www.acmeunited.com
ACMI Circon	www.circon.com
Acromed Corp.	www.johnsonandjohnson.com
ACS (Applied Cardiac Systems)	www.acsholter.com
Action Products, Inc.	www.actionproducts.com
Acuson, Inc.	www.acuson.com
Adenna, Inc.	www.adenna.com
Advanced Bionics Cor.	www.bionicear.com
Advanced Neuromodulation Systems	www.ans-medical.com
Advanced Ortho Systems	www.advanced-ortho.net
AdvantaJet	www.advantajet.com
Aesculap, Inc.	www.aesculap.de
Alcon Surgical, Inc.	www.alconlabs.com
Aldrich Chemical Co.	www.sigma-aldrich.com
Alimed, Inc.	www.alimed.com
Allegiance Healthcare Corp.	www.allegiance.net
Allergan Inc.	www.allergan.com
Allied Healthcare	www.alliedhpi.com
Alltech Associates, Inc.	www.alltechweb.com
AMAC Inc./Immunotech, Inc.	www.immunotech.com
American Endoscopy Services, Inc.	www.aesendo.com

American Endoscopy/Amersham Corp.	www.amersham.co.uk/
American Type Culture Collection	www.atcc.org
Amersham Corp.	www.amersham.com
AmerisourceBergen	www.amerisourcebergen.com
Angeion Corp.	www.angeion.com
Apple Medical Corp.	www.applemed.com
Applied Cardiac Systems, Inc. (ACS)	www.acsholter.com
Applied Imaging Corp.	www.cytovision.com
Arrow International, Inc.	www.arrowintl.com
Astra U.S.A., Inc.	www.astra.com
AstraZeneca International	www.astrazeneca.com
Atlas Surgical	www.sahaj.com
AVL Medical Instruments	www.avlmed.com
Bard, Inc., C. R.	www.crbard.com
Baxter Healthcare Corp.	www.baxter.com
Bayer Diagnostics	www.bayerdiag.com
BBL Microbiology Systems/Becton Dickinson	www.bd.com
Beckman Coulter, Inc. (Beckman Instruments)	www.beckmancoulter.com
Becton Dickinson and Co.	www.bd.com
Beere Precision Medical Instruments, Inc.	www.beeremedical.com
Beltone Electronics Corp.	www.beltone.com
Bennett X-Ray Corp.	www.bennettx-ray.com
Benson Medical	www.bensonmedical.ca
Biodex Medical Systems, Inc.	www.biodex.com
Bioject, Inc.	www.bioject.com
Bio-Logic Systems, Corp.	www.blsc.com
Bio-Lok International, Inc.	www.biolok.com
Bio-Med Devices, Inc.	www.biomeddevices.com
Bio-Medicus, Inc.	www.medtronic.com
Biomet, Inc.	www.biomet.com
Bio-Rad Laboratories Ltd.	www.bio-rad.com
Biosound, Inc.	www.biosound.com
Bird & Cronin Medical	www.birdcronin.com
Bird Life Design	www.trianim.com

Bledsoe Brace Systems	www.bledsoebrace.com
Boehringer Mannheim Corporation	www.boehringer.com
Boekel Scientific	www.boekelsci.com
Boston Scientific Corporation	www.bsci.com
Braintree Scientific, Inc.	www.braintreesci.com
Brasseler USA/Komer Medical	www.brasselerusa.com
Braun Medical Inc.	www.bbraunusa.com
Breas	www.breas.com
Bristol-Myers Co./Mead Johnson & Company	www.bms.com www.meadjohnson.com
Bristol-Myers Squibb Pharmaceutical	www.bms.com
Bruel & Kjaer Instruments, Inc.	www.bk.dk
Bruker Instruments	www.bruker.com
Burroughs Wellcome Co.	www.glaxowellcome.com
C.B. Fleet Co., Inc.	www.cbfleet.com
Cabot Medical Corporation	(See ACMI)
Carbomedics, Inc.	www.carbomedics.com
Cardiovascular Imaging Systems (CVIS)	www.bsci.com
Cardio-Vascular Innovations, Inc.	www.cvico.com
Cardiovascular Systems/3M Health Care	www.3m.com
Carolina Medical, Inc.	www.caromed.com
Carrington Laboratories, Inc.	www.carringtonlabs.com
Cavitron CO2 Laser Systems/Cooper Life Sciences, Inc.	(See CooperVision, Inc) www.cooper+smith.com
Cavitron Surgical Systems, Inc./ Valleylab, Inc.	www.valleylab.com
Cavitron/Syntel Division/Alcon Surgical	www.alconlabs.com
Cell Robotics	www.cellrobotics.com
Cetylite Industries, Inc.	www.cetylite.com
Chiron Corporation	www.chiron.com
Cho-Pat, Inc.	www.cho-pat.com
Chughtai	www.chughtaidental.com
Ciba Corning Diagnostics Corporation	(See Chiron Corp.)
Ciba Vision Corporation	www.cibavision.com
Cilco/Alcon Surgical	www.alconlabs.com
Cincinnati Surgical Company	www.cincinnatisurgical.com
Circon Corporation	www.acmicorp.com

Common Manufacturers & Web Sites

Clarus Medical Systems, Inc.	www.clarusmedical.com
Clinimed, Inc.	www.clinimed.com
Clinipad Corporation	www.clinipad.com
Cliniex Medical Corporation	www.clinitex.fr (French)
COBE Laboratories, Inc. (Gambro BCT)	www.cobebct.com
Codman & Shurtleff, Inc.	www.codmanjnj.com
Coherent, Inc.	www.cohr.com
Color Max Technologies	www.color-vision.com
Conmed	www.conmed.com
Cook Incorporated	www.cookgroup.com
Cook Urological, Inc.	www.cookmedical.com/uro/home.do
CooperSurgical, Inc.	www.coopercos.com
CooperVision, Inc.	www.coopervision.com
Cordis Corporation (Johnson & Johnson ultimate parent)	www.cordis.lu
Core Dynamics, Inc.	www.core-dynamics.com
Corpak, Inc.	www.bldmedical.com
Coulter Corporation	www.coulter.com
C. R. Bard, Inc.	www.crbard.com
Critikon, Inc.	www.dinamap.com
Cryomedics, Inc./Cabot Medical Corp.	www.circoncorp.com
Custom Ultrasonics, Inc.	www.customultrasonics.com
CVIS (Cardiovascular Imaging Systems)/InterTherapy, Inc.	www.cvico.com
Cypress Bioscience, Inc.	www.cypressbio.com
Dainabot Company (Japan)	(See Abbott Laboratories)
DAKO Corp	www.dakousa.com
Datascope Corp	www.datascope.com
Datex-Ohmeda	www.ohmeda.com
Davol, Inc.	www.davol.com
Denison Orthopedic Appliance Corp.	www.cddenison.com
Dentsply International, Inc.	www.dentsply.com
Denver Biomaterials, Inc.	www.denverbio.com
DeRoyal Industries. Inc.	www.deroyal.com
Diasonics	www.diasonics.com (GE Medical)
Dicon	www.dicon.com
Doran Instruments, Inc.	www.diagnosysllc.com

Dornier Medical Systems, Inc.	www.dornier.com
Dow Medical	www.dow.com
Draeger, Inc. Critical Care Systems	www.draeger.com
Du Pont Company	www.dupont.com
Dyna-Med	www.dynamed.com
Dyonics, Inc/Smith & Nephew Dyonics, Inc.	www.smithnephew.at
E-Z-EM, Inc.	www.ezem.com
EBI Medical Systems, Inc./Biomet, Inc.	www.biomet.com www.ebimedical.com
Eli Lilly	www.lilly.com
Endo Direct. Inc.	www.heartport.com
Erie Scientific Co.	www.eriesci.com
Ethicon Endo-Surgery	www.eesonline.com
Euro-Med/CooperSurgical	www.euromed.nl
Everest Medical Corp.	www.everestmedical.com
Fenwal Electronics, Inc.	www.fenwal.com
Fibra-Sonics, Inc.	www.fibrasonics.com
Fillauer Inc.	www.fillauer.com
Fischer Imaging Corporation	www.fischerimaging.com
Fisher Scientific Co.	www.fisher.co.uk
Flexiflo	www.ross.com/productHandbook/
Flowtronics, Inc.	www.techexpo.com
Freeman Manufacturing Company	www.freemanmfg.com
Fresenius USA, Inc.	www.fmcna.com
Gambro BCT	www.cobebct.com
Gaymar Industries Inc.	www.gaymar.com
Geiger Instrument Corp.	www.geigerinst.com
GE Medical Systems	www.gemedicals.com
General Electric CGR USA	www.ge.com
Genzyme Corporation	www.genzyme.com
GIBCO Laboratories/Life Technologies, Inc.	www.lifetech.com
Glaxo, Inc.	www.glaxowellcome.com
Global Medi-Tex, Inc.	www.globalmeditek.com
Gomco/Allied Health Care Products, Inc.	www.alliedhpi.com

Gore & Associates, Inc., W. L. (Gore-Tex)	www.gore.com
Gould Instrument Systems, Inc.	www.gould.co.uk
Graham-Field, Inc.	www.grahamfield.com
Greenwald Surgical Co., Inc.	www.greenwaldsurgical.com
Grieshaber & Company, Inc.	www.grieshaber.ch
Guidant Corp.	www.guidant.com
Healthdyne Technologies	(See Respironics)
Hemocue, Inc.	www.hemocue.se
Hemostatix Corp.	www.inductothermindustries.com
HemoTec, Inc.	www.braunbiosystems.com
Heraeus Lasersonics, Inc/.Heraeus Surgical, Inc.	www.laserscope.com
Hewlett-Packard Co.	www.hp.com
Hitachi Denshi America, Ltd.	www.hdal.com
Hoffman-La Roche, Inc./Roche Diagnostic Systems, Inc.	www.roche.com
Hollister, Inc.	www.hollister.com
Hologic, Inc.	www.hologic.com
Howmedica, Inc.	www.osteonics.com
Hu-Friedy Manufacturing Co., Inc.	www.hu-friedy.com
Hybritech (USA)	www.coulter.com
Hyclone Laboratories, Inc.	www.hyclone.com
Hydro-Med, Inc.	www.hydromed.com
Imex Medical Systems, Inc.	(See Nicolet Vascular, Inc.)
Immunotech Corp.	www.immunotech.com
Inamed Corp.	www.inamed.com
Incstar Corp.	www.diasorin.com
Infimed, Inc.	www.infimed.com
Infrasonics, Inc.	(See Puritan Bennett)
Invacare Corporation	www.invacare.com
Iolab Corp.	(See Johnson & Johnson)
Iovision, Inc.	www.iovision.com
Isotec Corporation	www.isotec.de
Jarit Instruments	www.jarit.com
Jay Medical Ltd.	(See Rehab Designs, Inc.)
Johnson & Johnson	www.johnsonandjohnson.com

Kapp Surgical Instrument, Inc.	www.kappsurgical.com
Karl Storz	www.karlstorz.com
Katena Products, Inc.	www.katena.com
Kendall Co.	www.kendallhq.com
Kerr Corporation	www.kerrdental.com
Kinamed, Inc.	www.kinamed.com
Kirschner Medical Corp.	(See Biomet Inc.)
Kirwan Surgical Products, Inc.	www.kirwans.com
Kleen Test Products Co.	(See Meridian Industries)
KMI, Inc.	www.kmiinc.com
Kodak Company	www.kodak.com
Kontron Instruments, Inc.	www.kontronmedical.com (French)
Kowa Optimed, Inc.	www.optimed.com
KT Medical, Inc.	www.ktmedical.com
Kurzweil Applied Intelligence, Inc.	www.kurzweiltech.com and www.voicerecognition.com
L & M Instruments, Inc.	www.lminstruments.com
Labconco Corp.	www.labconco.com
Laparomed Corp.	(See Imaging Medical Technologies, Inc.)
Laser Diagnostic Technologies, Inc.	www.laserdiagnostic.com
Laser Photonics, Inc.	www.lpg.man.ac.uk
Laserscope	www.laserscope.com
Leibinger L.P.	www.leibinger.de (German)
Leica Microsystems, Inc.	www.leica-microsystems.com
Leisegang Medical, Inc.	www.leisegang.com
Leisure Lift	www.leisurelift.com
Life Medical Technologies, Inc. (Life Medical Equipment)	www.lifemedicalequipment.com
Life Support Products, Inc.	(See Allied Healthcare)
Life-Tech, Inc.	www.life-tech.com
Link America, Inc.	www.linkorthopedics.com
Linvatec Corporation	www.linvatec.com
LKB Diagnostics, Inc./Wallace, Inc.	www.wallac.fi
Lone Star Medical Products	www.lsmp.com
Lorenz Surgical, Walter	www.lorenzsurgical.com
Lumex	www.lumex.com

Common Manufacturers & Web Sites

Lumiscope Company, Inc.	www.lumiscope.net
Luxtec Corp.	www.luxtec.com
Machida, Inc.	www.machidascope.com
Mallinckrodt Medical, Inc.	www.mallinckrodt.com
Mansfield/Boston Scientific Corp.	www.bsci.com
Maramed Orthopedic Systems	www.maramed.com
Marco Ophthalmic, Inc.	www.marcooph.com
Marquette Electronics Inc., (USA)	www.gemedicals.com
Maxxim Medical	www.maxximmedical.com
Medical Graphics Corporation	www.mbbnet.umn.edu
Medical Devices International	www.cprmicroshield.com
Medical Innovations Corporation	www.aedi.com
M.E. Meditek Co., Ltd.	www.devicelink.com
Medline Industries, Inc.	www.medline.com
Medrad, Inc.	www.medrad.com
Medtronic Heart Valves, Inc.	www.medtronic.com
Medtronic, Inc.	www.medtronic.com
Medtronic Ophthalmics	www.medtronicophthalmics.com
Mennen Medical Corp.	www.mennenmedical.com
Mentor Corp.	www.mentorcorp.com
Mead Johnson Nutritionals	www.meadjohnson.com
Meridian Industries	www.meridiancompanies.com
Merck & Co., Inc.	www.merck.com
Micro-Aire Surgical Instruments, Inc.	www.microaire.com
Micro-Bio-Logics	www.microbiologics.com
Micromedics, Inc.	www.micromedics-usa.com
Microtek Medical, Inc.	www.microtekmed.com
Microvasive/Boston Scientific Corp.	www.bsci.com
Midas Rex Pneumatic Tools	www.midasrexlp.com
Midmark Corporation	www.midmark.com
Milex Products, Inc.	www.milexproducts.com
Mill-Rose Laboratories, Inc.	www.mrlabsinc.com
Millar Instruments, Inc.	www.millarinstruments.com
Minntech Corporation	www.minntech.com
	www.mbbnet.umn.edu/company _folder/mnn.html
Mityvac/Neward Enterprises, Inc.	www.mityvac.com

Nautilus	www.nautilus.com
Nellcor, Inc.	www.mallinckrodt.com
Neostar Medical Technologies, Inc. (formerly Akcess Med-Prods., Inc.)	(See Horizon Medical Products, Inc.)
New World Medical, Inc.	www.ahmedvalve.com
Ney Company, J. M.	www.jmney.com
Nichols Institute	www.nicholsdiag.com
Nicolet Vascular	www.nicoletvascular.com
Nihon Kohden (America), Inc.	www.nkusa.com
Nomos Corporation	www.nomos.com
Nordic Track	www.nordictrak.com
Nova Biomedical Corporation	www.nova.ch
Nova Ortho-Med,Inc.	www.novaortho-med.com
Novartis	www.novartis.com
Novo Industries A/S	www.novo.dk
Nuaire, Inc.	www.nuaire.com
Nalge Nunc International	www.nalgenunc.com
Oculus of America/Insight Instruments. Inc.	www.insightinstruments.com
OEM Medical	www.bigskylaser.com
Ohmeda (Datex-Ohmeda)	www.ohmeda.com
Olympus America, Inc.	www.olympus.com
Onyx Medical Corp.	www.onyxmedical.com
Optima Worldwide, Ltd.	www.optimacompany.com
Ormco Corp.	www.ormco.com
Ortho-Care, Inc.	www.ortho-care.com
Ortho Diagnostic Systems, Inc.	www.pslgroup.com
Ortho Med, Inc.	www.novaortho-med.com
Osada Electric Co., Inc.	www.osadausa.com
Osteotech, Inc.	www.osteotech.com
Ote Biomedica	www.modulusa.net
Oto-Med, Inc.	www.otomed.com
Palco Laboratories	www.palcolabs.com
Pall Biomedical Products Company	www.pall.com
Palumbo Orthopaedics	www.brace4u.com/palumbo/
Paramedical Distributors	(See Tyco Healthcare)
Pascal Company, Inc.	www.pascaldental.com

Common Manufacturers & Web Sites

Passy-Muir, Inc.	www.passy-muir.com
Peace Medical	(See Global Medi-Tek, Inc.)
Pentax Precision Instrument Corp.	www.pentaxmedical.com
Perma-Type Co., Inc.	www.perma-type.com
Perkin-Elmer Corp., Nelson Analytical	www.perkin-elmer.com
	www.galactic.com/instruments/
	nelson-analytical.htm
Philips Medical Systems North America	www.medical.philips.com
Physitemp Instruments, Inc.	www.physitemp.com
Pie Medical USA	www.piemedical.com
Pilling Weck, Inc.	www.pillingweck.com
Pioneer Medical, Inc.	www.pioneermed.com
Plastron	www.plastron.com
PLC Medical Systems	www.plcmed.com
PML Microbiologicals	www.pmlmicro.com
PMT Corp.	www.pmtcorp.com
Polaron Instruments, Inc./	www.bio-rad.com
Bio-Rad, Microscience Division	
Poly Vac, Inc.	www.polyvac.com
Popper & Sons, Inc.	www.popperandsons.com
Possis Medical, Inc.	www.possis.com
Pozzi Dental Products	www.americantooth.com/pozzi.htm
Precision Medical, Inc.	www.beeremedical.com
Premier Dental Products Co.	www.premusa.com
Proctor & Gamble	www.pg.com
Propper Manufacturing Co., Inc.	www.proppermfg.com
Puritan Bennett Corp. (Nellcor	www.cpapman.com
Puritan Bennett)	
PyMaH Corp. (Acquired by 3M in 1996)	www.3m.com
Quest Medical, Inc.	(See Advanced Neuromodulation
	Systems)
Ramvac Corporation	www.ramvac.com
Rayfield Technology, Inc.	www.rayglobe.com
Redfield Corporation	www.redfieldcorp.com
Rehab Designs, Inc.	www.rehabdesigns.com
Rehabilicare	www.rehabilicare.com
Respironics	www.respironics.com

Ricca Chemical Company	www.riccachemical.com
RJL Systems, Inc.	www.rjlsystems.com
Roche Diagnostic Systems, Inc.	www.roche.ch
Rocky Mountain/Orthodontics	www.rmortho.com
Roho, Inc.	www.rohoinc.com
Ross Laboratories/Ross Products Division	www.rosslaboratories.com www.ross.com
Rush-Berivon, Inc.	www.netdoor.com/com/berivon
Sammons Inc. (Fred Sammons, Inc.)	www.sammonspreston.com
Sanderson-Macleod, Inc.	www.smbrushes.com
Sandoz Pharmaceutical Corporation	(See Novartis)
Sargent-Welch Scientific Co.	www.sargentwelch.com
Scanlan International, Inc.	www.scanlangroup.com
Schering-Plough Corporation	www.schering-plough.com
Schlueter Instruments, Corp.	www.iscpubs.com/bg/us/manu/ manu1978.html
Schott Fibre Optics, Inc.	www.schott.co.uk
Schuco	www.schuco.co.uk
Sechrist Industries, Inc.	www.sechristind.com
Seitz Corporation	www.seitzcorp.com
SensorMedics Corp	www.sensormedics.com
Shandon Lipshaw, Inc.	http://guide.labanimal.com/ product/6/5.html
Sharplan Lasers, Inc.	www.escmed.com
Sharpoint/Surgical Specialties Corp.	www.sharpoint.com
Sherwood Medical Company	www.sherwood.de
Shimadzu Precision Instr. Inc./ Med. Systems	www.shimadzu.com
Shippert Medical Technologies Corp.	www.shippertmedical.com
Siemens Corporation	www.siemens.com
Siemens Elema	www.siemens.fi
Sigma Diagnostics	www.sigma-aldrich.com
Sil-Med Corporation	www.silmed.com
Silipos	www.silipos.com
Sklar Instrument Company	www.sklarcorp.com
SMI	www.smi.de
Smith and Nephew DonJoy, Inc.	www.donjoy.com
Smith & Nephew Dyonics, Inc.	www.smithnephew.com

Smith and Nephew Richards, Inc.	www.smithnephew.com
Smith and Nephew Rolyan, Inc.	www.easyliving.com
SmithKline Beecham	www.sb.com
Snowden-Pencer	www.snowdenpencer.com
Sodem Systems	www.sodem.ch
Sola Optical USA Inc./Sola Ophthalmics	www.sola.com
Sontec Instruments, Inc.	www.sontecinstruments.com
Sony Electronics, Inc., Medical Systems	www.sony.com
Sony	www.ultrasoundsales.com
	www.medelex.com
	www.avsupply.com/sonymed.htm
SpaceLabs Medical, Inc.	www.spacelabs.com
Spectrum Surgical Instruments Co.	www.spectrumsurgical.com
Spencer Technologies	www.spencertechnologies.com
STAAR Surgical Co.	www.staar.com
Stephens Instruments, Inc.	www.stephensinst.com
Sterion, Inc.	www.sterion.com
St. Jude Medical Co.	www.sjm.com
Stortz Instrument Co.	www.elmed.com
Stryker Corporation, Medical Division	www.strykercorp.com
Sulzer Carbomedics, Inc.	www.carbomedics.com
Sun-Med, Inc.	www.sunmedica.com
Surgidyne, Inc.	(See Sterion)
Surgilase, Inc.	www.laserengineering.com
Surgitek	www.circoncorp.com
Sutter Corp.	www.sutter.com
Synectic Engineering, Inc.	www.synectic.net
Tartan Orthopedics, Ltd.	www.tartanortho.com
Taut, Inc.	www.taut.com
Telectronics Pacing Systems, Inc.	(See St. Jude Medical)
Teledyne, Inc.	www.waterpik.com
Terumo Cardiovascular Systems.	www.terumo-us.com
Texas Medical Products, Inc.	www.surgimedics.com
Thermo Electron Corp.	www.thermo.com
Thomas Scientific	www.thomassci.com
Thoratec Laboratories Corp.	www.thoratec.com
Tidi Products Inc., National	www.bantahealthcare.com

Toolmex Corp.	www.toolmex-polmach.co.uk
TomTec	www.tomtec.de
Toshiba America Medical Systems	www.toshiba.com
Trimedyne, Inc.	www.trimedyne.com
Truform Orthotics & Prosthetics	www.truform-otc.com
Tulip Company, The	www.tulipmedical.com
Tyco International	www.tycoint.com
United States Catheter & Instrument Co./Bard Inc. (USCI)	www.crbard.com
United States Surgical Corp.	(See AUTO SUTURE)
Urocare Products, Inc.	www.urocare.com
U.S. Endoscopy Group	www.usendoscopy.com
U.S. Orthotics, Inc.	www.usendoscopy.com
USCI (United States Catheter and Instrument Co./Bard, Inc.)	www.crbard.com
US Surgical	www.ussurg.com
Vacumed	www.vacumed.com
Valley Forge Scientific Corp.	www.vfsc.com
Valleylab, Inc.	www.valleylab.com
Vance Products Inc.	www.cookgroup.com
Varian	www.varian.com
Velcro USA, Inc.	www.velcro.com
Veratex Corp.	www.veratex.com
Vicon Industries, Inc.	www.vicon-cctv.com
Victoreen, Inc.	www.victoreen.com
Vingmed U.S.A.	www.vingmed.se
Vision Sciences	www.visionscience.com
Visitec Co.	www.visitec.com
Vistec, Inc.	www.vistec.net
Visx, Inc.	www.visx.com
Vital Signs, Inc.	www.vital-signs.com
Volk Optical	www.volk.com
Vygon Corp.	www.vygonusa.com
Wampole Laboratories	www.wampolelabs.com
Weck & Co., Inc., Edward	www.weckclosure.com
Welch Allyn, Inc.	www.welchallyn.com
Wells Johnson Co.	www.wellsgrp.com

Common Manufacturers & Web Sites

Wilson Cook Medical, Inc.	www.cookgroup.com/wilson_cook/
Wisap USA	www.wisap.com
Wolf Medical Instruments Corp., Richard	www.richard-wolf.com
Wyeth-Ayerst Laboratories, Inc.	www.ahp.com/wyeth_labs.htm
Xomed Surgical Products	www.xomed.com
Zeiss Humphrey Systems	www.humphrey.com
Zeiss, Inc., Carl	www.zeiss.com
Zimmer, Inc.	www.zimmer.com
Zoll Medical Corp.	www.zoll.com